THE
CORINNE T. NETZER

ENCYCLOPEDIA
OF
FOOD VALUES

A DELL BOOK

A DELL HARDCOVER

Published by
Dell Publishing
a division of
Bantam Doubleday Dell Publishing Group, Inc.
666 Fifth Avenue
New York, New York 10103

Library of Congress Cataloging in Publication Data

Netzer, Corinne T.
  [Encyclopedia of food values]
  The Corinne T. Netzer encyclopedia of food values.
      p.   cm.
  ISBN 0-440-50367-1
  1. Food: Analysis Tables.   I. Title.   II. Title. Encyclopedia of
food values.
TX551.N42   1992
641.1—dc20   91-36727   CIP

Printed in the United States of America

Published simultaneously in Canada

February 1992

10   9   8   7   6   5   4   3   2   1

RRH

Contents

A special thanks . . .

to the men and women of the food industry for their cooperation in obtaining data;

to the United States Department of Agriculture;

to the Human Nutrition Information Service, and in particular, Barbara Anderson;

to my assistant, Margaret Sullivan, for her tireless and dedicated efforts on this project;

to my researchers, Leah Chaback and Susan Waggoner;

to Joy Stevens for her helpful suggestions;

to the best editor in the world: Elaine Wittman Chaback;

and to Leslie Schnur for her support, encouragement, and terrific sense of humor.

Foreword

The Encyclopedia of Food Values is the culmination of my many years of research and writing about food and food counts. It is the most comprehensive volume of nutritional data ever collected.

Whether you want to lose weight, restrict dietary cholesterol or sodium, cut fat, or boost fiber intake, my *Encyclopedia* makes it easy for you to take charge of your diet because it's *all* here—all the information currently available, and all in one place. This is not a handy take-it-with-you book, but a reference volume to be kept in the home and/or office and referred to as you would a dictionary.

Beginning with the Introduction (page ix), you will find everything you need to know to start eating healthfully and happily. In straightforward layman's terms I've explained calories and the essential nutrients of food: protein, carbohydrates, fat (and saturated fat), cholesterol, sodium, and fiber. I've supplied you with all the latest dietary guidelines and discussed how each nutrient can affect your health.

You need never again be confused about what you are eating, because following the Introduction is the fullest listing in existence of the eight food values. Included are more than just common foods like apples and oranges; exotic tasties are represented as well, such as fish-paste cakes, amaranth, and beefalo—plus thousands of brand-name items, including health foods and fast foods.

Because vitamins and minerals are an important part of good nutrition, I've added a special section at the back of the book. Starting on page 691, you'll find a quick guide to the way the body uses these essential nutrients and a listing of basic foods and sixteen important vitamins and minerals they contain.

Now, with my *Encyclopedia of Food Values* to help you, it's easy to calculate—and control—what's in your diet!

Good luck and good eating,
C.T.N.

Introduction

Are you really what you eat? Think about these facts:

- In America, where the typical diet is high in fat, breast cancer is relatively common; in Japan, where people eat much less fat, breast cancer is rare.
- High blood pressure, a disorder that affects a large number of Americans, is uncommon in countries where salt intake is low.
- As American's fat and cholesterol intake drops, so does the heart attack rate.

Are you what you eat? As far as your physical well-being is concerned, of course you are. So am I, and so is everyone else on this planet.

In many parts of the world, good health means finding enough to eat. But in the wealthier West, longevity often means *not* getting too much of a good thing. As my friend, Pat, often says, "No matter how hard I try to avoid it, wherever I go there's a candy bar or a pizza with my name on it."

Most of us can identify with Pat's problem. I certainly can. For years I believed feeling empty and starved was simply the price one paid for a slim body. I tried every fad diet that came along, always looking for a magic solution to the eternal diet dilemma. Then I got smart and became an informed consumer in the truest sense of the word. I began to study the basics of sound nutrition. To my surprise, I found I could control my weight without going hungry—and without giving up my favorite foods.

Far too many of us have made the scale our only measure of success, forgetting about nutrition entirely. A bulimic (a binge eater who compensates by regurgitating) might maintain a seemingly healthy weight, but would most likely be poorly nourished. An even more serious disorder born of the "think thin" mania is anorexia, in which the person stops eating almost completely. Of course, if you are overweight, taking off those extra pounds is important. But you don't have to starve to be slim and healthy. I can assure you that it's possible to have a full and satisfying diet without going overboard on fat, cholesterol, sodium, or calories. My own experience is proof that with the proper information you can make the proper food choices.

For most of us the key to good nutrition is being aware of what we're eating. To help us, the federal government has established general guidelines for an acceptable diet.

If you want to maintain or improve your health through nutrition, which includes maintaining a healthy weight, you can start by determining how many calories you need per day. The next—and most important—step is to learn to spend your calories wisely. Your average daily diet should look like this:

Guidelines for a Healthy Diet[1]
- 55%–58% total calories from carbohydrates—but no more than 10% of total calories from refined carbohydrates
- 12%–15% total calories from protein
- 30% total calories from fats (maximum)—but no more than 10% of total calories from saturated fats

Translating this formula into lunch may seem complicated, but it's really an easy and effective way to determine how your daily calories are best spent.

Following is a brief look at the major components of our daily diet—starting with calories, the basic unit of nourishment.

Calories

Calories are found in virtually all foods. They're the fuel that makes life possible, but too many can weigh the body down with stored fat.

Most of us think of fat as a social liability, and feeling fat can change your entire outlook on life. Being overweight can limit your choice of clothes, activities, and even jobs, but obesity is more than just a social liability—it's a health hazard. Excessive body weight is a risk factor for cardiovascular disease, high blood pressure, diabetes, and some forms of cancer.

How many calories do you need to maintain your healthy body weight? That's not a simple question to answer. There are many people who claim to gain weight on very little food, and all of us have run across that someone who seems able to eat anything without ever gaining an ounce. Is the difference just a matter of perception? Not really. Recent studies indicate that different individuals are likely to have very different caloric needs.

To begin to understand how many calories you need each day, refer to the Healthy Weight Chart (page xx), then use this equation:

$$\textit{Desirable weight in pounds} \times 12 = \textit{Daily Caloric Intake}$$

In this equation, twelve is the *average* number of calories needed daily by a low-activity person to sustain each pound of body weight. If you are moderately active, the number of calories needed per pound may be fifteen, while people who are very active may require twenty to twenty-five calories per pound. I have taken the lowest number as an average because, unfortunately, that's where most Americans fall on the activity scale. Between

1. Based on U.S. Government recommendations.

sedentary jobs and a car-oriented society, most of us just don't get enough exercise.

Suppose you currently weigh 154 pounds and you would like to reach your healthy weight of 120 pounds. Since $120 \times 12 = 1440$, you know that you must limit your daily caloric intake to 1440 to reach your goal.

Yet helpful as the question is, it isn't written in stone. How your body handles calories can be influenced by any number of factors, including:

- *Age:* The older you are, the fewer calories you need.
- *Sex:* Men generally need more calories than women.
- *Activity level:* Physically active people burn more calories than inactive people, both during physical exertion and at rest.
- *Body composition:* If two people are the same weight, the person with more muscle will burn more calories than the person with more fat. The reason: muscle burns calories, fat *is* calories.
- *Genetics:* Sad but true—it is possible to inherit a predisposition to gain weight.

The number of calories you need to reach and maintain your healty weight is dependent on *all* these factors. You may have to experiment to find the right number for you. Begin with the equation above and adjust your intake as needed.

If you want to lose weight, the slow-but-steady approach is best: the loss of a pound or so a week will produce longer-lasting results than crash diets, which encourage rebound weight gain. And gradually increasing your activity level (under a doctor's supervision if you are overweight, over thirty-five years old, or have a preexisting medical condition) will speed up weight loss.

Once you have established what your daily caloric intake should be, the information in this book will let you pick and choose how you'll use those calories.

Protein

Protein, needed by virtually every cell in the body, is made of various amino acids. Some are manufactured by the body, but nine are not. To get these nine additional—and essential—amino acids, we must consume protein.

Like me, you were probably raised to think that the more protein you eat, the better off you are. Unfortunately, this is not the case, because the foods that contain the most protein—meat, eggs, and dairy products—are also high in fat and cholesterol. These animal proteins are considered "complete" because they contain all nine essential amino acids. The government does not recommend eliminating them, just limiting your intake to 12%–15% of your daily diet.

Plant protein sources are not considered "complete" because individually they do not contain all the amino acids we need. They have to be eaten in combinations with each other to be complete. However, protein derived in this manner is generally low in fat and high in fiber. To combine plant protein you might follow this general formula:

Legumes + Grains = Complete Protein

Legumes include dried peas and beans, such as black-eyed peas, chick-peas (also known as garbanzo beans), kidney beans, lentils, lima beans, navy beans, and soybeans. Nuts are also in this category, but beware: they contain high amounts of fat. Grains include barley, corn, oats, rice, sesame seeds, sunflower seeds, and wheat. Just a few of the combinations that make complete proteins are peanut butter on whole wheat bread, beans and rice, and noodles with tofu (soybean curd).

To see how your daily protein intake fits the guidelines for a healthy diet (page x), multiply the number of calories you need to maintain your desirable weight by 15%, the maximum recommended protein calories per day. If your daily caloric intake should be 1200, $1200 \times .15 = 180$. Since there are 4 calories in every gram of protein, all you need to do now is divide 180 by 4: $180 \div 4 = 45$. You now know that you need to eat an average of 45 grams of protein daily to meet the government's recommended guidelines.

My book will give you the information you need to make the choices that will enable you to stay within these guidelines and still enjoy eating. Remember that 12%–15% of your diet means your *total* diet for one day—not just one meal. You might decide to splurge on lunch and stint on dinner and still stay within the limits.

Carbohydrates

If they gave an award for the most misunderstood nutrient, carbohydrates would definitely win. For years we were encouraged to eat protein and avoid starch, and dieters conscientiously shunned baked potatoes, bread, and pasta because they believed that's where the trouble was. Times change, new information is discovered, and we now realize that the calories aren't in the baked potato, they're in the butter and sour cream that goes on the potato. We now know that bread is not a culprit, and that a cup of pasta can be the centerpiece of a low-calorie meal.

Learning to enjoy carbohydrates without adding a ton of topping or sauce is one of the best diet moves you can make because, for most people, meals that are high in carbohydrates provide a sense of satisfaction and fullness.

Carbos are made of various types of starches and sugars, which the body uses for energy as well as for the building and repair of tissues. A no-carbohydrate diet will help you lose weight, but it may also make you lose muscle tissue and leave you feeling fatigued. Therefore, even if you want to lose weight, you need to make room for this nutrient in your diet.

The important thing to keep in mind is making room for the *right* carbohydrates, and that means mostly *complex carbohydrates*; those found in plants, fruits, vegetables, and whole grains. These foods provide a good ratio of nutrients to calories and should make up 45%–48% of your daily caloric intake.

Refined carbohydrates come to us in foods that have been highly processed and pack much less of a nutritional wallop—sugar, candy, and cakes. I'm not saying you have to give up sweets entirely. You can indulge once in a while—just remember to keep it under 10% of your total daily caloric intake.

You can find out if your carbo intake complies with government guidelines very easily. Suppose you have calculated that you should eat 1200 calories a day, 45% of which should come from complex carbohydrates. By multiplying 1200 by .45, you discover that you should eat some 540 calories worth of complex carbohydrates. When you divide 540 by 4 (the number of calories in each gram of carbohydrate) the result—135—is the number of grams of complex carbohydrates you should eat. (You can use the same equation, substituting .10 for .45, to determine how many grams of refined carbohydrates you may eat each day.)

Fat and Saturated Fat

Protein and carbohydrates both contain four calories per gram, but fat contains *nine calories per gram*—more than twice as many calories as the other two nutrients. Not surprisingly, fat is the most fattening nutrient there is!

The Encyclopedia of Food Values has two listings for the fat content of foods. The first is for *total fat*. The second listing is for *saturated fat*. I've separated saturated fat from the total fat, but I have not given individual figures for *un*saturated fats (polyunsaturated and monounsaturated) because while 30% or less of our calories may come from total fat, the government has stressed that only 10% of our total calories should come from saturated fat.

While these are the recommended maximums, lower amounts are preferable. This is bad news for most of us because, quite simply, fat tastes good. It adds flavor to fried foods and gives a creamy, rich texture to many others. If you find fat-rich foods irresistible, remind yourself of some simple facts. Not only is fat high in calories, but numerous studies indicate that saturated fat contributes to high cholesterol levels (see Cholesterol, page xiv). A diet high in saturated fats is considered to be a risk factor for heart attack as well as stroke, and *both* saturated and unsaturated fats have been cited as risk factors for several forms of cancer, including cancer of the breast, ovary, uterus, and colon. Cancer of the breast and colon are especially common in America and account for thousands of deaths each year. Because fat of all types has been linked to disease, the U.S. Surgeon General has recommended that Americans *reduce their intake of all fats in general and of saturated fats in particular.*

Your body's actual need for fat is far less than the government guidelines maximum allowance. The truth is, we don't need *any* saturated fats at all, and our need for unsaturated fats would be adequately met if they made up just 10% of our calories.

You can keep track of your intake of all fats by checking the *Encyclopedia*. However, it may help to remind yourself that the highest levels of saturated fat are usually animal fats, and that unsaturated fat is usually a vegetable fat, like corn oil. But there are major exceptions to this—tropical oils, such as coconut and palm, though vegetable fats, are both highly saturated.

Another way to distinguish saturated from unsaturated fat is to check their consistency at room temperature. Saturated fats, like butter and coconut oil, will remain firm at room temperature while an unsaturated fat, such as safflower oil, will be liquid.

You will find that all oil, including those considered unsaturated, contain some saturated fat. Even canola oil, thought to be the least saturated of all, still has 7% saturated fat. And many raw vegetables have measurable quantities of saturated fat—they have no cholesterol whatsoever, but they do contain some of the enemy fat (see also Cholesterol, below).

As with carbohydrates, fat values are given in the *Encyclopedia* in grams. To calculate your maximum daily allowance, determine how many calories you need to maintain a healthy body weight, then multiply this number by .3 (because 30% is the percentage of calories that may come from dietary fats). If your daily calorie intake is 1200, $1200 \times .3 = 360$, the number of fat calories you may eat on an average day. Now you need to convert this number to grams. Since there are 9 calories in each gram of fat, $360 \div 9 = 40$. But keep in mind that while 40 grams is your maximum *total* fat intake for the day, only 10%—or 4 grams—should be saturated. I can't stress often enough that for adults it's preferable to eat less than these "outer limits" of fat.

Cholesterol

What's all the fuss about cholesterol, and does it really contribute to heart disease?

Although the body does need cholesterol, it produces a complete supply daily (one thousand milligrams, on the average). You could eat a diet containing no cholesterol and never experience deficiency. Therefore, the amount of cholesterol you get in food—*dietary cholesterol*—is all extra. The body somewhat decreases its own production to compensate, but it generally doesn't decrease it enough to keep things in balance. That's when you could end up with too much cholesterol in your system. The excess cholesterol goes into the blood supply, where it can build up inside the arteries. When an artery of the heart becomes clogged with these deposits, the result can be a heart attack. When an artery supplying blood to the brain becomes clogged, the result can be a stroke.

While there is no irrefutable proof that eating over three hundred grams of cholesterol a day (the government's suggested maximum) will result in a heart attack, studies indicate that people with high cholesterol levels have higher rates of arterial disease than people whose cholesterol is within the acceptable limit. Therefore, excessive dietary cholesterol has been identified as a probable risk factor for both heart attacks and strokes.

According to government guidelines, an acceptable count for adults is two hundred or below. If your count is higher, you should act on the advice of your family physician, who will most likely suggest you lower your cholesterol intake.

Cholesterol is found only in animal sources, such as meat, poultry, fish, and dairy. Though these products are often high in fat, it is important to know that fat and cholesterol are *not* the same thing. You might ingest a food that is cholesterol-free and still raise your cholesterol level because it contains a great deal of saturated fat.

Conversely, just as cholesterol-free doesn't necessarily mean fat-free, some low-fat foods—certain shellfish, for example—contain high amounts of cholesterol. Also, remember to check the cholesterol content of low-fat and calorie-reduced animal products—low-fat cottage cheese contains about 60% less fat than the regular type, but only 33% less cholesterol.

The good news is that dietary fiber (see page xvi), eaten regularly, can help lower blood cholesterol levels to some degree. A lot of attention has been given to oat bran, but all kinds of bran (corn and rice, for example) are equally effective, as are other high-fiber sources, such as beans.

Sodium

What can damage your health even though it's fat-free, cholesterol-free, and low-calorie? Sodium, which most people think of as salt. (Salt and sodium are not the same, but since salt contains high amounts of sodium, we often speak of them as if they were.)

The biggest problem with eating too much sodium is that it can contribute to high blood pressure, which, in turn, is linked to stroke, heart attack, and kidney failure. In cultures where average salt consumption is low, so is the percentage of population that suffers from high blood pressure. In northern Japan, where the diet is high in salty foods like pickled vegetables, fermented soy products, and preserved fish, there is almost a 40% incidence of high blood pressure.

According to the government's recommended daily dietary allowances, adults may consume a *maximum* of from 1100 to 3300 milligrams of sodium per day. Most of us, however, don't need this much because we're sedentary and therefore don't have to replace sodium lost through perspiration.

Although we need less salt than the RDA calls for, we usually ingest far more. Health professionals estimate that the average American consumes from two to four teaspoons of salt a day. Since each teaspooon of salt contains 2132 milligrams of sodium, you can see why so many of us might end up with high blood pressure.

A young friend of mine recently said she didn't worry about getting too much salt because she never cooked with it or shook it on at mealtime. But when she used the prepublication *Encyclopedia* research to keep track of her diet, she discovered she was getting much more sodium than she thought. What she didn't realize was that most foods contain natural amounts of sodium. Even a stalk of raw celery contains 35 milligrams of sodium.

Additional amounts get into our diet because salt, an excellent preservative and flavor enhancer, is added to almost every preprepared food item on the market, from canned vegetables to whole-grain cereals. If you're concerned about sodium in your diet, be sure to use this book to find what your sodium intake *really* is.

Your craving for salt is acquired, and as you reduce your salt intake you will gradually notice that it takes less to satisfy you. While your taste buds are making the adjustment, perk up your food with herbs and spices. I even know reformed salt junkies who complain that food prepared by most other people is "too salty" for them!

Fiber

We never do anything by halves, so it shouldn't be surprising that we've jumped wholeheartedly aboard the fiber bandwagon. Are we helping ourselves to better health or simply embracing another fashionable fad?

So much has been written about oat bran that many people think it's the only way to get fiber into the diet. Not true at all. First of all, there are as many kinds of bran as there are types of grain, and all are good sources of fiber. Also, fiber can be found in a wide variety of foods besides bran.

Fiber, which our grandmothers called roughage, comes from plants. Whole grains, fruits, and vegetables are the most common sources of fiber in our diet. We also get some (although in much smaller amounts) when the pectins, gums, and thickeners derived from plants are added to foods to improve texture and taste.

Different types of food are digested in different parts of the body. Sugar literally "melts in your mouth," which is why you can eat so much without feeling full! Fiber, however, cannot be digested by saliva. Nor can it be digested by the enzymes in the stomach. It goes into the intestines "as is," which is why high-fiber foods provide a satisfying feeling of fullness.

The key health benefit of fiber is that it helps the intestinal tract function, and many studies indicate that a high-fiber diet may prevent a number of common intestinal ailments. Hemorrhoids and constipation both have been linked to low-fiber diets. The reason: when stools are small, hard, and lack bulk, the system must strain to eliminate them.

A more serious ailment is diverticulitis, a condition in which pockets form on the walls of the large intestine. When these pockets become inflamed, medical intervention and sometimes surgery are necessary.

Another disease implicated in low-fiber diets is cancer of the colon. Although definitive studies are not yet available, researchers speculate that fiber can help protect against this form of cancer in two ways. First, it speeds waste products through the system, reducing your exposure to carcinogenic substances. Second, fiber dilutes the concentration of these carcinogens and may even prevent their formation during digestion.

It's also thought that by replacing fatty foods in the diet (oat bran for breakfast instead of bacon) and promoting efficient digestion, fiber can be of help in fighting high cholesterol. The oat bran craze was started when a best seller touted it, but further investigation has shown that any high-fiber food, eaten regularly, will do the job. Fiber is essentially a *preventative*, not a *cure*. If you think you may have any of the health problems described above, you need your physician's help and advice.

Remember that fiber is supposed to replace the overabundance of fats and refined carbohydrates in your diet—it isn't an antidote for a diet rich in saturated fats and cholesterol. Since Americans like a little fat and salt with their nutrition, many of us have opted for "fiber" in the form of bran muffins and breakfast cereals. While items like these can be quite healthy, be sure to check the *Encyclopedia* to make sure you aren't getting far less fiber and far more fat, sugar, and salt than you think.

You'll notice that fiber listings in the *Encyclopedia* are accompanied by a *c* or a *d*. This tells you whether the count is for *crude fiber* (c), or *dietary fiber* (d). Until recently, it was difficult for scientists to determine the fiber content of foods. For a long time a crude method of analysis was used—the results of that analysis are known as *crude fiber*. However, this process failed to detect much of the actual fiber in food. An improved method of analysis was found, and the results from this process yield values known as *dietary fiber*. Dietary fiber listings are not yet available for all foods. I have given you the dietary fiber listings whenever they are available because they are a more accurate indication of the amount of fiber you are actually eating.

The government has yet to establish strict guidelines for daily fiber intake. You don't want to go overboard and eat nothing but fiber, but you don't want to get too little either. Nutritionists suggest that a healthy goal to aim for is an average intake of 25–35 grams of fiber per day.

How to Use This Book

The food counts in this book are the latest currently available, drawn from sources supplied by the United States, Japanese, and Caribbean governments and from the food manufacturers and purveyors themselves. Although the *Encyclopedia* is as complete and accurate as possible, please remember that the food industry frequently changes and improves recipes, adds new products, and discontinues old ones.

To make *The Encyclopedia of Food Values* easy to use, I've listed foods alphabetically. For convenience, similar foods are grouped together under categories—bread, cheese, candy, cereal—and all foods and beverages available at fast-food restaurants are listed together under the name of the specific restaurant.

Keep in mind as you use the *Encyclopedia:*

- **Don't assume.** Always look up the item you're interested in. For example, don't assume that dry-roasted nuts are dramatically less fattening than oil-roasted nuts; don't assume that "no cholesterol" means no-fat or low-fat, because that isn't necessarily the case.
- **Realize that figures may be rounded off.** When manufacturers print food values on their packages, government regulations allow them to round off the figures. For example, a food value of .2 may appear on the label as 0. If figures in the *Encyclopedia* differ from package labels, it's because I have used the actual data for these foods whenever available. In the case of basic foods, where small fractions are given, I've rounded off the figures for your convenience—26.792 will be 26.8, and so on.
- **Understand that figures represent an average.** Food is produced during different growing seasons and in many different areas. These regional and seasonal differences can affect the nutrients found in foods.
- **Pay attention to package and serving sizes.** Notice that sizes and measurements differ according to the manufacturer. To be as accurate as possible, I have given you figures based on the manufacturer's serving size rather than multiplying or dividing to make sizes and amounts the same. If you are comparing products, be sure to check the portion size before you make your choice. It's difficult to make comparisons between food items if the values given are for different serving sizes. For example, what's considered a single serving of cake can vary quite a lot. Some manufacturers consider it 1/12 of the package, some consider it 1/9, and others consider it a 2″ × 2″ piece. If you compare food values in this case, you'll be misled. Also, remember not to compare measurements of capacity to measurements of weight. For instance, four ounces is not a half cup or four fluid ounces; four ounces is a weight and may be more or less than half of a cup.

However, you can compare unequal serving sizes if the foods are listed in *similar* measure—by weight or by capacity. For example, if the food values for one type of sauce are listed by the tablespoon and values for another type of sauce are given per fluid-ounce serving, you can compare them if you do a bit of math first. Simply divide the food values for the fluid-ounce listing by two (because one fluid ounce is equal to two tablespoons). If you aren't sure about converting foods of similar measures, see the Equivalency Chart on page xx.

SUMMARY OF NUTRITIONAL SUGGESTIONS
RECOMMENDED DAILY INTAKE[1]

Total Calories Daily
Sedentary lifestyle: Desired weight × 12
Moderately active lifestyle: Desired weight × 15
Very active lifestyle: Desired weight × 20–25

Protein
12%–15% of calories

Carbohydrates
55%–58% of calories
(Less than 10% of calories from refined carbohydrates)

Fat
Less than 30% of calories
(No more than 10% of calories from saturated fat)

Cholesterol
Under 300 grams daily

Sodium
1110–3300 milligrams per day maximum

Fiber
25–35 grams daily

1. Recommendations are those of the U.S. government, except in the case of fiber, where guidelines have yet to be established. The fiber recommendations are based on suggestions from professional nutritionists.

Healthy Weight Chart

Height (without shoes)	Weight in pounds (without clothes)[1]	
	19 to 34 years	35 years and over
5'0"	97–128	108–138
5'1"	101–132	111–143
5'2"	104–137	115–148
5'3"	107–141	119–152
5'4"	111–146	122–157
5'5"	114–150	126–162
5'6"	118–155	130–167
5'7"	121–160	134–172
5'8"	125–164	138–178
5'9"	129–169	142–183
5'10"	132–174	146–188
5'11"	136–179	151–194
6'0"	140–184	155–190
6'1"	144–189	159–205
6'2"	148–195	164–210
6'3"	152–200	168–216
6'4"	156–205	173–222

1. Suggested healthy weights for men and women. The lower weights generally apply to women, the higher weights to men.

SOURCE: *Report of the Dietary Guidelines Advisory Committee on the Dietary Guidelines for Americans, 1990.*

Equivalency Chart

EQUIVALENTS BY CAPACITY
(All measurements level)

1 quart = 4 cups
1 cup = 8 fluid ounces
= ½ pint
= 16 tablespoons
2 tablespoons = 1 fluid ounce
1 tablespoon = 3 teaspoons

EQUIVALENTS BY WEIGHT

1 pound = 16 ounces
3.57 ounces = 100 grams
1 ounce = 28.35 grams

Abbreviations and Symbols

approx.	approximately
c	crude fiber[1]
Ca	calcium
cal.	calories
carbo.	carbohydrates
chol.	cholesterol
cont.	container
d	dietary fiber
diam.	diameter
fl.	fluid
Fol	folacin
gms	grams
"	inch
I.U.	International Units
Fe	iron
<	less than
(0)	may contain trace amount
Mag	magnesium
Man	manganese
m.q.	measurable quantity[2]
mcg	microgram
mgs	milligrams
lb.	pound(s)
n.a.	not available
oz.	ounce(s)
pkg.	package
pkt.	packet
Pho	phosphorus
Pot	potassium
prot.	protein
Rib	riboflavin
sat.	saturated
Sod.	sodium
tbsp.	tablespoon
tsp.	teaspoon
Thi	thiamin
tot.	total
tr.	trace
w/	with
Zn	zinc

1. Crude method of analysis; actual content may be higher.
2. Believed to contain measurable quantities, but data unavailable at this time. (*Note:* A "measurable quantity" may range from a trace to substantial amounts.)

FOOD VALUES

CALORIES

◆

PROTEIN

◆

CARBOHYDRATES

◆

TOTAL FAT

◆

SATURATED FAT

◆

CHOLESTEROL

◆

SODIUM

◆

FIBER

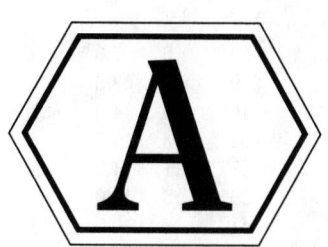

Food and Measure	cal.	prot. (gms)	carbo. (gms)	tot. fat (gms)	sat. fat (gms)	chol. (mgs)	sod. (mgs)	fiber (gms)
ABALONE, meat only:								
raw, 1 lb.	474	77.6	27.3	3.4	.7	384	1363	0
raw, 1 oz.	30	4.8	1.7	.2	<.1	24	85	0
fried[1], 4 oz.	214	22.3	12.5	7.7	1.9	107	670	.1 c
ABALONE MUSHROOM, see								
"Mushroom, oyster"								
ACAPULCO DIP:								
(*Ortega*), 1 oz.	8	0	2.0	0	0	0	0	n.a.
ACEROLA:								
untrimmed, 1 lb.	114	1.5	27.9	1.1	n.a.	0	26	1.5 c
trimmed, 1 oz.	9	.1	2.2	.1	(0)	0	2	.1 c
trimmed, ½ cup	16	.2	3.8	.1	(0)	0	4	.2 c
1 medium, approx. .2 oz.	2	<.1	.4	<.1	(0)	0	tr.	<.1 c
ACEROLA JUICE:								
1 fl. oz.	6	.1	1.5	.1	(0)	0	1	.1 c
6 fl. oz.	36	.7	8.7	.5	(0)	0	6	.5 c
ACKEE:								
trimmed, 1 oz.	51	1.2	1.6	4.9	n.a.	0	n.a.	.1 c
ACORN:								
raw, in shell, 1 lb.	1037	17.3	114.6	67.1	8.7	0	1515	7.2 c
raw, shelled, 1 oz.	105	1.8	11.8	6.8	.9	0	153	.7 c
dried, in shell, 1 lb.	1432	22.8	150.9	88.3	11.5	0	1995	9.5 c
dried, shelled, 1 oz.	145	2.3	15.2	8.9	1.2	0	201	1.0 c
ACORN FLOUR:								
full-fat, 1 oz.	142	2.1	15.2	8.6	1.1	0	202	.8 c
ACORN SQUASH:								
raw:								
untrimmed, 1 lb.	138	2.8	35.9	.3	.1	0	11	4.8 c
trimmed, 1 oz.	11	.2	3.0	<.1	tr.	0	1	.4 c
1 medium, 4⅓" × 4" diam.,								
approx. 1.3 lb.	172	3.5	44.9	.4	.1	0	14	6.0 c

1. *Dipped in flour and salted before frying.*

Food and Measure	cal.	prot. (gms)	carbo. (gms)	tot. fat (gms)	sat. fat (gms)	chol. (mgs)	sod. (mgs)	fiber (gms)
ACORN SQUASH, RAW *(cont.)*								
cubed, ½ cup	28	.6	7.3	.1	<.1	0	3	1.0 c
(*Frieda* of California), 1 lb.	249	8.6	63.5	.5	n.a.	0	45	m.q.
(*Frieda* of California), 1 oz.	16	.5	4.0	<.1	tr.	0	3	m.q.
baked, 4 oz.	64	1.3	16.5	.2	<.1	0	5	2.2 c
baked, cubed, ½ cup	57	1.1	14.9	.1	<.1	0	4	2.0 c
boiled, mashed, 4 oz.	39	.8	10.0	.1	<.1	0	3	1.3 c
boiled, mashed, ½ cup	41	.8	10.7	.1	<.1	0	3	1.4 c
ADZUKI BEAN:								
raw:								
1 oz.	93	5.6	17.8	.2	tr.	0	1	1.5 c
½ cup	323	19.5	61.7	.5	tr.	0	5	5.2 c
(*Arrowhead Mills*), 2 oz.	190	13.0	35.0	1.0	tr.	0	3	14.3 d
boiled, 4 oz.	145	8.5	28.1	.1	tr.	0	9	2.3 c
boiled, ½ cup	147	8.7	28.5	.1	tr.	0	9	2.3 c
ADZUKI BEAN, CANNED:								
sweetened, 4 oz.	269	4.3	62.4	<.1	(0)	0	247	1.7 c
sweetened, ½ cup	351	5.6	81.4	<.1	(0)	0	323	2.3 c
ADZUKI BEAN, YOKAN, see "Yokan"								
AGAR, see "Seaweed"								
AHI, see "Tuna, yellowfin"								
AKU, see "Tuna, skipjack"								
ALBACORE, see "Tuna, canned"								
ALCOHOLIC BEVERAGES, see specific listings								
ALE, see "Beer, ale, and malt liquor"								
ALFALFA SEEDS:								
(*Arrowhead Mills*), 1 cup	40	5.0	4.0	1.0	n.a.	0	n.a.	m.q.
ALFALFA SEEDS, SPROUTED, raw:								
1 lb.	132	18.1	17.1	3.1	.3	0	29	10.0 d
1 oz.	8	1.1	1.1	.2	<.1	0	2	.6 d
½ cup	5	.7	.6	.1	<.1	0	1	.4 d
1 tbsp.	1	.1	.1	<.1	tr.	0	tr.	.1 d
ALFREDO SAUCE:								
canned (*Progresso* Authentic Pasta Sauces), ½ cup	340	13.0	6.0	30.0	19.0	95	1080	n.a.
refrigerated (*Contadina Fresh*), 6 oz.	540	9.0	10.0	53.0	m.q.	85	620	n.a.
ALFREDO SAUCE MIX:								
(*French's Pasta Toss*), 2 tsp. dry	25	1.0	2.0	2.0	n.a.	n.a.	310	n.a.
(*Lawry's* Pasta Alfredo), 1 pkg.	226	8.0	19.2	13.3	m.q.	n.a.	3222	.6 c
ALGAE, see "Seaweed"								
ALLSPICE, ground:								
1 oz.	75	1.7	20.4	2.5	.7	0	22	6.1 c
1 tbsp.	16	.4	4.3	.5	.2	0	5	1.3 c
1 tsp.	5	.1	1.4	.2	.1	0	1	.4 c

Food and Measure	cal.	prot. (gms)	carbo. (gms)	tot. fat (gms)	sat. fat (gms)	chol. (mgs)	sod. (mgs)	fiber (gms)
(*Spice Islands*), 1 tsp.	6	.1	1.3	.1	tr.	0	1	.4 c
(*Tone's*), 1 tsp.	5	.1	1.4	.2	.1	0	2	.4 d
ALMOND[1]:								
(*Beer Nuts*), 1 oz.	180	5.0	7.0	14.4	m.q.	0	51	m.q.
(*Dole*), 1 oz.	170	6.0	12.0	14.0	m.q.	0	4	m.q.
dried:								
in shell, 1 lb.	1069	36.2	37.0	94.7	9.0	0	19	4.9 c
1 oz., approx. 24 whole kernels . .	167	5.7	5.8	14.8	1.4	0	3	8.6 d
whole kernels, 1 cup	837	28.3	29.0	74.1	7.0	0	15	6.7 d
chopped, 1 cup	766	25.9	26.5	67.9	6.4	0	14	6.1 d
sliced or diced, 1 cup	554	18.8	19.2	49.1	4.7	0	10	4.4 d
slivered, 1 cup packed	795	26.9	27.5	70.5	6.7	0	15	6.4 d
dried, blanched:								
1 oz.	166	5.8	5.3	14.9	1.4	0	3	.7 c
whole kernels, 1 cup	850	29.6	26.9	76.2	7.2	0	15	3.3 c
sliced, 1 cup	615	21.4	19.5	55.2	5.2	0	11	2.4 c
whole, sliced, or slivered								
(*Planters*), 1 oz.	170	6.0	6.0	15.0	2.0	0	0	m.q.
dry-roasted:								
1 oz.	167	4.6	6.9	14.7	1.4	0	3	1.4 c
whole kernels, 1 cup	810	22.5	33.4	71.2	6.8	0	15	6.8 c
salted, 1 oz.	167	4.6	6.9	14.7	1.4	0	221	1.4 c
salted, whole kernels, 1 cup	810	22.5	33.4	71.2	6.8	0	1076	6.8 c
(*Planters*), 1 oz.	170	6.0	6.0	15.0	2.0	0	200	m.q.
oil-roasted:								
1 oz., approx. 22 whole kernels . .	176	5.8	4.5	16.4	1.6	0	3	3.2 d
whole kernels, 1 cup	970	32.0	24.9	90.5	8.6	0	16	17.6 d
salted, 1 oz., approx. 22 whole								
kernels	176	5.8	4.5	16.4	1.6	0	221	3.2 d
salted, whole kernels, 1 cup	970	32.0	24.9	90.5	8.6	0	1223	17.6 d
oil-roasted, blanched:								
1 oz., approx. 24 whole kernels . .	174	5.4	5.1	16.1	1.5	0	3	3.2 d
whole kernels, 1 cup	870	27.0	25.6	80.3	7.6	0	17	15.9 d
salted, 1 oz., approx. 24 whole								
kernels	174	5.4	5.1	16.1	1.5	0	220	3.2 d
salted, whole kernels, 1 cup	870	27.0	25.6	80.3	7.6	0	1120	15.9 d
toasted, 1 oz.	167	5.8	6.5	14.4	1.4	0	3	1.4 c
ALMOND BUTTER:								
plain:								
1 oz.	179	4.3	6.0	16.8	1.6	0	3	.4 c
½ cup	791	18.9	26.5	73.9	7.0	0	14	1.9 c
1 tbsp.	101	2.4	3.4	9.5	.9	0	2	.2 c
raw (*Hain* Natural), 2 tbsp.	190	8.0	3.0	18.0	2.0	0	5	m.q.
blanched, toasted (*Hain*), 2 tbsp.	220	8.0	3.0	19.0	2.0	0	10	m.q.
smooth (*Westbrae Natural*),								
2 tbsp.	190	7.0	7.0	17.0	m.q.	0	0	m.q.
salted:								
1 oz.	179	4.3	6.0	16.8	1.6	0	128	.4 c

1. *Shelled, except as noted.*

Food and Measure	cal.	prot. (gms)	carbo. (gms)	tot. fat (gms)	sat. fat (gms)	chol. (mgs)	sod. (mgs)	fiber (gms)
ALMOND BUTTER, SALTED *(cont.)*								
1 cup	791	18.9	26.5	73.9	7.0	0	563	1.9 c
1 tbsp.	101	2.4	3.4	9.5	.9	0	72	.2 c
honey and cinnamon:								
1 oz.	171	4.5	7.6	14.8	1.4	0	3	.4 c
½ cup	753	19.8	33.7	65.3	6.2	0	14	1.9 c
1 tbsp.	96	2.5	4.3	8.4	.8	0	2	.2 c
salted:								
1 oz.	171	4.5	7.6	14.8	1.4	0	48	.4 c
½ cup	753	19.8	33.7	65.3	6.2	0	213	1.9 c
1 tbsp.	96	2.5	4.3	8.4	.8	0	27	.2 c
ALMOND MEAL, partially defatted:								
4 oz.	463	44.8	32.8	20.8	2.0	0	8	2.6 c
1 oz.	116	11.2	8.2	5.2	.5	0	2	.7 c
salted, 4 oz.	463	44.8	32.8	20.8	2.0	0	846	2.6 c
salted, 1 oz.	116	11.2	8.2	5.2	.5	0	211	.7 c
ALMOND OIL:								
1 oz.	251	0	0	28.4	2.3	0	0	0
½ cup	964	0	0	109.0	9.0	0	0	0
1 tbsp.	120	0	0	13.6	1.1	0	0	0
(Hain), 1 tbsp.	120	0	0	14.0	1.0	0	0	0
ALMOND PASTE:								
4 oz.	506	13.4	49.4	30.8	2.9	0	10	6.8 c
1 oz.	127	3.4	12.4	7.2	.7	0	3	1.7 c
1 cup packed	1012	26.9	98.9	61.7	5.9	0	21	13.6 c
ALMOND POWDER:								
full-fat:								
4 oz.	671	22.5	25.4	58.6	5.6	0	7	2.2 c
1 oz.	168	5.6	6.4	14.7	1.4	0	2	.5 c
1 cup not packed	385	12.9	14.5	33.6	3.2	0	4	1.2 c
partially defatted[1]:								
4 oz.	446	42.5	36.1	18.1	1.7	0	11	3.2 c
1 oz.	112	10.6	9.0	4.5	.4	0	3	.8 c
1 cup not packed	255	24.4	20.7	10.4	1.0	0	6	1.8 c
AMARANTH:								
raw:								
untrimmed, 1 lb.	110	10.5	17.2	1.4	.4	0	83	4.2 c
trimmed, 1 oz.	7	.7	1.1	.1	<.1	0	6	.3 c
trimmed, ½ cup	4	.3	.6	<.1	<.1	0	3	.1 c
1 leaf, approx. .5 oz.	4	.3	.6	.1	<.1	0	3	.1 c
boiled, drained, 4 oz.	24	2.4	4.7	.2	.1	0	24	1.5 c
boiled, drained, ½ cup	14	1.4	2.7	.1	<.1	0	14	.9 c
AMARANTH, WHOLE GRAIN:								
1 oz.	106	4.1	18.8	1.8	.5	0	6	4.3 d
1 cup	729	28.2	129.0	12.7	3.2	0	42	29.6 d
AMARANTH DINNER, canned:								

1. *Made from blanched almonds.*

Food and Measure	cal.	prot. (gms)	carbo. (gms)	tot. fat (gms)	sat. fat (gms)	chol. (mgs)	sod. (mgs)	fiber (gms)
w/garden vegetables (*Health Valley*								
Fast Menu), 7½ oz.	120	8.0	16.0	3.0	m.q.	0	138	8.3 d
AMARANTH FLOUR:								
(*Arrowhead Mills*), 2 oz.	200	8.0	35.0	3.0	m.q.	0	<1	3.9 d
AMARANTH SEED:								
(*Arrowhead Mills*), 2 oz.	200	8.0	35.0	3.0	m.q.	0	1	3.9 d
AMBERJACK, meat only:								
raw, 1 lb.	386	82.1	0	4.1	m.q.	m.q.	m.q.	0
raw, 1 oz.	24	5.1	0	.3	tr.	m.q.	m.q.	0
ANASAZI BEAN:								
raw (*Arrowhead Mills*), 2 oz.	200	13.0	35.0	1.0	n.a.	0	3	12.1 d
ANCHOVY, European, meat only:								
raw, 1 lb.	592	92.3	0	22.0	5.8	m.q.	471	0
raw, 1 oz.	37	5.8	0	1.4	.4	m.q.	29	0
ANCHOVY, CANNED, in olive oil,								
drained:								
1 oz.	60	8.2	0	2.8	.6	m.q.	1040	0
1.6 oz., yield from 2-oz. can	95	13.0	0	4.4	1.0	m.q.	1651	0
5 medium, approx. .7 oz.	42	5.8	0	1.9	.4	m.q.	734	0
ANGEL HAIR PASTA, see "Pasta"								
ANISE SEED:								
1 oz.	95	5.0	14.2	4.5	n.a.	0	5	4.1 c
1 tbsp.	23	1.2	3.4	1.1	n.a.	0	1	1.0 c
1 tsp.	7	.4	1.1	.3	n.a.	0	tr.	.3 c
(*Tone's*), 1 tsp.	7	.4	1.1	.3	n.a.	0	2	.3 d
ANTELOPE, meat only:								
raw, 1 oz.	32	6.4	0	.6	.2	27	14	0
roasted[1]:								
12 oz., yield from 1 lb. boneless	510	100.2	0	9.1	3.3	427	183	0
4 oz.	170	33.4	0	3.0	1.1	143	61	0
diced, 1 cup, approx. 4.9 oz.	210	41.2	0	3.7	1.4	176	76	0
APIO ROOT, see "Celeriac"								
APPLE:								
raw, untrimmed, 1 lb.	244	.8	63.7	1.5	.2	0	2	9.2 d
raw, cored, unpeeled:								
1 oz.	17	.1	4.3	.1	<.1	0	tr.	.6 d
1 medium, 2¾" diam., approx.								
3 per lb.	81	.3	21.1	.5	.1	0	1	3.0 d
sliced, ½ cup	32	.1	8.4	.2	<.1	0	tr.	1.2 d
raw, cored, peeled:								
1 oz.	16	<.1	4.2	.1	<.1	0	tr.	.5 d
1 medium, 2¾" diam., approx.								
3 per lb.	72	.2	19.0	.4	.1	0	tr.	2.4 d
sliced, ½ cup	31	.1	8.2	.2	<.1	0	tr.	1.0 d
boiled, peeled, 4 oz.	60	.3	15.5	.4	.1	0	1	2.2 d
boiled, peeled, sliced, ½ cup	46	.2	11.7	.3	.1	0	1	1.6 d
microwaved, peeled, 4 oz.	64	.3	16.3	.5	.1	0	1	2.7 d
microwaved, peeled, sliced, ½ cup	48	.2	12.3	.4	.1	0	1	2.0 d

1. *Without added ingredients.*

Food and Measure	cal.	prot. (gms)	carbo. (gms)	tot. fat (gms)	sat. fat (gms)	chol. (mgs)	sod. (mgs)	fiber (gms)
APPLE, CANNED:								
baked, whole (*Lucky Leaf/ Musselman's*), 1 apple	110	0	28.0	0	0	0	35	m.q.
baked style (*White House*), 3.5 oz. ...	118	0	29.0	0	0	0	11	m.q.
chipped (*Lucky Leaf/Musselman's*), 4 oz.	50	0	12.0	0	0	0	10	m.q.
chipped, in water (*White House*), 4 oz.	50	0	12.0	0	0	0	5	m.q.
diced (*Lucky Leaf/Musselman's*), 4 oz.	50	0	12.0	0	0	0	10	m.q.
rings, spiced (*White House*), 3.5 oz.	180	0	44.0	0	0	0	25	m.q.
rings, spiced, red/green (*Lucky Leaf/ Musselman's*), 4 oz.	100	0	24.0	0	0	0	20	m.q.
sliced:								
dessert (*Lucky Leaf/Musselman's*), 4 oz.	70	0	16.0	0	0	0	25	m.q.
sweetened:								
unheated, 4 oz.	76	.2	18.9	.6	.1	0	3	2.1 d
unheated, ½ cup	68	.2	17.0	.5	.1	0	3	1.8 d
heated, 4 oz.	76	.2	19.1	.5	.1	0	3	2.3 d
heated, ½ cup	68	.2	17.2	.4	.1	0	3	2.1 d
(*White House*), 4 oz.	54	0	14.0	0	0	0	10	m.q.
in syrup (*Lucky Leaf/ Musselman's*), 4 oz.	50	0	13.0	0	0	0	35	m.q.
in water (*Lucky Leaf/ Musselman's*), 4 oz.	50	0	12.0	0	0	0	10	m.q.
in water (*White House*), 4 oz.	40	0	12.0	0	0	0	5	m.q.
unpeeled (*Lucky Leaf/ Musselman's*), 4 oz.	90	0	22.0	0	0	0	15	m.q.
whole, peeled, cored (*Lucky Leaf/ Musselman's*), 1 apple	90	0	21.0	0	0	0	10	m.q.
APPLE, DEHYDRATED, sulfured[1]:								
uncooked, 4 oz.	392	1.5	111.7	.7	.1	0	141	4.6 c
uncooked, ½ cup	104	.4	28.1	.2	<.1	0	37	1.2 c
cooked, 4 oz.	84	.3	22.6	.1	<.1	0	29	1.0 c
cooked, ½ cup	71	.3	19.3	.1	<.1	0	25	.8 c
chips (*Weight Watchers*), .75-oz. pkg.	70	0	19.0	0	0	0	200	4.0 d
APPLE, DRIED:								
chunks (*Sun-Maid/Sunsweet*). 2 oz.	150	1.0	42.0	0	0	0	<40	m.q.
sliced, uncooked (*Del Monte*), 2 oz.	140	0	37.0	0	0	0	<50	m.q.
sulfured[1], uncooked:								
4 oz.	276	1.1	74.7	.4	.1	0	99	3.3 c
10 rings, approx. 2.3 oz.	155	.6	42.2	.2	<.1	0	56	1.8 c
½ cup	105	.4	28.3	.1	<.1	0	38	1.2 c
sulfured[1], cooked:								
unsweetened, 4 oz.	65	.2	17.4	.1	<.1	0	23	.8 c

1. *Sodium bisulfite used to preserve color; unsulfured product would contain lower levels of sodium.*

Food and Measure	cal.	prot. (gms)	carbo. (gms)	tot. fat (gms)	sat. fat (gms)	chol. (mgs)	sod. (mgs)	fiber (gms)
unsweetened, ½ cup	72	.3	19.6	.1	<.1	0	26	.9 c
sweetened, 4 oz.	94	.2	23.5	.1	<.1	0	22	.7 c
sweetened, ½ cup	116	.3	29.0	.1	<.1	0	27	.9 c
APPLE, ESCALLOPED, frozen:								
(*Stouffer's*), 4 oz.	130	0	27.0	2.0	m.q.	n.a.	15	n.a.
APPLE, FROZEN, unsweetened:								
4 oz.	54	.3	14.0	.4	.1	0	3	2.3 d
sliced, ½ cup	41	.2	10.6	.3	<.1	0	3	1.8 d
heated, 4 oz.	53	.3	13.6	.4	.1	0	3	2.2 d
heated, sliced, ½ cup	48	.3	12.4	.3	.1	0	3	2.0 d
APPLE, GLAZED, frozen:								
in raspberry sauce (*The Budget*								
Gourmet Side Dish), 5 oz.	110	0	22.0	3.0	m.q.	10	210	m.q.
APPLE BUTTER:								
(*Bama*), 2 tbsp.	25	0	6.0	0	0	0	5	m.q.
(*Lucky Leaf/Musselman's*), 4 oz. . . .	200	0	49.0	1.0	(0)	0	15	m.q.
(*Smucker's* Autumn Harvest/Simply								
Fruit), 1 tsp.	12	0	3.0	0	0	0	0	m.q.
(*Tap'n Apple*), 1 oz.	45	<1.0	13.2	<.1	(0)	0	<1	.5 d
(*White House*), 1 oz.	50	0	12.0	0	0	0	5	m.q.
natural or cider (*Smucker's*), 1 tsp.	12	0	3.0	0	0	0	0	m.q.
APPLE CAKE, see "Cake"								
APPLE CHIPS, see "Apple,								
dehydrated"								
APPLE CIDER, 6 fl. oz.:								
canned or bottled:								
(*Indian Summer*)	80	<1.0	20.0	<1.0	(0)	0	10	m.q.
(*Lucky Leaf/Musselman's*)	90	0	21.0	0	0	0	0	m.q.
cinnamon (*Indian Summer*)	90	<1.0	21.0	<1.0	(0)	0	10	m.q.
sparkling (*Lucky Leaf*)	80	0	18.0	0	0	0	45	m.q.
canned or frozen[1] (*Tree Top*)	90	0	22.0	0	0	0	10	n.a.
APPLE COBBLER, see "Cobbler"								
APPLE CRISP, frozen:								
(*Pepperidge Farm* Berkshire),								
1 ramekin	250	2.0	43.0	8.0	4.0	4.0	130	1.0 d
(*Weight Watchers*), ½ pkg. or 3.5 oz.	190	1.0	40.0	5.0	<1.0	n.a.	190	m.q.
APPLE DANISH, see "Danish								
pastry"								
APPLE DRINK:								
(*Hi-C* Candy Apple Cooler),								
8.45 fl. oz.	132	<.1	32.6	<.1	0	0	25	(0)
(*Hi-C* Candy Apple Cooler), 6 fl. oz.	94	<.1	23.1	<.1	0	0	17	(0)
APPLE DUMPLING, frozen:								
(*Pepperidge Farm*), 3 oz.	260	2.0	33.0	13.0	m.q.	n.a.	230	m.q.
APPLE FRITTER, frozen:								
(*Mrs. Paul's*), 2 pieces	240	4.0	35.0	9.0	m.q.	5	500	n.a.
APPLE FRUIT ROLL, see "Fruit								
snack"								

1. *Diluted according to package directions.*

Food and Measure	cal.	prot. (gms)	carbo. (gms)	tot. fat (gms)	sat. fat (gms)	chol. (mgs)	sod. (mgs)	fiber (gms)
APPLE FRUIT SQUARE, frozen:								
(*Pepperidge Farm*), 1 piece	220	2.0	27.0	12.0	m.q.	n.a.	170	m.q.
APPLE JUICE, 6 fl. oz., except as noted:								
canned, bottled or boxed:								
1 fl. oz.	15	<.1	3.6	<.1	tr.	0	1	.1 c
6 fl. oz.	87	.1	21.7	.2	<.1	0	6	.4 c
(*IGA* Unsweetened)	74	0	18.0	0	0	0	10	m.q.
(*Indian Summer*)	90	<1.0	21.0	<1.0	(0)	0	10	m.q.
(*Kraft* Pure 100%)	80	0	20.0	0	0	0	5	m.q.
(*Lucky Leaf/Musselman's* Regular or 100% Vitamin C Enriched) ..	90	0	21.0	0	0	0	0	m.q.
(*Lucky Leaf/Musselman's* Individual Portion Control), 3.8 fl. oz.	60	0	14.0	0	0	0	0	m.q.
(*Minute Maid*), 8.45 fl. oz.	128	.2	31.9	.3	(0)	0	32	m.q.
(*Minute Maid* Juices to Go), 11.5 fl. oz.	174	.2	43.4	.4	(0)	0	44	m.q.
(*Minute Maid* Juices to Go), 9.6 fl. oz.	145	.2	35.3	.3	(0)	0	37	m.q.
(*Minute Maid On The Go*), 10 fl. oz.	152	.2	37.8	.4	(0)	0	38	m.q.
(*Mott's*), 10 oz.	148	0	37.0	0	0	0	22	m.q.
(*Mott's*), 9.5 fl. oz.	141	0	35.0	0	0	0	20	m.q.
(*Mott's*)	88	0	22.0	0	0	0	13	m.q.
(*Mott's* Aseptic), 8.45 fl. oz.	124	0	31.0	0	0	0	18	m.q.
(*Mott's* Natural Style)	76	0	19.0	0	0	0	28	m.q.
(*Ocean Spray*)	90	0	23.0	0	0	0	14	m.q.
(*Red Cheek* Natural)	97	.2	24.0	0	0	0	16	m.q.
(*Red Cheek* 100% Pure)	97	.2	24.0	0	0	0	7	m.q.
(*S&W* 100% Pure Unsweetened)	85	0	20.0	0	0	0	5	m.q.
(*Tree Top*)	90	0	22.0	0	0	0	10	.2 c
(*TreeSweet*)	90	0	22.0	0	0	0	15	m.q.
(*Tropicana* 100% Pure), 8 fl. oz.	116	(0)	28.5	0	0	0	17	m.q.
(*Veryfine* 100%), 8 fl. oz.	107	.2	27.0	0	0	0	<10	m.q.
(*White House*)	87	0	22.0	0	0	0	5	m.q.
blend (*Libby's Juicy Juice*)	90	0	21.0	0	0	0	5	m.q.
sparkling (*Welch's*)	100	0	24.0	0	0	0	5	0
chilled or frozen[1]:								
(*Minute Maid*)	91	.1	22.7	.2	0	0	23	m.q.
(*Sunkist*), 8 fl. oz.	79	.2	19.4	.2	0	0	12	m.q.
(*Tree Top*)	90	0	22.0	0	0	0	10	m.q.
frozen[2]:								
undiluted	349	1.1	86.5	.8	.1	0	54	m.q.
6 fl. oz.	84	.3	20.7	.2	<.1	0	13	.6 c
(*A&P*)	90	<1.0	22.0	<1.0	(0)	0	0	m.q.
APPLE JUICE COCKTAIL:								
(*Welch's Orchard*), 10 fl. oz.	170	0	42.0	0	0	0	95	0

1. *Diluted according to package directions.*
2. *Diluted according to package directions, except as noted.*

Food and Measure	cal.	prot. (gms)	carbo. (gms)	tot. fat (gms)	sat. fat (gms)	chol. (mgs)	sod. (mgs)	fiber (gms)
APPLE PASTRY POCKET:								
(*Tastykake*), 3 oz.	323	4.3	38.3	17.6	4.0	11	222	1.5 d
APPLE PIE, see "Pie"								
APPLE PIE FILLING, see "Pie filling"								
APPLE PIE SPICE:								
(*Tone's*), 1 tsp.	9	.2	2.4	.2	.1	0	1	.7 d
APPLE PUNCH:								
(*Red Cheek*), 6 fl. oz.	113	.3	28.0	0	0	0	7	(0)
APPLE RINGS, SPICED, see "Apple, canned"								
APPLE STICKS, frozen:								
breaded, fried (*Farm Rich*), 4 oz. ...	260	2.0	44.0	8.0	m.q.	0	565	m.q.
APPLE TURNOVER, see "Turnover, frozen" and "Turnover, refrigerated"								
APPLE-APRICOT SAUCE:								
(*Lucky Leaf/Musselman's* Fruit n' Sauce), 4 oz.	90	0	22.0	0	0	0	<20	m.q.
APPLE-CHERRY CIDER:								
(*Indian Summer*), 6 fl. oz.	100	<1.0	25.0	<1.0	(0)	0	10	m.q.
APPLE-CHERRY JUICE:								
(*Musselman's* Breakfast Cocktail), 6 fl. oz.	100	1.0	26.0	0	0	0	5	m.q.
(*Red Cheek*), 6 fl. oz.	113	.2	28.0	0	0	0	11	m.q.
APPLE-CHERRY SAUCE:								
(*Lucky Leaf/Musselman's* Fruit n' Sauce), 4 oz.	100	0	24.0	0	0	0	<20	m.q.
APPLE-CHERRY-BERRY DRINK:								
(*Veryfine*), 8 fl. oz.	130	.1	33.0	0	0	0	<25	m.q.
APPLE-CITRUS JUICE:								
canned or frozen[1] (*Tree Top*), 6 fl. oz.	90	1.0	22.0	0	0	0	10	m.q.
APPLE-CRANBERRY CIDER:								
(*Indian Summer*), 6 fl. oz.	100	<1.0	24.0	<1.0	(0)	0	10	m.q.
APPLE-CRANBERRY DRINK:								
(*Mott's*), 10 oz.	176	0	44.0	0	0	0	3	(0)
(*Mott's*), 9.5 oz.	167	0	42.0	0	0	0	3	(0)
APPLE-CRANBERRY JUICE:								
(*Apple & Eve*), 6 fl. oz.	80	0	19.0	0	0	0	5	m.q.
(*Lucky Leaf*), 6 fl. oz.	130	0	32.0	0	0	0	10	m.q.
(*Mott's*), 9.5 oz.	147	0	38.0	0	0	0	27	m.q.
(*Mott's*), 6 fl. oz.	83	0	24.0	0	0	0	17	m.q.
(*Mott's* Aseptic), 8.45 fl. oz.	136	0	34.0	0	0	0	24	m.q.
canned or frozen[1] (*Tree Top*), 6 fl. oz.	100	0	25.0	0	0	0	10	m.q.
APPLE-CRANBERRY JUICE COCKTAIL:								
(*Veryfine*), 8 fl. oz.	130	.1	33.0	0	0	0	<10	(0)

1. *Diluted according to package directions.*

Food and Measure	cal.	prot. (gms)	carbo. (gms)	tot. fat (gms)	sat. fat (gms)	chol. (mgs)	sod. (mgs)	fiber (gms)
APPLE-CRANBERRY JUICE DRINK:								
(*Tropicana* Single Serve), 10 fl. oz.	175	(0)	43.0	0	0	0	<3	(0)
APPLE-CRANBERRY SAUCE:								
(*Lucky Leaf*), 4 oz.	80	0	19.0	0	0	0	15	(0)
APPLE-GRAPE JUICE:								
(*Libby's Juicy Juice*), 6 fl. oz.	90	0	22.0	0	0	0	10	m.q.
(*Mott's*), 9.5 fl. oz. can	139	0	37.0	0	0	0	27	m.q.
(*Mott's*), 6 fl. oz.	86	0	23.0	0	0	0	17	m.q.
(*Mott's* Aseptic), 8.45 fl. oz.	128	0	32.0	0	0	0	24	m.q.
(*Red Cheek*), 6 fl. oz.	109	.3	27.0	0	0	0	9	m.q.
canned or frozen[1] (*Tree Top*), 6 fl. oz.	100	0	25.0	0	0	0	10	m.q.
APPLE-GRAPE JUICE COCKTAIL:								
(*Musselman's* Breakfast), 6 fl. oz. ..	110	0	28.0	0	0	0	5	(0)
(*Welch's Orchard*), 6 fl. oz.	110	0	27.0	0	0	0	20	(0)
(*Welch's Orchard* Cocktails-In-A-Box), 8.45 fl. oz.	150	0	38.0	0	0	0	20	(0)
frozen[1] (*Welch's* Orchard), 6 fl. oz.	110	0	27.0	0	0	0	10	(0)
APPLE-GRAPE-CHERRY JUICE COCKTAIL:								
(*Welch's Orchard*), 6 fl. oz.	110	0	27.0	0	0	0	20	(0)
(*Welch's Orchard* Cocktails-In-A-Box), 8.45 fl. oz.	150	0	38.0	0	0	0	20	(0)
frozen[1] (*Welch's Orchard*), 6 fl. oz. ...	90	0	22.0	0	0	0	10	(0)
APPLE-GRAPE-RASPBERRY JUICE COCKTAIL:								
(*Welch's Orchard*), 6 fl. oz.	100	0	26.0	0	0	0	20	(0)
(*Welch's Orchard* Cocktails-In-A-Box), 8.45 fl. oz.	140	0	35.0	0	0	0	20	(0)
frozen[1] (*Welch's* Orchard), 6 fl. oz.	90	0	22.0	0	0	0	10	(0)
APPLE-ORANGE-PINEAPPLE JUICE COCKTAIL:								
(*Welch's Orchard Tropicals*), 10 fl. oz.	180	0	45.0	0	0	0	0	(0)
(*Welch's Orchard Tropicals* Cocktails-In-A-Box), 8.45 fl. oz.	140	0	35.0	0	0	0	20	(0)
bottled or frozen[1] (*Welch's Orchard Tropicals*), 6 fl. oz.	100	0	25.0	0	0	0	20	(0)
APPLE-PEACH SAUCE:								
(*Lucky Leaf/Musselman's* Fruit n' Sauce), 4 oz.	90	0	22.0	0	0	0	<20	m.q.
APPLE-PEAR JUICE:								
canned or frozen[1] (*Tree Top*), 6 fl. oz.	90	0	22.0	0	0	0	10	m.q.
APPLE-PINEAPPLE SAUCE:								
(*Lucky Leaf/Musselman's* Fruit n' Sauce), 4 oz.	110	0	26.0	0	0	0	<20	m.q.

1. *Diluted according to package directions.*

Food and Measure	cal.	prot. (gms)	carbo. (gms)	tot. fat (gms)	sat. fat (gms)	chol. (mgs)	sod. (mgs)	fiber (gms)
APPLE-RASPBERRY DRINK:								
(*Mott's*), 10 oz.	158	0	40.0	0	0	0	17	(0)
(*Mott's*), 9.5 fl. oz.	150	0	38.0	0	0	0	16	(0)
APPLE-RASPBERRY JUICE:								
(*Mott's*), 9.5 fl. oz.	134	0	35.0	0	0	0	76	m.q.
(*Mott's*), 6 fl. oz.	83	0	22.0	0	0	0	48	m.q.
(*Mott's* Aseptic), 8.45 fl. oz.	124	0	31.0	0	0	0	67	m.q.
(*Red Cheek*), 6 fl. oz.	113	.3	28.0	0	0	0	8	m.q.
canned or frozen[1] (*Tree Top*), 6 fl. oz.	80	0	21.0	0	0	0	10	m.q.
APPLE-RASPBERRY JUICE COCKTAIL:								
(*Veryfine*), 8 fl. oz.	110	0	27.0	0	0	0	<15	(0)
APPLE-STRAWBERRY SAUCE:								
(*Lucky Leaf/Musselman's* Fruit n' Sauce), 4 oz.	100	0	24.0	0	0	0	<20	m.q.
APPLE-WHITE GRAPE JUICE COCKTAIL, frozen[1]:								
(*Welch's* No Sugar Added), 6 fl. oz.	40	0	10.0	0	0	0	5	(0)
APPLESAUCE, canned or in jars:								
4 oz.	86	.2	22.6	.2	<.1	0	32	1.4 d
½ cup	97	.2	25.5	.2	<.1	0	32	1.5 d
no salt added, 4 oz.	86	.2	22.6	.2	<.1	0	3	1.3 d
no salt added, ½ cup	97	.2	25.5	.2	<.1	0	4	1.4 d
(*A&P*), ½ cup	110	<1.0	25.0	<1.0	(0)	0	15	m.q.
(*A&P* Unsweetened), ½ cup	50	<1.0	10.0	<1.0	(0)	0	0	m.q.
(*Del Monte*), ½ cup	90	0	24.0	0	0	0	<5	m.q.
(*Del Monte Lite*), ½ cup	50	0	13.0	0	0	0	<10	m.q.
(*Featherweight*), ½ cup	50	0	12.0	0	0	0	<3	m.q.
(*Finast*), ½ cup	105	0	25.0	0	0	0	10	m.q.
(*Finast* Unsweetened), ½ cup	56	.4	15.0	.2	(0)	0	n.a.	m.q.
(*Hunt's Snack Pack*), 4.25 oz.	80	0	19.0	0	0	0	n.a.	m.q.
(*Lucky Leaf/Musselman's*), 4 oz. ...	80	0	20.0	0	0	0	20	m.q.
(*Lucky Leaf/Musselman's* Juice Pack), 4 oz.	50	0	12.0	0	0	0	0	m.q.
(*Lucky Leaf/Musselman's* Individual Portion Control, Regular), 4 oz.	80	0	20	0	0	0	0	m.q.
(*Lucky Leaf/Musselman's* Individual Portion Control, Natural), 4 oz.	50	0	13.0	0	0	0	0	m.q.
(*Lucky Leaf/Musselman's* Unsweetened), 4 oz.	50	0	12.0	0	0	0	0	m.q.
(*Mott's*), 6 oz.	150	0	36.0	0	0	0	<1	m.q.
(*Mott's* Chunky), 6 oz.	86	0	21.0	0	0	0	11	m.q.
(*Mott's* Natural), 6 oz.	80	0	20.0	0	0	0	3	m.q.
(*Mott's* Natural Single Serve), 4 oz.	53	0	13.0	0	0	0	2	m.q.
(*Mott's* Single Serve), 4 oz.	100	0	24.0	0	0	0	<1	m.q.
(*S&W*), ½ cup	90	0	24.0	0	0	0	10	m.q.
(*S&W* Unsweetened) ½ cup	55	0	14.0	0	0	0	5	m.q.

1. *Diluted according to package directions.*

Food and Measure	cal.	prot. (gms)	carbo. (gms)	tot. fat (gms)	sat. fat (gms)	chol. (mgs)	sod. (mgs)	fiber (gms)
APPLESAUCE *(cont.)*								
(S&W/Nutradiet), ½ cup	55	0	14.0	0	0	0	10	m.q.
(Stokely), ½ cup	90	0	23.0	0	0	0	30	m.q.
(Stokely Unsweetened), ½ cup	45	0	12.0	0	0	0	5	m.q.
(Tree Top Original), ½ cup	80	0	21.0	0	0	0	0	m.q.
(White House Regular or Chunky),								
4 oz.	80	0	22.0	0	0	0	5	m.q.
(White House Unsweetened), 4 oz.	50	0	12.0	0	0	0	5	m.q.
in apple juice *(White House)*, 4 oz. ..	50	0	13.0	0	0	0	5	m.q.
chunky *(Lucky Leaf/Musselman's)*,								
4 oz.	80	0	20.0	0	0	0	20	m.q.
cinnamon *(Mott's)*, 6 oz.	152	0	36.0	0	0	0	<1	m.q.
cinnamon *(Mott's* Single Serve), 4 oz.	101	0	24.0	0	0	0	<1	m.q.
unsweetened (see also specific								
brands):								
4 oz.	49	.2	12.8	.1	tr.	0	2	1.7 d
½ cup	53	.2	13.8	.1	<.1	0	2	1.8 d
APRICOT:								
untrimmed, 1 lb.	202	5.9	46.9	1.7	.1	0	2	5.6 d
pitted, 1 oz.	14	.4	3.2	.1	tr.	0	<1	.4 d
3 medium, approx. 4 oz. or								
12 per lb.	51	1.5	11.8	.4	<.1	0	1	1.4 d
halves, ½ cup	37	1.1	8.6	.3	<.1	0	1	1.0 d
APRICOT, CANNED, ½ cup,								
except as noted:								
½ cup	80	0	20.0	0	0	0	5	m.q.
whole, peeled *(Del Monte)*	100	0	27.0	0	0	0	<10	m.q.
halves, unpeeled *(Del Monte)*	100	0	26.0	0	0	0	<10	m.q.
halves, unpeeled *(Del Monte Lite)* ..	60	0	16.0	0	0	0	<10	m.q.
in water, unpeeled:								
4 oz.	31	.8	7.2	.2	<.1	0	3	.5 c
halves	33	.9	7.8	.2	<.1	0	4	.5 c
3 halves and 1¾ tbsp. liquid	22	.6	5.4	.1	tr.	0	2	.4 c
halves *(S&W)*	35	0	9.0	0	0	0	5	m.q.
halves *(S&W/Nutradiet)*	35	0	9.0	0	0	0	5	m.q.
in water, peeled:								
4 oz. or ½ cup	25	.8	6.2	<.1	tr.	0	12	.4 c
2 apricots and 2 tbsp. liquid	20	.6	4.9	<.1	tr.	0	10	.3 c
whole *(S&W/Nutradiet)*	28	0	7.0	0	0	0	5	m.q.
in juice *(Featherweight)*	50	1.0	12.0	0	0	0	<10	m.q.
in juice, unpeeled:								
4 oz.	54	.7	14.0	<.1	tr.	0	5	.5 d
halves	60	.8	15.3	<.1	tr.	0	5	.6 d
3 halves and 1¾ tbsp. liquid	40	.5	10.4	<.1	tr.	0	3	.4 d
(Libby Lite)	60	0	17.0	0	0	0	5	m.q.
in extra light syrup, unpeeled:								
4 oz.	56	.7	14.2	.1	tr.	0	2	.5 c
halves	61	.7	15.4	.1	tr.	0	3	.5 c
3 halves and 1¾ tbsp. liquid	41	.5	10.5	.1	tr.	0	2	.4 c

Food and Measure	cal.	prot. (gms)	carbo. (gms)	tot. fat (gms)	sat. fat (gms)	chol. (mgs)	sod. (mgs)	fiber (gms)
in light syrup, unpeeled:								
4 oz.	71	.6	18.7	.1	tr.	0	5	.5 c
halves	80	.7	20.9	.1	tr.	0	5	.5 c
3 halves and 1¾ tbsp. liquid	54	.5	14.0	<.1	tr.	0	3	.4 c
halves (*Pathmark* No Frills)	80	0	20.0	0	0	0	5	m.q.
in heavy syrup, unpeeled:								
4 oz.	94	.6	24.3	.1	tr.	0	5	.5 c
halves	107	.7	27.7	.1	tr.	0	5	.5 c
3 halves and 1¾ tbsp. liquid	70	.5	18.3	.1	tr.	0	3	.3 c
(*A&P*), ½ cup	110	<1.0	28.0	1.0	n.a.	0	15	m.q.
halves (*IGA*), 1 cup	220	1.0	56.0	0	0	0	15	m.q.
halves (*S&W*)	110	0	28.0	0	0	0	15	m.q.
in heavy syrup, peeled:								
4 oz.	94	.6	24.3	.1	tr.	0	12	.4 c
whole	107	.7	27.7	.1	tr.	0	14	.5 c
2 apricots and 2 tbsp. liquid	75	.5	19.3	.1	tr.	0	9	.3 c
whole (*S&W*)	100	0	26.0	0	0	0	15	m.q.
in extra heavy syrup, peeled:								
4 oz.	109	.6	28.2	<.1	tr.	0	15	.4 c
whole	118	.7	30.6	.1	tr.	0	16	.4 c
2 apricots and 2 tbsp. liquid	87	.5	22.4	<.1	tr.	0	12	.3 c
APRICOT, DEHYDRATED, sulfured[1]:								
uncooked, 4 oz.	363	5.6	94.0	.7	<.1	0	15	4.5 c
uncooked, ½ cup	192	2.9	49.7	.4	<.1	0	8	2.4 c
cooked, 4 oz.	143	2.2	37.0	.3	<.1	0	6	1.8 c
cooked, ½ cup	156	2.4	40.5	.3	<.1	0	6	1.9 c
APRICOT, DRIED:								
(*Del Monte*), 2 oz.	140	2.0	35.0	0	0	0	<10	m.q.
(*Sun Maid/Sunsweet*), 2 oz.	140	2.0	35.0	0	0	0	<10	m.q.
sulfured, uncooked:								
4 oz.	270	4.1	70.0	.5	<.1	0	11	8.8 d
10 halves, 1.2 oz.	83	1.3	21.6	.2	<.1	0	3	2.7 d
halves, ½ cup	155	2.4	40.1	.3	<.1	0	7	5.1 d
sulfured, cooked:								
unsweetened, 4 oz.	96	1.5	24.8	.2	<.1	0	3	1.2 c
unsweetened, halves, ½ cup	106	1.6	27.4	.2	<.1	0	4	1.3 c
sweetened, 4 oz.	128	1.3	33.2	.2	<.1	0	3	1.1 c
sweetened, halves, ½ cup	153	1.6	39.5	.2	<.1	0	4	1.3 c
APRICOT, FROZEN, sweetened:								
4 oz.	111	.8	28.5	.1	tr.	0	5	.7 c
½ cup	119	.9	30.4	.1	tr.	0	5	.7 c
APRICOT FRUIT SNACK, see "Fruit snack"								
APRICOT KERNEL OIL:								
1 oz.	251	0	0	28.4	1.8	0	0	0
½ cup	964	0	0	109.0	6.9	0	0	0
1 tbsp.	120	0	0	13.6	.9	0	0	0
(*Hain*), 1 tbsp.	120	0	0	14.0	1.0	0	0	0

1. *If sodium bisulfite is used to preserve color, sodium value will be much higher.*

Food and Measure	cal.	prot. (gms)	carbo. (gms)	tot. fat (gms)	sat. fat (gms)	chol. (mgs)	sod. (mgs)	fiber (gms)
APRICOT NECTAR, canned or bottled:								
1 fl. oz.	18	.1	4.5	<.1	tr.	0	1	.2 d
6 fl. oz.	106	.7	27.1	.2	tr.	0	6	1.1 d
(*Del Monte*), 6 fl. oz.	100	1.0	26.0	0	0	0	<10	m.q.
(*Libby's*), 6 fl. oz.	110	0	26.0	0	0	0	0	m.q.
(*S&W*), 6 fl. oz.	100	0	26.0	0	0	0	10	m.q.
APRICOT-PINEAPPLE NECTAR:								
(*S&W/Nutradiet*), 4 fl. oz.	35	0	12.0	0	0	0	20	m.q.
ARBY'S:								
sandwiches, 1 serving:								
beef 'n cheddar, 7 oz.	455	25.7	27.7	26.8	7.6	63	955	m.q.
chicken breast, 6.5 oz.	493	23.0	47.9	25.0	5.1	91	1019	m.q.
ham 'n cheese, 5.5 oz.	292	22.9	19.2	13.7	4.7	45	1350	m.q.
roast beef, regular, 5.2 oz.	353	22.2	31.6	14.8	7.3	39	588	m.q.
roast beef, super, 8.3 oz.	501	25.1	50.4	22.1	8.5	40	798	m.q.
roast chicken club, 8.3 oz.	610	31.0	40.0	33.0	8.0	80	1500	m.q.
turkey deluxe, 7 oz.	375	23.8	32.5	16.6	4.1	39	1047	m.q.
french fries, 2.5 oz.	246	2.1	29.8	13.2	3.0	0	114	m.q.
potato cakes, 3 oz.	204	1.8	19.8	12.0	2.2	0	397	m.q.
shake, Jamocha, 11.5 oz.	368	9.3	59.1	10.5	2.5	35	262	(0)
ARROWHEAD:								
raw:								
untrimmed, 1 lb.	337	18.2	68.8	1.0	n.a.	0	75	2.8 c
trimmed, 1 oz.	28	1.5	5.7	.1	(0)	0	6	.2 c
1 large corm, 3½″ diam., approx. 1.2 oz.	26	1.3	5.1	.1	(0)	0	6	.2 c
1 medium corm, 2⅝″ diam., approx. .6 oz.	12	.6	2.4	<.1	(0)	0	3	.1 c
boiled, drained, 4 oz.	88	5.1	18.3	.1	(0)	0	20	1.7 c
boiled, drained, 1 medium corm	9	.5	1.9	<.1	(0)	0	2	.2 c
ARROWROOT, powdered:								
(*Tone's*), 1 tsp.	10	0	2.3	0	0	0	1	0
ARROWROOT FLOUR:								
1 oz.	101	.1	25.0	<.1	tr.	0	1	1.0 d
1 cup	457	.4	112.8	.1	<.1	0	2	4.4 d
ARTHUR TREACHER'S:								
chicken, 2 patties, 4.8 oz.	369	27.1	16.5	21.6	3.5	65	495	m.q.
chicken sandwich, 5.5 oz.	413	16.2	44.0	19.2	2.8	32	708	m.q.
chips, 4 oz.	276	4.0	34.9	13.2	2.3	<85	39	m.q.
cod tail shape, bake 'n broil, 5 oz.	245	19.6	9.7	14.2	m.q.	m.q.	144	m.q.
coleslaw, 3 oz.	123	1.0	11.1	8.2	1.1	7	266	m.q.
fish, 2 pieces, 5.2 oz.	355	19.2	25.4	19.8	2.8	56	450	m.q.
fish sandwich, 5.5 oz.	440	16.4	39.4	24.0	4.2	42	836	m.q.
Krunch Pup, 2-oz. piece	203	5.4	12.0	14.8	3.7	25	446	m.q.
Lemon Luv, 3-oz. piece	276	2.6	35.1	13.9	2.2	<1	314	m.q.
shrimp, 7 pieces, 4.1 oz.	381	13.1	27.2	24.4	3.3	93	538	m.q.

Food and Measure	cal.	prot. (gms)	carbo. (gms)	tot. fat (gms)	sat. fat (gms)	chol. (mgs)	sod. (mgs)	fiber (gms)
ARTICHOKE, globe:								
raw:								
untrimmed, 1 lb.	85	5.9	19.1	.3	.1	0	171	9.4 d
1 medium, approx. 11.3 oz.	60	4.2	13.5	.2	<.1	0	121	6.7 d
1 large, approx. 14.3 oz.	76	5.3	17.0	.2	.1	0	153	8.4 d
boiled, drained:								
untrimmed, 4 oz.	23	1.6	5.1	.1	<.1	0	43	.6 c
1 medium, approx. 10.6 oz.	60	4.2	13.4	.2	<.1	0	114	1.5 c
trimmed or hearts, 4 oz.	57	3.9	12.7	.2	<.1	0	108	1.4 c
hearts, ½ cup	42	2.9	9.4	.1	<.1	0	80	1.1 c
ARTICHOKE, JERUSALEM, see								
"Jerusalem artichoke"								
ARTICHOKE HEARTS,								
CANNED:								
marinated (*S&W*), 3.5 oz.	225	2.0	6.0	26.0	m.q.	0	15	m.q.
ARTICHOKE HEARTS,								
FROZEN:								
9-oz. pkg.	96	6.7	19.8	1.1	.3	0	120	2.0 c
boiled, drained, 4 oz.	51	3.5	10.4	.6	.1	0	60	1.0 c
(*Birds Eye* Deluxe), 3 oz.	30	2.0	7.0	0	0	0	40	m.q.
(*Seabrook*), 3 oz.	25	3.0	4.0	0	0	0	6	1.0 c
ARUGULA:								
(*Frieda* of California), 1 lb.	104	10.0	17.7	1.4	n.a.	0	68	4.1 d
(*Frieda* of California), 1 oz.	7	.6	1.1	<.1	(0)	0	4	.3 d
ASPARAGUS:								
raw:								
untrimmed, 1 lb.	54	7.3	8.9	.5	.1	0	5	2.4 d
trimmed, 1 oz.	6	.9	1.0	.1	<.1	0	1	.3 d
4 spears, approx. 3.8 oz.	13	1.8	2.1	.1	<.1	0	1	.6 d
cuts and spears, ½ cup	15	2.1	2.5	.2	<.1	0	1	.7 d
boiled, drained:								
4 spears, ½" diam. at base	15	1.6	2.6	.2	<.1	0	3	.5 c
cuts and spears, 4 oz.	28	2.9	5.0	.4	.1	0	5	.9 c
cuts and spears, ½ cup	22	2.3	4.0	.3	.1	0	4	.8 c
ASPARAGUS, CANNED, ½ cup,								
except as noted:								
w/liquid:								
4 oz.	16	2.0	2.6	.2	<.1	0	395	.6 c
½ cup	17	2.2	2.8	.2	.1	0	425	.6 c
low-sodium, 4 oz.	16	2.0	2.6	.2	<.1	0	5	.6 c
low-sodium	17	2.2	2.8	.2	.1	0	5	.6 c
(*Green Giant* 50% Less Salt)	20	2.0	3.0	0	0	0	210	1.0 d
green (*Green Giant*)	20	2.0	3.0	0	0	0	420	1.0 d
green tipped (*Del Monte*)	20	2.0	3.0	0	0	0	355	m.q.
white (*Green Giant*)	16	2.0	3.0	0	0	0	410	1.0 d
spears:								
all green, and tips (*Del Monte*)	20	2.0	3.0	0	0	0	355	m.q.
all green (*S&W* Fancy)	18	2.0	3.0	0	0	0	320	m.q.
colossal, all green (*S&W* Fancy)	20	2.0	4.0	0	0	0	320	m.q.

Food and Measure	cal.	prot. (gms)	carbo. (gms)	tot. fat (gms)	sat. fat (gms)	chol. (mgs)	sod. (mgs)	fiber (gms)
ASPARAGUS, CANNED *(cont.)*								
drained, 4 oz.	22	2.4	2.8	.7	.2	0	m.q.	m.q.
drained, spears	24	2.6	3.0	.8	.2	0	m.q.	m.q.
(*Stokely*)	20	2.0	3.0	0	0	0	380	m.q.
(*Stokely* No Salt or Sugar Added) ...	20	2.0	3.0	0	0	0	5	m.q.
spears, cut, green (*Pathmark*)	20	3.0	2.0	0	0	0	450	m.q.
spears, cut, green (*Pathmark* No Salt Added)	20	3.0	2.0	0	0	0	5	m.q.
points, all green (*S&W/Nutradiet*) ..	17	4.0	3.0	0	0	0	10	m.q.
cuts and tips (*Finast*), 1 cup	35	4.0	6.0	0	0	0	720	m.q.
ASPARAGUS, FROZEN:								
cuts and spears, 10-oz. pkg.	69	9.2	11.7	.7	.1	0	24	2.5 c
boiled, drained, cuts and spears, 4 oz.	32	3.3	5.5	.5	.1	0	5	1.0 c
boiled, drained, 4 spears, approx. 2.1 oz.	17	1.8	2.9	.3	.1	0	2	.5 c
spears:								
(*Birds Eye*), 3.3 oz.	25	3.0	4.0	0	0	0	0	m.q.
(*Finast*), 3.3 oz.	25	3.0	4.0	0	0	0	5	m.q.
(*Frosty Acres*), 3.3 oz.	25	3.0	4.0	0	0	0	4	1.0 c
(*Seabrook*), 3.3 oz.	25	3.0	4.0	0	0	0	4	1.0 c
(*Southern*), 3.5 oz.	27	3.3	4.1	.2	0	0	20	m.q.
cuts:								
(*Birds Eye*), 3.3 oz.	25	3.0	4.0	0	0	0	5	m.q.
(*Green Giant Harvest Fresh*) ½ cup	25	3.0	4.0	0	0	.0	95	2.0 d
(*Seabrook*), 3.3 oz.	25	3.0	4.0	0	0	0	6	m.q.
cuts and spears (*Frosty Acres*), 3.3 oz.	25	3.0	4.0	0	0	0	6	m.q.
ASPARAGUS BEAN, see "Yardlong bean"								
ASPARAGUS PILAF, frozen:								
(*Green Giant* Microwave Garden Gourmet), 1 pkg.	190	5.0	37.0	4.0	2.0	10	610	3.0 d
AU JUS GRAVY:								
canned:								
¼ cup	10	.7	1.5	.1	.1	<1	m.q.	n.a.
(*Franco-American*), 2 oz.	10	0	2.0	0	0	0	330	n.a.
(*Heinz* HomeStyle), 2 oz. or ¼ cup	18	0	2.0	1.0	n.a.	n.a.	350	n.a.
mix[1]:								
.8-oz. pkt. dry	79	3.0	9.9	3.3	1.7	4	2392	.1 c
¼ cup	8	.3	1.0	.3	.2	<1	241	tr.c
(*French's*), ¼ cup	10	0	2.0	0	0	0	260	n.a.
(*Lawry's*), 1 cup	84	6.3	11.1	1.6	m.q.	n.a.	3454	.2 c
(*McCormick/Shilling*), ¼ cup	20	1.0	3.5	.3	n.a.	n.a.	786	n.a.
(*Tone's*), 1 tsp. dry	10	.4	1.0	.5	.1	<1	680	tr.d
AUBERGINE, see "Eggplant"								

---

1. *Prepared according to package directions, except as noted.*

Food and Measure	cal.	prot. (gms)	carbo. (gms)	tot. fat (gms)	sat. fat (gms)	chol. (mgs)	sod. (mgs)	fiber (gms)
AVOCADO:								
all varieties:								
untrimmed, 1 lb.	540	6.7	24.8	51.4	8.2	0	35	7.1 c
trimmed, 1 oz.	46	.6	2.1	4.3	.7	0	3	.6 c
1 medium, approx. 9.6 oz.	324	4.0	14.9	30.8	4.9	0	21	4.2 c
pureed, ½ cup	185	2.3	8.5	17.6	2.8	0	12	2.4 c
California:								
untrimmed, 1 lb.	610	7.3	23.8	59.8	8.9	0	42	9.3 d
trimmed, 1 oz.	50	.6	2.0	4.9	.7	0	3	.8 d
1 medium, approx. 8 oz.	306	3.6	12.0	30.0	4.5	0	21	4.7 d
pureed, ½ cup	204	2.4	8.0	19.9	3.0	0	14	3.1 d
Florida:								
untrimmed, 1 lb.	339	4.8	27.1	26.9	5.3	0	14	6.4 c
trimmed, 1 oz.	32	.5	2.5	2.5	.5	0	1	.6 c
1 medium, approx. 1 lb.	339	4.8	27.1	27.0	5.3	0	14	6.4 c
pureed, ½ cup	129	1.8	10.3	10.2	2.0	0	6	2.4 c
AVOCADO DIP:								
(*Kraft*), 2 tbsp.	50	1.0	3.0	4.0	2.0	0	210	n.a.
AVOCADO OIL:								
1 oz.	251	0	0	28.4	3.3	0	0	0
½ cup	964	0	0	109.0	12.6	0	0	0
1 tbsp.	124	0	0	14.0	1.6	0	0	0
(*Hain*), 1 tbsp.	120	0	0	14.0	1.0	0	0	0

AWA, see "Milkfish"

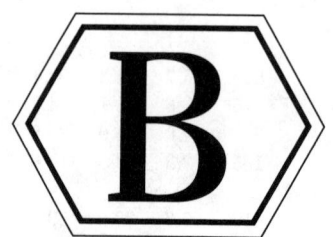

Food and Measure	cal.	prot. (gms)	carbo. (gms)	tot. fat (gms)	sat. fat (gms)	chol. (mgs)	sod. (mgs)	fiber (gms)
BABASSU OIL:								
1 oz.	251	0	0	28.4	23.0	0	0	0
½ cup	964	0	0	109.0	88.5	0	0	0
1 tbsp.	120	0	0	13.6	11.0	0	0	0
BABY FOOD, in jars:								
apple (*Earth's Best*), 4.5 oz.	60	0	14.0	1.0	(0)	0	5	m.q.
apple, Dutch, dessert:								
(*Beech-Nut Stages* 2), 4.5 oz.	100	0	24.0	0	0	0	15	m.q.
strained (*Gerber*), 4.5 oz.	100	0	21.0	2.0	n.a.	4	18	m.q.
junior (*Gerber*), 6 oz.	130	0	29.0	2.0	n.a.	7	24	m.q.
apple betty:								
strained, 4.8-oz. jar	97	.5	26.5	0	0	0	14	m.q.
strained, 1 oz.	20	.1	5.6	0	0	0	3	m.q.
junior, 7.8-oz. jar	153	.8	41.7	0	0	0	19	m.q.
junior, 1 oz.	20	.1	5.4	0	0	0	2	m.q.
apple juice:								
4.2-fl.-oz. jar	61	0	15.2	.1	(0)	0	4	m.q.
1 fl. oz.	14	0	3.6	tr.	(0)	0	1	m.q.
(*Beech-Nut Stages* 1), 4.2 fl. oz. ..	60	0	14.0	0	0	0	5	m.q.
(*Earth's Best*), 4.2 fl. oz.	60	0	14.0	0	0	0	20	m.q.
strained (*Gerber*), 4.2 fl. oz.	60	0	15.0	0	0	0	2	m.q.
apple-apricot (*Earth's Best*), 4.5 oz.	70	0	15.0	1.0	(0)	0	5	m.q.
apple-banana (*Earth's Best*), 4.5 oz.	80	0	18.0	1.0	(0)	0	15	m.q.
apple-banana juice (*Earth's Best*),								
4.2 fl. oz.	60	0	14.0	0	0	0	2	m.q.
apple-banana juice, strained (*Gerber*),								
4.2 fl. oz.	70	0	16.0	1.0	(0)	0	4	m.q.
apple-blueberry:								
(*Earth's Best*), 4.5 oz.	60	0	14.0	1.0	(0)	0	n.a.	m.q.
strained:								
4.8-oz. jar	82	.3	22.0	.3	(0)	0	2	.3 c

Food and Measure	cal.	prot. (gms)	carbo. (gms)	tot. fat (gms)	sat. fat (gms)	chol. (mgs)	sod. (mgs)	fiber (gms)
1 oz.	17	.1	4.6	.1	(0)	0	<1	.1 c
(Gerber), 4.5 oz.	60	0	14.0	1.0	(0)	0	1	m.q.
junior:								
7.8-oz. jar	137	.4	36.5	.4	(0)	0	28	.4 c
1 oz.	18	.1	4.7	.1	(0)	0	4	.1 c
(Gerber), 6 oz.	80	0	19.0	1.0	(0)	0	2	m.q.
apple-cherry juice:								
4.2-fl.-oz. jar	53	.2	12.9	.3	(0)	0	4	m.q.
1 fl. oz.	13	tr.	3.1	.1	(0)	0	1	m.q.
(Beech-Nut Stages 2), 4 fl. oz. ...	60	0	14.0	0	0	0	5	m.q.
strained (Gerber), 4.2 fl. oz.	60	0	15.0	0	0	0	5	m.q.
apple-cranberry juice (Beech-Nut								
Stages 2), 4 fl. oz.	60	0	14.0	0	0	0	5	m.q.
apple-grape juice:								
4.2-fl.-oz. jar	60	.1	14.8	.2	(0)	0	4	m.q.
1 fl. oz.	14	tr.	3.5	.1	(0)	0	1	m.q.
(Beech-Nut Stages 2), 4 fl. oz. ...	70	0	16.0	0	0	0	15	m.q.
(Earth's Best), 4.2 fl. oz.	60	0	14.0	0	0	0	15	m.q.
strained (Gerber), 4.2 fl. oz.	60	0	15.0	0	0	0	5	m.q.
apple-peach juice:								
4.2-fl.-oz. jar	55	.2	13.5	.1	(0)	0	n.a.	m.q.
1 fl. oz.	13	tr.	3.2	tr.	(0)	0	n.a.	m.q.
strained (Gerber), 4.2 fl. oz.	60	0	14.0	0	0	0	5	m.q.
apple, peaches, and strawberries								
(Beech-Nut Stages 2), 4.5 oz. ..	100	0	24.0	0	0	0	0	m.q.
apple, pears, and bananas (Beech-Nut								
Stages 2), 4.5 oz.	100	0	24.0	0	0	0	0	m.q.
apple-plum (Earth's Best), 4.5 oz. ..	70	0	16.0	1.0	(0)	0	10	m.q.
apple-plum juice:								
4.2-fl.-oz. jar	63	.1	16.0	0	0	0	n.a.	m.q.
1 fl. oz.	15	tr.	3.8	0	0	0	n.a.	m.q.
strained (Gerber), 4.2 fl. oz.	60	0	15.0	0	0	0	6	m.q.
apple-prune juice:								
4.2-fl.-oz. jar	94	.3	23.4	.2	(0)	0	7	m.q.
1 fl. oz.	23	.1	5.6	tr.	(0)	0	2	m.q.
strained (Gerber), 4.2 fl. oz.	70	0	17.0	0	0	0	5	m.q.
apple-raspberry, sweetened:								
strained, 4.8-oz. jar	79	.3	21.2	.2	(0)	0	3	m.q.
strained, 1 oz.	17	.1	4.5	tr.	(0)	0	1	m.q.
junior, 7.8-oz. jar	127	.4	34.1	.4	(0)	0	4	m.q.
junior, 1 oz.	16	.1	4.4	tr.	(0)	0	<1	m.q.
apple and strawberries (Beech-Nut								
Stages 2), 4.5 oz.	90	0	22.0	0	0	0	0	m.q.
applesauce:								
(Beech-Nut Stages 3), 6 oz.	90	0	22.0	0	0	0	0	m.q.
(Gerber First Foods), 2.5-oz. jar ..	40	0	9.0	0	0	0	1	m.q.
strained:								
4.5-oz. jar	53	.2	14.0	.2	(0)	0	3	.7 c
1 oz.	12	.1	3.1	tr.	(0)	0	1	.2 c
(Gerber), 4.5 oz.	60	0	14.0	1.0	(0)	0	3	m.q.

Food and Measure	cal.	prot. (gms)	carbo. (gms)	tot. fat (gms)	sat. fat (gms)	chol. (mgs)	sod. (mgs)	fiber (gms)
BABY FOOD, APPLESAUCE *(cont.)*								
junior:								
7.5-oz. jar	79	.1	21.9	0	0	0	5	1.2 c
1 oz.	11	tr.	2.9	0	0	0	1	.2 c
(Gerber), 6 oz.	90	0	20.0	1.0	(0)	0	3	m.q.
and apricots:								
strained, 4.8-oz. jar	60	.3	15.7	.3	(0)	0	4	.9 c
strained, 1 oz.	13	.1	3.3	.1	(0)	0	1	.2 c
strained *(Gerber)*, 4.5 oz.	70	0	15.0	1.0	(0)	0	3	m.q.
junior, 7.8-oz. jar	104	.5	27.3	.5	(0)	0	6	1.5 c
junior, 1 oz.	13	.1	3.5	.1	(0)	0	1	.2 c
(Beech-Nut Stages 2), 4.5 oz. . .	80	0	19.0	0	0	0	0	m.q.
and bananas *(Beech-Nut Stages 3)*,								
6 oz.	100	0	25.0	0	0	0	0	m.q.
and bananas *(Beech-Nut Stages 2)*,								
4.5 oz.	80	0	18.0	0	0	0	0	m.q.
and cherries:								
strained, 4.8-oz. jar	65	.4	17.7	0	0	0	3	m.q.
strained or junior, 1 oz.	14	.1	3.7	0	0	0	1	m.q.
junior, 7.8-oz. jar	106	.6	28.8	0	0	0	6	m.q.
(Beech-Nut Stages 3), 6 oz.	100	0	24.0	0	0	0	0	m.q.
(Beech-Nut Stages 2), 4.5 oz. . .	70	0	18.0	0	0	0	5	m.q.
golden delicious *(Beech-Nut*								
Stages 1), 2.8 oz.	50	0	13.0	0	0	0	0	m.q.
golden delicious *(Beech-Nut*								
Stages 1), 4.5 oz.	70	0	17.0	0	0	0	0	m.q.
and pineapple:								
strained, 4.5-oz. jar	48	.1	12.9	.1	(0)	0	3	m.q.
strained, 1 oz.	11	tr.	2.9	tr.	(0)	0	1	m.q.
junior, 7.5-oz. jar	83	.2	22.3	.2	(0)	0	4	m.q.
junior, 1 oz.	11	tr.	3.0	tr.	(0)	0	1	m.q.
apricot:								
w/pears *(Beech-Nut Stages 3)*,								
6 oz.	120	1.0	27.0	0	0	0	0	m.q.
w/pears and applesauce *(Beech-*								
Nut Stages 2), 4.5 oz.	90	0	21.0	0	0	0	0	m.q.
w/tapioca:								
strained:								
4.8-oz. jar	80	.4	22.0	0	0	0	11	.4 c
1 oz.	17	.1	4.6	0	0	0	2	.1 c
(Gerber), 4.5 oz.	90	0	20.0	1.0	(0)	0	8	m.q.
junior:								
7.8-oz. jar	139	.6	38.0	0	0	0	14	1.0 c
1 oz.	18	.1	4.9	0	0	0	2	.1 c
(Gerber), 6 oz.	130	1.0	29.0	1.0	(0)	0	9	m.q.
banana:								
(Earth's Best), 4.5 oz.	100	2.0	22.0	0	0	0	60	m.q.
(Gerber First Foods), 2.5 oz.	60	1.0	15.0	0	0	0	3	m.q.

Food and Measure	cal.	prot. (gms)	carbo. (gms)	tot. fat (gms)	sat. fat (gms)	chol. (mgs)	sod. (mgs)	fiber (gms)
Chiquita (*Beech-Nut Stages* 1), 2.8 oz.	70	0	16.0	0	0	0	0	m.q.
Chiquita (*Beech-Nut Stages* 1), 4.5 oz.	110	1.0	26.0	0	0	0	0	m.q.
w/pears and apples (*Beech-Nut Stages* 3), 6 oz.	130	0	31.0	0	0	0	0	m.q.
w/pears and applesauce (*Beech-Nut Stages* 2), 4.5 oz.	100	0	24.0	0	0	0	0	m.q.
and pineapple, w/tapioca:								
strained:								
4.8-oz. jar	91	.3	24.8	.1	(0)	0	10	m.q.
1 oz.	19	.1	5.2	tr.	(0)	0	2	m.q.
(*Gerber*), 4.5 oz.	60	1.0	15.0	0	0	0	5	m.q.
junior:								
7.8-oz. jar	143	.5	39.3	0	0	0	13	m.q.
1 oz.	18	.1	5.1	0	0	0	2	m.q.
(*Gerber*), 6 oz.	90	1.0	20.0	1.0	(0)	0	7	m.q.
w/tapioca:								
strained:								
4.8-oz. jar	77	.5	20.6	.1	(0)	0	12	.2 c
1 oz.	16	.1	4.3	tr.	(0)	0	3	tr.c
(*Gerber*), 4.5 oz.	110	1.0	24.0	1.0	(0)	0	12	m.q.
junior:								
7.8-oz. jar	147	.8	39.1	.4	(0)	0	21	.4 c
1 oz.	19	.1	5.0	tr.	(0)	0	3	.1 c
(*Gerber*), 6 oz.	140	1.0	31.0	1.0	(0)	0	15	m.q.
banana yogurt (*Beech-Nut Stages* 2), 4.5 oz.	120	1.0	26.0	2.0	m.q.	m.q.	30	m.q.
banana-apple dessert, strained (*Gerber*), 4.5 oz.	90	0	20.0	1.0	(0)	0	9	m.q.
banana-pineapple dessert (*Beech-Nut Stages* 2), 4.5 oz.	110	0	27.0	0	0	0	15	m.q.
beans, green:								
(*Beech-Nut Stages* 1), 4.5 oz.	35	1.0	8.0	0	0	0	0	m.q.
(*Beech-Nut Stages* 3), 6 oz.	45	2.0	10.0	0	0	0	80	m.q.
(*Gerber First Foods*), 2.5 oz.	20	1.0	5.0	0	0	0	1	m.q.
strained:								
4.5-oz. jar	32	1.7	7.6	.1	(0)	0	2	1.3 c
1 oz.	7	.4	1.7	tr.	(0)	0	1	.3 c
(*Gerber*), 4.5 oz.	50	2.0	8.0	1.0	(0)	0	1	m.q.
junior, 7.3-oz. jar	51	2.5	11.8	.3	(0)	0	3	2.0 c
junior, 1 oz.	7	.3	1.6	tr.	(0)	0	tr.	.3 c
buttered:								
strained, 4.5-oz. jar	42	1.6	8.5	1.0	n.a.	n.a.	4	m.q.
strained, 1 oz.	9	.3	1.9	.2	n.a.	n.a.	1	m.q.
junior, 7.3-oz. jar	67	2.7	12.5	1.8	n.a.	n.a.	4	m.q.
junior, 1 oz.	9	.4	1.7	.3	n.a.	n.a.	1	m.q.
creamed, junior:								
7.5-oz. jar	68	2.1	15.3	.9	n.a.	n.a.	26	m.q.

Food and Measure	cal.	prot. (gms)	carbo. (gms)	tot. fat (gms)	sat. fat (gms)	chol. (mgs)	sod. (mgs)	fiber (gms)
BABY FOOD, BEANS, GREEN, CREAMED *(cont.)*								
1 oz.	9	.3	2.0	.1	n.a.	n.a.	3	m.q.
(*Gerber*), 6 oz.	80	3.0	16.0	1.0	n.a.	n.a.	14	m.q.
and rice (*Earth's Best*), 4.5 oz. ..	70	2.0	14.0	0	0	0	0	m.q.
beef:								
(*Beech-Nut Stages* 1), 2.8 oz.	90	10.0	0	5.0	m.q.	m.q.	40	0
junior (*Gerber*), 2.5 oz.	80	11.0	1.0	4.0	m.q.	20	38	0
and egg yolks:								
strained, 3.5-oz. jar	106	13.5	0	5.3	2.6	m.q.	80	0
strained, 1 oz.	30	3.9	0	1.5	.7	m.q.	23	0
strained (*Gerber*), 2.5 oz.	80	10.0	0	4.0	m.q.	21	38	0
junior, 3.5-oz. jar	105	14.3	0	4.9	2.6	m.q.	65	0
junior, 1 oz.	30	4.1	0	1.4	.7	m.q.	19	0
w/beef heart, strained,								
3.5-oz. jar	93	12.6	0	4.4	2.1	m.q.	62	.1 c
w/beef heart, strained, 1 oz. ..	27	3.6	0	1.2	.6	m.q.	18	tr.c
beef dinner:								
and egg noodle:								
(*Beech-Nut Stages* 2), 4.5 oz. ..	90	2.0	11.0	4.0	m.q.	m.q.	35	m.q.
(*Beech-Nut Stages* 3), 6 oz.	150	6.0	14.0	8.0	m.q.	m.q.	45	m.q.
strained:								
4.5-oz. jar	68	2.9	9.0	2.2	m.q.	m.q.	37	.4 c
1 oz.	15	.6	2.0	.5	m.q.	m.q.	8	.1 c
(*Gerber*), 4.5 oz.	90	3.0	12.0	3.0	m.q.	6	14	m.q.
junior:								
7.5-oz. jar	122	5.4	15.7	4.0	m.q.	m.q.	37	.4 c
1 oz.	16	.7	2.1	.5	m.q.	m.q.	5	.1 c
(*Gerber*), 6 oz.	120	5.0	16.0	4.0	m.q.	10	27	m.q.
and rice, toddler, 6.2-oz. jar	146	8.9	15.5	5.1	m.q.	m.q.	632	.5 c
and rice, toddler, 1 oz.	23	1.4	2.5	.8	m.q.	m.q.	101	.1 c
supreme (*Beech-Nut Stages* 2),								
4.5 oz.	120	3.0	13.0	6.0	m.q.	m.q.	40	n.a.
w/vegetables, high meat:								
strained, 4.5-oz. jar	96	7.3	5.3	5.3	m.q.	m.q.	46	.4 c
strained, 1 oz.	21	1.6	1.2	1.2	m.q.	m.q.	10	.1 c
junior, 4.5-oz. jar	108	8.1	6.7	5.9	m.q.	m.q.	42	.3 c
junior, 1 oz.	24	1.8	1.5	1.3	m.q.	m.q.	9	.1 c
w/vegetables, lean meat, strained								
(*Gerber*), 4.5 oz.	90	7.0	9.0	3.0	m.q.	11	32	m.q.
w/vegetables, lean meat, junior								
(*Gerber*), 4.5 oz.	100	8.0	10.0	3.0	m.q.	12	29	m.q.
beef stew:								
toddler, 6.2-oz. jar	90	9.1	9.6	2.1	1.0	22	611	.5 c
toddler, 1 oz.	14	1.4	1.5	.3	.2	4	98	.1 c
(*Beech-Nut Stages* Table Time),								
6 oz.	150	10.0	16.0	6.0	m.q.	m.q.	380	m.q.
beets, strained:								
4.5-oz. jar	43	1.7	9.8	.1	n.a.	0	106	1.0 c

Food and Measure	cal.	prot. (gms)	carbo. (gms)	tot. fat (gms)	sat. fat (gms)	chol. (mgs)	sod. (mgs)	fiber (gms)
1 oz.	10	.4	2.2	tr.	n.a.	0	24	.2 c
(*Gerber*), 4.5 oz.	60	1.0	11.0	1.0	n.a.	0	115	m.q.
biscuit[1], teething, 1 oz.	111	3.0	21.7	1.2	n.a.	n.a.	103	.1 c
biscuit[1], teething, 1 biscuit, .4 oz. ...	43	1.2	8.4	.5	n.a.	n.a.	40	.1 c
broccoli, carrots, and cheese, junior								
(*Gerber*), 6 oz.	50	1.0	10.0	1.0	n.a.	7	78	m.q.
carrots:								
(*Beech-Nut Stages* 3), 6 oz.	60	1.0	13.0	0	0	0	170	m.q.
(*Earth's Best*), 4.5 oz.	40	1.0	7.0	1.0	0	0	70	m.q.
(*Gerber First Foods*), 2.5 oz.	40	1.0	6.0	1.0	0	0	19	m.q.
strained:								
4.5-oz. jar	34	1.0	7.7	.2	0	0	48	1.0 c
1 oz.	8	.2	1.7	tr.	0	0	11	.2 c
(*Gerber*), 4.5 oz.	35	1.0	8.0	0	0	0	46	m.q.
junior:								
7.5-oz. jar	67	1.7	15.4	.4	0	0	104	1.7 c
1 oz.	9	.2	2.1	tr.	0	0	14	.2 c
(*Gerber*), 6 oz.	80	3.0	16.0	1.0	n.a.	0	83	m.q.
buttered:								
strained, 4.5-oz. jar	46	1.1	9.4	.8	n.a.	n.a.	24	m.q.
junior, 1 oz.	10	.2	2.1	.2	n.a.	n.a.	5	m.q.
junior, 7.5-oz. jar	70	1.7	14.3	1.2	n.a.	n.a.	34	m.q.
junior, 1 oz.	9	.2	1.9	.2	n.a.	n.a.	5	m.q.
regal Imperial (*Beech-Nut*								
Stages 1), 2.8 oz.	30	0	7.0	0	0	0	80	m.q.
regal Imperial (*Beech-Nut*								
Stages 1), 4.5 oz.	40	1.0	9.0	0	0	0	130	m.q.
cereal:								
barley:								
dry, .5 oz.	52	1.6	10.7	.5	(0)	0	7	.2 c
dry, 1 tbsp.	9	.3	1.8	.1	(0)	0	1	tr.c
prepared[2], 1 oz.	31	1.3	4.6	.9	m.q.	m.q.	14	.1 c
(*Beech-Nut Stages* 1), .5 oz. dry	50	1.0	11.0	0	0	0	15	m.q.
(*Beech-Nut Stages* 1), prepared[3]	100	2.0	16.0	3.0	m.q.	m.q.	35	m.q.
(*Gerber*), .5 oz. dry	60	1.0	11.0	1.0	(0)	0	n.a.	m.q.
(*Gerber*), prepared[4]	100	3.0	14.0	4.0	m.q.	m.q.	n.a.	m.q.
and egg yolks:								
strained, 4.5-oz. jar	66	2.5	9.0	2.3	.8	81	42	.2 c
strained, 1 oz.	15	.5	2.0	.5	.2	18	9	tr.c
junior, 7.5-oz. jar	110	4.1	15.1	3.8	1.3	m.q.	70	.2 c
junior, 1 oz.	15	.5	2.0	.5	.2	m.q.	9	tr.c
and bacon, strained, 4.5-oz. jar	101	3.2	8.0	6.4	m.q.	m.q.	62	m.q.
and bacon, strained, 1 oz.	22	.7	1.8	1.4	m.q.	m.q.	14	m.q.
and bacon, junior, 7.5-oz. jar ..	178	5.4	15.1	11.0	m.q.	m.q.	97	m.q.
and bacon, junior, 1 oz.	24	.7	2.0	1.5	m.q.	m.q.	13	m.q.

1. *Made with enriched flour.*
2. *Prepared according to package directions, with whole milk.*
3. *Prepared with ½ oz. cereal and 2.4 fl. oz. formula.*
4. *Prepared with ½ oz. cereal and 2.4 fl. oz. whole milk.*

Food and Measure	cal.	prot. (gms)	carbo. (gms)	tot. fat (gms)	sat. fat (gms)	chol. (mgs)	sod. (mgs)	fiber (gms)
BABY FOOD, CEREAL (cont.)								
high protein:								
dry, .5 oz.	51	5.1	6.6	.8	(0)	0	7	.3 c
dry, 1 tbsp.	9	.9	1.1	.1	(0)	0	1	.1 c
prepared[1], 1 oz.	31	2.5	3.3	1.1	m.q.	m.q.	14	.1 c
(Gerber), .5 oz. dry	50	5.0	6.0	1.0	(0)	0	n.a.	m.q.
(Gerber), prepared[2]	100	7.0	9.0	4.0	m.q.	m.q.	n.a.	m.q.
w/apple and orange:								
dry, .5 oz.	53	3.6	8.2	.9	(0)	0	15	.2 c
dry, 1 tbsp.	9	.6	1.4	.2	(0)	0	2	tr.c
prepared[1], 1 oz.	32	2.0	3.8	1.1	m.q.	m.q.	16	.1 c
(Gerber), .5 oz. dry	60	4.0	8.0	1.0	(0)	0	n.a.	m.q.
(Gerber), prepared[2]	100	6.0	11.0	4.0	m.q.	m.q.	n.a.	m.q.
mixed:								
dry, .5 oz.	54	1.7	10.4	.6	(0)	0	6	.1 c
dry, 1 tbsp.	9	.3	1.8	.1	(0)	0	1	tr.c
prepared[1], 1 oz.	32	1.3	4.5	1.0	m.q.	m.q.	13	tr.c
(Beech-Nut Stages 2), .5 oz. dry	50	1.0	10.0	1.0	(0)	0	15	m.q.
(Beech-Nut Stages 2), prepared[2]	100	4.0	14.0	3.0	m.q.	m.q.	50	m.q.
(Earth's Best), .5 oz. dry	60	2.0	11.0	0	0	0	0	m.q.
(Earth's Best), prepared[3]	110	3.0	16.0	3.0	m.q.	n.a.	15	m.q.
(Gerber), .5 oz. dry	50	1.0	10.0	1.0	(0)	0	n.a.	m.q.
(Gerber), prepared[2]	100	3.0	13.0	4.0	m.q.	m.q.	n.a.	m.q.
w/applesauce and bananas:								
strained, 4.8-oz. jar	111	1.6	24.2	.7	(0)	0	3	.4 c
strained, 1 oz.	23	.3	5.1	.1	(0)	0	1	.1 c
strained (Gerber), 4.5 oz. ...	100	1.0	22.0	1.0	(0)	0	4	m.q.
junior, 7.8-oz. jar	183	2.6	40.5	.9	(0)	0	78	.6 c
junior, 1 oz.	24	.3	5.2	.1	(0)	0	10	.1 c
junior (Gerber), 6 oz.	140	2.0	29.0	2.0	(0)	0	5	m.q.
(Beech-Nut Stages 2), 4.5 oz.	90	2.0	19.0	1.0	(0)	0	0	m.q.
w/bananas:								
dry, .5 oz	56	1.5	10.9	.7	(0)	0	17	.1 c
dry, 1 tbsp.	9	.3	1.9	.1	(0)	0	3	tr.c
prepared w/whole milk, 1 oz.	33	1.3	4.7	1.0	m.q.	m.q.	17	tr.c
(Gerber), .5 oz. dry	60	1.0	11.0	1.0	(0)	0	n.a.	m.q.
(Gerber), prepared[2]	100	3.0	14.0	4.0	m.q.	m.q.	n.a.	m.q.
w/honey:								
dry, .5 oz.	55	2.0	10.4	.7	(0)	0	6	m.q.
dry, 1 tbsp.	9	.3	1.8	.1	(0)	0	1	m.q.
prepared[1], 1 oz.	33	1.4	4.5	1.0	m.q.	m.q.	14	m.q.
oatmeal:								
dry, .5 oz.	56	1.9	9.8	1.1	(0)	0	5	.2 c
dry, 1 tbsp.	10	.3	1.7	.2	(0)	0	1	tr.c
prepared[1], 1 oz.	33	1.4	4.3	1.2	m.q.	m.q.	13	.1 c
(Beech-Nut Stages 1), .5 oz. dry	60	2.0	10.0	1.0	(0)	0	15	m.q.

1. Prepared according to package directions, with whole milk.
2. Prepared with 1/2 oz. cereal and 2.4 fl. oz. milk.
3. Prepared with 1/2 oz. cereal and 2.5 fl. oz. formula.

Food and Measure	cal.	prot. (gms)	carbo. (gms)	tot. fat (gms)	sat. fat (gms)	chol. (mgs)	sod. (mgs)	fiber (gms)
(*Beech-Nut Stages* 1), prepared[1]	100	3.0	15.0	4.0	m.q.	m.q.	35	m.q.
(*Gerber*), .5 oz. dry	60	2.0	10.0	1.0	(0)	0	n.a.	m.q.
(*Gerber*), prepared[2]	100	4.0	13.0	4.0	m.q.	m.q.	n.a.	m.q.
whole grain, instant (*Earth's Best*), .5 oz. dry	60	2.0	12.0	0	0	0	0	m.q.
whole grain, instant (*Earth's Best*), prepared[3]	110	3.0	17.0	3.0	m.q.	n.a.	15	m.q.
w/applesauce and bananas:								
strained, 4.8-oz. jar	99	1.8	20.8	.9	(0)	0	2	1.0 c
strained, 1 oz.	21	.4	4.4	.2	(0)	0	1	.2 c
strained (*Gerber*), 4.5 oz. ...	100	1.0	21.0	1.0	(0)	0	4	m.q.
junior, 7.8-oz. jar	165	2.9	34.6	1.6	(0)	0	69	.9 c
junior, 1 oz.	21	.4	4.5	.2	(0)	0	9	.1 c
junior (*Gerber*), 6 oz.	130	2.0	27.0	2.0	(0)	0	7	m.q.
(*Beech-Nut Stages* 2), 4.5 oz.	90	2.0	17.0	1.0	(0)	0	5	m.q.
w/bananas:								
dry, .5 oz.	56	1.7	10.4	.9	(0)	0	17	.1 c
dry, 1 tbsp.	9	.3	1.8	.1	(0)	0	3	tr.c
prepared[4], 1 oz.	33	1.3	4.5	1.1	m.q.	m.q.	17	tr.c
(*Beech-Nut Stages* 2), .5 oz. dry	60	1.0	11.0	1.0	(0)	0	15	m.q.
(*Beech-Nut Stages* 2), prepared[2]	100	4.0	15.0	4.0	m.q.	m.q.	50	m.q.
(*Gerber*), .5 oz. dry	60	2.0	11.0	1.0	(0)	0	n.a.	m.q.
(*Gerber*), prepared[2]	110	4.0	14.0	4.0	m.q.	m.q.	n.a.	m.q.
w/honey:								
dry, .5 oz.	55	1.9	9.8	1.0	(0)	0	7	m.q.
dry, 1 tbsp.	9	.3	1.7	.2	(0)	0	1	m.q.
prepared[4], 1 oz.	33	1.4	4.3	1.1	m.q.	m.q.	14	m.q.
rice:								
dry, .5 oz.	56	1.0	11.0	.7	(0)	0	5	.1 c
dry, 1 tbsp.	9	.2	1.9	.1	(0)	0	1	tr.c
prepared[4], 1 oz.	33	1.1	4.7	1.0	m.q.	m.q.	13	tr.c
(*Beech-Nut Stages* 1), .5 oz. dry	60	1.0	12.0	0	0	0	15	m.q.
(*Beech-Nut Stages* 1), prepared[1]	110	2.0	17.0	3.0	m.q.	n.a.	30	m.q.
(*Gerber*), .5 oz. dry	60	1.0	11.0	1.0	(0)	0	n.a.	m.q.
(*Gerber*), prepared[2]	100	3.0	14.0	4.0	m.q.	m.q.	n.a.	m.q.
brown:								
(*Health Valley*), .5 oz. or 1 tbsp. dry	60	1.0	10.0	1.0	(0)	0	5	.7 d
instant (*Earth's Best*), .5 oz. dry	60	1.0	12.0	0	0	0	0	m.q.
instant (*Earth's Best*), prepared[3]	110	2.0	17.0	3.0	m.q.	n.a.	15	m.q.
w/apples (*Beech-Nut Stages* 2), .5 oz. dry	60	0	13.0	0	0	0	15	m.q.

1. *Prepared with ½ oz. cereal and 2.4 fl. oz. formula.*
2. *Prepared with ½ oz. cereal and 2.4 fl. oz. whole milk.*
3. *Prepared with ½ oz. cereal and 2.5 fl. oz. formula.*
4. *Prepared according to package directions, with whole milk.*

Food and Measure	cal.	prot. (gms)	carbo. (gms)	tot. fat (gms)	sat. fat (gms)	chol. (mgs)	sod. (mgs)	fiber (gms)
BABY FOOD, CEREAL, RICE *(cont.)*								
w/apples (*Beech-Nut Stages* 2),								
prepared [1]	110	3.0	17.0	3.0	m.q.	n.a.	50	m.q.
w/applesauce and bananas:								
strained, 4.8-oz. jar	107	1.6	23.1	.5	(0)	0	38	.2 c
strained, 1 oz.	23	.3	4.9	.1	(0)	0	8	tr.c
strained (*Gerber*), 4.5 oz. ...	100	1.0	23.0	1.0	(0)	0	14	m.q.
(*Beech-Nut Stages* 2), 4.5 oz.	100	2.0	24.0	0	0	0	25	m.q.
w/bananas:								
dry, .5 oz.	57	1.2	11.3	.6	(0)	0	14	.1 c
dry, 1 tbsp.	10	.2	1.9	.1	(0)	0	2	tr.c
prepared,[2] 1 oz.	33	1.2	4.8	1.0	m.q.	m.q.	16	tr.c
(*Beech-Nut Stages* 2), .5 oz.								
dry	60	1.0	13.0	0	0	0	15	m.q.
(*Beech-Nut Stages* 2),								
prepared [1]	100	3.0	17.0	3.0	m.q.	m.q.	50	m.q.
(*Gerber*), .5 oz. dry	50	1.0	12.0	0	0	0	n.a.	m.q.
(*Gerber*), prepared [1]	100	3.0	15.0	3.0	m.q.	m.q.	n.a.	m.q.
w/honey:								
dry, .5 oz.	56	1.0	11.4	.4	(0)	0	7	m.q.
dry, 1 tbsp.	9	.2	1.9	.1	(0)	0	1	m.q.
prepared,[2] 1 oz.	33	1.1	4.9	.9	m.q.	m.q.	14	m.q.
w/mixed fruit, junior:								
7.8-oz. jar	186	2.3	41.0	.5	(0)	0	24	.5 c
1 oz.	24	.3	5.3	1	(0)	0	3	.1 c
(*Gerber*), 6 oz.	140	1.0	31.0	1.0	(0)	0	17	m.q.
sprouted (*Health Valley*), .5 oz. or								
1 tbsp. dry	60	1.0	10.0	1.0	(0)	0	5	2.1 d
chicken:								
(*Beech-Nut Stages* 1), 2.8 oz.	80	10.0	0	4.0	m.q.	m.q.	55	0
junior (*Gerber*), 2.5 oz.	110	11.0	1.0	.7.0	m.q.	42	28	0
and egg yolks:								
strained, 3.5-oz. jar	128	13.6	.1	7.8	2.0	m.q.	47	0
strained, 1 oz.	37	3.9	tr.	2.2	.6	m.q.	13	0
strained (*Gerber*), 2.5 oz.	110	10.0	1.0	7.0	m.q.	44	28	0
junior, 3.5-oz. jar	148	14.6	0	9.5	2.4	m.q.	50	0
junior, 1 oz.	42	4.2	0	2.7	.7	m.q.	14	0
sticks and egg yolks, junior,								
2.5-oz. jar	134	10.4	1.0	10.2	m.q.	m.q.	340	.1 c
sticks and egg yolks, junior, .4-oz.								
stick	19	1.5	.1	1.4	m.q.	m.q.	48	tr.c
chicken dinner:								
and noodle:								
(*Beech-Nut Stages* 2), 4.5 oz. ..	90	2.0	14.0	3.0	m.q.	m.q.	55	m.q.
(*Beech-Nut Stages* 3), 6 oz.	100	7.0	12.0	2.0	m.q.	m.q.	55	m.q.

1. *Prepared with ½ oz. cereal and 2.4 fl. oz. whole milk.*
2. *Prepared according to package directions, with whole milk.*

Food and Measure	cal.	prot. (gms)	carbo. (gms)	tot. fat (gms)	sat. fat (gms)	chol. (mgs)	sod. (mgs)	fiber (gms)
strained:								
4.5-oz. jar	67	2.7	9.6	1.9	m.q.	m.q.	20	.4 c
1 oz.	15	.6	2.1	.4	m.q.	m.q.	5	.1 c
(Gerber), 4.5 oz.	90	3.0	12.0	3.0	m.q.	10	17	m.q.
junior:								
7.5-oz. jar	109	4.1	16.1	3.0	m.q.	m.q.	36	1.3 c
1 oz.	15	.5	2.1	.4	m.q.	m.q.	5	.2 c
(Gerber), 6 oz.	100	4.0	15.0	3.0	m.q.	14	20	m.q.
and rice (Beech-Nut Stages 2),								
4.5 oz.	80	2.0	11.0	3.0	m.q.	m.q.	40	m.q.
w/vegetables, high meat:								
strained, 4.5-oz. jar	100	8.0	7.6	4.6	m.q.	m.q.	35	.3 c
strained, 1 oz.	22	1.8	1.7	1.0	m.q.	m.q.	8	.1 c
junior, 4.5-oz. jar	117	9.0	5.4	7.0	m.q.	m.q.	33	.3 c
junior, 1 oz.	26	2.0	1.2	1.6	m.q.	m.q.	7	.1 c
w/vegetables, lean meat, strained								
(Gerber) 4.5 oz.	90	7.0	8.0	3.0	m.q.	18	31	m.q.
w/vegetables, lean meat, junior								
(Gerber), 4.5 oz.	90	7.0	10.0	3.0	m.q.	19	32	m.q.
chicken soup:								
strained, 4.5-oz. jar	64	2.0	9.2	2.2	m.q.	m.q.	20	(0)
strained, 1 oz.	14	.4	2.0	.5	m.q.	m.q.	5	(0)
cream of, strained, 4.5-oz. jar ...	74	3.2	10.8	2.0	m.q.	m.q.	24	.4 c
cream of, strained, 1 oz.	16	.7	2.4	.5	m.q.	m.q.	5	.1 c
hearty, w/stars (Beech-Nut Stages								
Table Time), 6 oz.	180	4.0	20.0	9.0	m.q.	m.q.	350	m.q.
chicken stew, toddler, 6-oz. jar	132	8.9	10.9	6.4	1.9	49	683	.5 c
chicken stew, toddler, 1 oz.	22	1.5	1.8	1.1	.3	8	114	.1 c
cookie[1]:								
plain, 1 oz.	123	3.3	19.0	3.7	1.1	n.a.	55	.1 c
plain, 1 cookie, .2 oz.	28	.8	4.4	.9	.2	n.a.	12	tr.c
arrowroot, 1 oz.	125	2.2	20.2	4.0	.9	<1	105	m.q.
arrowroot, 1 cookie, .2 oz.	24	.4	4.3	.9	.2	<1	22	m.q.
zwieback, 1 oz.	121	2.9	21.0	2.8	1.1	6	66	.1 c
zwieback, 1 cookie, .2 oz.	30	.7	5.2	.7	.3	2	16	tr.c
corn, creamed:								
strained, 4.5-oz. jar	73	1.8	18.1	.5	n.a.	n.a.	55	.4 c
strained, 1 oz.	16	.4	4.0	.1	n.a.	n.a.	12	.1 c
strained (Gerber), 4.5 oz.	80	2.0	16.0	1.0	n.a.	n.a.	12	m.q.
junior, 7.5-oz. jar	138	3.1	34.7	.8	n.a.	n.a.	111	.2 c
junior, 1 oz.	18	.4	4.6	.1	n.a.	n.a.	15	tr.c
(Beech-Nut Stages 2), 4.5 oz.	100	2.0	20.0	1.0	n.a.	n.a.	25	m.q.
cottage cheese, w/pineapple:								
strained, 4.8-oz. jar	94	4.0	17.8	1.1	m.q.	m.q.	70	1.7 c
strained, 1 oz.	20	.8	3.7	.2	m.q.	m.q.	15	.4 c
junior, 7.8-oz. jar	172	6.5	35.1	1.5	m.q.	m.q.	113	2.1 c
junior, 1 oz.	22	.8	4.5	.2	m.q.	m.q.	15	.3 c

1. Made with enriched flour.

Food and Measure	cal.	prot. (gms)	carbo. (gms)	tot. fat (gms)	sat. fat (gms)	chol. (mgs)	sod. (mgs)	fiber (gms)
BABY FOOD, COTTAGE CHEESE, W/PINEAPPLE *(cont.)*								
high cheese, strained, 4.8-oz. jar	157	8.5	25.4	3.0	m.q.	m.q.	201	1.2 c
high cheese, strained, 1 oz.	33	1.8	5.3	.6	m.q.	m.q.	42	.3 c
(*Beech-Nut Stages* 2), 4.5 oz.	130	2.0	26.0	1.0	m.q.	m.q.	15	m.q.
(*Beech-Nut Stages* 3), 6 oz.	170	3.0	36.0	2.0	m.q.	m.q.	20	m.q.
egg yolks, strained:								
3.3-oz. jar	191	9.4	.9	16.3	4.9	739	37	0
1 oz.	58	2.8	.3	4.9	1.5	223	11	0
(*Gerber*), 2.25 oz.	130	6.0	1.0	11.0	m.q.	398	27	0
fruit dessert:								
(*Beech-Nut Stages* 2), 4.5 oz.	80	0	20.0	0	0	0	0	m.q.
(*Beech-Nut Stages* 3), 6 oz.	120	0	28.0	0	0	0	5	m.q.
strained:								
4.8-oz. jar	79	.4	21.6	0	0	0	18	.3 c
1 oz.	17	.1	4.5	0	0	0	4	.1 c
(*Gerber*), 4.5 oz.	100	0	24.0	1.0	(0)	0	13	m.q.
junior:								
7.8-oz. jar	138	.6	37.9	0	0	0	29	.7 c
1 oz.	18	.1	4.9	0	0	0	4	.1 c
(*Gerber*), 6 oz.	130	0	30.0	1.0	(0)	0	12	m.q.
tropical, junior, 7.8-oz. jar	131	.4	36.1	0	0	0	16	m.q.
tropical, junior, 1 oz.	17	.1	4.7	0	0	0	2	m.q.
fruit juice, mixed:								
4.2-fl.-oz. jar	61	.2	15.1	.1	(0)	0	5	m.q.
1 fl. oz.	14	tr.	3.6	tr.	(0)	0	1	m.q.
(*Beech-Nut Stages* 2), 4 fl. oz. ...	60	0	15.0	0	0	0	5	m.q.
strained (*Gerber*), 4.2 fl. oz.	70	0	15.0	1.0	n.a.	0	2	m.q.
tropical blend (*Beech-Nut*								
Stages 2), 4 fl. oz.	70	0	17.0	0	0	0	5	m.q.
fruit, mixed:								
and yogurt (*Beech-Nut Stages* 2),								
4.5 oz.	130	1.0	28.0	1.0	m.q.	m.q.	20	m.q.
and yogurt (*Beech-Nut Stages* 3),								
6 oz.	160	1.0	36.0	2.0	m.q.	m.q.	30	m.q.
tropical, w/tapioca, strained								
(*Gerber*), 4.5 oz.	80	0	20.0	0	0	0	6	m.q.
grape juice, white (*Beech-Nut*								
Stages 1), 4.2 fl. oz.	80	0	20.0	0	0	0	10	m.q.
grape juice, white, strained (*Gerber*),								
4.2 fl. oz.	80	0	21.0	0	0	0	5	m.q.
guava:								
and papaya, w/tapioca, strained								
4.5-oz. jar	80	.3	21.8	.1	(0)	0	5	.7 c
and papaya, w/tapioca, strained,								
1 oz.	18	.1	4.8	tr.	(0)	0	1	.2 c
w/tapioca, strained:								
4.5-oz. jar	86	.4	23.4	0	0	0	2	1.3 c
1 oz.	19	.1	5.2	0	0	0	1	.3 c
(*Gerber*), 4.5 oz.	90	0	20.0	1.0	n.a.	0	3	m.q.

Food and Measure	cal.	prot. (gms)	carbo. (gms)	tot. fat (gms)	sat. fat (gms)	chol. (mgs)	sod. (mgs)	fiber (gms)
tropical fruit dessert (*Beech-Nut*								
Stages 2), 4.5 oz.	100	0	24.0	0	0	0	10	m.q.
ham, junior (*Gerber*), 2.5 oz.	90	11.0	0	5.0	m.q.	21	30	0
ham and egg yolks:								
strained:								
3.5-oz. jar	110	13.7	0	5.7	1.9	m.q.	40	0
1 oz.	32	3.9	0	1.6	.6	m.q.	12	0
(*Gerber*), 2.5 oz.	90	10.0	1.0	5.0	m.q.	17	30	0
junior, 3.5-oz. jar	123	14.9	0	6.6	2.2	m.q.	66	0
junior, 1 oz.	35	4.3	0	1.9	.6	m.q.	19	0
ham w/vegetables dinner:								
high meat:								
strained, 4.5-oz. jar	97	8.0	7.1	4.4	1.5	m.q.	29	.3 c
strained, 1 oz.	21	1.8	1.6	1.0	.3	m.q.	6	.1 c
junior, 4.5-oz. jar	98	8.2	7.9	4.2	1.4	23	28	.2 c
junior, 1 oz.	22	1.8	1.7	.9	.3	5	6	.1 c
lean meat, strained (*Gerber*),								
4.5 oz.	100	7.0	10.0	4.0	m.q.	12	26	m.q.
lean meat, junior (*Gerber*), 4.5 oz.	110	8.0	11.0	4.0	m.q.	11	27	m.q.
Hawaiian delight dessert, strained								
(*Gerber*), 4.5 oz.	120	2.0	25.0	1.0	n.a.	2	23	m.q.
Hawaiian delight dessert, junior								
(*Gerber*), 6 oz.	150	2.0	33.0	1.0	n.a.	3	32	m.q.
Juice Plus (*Beech-Nut Stages* 2),								
4 fl. oz.	80	0	20.0	0	0	0	10	m.q.
lamb:								
(*Beech-Nut Stages* 1), 2.8 oz.	70	9.0	0	3.0	m.q.	m.q.	50	0
and egg yolks:								
strained, 3.5-oz. jar	102	13.9	.1	4.7	2.3	m.q.	62	0
strained, 1 oz.	29	4.0	tr.	1.3	.7	m.q.	18	0
strained (*Gerber*), 2.5 oz.	70	10.0	1.0	3.0	m.q.	27	36	0
junior, 3.5-oz. jar	111	15.0	0	5.2	2.5	m.q.	73	0
junior, 1 oz.	32	4.3	0	1.5	.7	m.q.	21	0
lamb and noodles dinner, junior,								
7.5-oz. jar	138	4.8	18.6	4.7	m.q.	m.q.	39	m.q.
lamb and noodles dinner, junior,								
1 oz.	18	.6	2.5	.6	m.q.	m.q.	5	m.q.
lasagna, beef, dinner, toddler,								
6.2-oz. jar	137	7.4	17.7	3.8	m.q.	m.q.	804	.4 c
lasagna, beef, dinner, toddler, 1 oz.	22	1.2	2.8	.6	m.q.	m.q.	129	.1 c
liver and egg yolks, strained,								
3.5-oz. jar	100	14.2	1.4	3.7	1.4	182	73	0
liver and egg yolks, strained, 1 oz.	29	4.1	.4	1.1	.4	52	21	0
macaroni dinner:								
and bacon, junior, 7.5-oz. jar	160	5.4	18.2	7.1	m.q.	m.q.	166	m.q.
and bacon, junior, 1 oz.	21	.7	2.4	.9	m.q.	m.q.	22	m.q.
and beef (*Beech-Nut Stages* 2),								
4.5 oz.	90	2.0	13.0	4.0	m.q.	m.q.	40	m.q.

Food and Measure	cal.	prot. (gms)	carbo. (gms)	tot. fat (gms)	sat. fat (gms)	chol. (mgs)	sod. (mgs)	fiber (gms)
BABY FOOD, MACARONI DINNER *(cont.)*								
and beef *(Beech-Nut Stages 3)*,								
6 oz.	160	6.0	17.0	8.0	m.q.	m.q.	85	m.q.
and cheese:								
strained, 4.5-oz. jar	76	3.3	9.6	2.7	m.q.	m.q.	93	.1 c
strained, 1 oz.	17	.7	2.1	.6	m.q.	m.q.	21	tr.c
strained *(Gerber)*, 4.5 oz.	90	4.0	12.0	3.0	m.q.	4	108	m.q.
junior, 7.5-oz. jar	130	5.5	17.5	4.3	m.q.	m.q.	163	.2 c
junior, 1 oz.	17	.7	2.3	.6	m.q.	m.q.	22	tr.c
and ham, junior, 7.5-oz. jar	127	6.8	18.0	2.9	m.q.	m.q.	101	m.q.
and ham, junior, 1 oz.	17	.9	2.4	.4	m.q.	m.q.	13	m.q.
tomato and beef:								
strained:								
4.5-oz. jar	71	2.9	11.3	1.4	m.q.	m.q.	21	.5 c
1 oz.	16	.6	2.5	.3	m.q.	m.q.	5	.1 c
(Gerber), 4.5 oz.	80	3.0	12.0	2.0	m.q.	3	41	m.q.
junior:								
7.5-oz. jar	125	5.3	20.1	2.4	m.q.	m.q.	35	.6 c
1 oz.	17	.7	2.7	.3	m.q.	m.q.	5	.1 c
(Gerber), 6 oz.	110	4.0	18.0	2.0	m.q.	6	27	m.q.
mango:								
w/tapioca, strained, 4.8-oz. jar ...	109	.4	29.2	.3	(0)	0	6	.2 c
w/tapioca, strained, 1 oz.	23	.1	6.1	.1	(0)	0	1	tr.c
w/tapioca, strained *(Gerber)*,								
4.5 oz.	90	0	21.0	1.0	(0)	0	4	m.q.
tropical fruit dessert *(Beech-Nut*								
Stages 2), 4.5 oz.	100	0	25.0	0	0	0	15	m.q.
mango, banana, and passion fruit								
juice, w/tapioca, strained								
(Gerber), 4.5 oz.	100	0	25.0	0	0	0	12	m.q.
meat sticks and egg yolks, junior,								
2.5-oz. jar	130	9.5	.8	10.4	4.1	m.q.	388	.1 c
meat sticks and egg yolks, junior,								
.4-oz. stick	18	1.3	.1	1.5	.6	m.q.	55	tr.c
orange juice:								
4.2-fl.-oz. jar	58	.8	13.3	.3	(0)	0	2	m.q.
1 fl. oz.	14	.2	3.2	.1	(0)	0	<1	m.q.
(Beech-Nut Stages 3), 4 fl. oz. ...	60	0	14.0	0	0	0	0	m.q.
strained *(Gerber)*, 4.2 fl. oz.	70	1.0	14.0	1.0	(0)	0	5	m.q.
orange-apple juice, 4.2-fl.-oz. jar ...	56	.5	13.2	.3	(0)	0	4	m.q.
orange-apple juice, 1 fl. oz.	13	.1	3.1	.1	(0)	0	1	m.q.
orange-apple-banana juice,								
4.2-fl.-oz. jar	61	.5	15.0	.1	(0)	0	6	m.q.
orange-apple-banana juice, 1 fl. oz.	15	.1	3.6	tr.	(0)	0	1	m.q.
orange-apricot juice, 4.2-fl.-oz. jar ..	60	1.0	14.2	.1	(0)	0	7	m.q.
orange-apricot juice, 1 fl. oz.	14	.2	3.4	tr.	(0)	0	2	m.q.
orange-banana juice, 4.2-fl.-oz. jar ..	65	.9	15.4	.1	(0)	0	4	m.q.
orange-banana juice, 1 fl.-oz.	15	.2	3.7	tr.	(0)	0	1	m.q.
orange-pineapple juice, 4.2-fl.-oz. jar	63	.7	15.2	.1	(0)	0	2	m.q.

Food and Measure	cal.	prot. (gms)	carbo. (gms)	tot. fat (gms)	sat. fat (gms)	chol. (mgs)	sod. (mgs)	fiber (gms)
orange-pineapple juice, 1 fl. oz.	15	.2	3.6	tr.	(0)	0	1	m.q.
papaya:								
and applesauce, w/tapioca,								
strained, 4.5 oz.	89	.3	24.2	.1	(0)	0	6	.5 c
and applesauce, w/tapioca,								
strained, 1 oz.	20	.1	5.4	tr.	(0)	0	1	.1 c
w/tapioca, strained (*Gerber*),								
4.5 oz.	80	0	19.0	1.0	(0)	0	9	m.q.
tropical fruit dessert (*Beech-Nut*								
Stages 2), 4.5 oz.	100	0	24.0	0	0	0	15	m.q.
peach:								
(*Beech-Nut Stages* 3), 6 oz.	90	1.0	22.0	0	0	0	0	m.q.
(*Gerber First Foods*), 2.5 oz.	30	0	8.0	0	0	0	3	m.q.
strained:								
sweetened, 4.8-oz. jar	96	.7	25.5	.2	(0)	0	8	1.0 c
sweetened, 1 oz.	20	.1	5.4	tr.	(0)	0	2	.2 c
(*Gerber*), 4.5 oz.	90	1.0	19.0	1.0	(0)	0	4	m.q.
junior:								
sweetened, 7.8-oz. jar	157	1.2	41.6	.4	(0)	0	10	1.6 c
sweetened, 1 oz.	20	.2	5.4	tr.	(0)	0	1	.2 c
(*Gerber*), 6 oz.	110	1.0	25.0	1.0	(0)	0	5	m.q.
and mango, w/tapioca, strained								
(*Gerber*), 4.5 oz.	100	0	24.0	1.0	(0)	0	9	m.q.
melba:								
strained, 4.8-oz. jar	81	.3	22.3	0	0	0	12	m.q.
strained, 1 oz.	17	.1	4.7	0	0	0	2	m.q.
junior, 7.8-oz. jar	132	.6	36.1	0	0	0	19	m.q.
junior, 1 oz.	17	.1	4.6	0	0	0	2	m.q.
w/oatmeal and banana (*Earth's*								
Best), 4.5 oz.	70	2.0	15.0	1.0	n.a.	0	5	m.q.
yellow cling (*Beech-Nut Stages* 1),								
2.8 oz.	50	0	12.0	0	0	0	0	m.q.
yellow cling (*Beech-Nut Stages* 1),								
4.5 oz.	70	0	15.0	0	0	0	0	m.q.
and yogurt (*Beech-Nut Stages* 2),								
4.5 oz.	120	1.0	25.0	2.0	m.q.	m.q.	30	m.q.
peach cobbler, strained (*Gerber*),								
4.5 oz.	100	1.0	23.0	1.0	(0)	0	9	m.q.
peach cobbler, junior (*Gerber*), 6 oz.	130	1.0	30.0	1.0	(0)	0	15	m.q.
pear:								
(*Earth's Best*), 4.5 oz.	60	0	14.0	0	0	0	11	m.q.
(*Gerber First Foods*), 2.5 oz.	40	0	11.0	0	0	0	2	m.q.
strained:								
4.5-oz. jar	53	.4	13.9	.2	(0)	0	3	m.q.
1 oz.	12	.1	3.1	tr.	(0)	0	1	m.q.
(*Gerber*), 4.5 oz.	80	1.0	16.0	1.0	(0)	0	3	m.q.
junior:								
7.5-oz. jar	93	.6	24.7	.2	(0)	0	4	m.q.
1 oz.	12	.1	3.3	tr.	(0)	0	1	m.q.

Food and Measure	cal.	prot. (gms)	carbo. (gms)	tot. fat (gms)	sat. fat (gms)	chol. (mgs)	sod. (mgs)	fiber (gms)
BABY FOOD, PEAR *(cont.)*								
(Gerber), 6 oz.	100	1.0	21.0	1.0	(0)	0	2	m.q.
Bartlett:								
(Beech-Nut Stages 1), 2.8 oz. ...	50	0	13.0	0	0	0	0	m.q.
(Beech-Nut Stages 1), 4.5 oz. ...	70	0	18.0	0	0	0	0	m.q.
(Beech-Nut Stages 3), 6 oz.	100	0	24.0	0	0	0	5	m.q.
and pineapple *(Beech-Nut*								
Stages 2), 4.5 oz.	90	0	21.0	0	0	0	0	m.q.
and applesauce *(Beech-Nut*								
Stages 2), 4.5 oz.	80	0	20.0	0	0	0	0	m.q.
and pineapple:								
strained:								
4.5-oz. jar	52	.4	13.9	.1	(0)	0	5	.3 c
1 oz.	12	.1	3.1	tr.	(0)	0	1	.1 c
(Gerber), 4.5 oz.	80	1.0	16.0	1.0	(0)	0	3	m.q.
junior:								
7.5-oz. jar	93	.6	24.4	.4	(0)	0	2	.5 c
1 oz.	12	.1	3.2	.1	(0)	0	<1	.1 c
(Gerber), 6 oz.	100	1.0	21.0	1.0	(0)	0	3	m.q.
pear juice:								
(Beech-Nut Stages 1), 4 fl. oz. ...	60	0	15.0	0	0	0	5	m.q.
(Earth's Best), 4.2 fl. oz.	60	0	15.0	0	0	0	0	m.q.
strained *(Gerber)*, 4.2 fl. oz.	60	0	16.0	0	0	0	6	m.q.
peas:								
(Gerber First Foods), 2.5 oz.	40	2.0	6.0	1.0	(0)	0	2	m.q.
strained:								
4.5-oz. jar	52	4.5	10.4	.4	(0)	0	5	1.5 c
1 oz.	11	1.0	2.3	.1	(0)	0	1	.3 c
(Gerber), 4.5 oz.	60	4.0	10.0	1.0	(0)	0	6	m.q.
junior *(Gerber)*, 6 oz.	90	5.0	16.0	1.0	(0)	0	5	m.q.
buttered:								
strained, 4.5-oz. jar	72	4.7	13.6	1.4	n.a.	n.a.	10	m.q.
strained, 1 oz.	16	1.0	3.0	.3	n.a.	n.a.	2	m.q.
junior, 7.3-oz. jar	123	7.3	23.3	2.6	n.a.	n.a.	11	m.q.
junior, 1 oz.	17	1.0	3.2	.4	n.a.	n.a.	2	m.q.
creamed, strained, 4.5-oz. jar ...	68	2.8	11.4	2.4	n.a.	n.a.	18	.5 c
creamed, strained, 1 oz.	15	.6	2.5	.5	n.a.	n.a.	4	.1 c
tender, sweet *(Beech-Nut*								
Stages 1), 2.8 oz.	40	2.0	6.0	0	0	0	0	m.q.
tender, sweet *(Beech-Nut*								
Stages 1), 4.5 oz.	60	4.0	10.0	0	0	0	0	m.q.
peas, split and ham dinner, junior,								
7.5-oz. jar	152	7.0	24.1	2.8	m.q.	m.q.	30	.6 c
peas, split and ham dinner, junior,								
1 oz.	20	.9	3.2	.4	m.q.	m.q.	4	.1 c
peas and brown rice *(Earth's Best)*,								
4.5 oz.	80	4.0	12.0	2.0	n.a.	0	0	m.q.
peas and carrots *(Beech-Nut*								
Stages 2), 4.5 oz.	60	2.0	11.0	0	0	0	35	m.q.

Food and Measure	cal.	prot. (gms)	carbo. (gms)	tot. fat (gms)	sat. fat (gms)	chol. (mgs)	sod. (mgs)	fiber (gms)
pineapple orange dessert, strained,								
4.5-oz. jar	89	.3	24.4	0	0	0	13	m.q.
pineapple orange dessert, strained,								
1 oz.	20	.1	5.4	0	0	0	3	m.q.
plum:								
w/bananas and rice (*Earth's Best*),								
4.5 oz.	90	2.0	19.0	0	0	0	15	m.q.
w/rice (*Beech-Nut Stages* 2),								
4.5 oz.	150	1.0	34.0	0	0	0	0	m.q.
w/tapioca:								
strained:								
4.8-oz. jar	96	.2	26.6	0	0	0	8	m.q.
1 oz.	20	tr.	5.6	0	0	0	2	m.q.
(*Gerber*), 4.5 oz.	90	0	22.0	0	0	0	5	m.q.
junior:								
7.8-oz. jar	163	.3	45.0	0	0	0	18	m.q.
1 oz.	21	tr.	5.8	0	0	0	2	m.q.
(*Gerber*), 6 oz.	130	1.0	30.0	1.0	(0)	0	3	m.q.
pork and egg yolks, strained,								
3.5-oz. jar	123	13.8	0	7.1	2.4	m.q.	42	0
pork and egg rolls, strained, 1 oz. ...	35	4.0	0	2.0	.7	m.q.	12	0
pretzel[1], 1 oz.	113	3.1	23.3	.6	(0)	n.a.	76	.1 c
pretzel[1], 1 piece, .2 oz.	24	.7	4.9	.1	(0)	n.a.	16	tr.c
prune:								
(*Gerber First Foods*), 2.5 oz.	70	1.0	16.0	0	0	0	4	m.q.
w/oatmeal (*Earth's Best*), 4.5 oz.	100	1.0	24.0	0	0	0	20	m.q.
w/pears (*Beech-Nut Stages* 2),								
4.5 oz.	90	0	22.0	0	0	0	0	m.q.
w/tapioca:								
strained, 4.8-oz. jar	94	.8	25.0	.1	(0)	0	6	.4 c
strained, 1 oz.	20	.2	5.2	tr.	(0)	0	1	.1 c
strained (*Gerber*), 4.5 oz.	100	1.0	22.0	1.0	(0)	0	5	m.q.
junior, 7.8-oz. jar	155	1.3	41.2	.2	(0)	0	5	.7 c
junior, 1 oz.	20	.2	5.3	tr.	(0)	0	1	.1 c
prune-orange juice, 4.2-fl.-oz. jar ..	91	.8	21.8	.4	(0)	0	2	m.q.
prune-orange juice, 1 fl. oz.	22	.2	5.2	.1	(0)	0	1	m.q.
pudding:								
caramel:								
strained, 4.8-oz. jar	104	1.8	23.2	.9	n.a.	n.a.	37	n.a.
strained, 1 oz.	22	.4	4.9	.2	n.a.	n.a.	8	n.a.
junior, 7.5-oz. jar	167	2.9	36.2	1.9	n.a.	n.a.	60	n.a.
junior, 1 oz.	22	.4	4.8	.3	n.a.	n.a.	8	n.a.
cherry vanilla:								
strained:								
4.8-oz. jar	91	.3	24.1	.4	n.a.	n.a.	22	.2 c
1 oz.	19	.1	5.1	.1	n.a.	n.a.	5	tr.c
(*Gerber*), 4.5 oz.	90	0	21.0	1.0	n.a.	3	12	m.q.
junior, 7.8-oz. jar	152	.4	40.5	.4	n.a.	n.a.	32	.3 c

1. *Made with enriched flour.*

Food and Measure	cal.	prot. (gms)	carbo. (gms)	tot. fat (gms)	sat. fat (gms)	chol. (mgs)	sod. (mgs)	fiber (gms)
BABY FOOD, PUDDING, CHERRY VANILLA *(cont.)*								
junior, 1 oz.	20	.1	5.2	.1	n.a.	n.a.	4	tr.c
chocolate custard:								
strained, 4.5-oz. jar	107	2.4	20.6	2.1	n.a.	n.a.	30	n.a.
strained, 1 oz.	24	.5	4.6	.5	n.a.	n.a.	7	n.a.
junior, 7.8-oz. jar	195	4.2	38.3	3.5	n.a.	n.a.	55	n.a.
junior, 1 oz.	25	.5	4.9	.5	n.a.	n.a.	7	n.a.
orange, strained, 4.8-oz. jar	108	1.5	23.8	1.2	n.a.	n.a.	n.a.	.5 c
orange, strained, 1 oz.	23	.3	5.0	.3	n.a.	n.a.	n.a.	.1 c
pineapple:								
strained, 4.5-oz. jar	104	1.6	26.0	.4	n.a.	n.a.	24	.9 c
strained, 1 oz.	23	.4	5.8	.1	n.a.	n.a.	5	.2 c
junior, 7.8-oz. jar	192	3.1	47.4	.9	n.a.	n.a.	48	1.7 c
junior, 1 oz.	25	.4	6.1	.1	n.a.	n.a.	6	.2 c
vanilla custard:								
strained:								
4.5-oz. jar	109	2.0	20.6	2.5	1.3	n.a.	36	n.a.
1 oz.	24	.4	4.6	.6	.3	n.a.	8	n.a.
(*Gerber*), 4.5 oz.	100	2.0	22.0	1.0	m.q.	14	32	n.a.
junior:								
7.8-oz. jar	196	3.5	35.7	5.0	2.6	n.a.	64	n.a.
1 oz.	25	.5	4.6	.7	.3	n.a.	8	n.a.
(*Gerber*), 6 oz.	150	3.0	31.0	2.0	m.q.	23	41	n.a.
(*Beech-Nut Stages* 2), 4.5 oz. ..	140	2.0	24.0	4.0	m.q.	n.a.	60	n.a.
(*Beech-Nut Stages* 3), 6 oz.	180	3.0	30.0	5.0	m.q.	n.a.	80	n.a.
spaghetti dinner:								
and beef (*Beech-Nut Stages* 3),								
6 oz.	170	6.0	17.0	8.0	m.q.	m.q.	75	m.q.
tomato and meat:								
junior, 7.5 oz. jar	135	5.4	21.6	2.7	m.q.	m.q.	42	.9 c
junior, 1 oz.	18	.7	2.9	.4	m.q.	m.q.	6	.1 c
toddler, 6.2-oz. jar	133	9.4	19.1	1.8	m.q.	m.q.	634	.7 c
toddler, 1 oz.	21	1.5	3.1	.3	m.q.	m.q.	101	.1 c
tomato sauce and beef, junior								
(*Gerber*), 6 oz.	120	5.0	19.0	3.0	m.q.	7	41	m.q.
spaghetti rings in meat sauce (*Beech-Nut Stages* Table Time), 6 oz.	160	7.0	22.0	4.0	m.q.	m.q.	390	m.q.
spinach, creamed								
strained:								
4.5-oz. jar	48	3.2	7.3	1.7	n.a.	n.a.	62	.6 c
1 oz.	11	.7	1.6	.4	n.a.	n.a.	14	.1 c
(*Gerber*), 4.5 oz.	60	4.0	9.0	1.0	n.a.	n.a.	73	m.q.
junior, 7.5-oz. jar	90	6.4	13.7	3.0	n.a.	n.a.	117	1.1 c
junior, 1 oz.	12	.9	1.8	.4	n.a.	n.a.	16	.1 c
squash:								
(*Gerber First Foods*), 2.5 oz.	20	1.0	5.0	0	0	0	2	m.q.
strained:								
4.5-oz. jar	30	1.1	7.2	.2	(0)	0	3	.9 c
1 oz.	7	.2	1.6	.1	(0)	0	1	.2 c

Food and Measure	cal.	prot. (gms)	carbo. (gms)	tot. fat (gms)	sat. fat (gms)	chol. (mgs)	sod. (mgs)	fiber (gms)
(*Gerber*), 4.5 oz.	35	1.0	8.0	0	0	0	3	m.q.
junior:								
7.5-oz. jar	51	1.8	12.0	.4	(0)	0	3	1.5 c
1 oz.	7	.2	1.6	.1	(0)	0	<1	.2 c
(*Gerber*), 6 oz.	60	1.0	11.0	1.0	(0)	0	3	m.q.
buttered:								
strained, 4.5-oz. jar	37	.8	8.8	.4	n.a.	n.a.	2	m.q.
strained, 1 oz.	8	.2	1.9	.1	n.a.	n.a.	<1	m.q.
junior, 7.5-oz. jar	63	1.5	13.7	1.3	n.a.	n.a.	3	m.q.
junior, 1 oz.	8	.2	1.8	.2	n.a.	n.a.	<1	m.q.
butternut (*Beech-Nut Stages* 1),								
2.8 oz.	30	0	7.0	0	0	0	0	m.q.
butternut (*Beech-Nut Stages* 1),								
4.5 oz.	50	1.0	11.0	0	0	0	0	m.q.
winter (*Earth's Best*), 4.5 oz.	50	1.0	12.0	0	0	0	10	m.q.
sweet potato:								
(*Beech-Nut Stages* 1), 2.8 oz.	60	0	14.0	0	0	0	10	m.q.
(*Beech-Nut Stages* 1), 4.5 oz.	90	1.0	20.0	0	0	0	80	m.q.
(*Beech-Nut Stages* 3), 6 oz.	110	1.0	26.0	0	0	0	80	m.q.
(*Earth's Best*), 4.5 oz.	60	1.0	12.0	1.0	(0)	0	15	m.q.
(*Gerber First Foods*), 2.5 oz.	50	1.0	11.0	0	0	0	11	m.q.
strained:								
4.8-oz. jar	77	1.5	17.8	.2	(0)	0	27	.9 c
1 oz.	16	.3	3.7	tr.	(0)	0	6	.2 c
(*Gerber*), 4.5 oz.	80	1.0	18.0	1.0	(0)	0	22	m.q.
junior:								
7.8-oz. jar	133	2.4	30.7	.3	(0)	0	49	1.4 c
1 oz.	17	.3	4.0	tr.	(0)	0	6	.2 c
(*Gerber*), 6 oz.	110	1.0	24.0	1.0	(0)	0	39	m.q.
buttered:								
strained, 4.8-oz. jar	76	1.3	15.9	1.0	n.a.	n.a.	11	m.q.
strained, 1 oz.	16	.3	3.3	.2	n.a.	n.a.	2	m.q.
junior, 7.8-oz. jar	126	1.8	26.8	1.6	n.a.	n.a.	17	m.q.
junior, 1 oz.	16	.2	3.5	.2	n.a.	n.a.	2	m.q.
turkey:								
(*Beech-Nut Stages* 1), 2.8 oz.	100	9.0	0	6.0	m.q.	m.q.	50	0
junior (*Gerber*), 2.5 oz.	100	10.0	1.0	6.0	m.q.	38	37	0
and egg yolks:								
strained:								
3.5-oz. jar	113	14.1	.1	5.8	1.9	m.q.	54	0
1 oz.	32	4.0	tr.	1.7	.5	m.q.	16	0
(*Gerber*), 2.5 oz.	100	10.0	1.0	6.0	m.q.	42	38	0
junior, 3.5-oz. jar	128	15.2	0	7.0	2.3	m.q.	72	0
junior, 1 oz.	37	4.4	0	2.0	.7	m.q.	20	0
sticks and egg yolks, junior,								
2.5-oz. jar	129	9.7	1.0	10.1	m.q.	m.q.	343	.4 c
sticks and egg yolks, junior,								
.4-oz. stick	18	1.4	.1	1.4	m.q.	m.q.	48	tr.c

Food and Measure	cal.	prot. (gms)	carbo. (gms)	tot. fat (gms)	sat. fat (gms)	chol. (mgs)	sod. (mgs)	fiber (gms)
BABY FOOD *(cont.)*								
turkey dinner:								
and rice:								
(*Beech-Nut Stages* 2), 4.5 oz. ...	70	2.0	12.0	2.0	m.q.	m.q.	35	m.q.
(*Beech-Nut Stages* 3), 6 oz.	110	6.0	14.0	4.0	m.q.	m.q.	65	m.q.
strained:								
4.5-oz. jar	63	2.4	9.4	1.7	.5	13	21	.1 c
1 oz.	14	.5	2.1	.4	.1	3	5	tr.c
(*Gerber*), 4.5 oz.	80	3.0	10.0	3.0	m.q.	15	20	m.q.
junior:								
7.5-oz. jar	104	3.8	15.3	2.9	.9	m.q.	33	.4 c
1 oz.	14	.5	2.0	.4	.1	m.q.	4	.1 c
(*Gerber*), 6 oz.	110	4.0	14.0	4.0	m.q.	19	34	m.q.
supreme (*Beech-Nut Stages* 2),								
4.5 oz.	120	4.0	11.0	6.0	m.q.	m.q.	35	m.q.
w/vegetables, high meat:								
strained, 4.5-oz. jar	111	7.2	7.7	6.1	m.q.	m.q.	38	.1 c
strained, 1 oz.	25	1.6	1.7	1.4	m.q.	m.q.	8	tr.c
junior, 4.5-oz. jar	115	7.6	7.5	6.4	m.q.	m.q.	56	.3 c
junior, 1 oz.	25	1.7	1.7	1.4	m.q.	m.q.	12	.1 c
w/vegetables, lean meat, strained								
(*Gerber*), 4.5 oz.	100	7.0	9.0	4.0	m.q.	17	31	m.q.
w/vegetables, lean meat, junior								
(*Gerber*), 4.5 oz.	100	7.0	10.0	4.0	m.q.	16	31	m.q.
veal:								
(*Beech-Nut Stages* 1), 2.8 oz.	60	10.0	0	2.0	m.q.	m.q.	50	0
junior (*Gerber*), 2.5 oz.	80	11.0	0	4.0	m.q.	19	39	0
and egg yolks:								
strained:								
3.5-oz. jar	100	13.4	0	4.7	2.3	m.q.	64	0
1 oz.	29	3.8	0	1.4	.7	m.q.	18	0
(*Gerber*), 2.5 oz.	80	10.0	1.0	4.0	m.q.	18	38	0
junior, 3.5-oz. jar	109	15.1	0	4.9	2.4	m.q.	68	0
junior, 1 oz.	31	4.3	0	1.4	.7	m.q.	19	0
veal w/vegetables dinner, high meat:								
strained, 4.5-oz. jar	89	7.6	7.8	3.4	m.q.	m.q.	30	.4 c
strained, 1 oz.	20	1.7	1.7	.8	m.q.	m.q.	7	.1 c
junior, 4.5-oz. jar	93	7.8	7.4	4.0	m.q.	m.q.	32	.2 c
junior, 1 oz.	21	1.7	1.6	.9	m.q.	m.q.	7	.1 c
vegetable dinner:								
and bacon:								
strained:								
4.5-oz. jar	88	2.0	11.0	4.2	1.5	4	55	.5 c
1 oz.	19	.4	2.4	.9	.3	1	12	.1 c
(*Gerber*), 4.5 oz.	100	2.0	11.0	5.0	m.q.	4	68	m.q.
junior:								
7.5-oz. jar	150	3.9	16.1	8.2	3.0	m.q.	96	.4 c
1 oz.	20	.5	2.1	1.1	.4	m.q.	13	.1 c
(*Gerber*), 6 oz.	140	4.0	17.0	6.0	m.q.	6	105	m.q.

Food and Measure	cal.	prot. (gms)	carbo. (gms)	tot. fat (gms)	sat. fat (gms)	chol. (mgs)	sod. (mgs)	fiber (gms)
and beef:								
strained:								
4.5-oz. jar	67	2.5	9.0	2.6	m.q.	m.q.	27	.3 c
1 oz.	15	.6	2.0	.6	m.q.	m.q.	6	.1 c
(*Gerber*), 4.5 oz.	90	3.0	11.0	4.0	m.q.	5	17	m.q.
junior:								
7.5-oz. jar	113	5.0	15.8	3.6	m.q.	m.q.	52	.4 c
1 oz.	15	.7	2.1	.5	m.q.	m.q.	7	.1 c
(*Gerber*), 6 oz.	110	4.0	16.0	3.0	m.q.	7	31	m.q.
and chicken:								
strained:								
4.5-oz. jar	55	2.5	8.5	1.4	m.q.	m.q.	14	.3 c
1 oz.	12	.6	1.9	.3	m.q.	m.q.	3	.1 c
(*Gerber*), 4.5 oz.	80	3.0	12.0	2.0	m.q.	7	12	m.q.
junior:								
7.5-oz. jar	106	4.0	18.0	2.3	m.q.	m.q.	18	.4 c
1 oz.	14	.5	2.4	.3	m.q.	m.q.	2	.1 c
(*Gerber*), 6 oz.	100	3.0	15.0	3.0	m.q.	13	20	m.q.
w/dumplings and beef:								
strained, 4.5-oz. jar	61	2.6	9.8	1.2	m.q.	m.q.	62	m.q.
strained, 1 oz.	14	.6	2.2	.3	m.q.	m.q.	14	m.q.
junior, 7.5-oz. jar	103	4.4	17.0	1.7	m.q.	m.q.	110	m.q.
junior, 1 oz.	14	.6	2.3	.2	m.q.	m.q.	15	m.q.
and ham:								
strained:								
4.5-oz. jar	62	2.2	8.8	2.2	m.q.	m.q.	15	.2 c
1 oz.	14	.5	1.9	.5	m.q.	m.q.	3	.1 c
(*Gerber*), 4.5 oz.	80	2.0	11.0	3.0	m.q.	4	14	m.q.
junior:								
7.5-oz. jar	110	5.2	14.9	3.6	m.q.	m.q.	37	.4 c
1 oz.	15	.7	2.0	.5	m.q.	m.q.	5	.1 c
(*Gerber*), 6 oz.	120	3.0	17.0	4.0	m.q.	7	24	m.q.
toddler, 6.2-oz. jar	128	7.4	13.9	5.2	1.9	14	531	m.q.
toddler, 1 oz.	21	1.2	2.2	.8	.3	2	85	m.q.
and lamb:								
strained, 4.5-oz. jar	67	2.5	8.9	2.6	m.q.	m.q.	26	.4 c
strained, 1 oz.	15	.6	2.0	.6	m.q.	m.q.	6	.1 c
junior, 7.5-oz. jar	108	4.4	15.1	3.7	m.q.	m.q.	28	.4 c
junior, 1 oz.	14	.6	2.0	.5	m.q.	m.q.	4	.1 c
and liver:								
strained, 4.5-oz. jar	50	2.8	8.8	.6	m.q.	m.q.	24	.2 c
strained, 1 oz.	11	.6	1.9	.1	m.q.	m.q.	5	.1 c
junior, 7.5-oz. jar	93	3.9	17.5	1.2	m.q.	m.q.	27	.6 c
junior, 1 oz.	12	.5	2.3	.2	m.q.	m.q.	4	.1 c
mixed:								
strained, 4.5-oz. jar	52	1.5	12.2	.1	(0)	(0)	10	m.q.
strained, 1 oz.	11	.3	2.7	tr.	(0)	(0)	2	m.q.
junior, 7.5-oz. jar	71	2.1	16.8	.1	(0)	(0)	19	m.q.
junior, 1 oz.	9	.3	2.2	tr.	(0)	(0)	2	m.q.

Food and Measure	cal.	prot. (gms)	carbo. (gms)	tot. fat (gms)	sat. fat (gms)	chol. (mgs)	sod. (mgs)	fiber (gms)
BABY FOOD, VEGETABLE DINNER *(cont.)*								
noodles and chicken:								
strained, 4.5-oz. jar	81	2.6	10.1	3.3	m.q.	m.q.	26	.2 c
strained, 1 oz.	18	.6	2.2	.7	m.q.	m.q.	6	.1 c
junior, 7.5-oz. jar	137	3.7	19.4	4.8	m.q.	m.q.	54	.4 c
junior, 1 oz.	18	.5	2.6	.6	m.q.	m.q.	7	.1 c
noodles and turkey:								
strained, 4.5 oz.	56	1.5	8.7	1.6	m.q.	m.q.	27	.3 c
strained, 1 oz.	12	.3	1.9	.4	m.q.	m.q.	6	.1 c
junior, 7.5 oz.	110	3.9	16.1	3.2	m.q.	m.q.	37	.5 c
junior, 1 oz.	15	.5	2.1	.4	m.q.	m.q.	5	.1 c
and turkey:								
strained:								
4.5-oz. jar	54	2.1	8.4	1.5	m.q.	m.q.	17	.3 c
1 oz.	12	.5	1.9	.3	m.q.	m.q.	4	.1 c
(Gerber), 4.5 oz.	70	2.0	10.0	2.0	m.q.	12	17	m.q.
junior:								
7.5-oz. jar	101	3.6	16.4	2.7	m.q.	m.q.	36	.4 c
1 oz.	13	.5	2.2	.4	m.q.	m.q.	5	.1 c
(Gerber), 6 oz.	100	3.0	15.0	3.0	m.q.	19	24	m.q.
toddler, 6.2-oz. jar	141	8.5	14.2	6.1	m.q.	m.q.	591	.9 c
toddler, 1 oz.	23	1.4	2.3	1.0	m.q.	m.q.	95	.1 c
vegetable entree:								
beef *(Beech-Nut Stages* 2), 4.5 oz.	90	2.0	10.0	4.0	m.q.	m.q.	35	m.q.
beef *(Beech-Nut Stages* 3), 6 oz. . .	160	6.0	16.0	7.0	m.q.	m.q.	70	m.q.
chicken *(Beech-Nut Stages* 2),								
4.5 oz.	90	3.0	14.0	3.0	m.q.	m.q.	65	m.q.
chicken *(Beech-Nut Stages* 3),								
6 oz.	90	7.0	13.0	2.0	m.q.	m.q.	70	m.q.
ham *(Beech-Nut Stages* 2), 4.5 oz.	80	3.0	12.0	3.0	m.q.	m.q.	30	m.q.
lamb *(Beech-Nut Stages* 2), 4.5 oz.	90	2.0	13.0	4.0	m.q.	m.q.	40	m.q.
vegetable stew, w/chicken *(Beech-*								
Nut Stages Table Time), 6 oz.	190	5.0	23.0	8.0	m.q.	m.q.	340	m.q.
vegetables:								
garden:								
(Beech-Nut Stages 2), 4.5 oz. . .	60	2.0	11.0	0	0	0	35	m.q.
strained:								
4.5-oz. jar	48	2.9	8.7	.3	(0)	0	45	1.2 c
1 oz.	11	.7	1.9	.1	(0)	0	10	.3 c
(Gerber), 4.5 oz.	50	3.0	8.0	1.0	(0)	0	26	m.q.
mixed:								
(Beech-Nut Stages 2), 4.5 oz. . .	50	1.0	12.0	0	0	0	30	m.q.
strained:								
4.5-oz. jar	52	1.6	10.2	.6	(0)	0	16	.5 c
1 oz.	11	.3	2.3	.1	(0)	0	4	.1 c
(Gerber), 4.5 oz.	60	1.0	11.0	1.0	(0)	0	15	m.q.
junior:								
7.5-oz. jar	88	3.1	17.4	.8	(0)	0	77	1.1 c
1 oz.	12	.4	2.3	.1	(0)	0	10	.1 c
(Gerber), 6 oz.	70	2.0	14.0	1.0	(0)	0	32	m.q.

Food and Measure	cal.	prot. (gms)	carbo. (gms)	tot. fat (gms)	sat. fat (gms)	chol. (mgs)	sod. (mgs)	fiber (gms)
BACKFAT, see "Pork backfat"								
BACON:								
raw:								
1 oz.	158	2.5	<.1	16.3	6.0	19	194	0
1 thick slice, approx. 1.3 oz.	211	3.3	<.1	21.9	8.1	26	260	0
(*JM*), 2 slices	280	4.0	1.0	29.0	m.q.	38	530	0
(*JM* Lower Sodium), 2 slices	290	5.0	1.0	30.0	m.q.	m.q.	250	0
(*Jones Dairy Farm*), 1 slice	165	2.3	tr.	17.0	m.q.	25	187	0
cooked:								
4.5 oz., yield from 1 lb. raw	732	38.7	.8	62.5	22.1	107	2026	0
3 slices, 20 slices per lb.	109	5.8	.1	9.4	3.3	16	303	0
(*Black Label* Sliced), 2 slices	60	4.0	0	5.0	m.q.	m.q.	298	0
(*JM*), 2 slices	100	4.0	1.0	9.0	m.q.	12	370	0
(*JM* Lower Sodium), 2 slices	100	4.0	1.0	9.0	m.q.	m.q.	260	0
(*Kahn's American Beauty*),								
2 slices	100	5.0	n.a.	9.0	m.q.	m.q.	m.q.	0
(*Oscar Mayer*), 5 oz., approx. yield								
from 16-oz. pkg. raw	784	47.1	3.0	64.9	25.8	127	3236	0
(*Oscar Mayer*), 1 slice, approx.								
.2 oz.	33	2.0	.1	2.8	1.2	5	138	0
(*Oscar Mayer* Center Cut), 6 oz.,								
approx. yield from 1 lb. raw . . .	852	68.8	3.5	62.5	27.5	189	3813	0
(*Oscar Mayer* Center Cut), 1 slice,								
approx. .2 oz.	25	2.0	.1	1.8	.8	6	113	0
(*Oscar Mayer* Lower Salt), 5.6 oz.,								
approx. yield from 1 lb. raw . . .	870	57.2	2.3	70.3	25.1	170	2768	0
(*Oscar Mayer* Lower Salt), 1 slice,								
approx. .2 oz.	33	2.2	.1	2.6	.9	6	104	0
(*Range Brand* Sliced), 2 slices . . .	110	6.0	0	9.0	m.q.	m.q.	392	0
(*Red Label*), 3 slices	110	6.0	0	10.0	m.q.	m.q.	m.q.	0
thick sliced (*Oscar Mayer*), 5 oz.,								
approx. yield from 1 lb. raw . . .	811	50.6	1.1	67.1	25.8	123	3656	0
thick sliced (*Oscar Mayer*), 1 slice,								
approx. .4 oz.	58	3.6	.1	4.8	1.9	9	259	0
BACON, CANADIAN-STYLE:								
unheated, 1-oz slice	45	5.9	.5	2.0	.6	14	399	0
unheated (*Jones Dairy Farm*), 1 slice	25	3.2	tr.	1.0	m.q.	7	144	0
grilled, 4.9 oz., yield from 6-oz. pkg.								
unheated	257	33.7	1.9	11.7	4.0	80	2149	0
grilled, 2 slices, yield from								
2 unheated 1-oz. slices	86	11.3	.6	3.9	1.3	27	719	0
(*Hormel* Sliced), 1 oz.	45	6.0	0	2.0	m.q.	m.q.	315	0
(*Light & Lean*), 2 slices	35	6.0	0	1.0	m.q.	m.q.	m.q.	0
(*Oscar Mayer*), .8-oz. slice	28	4.7	.1	1.0	.3	11	305	0
BACON, SUBSTITUTE:								
beef, raw or unheated, 1 oz.	115	2.8	.2	11.0	4.5	23	271	0
beef, raw (*JM*), 2 slices	200	9.0	1.0	18.0	m.q.	53	430	0
beef, heated:								
6 oz., yield from 12-oz. pkg. raw	764	53.2	2.4	58.5	24.4	202	700	0

Food and Measure	cal.	prot. (gms)	carbo. (gms)	tot. fat (gms)	sat. fat (gms)	chol. (mgs)	sod. (mgs)	fiber (gms)
BACON, SUBSTITUTE, BEEF, HEATED *(cont.)*								
(*JM*), 2 slices	100	7.0	1.0	7.0	m.q.	20	320	0
(*Sizzlean*), 2 strips	70	6.0	0	5.0	m.q.	m.q.	480	0
pork, raw or unheated, 1 oz.	110	3.3	.2	10.5	3.7	20	280	0
pork, heated:								
6 oz., yield from 12-oz. pkg. raw	780	49.2	1.8	62.4	21.7	179	3568	0
(*Sizzlean*), 2 strips	90	6.0	0	8.0	m.q.	m.q.	530	0
brown sugar cured (*Sizzlean*),								
2 strips	110	6.0	2.0	9.0	m.q.	m.q.	490	0
turkey, heated (*Louis Rich*), 1 slice	32	2.4	.3	2.4	.7	10	186	0
"BACON," VEGETARIAN:								
1 oz.	88	3.0	1.8	8.4	1.3	0	415	.2 d
1 strip, approx. .28 oz.	25	.9	.5	2.4	.4	0	117	tr.d
frozen (*Morningstar Farms* Breakfast								
Strips), 3 strips, approx. .9 oz.	80	3.0	4.0	6.0	1.0	0	350	n.a.
frozen (*Worthington Stripples*),								
4 strips, approx. 1.2 oz.	120	4.0	6.0	9.0	1.0	0	460	n.a.
BACON BITS:								
(*Hormel*), 1 tbsp.	30	3.0	0	2.0	n.a.	n.a.	313	0
(*Libby's Bacon Crumbles*), 1 tbsp. ...	25	2.0	2.0	1.0	n.a.	n.a.	m.q.	0
(*Oscar Mayer*), 3-oz. can	248	31.6	2.5	12.4	4.3	67	2224	0
(*Oscar Mayer*), ¼ oz.	20	2.6	.2	1.0	.3	6	183	0
BACON BITS, IMITATION:								
(*Bac*Os*), 2 tsp.	25	2.0	2.0	1.0	n.a.	0	90	n.a.
(*McCormick/Shilling* Bac'N Pieces),								
1 tsp.	26	2.0	2.0	.4	n.a.	n.a.	51	n.a.
(*Tone's*), 1 tsp.	7	.8	.4	.3	0	0	59	n.a.
BACON AND HORSERADISH DIP:								
(*Breakstone's*), 2 tbsp.	70	1.0	2.0	6.0	3.0	15	270	n.a.
(*Kraft*), 2 tbsp.	60	1.0	3.0	5.0	3.0	0	200	n.a.
(*Kraft* Premium), 2 tbsp.	50	1.0	2.0	5.0	3.0	15	270	n.a.
(*Sealtest*), 2 tbsp.	70	1.0	2.0	6.0	3.0	15	270	n.a.
BACON AND ONION DIP:								
(*Breakstone's* Gourmet), 2 tbsp.	70	1.0	2.0	6.0	3.0	15	210	n.a.
(*Kraft* Premium), 2 tbsp.	60	1.0	2.0	5.0	3.0	15	170	n.a.
BAGEL:								
raisin-honey cinnamon (*Finast*),								
2½ oz., approx. 1 piece	200	8.0	40.0	1.0	n.a.	0	305	m.q.
BAGEL, FROZEN, 1 piece:								
plain:								
(*Lender's*), 2 oz.	150	6.0	30.0	1.0	n.a.	0	320	m.q.
(*Lender's* Bagelettes), .9 oz.	70	3.0	13.0	<1.0	n.a.	0	170	m.q.
(*Lender's* Big'n Crusty), 3⅛ oz. ..	240	9.0	47.0	1.0	n.a.	0	450	m.q.
(*Sara Lee*), 3.1 oz.	230	9.0	46.0	1.0	n.a.	0	580	m.q.
(*Sara Lee*), 2.5 oz.	190	8.0	38.0	1.0	n.a.	0	460	m.q.
blueberry (*Lender's*), 2.5 oz.	190	7.0	38.0	1.0	n.a.	0	250	m.q.
cinnamon raisin (*Sara Lee*), 2.5 oz.	200	7.0	39.0	2.0	m.q.	0	230	m.q.

Food and Measure	cal.	prot. (gms)	carbo. (gms)	tot. fat (gms)	sat. fat (gms)	chol. (mgs)	sod. (mgs)	fiber (gms)
cinnamon'n raisin (*Lender's* Big'n								
Crusty), 3⅛ oz.	250	8.0	49.0	2.0	m.q.	0	370	m.q.
cinnamon and raisin (*Sara Lee*),								
3.1 oz.	240	8.0	48.0	2.0	m.q.	0	280	m.q.
egg:								
(*Lender's*), 2 oz.	150	7.0	29.0	1.0	n.a.	5	360	m.q.
(*Lender's* Big'n Crusty), 3⅛ oz. . . .	250	9.0	47.0	2.0	m.q.	15	380	m.q.
(*Sara Lee*), 3.1 oz.	250	9.0	48.0	2.0	m.q.	20	450	m.q.
(*Sara Lee*), 2.5 oz.	200	8.0	38.0	2.0	m.q.	15	360	m.q.
garlic (*Lender's*), 2 oz.	160	6.0	32.0	1.0	n.a.	0	340	m.q.
garlic (*Lender's* Big'n Crusty),								
3⅛ oz.	250	9.0	50.0	1.0	n.a.	0	530	m.q.
oat bran:								
(*Lender's*), 2.5 oz.	170	7.0	36.0	2.0	m.q.	0	290	3.0 d
(*Sara Lee*), 3 oz.	220	9.0	47.0	1.0	n.a.	0	450	m.q.
(*Sara Lee*), 2.5 oz.	180	8.0	38.0	1.0	n.a.	0	360	m.q.
onion:								
(*Lender's*), 2 oz.	160	7.0	31.0	1.0	n.a.	0	290	m.q.
(*Lender's* Bagelettes), .9 oz.	70	3.0	14.0	<1.0	n.a.	0	135	<.1 d
(*Lender's* Big'n Crusty), 3⅛ oz. . . .	230	9.0	46.0	1.0	n.a.	0	480	m.q.
(*Sara Lee*), 3.1 oz.	230	9.0	45.0	1.0	n.a.	0	560	m.q.
(*Sara Lee*), 2.5 oz.	190	7.0	37.0	1.0	n.a.	0	450	m.q.
poppy (*Lender's*), 2 oz.	160	7.0	29.0	1.0	n.a.	0	370	m.q.
poppy seed (*Sara Lee*), 3.1 oz.	230	9.0	46.0	1.0	n.a.	n.a.	560	m.q.
poppy seed (*Sara Lee*), 2.5 oz.	190	8.0	37.0	1.0	n.a.	0	450	m.q.
pumpernickel (*Lender's*), 2 oz.	160	6.0	31.0	1.0	n.a.	0	330	m.q.
raisin (*Lender's* Bagelettes), .9 oz.	70	2.0	14.0	<1.0	n.a.	0	110	m.q.
raisin'n honey (*Lender's*), 2.5 oz. . . .	200	8.0	40.0	1.0	n.a.	0	310	m.q.
rye (*Lender's*), 2 oz.	150	6.0	30.0	1.0	n.a.	0	310	m.q.
sesame (*Lender's*), 2 oz.	160	7.0	31.0	1.0	n.a.	0	320	m.q.
sesame seed (*Sara Lee*), 3.1 oz. . . .	240	9.0	46.0	2.0	m.q.	0	550	m.q.
sesame seed (*Sara Lee*), 2.5 oz. . . .	190	8.0	37.0	1.0	n.a.	0	440	m.q.
soft (*Lender's*), 2.5 oz.	210	7.0	36.0	3.0	m.q.	12	350	m.q.
wheat'n raisin (*Lender's*), 2.5 oz. . . .	190	6.0	39.0	1.0	n.a.	0	310	m.q.
BAKED BEANS, canned (see also								
specific bean listings):								
(*Allens*), ½ cup	170	6.0	21.0	6.0	m.q.	n.a.	330	m.q.
(*Campbell's* Home Style), 8 oz.	220	11.0	48.0	4.0	m.q.	n.a.	820	m.q.
(*Grandma Brown's*), 1 cup	301	14.6	53.9	3.0	m.q.	<1	655	15.5 d
(*Grandma Brown's* Saucepan), 1 cup	307	13.7	52.3	4.8	m.q.	<1	592	14.8 d
(*Green Giant*), ½ cup	150	5.0	28.0	2.0	n.a.	n.a.	670	n.a.
(*S&W* Brick Oven), ½ cup	160	7.0	28.0	2.0	m.q.	n.a.	560	m.q.
(*Van Camp's*), 1 cup	260	11.0	52.0	2.0	m.q.	n.a.	1020	m.q.
(*Van Camp's* Deluxe), 1 cup	320	13.0	57.0	4.0	m.q.	n.a.	970	m.q.
plain or vegetarian:								
4 oz.	105	5.4	23.3	.5	.1	0	450	8.7 d
½ cup	118	6.1	26.1	.6	.1	0	504	9.8 d
(*A&P*), ½ cup	130	7.0	25.0	<1.0	n.a.	0	420	m.q.
(*Allens*), ½ cup	110	6.0	19.0	1.0	n.a.	0	380	m.q.

Food and Measure	cal.	prot. (gms)	carbo. (gms)	tot. fat (gms)	sat. fat (gms)	chol. (mgs)	sod. (mgs)	fiber (gms)
BAKED BEANS, PLAIN OR VEGETARIAN *(cont.)*								
(*B&M*), 8 oz.	230	14.0	50.0	3.0	m.q.	0	370	11.0 d
(*Campbell's*), 7¾ oz.	170	11.0	40.0	1.0	n.a.	0	780	m.q.
(*Van Camp's* Vegetarian Style),								
1 cup	206	10.0	42.0	.6	n.a.	0	950	m.q.
w/miso (*Health Valley* Vegetarian),								
4 oz.	90	6.0	19.0	1.0	n.a.	0	134	6.5 d
barbecue (*B&M*), 8 oz.	260	15.0	48.0	6.0	m.q.	5	1000	11.0 d
barbecue (*Campbell's*), 7⅞ oz.	210	10.0	43.0	4.0	m.q.	n.a.	900	m.q.
w/beef, 4 oz.	137	7.2	19.2	3.9	1.9	25	539	1.2 c
w/beef, ½ cup	161	8.5	22.5	4.6	2.3	29	632	1.4 c
Boston (*Health Valley*), 4 oz.	213	11.0	43.0	1.0	n.a.	0	74	22.3 d
Boston (*Health Valley* No Salt								
Added), 4 oz.	213	11.0	43.0	1.0	n.a.	0	25	22.3 d
brown sugar (*Van Camp's*), 1 cup	284	11.6	47.8	5.1	m.q.	n.a.	692	3.2 c
w/franks:								
4 oz.	161	7.7	17.5	7.5	2.7	7	488	7.8 d
½ cup	182	8.6	19.7	8.4	3.0	8	551	8.8 d
(*Van Camp's Beanee Weenee*),								
1 cup	326	15.2	31.7	15.4	5.0	15	990	7.0 d
honey (*B&M*), 8 oz.	240	15.0	50.0	2.0	m.q.	0	940	11.0 d
hot N spicy (*B&M*), 8 oz.	240	14.0	50.0	3.0	1.0	3	990	12.0 d
maple (*B&M/Friends*), 8 oz.	240	14.0	52.0	2.0	1.0	<5	890	11.0 d
in molasses and brown sugar sauce								
(*Campbell's* Old Fashioned), 8 oz.	230	11.0	49.0	3.0	m.q.	n.a.	730	m.q.
pea (*B&M*), 8 oz.	270	14.0	50.0	6.0	m.q.	5	750	11.0 d
pea, small (*Friends*), 8 oz.	360	17.0	62.0	4.0	3.0	6	1040	15.0 d
w/pork:								
4 oz.	120	5.9	22.7	1.8	.7	8	469	2.9 d
½ cup	133	6.5	25.2	2.0	.8	9	522	3.3 d
(*A&P*), ½ cup	150	7.0	25.0	2.0	m.q.	m.q.	440	m.q.
(*Allens* Extra Fancy), ½ cup	125	5.0	24.0	1.0	m.q.	m.q.	540	m.q.
(*Allens* Extra Standard), ½ cup	90	5.0	15.0	1.0	m.q.	m.q.	350	m.q.
(*Allens* Fancy), ½ cup	110	6.0	18.0	1.0	m.q.	m.q.	430	m.q.
(*Hormel Micro-Cup*), 7.5 oz.	254	11.0	41.0	5.0	m.q.	30	650	m.q.
(*Hunt's*), 4 oz.	140	6.0	26.0	1.0	m.q.	m.q.	400	m.q.
(*S&W*), ½ cup	130	5.0	22.0	2.0	m.q.	m.q.	135	m.q.
(*Van Camp's*), 1 cup	216	10.9	41.0	1.9	1.0	m.q.	1000	9.9 d
in sweet sauce, 4 oz.	126	6.0	23.8	1.7	.6	8	381	6.2 d
in sweet sauce, ½ cup	140	6.7	26.5	1.8	.7	9	423	6.9 d
in tomato sauce:								
4 oz.	111	5.9	22.0	1.2	.4	8	499	6.2 d
½ cup	123	6.5	24.4	1.3	.5	9	554	6.9 d
(*B&M*), 8 oz.,	230	12.0	48.0	3.0	1.0	1	1010	10.0 d
(*Campbell's*), 8 oz.	200	10.0	43.0	3.0	m.q.	n.a.	770	m.q.
(*Finast*, 40 oz.), ½ cup	120	7.0	21.0	1.0	n.a.	n.a.	930	m.q.
(*Finast*, 16 oz.), 1 cup	270	13.0	50.0	3.0	m.q.	n.a.	1180	m.q.
(*Pathmark*), ½ cup	150	7.0	23.0	2.0	m.q.	n.a.	440	m.q.
(*Pathmark* No Frills), ½ cup	160	7.0	28.0	2.0	m.q.	n.a.	390	m.q.

Food and Measure	cal.	prot. (gms)	carbo. (gms)	tot. fat (gms)	sat. fat (gms)	chol. (mgs)	sod. (mgs)	fiber (gms)
vegetarian, see "plain or vegetarian," above								
BAKING POWDER:								
(*Davis*), 1 tsp.	8	0	2.0	0	0	0	330	0
(*Featherweight* Low Salt), 1 tsp.	8	0	2.0	0	0	0	2'	0
(*Tone's*), 1 tsp.	5	0	1.0	0	0	0	290	0
BAKING SODA:								
(*Tone's*), 1 tsp.	0	0	0	0	0	0	821	0
BALSAM PEAR, LEAFY TIPS:								
raw:								
untrimmed, 1 lb.	52	9.1	5.7	1.2	n.a.	0	18	3.9 c
trimmed, 1 oz.	9	1.5	.9	.2	(0)	0	3	.6 c
trimmed, ½ cup	7	1.3	.8	.2	(0)	0	3	.6 c
1 leaf, approx. .1 oz.	1	.2	.1	<.1	(0)	0	tr.	.1 c
boiled, drained, 4 oz.	40	4.1	7.7	.2	(0)	0	15	2.1 c
boiled, drained, ½ cup	10	1.0	2.0	.1	(0)	0	4	.5 c
BALSAM PEAR, PODS:								
raw:								
untrimmed, 1 lb.	64	3.8	13.9	.6	n.a.	0	20	5.3 c
trimmed, 1 oz.	5	.3	1.1	.1	(0)	0	1	.4 c
1 pod, 9⅜″ × 1½″, approx.								
5.3 oz.	21	1.2	4.6	.2	(0)	0	6	1.7 c
½″ pieces, ½ cup	8	.5	1.7	.1	(0)	0	3	.7 c
boiled, drained, 4 oz.	22	1.0	4.9	.2	(0)	0	7	1.2 c
boiled, drained, ½″ pieces, ½ cup ..	12	.5	2.7	.1	(0)	0	4	.7 c
BAMBOO SHOOTS:								
raw:								
w/sheath, 1 lb.	36	3.4	6.8	.4	.1	0	6	3.4 d
trimmed, 1 oz.	8	.7	1.5	.1	.1	0	1	.7 d
½″ slices, ½ cup	21	2.0	4.0	.2	.1	0	3	2.0 d
boiled, drained:								
4 oz.	14	1.7	2.2	.2	.1	0	5	.7 c
1 shoot, approx. 5.1 oz.	18	2.2	2.8	.3	.1	0	6	.9 c
½″ slices, ½ cup	8	.9	1.2	.1	<.1	0	3	.4 c
BAMBOO SHOOTS, CANNED:								
drained, 4 oz.	22	2.0	3.7	.5	.1	0	8	.8 c
drained, ⅛″ slices, ½ cup	13	1.1	2.1	.3	.1	0	5	.4 c
(*La Choy*), 1.5 oz.	8	.7	1.4	.2	n.a.	0	3	m.q.
BANANA:								
unpeeled, 1 lb.	271	3.1	69.1	1.4	.5	0	3	4.7 d
peeled, 1 oz.	26	.3	6.6	.1	.1	0	<1	.5 d
1 medium, 8¾″ × 1¹³⁄₃₂″, approx.								
6.2 oz.	105	1.2	26.7	.6	<.1	0	1	1.8 d
mashed, ½ cup	104	1.2	26.4	.5	<.1	0	1	1.8 d
BANANA, BAKING, see "Plantain"								
BANANA, DEHYDRATED or								
powdered:								
1 oz.	98	1.1	25.0	.5	.2	0	1	.5 c
¼ cup	87	1.0	22.1	.5	.2	0	1	.5 c

Food and Measure	cal.	prot. (gms)	carbo. (gms)	tot. fat (gms)	sat. fat (gms)	chol. (mgs)	sod. (mgs)	fiber (gms)
BANANA, DEHYDRATED *(cont.)*								
1 tbsp.	21	.2	5.5	.1	<.1	0	tr.	.1 c
BANANA, RED:								
1 medium, 7¼″ × 1¹⁷⁄₃₂″	118	1.6	30.7	.3	n.a.	0	1	m.q.
sliced, ½ cup	68	.9	17.6	.2	n.a.	0	1	m.q.
BANANA CHIP, freeze-dried:								
(*Mountain House*), ½ cup[1]	248	2.0	15.0	8.0	m.q.	0	n.a.	m.q.
BANANA NECTAR:								
(*Libby's*), 6 fl. oz.	110	0	26.0	0	0	0	15	m.q.
BANANA SQUASH, baked:								
(*Frieda* of California), 1 lb.	286	8.2	69.9	1.8	n.a.	0	45	m.q.
(*Frieda* of California), 1 oz.	18	.5	4.4	.1	n.a.	0	3	m.q.
BANNER BEAN SEED, dried:								
whole, 1 oz.	95	6.3	17.4	.3	n.a.	0	n.a.	2.2 c
BARBADOS CHERRY, see "Acerola"								
BARBECUE LOAF:								
1 oz.	49	4.5	1.8	2.5	.9	11	378	0
1 slice, 5⅞″ × 3½″ × ¹⁄₁₆″, approx. .8 oz.	40	3.6	1.5	2.1	.7	9	307	0
(*Oscar Mayer*), 1-oz. slice	46	4.5	1.7	2.3	1.0	14	333	0
BARBECUE SAUCE:								
1 tbsp.	12	.3	2.0	.3	<.1	0	130	.1 c
(*Enrico's* Original), 1 tbsp.	18	1.0	3.0	1.0	n.a.	0	4	n.a.
(*Estee*), 1 tbsp.	18	<1.0	3.0	<1.0	<1.0	0	5	n.a.
(*Heinz* Old Fashioned), 1 tbsp.	18	.2	4.1	.1	(0)	0	180	tr. c
(*Heinz* Select), 1 tbsp.	18	.2	4.2	.1	(0)	0	60	.1 c
(*Heinz* Thick and Rich), 1 tbsp.	20	0	5.0	0	0	0	230	n.a.
(*Heinz* Thick and Rich Chunky), 1 tbsp.	20	0	5.0	0	0	0	230	n.a.
(*Hunt* Original), 1 tbsp.	20	0	5.0	0	0	0	190	n.a.
(*Kraft*), 2 tbsp.	45	0	10.0	1.0	0	0	460	n.a.
(*Kraft Thick'n Spicy* Original), 2 tbsp.	50	0	12.0	1.0	0	0	430	n.a.
(*Maull's* Genuine), 1 tbsp.	20	<1.0	4.8	<1.0	n.a.	<1	160	<1.0 d
(*Maull's* Lite), 1 tbsp.	12	1.0	3.0	<1.0	n.a.	<1	105	<1.0 d
(*Ott's*), 1 tbsp.	14	.2	3.2	.1	n.a.	<1	147	.1 d
beer flavor (*Maull's*), 1 tbsp.	20	<1.0	4.0	<1.0	n.a.	<1	129	<1.0 d
Cajun style (*Golden Dipt*), 1 fl. oz. ..	90	0	5.0	8.0	1.0	0	360	n.a.
Cajun (*Heinz*), 1 tbsp.	15	.3	3.4	.1	(0)	n.a.	108	.1 c
chunky (*Kraft Thick'n Spicy*), 2 tbsp.	60	0	13.0	1.0	0	0	420	n.a.
Dijon and honey (*Lawry's*), ½ cup ..	203	4.7	27.0	1.2	n.a.	n.a.	1768	.4 c
garlic (*Kraft*), 2 tbsp.	40	0	9.0	0	0	0	420	n.a.
Hawaiian style (*Heinz*), 1 tbsp.	19	.2	4.4	.1	(0)	n.a.	108	.1 c
hickory smoke:								
(*Heinz*), 1 tbsp.	19	.3	4.4	.1	(0)	n.a.	56	.1 c
(*Heinz* Thick and Rich), 1 tbsp. ..	20	0	5.0	0	0	0	220	n.a.

1. *Prepared according to package directions.*

Food and Measure	cal.	prot. (gms)	carbo. (gms)	tot. fat (gms)	sat. fat (gms)	chol. (mgs)	sod. (mgs)	fiber (gms)
(*Kraft*), 2 tbsp.	45	0	10.0	1.0	0	0	440	n.a.
(*Kraft Thick'n Spicy*), 2 tbsp.	50	0	12.0	1.0	0	0	430	n.a.
onion bits (*Kraft*), 2 tbsp.	50	0	11.0	1.0	0	0	340	n.a.
honey (*Hain*), 1 tbsp.	14	0	1.0	1.0	n.a.	0	120	n.a.
w/honey (*Kraft Thick'n Spicy*), 2 tbsp.	60	0	13.0	1.0	0	0	340	n.a.
hot:								
(*Heinz* Thick and Rich), 1 tbsp. ..	20	0	5.0	0	0	0	220	n.a.
(*Kraft*), 2 tbsp.	45	0	9.0	1.0	0	0	520	n.a.
hickory smoke (*Kraft*), 2 tbsp.	45	0	9.0	1.0	0	0	360	n.a.
Italian seasonings (*Kraft*), 2 tbsp. ..	50	0	10.0	1.0	0	0	280	n.a.
Kansas City style (*Kraft*), 2 tbsp. ..	50	0	11.0	1.0	0	0	270	n.a.
Kansas City style (*Kraft Thick'n Spicy*), 2 tbsp.	60	0	13.0	1.0	0	0	270	n.a.
mesquite:								
(*Enrico's*), 1 tbsp.	18	1.0	3.0	1.0	n.a.	0	4	n.a.
smoke (*Kraft*), 2 tbsp.	45	0	10.0	1.0	0	0	410	n.a.
smoke (*Kraft Thick'n Spicy*), 2 tbsp.	50	0	12.0	1.0	0	0	430	n.a.
mild (*French's Cattleman's*), 1 tbsp.	25	0	5.0	0	0	0	260	n.a.
mushroom (*Heinz*), 1 tbsp.	14	.3	3.2	.1	(0)	n.a.	219	.1 c
mushroom (*Heinz* Thick and Rich), 1 tbsp.	20	0	5.0	0	0	0	220	n.a.
onion:								
(*Heinz*), 1 tbsp.	15	.3	3.4	.1	(0)	n.a.	255	.1 c
(*Heinz* Thick and Rich), 1 tbsp. ..	20	0	5.0	0	0	0	200	n.a.
(*Maull's*), 1 tbsp.	20	<1.0	4.0	<1.0	n.a.	<1	135	<1.0 d
bits (*Kraft*), 2 tbsp.	50	0	11.0	1.0	0	0	340	n.a.
w/orange juice (*Lawry's* California Grill), ¼ cup	34	3.8	3.4	.7	n.a.	n.a.	3846	.1 c
Oriental (*La Choy*), 1 tbsp.	16	.7	3.8	<.1	tr.	0	304	<.1 d
sloppy Joe, w/beef (*Libby's*), ⅓ cup	110	5.0	7.0	7.0	m.q.	m.q.	190	n.a.
smoky:								
(*French's Cattleman's*), 1 tbsp. ...	25	0	5.0	0	0	0	300	n.a.
(*Maull's*), 1 tbsp.	20	<1.0	4.0	<1.0	n.a.	<1	139	<.7 c
(*Ott's*), 1 tbsp.	14	.2	3.3	.1	n.a.	<1	149	.1 d
sweet:								
(*Maull's* Sweet & Mild), 1 tbsp. ...	27	<1.0	5.0	<1.0	n.a.	<1	125	<1.0 d
(*Maull's* Sweet & Smokey), 1 tbsp.	25	<1.0	6.0	<1.0	n.a.	<1	140	<1.0 d
teriyaki marinade, see "Teriyaki sauce"								
Texas style, hot (*Heinz*), 1 tbsp. ...	15	.3	3.2	.2	(0)	n.a.	210	.2 c
BARBECUE SPICE:								
(*Tone's*), 1 tsp.	9	.3	1.4	.4	<.1	0	713	.3 d
BARLEY:								
raw, 1 oz.	100	3.5	20.8	.7	.1	0	3	4.9 d
raw, 1 cup	651	23.0	135.2	4.2	.9	0	22	31.8 d

Food and Measure	cal.	prot. (gms)	carbo. (gms)	tot. fat (gms)	sat. fat (gms)	chol. (mgs)	sod. (mgs)	fiber (gms)
BARLEY *(cont.)*								
cooked *(Tone's)*, 1 tsp.	8	.2	1.8	.1	<.1	0	tr.	.2 d
flaked, see "Barley flakes"								
pearled, raw:								
1 oz.	100	2.8	22.0	.3	.1	0	3	4.4 d
1 cup	704	19.8	155.5	2.3	.9	0	18	31.2 d
(Arrowhead Mills), 2 oz.	200	5.0	45.0	1.0	n.a.	0	1	7.2 d
medium *(Quaker Scotch* Brand),								
1.7 oz., approx. ¼ cup	172	5.0	36.3	.5	n.a.	0	0	5.0 d
quick *(Quaker Scotch Brand)*,								
⅓ cup	172	5.5	36.3	.5	n.a.	0	0	5.0 d
pearled, cooked:								
4 oz.	139	2.6	32.0	.5	.1	0	1	.3 c
1 cup	193	3.6	44.3	.7	.1	0	5	.4 c
(Tone's), 1 tsp.	8	.2	1.8	<.1	tr.	0	<1	.2 d
BARLEY FLAKES:								
(Arrowhead Mills), 2 oz.	200	5.0	45.0	1.0	n.a.	0	1	7.2 d
BARLEY FLOUR:								
(Arrowhead Mills), 2 oz.	200	7.0	35.0	1.0	n.a.	0	1	7.2 d
BARRACUDA, meat only, raw:								
1 lb.	426	89.4	0	5.0	m.q.	m.q.	m.q.	0
1 oz.	27	5.6	0	.3	m.q.	m.q.	m.q.	0
BASELLA, see "Vine spinach"								
BASIL, dried, crumbled:								
1 oz.	71	4.1	17.3	1.1	(0)	0	10	5.0 c
1 tbsp.	11	.7	2.7	.2	(0)	0	2	.8 c
1 tsp.	4	.2	.9	.1	(0)	0	tr.	.3 c
(Spice Islands), 1 tsp.	3	.1	.7	<.1	(0)	0	<1	.2 c
(Tone's), 1 tsp.	4	.2	.9	.1	(0)	0	1	.3 d
BASS, FRESHWATER, mixed								
species, meat only, raw:								
1 lb.	516	85.5	0	16.7	3.5	308	317	0
1 oz.	32	5.3	0	1.0	.2	19	20	0
1 fillet, approx. 5.6 oz., yield from								
1-lb. whole fish	90	14.9	0	2.9	.6	54	55	0
BASS, SEA see "Sea bass"								
BASS, STRIPED, meat only, raw:								
1 lb.	439	80.4	0	10.6	2.3	363	313	0
1 oz.	27	5.0	0	.7	.1	23	23	0
1 fillet, approx. 5.6 oz., yield from								
2-lb. whole fish	154	28.2	0	3.7	.8	127	110	0
BATTER MIX (see also specific								
listings):								
(Golden Dipt), 1 oz.	100	3.0	21.0	0	0	0	740	m.q.
BAY LEAF, dried, crumbled:								
1 oz.	89	2.2	21.3	2.4	.6	0	7	7.4 c
1 tbsp.	6	.1	1.4	.2	<.1	0	tr.	.5 c
1 tsp.	2	<.1	.2	<.1	tr.	0	tr.	.2 c
(Spice Islands), 1 tsp.	5	.1	.3	.1	n.a.	0	<1	.3 c

Food and Measure	cal.	prot. (gms)	carbo. (gms)	tot. fat (gms)	sat. fat (gms)	chol. (mgs)	sod. (mgs)	fiber (gms)
(*Tone's*), 1 tsp.	2	.1	.5	.1	<.1	0	0	.2 d
BEAN CURD, see "Tofu"								
BEAN DIP (see also specific listings):								
hot (*Hain*), 4 tbsp.	70	4.0	10.0	1.0	n.a.	5	250	m.q.
BEAN MIX (see also specific bean listings):								
Cajun, and sauce (*Lipton*),								
¼ pkg. dry	130	5.0	28.0	<1.0	n.a.	n.a.	400	m.q.
Cajun, and sauce (*Lipton*), ½ cup[1] . .	160	5.0	28.0	3.0	m.q.	m.q.	440	m.q.
chicken, and sauce (*Lipton*),								
¼ pkg. dry	120	6.0	26.0	1.0	n.a.	n.a.	470	m.q.
chicken, and sauce (*Lipton*), ½ cup[1]	150	6.0	26.0	4.0	m.q.	m.q.	500	m.q.
BEAN SALAD, canned:								
four bean (*Joan of Arc/Read*), ½ cup	100	3.0	23.0	1.0	n.a.	0	660	3.3 d
green bean, German-style (*Joan of Arc/Read*), 1 cup	180	3.0	27.0	7.0	m.q.	n.a.	920	3.6 d
three bean (*Green Giant*), ½ cup . . .	70	2.0	18.0	<1.0	0	0	470	3.0 d
three bean (*Joan of Arc/Read*),								
½ cup	90	2.0	22.0	0	0	0	710	3.0 d
BEAN SPROUTS, see specific bean listings								
BEAN SPROUTS, CANNED:								
(*La Choy*), 2 oz.	6	.7	1.4	.1	n.a.	0	17	.7 d
BEANS, see specific listings								
BEANS, BAKED, see "Baked beans"								
BEANS AND FRANKFURTER DINNER, frozen:								
(*Banquet*), 10 oz.	520	17.0	57.0	25.0	m.q.	35	1230	m.q.
(*Morton*), 10 oz.	350	11.0	46.0	13.0	m.q.	30	1490	m.q.
(*Swanson*), 10½ oz.	440	14.0	53.0	19.0	m.q.	m.q.	900	m.q.
BEANS, REFRIED, see "Refried beans"								
BEANS, SNAP, see "Green bean"								
BEAR, meat only:								
raw, 1 oz.	46	5.7	0	2.4	m.q.	m.q.	m.q.	0
simmered[2]:								
9.8 oz., yield from 1 lb. boneless	717	89.7	0	37.0	m.q.	m.q.	m.q.	0
4 oz.	294	36.8	0	15.2	m.q.	m.q.	m.q.	0
diced, 1 cup, approx. 4.9 oz.	363	45.4	0	18.7	m.q.	m.q.	m.q.	0
BEARNAISE SAUCE:								
(*Great Impressions*), 2 tbsp.	192	.5	.2	21.0	m.q.	48	148	n.a.
mix, dry, .9-oz. pkt.	90	3.5	14.8	2.2	.3	tr.	841	.1 c
mix, ½ cup[3]	351	4.2	8.8	34.1	20.9	95	633	<.1 c

1. *Prepared according to package directions, with 1 tbsp. butter.*
2. *Without added ingredients.*
3. *Prepared according to package directions, with milk and butter.*

Food and Measure	cal.	prot. (gms)	carbo. (gms)	tot. fat (gms)	sat. fat (gms)	chol. (mgs)	sod. (mgs)	fiber (gms)
BEAVER, meat only:								
raw, 1 oz.	41	6.8	0	1.4	m.q.	m.q.	14	0
roasted[1]:								
14.1 oz., yield from 1 lb. raw								
boneless	662	109.1	0	21.8	m.q.	m.q.	185	0
4 oz.	188	31.0	0	6.2	m.q.	m.q.	52	0
diced, 1 cup, approx. 4.9 oz.	232	38.3	0	7.6	m.q.	m.q.	64	0
BEECHNUT, dried:								
in shell, 1 lb.	1595	17.2	92.7	138.4	15.8	0	m.q.	10.2 c
shelled, 1 oz.	164	1.8	9.5	14.2	1.6	0	m.q.	1.1 c
BEEF[2], retail trim[3], meat only:								
brisket, whole, all grades:								
separable lean and fat, trimmed to								
¼" fat:								
raw, 1 oz.	88	4.8	0	7.5	3.0	21	18	0
braised, 11.6 oz., yield from								
1 lb. raw	1271	77.6	0	104.1	40.8	309	200	0
braised, 4 oz.	437	26.6	0	35.8	14.0	107	69	0
separable lean and fat, trimmed to								
0" fat:								
braised, 11.1 oz., yield from								
1 lb. raw	913	84.2	0	61.4	23.7	294	204	0
braised, 4 oz.	330	30.4	0	22.1	8.5	105	74	0
separable lean only, trimmed to								
¼" fat:								
braised, 8.2 oz., yield from 1 lb.								
raw w/fat	561	69.0	0	29.6	10.6	215	163	0
braised, 4 oz.	274	33.7	0	14.5	5.2	105	79	0
separable lean only, trimmed to								
0" fat:								
braised, 9.3 oz., yield from 1 lb.								
raw w/fat	574	78.4	0	26.6	9.6	245	185	0
braised, 4 oz.	247	33.7	0	11.4	4.1	105	79	0
brisket, flat half, all grades:								
separable lean and fat, trimmed to								
¼" fat:								
raw, 1 oz.	82	5.1	0	6.7	2.7	20	18	0
braised, 11.5 oz., yield from								
1 lb. raw	1189	81.2	0	93.1	36.0	310	183	0
braised, 4 oz.	413	28.4	0	32.3	12.5	108	64	0
separable lean and fat, trimmed to								
0" fat:								
braised, 11.5 oz., yield from								
1 lb. raw	702	99.5	0	30.7	10.9	310	202	0
braised, 4 oz.	244	34.6	0	10.7	3.8	108	70	0

1. *Without added ingredients.*
2. *Cooked meats are prepared without added ingredients, except as noted.*
3. *Meat trimmed to 0" or ¼" fat refers to the amount of fat present during cooking. For "lean only" listings, all visible fat is trimmed after cooking. (Bear in mind that a small amount of fat is always present, even in meat trimmed to 0" fat before cooking.)*

Food and Measure	cal.	prot. (gms)	carbo. (gms)	tot. fat (gms)	sat. fat (gms)	chol. (mgs)	sod. (mgs)	fiber (gms)
separable lean only, trimmed to ¼″ fat:								
braised, 7.9 oz., yield from 1 lb.								
raw w/fat	500	71.0	0	21.9	7.1	214	142	0
braised, 4 oz.	252	35.7	0	11.0	3.6	108	71	0
separable lean only, trimmed to 0″ fat:								
braised, 10.9 oz., yield from								
1 lb. raw w/fat	591	97.8	0	19.2	6.3	295	195	0
braised, 4 oz.	217	35.7	0	7.0	2.3	108	71	0
brisket, point half, all grades:								
separable lean and fat, trimmed to ¼″ fat:								
raw, 1 oz.	94	4.6	0	8.2	3.4	22	18	0
braised, 11.6 oz., yield from								
1 lb. raw	1323	72.6	0	112.4	44.5	303	212	0
braised, 4 oz.	458	25.1	0	38.9	15.4	104	74	0
separable lean and fat, trimmed to 0″ fat:								
braised, 11.1 oz., yield from								
1 lb. raw	1124	73.9	0	89.6	35.3	289	213	0
braised, 4 oz.	406	26.7	0	32.3	12.7	104	77	0
separable lean only, trimmed to ¼″ fat:								
braised, 7.6 oz., yield from 1 lb.								
raw w/fat	563	60.4	0	33.8	12.7	196	166	0
braised, 4 oz.	296	31.8	0	17.8	6.7	103	87	0
separable lean only, trimmed to 0″ fat:								
braised, 8.2 oz., yield from 1 lb.								
raw w/fat	566	65.0	0	32.0	12.0	211	178	0
braised, 4 oz.	277	31.8	0	15.6	5.9	103	87	0
chuck, arm pot roast, separable lean and fat:								
choice grade, trimmed to ¼″ fat								
raw, 1 oz.	72	5.2	0	5.5	2.2	20	17	0
braised, 9.1 oz., yield from 1 lb.								
raw w/bone	894	69.4	0	66.3	26.1	256	152	0
braised, 4 oz.	395	30.6	0	29.2	11.5	112	67	0
choice grade, trimmed to 0″ fat:								
braised, 8.8 oz., yield from 1 lb.								
raw w/bone	730	73.4	0	46.3	18.0	249	155	0
braised, 4 oz.	332	33.4	0	21.0	8.2	113	70	0
select grade, trimmed to ¼″ fat:								
raw, 1 oz.	66	5.3	0	4.8	2.0	19	17	0
braised, 9 oz., yield from 1 lb.								
raw w/bone	800	70.8	0	55.2	21.8	253	153	0
braised, 4 oz.	357	31.6	0	24.6	9.7	113	68	0

Food and Measure	cal.	prot. (gms)	carbo. (gms)	tot. fat (gms)	sat. fat (gms)	chol. (mgs)	sod. (mgs)	fiber (gms)
BEEF, CHUCK, ARM POT ROAST *(cont.)*								
select grade, trimmed to 0″ fat:								
braised, 8.8 oz., yield from 1 lb.								
raw w/bone	649	75.0	0	36.4	14.2	250	156	0
braised, 4 oz.	295	34.1	0	16.6	6.5	113	71	0
chuck, arm pot roast, separable lean only:								
choice grade, trimmed to ¼″ fat:								
braised, 6.6 oz., yield from 1 lb.								
raw w/bone and fat	421	61.8	0	17.4	6.3	189	124	0
braised, 4 oz.	255	37.4	0	10.5	3.8	115	75	0
choice grade, trimmed to 0″ fat:								
braised, 7.3 oz., yield from 1 lb.								
raw w/bone and fat	453	68.2	0	18.0	6.5	209	136	0
braised, 4 oz.	248	37.4	0	10.0	3.6	115	75	0
select grade, trimmed to ¼″ fat:								
braised, 6.9 oz., yield from 1 lb.								
raw w/bone and fat	405	65.0	0	14.2	5.1	199	130	0
braised, 4 oz.	234	37.4	0	8.2	3.0	115	75	0
select grade, trimmed to 0″ fat:								
braised, 7.6 oz., yield from 1 lb.								
raw w/bone and fat	427	71.2	0	13.6	4.9	218	142	0
braised, 4 oz.	225	37.4	0	7.1	2.6	115	75	0
chuck, blade roast, separable lean and fat:								
choice grade, trimmed to ¼″ fat:								
raw, 1 oz.	77	4.8	0	6.3	2.5	20	19	0
braised, 8.7 oz., yield from 1 lb.								
raw w/bone	899	64.9	0	69.0	27.5	256	158	0
braised, 4 oz.	412	29.7	0	31.5	12.6	117	73	0
choice grade, trimmed to 0″ fat:								
braised, 8.4 oz., yield from 1 lb.								
raw w/bone	828	64.2	0	61.4	24.4	247	155	0
braised, 4 oz.	395	30.6	0	29.3	11.6	118	74	0
select grade, trimmed to ¼″ fat:								
raw, 1 oz.	67	4.9	0	5.1	2.1	20	19	0
braised, 8.7 oz., yield from 1 lb.								
raw w/bone	808	66.9	0	57.9	23.1	257	161	0
braised, 4 oz.	370	30.6	0	26.5	10.5	118	74	0
select grade, trimmed to 0″ fat:								
braised, 8.3 oz., yield from 1 lb.								
raw w/bone	736	64.8	0	50.9	20.2	245	155	0
braised, 4 oz.	355	31.3	0	24.6	9.8	118	75	0
chuck, blade roast, separable lean only:								
choice grade, trimmed to ¼″ fat:								
braised, 6.6 oz., yield from 1 lb.								
raw w/bone and fat	491	58.1	0	26.9	10.4	198	133	0
braised, 4 oz.	298	35.2	0	16.3	6.3	120	81	0

Food and Measure	cal.	prot. (gms)	carbo. (gms)	tot. fat (gms)	sat. fat (gms)	chol. (mgs)	sod. (mgs)	fiber (gms)
choice grade, trimmed to 0″ fat:								
braised, 6.7 oz., yield from 1 lb.								
raw w/bone and fat	507	59.3	0	28.1	10.9	202	136	0
braised, 4 oz.	301	35.2	0	16.7	6.5	120	81	0
select grade, trimmed to ¼″ fat:								
braised, 7 oz., yield from 1 lb.								
raw w/bone and fat	475	62.1	0	23.2	9.0	212	142	0
braised, 4 oz.	269	35.2	0	13.2	5.1	120	81	0
select grade, trimmed to 0″ fat:								
braised, 6.8 oz., yield from 1 lb.								
raw w/bone and fat	462	60.3	0	22.7	8.8	206	138	0
braised, 4 oz.	270	35.2	0	13.3	5.1	120	81	0
flank, choice grade, trimmed to 0″ fat:								
separable lean and fat:								
raw, 1 oz.	51	5.6	0	3.0	1.3	15	20	0
braised, 9.2 oz., yield from 1 lb.								
raw	691	70.8	0	43.1	18.1	190	184	0
braised, 4 oz.	298	30.6	0	18.6	7.8	82	79	0
broiled, 11.7 oz., yield from								
1 lb. raw	753	88.1	0	41.8	17.7	226	270	0
broiled, 4 oz.	256	30.0	0	14.2	6.0	77	92	0
separable lean only:								
braised, 8.7 oz., yield from 1 lb.								
raw w/fat	583	69.0	0	32.0	13.6	175	177	0
braised, 4 oz.	269	31.8	0	14.7	6.3	81	82	0
broiled, 11.3 oz., yield from								
1 lb. raw w/fat	662	86.6	0	32.4	13.9	213	265	0
broiled, 4 oz.	235	30.7	0	11.5	4.9	76	94	0
ground, extra lean:								
raw, 1 oz.	66	5.3	0	4.8	1.9	19	19	0
baked:								
medium, 12.2 oz., yield from								
1 lb. raw	863	84.4	0	55.7	21.9	283	170	0
medium, 4 oz.	284	27.7	0	18.3	7.2	93	56	0
well done, 9.5 oz., yield from								
1 lb. raw	733	81.2	0	42.8	16.8	286	172	0
well done, 4 oz.	311	34.4	0	18.1	7.1	121	73	0
broiled:								
medium, 11.9 oz., yield from								
1 lb. raw	859	85.3	0	54.9	21.6	281	234	0
medium, 4 oz.	290	28.8	0	18.5	7.3	95	79	0
well done, 9.9 oz., yield from								
1 lb. raw	744	80.3	0	44.4	17.4	277	230	0
well done, 4 oz.	301	32.4	0	17.9	7.0	112	93	0
pan-fried:								
medium, 12 oz., yield from 1 lb.								
raw	866	84.9	0	55.8	21.9	274	238	0
medium, 4 oz.	289	28.3	0	18.6	7.3	92	79	0

Food and Measure	cal.	prot. (gms)	carbo. (gms)	tot. fat (gms)	sat. fat (gms)	chol. (mgs)	sod. (mgs)	fiber (gms)
BEEF, GROUND, EXTRA LEAN, PAN-FRIED *(cont.)*								
well done, 10.4 oz., yield from								
1 lb. raw	777	82.6	0	47.1	18.5	275	238	0
well done, 4 oz.	298	31.7	0	18.1	7.1	105	92	0
ground, lean:								
raw, 1 oz.	75	5.0	0	5.9	2.4	21	20	0
baked:								
medium, 11.9 oz., yield from								
1 lb. raw	899	80.4	0	61.6	24.2	262	187	0
medium, 4 oz.	304	27.1	0	20.8	8.2	88	64	0
well done, 9.3 oz., yield from								
1 lb. raw	768	77.9	0	48.3	19.0	261	187	0
well done, 4 oz.	331	33.6	0	20.8	8.2	112	81	0
broiled:								
medium, 11.4 oz., yield from								
1 lb. raw	876	79.6	0	59.4	23.4	280	248	0
medium, 4 oz.	308	28.0	0	20.9	8.2	99	87	0
well done, 9.9 oz., yield from								
1 lb. raw	785	79.2	0	49.6	19.5	283	250	0
well done, 4 oz.	318	32.0	0	20.0	7.9	115	101	0
pan-fried:								
medium, 11.5 oz., yield from								
1 lb. raw	901	79.2	0	62.3	24.5	275	251	0
medium, 4 oz.	312	27.5	0	21.6	8.5	95	87	0
well done, 10.1 oz., yield from								
1 lb. raw	791	78.8	0	50.5	19.9	273	249	0
well done, 4 oz.	314	31.3	0	20.0	7.9	108	99	0
ground, regular:								
raw, 1 oz.	88	4.7	0	7.5	3.1	24	19	0
baked:								
medium, 11.2 oz., yield from								
1 lb. raw	913	73.2	0	66.6	26.2	276	191	0
medium, 4 oz.	325	26.1	0	23.7	9.3	99	68	0
well done, 9 oz., yield from 1 lb.								
raw	804	73.2	0	54.5	21.4	274	189	0
well done, 4 oz.	359	3.9	0	24.3	9.6	122	85	0
broiled:								
medium, 10.7 oz., yield from								
1 lb. raw	880	73.2	0	62.9	24.7	273	251	0
medium, 4 oz.	328	27.3	0	23.5	9.2	102	94	0
well done, 9.6 oz., yield from								
1 lb. raw	793	74.0	0	52.9	20.8	274	252	0
well done, 4 oz.	331	30.8	0	22.1	8.7	115	105	0
pan-fried:								
medium, 10.9 oz., yield from								
1 lb. raw	941	73.7	0	69.5	27.3	273	258	0
medium, 4 oz.	347	27.1	0	25.6	10.0	101	95	0
well done, 9.8 oz., yield from								
1 lb. raw	792	74.8	0	52.4	20.6	272	257	0
well done, 4 oz.	324	30.6	0	21.5	8.4	111	105	0

Food and Measure	cal.	prot. (gms)	carbo. (gms)	tot. fat (gms)	sat. fat (gms)	chol. (mgs)	sod. (mgs)	fiber (gms)
ground, frozen patties:								
raw, 4-oz patty	319	19.3	0	26.2	10.6	89	77	0
raw, 3-oz. patty	240	14.5	0	19.7	8.0	67	58	0
broiled, medium, 11 oz., yield								
from 1 lb. raw	882	76.7	0	61.5	24.2	294	242	0
broiled, medium, 4 oz.	320	27.8	0	22.3	8.8	106	87	0
lean cuts, raw, 4 oz.:								
(Brae Beef)	120	26.0	0	2.0	.7	57	60	0
cube steak (Lean and Free)	109	23.8	0	1.0	m.q.	m.q.	61	0
ground (Lean and Free)	161	21.5	0	7.5	m.q.	m.q.	67	0
ribeye (Lean and Free)	121	24.7	0	2.6	m.q.	59	71	0
roast, rolled (Lean and Free)	125	25.4	0	2.8	m.q.	60	m.q.	0
round steak (Lean and Free)	111	25.7	0	1.1	m.q.	60	m.q.	0
sirloin steak (Lean and Free)	111	24.2	0	1.8	m.q.	67	66	0
sirloin tip (Lean and Free)	110	23.2	0	1.2	m.q.	62	66	0
steakburger (Lean and Free)	174	22.5	0	9.3	m.q.	64	77	0
strip loin steak (Lean and Free) ..	113	25.2	0	1.8	m.q.	61	67	0
T-bone (Lean and Free)	125	25.5	0	2.7	m.q.	54	m.q.	0
tenderloin fillet steak (Lean and								
Free)	116	23.6	0	2.4	m.q.	68	61	0
top round (Lean Limousin)	134	24.6	0	4.5	m.q.	m.q.	49	0
porterhouse steak, choice grade,								
trimmed to ¼″ fat:								
separable lean and fat:								
raw, 1 oz.	77	5.0	0	6.2	2.5	19	14	0
broiled, 9 oz., yield from 1 lb.								
raw w/bone	776	63.1	0	56.2	22.6	210	156	0
broiled, 4 oz.	346	28.2	0	25.1	10.1	94	69	0
separable lean only:								
broiled, 7.3 oz., yield from 1 lb.								
raw w/bone and fat	448	58.0	0	22.3	8.9	165	136	0
broiled, 4 oz.	247	31.9	0	12.2	4.9	91	75	0
rib, whole (ribs 6–12), separable lean								
and fat, trimmed to ¼″ fat:								
choice grade:								
raw, 1 oz.	94	4.6	0	8.3	3.4	20	15	0
broiled, 9.5 oz., yield from 1 lb.								
raw w/bone	968	59.1	0	79.4	32.2	221	168	0
broiled, 4 oz.	408	24.9	0	33.5	13.6	93	70	0
roasted, 10.2 oz., yield from								
1 lb. raw w/bone	1091	64.3	0	90.5	36.5	245	182	0
roasted, 4 oz.	426	25.1	0	35.4	14.3	96	71	0
prime grade:								
raw, 1 oz.	103	4.5	0	9.3	3.9	21	15	0
broiled, 9.7 oz., yield from 1 lb.								
raw w/bone	1080	59.9	0	91.4	37.8	234	170	0
broiled, 4 oz.	445	24.6	0	37.6	15.6	96	70	0
roasted, 9.8 oz., yield from 1 lb.								
raw w/bone	1143	62.1	0	97.3	40.3	237	179	0
roasted, 4 oz.	464	25.2	0	41.9	17.7	98	71	0

Food and Measure	cal.	prot. (gms)	carbo. (gms)	tot. fat (gms)	sat. fat (gms)	chol. (mgs)	sod. (mgs)	fiber (gms)
BEEF, RIB, WHOLE, LEAN AND FAT *(cont.)*								
select grade:								
raw, 1 oz.	84	4.7	0	7.1	2.9	20	16	0
broiled, 9.3 oz., yield from 1 lb.								
raw w/bone	857	59.7	0	66.7	27.1	217	168	0
broiled, 4 oz.	366	25.5	0	28.5	11.6	93	71	0
roasted, 10.2 oz., yield from								
1 lb. raw w/bone	975	66.3	0	76.7	30.9	243	186	0
roasted, 4 oz.	381	25.9	0	30.0	12.1	95	73	0
rib, whole (ribs 6–12), separable lean only, trimmed to ¼″ fat:								
choice grade:								
broiled, 6.8 oz., yield from 1 lb.								
raw w/bone and fat	460	51.1	0	26.8	10.9	150	137	0
broiled, 4 oz.	269	29.9	0	15.7	6.4	87	81	0
roasted, 7.2 oz., yield from 1 lb.								
raw w/bone and fat	492	55.2	0	28.4	11.3	162	147	0
roasted, 4 oz.	276	30.9	0	15.9	6.4	91	82	0
prime grade:								
broiled, 6.9 oz., yield from 1 lb.								
raw w/bone and fat	551	51.3	0	36.8	15.7	160	137	0
broiled, 4 oz.	318	29.5	0	21.2	9.0	92	79	0
roasted, 6.9 oz., yield from 1 lb.								
raw w/bone and fat	571	53.2	0	38.1	16.3	158	144	0
roasted, 4 oz.	331	30.9	0	22.1	9.4	92	84	0
select grade:								
broiled, 7.1 oz., yield from 1 lb.								
raw w/bone and fat	414	52.9	0	20.9	8.5	155	142	0
broiled, 4 oz.	234	29.9	0	11.8	4.8	87	81	0
roasted, 7.5 oz., yield from 1 lb.								
raw w/bone and fat	454	58.1	0	22.9	9.1	171	154	0
roasted, 4 oz.	242	30.9	0	12.2	4.8	91	82	0
rib, large end (ribs 6–9), separable lean and fat:								
choice grade, trimmed to ¼″ fat:								
raw, 1 oz.	98	4.5	0	8.7	3.6	21	15	0
broiled, 9.5 oz., yield from 1 lb.								
raw w/bone	988	56.4	0	82.8	33.7	219	169	0
broiled, 4 oz.	416	23.8	0	34.9	14.2	92	71	0
roasted, 10.5 oz., yield from								
1 lb. raw w/bone	1139	66.2	0	94.9	38.3	253	187	0
roasted, 4 oz.	434	25.3	0	36.2	14.6	96	71	0
choice grade, trimmed to 0″ fat:								
roasted, 10.2 oz., yield from								
1 lb. raw w/bone	1080	66.1	0	88.4	35.7	246	186	0
roasted, 4 oz.	422	25.9	0	34.6	13.9	96	73	0
prime grade, trimmed to ¼″ fat:								
raw, 1 oz.	107	4.4	0	9.8	4.1	21	15	0

Food and Measure	cal.	prot. (gms)	carbo. (gms)	tot. fat (gms)	sat. fat (gms)	chol. (mgs)	sod. (mgs)	fiber (gms)
broiled, 9.8 oz., yield from 1 lb.								
raw w/bone	1154	56.7	0	101.1	41.9	240	170	0
broiled, 4 oz.	468	23.0	0	41.1	17.0	98	69	0
roasted, 10 oz., yield from 1 lb.								
raw w/bone	1137	63.6	0	96.0	39.8	241	179	0
roasted, 4 oz.	456	25.5	0	38.5	15.9	96	71	0
select grade, trimmed to ¼" fat:								
raw, 1 oz.	86	4.6	0	7.4	3.0	20	16	0
broiled, 9.5 oz., yield from 1 lb.								
raw w/bone	873	57.9	0	69.3	28.1	216	173	0
broiled, 4 oz.	367	24.4	0	29.2	11.9	91	73	0
roasted, 10.3 oz., yield from								
1 lb. raw w/bone	996	67.8	0	78.3	31.6	248	190	0
roasted, 4 oz.	386	26.2	0	30.3	12.2	96	74	0
select grade, trimmed to 0" fat:								
roasted, 10.1 oz., yield from								
1 lb. raw w/bone	946	67.2	0	73.1	29.5	241	187	0
roasted, 4 oz.	375	26.6	0	29.0	11.7	95	74	0
rib, large end (ribs 6–9), separable lean only:								
choice grade, trimmed to ¼" fat:								
broiled, 6.7 oz., yield from 1 lb.								
raw w/bone and fat	458	48.1	0	28.0	11.4	144	137	0
broiled, 4 oz.	272	28.5	0	16.6	6.8	86	82	0
roasted, 7.2 oz., yield from 1 lb.								
raw w/bone and fat	508	55.9	0	29.8	11.9	164	148	0
roasted, 4 oz.	284	31.2	0	16.7	6.7	92	83	0
choice grade, trimmed to 0" fat:								
roasted, 7.3 oz., yield from 1 lb.								
raw w/bone and fat	523	57.0	0	31.1	12.4	168	151	0
roasted, 4 oz.	287	31.2	0	17.0	6.8	92	83	0
prime grade, trimmed to ¼" fat:								
broiled, 6.8 oz., yield from 1 lb.								
raw w/bone and fat	569	47.8	0	40.5	17.3	159	136	0
broiled, 4 oz.	333	27.9	0	23.7	10.1	93	79	0
roasted, 6.9 oz., yield from 1 lb.								
raw w/bone and fat	555	54.0	0	36.0	15.4	159	143	0
roasted, 4 oz.	321	31.2	0	20.8	8.9	92	83	0
select grade, trimmed to ¼" fat:								
broiled, 7.2 oz., yield from 1 lb.								
raw w/bone and fat	420	51.3	0	22.3	9.1	154	147	0
broiled, 4 oz.	234	28.6	0	12.4	5.0	86	82	0
roasted, 7.7 oz., yield from 1 lb.								
raw w/bone and fat	478	59.7	0	24.7	9.9	176	158	0
roasted, 4 oz.	249	31.2	0	12.9	5.2	92	83	0
select grade, trimmed to 0" fat:								
roasted, 7.7 oz., yield from 1 lb.								
raw w/bone and fat	478	59.7	0	24.7	9.9	176	158	0
roasted, 4 oz.	249	31.2	0	12.9	5.2	92	83	0

Food and Measure	cal.	prot. (gms)	carbo. (gms)	tot. fat (gms)	sat. fat (gms)	chol. (mgs)	sod. (mgs)	fiber (gms)
BEEF *(cont.)*								
rib, shortrib, choice grade:								
separable lean and fat:								
raw, 1 oz.	110	4.1	0	10.3	4.5	22	14	0
braised, 8 oz., yield from 1 lb.								
raw w/bone	1064	48.7	0	94.9	40.2	212	114	0
braised, 4 oz.	534	24.5	0	47.6	20.2	107	57	0
separable lean only:								
raw, 1 oz.	49	5.4	0	2.9	1.2	17	18	0
braised, 4.3 oz., yield from 1 lb.								
raw w/bone and fat	363	37.8	0	22.3	9.5	114	72	0
braised, 4 oz.	335	34.9	0	20.6	8.7	105	66	0
rib, small end (ribs 10–12), separable lean and fat:								
choice grade, trimmed to ¼" fat:								
raw, 1 oz.	89	4.7	0	7.7	3.2	20	15	0
broiled, 9.6 oz., yield from 1 lb.								
raw w/bone	951	64.0	0	75.1	30.4	228	168	0
broiled, 4 oz.	376	26.7	0	31.3	12.7	95	70	0
roasted, 9.8 oz., yield from 1 lb.								
raw w/bone	1023	61.3	0	84.4	34.0	233	174	0
roasted, 4 oz.	416	24.9	0	34.3	13.8	95	70	0
choice grade, trimmed to 0" fat:								
broiled, 9.6 oz., yield from 1 lb.								
raw w/bone	848	67.3	0	62.1	25.1	225	173	0
broiled, 4 oz.	354	28.0	0	25.9	10.4	94	73	0
prime grade, trimmed to ¼" fat:								
raw, 1 oz.	97	4.7	0	8.5	3.5	20	15	0
broiled, 9.6 oz., yield from 1 lb.								
raw w/bone	982	65.0	0	78.1	32.2	228	170	0
broiled, 4 oz.	409	27.1	0	32.5	13.4	95	70	0
roasted, 9.7 oz., yield from 1 lb.								
raw w/bone	1151	60.5	0	98.9	40.9	233	179	0
roasted, 4 oz.	473	24.8	0	40.7	16.8	95	74	0
select grade, trimmed to ¼" fat:								
raw, 1 oz.	81	4.8	0	6.7	2.8	20	15	0
broiled, 9.3 oz., yield from 1 lb.								
raw w/bone	850	63.2	0	64.3	26.0	222	165	0
broiled, 4 oz.	364	27.1	0	27.5	11.1	95	70	0
roasted, 10.1 oz., yield from 1 lb. raw w/bone	948	64.3	0	74.7	30.0	238	181	0
roasted, 4 oz.	375	25.5	0	29.6	11.9	94	71	0
select grade, trimmed to 0" fat:								
broiled, 9.3 oz., yield from 1 lb.								
raw w/bone	755	66.0	0	52.5	21.2	219	169	0
broiled, 4 oz.	323	28.2	0	22.4	9.1	94	73	0

Food and Measure	cal.	prot. (gms)	carbo. (gms)	tot. fat (gms)	sat. fat (gms)	chol. (mgs)	sod. (mgs)	fiber (gms)
rib, small end (ribs 10–12), separable lean only:								
choice grade, trimmed to ¼″ fat:								
broiled, 7.1 oz., yield from 1 lb.								
raw w/bone and fat	469	56.4	0	25.3	10.2	161	139	0
broiled, 4 oz.	264	31.8	0	14.3	5.8	91	78	0
roasted, 6.9 oz., yield from 1 lb.								
raw w/bone and fat	456	52.6	0	25.6	10.2	154	140	0
roasted, 4 oz.	263	30.4	0	14.8	5.9	90	81	0
choice grade, trimmed to 0″ fat:								
broiled, 7.8 oz., yield from 1 lb.								
raw w/bone and fat	496	61.7	0	25.7	10.4	176	152	0
broiled, 4 oz.	255	31.8	0	13.3	5.4	91	78	0
prime grade, trimmed to ¼″ fat:								
raw, 1 oz.	57	5.7	0	3.6	1.5	17	18	0
broiled, 7.3 oz., yield from 1 lb.								
raw w/bone and fat	540	58.3	0	32.3	13.7	166	144	0
broiled, 4 oz.	295	31.8	0	17.6	7.5	91	78	0
roasted, 6.8 oz., yield from 1 lb.								
raw w/bone and fat	584	51.3	0	40.5	17.2	154	144	0
roasted, 4 oz.	345	30.3	0	23.9	10.1	91	85	0
select grade, trimmed to ¼″ fat:								
broiled, 7.1 oz., yield from 1 lb.								
raw w/bone and fat	416	56.4	0	19.5	7.9	161	139	0
broiled, 4 oz.	235	31.8	0	11.0	4.4	91	78	0
roasted, 7.4 oz., yield from 1 lb.								
raw w/bone and fat	425	56.4	0	20.5	8.1	165	150	0
roasted, 4 oz.	230	30.4	0	11.1	4.3	90	81	0
select grade, trimmed to 0″ fat:								
broiled, 7.8 oz., yield from 1 lb.								
raw w/bone and fat	436	61.7	0	19.1	7.7	176	152	0
broiled, 4 oz.	225	31.8	0	9.9	4.0	91	78	0
rib eye, small end (ribs 10–12), choice grade, trimmed to ¼″ fat:								
separable lean and fat:								
raw, 1 oz.	78	5.0	0	6.3	2.6	19	16	0
broiled, 11.9 oz., yield from 1 lb. raw	1035	83.9	0	75.0	30.4	279	216	0
broiled, 4 oz.	348	28.2	0	25.2	10.2	94	73	0
separable lean only:								
broiled, 9.7 oz., yield from 1 lb.								
raw w/fat	622	77.4	0	32.3	13.1	221	190	0
broiled, 4 oz.	255	31.8	0	13.3	5.4	91	78	0
round, full cut, separable lean and fat, trimmed to ¼″ fat:								
choice grade:								
raw, 1 oz.	57	5.8	0	3.6	1.4	18	15	0

Food and Measure	cal.	prot. (gms)	carbo. (gms)	tot. fat (gms)	sat. fat (gms)	chol. (mgs)	sod. (mgs)	fiber (gms)
BEEF, ROUND, FULL CUT, LEAN AND FAT *(cont.)*								
broiled, 11 oz., yield from 1 lb.								
raw w/bone	750	85.6	0	42.6	16.1	249	192	0
broiled, 4 oz.	272	31.0	0	15.4	5.9	91	69	0
select grade:								
raw, 1 oz.	54	5.8	0	3.3	1.3	18	15	0
broiled, 11 oz., yield from 1 lb.								
raw w/bone	697	85.7	0	36.7	12.9	173	193	0
broiled, 4 oz.	253	31.1	0	13.3	4.7	62	70	0
round, full cut, separable lean only, trimmed to ¼″ fat:								
choice grade:								
broiled, 10.1 oz., yield from 1 lb. raw w/bone and fat	540	82.7	0	20.7	7.3	220	180	0
broiled, 4 oz.	217	33.1	0	8.3	2.9	88	73	0
select grade:								
broiled, 10 oz., yield from 1 lb. raw w/bone and fat	485	82.5	0	14.7	5.2	219	180	0
broiled, 4 oz.	195	33.2	0	5.9	2.1	88	73	0
round, bottom, separable lean and fat:								
choice grade, trimmed to ¼″ fat:								
raw, 1 oz.	62	5.7	0	4.2	1.6	18	16	0
braised, 9.9 oz., yield from 1 lb.								
raw	801	80.8	0	50.6	19.0	270	140	0
braised, 4 oz.	322	32.5	0	20.3	7.6	109	57	0
roasted, 11.9 oz., yield from 1 lb. raw	880	89.3	0	55.3	20.8	270	212	0
roasted, 4 oz.	295	30.0	0	18.5	7.0	91	71	0
choice grade, trimmed to 0″ fat:								
braised, 9.7 oz., yield from 1 lb.								
raw	627	85.5	0	29.1	10.2	265	140	0
braised, 4 oz.	257	35.1	0	12.0	4.2	109	58	0
roasted, 12 oz., yield from 1 lb.								
raw	691	96.9	0	30.7	10.7	266	223	0
roasted, 4 oz.	230	32.2	0	10.2	3.5	88	74	0
select grade, trimmed to ¼″ fat:								
raw, 1 oz.	55	5.8	0	3.4	1.3	18	16	0
braised, 10 oz., yield from 1 lb.								
raw	731	81.4	0	42.5	16.1	270	140	0
braised, 4 oz.	294	32.7	0	17.1	6.5	109	57	0
roasted, 11.7 oz., yield from 1 lb. raw	790	90.5	0	44.8	16.9	269	214	0
roasted, 4 oz.	265	30.4	0	15.0	5.7	91	71	0
select grade, trimmed to 0″ fat:								
braised, 9.7 oz., yield from 1 lb.								
raw	556	86.0	0	20.9	7.3	265	140	0
braised, 4 oz.	228	35.3	0	8.6	3.0	109	58	0
roasted, 12 oz., yield from 1 lb.								

Food and Measure	cal.	prot. (gms)	carbo. (gms)	tot. fat (gms)	sat. fat (gms)	chol. (mgs)	sod. (mgs)	fiber (gms)
raw	602	97.5	0	20.6	7.0	265	224	0
roasted, 4 oz.	201	32.4	0	6.8	2.3	88	75	0
round, bottom, separable lean only:								
choice grade, trimmed to ¼″ fat:								
braised, 8.5 oz., yield from 1 lb.								
raw w/fat	529	76.1	0	22.7	7.7	231	123	0
braised, 4 oz.	249	35.8	0	10.7	3.6	109	58	0
roasted, 10.3 oz., yield from								
1 lb. raw w/fat	579	84.3	0	24.3	8.3	227	193	0
roasted, 4 oz.	225	32.6	0	9.4	3.2	88	75	0
choice grade, trimmed to 0″ fat:								
braised, 9.4 oz., yield from 1 lb.								
raw w/fat	570	84.3	0	23.2	7.8	256	136	0
braised, 4 oz.	242	35.8	0	9.9	3.3	109	58	0
roasted, 11.8 oz., yield from								
1 lb. raw w/fat	644	96.1	0	25.9	8.7	259	220	0
roasted, 4 oz.	219	32.6	0	8.8	3.0	88	75	0
select grade, trimmed to ¼″ fat:								
braised, 8.6 oz., yield from 1 lb.								
raw w/fat	479	77.1	0	16.6	5.6	234	124	0
braised, 4 oz.	222	35.8	0	7.7	2.6	109	58	0
roasted, 10.5 oz., yield from								
1 lb. raw w/fat	534	86.0	0	18.5	6.3	232	197	0
roasted, 4 oz.	203	32.6	0	7.0	2.4	88	75	0
select grade, trimmed to 0″ fat:								
braised, 9.5 oz., yield from 1 lb.								
raw w/fat	518	85.3	0	17.0	5.7	259	138	0
braised, 4 oz.	218	35.8	0	7.1	2.4	109	58	0
roasted, 11.9 oz., yield from								
1 lb. raw w/fat	580	97.2	0	18.2	6.0	262	223	0
roasted, 4 oz.	194	32.6	0	6.1	2.0	88	75	0
round, eye of, separable lean and fat:								
choice grade, trimmed to ¼″ fat:								
raw, 1 oz.	62	5.6	0	4.2	1.7	17	14	0
roasted, 11.7 oz., yield from								
1 lb. raw	802	88.6	0	47.0	18.3	241	197	0
roasted, 4 oz.	273	30.2	0	16.0	6.2	82	67	0
choice grade, trimmed to 0″ fat:								
roasted, 11.7 oz., yield from								
1 lb. raw	600	95.9	0	21.1	7.8	231	206	0
roasted, 4 oz.	204	32.7	0	7.2	2.6	78	70	0
select grade, trimmed to ¼″ fat:								
raw, 1 oz.	57	5.6	0	3.7	1.5	17	14	0
roasted, 11.7 oz., yield from								
1 lb. raw	723	89.8	0	37.6	14.7	239	199	0
roasted, 4 oz.	246	30.6	0	12.8	5.0	82	68	0
select grade, trimmed to 0″ fat:								
roasted, 11.7 oz., yield from								
1 lb. raw	535	95.9	0	13.9	5.1	231	206	0

Food and Measure	cal.	prot. (gms)	carbo. (gms)	tot. fat (gms)	sat. fat (gms)	chol. (mgs)	sod. (mgs)	fiber (gms)
BEEF, ROUND, EYE OF, LEAN AND FAT *(cont.)*								
roasted, 4 oz.	183	32.7	0	4.7	1.7	78	70	0
round, eye of, separable lean only:								
choice grade, trimmed to ¼″ fat:								
roasted, 10.3 oz., yield from								
1 lb. raw w/fat	513	84.9	0	16.7	6.1	202	182	0
roasted, 4 oz.	198	32.9	0	6.5	2.3	78	70	0
choice grade, trimmed to 0″ fat:								
roasted, 11.7 oz., yield from								
1 lb. raw w/1% fat	580	96.0	0	18.9	6.8	228	205	0
roasted, 4 oz.	198	32.9	0	6.5	2.3	78	70	0
select grade, trimmed to ¼″ fat:								
roasted, 10.3 oz., yield from								
1 lb. raw w/fat	468	84.9	0	11.7	4.3	202	182	0
roasted, 4 oz.	181	32.9	0	4.5	1.6	78	70	0
select grade, trimmed to 0″ fat:								
roasted, 10.4 oz., yield from								
1 lb. raw w/1% fat	460	85.8	0	10.4	3.8	204	184	0
roasted, 4 oz.	176	32.9	0	4.0	1.4	78	70	0
round, tip, separable lean and fat:								
choice grade, trimmed to ¼″ fat:								
raw, 1 oz.	60	5.4	0	4.1	1.6	19	16	0
roasted, 11.3 oz., yield from								
1 lb. raw	792	84.9	0	47.6	18.1	265	199	0
roasted, 4 oz.	280	30.1	0	16.9	6.4	94	70	0
choice grade, trimmed to 0″ fat:								
roasted, 11.6 oz., yield from								
1 lb. raw	661	92.4	0	29.6	10.9	269	212	0
roasted, 4 oz.	227	31.7	0	10.2	3.7	93	73	0
prime grade, trimmed to ¼″ fat:								
raw, 1 oz.	61	5.5	0	4.1	1.6	18	16	0
roasted, 11.5 oz., yield from								
1 lb. raw	895	86.1	0	58.5	22.6	270	202	0
roasted, 4 oz.	311	29.0	0	20.3	7.8	94	70	0
select grade, trimmed to ¼″ fat:								
raw, 1 oz.	53	5.6	0	3.2	1.3	18	16	0
roasted, 11.4 oz., yield from								
1 lb. raw	728	87.5	0	39.3	14.9	266	203	0
roasted, 4 oz.	255	30.7	0	13.8	5.2	93	71	0
select grade, trimmed to 0″ fat:								
roasted, 11.6 oz., yield from								
1 lb. raw	613	93.0	0	23.9	8.8	269	212	0
roasted, 4 oz.	211	31.9	0	8.2	3.0	92	73	0
round, tip, separable lean only:								
choice grade, trimmed to ¼″ fat:								
roasted, 9.9 oz., yield from 1 lb.								
raw w/fat	531	81.0	0	20.0	7.2	228	183	0
roasted, 4 oz.	213	32.6	0	8.3	2.9	92	74	0

Food and Measure	cal.	prot. (gms)	carbo. (gms)	tot. fat (gms)	sat. fat (gms)	chol. (mgs)	sod. (mgs)	fiber (gms)
choice grade, trimmed to 0″ fat:								
roasted, 11.3 oz., yield from								
1 lb. raw w/fat	577	91.9	0	20.5	7.2	259	208	0
roasted, 4 oz.	204	32.6	0	7.3	2.5	92	74	0
prime grade, trimmed to ¼″ fat:								
roasted, 9.9 oz., yield from 1 lb.								
raw w/fat	610	82.1	0	28.0	10.6	231	186	0
roasted, 4 oz.	242	32.6	0	11.4	4.2	92	74	0
select grade, trimmed to ¼″ fat:								
roasted, 10.3 oz., yield from								
1 lb. raw w/fat	528	84.1	0	18.8	6.6	237	190	0
roasted, 4 oz.	204	32.6	0	7.3	2.5	92	74	0
select grade, trimmed to 0″ fat:								
roasted, 11.3 oz., yield from								
1 lb. raw w/fat	545	91.9	0	17.0	5.9	259	208	0
roasted, 4 oz.	193	32.6	0	6.0	2.1	92	74	0
round, top, separable lean and fat:								
choice grade, trimmed to ¼″ fat:								
raw, 1 oz.	51	6.1	0	2.8	1.1	17	14	0
braised, 10.2 oz., yield from								
1 lb. raw	750	97.0	0	37.2	14.1	262	129	0
braised, 4 oz.	295	38.1	0	14.6	5.5	102	51	0
broiled, 11.5 oz., yield from								
1 lb. raw	730	98.4	0	34.4	12.8	276	194	0
broiled, 4 oz.	254	34.2	0	12.0	4.5	96	68	0
pan-fried in vegetable oil,								
10 oz., yield from 1 lb. raw ..	783	91.6	0	43.5	15.0	274	192	0
pan-fried in vegetable oil, 4 oz.	314	36.7	0	17.4	6.0	110	77	0
choice grade, trimmed to 0″ fat:								
braised, 9.4 oz., yield from 1 lb.								
raw	577	95.1	0	18.9	6.7	241	120	0
braised, 4 oz.	245	40.4	0	8.0	2.9	102	51	0
prime grade, trimmed to ¼″ fat:								
raw, 1 oz.	51	6.3	0	2.7	1.0	17	14	0
broiled, 11.6 oz., yield from								
1 lb. raw	754	102.2	0	35.3	12.7	277	199	0
broiled, 4 oz.	260	35.2	0	12.1	4.4	95	68	0
select grade, trimmed to ¼″ fat:								
raw, 1 oz.	47	6.1	0	2.3	.9	17	14	0
broiled, 11.6 oz., yield from								
1 lb. raw	676	99.3	0	28.0	10.7	279	196	0
broiled, 4 oz.	234	34.2	0	9.7	3.7	96	68	0
select grade, trimmed to 0″ fat:								
braised, 9.4 oz., yield from 1 lb.								
raw	534	95.1	0	14.2	5.1	241	120	0
braised, 4 oz.	227	40.4	0	6.0	2.2	102	51	0

Food and Measure	cal.	prot. (gms)	carbo. (gms)	tot. fat (gms)	sat. fat (gms)	chol. (mgs)	sod. (mgs)	fiber (gms)
BEEF *(cont.)*								
round, top, separable lean only:								
choice grade, trimmed to ¼″ fat:								
braised, 9.2 oz., yield from 1 lb.								
raw w/fat	553	93.9	0	16.9	5.8	234	117	0
braised, 4 oz.	242	41.0	0	7.4	2.5	102	51	0
broiled, 9.1 oz., yield from 1 lb.								
raw w/fat	485	81.41	0	15.2	5.2	216	157	0
broiled, 4 oz.	214	35.9	0	6.7	2.3	95	69	0
pan-fried in vegetable oil,								
8.9 oz., yield from 1 lb. raw								
w/fat	571	88.2	0	21.6	6.1	244	179	0
pan-fried in vegetable oil, 4 oz.	257	39.8	0	9.7	2.7	110	81	0
choice grade, trimmed to 0″ fat:								
braised, 9.2 oz., yield from 1 lb.								
raw w/fat	539	94.3	0	15.1	5.2	235	117	0
braised, 4 oz.	235	41.0	0	6.6	2.3	102	51	0
prime grade, trimmed to ¼″ fat:								
broiled, 11.25 oz., yield from								
1 lb. raw w/fat	687	101.1	0	28.3	9.9	268	195	0
broiled, 4 oz.	244	35.9	0	10.1	3.5	95	69	0
select grade, trimmed to ¼″ fat:								
braised, 9.2 oz., yield from 1 lb.								
raw w/fat	513	94.7	0	12.1	4.1	236	118	0
braised, 4 oz.	222	41.0	0	5.2	1.8	102	51	0
broiled, 9.2 oz., yield from 1 lb.								
raw w/fat	439	82.45	0	9.6	3.3	218	159	0
broiled, 4 oz.	192	35.9	0	4.2	1.4	95	69	0
select grade, trimmed to 0″ fat:								
braised, 9.2 oz., yield from 1 lb.								
raw w/fat	497	94.3	0	10.4	3.6	235	117	0
braised, 4 oz.	215	41.0	0	4.5	1.6	102	51	0
shank crosscuts, choice grade,								
trimmed to ¼″ fat:								
separable lean and fat:								
raw, 1 oz.	50	5.8	0	2.8	1.1	13	17	0
simmered, 6.8 oz., yield from								
1 lb. raw w/bone	511	59.5	0	28.5	11.1	156	118	0
simmered, 4 oz.	298	34.8	0	16.6	6.5	91	69	0
separable lean only:								
simmered, 6 oz., yield from								
1 lb. raw w/bone and fat	341	57.1	0	10.8	3.9	132	109	0
simmered, 4 oz.	228	38.2	0	7.2	2.6	88	73	0
short loin, see "porterhouse steak,"								
"T-bone steak," and "top loin"								
sirloin, top, separable lean and fat:								
choice grade, trimmed to ¼″ fat:								
raw, 1 oz.	64	5.4	0	4.6	1.8	19	15	0
broiled, 10.8 oz., yield from								

Food and Measure	cal.	prot. (gms)	carbo. (gms)	tot. fat (gms)	sat. fat (gms)	chol. (mgs)	sod. (mgs)	fiber (gms)
1 lb. raw	822	84.5	0	51.2	20.4	275	191	0
broiled, 4 oz.	305	31.3	0	19.0	7.6	102	70	0
pan-fried in vegetable oil,								
10.8 oz., yield from 1 lb. raw	1000	86.2	0	70.1	27.3	301	214	0
pan-fried in vegetable oil, 4 oz.	370	31.9	0	25.9	10.1	111	79	0
choice grade, trimmed to 0″ fat:								
broiled, 10.8 oz., yield from								
1 lb. raw	698	89.0	0	35.2	13.9	273	713	0
broiled, 4 oz.	260	33.1	0	13.1	5.2	101	73	0
select grade, trimmed to ¼″ fat:								
raw, 1 oz.	59	5.5	0	3.9	1.6	19	15	0
broiled, 10.75 oz., yield from								
1 lb. raw	749	85.7	0	42.5	17.0	275	193	0
broiled, 4 oz.	278	31.8	0	15.8	6.3	102	71	0
select grade, trimmed to 0″ fat:								
broiled, 10.75 oz., yield from								
1 lb. raw	595	90.6	0	23.1	9.1	272	198	0
broiled, 4 oz.	221	33.7	0	8.6	3.4	101	74	0
sirloin, top, separable lean only:								
choice grade, trimmed to ¼″ fat:								
broiled, 9.3 oz., yield from 1 lb.								
raw w/fat	533	80.2	0	21.1	8.2	235	174	0
broiled, 4 oz.	229	34.4	0	9.1	3.5	101	75	0
pan-fried in vegetable oil,								
8.7 oz., yield from 1 lb. raw								
w/fat	588	80.3	0	27.1	9.9	245	190	0
pan-fried in vegetable oil, 4 oz.	270	36.8	0	12.4	4.6	112	87	0
choice grade, trimmed to 0″ fat:								
broiled, 10 oz., yield from 1 lb.								
raw w/fat	572	86.9	0	22.3	8.7	225	189	0
broiled, 4 oz.	227	34.4	0	8.8	3.4	101	75	0
select grade, trimmed to ¼″ fat:								
broiled, 9.4 oz., yield from 1 lb.								
raw w/fat	496	81.1	0	16.6	6.4	238	176	0
broiled, 4 oz.	211	34.4	0	7.0	2.7	101	75	0
select grade, trimmed to 0″ fat:								
broiled, 10.4 oz., yield from								
1 lb. raw w/fat	532	89.6	0	16.5	6.4	263	195	0
broiled, 4 oz.	204	34.4	0	6.4	2.5	101	75	0
T-bone steak, choice grade, trimmed								
to ¼″ fat:								
separable lean and fat:								
raw, 1 oz.	77	5.0	0	6.2	2.5	19	14	0
broiled, 9 oz., yield from 1 lb.								
raw w/bone	729	61.2	0	51.9	20.9	203	151	0
broiled, 4 oz.	338	28.3	0	24.0	9.7	94	69	0
separable lean only:								
broiled, 7.1 oz., yield from 1 lb.								
raw w/bone and fat	430	56.7	0	20.9	8.4	161	133	0

Food and Measure	cal.	prot. (gms)	carbo. (gms)	tot. fat (gms)	sat. fat (gms)	chol. (mgs)	sod. (mgs)	fiber (gms)
BEEF, T-BONE STEAK, LEAN ONLY *(cont.)*								
broiled, 4 oz.	243	31.9	0	11.8	4.7	91	75	0
tenderloin, separable lean and fat:								
choice grade, trimmed to ¼" fat:								
raw, 1 oz.	82	5.0	0	6.7	2.7	20	14	0
broiled, 4.1 oz., yield from								
6.1-oz. raw steak	356	29.4	0	25.6	10.0	101	69	0
broiled, 4 oz.	345	28.4	0	24.8	9.7	98	67	0
roasted, 11.6 oz., yield from								
1 lb. raw	1115	77.7	0	86.0	34.3	282	212	0
roasted, 4 oz.	384	26.8	0	29.9	11.8	98	74	0
choice grade, trimmed to 0" fat:								
broiled, 3.2 oz., yield from								
4.75 oz. raw steak	225	24.9	0	13.2	5.1	78	57	0
broiled, 4 oz.	277	30.6	0	16.2	6.2	96	69	0
prime grade, trimmed to ¼" fat:								
raw, 1 oz.	81	5.1	0	6.5	2.7	20	14	0
broiled, 4.2 oz., yield from								
6.1-oz. raw steak	381	29.9	0	28.1	11.2	103	71	0
broiled, 4 oz.	359	28.2	0	26.5	10.6	98	67	0
roasted, 11.5 oz., yield from								
1 lb. raw	1149	77.2	0	90.9	36.3	287	179	0
roasted, 4 oz.	400	26.8	0	31.6	12.6	100	62	0
select grade, trimmed to ¼" fat:								
raw, 1 oz.	79	5.0	0	6.4	2.6	20	14	0
broiled, 4.1 oz., yield from								
6.1-oz. raw steak	317	30.0	0	21.0	8.2	100	70	0
broiled, 4 oz.	307	29.0	0	20.3	8.0	98	68	0
roasted, 11.7 oz., yield from								
1 lb. raw	1071	78.1	0	81.7	32.4	283	186	0
roasted, 4 oz.	367	26.8	0	28.0	11.1	98	64	0
select grade, trimmed to 0" fat:								
broiled, 3.3 oz., yield from								
4.75-oz. raw steak	213	25.3	0	11.6	4.5	79	57	0
broiled, 4 oz.	260	30.8	0	14.2	5.4	96	70	0
tenderloin, separable lean only:								
choice grade, trimmed to ¼" fat:								
broiled, 3.4 oz., yield from								
6.1-oz. raw steak w/fat	213	27.1	0	10.8	4.0	81	60	0
broiled, 4 oz.	252	32.0	0	12.7	4.8	95	71	0
roasted, 8.8 oz., yield from 1 lb.								
raw w/fat	578	69.3	0	31.3	11.8	207	180	0
roasted, 4 oz.	262	31.4	0	14.2	5.4	94	82	0
choice grade, trimmed to 0" fat:								
broiled, 3 oz., yield from								
4.75-oz. raw steak w/fat	180	24.0	0	8.6	3.2	71	54	0
broiled, 4 oz.	240	32.0	0	11.5	4.3	95	71	0
prime grade, trimmed to ¼" fat:								
broiled, 3.5 oz., yield from								
6.1-oz. raw steak w/fat	227	27.7	0	12.1	4.7	82	62	0

Food and Measure	cal.	prot. (gms)	carbo. (gms)	tot. fat (gms)	sat. fat (gms)	chol. (mgs)	sod. (mgs)	fiber (gms)
broiled, 4 oz.	263	32.0	0	14.0	5.5	95	71	0
roasted, 8.8 oz., yield from 1 lb.								
raw w/fat	638	68.8	0	38.2	14.9	215	148	0
roasted, 4 oz.	289	31.2	0	17.3	6.8	98	67	0
select grade, trimmed to ¼″ fat:								
broiled, 3.5 oz., yield from								
6.1-oz. raw steak w/fat	197	28.0	0	8.6	3.2	83	62	0
broiled, 4 oz.	226	32.0	0	9.9	3.7	95	71	0
roasted, 8.9 oz., yield from 1 lb.								
raw w/fat	531	69.6	0	25.9	9.8	208	154	0
roasted, 4 oz.	239	31.4	0	11.7	4.4	94	69	0
select grade, trimmed to 0″ fat:								
broiled, 3.1 oz., yield from								
4.75-oz. raw steak w/fat	174	24.6	0	7.7	2.9	73	55	0
broiled, 4 oz.	227	32.0	0	10.0	3.7	95	71	0
top loin, separable lean and fat:								
choice grade, trimmed to ¼″ fat:								
raw, 1 oz.	74	5.3	0	5.7	2.3	19	15	0
broiled, 6.3 oz., yield from								
9.2-oz. raw steak	536	45.7	0	37.8	15.0	143	114	0
broiled, 4 oz.	338	28.8	0	23.8	9.4	90	71	0
choice grade, trimmed to 0″ fat:								
broiled, 5.5 oz., yield from								
7.9-oz. raw steak	353	43.2	0	18.7	7.2	119	104	0
broiled, 4 oz.	259	31.6	0	13.6	5.3	87	76	0
prime grade, trimmed to ¼″ fat:								
raw, 1 oz.	86	5.2	0	7.1	2.9	20	15	0
broiled, 6.3 oz., yield from								
9.2-oz. raw steak	582	45.7	0	42.9	17.3	143	114	0
broiled, 4 oz.	366	28.8	0	27.0	10.9	90	71	0
select grade, trimmed to ¼″ fat:								
raw, 1 oz.	65	5.4	0	4.7	1.9	19	15	0
broiled, 6.3 oz., yield from								
9.2-oz. raw steak	473	46.1	0	30.6	12.1	140	114	0
broiled, 4 oz.	302	29.4	0	19.5	7.7	90	73	0
select grade, trimmed to 0″ fat:								
broiled, 5.5 oz., yield from								
7.9-oz. raw steak	309	43.5	0	13.6	5.3	119	104	0
broiled, 4 oz.	226	31.8	0	10.0	3.9	87	76	0
top loin, separable lean only:								
choice grade, trimmed to ¼″ fat:								
broiled, 5.2 oz., yield from								
9.2-oz. raw steak w/fat	314	42.1	0	14.9	5.7	112	100	0
broiled, 4 oz.	243	32.5	0	11.5	4.4	86	77	0
choice grade, trimmed to 0″ fat:								
broiled, 5.25 oz., yield from								
7.9-oz. raw steak w/fat	311	42.6	0	14.3	5.5	113	101	0
broiled, 4 oz.	237	32.5	0	10.9	4.2	86	77	0

Food and Measure	cal.	prot. (gms)	carbo. (gms)	tot. fat (gms)	sat. fat (gms)	chol. (mgs)	sod. (mgs)	fiber (gms)
BEEF, TOP LOIN, LEAN ONLY *(cont.)*								
prime grade, trimmed to ¼″ fat:								
broiled, 5.2 oz., yield from								
9.2-oz. raw steak w/fat	360	42.1	0	20.0	8.0	112	100	0
broiled, 4 oz.	278	32.5	0	15.4	6.2	86	77	0
select grade, trimmed to ¼″ fat:								
broiled, 5.3 oz., yield from								
9.2-oz. raw steak w/fat	291	43.2	0	11.8	4.5	115	103	0
broiled, 4 oz.	219	32.5	0	8.8	3.4	86	77	0
select grade, trimmed to 0″ fat:								
broiled, 5.4 oz., yield from								
7.9-oz. raw steak w/fat	280	43.5	0	10.5	4.0	116	103	0
broiled, 4 oz.	209	32.5	0	7.8	3.0	86	77	0
BEEF, CORNED:								
(*Eckrich* Slender Sliced), 1 oz.	40	6.0	1.0	1.0	m.q.	m.q.	270	0
(*Healthy Deli*), 1 oz.	35	5.7	.7	1.0	m.q.	11	210	0
(*Healthy Deli* St. Paddy's), 1 oz.	24	3.9	1.1	.4	m.q.	7	290	0
(*Hillshire Farm*), 1 oz.	31	6.0	<1.0	.4	m.q.	m.q.	230	0
(*Oscar Mayer*), .6-oz. slice	17	3.4	.1	.3	.2	8	204	0
brisket, cured:								
raw, 1 oz.	56	4.2	<.1	4.2	1.3	15	345	0
cooked, 11.3 oz., yield from 1 lb.								
raw	802	58.1	1.5	60.7	20.3	314	3628	0
cooked, 4 oz.	285	20.6	.5	21.5	7.2	111	1286	0
loaf, jellied, 1-oz. slice	46	6.7	0	1.9	.8	12	294	0
canned:								
1 oz.	71	7.7	0	4.2	1.8	24	285	0
(*Dinty Moore*), 2 oz.	130	15.0	0	8.0	m.q.	m.q.	m.q.	0
(*Libby's*, 7 oz.), 2.3 oz.	160	17.0	2.0	9.0	m.q.	m.q.	720	0
(*Libby's*, 12 oz.), 2.4 oz.	160	17.0	2.0	9.0	m.q.	m.q.	750	0
BEEF, CORNED, HASH, canned:								
(*Libby's*, 24 oz.), 8 oz.	420	19.0	21.0	28.0	m.q.	m.q.	1330	m.q.
(*Libby's*, 15 oz.), 7½ oz.	400	18.0	20.0	27.0	m.q.	m.q.	1260	m.q.
(*Mary Kitchen*, 25 oz.), 8⅓ oz.	400	22.0	19.0	27.0	m.q.	m.q.	1429	m.q.
(*Mary Kitchen*, 15 oz.), 7½ oz.	360	20.0	19.0	24.0	m.q.	m.q.	1386	m.q.
(*Nalley's*), 8 oz.	420	17.0	27.0	27.0	m.q.	m.q.	940	m.q.
(*Pathmark* No Frills), 7½ oz.	410	16.0	27.0	26.0	m.q.	m.q.	1250	m.q.
BEEF, CORNED, SPREAD:								
canned (*Hormel*), ½ oz.	35	2.0	0	3.0	m.q.	m.q.	m.q.	(0)
BEEF, DRIED:								
cured, 1 oz.	47	8.3	.4	1.1	.5	m.q.	984	0
BEEF, GROUND, see "Beef"								
BEEF, ROAST, see "Beef" and								
"Beef luncheon meat"								
BEEF, ROAST, HASH:								
canned (*Mary Kitchen*), 7½ oz.	350	20.0	18.0	22.0	m.q.	m.q.	1142	m.q.
frozen (*Stouffer's*), 10 oz.	380	30.0	16.0	22.0	m.q.	m.q.	1340	m.q.
BEEF, ROAST, SPREAD, canned:								
(*Hormel*), ½ oz.	31	2.0	0	2.0	m.q.	m.q.	m.q.	0

Food and Measure	cal.	prot. (gms)	carbo. (gms)	tot. fat (gms)	sat. fat (gms)	chol. (mgs)	sod. (mgs)	fiber (gms)
(*Underwood*), 2⅛ oz.	140	9.0	<1.0	11.0	5.0	45	360	n.a.
(*Underwood* Light), 2⅛ oz.	90	9.0	2.0	6.0	2.0	30	210	n.a.
mesquite smoked (*Underwood*), 2⅛ oz.	126	9.0	<1.0	11.0	5.0	45	300	n.a.
BEEF, VARIETY MEATS, see specific listings								
"BEEF," VEGETARIAN:								
canned:								
slices (*Worthington* Savory Slices), 2 slices, approx. 2 oz.	100	8.0	4.0	6.0	m.q.	0	340	m.q.
steak (*Worthington Prime Stakes*), 3.25-oz. piece	160	10.0	7.0	10.0	m.q.	0	410	m.q.
steak (*Worthington Vegetable Steaks*), 2½ pieces, approx. 3.2 oz.	110	17.0	5.0	2.0	m.q.	0	400	m.q.
stew (*Worthington* Country Stew), 9.5 oz.	220	10.0	23.0	10.0	1.0	0	760	m.q.
frozen:								
(*Worthington Stakelets*), 2.5-oz. piece	150	13.0	7.0	8.0	1.0	0	460	m.q.
corned, slices (*Worthington*), 4 slices or 2 oz.	120	9.0	8.0	6.0	1.0	0	740	m.q.
corned, roll (*Worthington*), 2.5 oz.	150	12.0	9.0	7.0	1.0	0	660	m.q.
pie (*Worthington*), 8-oz. pie	360	9.0	44.0	16.0	m.q.	0	1940	m.q.
roll (*Worthington*), 4 slices, 2.5 oz.	130	12.0	7.0	6.0	m.q.	0	750	m.q.
roll, smoked (*Worthington*), 3 slices or 2 oz.	120	10.0	7.0	6.0	m.q.	0	790	m.q.
BEEF CASSEROLE, see "Beef entree, frozen"								
BEEF DINNER, frozen:								
(*Banquet Extra Helping*), 16 oz.	870	34.0	50.0	61.0	m.q.	120	810	m.q.
(*Swanson*), 11.25 oz.	310	26.0	38.0	6.0	m.q.	m.q.	770	m.q.
in barbecue sauce (*Swanson*), 11 oz.	460	30.0	51.0	17.0	m.q.	m.q.	860	m.q.
chopped (*Banquet*), 11 oz.	420	21.0	14.0	32.0	m.q.	80	600	m.q.
chopped steak (*Swanson Hungry Man*), 16.75 oz.	640	35.0	41.0	37.0	m.q.	m.q.	1600	m.q.
enchilada, see "Enchilada dinner"								
meat loaf, see "Meat loaf dinner"								
Mexicana (*The Budget Gourmet*), 12.8 oz.	560	33.0	56.0	23.0	m.q.	50	1290	m.q.
patty, charbroiled (*Freezer Queen*), 10 oz.	300	17.0	20.0	17.0	m.q.	m.q.	1260	m.q.
patty, cheese, sandwich (*Kid Cuisine*), 6.25 oz.	400	12.0	47.0	19.0	m.q.	40	550	m.q.
pepper steak:								
(*Armour Classics Lite*), 11.25 oz.	220	17.0	29.0	4.0	m.q.	35	970	m.q.
(*Healthy Choice*), 11 oz.	290	24.0	35.0	6.0	3.0	65	530	m.q.
(*Le Menu*), 11.5 oz.	370	26.0	36.0	13.0	m.q.	m.q.	1020	m.q.

Food and Measure	cal.	prot. (gms)	carbo. (gms)	tot. fat (gms)	sat. fat (gms)	chol. (mgs)	sod. (mgs)	fiber (gms)
BEEF DINNER, FROZEN *(cont.)*								
pot roast, Yankee:								
(*Armour Classics*), 10 oz.	310	25.0	26.0	12.0	m.q.	85	670	m.q.
(*The Budget Gourmet*), 11 oz. . . .	380	27.0	22.0	21.0	m.q.	70	690	m.q.
(*Healthy Choice*), 11 oz.	260	19.0	36.0	4.0	2.0	45	310	m.q.
(*Le Menu*), 10 oz.	330	26.0	27.0	13.0	m.q.	m.q.	700	m.q.
Salisbury steak:								
(*Armour Classics*), 11.25 oz.	350	22.0	26.0	17.0	m.q.	55	1430	m.q.
(*Armour Classics Lite*), 11.5 oz.	300	21.0	29.0	2.0	m.q.	35	1020	m.q.
(*Banquet*), 11 oz.	500	23.0	26.0	34.0	m.q.	80	600	m.q.
(*Banquet Extra Helping*), 18 oz. . .	910	50.0	49.0	60.0	m.q.	175	740	m.q.
(*Freezer Queen*), 10 oz.	380	18.0	28.0	22.0	m.q.	m.q.	1260	m.q.
(*Healthy Choice*), 11.5 oz.	300	19.0	41.0	7.0	3.0	50	480	m.q.
(*Le Menu*), 10.5 oz.	370	20.0	28.0	20.0	m.q.	m.q.	880	m.q.
(*Le Menu* Lightstyle), 10 oz. . . .	280	18.0	31.0	9.0	m.q.	m.q.	400	m.q.
(*Morton*), 10 oz.	300	12.0	23.0	17.0	m.q.	40	1420	m.q.
(*Swanson*), 10.75 oz.	400	18.0	43.0	17.0	m.q.	m.q.	880	m.q.
(*Swanson Hungry Man*), 16.5 oz.	680	41.0	37.0	41.0	m.q.	m.q.	1730	m.q.
w/gravy and mushrooms (*Stouffer's Dinner Supreme*), 11⅝ oz.	400	25.0	24.0	23.0	m.q.	m.q.	1230	m.q.
w/mushroom gravy (*Banquet Extra Helping*), 18 oz.	890	51.0	48.0	58.0	m.q.	169	685	m.q.
parmigiana (*Armour Classics*), 11.5 oz.	410	22.0	32.0	21.0	m.q.	60	1120	m.q.
sirloin (*The Budget Gourmet*), 11.5 oz.	410	26.0	28.0	22.0	m.q.	105	890	m.q.
short ribs, boneless (*Armour Classics*), 9.75 oz.	380	24.0	34.0	16.0	m.q.	90	790	m.q.
sirloin:								
chopped (*Le Menu*), 12.25 oz. . . .	430	25.0	28.0	24.0	m.q.	m.q.	1010	m.q.
chopped (*Swanson*), 10.75 oz. . . .	340	20.0	28.0	16.0	m.q.	m.q.	790	m.q.
roast (*Armour Classics*) 10.45 oz.	190	19.0	21.0	4.0	m.q.	55	970	m.q.
tips:								
(*Armour Classics*), 10.25 oz. . .	230	22.0	20.0	7.0	m.q.	70	820	m.q.
(*Healthy Choice*), 11.75 oz.	290	25.0	33.0	6.0	3.0	70	350	m.q.
(*Le Menu*), 11.5 oz.	400	30.0	29.0	18.0	m.q.	m.q.	760	m.q.
in Burgundy sauce (*The Budget Gourmet*), 11 oz.	310	24.0	28.0	11.0	m.q.	65	720	m.q.
sliced:								
(*Morton*), 10 oz.	220	24.0	20.0	5.0	m.q.	65	950	m.q.
(*Swanson Hungry Man*), 15.25 oz.	450	37.0	49.0	12.0	m.q.	m.q.	1060	m.q.
gravy and (*Freezer Queen*), 10 oz.	210	18.0	18.0	7.0	m.q.	m.q.	1010	m.q.
steak Diane (*Armour Classics Lite*), 10 oz.	290	27.0	25.0	9.0	m.q.	80	440	m.q.
Stroganoff (*Armour Classics Lite*), 11.25 oz.	250	18.0	33.0	6.0	m.q.	55	510	m.q.
Stroganoff (*Le Menu*), 10 oz.	430	26.0	28.0	24.0	m.q.	m.q.	980	m.q.
Swiss steak (*The Budget Gourmet*), 11.2 oz.	450	23.0	40.0	22.0	m.q.	70	1110	m.q.

Food and Measure	cal.	prot. (gms)	carbo. (gms)	tot. fat (gms)	sat. fat (gms)	chol. (mgs)	sod. (mgs)	fiber (gms)
Swiss steak (*Swanson*), 10 oz.	350	26.0	37.0	11.0	m.q.	m.q.	700	m.q.
tamale, see "Tamale dinner"								
BEEF ENTREE, CANNED:								
chow mein (*La Choy* Bi-Pack),								
¾ cup	70	7.0	8.0	1.0	m.q.	20	840	1.0 d
pepper Oriental (*La Choy* Bi-Pack),								
¾ cup	80	7.0	10.0	2.0	m.q.	18	950	1.0 d
stew:								
(*Dinty Moore*, 40 oz.), 8 oz.	210	13.0	16.0	11.0	m.q.	m.q.	971	m.q.
(*Dinty Moore*, 24 oz.), 8 oz.	220	12.0	15.0	12.0	m.q.	m.q.	980	m.q.
(*Estee*), 7.5 oz.	210	14.0	15.0	11.0	5.0	30	65	m.q.
(*Featherweight*), 7.5 oz.	160	17.0	17.0	3.0	m.q.	35	400	m.q.
(*Hormel/Dinty Moore Micro-Cup*),								
7.5 oz.	190	10.0	17.0	9.0	m.q.	50	860	m.q.
(*Libby's*, 24 oz.), 8 oz.	170	12.0	19.0	6.0	m.q.	m.q.	930	m.q.
(*Libby's*, 15 oz.), 7.5 oz.	160	12.0	18.0	5.0	m.q.	m.q.	870	m.q.
(*Nalley's* Big Chunk), 7.5 oz.	200	10.0	24.0	7.0	m.q.	m.q.	790	m.q.
(*Nalley's* Homestyle), 8 oz.	180	11.0	22.0	5.0	m.q.	m.q.	810	m.q.
(*Pathmark* No Frills), 8 oz.	190	10.0	25.0	4.0	m.q.	m.q.	625	m.q.
(*Wolf* Brand), scant cup, 7.75 oz.	179	9.6	18.3	7.5	m.q.	m.q.	1043	.6 c
BEEF ENTREE, FREEZE-								
DRIED, 1 cup[1]:								
and rice, w/onions (*Mountain House*)	330	11.0	42.0	12.0	m.q.	m.q.	265	m.q.
stew (*Mountain House*)	260	16.0	26.0	9.0	m.q.	m.q.	75	m.q.
Stroganoff (*Mountain House*)	270	10.0	26.0	13.0	m.q.	m.q.	118	n.a.
BEEF ENTREE, FROZEN:								
(*Banquet* Platters), 10 oz.	460	22.0	20.0	34.0	m.q.	75	630	m.q.
and broccoli, w/rice (*La Choy Fresh*								
& Lite), 11 oz.	260	17.0	42.0	5.0	m.q.	51	1299	5.2 d
burrito, see "Burrito entree"								
casserole (*Pillsbury Microwave*								
Classic), 1 pkg.	430	16.0	34.0	25.0	m.q.	m.q.	1100	m.q.
champignon (*Tyson Gourmet*								
Selection), 10.5 oz.	370	27.0	31.0	15.0	m.q.	m.q.	830	m.q.
cheeseburger (*MicroMagic*),								
4.75 oz.	450	17.0	29.0	25.0	m.q.	80	790	m.q.
chop suey, w/rice (*Stouffer's*), 12 oz.	300	16.0	38.0	9.0	m.q.	m.q.	1170	m.q.
creamed, chipped:								
(*Banquet Cookin' Bags*), 4 oz. ...	100	7.0	9.0	4.0	m.q.	m.q.	m.q.	n.a.
(*Freezer Queen Cook-In-Pouch*),								
5 oz.	80	5.0	11.0	2.0	m.q.	m.q.	500	m.q.
(*Myers*), 3.5 oz.	136	9.0	7.0	8.0	m.q.	m.q.	863	n.a.
(*Stouffer's*), 5.5 oz.	230	12.0	9.0	16.0	m.q.	m.q.	850	n.a.
Dijon, w/pasta and vegetables (*Right*								
Course), 9.5 oz.	290	20.0	31.0	9.0	2.0	40	580	m.q.
enchilada, see "Enchilada entree"								
fiesta, w/corn pasta (*Right Course*),								
8⅞ oz.	270	18.0	33.0	7.0	2.0	30	590	m.q.
hamburger (*MicroMagic*), 4 oz.	350	13.0	26.0	18.0	m.q.	55	500	m.q.

1. *Prepared according to package directions.*

Food and Measure	cal.	prot. (gms)	carbo. (gms)	tot. fat (gms)	sat. fat (gms)	chol. (mgs)	sod. (mgs)	fiber (gms)
BEEF ENTREE, FROZEN *(cont.)*								
London broil, in mushroom sauce								
(*Weight Watchers*), 7.37 oz.	140	18.0	9.0	3.0	1.0	40	510	n.a.
meat loaf, see "Meat loaf entree"								
Oriental (*The Budget Gourmet* Slim								
Selects), 10 oz.	290	17.0	36.0	9.0	m.q.	25	690	m.q.
Oriental, w/vegetables and rice								
(*Lean Cuisine*), 8⅝ oz.	250	18.0	28.0	7.0	2.0	45	900	m.q.
patty:								
charbroiled, mushroom gravy and:								
(*Banquet Cookin' Bags*), 5 oz.	210	9.0	8.0	15.0	m.q.	m.q.	m.q.	n.a.
(*Banquet Family Entrees*), 8 oz.	290	13.0	13.0	21.0	m.q.	m.q.	m.q.	n.a.
(*Freezer Queen Cook-In-Pouch*),								
5 oz.	90	10.0	7.0	3.0	m.q.	m.q.	900	n.a.
(*Freezer Queen Family Suppers*),								
7 oz.	180	12.0	9.0	11.0	m.q.	m.q.	1050	n.a.
onion gravy and (*Banquet Family*								
Entrees), 8 oz.	300	12.0	14.0	21.0	m.q.	m.q.	m.q.	n.a.
onion gravy and (*Freezer Queen*								
Family Suppers), 7 oz.	200	13.0	10.0	12.0	m.q.	m.q.	960	n.a.
and peppers in sauce, w/rice (*Freezer*								
Queen Single Serve), 9 oz.	260	21.0	38.0	3.0	m.q.	m.q.	810	m.q.
pepper Oriental (*Chun King*), 13 oz.	310	17.0	53.0	3.0	m.q.	m.q.	1300	m.q.
pepper steak:								
(*Dining Lite*), 9 oz.	260	18.0	33.0	6.0	m.q.	40	1050	m.q.
(*Healthy Choice*), 9.5 oz.	250	18.0	36.0	4.0	2.0	40	340	m.q.
(*Tyson Gourmet Selection*),								
11.25 oz.	330	20.0	38.0	11.0	m.q.	m.q.	1130	m.q.
green, w/rice (*Stouffer's*), 10.5 oz.	330	21.0	36.0	11.0	m.q.	m.q.	1440	m.q.
w/rice (*The Budget Gourmet*),								
10 oz.	300	15.0	39.0	9.0	m.q.	25	800	m.q.
w/rice and vegetables (*La Choy*								
Fresh & Lite), 10 oz.	280	21.0	33.0	8.0	m.q.	36	1082	2.0 d
pie:								
(*Banquet*), 7 oz.	510	12.0	39.0	33.0	m.q.	25	870	m.q.
(*Banquet* Supreme Microwave),								
7 oz.	440	14.0	30.0	29.0	m.q.	35	730	m.q.
(*Morton*), 7 oz.	430	11.0	27.0	31.0	m.q.	30	740	m.q.
(*Myers*), 3.5 oz.	123	7.0	10.0	6.0	m.q.	m.q.	343	m.q.
(*Stouffer's*), 10 oz.	500	20.0	33.0	32.0	m.q.	m.q.	1300	m.q.
(*Swanson* Pot Pie), 7 oz.	370	12.0	36.0	19.0	m.q.	m.q.	730	m.q.
(*Swanson Hungry Man* Pot Pie),								
16 oz.	610	24.0	58.0	31.0	m.q.	m.q.	1360	m.q.
pot roast, homestyle (*Right Course*),								
9.25 oz.	220	17.0	22.0	7.0	2.0	35	550	m.q.
ragout, w/rice pilaf (*Right Course*),								
10 oz.	300	19.0	38.0	8.0	2.0	50	550	m.q.
Salisbury steak:								
(*Dining Lite*), 9 oz.	200	18.0	14.0	8.0	m.q.	55	1000	n.a.

Food and Measure	cal.	prot. (gms)	carbo. (gms)	tot. fat (gms)	sat. fat (gms)	chol. (mgs)	sod. (mgs)	fiber (gms)
(*Swanson* Homestyle Recipe),								
10 oz.	320	21.0	22.0	16.0	m.q.	m.q.	980	m.q.
charbroiled, w/vegetable medley								
(*Freezer Queen* Single Serve),								
9 oz.	330	22.0	14.0	22.0	m.q.	m.q.	990	m.q.
gravy and:								
(*Banquet Cookin' Bags*), 5 oz.	190	9.0	8.0	14.0	m.q.	m.q.	m.q.	n.a.
(*Banquet Family Entrees*), 8 oz.	300	13.0	12.0	22.0	m.q.	m.q.	m.q.	n.a.
(*Freezer Queen Cook-In-Pouch*),								
5 oz.	160	9.0	7.0	11.0	m.q.	m.q.	850	n.a.
(*Freezer Queen Family Suppers*),								
7 oz.	200	13.0	9.0	13.0	m.q.	m.q.	1110	n.a.
in gravy (*Stouffer's*), 9⅞ oz.	250	21.0	9.0	14.0	m.q.	m.q.	1070	n.a.
w/Italian style sauce and								
vegetables (*Lean Cuisine*),								
9.5 oz.	280	25.0	12.0	15.0	5.0	100	840	m.q.
Romana (*Weight Watchers*),								
8.75 oz.	190	20.0	13.0	7.0	2.0	40	470	m.q.
sirloin (*The Budget Gourmet* Slim								
Selects), 9 oz.	280	21.0	31.0	8.0	m.q.	75	870	m.q.
supreme (*Tyson Gourmet*								
Selection), 10 oz.	430	16.0	34.0	26.0	m.q.	m.q.	810	m.q.
short ribs (*Tyson Gourmet Selection*),								
11 oz.	470	25.0	38.0	24.0	m.q.	m.q.	950	m.q.
short ribs, in gravy (*Stouffer's*), 9 oz.	350	30.0	12.0	20.0	m.q.	m.q.	900	n.a.
sirloin:								
in herb sauce (*The Budget*								
Gourmet Slim Selects), 10 oz.	290	19.0	27.0	12.0	m.q.	25	770	m.q.
roast (*The Budget Gourmet*),								
9.5 oz.	330	13.0	36.0	14.0	m.q.	85	700	m.q.
tips:								
in Burgundy sauce (*Swanson*								
Homestyle Recipe), 7 oz. . . .	160	12.0	16.0	5.0	m.q.	m.q.	550	m.q.
w/country style vegetables (*The*								
Budget Gourmet), 10 oz.	310	16.0	21.0	18.0	m.q.	40	570	m.q.
and mushrooms, in wine sauce								
(*Weight Watchers*), 7.5 oz. . . .	220	20.0	19.0	7.0	3.0	50	540	m.q.
sliced:								
barbecue sauce and (*Banquet*								
Cookin' Bags), 4 oz.	100	9.0	11.0	2.0	m.q.	m.q.	m.q.	n.a.
gravy and:								
(*Banquet Cookin' Bags*), 4 oz.	100	8.0	5.0	5.0	m.q.	m.q.	m.q.	n.a.
(*Banquet Family Entrees*), 8 oz.	160	20.0	8.0	5.0	m.q.	m.q.	m.q.	m.q.
(*Freezer Queen Cook-In-Pouch*),								
4 oz.	60	9.0	4.0	1.0	m.q.	m.q.	500	n.a.
(*Freezer Queen Deluxe Family*								
Suppers), 7 oz.	130	15.0	10.0	3.0	m.q.	m.q.	870	n.a.
steak, breaded (*Hormel*), 4 oz.	370	14.0	13.0	30.0	m.q.	m.q.	m.q.	m.q.

Food and Measure	cal.	prot. (gms)	carbo. (gms)	tot. fat (gms)	sat. fat (gms)	chol. (mgs)	sod. (mgs)	fiber (gms)
BEEF ENTREE, FROZEN *(cont.)*								
steak, Ranchero (*Lean Cuisine*),								
9.25 oz.	270	16.0	30.0	9.0	3.0	40	950	m.q.
stew (*Banquet Family Entrees*), 7 oz.	140	6.0	18.0	5.0	m.q.	m.q.	m.q.	m.q.
stew (*Freezer Queen Family Suppers*),								
7 oz.	150	9.0	15.0	6.0	m.q.	m.q.	820	m.q.
Stroganoff:								
(*The Budget Gourmet* Slim								
Selects), 8.75 oz.	280	18.0	29.0	10.0	m.q.	60	560	m.q.
(*Myers*), 3.5 oz.	112	8.0	7.0	6.0	m.q.	m.q.	346	n.a.
(*Weight Watchers*), 8.5 oz.	290	22.0	26.0	9.0	4.0	25	600	m.q.
w/parsley noodles (*Stouffer's*),								
9.75 oz.	390	24.0	28.0	20.0	m.q.	m.q.	1090	m.q.
sauce with, and noodles (*Banquet*								
Family Entrees), 7 oz.	190	17.0	18.0	6.0	m.q.	m.q.	m.q.	m.q.
Szechuan (*Chun King*), 13 oz.	340	20.0	57.0	3.0	m.q.	m.q.	1810	m.q.
Szechwan, w/noodles and vegetables								
(*Lean Cuisine*), 9.25 oz.	260	20.0	22.0	10.0	3.0	100	680	m.q.
teriyaki:								
(*Chun King*), 13 oz.	380	22.0	68.0	2.0	m.q.	m.q.	2200	m.q.
(*Dining Lite*), 9 oz.	270	20.0	36.0	5.0	m.q.	45	850	m.q.
w/rice and vegetables (*La Choy*								
Fresh & Lite), 10 oz.	240	17.0	39.9	5.0	m.q.	57	1198	2.0 d
in sauce, w/rice and vegetables								
(*Stouffer's*), 9.75 oz.	290	22.0	33.0	8.0	m.q.	m.q.	1450	m.q.
tortellini, see "Tortellini dishes"								
BEEF ENTREE, PACKAGED,								
1 serving:								
pepper steak, Oriental (*Hormel Top*								
Shelf)	290	25.0	25.0	10.0	m.q.	45	1700	m.q.
ribs, boneless (*Hormel Top Shelf*) ...	440	28.0	29.0	24.0	m.q.	90	550	m.q.
roast, tender (*Hormel Top Shelf*)	240	27.0	18.0	7.0	m.q.	65	980	m.q.
Salisbury steak, w/potatoes (*Hormel*								
Top Shelf)	254	29.0	22.0	6.0	m.q.	88	1211	m.q.
Stroganoff (*Hormel Top Shelf*)	320	29.0	24.0	12.0	m.q.	48	1250	m.q.
sukiyaki (*Hormel Top Shelf*)	330	24.0	36.0	10.0	m.q.	45	1700	m.q.
BEEF ENTREE MIX:								
meat loaf, see "Meat loaf entree								
mix"								
stew, hearty (*Lipton Microeasy*),								
¼ pkg. dry	70	2.0	14.0	<1.0	n.a.	n.a.	730	m.q.
stew, hearty (*Lipton Microeasy*),								
¼ pkg.[1]	370	31.0	14.0	20.0	m.q.	m.q.	800	m.q.
BEEF GRAVY, canned:								
1 oz.	15	1.1	1.4	.7	.3	1	159	0
¼ cup	31	2.2	2.8	1.4	.7	2	326	0
(*Franco-American*), 2 oz.	25	0	4.0	1.0	m.q.	m.q.	340	n.a.

1. *Prepared according to package directions with 1½ lbs. beef stew meat.*

Food and Measure	cal.	prot. (gms)	carbo. (gms)	tot. fat (gms)	sat. fat (gms)	chol. (mgs)	sod. (mgs)	fiber (gms)
w/chunky beef (*Hormel Great Beginnings*), 5 oz.	136	12.0	7.0	7.0	m.q.	m.q.	904	n.a.
BEEF JERKY (see also "Sausage sticks"):								
(*Frito-Lay's*), .21 oz.	25	3.0	1.0	1.0	m.q.	10	200	0
(*Frito-Lay's* Tender), .7 oz.	120	5.0	2.0	10.0	m.q.	25	370	0
(*Hickory Farms*), 1 oz.	100	16.0	4.0	3.0	m.q.	73	1360	0
(*Hormel* Lumberjack), 1 oz.	101	5.0	0	9.0	m.q.	m.q.	304	0
(*Pemmican Arrowhead*), 1 piece, approx. .7 oz.	70	8.0	2.0	3.0	m.q.	m.q.	580	0
(*Pemmican Steakers*), 1 pouch, approx. 1.1 oz.	80	14.0	4.0	1.0	m.q.	m.q.	470	0
(*Pemmican Steakers*), 1 strip, approx. .37 oz.	40	5.0	2.0	1.0	m.q.	m.q.	160	0
(*Pemmican Tender Brave/Chief/Trail/ Tribe* Packs), 1 oz.	80	14.0	2.0	2.0	m.q.	m.q.	830	0
(*Pemmican Tender Tomahawk*), 1 piece, approx. .25 oz.	20	3.0	1.0	1.0	m.q.	m.q.	210	0
(*Slim Jim*), 1 piece, approx. .14 oz.	20	2.0	1.0	1.0	m.q.	m.q.	120	0
(*Slim Jim Big Jerk*), 1 piece, approx. .25 oz.	25	3.0	1.0	1.0	m.q.	m.q.	220	0
(*Slim Jim Giant Jerk*), 1 piece, approx. .63 oz.	60	7.0	2.0	2.0	m.q.	m.q.	510	0
natural, peppered, jalapeño, or *Tabasco*:								
(*Pemmican*), 1.1 oz.	90	13.0	4.0	2.0	m.q.	m.q.	960	0
(*Pemmican*), 1⁵⁄₁₆ oz. slab	110	16.0	5.0	3.0	m.q.	m.q.	1150	0
(*Pemmican*), ¼ oz. steak	25	3.0	1.0	1.0	m.q.	m.q.	220	0
natural style (*Pemmican*), 1 oz.	80	12.0	4.0	2.0	m.q.	m.q.	880	0
regular or *Tabasco* (*Slim Jim Super Jerk*), 1 piece, approx. .31 oz.	30	4.0	1.0	1.0	m.q.	m.q.	250	0
teriyaki, natural style:								
(*Pemmican*), 1 oz.	80	12.0	4.0	2.0	m.q.	m.q.	800	0
(*Pemmican*), 1⁵⁄₁₆ oz. slab	100	15.0	5.0	2.0	m.q.	m.q.	1030	0
(*Pemmican*), ¼ oz. steak	20	3.0	1.0	1.0	m.q.	m.q.	200	0
BEEF LUNCHEON MEAT:								
(*Eckrich* Slender Sliced), 1 oz.	35	6.0	1.0	1.0	m.q.	m.q.	270	0
corned, see "Beef, corned"								
loaf, 1 oz. slice, 4″ × 4″ × ³⁄₃₂″	87	4.1	.8	7.4	3.2	18	377	0
loaf, jellied (*Hormel* Perma-Fresh), 2 slices	90	14.0	0	4.0	m.q.	m.q.	900	0
roast:								
(*Healthy Deli*), 1 oz.	30	6.4	.2	.4	m.q.	13	130	0
(*Oscar Mayer* Thin Sliced), .4-oz. slice	14	2.4	.2	.4	.2	5	55	0
Italian (*Healthy Deli*), 1 oz.	31	6.2	.1	.6	m.q.	16	140	0
oven-roasted, cured (*Hillshire Farm* Deli Select), 1 oz.	31	6.0	<1.0	.5	m.q.	m.q.	270	0

Food and Measure	cal.	prot. (gms)	carbo. (gms)	tot. fat (gms)	sat. fat (gms)	chol. (mgs)	sod. (mgs)	fiber (gms)
BEEF LUNCHEON MEAT, ROAST *(cont.)*								
top round, oven-roasted (*Boar's*								
Head), 1 oz.	40	7.0	<1.0	1.0	m.q.	20	30	0
top round, oven-roasted (*Boar's*								
Head Deluxe), 1 oz.	45	7.0	<1.0	2.0	m.q.	20	40	0
sandwich steak (*Steak-Umm*), 2 oz.	180	9.0	0	16.0	m.q.	m.q.	50	0
sliced:								
1 oz.	35	6.2	.1	.9	.4	12	470	0
thin, 5 slices, approx. .75 oz.	26	4.6	.1	.7	.3	9	348	0
smoked:								
(*Hillshire Farm* Deli Select), 1 oz.	31	6.0	<1.0	.5	m.q.	m.q.	270	0
(*Oscar Mayer*), .5-oz. slice	14	2.7	.1	.3	.1	7	173	0
cured (*Hormel*), 1 oz.	50	5.0	0	2.0	m.q.	m.q.	315	0
cured, dried (*Hormel*), 1 oz.	45	8.0	0	1.0	m.q.	m.q.	822	0
BEEF MARINADE SEASONING MIX:								
(*Lawry's*), 1 pkg.	49	1.2	10.7	.2	n.a.	0	7284	<.1 c
BEEF PIE, see "Beef entree, frozen"								
BEEF POCKET SANDWICH, frozen:								
and broccoli (*Lean Pockets*), 1 pkg.	250	11.0	30.0	8.0	m.q.	m.q.	760	m.q.
'n cheddar (*Hot Pockets*), 5 oz.	370	17.0	36.0	17.0	m.q.	60	1390	m.q.
BEEF ROLL OR STICK, see "Beef jerky" and "Sausage sticks"								
BEEF SANDWICH, see "Beef pocket sandwich"								
BEEF SAUCE, see "Beef gravy"								
BEEF SEASONING MIX, dry:								
ground, w/onions (*French's*), ¼ pkg.	25	1.0	6.0	0	0	0	440	n.a.
BEEF STEW, see "Beef entree"								
BEEF STEW SEASONING MIX:								
(*French's*), ⅙ pkg.	25	0	5.0	0	0	0	770	n.a.
(*Lawry's*), 1 pkg.	131	5.4	25.7	.7	n.a.	0	3181	1.2 c
(*McCormick/Schilling*), ¼ pkg.	33	1.3	6.0	.3	n.a.	n.a.	806	n.a.
BEEF STROGANOFF SEASONING MIX:								
(*McCormick/Schilling*), ¼ pkg.	32	1.0	6.0	.3	n.a.	n.a.	1078	n.a.
BEEF SUET, see "Suet"								
BEEF TALLOW:								
1 oz.	256	0	0	28.4	14.1	31	0	0
½ cup	925	0	0	102.5	51.0	112	0	0
1 tbsp.	115	0	0	12.8	6.4	14	0	0
BEEFALO, composite cuts, meat only:								
raw, 1 oz.	41	6.6	0	1.4	.6	13	22	0
roasted[1]:								

1. *Without added ingredients.*

Food and Measure	cal.	prot. (gms)	carbo. (gms)	tot. fat (gms)	sat. fat (gms)	chol. (mgs)	sod. (mgs)	fiber (gms)
12 oz., yield from 1 lb. boneless	639	104.3	0	21.5	9.1	197	279	0
4 oz.	213	34.8	0	7.2	3.0	66	93	0
diced, 1 cup, approx. 4.9 oz.	263	42.9	0	8.8	3.8	81	115	0
BEER, ALE, AND MALT LIQUOR, 12 fl. oz.:								
(*Anheuser Marzen*)	168	2.3	15.2	0	0	0	12	0
(*Beck's*)	148	1.7	10.0	0	0	0	14	0
(*Bud Light*)	110	1.1	6.9	0	0	0	12	0
(*Budweiser*)	144	1.2	11.3	0	0	0	12	0
(*Busch*)	144	1.2	11.9	0	0	0	12	0
(*Carlsberg*)	149	1.2	11.9	0	0	0	12	0
(*Carlsberg* Light)	110	1.1	6.5	0	0	0	12	0
(*Coqui* Malt Liquor)	208	1.7	9.8	0	0	0	13	0
(*Dribeck's*)	94	1.0	7.0	0	0	0	14	0
(*Elephant* Imported Malt Liquor) ...	208	1.6	16.9	0	0	0	12	0
(*King Cobra* Malt Liquor)	182	1.4	15.2	0	0	0	12	0
(*Knickerbocker*)	140	.9	12.3	0	0	0	9	0
(*LA*)	114	.8	16.4	0	0	0	12	0
(*Lite*)	96	.8	2.8	0	0	0	6	0
(*Lite* Genuine Draft)	98	.8	3.5	0	0	0	6	0
(*Lowenbräu* Dark Special)	158	1.4	14.3	0	0	0	7	0
(*Lowenbräu* Special)	158	1.4	14.3	0	0	0	7	0
(*McSorley's* Ale)	166	1.7	14.7	0	0	0	6	0
(*Meister Brau*)	141	1.0	12.8	0	0	0	6	0
(*Meister Brau* Light)	98	.8	3.5	0	0	0	6	0
(*Michelob*)	156	1.5	13.6	0	0	0	12	0
(*Michelob* Classic Dark)	158	1.5	14.4	0	0	0	12	0
(*Michelob* Dry)	133	1.3	7.8	0	0	0	12	0
(*Michelob* Light)	134	1.2	11.9	0	0	0	12	0
(*Miller* Genuine Draft)	147	1.0	13.1	0	0	0	7	0
(*Miller High Life*)	147	1.0	13.1	0	0	0	7	0
(*Miller Magnum*)	162	1.3	10.2	0	0	0	8	0
(*Milwaukee's Best*)	133	.9	11.4	0	0	0	6	0
(*Milwaukee's Best* Light)	98	.8	3.5	0	0	0	6	0
(*Natural* Light)	110	1.1	6.6	0	0	0	12	0
(*Ortlieb's*)	140	.9	12.3	0	0	0	9	0
(*Prior* Double Dark)	171	1.4	15.4	0	0	0	10	0
(*Rheingold*)	148	1.0	12.9	0	0	0	9	0
(*Rheingold* Light)	96	.7	2.8	0	0	0	7	0
(*Rolling Rock* Light)	104	.4	8.0	0	0	0	<1	0
(*Rolling Rock* Premium)	145	.4	10.0	0	0	0	<1	0
(*Schmidt's*)	148	1.0	12.9	0	0	0	9	0
(*Schmidt's* Classic)	144	1.0	12.8	0	0	0	10	0
(*Schmidt's* Light)	96	.7	2.8	0	0	0	7	0
(*Sharp's*)	86	1.0	9.5	0	0	0	5	0
(*Tiger Head* Ale)	166	1.7	14.7	0	0	0	6	0
BEER BATTER MIX:								
(*Golden Dipt*), 1 oz.	100	2.0	22.0	0	0	0	650	n.a.

Food and Measure	cal.	prot. (gms)	carbo. (gms)	tot. fat (gms)	sat. fat (gms)	chol. (mgs)	sod. (mgs)	fiber (gms)
BEERWURST (see also "Salami, beer"):								
beef:								
1 oz.	92	3.5	.5	8.3	3.4	16	264	0
1 slice, 4" diam. × ⅛", approx.								
.8 oz.	75	2.8	.4	6.8	2.8	13	214	0
1 slice, 2¾" diam. × ¹⁄₁₆", approx.								
.2 oz.	19	.7	.1	1.8	.7	3	56	0
pork:								
1 oz.	67	4.0	.6	5.3	1.8	17	352	0
1 slice, 4" diam. × ⅛", approx.								
.8 oz.	55	3.3	.5	4.3	1.4	13	285	0
1 slice, 2¾" diam. × ¹⁄₁₆", approx.								
.2 oz.	14	.9	.1	1.1	.4	4	74	0
BEET:								
raw:								
untrimmed, 1 lb.	133	4.5	30.4	.4	.1	0	220	3.0 d
trimmed, 1 oz.	12	.4	2.8	<.1	tr.	0	20	.3 d
2 medium, 2" diam., approx.								
8.6 oz.	71	2.4	16.3	.2	<.1	0	118	1.6 d
sliced, ½ cup	30	1.0	6.8	.1	<.1	0	49	.7 d
boiled, drained:								
4 oz.	35	1.2	7.6	.1	tr.	0	56	1.0 c
2 medium, 2" diam., approx.								
3.5 oz.	31	1.1	6.7	.1	tr.	0	49	.9 c
sliced, ½ cup	26	.9	5.7	<.1	tr.	0	42	.7 c
BEET, CANNED, ½ cup, except as noted:								
w/liquid:								
4 oz.	33	.9	7.7	.1	<.1	0	298	1.2 d
½ cup	36	1.0	8.3	.1	<.1	0	324	1.4 d
low-sodium, 4 oz.	33	.9	7.7	.1	<.1	0	52	1.2 d
low-sodium	36	1.0	8.3	.1	<.1	0	57	1.4 d
drained, 4 oz.	35	1.0	8.2	.2	<.1	0	m.q.	1.9 d
drained, sliced	27	.8	6.1	.1	<.1	0	m.q.	1.4 d
(*Stokely* No Salt or Sugar Added) ...	40	1.0	8.0	0	0	0	40	m.q.
whole:								
(*IGA*)	40	1.0	9.0	0	0	0	275	m.q.
or sliced (*A&P*)	40	1.0	9.0	<1.0	(0)	0	300	m.q.
sliced or cut (*Stokely*)	40	1.0	8.0	0	0	0	300	m.q.
small (*S&W*)	40	1.0	9.0	0	0	0	270	m.q.
tiny or sliced, w/liquid (*Del Monte*)	35	1.0	8.0	0	0	0	290	m.q.
sliced:								
(*A&P* No Salt Added)	35	1.0	8.0	<1.0	(0)	0	50	m.q.
(*Featherweight*)	45	1.0	10.0	0	0	0	55	m.q.
(*Finast*)	40	1.0	9.0	0	0	0	390	m.q.
(*Finast* No Salt Added)	40	1.0	9.0	0	0	0	40	m.q.
(*Pathmark*)	45	1.0	10.0	0	0	0	330	m.q.
(*Pathmark* No Salt Added)	35	1.0	7.0	0	0	0	35	m.q.

Food and Measure	cal.	prot. (gms)	carbo. (gms)	tot. fat (gms)	sat. fat (gms)	chol. (mgs)	sod. (mgs)	fiber (gms)
(*S&W/Nutradiet*)	35	1.0	9.0	0	0	0	40	m.q.
w/liquid (*Del Monte* No Salt Added)	35	1.0	8.0	0	0	0	100	m.q.
small, tender (*S&W* Premium) ...	40	1.0	9.0	0	0	0	270	m.q.
diced or julienne (*S&W*)	40	1.0	9.0	0	0	0	270	m.q.
diced (*Stokely*)	35	1.0	7.0	0	0	0	300	m.q.
Harvard:								
w/liquid, 4 oz.	83	1.0	20.6	.1	<.1	0	184	m.q.
w/liquid, sliced	89	1.0	22.4	.1	<.1	0	199	m.q.
(*Stokely*)	70	1.0	18.0	0	0	0	135	m.q.
pickled:								
w/liquid, 4 oz. or ½ cup	74	.9	18.5	.1	<.1	0	299	.7 c
(*Stokely*)	100	1.0	25.0	0	0	0	400	m.q.
(*Stokely* Jars)	90	1.0	22.0	0	0	0	280	m.q.
whole, extra small (*S&W*)	70	1.0	16.0	0	0	0	215	m.q.
crinkle sliced, w/liquid (*Del Monte*)	80	1.0	19.0	0	0	0	375	m.q.
w/red wine vinegar, sliced (*S&W*								
Regular or Party)	70	1.0	16.0	0	0	0	215	m.q.
BEET GREENS:								
raw:								
untrimmed, 1 lb.	49	4.6	10.1	.2	<.1	0	510	3.3 c
trimmed, 1 oz.	5	.5	1.1	<.1	tr.	0	57	.4 c
1 leaf, approx. 2 oz.	6	.6	1.3	<.1	tr.	0	64	.4 c
1″ pieces, ½ cup	4	.4	.8	<.1	tr.	0	38	.3 c
boiled, drained, 4 oz.	31	2.9	6.2	.2	<.1	0	273	1.2 c
boiled, drained, 1″ pieces, ½ cup ...	20	1.9	3.9	.1	<.1	0	173	.8 c
BEET ROOT JUICE, bottled:								
(*Biotta*), 6 fl. oz.	75	1.8	15.9	.1	(0)	0	128	m.q.
BELLY, PORK, see "Pork belly"								
BERLINER, beef and pork:								
1 oz.	65	4.3	.7	4.9	1.7	13	368	0
1 slice, 2½″ diam. × ¼″, approx.								
.8 oz.	53	3.5	.6	4.0	1.4	11	298	0
BERRY DRINK (see also "Punch"):								
(*Hawaiian Punch* Very Berry),								
6 fl. oz.	90	0	22.0	0	0	0	30	(0)
wild (*Hi-C*), 8.45 fl. oz. box	129	.1	31.7	.1	(0)	0	24	(0)
wild (*Hi-C*), 6 fl. oz.	92	.1	22.5	.1	(0)	0	17	(0)
mix[1], 8 fl. oz.:								
(*Kool-Aid* Berry Blue								
Presweetened)	80	0	21.0	0	0	0	5	0
(*Kool-Aid* Berry Blue Sugar Free)	4	0	0	0	0	0	5	0
(*Kool-Aid* Sharkleberry Fin/Berry								
Blue)	100	0	25.0	0	0	0	0	0
(*Kool-Aid* Sharkleberry Fin								
Presweetened)	80	0	21.0	0	0	0	0	0
(*Kool-Aid* Sharkleberry Fin Sugar								
Free)	4	0	0	0	0	0	0	0

1. *Prepared according to package directions.*

Food and Measure	cal.	prot. (gms)	carbo. (gms)	tot. fat (gms)	sat. fat (gms)	chol. (mgs)	sod. (mgs)	fiber (gms)
BERRY DRINK, MIX *(cont.)*								
blend (*Crystal Light* Sugar Free)	4	0	0	0	0	0	0	0
BERRY JUICE, canned (see also specific listings):								
(*Libby's Juicy Juice*), 6 fl. oz.	90	0	22.0	0	0	0	10	m.q.
BERRY JUICE DRINK:								
(*Tropicana* Berries & Berries),								
10 fl. oz.	156	(0)	39.0	0	0	0	<3	(0)
wild (*Tropicana* Juice Sparkler),								
8 fl. oz.	110	(0)	27.0	0	0	0	15	(0)
BISCUIT, 1 piece, except as noted:								
(*Wonder*)	80	2.0	14.0	1.0	n.a.	n.a.	140	.6 d
country (*Awrey's 3"*), 2 oz.	160	4.0	23.0	5.0	1.0	0	530	1.0 d
round or square (*Awrey's 2"*), 1 oz.	80	2.0	12.0	3.0	1.0	0	260	0
sliced or unsliced (*Awrey's*), 2 oz. . .	160	4.0	23.0	5.0	1.0	0	520	1.0 d
square (*Awrey's 3"*), 2 oz.	160	4.0	23.0	5.0	1.0	0	520	1.0 d
BISCUIT, FROZEN:								
(*Bridgford*), 2 oz.	180	4.0	28.0	6.0	m.q.	1	632	m.q.
BISCUIT, REFRIGERATED,								
1 piece, except as noted:								
(*Ballard Ovenready*)	50	1.0	10.0	1.0	0	0	180	m.q.
(*Big Country Butter Tastin'*)	100	2.0	14.0	4.0	<1.0	0	320	m.q.
(*1869 Brand Butter Tastin'*)	100	2.0	12.0	5.0	1.0	0	300	m.q.
(*Pillsbury* Big Premium Heat 'n Eat),								
2 pieces	280	5.0	32.0	15.0	3.0	0	610	m.q.
(*Pillsbury* Country)	50	1.0	10.0	1.0	0	0	180	m.q.
(*Roman Meal*), 2 pieces	180	4.2	32.2	3.8	.9	0	456	1.4 d
baking powder (*1869 Brand*)	100	2.0	12.0	5.0	1.0	0	310	m.q.
butter (*Pillsbury*)	50	1.0	10.0	1.0	0	0	180	m.q.
buttermilk:								
(*Ballard Ovenready*)	50	1.0	10.0	1.0	n.a.	n.a.	180	m.q.
(*Big Country*)	100	2.0	14.0	4.0	<1.0	0	320	m.q.
(*1869 Brand*)	100	2.0	12.0	5.0	1.0	0	310	m.q.
(*Hungry Jack* Extra Rich)	50	1.0	9.0	1.0	<1.0	0	180	m.q.
(*Pillsbury*)	50	1.0	10.0	1.0	1.0	0	180	m.q.
(*Pillsbury* Heat 'n Eat), 2 pieces	170	4.0	27.0	5.0	1.0	0	530	m.q.
(*Pillsbury* Tender Layer)	50	1.0	9.0	1.0	0	0	170	m.q.
flaky (*Hungry Jack*)	90	2.0	12.0	4.0	<1.0	0	300	m.q.
fluffy (*Hungry Jack*)	90	2.0	12.0	4.0	1.0	0	280	m.q.
flaky:								
(*Hungry Jack*)	80	2.0	12.0	4.0	<1.0	0	300	m.q.
(*Hungry Jack Butter Tastin'*)	90	2.0	11.0	4.0	<1.0	0	280	m.q.
honey (*Hungry Jack Honey Tastin'*)	90	2.0	13.0	4.0	<1.0	0	290	m.q.
fluffy (*Pillsbury* Good 'n Buttery) . . .	90	1.0	11.0	5.0	1.0	0	270	m.q.
oat bran, honey nut (*Roman Meal*) . .	131	2.4	19.7	4.7	1.2	0	278	.9 d
Southern style (*Big Country*)	100	2.0	14.0	4.0	<1.0	0	320	m.q.
white (*Roman Meal* Premium)	127	2.4	18.8	4.7	1.2	0	308	m.q.
BISCUIT MIX:								
(*Arrowhead Mills*), 2 oz.	100	4.0	19.0	1.0	n.a.	0	96	m.q.

Food and Measure	cal.	prot. (gms)	carbo. (gms)	tot. fat (gms)	sat. fat (gms)	chol. (mgs)	sod. (mgs)	fiber (gms)
(*Bisquick*), ½ cup	240	4.0	37.0	8.0	2.0	0	700	m.q.
(*Martha White BixMix*), 1 piece[1] ...	100	2.0	15.0	3.0	m.q.	1	240	m.q.
(*Robin Hood/Gold Medal* Pouch Mix),								
⅛ mix, approx. .7-oz. piece[2] ..	90	2.0	14.0	3.0	1.0	0	270	m.q.
buttermilk (*Health Valley* Biscuit &								
Pancake), 1 oz.	100	4.0	20.0	1.0	n.a.	0	170	3.3 d
buttermilk (*Tone's*), 1 tsp.	<1	.1	<.1	tr.	n.a.	n.a.	<1	0
BISON, meat only:								
raw, 1 oz.	31	6.1	0	.5	.2	18	15	0
roasted[3]:								
12 oz., yield from 1 lb. raw								
boneless	487	96.8	0	8.2	3.1	279	193	0
4 oz.	162	32.3	0	2.7	1.0	93	65	0
diced, 1 cup, approx. 4.9 oz.	200	39.8	0	3.4	1.3	115	80	0
BITTER GOURD OR MELON,								
see "Balsam pear"								
BLACK BEAN (see also "Black								
turtle soup bean"):								
raw, 1 oz.	97	6.1	17.7	.4	.1	0	1	3.7 d
raw, ½ cup	330	21.0	60.5	1.4	.4	0	5	12.8 d
boiled, 4 oz.	150	10.0	26.9	.6	.2	0	1	4.8 d
boiled, ½ cup	113	7.6	20.4	.5	.1	0	1	3.6 d
BLACK BEAN, CANNED:								
(*Progresso*), ½ cup	90	9.0	19.0	1.0	n.a.	0	350	6.5 d
BLACK BEAN DINNER, canned:								
Western, w/garden vegetables								
(*Health Valley Fast Menu*),								
7½ oz.	120	13.0	14.0	1.0	n.a.	0	170	14.5 d
BLACK BEAN MIX:								
instant (*Fantastic Foods*), ½ cup[4] ...	157	10.0	28.0	2.0	m.q.	n.a.	400	m.q.
instant (*Fantastic Foods*), ½ cup[5] ...	207	10.0	28.0	8.0	m.q.	m.q.	469	m.q.
BLACK TURTLE BEAN:								
raw (*Arrowhead Mills*), 2 oz.	190	13.0	35.0	1.0	(0)	0	9	11.3 d
BLACK TURTLE SOUP BEAN:								
raw, 1 oz.	96	6.0	17.9	.3	.1	0	3	1.5 c
raw, ½ cup	312	19.6	58.2	.8	.2	0	8	4.9 c
boiled, 4 oz.	147	9.3	27.6	.4	.1	0	3	2.3 c
boiled, ½ cup	120	7.5	22.4	.3	.1	0	3	1.9 c
BLACK TURTLE SOUP BEAN,								
CANNED:								
w/liquid, 4 oz.	103	6.8	18.8	.3	.1	0	435	1.3 c
BLACKBERRY:								
untrimmed, 1 lb.	225	3.1	56.0	1.7	(0)	0	1	19.7 d
trimmed, 1 oz.	15	.2	3.6	.1	(0)	0	tr.	1.3 d
trimmed, ½ cup	37	.5	9.2	.3	(0)	0	tr.	3.3 d

1. *Prepared according to package directions.*
2. *Prepared with skim milk.*
3. *Without added ingredients.*
4. *Prepared according to package directions, without added ingredients.*
5. *Prepared with 2 tbsp. salted butter.*

Food and Measure	cal.	prot. (gms)	carbo. (gms)	tot. fat (gms)	sat. fat (gms)	chol. (mgs)	sod. (mgs)	fiber (gms)
BLACKBERRY, CANNED:								
in water (*Allens*), ½ cup	25	1.0	4.0	<1.0	(0)	0	15	m.q.
in heavy syrup, 4 oz.	104	1.5	26.2	.2	(0)	0	3	2.9 c
in heavy syrup, ½ cup	118	1.7	29.6	.2	(0)	0	3	3.3 c
BLACKBERRY, FROZEN, unsweetened:								
18-oz. pkg.	326	6.0	79.9	2.2	(0)	0	7	13.8 c
½ cup	49	.9	11.8	.3	(0)	0	1	2.0 c
BLACKBERRY COBBLER, see "Cobbler, frozen"								
BLACKBERRY PIE, see "Pie"								
BLACKENED REDFISH SEASONING, see "Fish seasoning and coating mix"								
BLACK-EYED PEAS, dried, see "Cowpea"								
BLACK-EYED PEAS, CANNED:								
fresh (*Allens*), ½ cup	100	7.0	18.0	<1.0	(0)	0	370	m.q.
fresh, w/snaps (*Allens*), ½ cup	100	5.0	20.0	<1.0	(0)	0	370	m.q.
mature:								
(*Allens*), ½ cup	105	5.0	20.0	<1.0	(0)	0	300	m.q.
(*Joan of Arc/Green Giant*), ½ cup	90	7.0	18.0	1.0	(0)	0	300	4.0 d
w/pork:								
(*A&P*), ½ cup	120	7.0	20.0	1.0	m.q.	m.q.	410	m.q.
(*Allens*), ½ cup	105	5.0	18.0	1.0	m.q.	m.q.	300	m.q.
(*Luck's*), 7.5 oz.	200	11.0	25.0	6.0	m.q.	m.q.	760	7.0 d
BLACK-EYED PEAS, FROZEN (see also "Cowpea, frozen"):								
(*Frosty Acres*), 3.3 oz.	130	9.0	23.0	1.0	(0)	0	6	1.0 c
(*Seabrook*), 3.3 oz.	130	9.0	23.0	1.0	(0)	0	6	1.0 c
(*Southern*), 3.5 oz.	136	8.9	24.2	.7	(0)	0	20	m.q.
BLINTZ, see "Cheese blintz"								
BLOOD SAUSAGE:								
1 oz.	107	4.1	.4	9.8	3.8	34	m.q.	0
1 slice, 5″ × 4⅝″ × 1/16″, approx. .9 oz.	95	3.7	.3	8.6	3.3	30	m.q.	0
BLOODY MARY[1]:								
1 fl. oz.	23	.2	1.0	tr.	tr.	0	67	(0)
BLOODY MARY MIX, bottled: (*Holland House* Smooth N' Spicy),								
1 fl. oz.	3	0	<1.0	0	0	0	329	(0)
BLUE CHEESE DIP, see "Cheese dip"								
BLUEBERRY:								
untrimmed, 1 lb.	250	3.0	62.8	1.7	(0)	0	27	10.2 d
untrimmed, 1 pint, approx. 14.5 oz.	226	2.7	56.8	1.5	(0)	0	24	9.2 d
trimmed, 1 oz.	16	.2	4.0	.1	(0)	0	2	.7 d
trimmed, ½ cup	41	.5	10.2	.3	(0)	0	5	1.7 d

1. *Recipe: 61.5% tomato juice, 28.3% vodka, 10.2% lemon juice.*

Food and Measure	cal.	prot. (gms)	carbo. (gms)	tot. fat (gms)	sat. fat (gms)	chol. (mgs)	sod. (mgs)	fiber (gms)
BLUEBERRY, CANNED:								
in water (*Lucky Leaf/Musselman's*),								
4 oz.	40	0	9.0	0	0	0	0	m.q.
in heavy syrup:								
4 oz.	100	.7	25.0	.4	(0)	0	3	1.0 c
½ cup	112	.8	28.2	.4	(0)	0	4	1.2 c
(*A&P*), ½ cup	110	<1.0	28.0	<1.0	(0)	0	25	m.q.
(*S&W*), ½ cup	111	0	30.0	0	0	0	<10	m.q.
BLUEBERRY, FROZEN:								
unsweetened, 20-oz. pkg.	287	2.4	69.0	3.6	(0)	0	5	18.1 d
unsweetened, ½ cup	39	.3	9.4	.5	(0)	0	1	2.5 d
sweetened, 10-oz. pkg.	231	1.1	62.4	.4	(0)	0	4	2.6 c
sweetened, ½ cup	94	.5	25.2	.2	(0)	0	2	1.0 c
BLUEBERRY COBBLER, see								
"Cobbler, frozen"								
BLUEBERRY PIE, see "Pie"								
BLUEBERRY PIE FILLING, see								
"Pie filling"								
BLUEBERRY SYRUP:								
(*Estee*), 1 tbsp.	4	0	1.0	0	0	0	20	(0)
(*Featherweight*), 1 tbsp.	16	0	4.0	0	0	0	35	(0)
BLUEFISH, meat only, raw:								
1 lb.	562	90.9	0	19.2	4.2	266	272	0
1 oz.	35	5.7	0	1.2	.3	17	17	0
1 fillet, approx. 5.3 oz., yield from								
1½-lb. whole fish	186	30.1	0	6.4	1.4	88	90	0
BOAR, WILD, meat only:								
raw, 1 oz.	35	6.1	0	1.0	.3	m.q.	m.q.	0
roasted[1]:								
12 oz., yield from 1 lb. raw								
boneless	546	96.3	0	14.9	4.4	m.q.	m.q.	0
4 oz.	181	32.1	0	5.0	1.5	m.q.	m.q.	0
diced, 1 cup, approx. 4.9 oz.	224	39.6	0	6.1	1.8	m.q.	m.q.	0
BOCKWURST[2], raw:								
1 oz.	87	3.8	.1	7.8	2.9	m.q.	m.q.	0
1 link, 7 links per lb.	200	8.7	.3	8.6	3.3	m.q.	m.q.	0
BOK CHOY, see "Cabbage,								
Chinese"								
BOLOGNA:								
(*Boar's Head* Lower Salt), 1 oz.	80	4.0	<1.0	m.q.	m.q.	20	210	0
(*Eckrich*), 1-oz. slice	100	3.0	1.0	9.0	m.q.	m.q.	240	0
(*Eckrich* German Brand), 1-oz. slice	80	4.0	1.0	7.0	m.q.	m.q.	300	0
(*Eckrich* Sandwich), 1-oz. slice	100	3.0	1.0	9.0	m.q.	m.q.	240	0
(*Eckrich Lean Supreme*), 1-oz. slice	70	4.0	1.0	6.0	m.q.	m.q.	240	0
(*Eckrich Smorgas Pac*), 1-oz. slice ..	100	3.0	1.0	9.0	m.q.	m.q.	240	0
(*Eckrich* Thick Sliced, 12 oz.),								
1.7-oz. slice	160	5.0	2.0	15.0	m.q.	m.q.	420	0

1. *Without added ingredients.*
2. *Pork, veal, milk, and eggs.*

Food and Measure	cal.	prot. (gms)	carbo. (gms)	tot. fat (gms)	sat. fat (gms)	chol. (mgs)	sod. (mgs)	fiber (gms)
BOLOGNA *(cont.)*								
(Eckrich Thick Sliced, 1 lb.), 1.8-oz.								
slice	170	5.0	2.0	15.0	m.q.	m.q.	430	0
(Hillshire Farm Large), 1 oz.	90	3.0	<1.0	8.0	m.q.	m.q.	m.q.	0
(Hillshire Farm Ring), 1 oz.	89	3.0	<1.0	8.0	m.q.	m.q.	m.q.	0
(Hormel Coarse Ground, 1 lb.), 2 oz.	160	8.0	1.0	14.0	m.q.	m.q.	578	0
(Hormel Fine Ground, 1 lb.), 2 oz. ...	170	7.0	1.0	16.0	m.q.	m.q.	596	0
(Hormel Perma-Fresh), 2 slices	180	7.0	0	16.0	m.q.	m.q.	599	0
(JM), 1-oz. slice	90	3.0	1.0	8.0	m.q.	m.q.	350	0
(JM German Brand), 1-oz. slice	70	4.0	1.0	6.0	m.q.	m.q.	270	0
(Kahn's Deluxe Club), 1 slice	90	3.0	1.0	8.0	m.q.	m.q.	290	0
(Kahn's Deluxe Club Family Pack),								
1 slice	70	2.0	1.0	6.0	m.q.	m.q.	220	0
(Kahn's Giant Deluxe), 1 slice	90	3.0	1.0	8.0	m.q.	m.q.	290	0
(Kahn's Giant Thick Deluxe), 1 slice	110	4.0	1.0	10.0	m.q.	m.q.	330	0
(Kahn's Thick Deluxe), 1 slice	140	5.0	1.0	13.0	m.q.	m.q.	450	0
(Kahn's Thin Sliced Deluxe), 1 slice	60	2.0	1.0	5.0	m.q.	m.q.	190	0
(Light & Lean), 2 slices	140	6.0	2.0	12.0	m.q.	m.q.	m.q.	0
(Light & Lean Thin Sliced), 2 slices	70	3.0	1.0	6.0	m.q.	m.q.	m.q.	0
(OHSE), 1 oz.	75	3.0	3.0	6.0	m.q.	m.q.	280	0
(OHSE 15% Chicken), 1 oz.	90	3.0	1.0	8.0	m.q.	m.q.	320	0
(Oscar Mayer), .53-oz. slice	48	1.7	.4	4.4	1.7	10	167	0
(Oscar Mayer), 1-oz. slice	90	3.1	.7	8.3	3.2	19	311	0
(Oscar Mayer), 1.6-oz. slice	144	5.0	1.1	13.3	5.1	30	500	0
(Oscar Mayer Light), 1-oz. slice	64	3.2	.7	5.4	1.8	11	310	0
(Pilgrim's Pride), 1-oz. slice	59	3.9	.6	4.4	m.q.	16	228	0
w/cheese *(Eckrich)*, 1-oz. slice	90	3.0	1.0	9.0	m.q.	m.q.	250	0
w/cheese *(Oscar Mayer)*, .8-oz. slice	74	2.7	.6	6.8	2.6	15	232	0
beef:								
1-oz. slice, 4½" diam. × ⅛"	89	3.3	.6	8.0	3.3	16	284	0
1 slice, 4" diam. × ⅛", approx.								
.8 oz.	72	2.7	.5	6.5	2.7	13	230	0
(Boar's Head), 1 oz.	74	4.0	<1.0	7.0	m.q.	17	270	0
(Eckrich), 1-oz. slice	90	3.0	1.0	8.0	m.q.	m.q.	230	0
(Eckrich Thick Sliced), 1.5-oz.								
slice	130	4.0	2.0	12.0	m.q.	m.q.	340	0
(Hebrew National Original Deli								
Style), 1 oz.	90	3.0	<1.0	3.0	m.q.	15	330	0
(Hormel Coarse Ground, 1 lb.),								
2 oz.	160	8.0	1.0	14.0	m.q.	m.q.	576	0
(Hormel Perma-Fresh), 2 slices ..	170	6.0	1.0	16.0	m.q.	m.q.	592	0
(JM), 1-oz. slice	90	3.0	1.0	8.0	m.q.	m.q.	350	0
(Kahn's/Kahn's Giant), 1 slice ...	90	3.0	1.0	8.0	m.q.	m.q.	300	0
(Kahn's Family Pack), 1 slice	70	2.0	1.0	6.0	m.q.	m.q.	230	0
(Kahn's Pounder), 1 slice	90	3.0	1.0	8.0	m.q.	m.q.	300	0
(OHSE), 1 oz.	85	3.0	1.0	8.0	m.q.	m.q.	310	0
(Oscar Mayer), .53-oz. slice	48	1.7	.3	4.4	1.9	10	163	0
(Oscar Mayer), 1-oz. slice	89	3.1	.6	8.2	3.7	19	304	0
(Oscar Mayer), 1.6-oz. slice	143	5.0	1.0	13.3	5.8	31	489	0

Food and Measure	cal.	prot. (gms)	carbo. (gms)	tot. fat (gms)	sat. fat (gms)	chol. (mgs)	sod. (mgs)	fiber (gms)
(*Oscar Mayer* Light), 1-oz. slice ..	64	3.5	.9	5.3	2.1	10	316	0
garlic flavored (*Oscar Mayer*),								
1 oz.	90	3.1	.7	8.3	3.5	18	301	0
Lebanon:								
1 oz.	64	5.6	.6	4.2	1.8	19	359	0
1 slice, 4″ diam. × ⅛″, approx.								
.8 oz.	52	4.5	.5	3.4	1.4	15	291	0
(*Oscar Mayer*), .8-oz. slice	46	4.7	.4	2.9	1.4	16	302	0
beef and cheddar (*Kahn's*), 1 slice ..	90	4.0	1.0	8.0	m.q.	m.q.	320	0
beef and pork:								
1-oz. slice, 4½″ diam. × ⅛″	89	3.3	.8	8.0	3.0	16	289	0
1 slice, 4″ diam. × ⅛″, approx.								
.8 oz.	73	2.7	.6	6.5	2.7	13	234	0
(*Healthy Deli*), 1 oz.	41	4.4	1.1	2.0	m.q.	9	200	0
chicken, see "Chicken bologna"								
garlic:								
(*Eckrich*), 1-oz. slice	90	3.0	1.0	9.0	m.q.	m.q.	230	0
(*JM*), 1-oz. slice	90	3.0	1.0	8.0	m.q.	m.q.	350	0
(*Kahn's*), 1 slice	90	3.0	1.0	8.0	m.q.	m.q.	290	0
ham (*Boar's Head*), 1 oz.	40	5.0	1.0	2.0	m.q.	15	m.q.	0
ham (*Kahn's*), 1 slice	90	3.0	1.0	8.0	m.q.	m.q.	330	0
pork:								
1-oz. slice, 4½″ diam. × ⅛″	70	4.3	.2	5.6	2.0	17	336	0
1 slice, 4″ diam. × ⅛″, approx.								
.8 oz.	57	3.5	.2	4.6	1.6	14	272	0
pork and beef (*Boar's Head*), 1 oz. .	80	4.0	<1.0	7.0	m.q.	15	250	0
turkey, see "Turkey bologna"								
"BOLOGNA," VEGETARIAN								
frozen (*Worthington Bolono*),								
2 slices, approx. 1.3 oz.	60	7.0	2.0	2.0	0	0	390	m.q.
BOLOGNESE SAUCE:								
canned (*Progresso* Authentic Pasta								
Sauces), ½ cup	150	10.0	12.0	8.0	2.0	20	520	2.6 d
refrigerated (*Contadina Fresh*),								
7.5 oz.	230	22.0	12.0	11.0	m.q.	50	600	m.q.
BONITO, CARIBBEAN, meat								
only, raw:								
1 lb.	626	106.6	0	19.1	m.q.	m.q.	m.q.	0
1 oz.	39	6.7	0	1.2	m.q.	m.q.	m.q.	0
BONITO, JAPANESE, meat only,								
raw:								
1 lb.	585	117.0	1.8	9.1	m.q.	m.q.	200	0
1 oz.	37	7.3	.1	.6	m.q.	m.q.	12	0
BORAGE:								
raw:								
untrimmed, 1 lb.	76	6.5	11.1	2.5	n.a.	0	290	3.3 c
trimmed, 1 oz.	6	.5	.9	.2	(0)	0	23	.3 c
1″ pieces, ½ cup	9	.8	1.4	.3	(0)	0	35	.4 c
boiled, drained, 4 oz.	28	2.4	4.0	.9	(0)	0	98	1.2 c

Food and Measure	cal.	prot. (gms)	carbo. (gms)	tot. fat (gms)	sat. fat (gms)	chol. (mgs)	sod. (mgs)	fiber (gms)
BOUILLON, see "Soup"								
BOUILLON, DEHYDRATED:								
beef flavor:								
1 cube	6	.6	.6	.1	.1	tr.	864	(0)
cube (*Steero*), 1 cube	6	<1.0	1.0	<1.0	n.a.	n.a.	930	(0)
cube (*Wyler's*), 1 cube	6	<1.0	1.0	<1.0	n.a.	n.a.	930	(0)
instant:								
(*Featherweight*), 1 tsp.	18	0	2.0	1.0	n.a.	5	10	(0)
(*Lite-Line* Low Sodium), 1 tsp.	12	<1.0	2.0	<1.0	n.a.	n.a.	5	(0)
(*Steero*), 1 tsp.	6	<1.0	1.0	<1.0	n.a.	n.a.	930	(0)
(*Weight Watchers* Broth Mix),								
1 pkt.	8	1.0	1.0	0	0	0	930	(0)
(*Wyler's*), 1 tsp.	6	<1.0	1.0	<1.0	n.a.	n.a.	930	(0)
brown (*G. Washington's* Seasoning &								
Broth), .14 oz.	6	0	1.0	0	0	0	1015	(0)
brown, kosher (*G. Washington's*								
Seasoning & Broth), .14 oz. ...	6	0	1.0	0	0	0	1110	(0)
chicken flavor:								
1 cube	9	.7	1.1	.2	.1	1	1152	(0)
cube (*Steero*), 1 cube	8	<1.0	1.0	<1.0	n.a.	n.a.	990	(0)
cube (*Wyler's*), 1 cube	8	<1.0	1.0	<1.0	n.a.	n.a.	900	(0)
instant:								
(*Featherweight*), 1 tsp.	18	0	2.0	1.0	n.a.	5	5	(0)
(*Lite-Line* Low Sodium), 1 tsp.	12	<1.0	2.0	<1.0	n.a.	n.a.	5	(0)
(*Steero*), 1 tsp.	8	<1.0	1.0	<1.0	n.a.	n.a.	990	(0)
(*Weight Watchers* Broth Mix),								
1 pkt.	8	1.0	1.0	0	0	0	990	(0)
(*Wyler's*), 1 tsp.	8	<1.0	1.0	<1.0	n.a.	n.a.	900	(0)
golden (*G. Washington's* Seasoning &								
Broth), .13 oz.	6	0	1.0	0	0	0	935	(0)
golden, kosher (*G. Washington's*								
Seasoning & Broth), .13 oz. ...	6	0	1.0	0	0	0	1015	(0)
onion (*G. Washington's* Seasoning &								
Broth), .18 oz.	12	1.0	2.0	0	0	0	695	(0)
onion flavor, instant (*Wyler's*), 1 tsp.	10	<1.0	1.0	<1.0	n.a.	0	670	(0)
vegetable (*G. Washington's*								
Seasoning & Broth), .18 oz. ...	12	1.0	2.0	0	0	0	715	(0)
vegetable flavor, instant (*Wyler's*),								
1 tsp.	6	<1.0	1.0	<1.0	(0)	0	910	(0)
BOURBON, see "Liquor"								
BOURBON AND SODA[1]:								
1 fl. oz.	26	tr.	0	0	0	0	4	0
BOYSENBERRY, see "Blackberry"								
BOYSENBERRY, CANNED:								
in heavy syrup, 4 oz.	100	1.1	25.3	.1	(0)	0	3	2.2 c
in heavy syrup, ½ cup	113	1.3	28.6	.2	(0)	0	4	2.4 c

1. *Recipe: 63.8% club soda, 36.2% bourbon.*

Food and Measure	cal.	prot. (gms)	carbo. (gms)	tot. fat (gms)	sat. fat (gms)	chol. (mgs)	sod. (mgs)	fiber (gms)
BOYSENBERRY, FROZEN,								
unsweetened:								
10-oz. pkg.	141	3.1	34.6	.8	(0)	0	4	7.7 c
½ cup	33	.7	8.1	.2	(0)	0	1	1.8 c
BOYSENBERRY JUICE:								
(*Smucker's* Naturally 100%), 8 fl. oz.	120	0	30.0	0	0	0	10	m.q.
BRAINS[1]:								
beef:								
raw, 1 oz.	36	2.8	0	2.6	.6	474	29	0
pan-fried in vegetable oil, 12.4 oz.,								
yield from 1 lb. raw	690	44.1	0	55.6	13.1	7003	555	0
pan-fried in vegetable oil, 4 oz. ..	222	14.3	0	18.0	4.2	2262	179	0
simmered, 13.8 oz., yield from								
1 lb. raw	627	43.3	0	49.0	11.4	8030	469	0
simmered, 4 oz.	181	12.6	0	14.2	3.3	2329	136	0
lamb:								
raw, 1 oz.	35	3.0	0	2.4	.6	384	32	0
braised, 12.25 oz., yield from 1 lb.								
raw	504	43.5	0	35.3	9.0	7083	463	0
braised, 4 oz.	164	14.2	0	11.5	2.9	2317	152	0
pan-fried in vegetable oil, 8.5 oz.,								
yield from 1 lb. raw	654	40.7	0	53.3	13.6	6009	377	0
pan-fried in vegetable oil, 4 oz. ..	310	19.2	0	25.2	6.4	2840	178	0
pork:								
raw, 1 oz.	36	2.9	0	2.6	.6	622	34	0
braised, 13.5 oz., yield from 1 lb.								
raw	526	46.4	0	36.3	8.2	9749	348	0
braised, 4 oz.	156	13.8	0	10.8	2.4	2894	103	0
veal:								
raw, 1 oz.	34	2.9	0	2.3	m.q.	1803	144	0
braised, 12 oz., yield from 1 lb.								
raw	460	38.9	0	32.6	m.q.	10,503	529	0
braised, 4 oz.	154	13.0	0	10.9	m.q.	3515	177	0
pan-fried in vegetable oil, 11.6 oz.,								
yield from 1 lb. raw	703	47.8	0	55.3	m.q.	6996	581	0
pan-fried in vegetable oil, 4 oz. ..	242	16.4	0	19.0	m.q.	2404	200	0
BRAN, see "Cereal" and specific								
bran listings								
BRANDY, unflavored, see "Liquor"								
BRATWURST:								
(*Eckrich*), 1 link	310	11.0	1.0	30.0	m.q.	m.q.	820	0
(*Hickory Farms* Brotwurst), 1 oz. ..	90	4.0	1.0	8.0	m.q.	8	277	0
(*Hillshire Farm* Fully Cooked), 2 oz.	170	7.0	1.0	16.0	m.q.	m.q.	380	0
(*Kahn's*), 1 link	190	7.0	2.0	17.0	m.q.	m.q.	490	0
cheddar (*Hickory Farms* Cheddy								
Brots), 1 oz.	98	4.0	1.0	9.0	m.q.	7	259	0
fresh (*Hillshire Farm*), 2 oz.	190	7.0	1.0	17.0	m.q.	m.q.	410	0

1. *Cooked meats are prepared without added ingredients, except as noted.*

Food and Measure	cal.	prot. (gms)	carbo. (gms)	tot. fat (gms)	sat. fat (gms)	chol. (mgs)	sod. (mgs)	fiber (gms)
BRATWURST *(cont.)*								
hot (*Hickory Farms* Hot Brots),								
1 oz.	96	4.0	1.0	9.0	m.q.	8	269	0
pork, cooked:								
1 oz.	85	4.0	.6	7.3	2.6	17	158	0
1 link, 3 oz., 4 links per 12-oz.								
pkg.	256	12.0	1.8	22.0	7.9	51	473	0
pork and beef[1]:								
1 oz.	92	4.0	.8	7.9	2.8	18	315	0
1 link, approx. 2.5 oz.	226	10.0	2.1	19.5	7.0	44	778	0
smoked (*Hillshire Farm*), 2 oz.	190	8.0	1.0	17.0	m.q.	m.q.	540	0
spicy (*Hillshire Farm*), 2 oz.	180	8.0	1.0	17.0	m.q.	m.q.	m.q.	0
BRAUNSCHWEIGER:								
(*Hormel*), 1 oz.	80	4.0	0	7.0	m.q.	m.q.	322	0
(*JM*), 1-oz. slice	80	3.0	2.0	6.0	m.q.	m.q.	260	0
(*Oscar Mayer* German Brand), 1 oz.	96	4.0	.5	8.7	3.0	45	329	0
(*Oscar Mayer* Slices), 1-oz. slice	96	3.9	.6	8.7	3.2	50	327	0
(*Oscar Mayer* Slices), .9-oz. slice	89	3.6	.5	8.0	2.9	47	303	0
(*Oscar Mayer* Tube), 1 oz.	97	3.9	.7	8.7	3.0	47	301	0
pork, 1 oz.	102	3.8	1.0	9.1	3.1	44	324	0
pork, 1 slice, 2½″ × ¼″, approx.								
.6 oz.	65	2.4	.6	5.8	2.0	28	206	0
BRAZIL NUT[2]:								
in shell, 1 lb.	1428	31.2	27.9	144.2	35.2	0	3	5.0 c
1 oz., approx. 6 large or 8 medium	186	4.1	3.6	18.8	4.6	0	tr.	.7 c
1 cup, approx. 32 large	919	20.1	17.9	92.7	22.6	0	2	3.2 c
BREAD, 1 slice, except as noted:								
apple walnut (*Arnold*)	64	2.1	12.6	1.3	n.a.	1	103	1.3 d
(*Arnold Bran'nola* Original)	85	3.9	17.5	1.4	n.a.	tr.	137	2.9 d
barbecue (*Colombo* Brand BBQ								
Loaf), 2 oz.	139	7.9	23.5	1.6	n.a.	n.a.	318	m.q.
bran:								
and oat (*Oatmeal Goodness* Light)	40	2.0	6.0	<1.0	n.a.	0	90	m.q.
whole (*Brownberry* Natural)	58	2.3	11.7	1.4	n.a.	0	167	2.1 d
(*Brownberry Bran'nola*)	85	3.9	17.5	1.4	n.a.	tr.	137	2.9 d
(*Brownberry* Health Nut)	71	2.3	12.4	2.6	m.q.	0	158	2.5 d
cinnamon:								
oatmeal (*Oatmeal Goodness*)	90	4.0	15.0	2.0	m.q.	0	140	1.0 d
raisin (*Arnold*)	67	2.1	12.9	1.4	n.a.	2	86	.8 d
raisin swirl (*Pepperidge Farm*)	90	2.0	16.0	2.0	0	0	100	2.0 d
swirl (*Pepperidge Farm*)	90	2.0	15.0	3.0	0	0	110	2.0 d
date nut roll (*Dromedary*), ½″ slice	80	1.0	13.0	2.0	m.q.	n.a.	160	m.q.
French:								
(*DiCarlo* Parisian)	70	3.0	13.0	1.0	n.a.	n.a.	180	.7 d
extra sour (*Colombo* Brand), 2 oz.	150	7.7	26.9	1.3	n.a.	0	311	m.q.
extra sour, sliced (*Colombo*								
Brand), 2 oz.	153	7.6	27.2	1.6	n.a.	0	310	m.q.

1. *Nonfat dry milk added.*
2. *Dried and unblanched; shelled, except as noted.*

Food and Measure	cal.	prot. (gms)	carbo. (gms)	tot. fat (gms)	sat. fat (gms)	chol. (mgs)	sod. (mgs)	fiber (gms)
style (*Pepperidge Farm* Hearth), 1 oz.	75	2.5	14.0	1.0	0	0	160	.5 d
sweet (*Colombo* Brand French Stick), 2 oz.	154	7.2	27.1	1.9	n.a.	n.a.	331	m.q.
twin (*Pepperidge Farm* Hearth), 1 oz.	80	3.0	15.0	1.0	n.a.	0	160	0
garlic (*Colombo* Brand), 2 oz.	185	6.2	17.3	10.1	m.q.	n.a.	331	m.q.
grain:								
mixed (*Roman Meal* Round Top) ..	67	2.9	13.2	.8	n.a.	0	140	1.2 d
mixed (*Roman Meal* Thin Sliced Sandwich)	55	2.4	10.7	.7	n.a.	0	114	1.0 d
multi (*Roman Meal* Sun Grain) ...	68	3.2	12.3	1.4	n.a.	0	140	1.7 d
multi (*Weight Watchers*)	40	2.0	9.0	<1.0	n.a.	0	100	m.q.
nutty (*Arnold Bran'nola*)	85	3.9	17.4	1.6	n.a.	tr.	144	3.0 d
nutty (*Brownberry Bran'nola* Nutty Grains)	85	3.9	17.4	1.6	n.a.	tr.	144	3.0 d
seven (*Pepperidge Farm* Hearty Slice), 2 slices	180	5.0	36.0	2.0	0	0	340	2.0 d
granola, oat and honey (*Pepperidge Farm*)	60	2.0	12.0	2.0	0	0	105	2.0 d
(*Hollywood* Dark)	70	3.0	13.0	1.0	n.a.	n.a.	160	.8 d
(*Hollywood* Light)	70	3.0	13.0	1.0	n.a.	n.a.	150	.7 d
honey bran (*Pepperidge Farm* 1½ lb.)	90	3.0	18.0	1.0	n.a.	0	160	1.0 d
Italian:								
(*Arnold* Francisco International), 1-oz. slice	72	2.9	14.1	1.1	n.a.	0	190	.8 d
(*Brownberry* Light)	44	2.3	9.9	.5	n.a.	tr.	89	2.0 d
(*Pepperidge Farm* Hearth), 1 oz. ..	80	2.0	14.0	1.0	n.a.	0	150	0
(*Wonder* Family)	70	2.0	13.0	1.0	n.a.	n.a.	160	.7 d
light (*Arnold* Bakery)	45	2.4	9.9	.5	n.a.	tr.	90	2.0 d
thick sliced (*Arnold* Francisco International)	66	2.3	13.7	.8	n.a.	0	111	.9 d
(*Monk's* Hi-Fibre)	70	3.0	13.0	1.0	n.a.	0	80	1.4 d
oat:								
(*Arnold Bran'nola* Country)	90	3.7	17.8	2.0	m.q.	tr.	166	2.8 d
(*Brownberry Bran'nola* Country),	90	3.7	17.8	2.0	m.q.	tr.	166	2.8 d
crunchy (*Pepperidge Farm*), 2 slices	190	8.0	34.0	4.0	1.0	0	290	3.0 d
oat bran:								
(*Awrey's*)	50	2.0	10.0	0	0	0	130	1.0 d
(*Roman Meal* Split-Top)	68	2.9	13.2	.9	n.a.	0	140	1.1 d
(*Weight Watchers*)	40	1.0	10.0	<1.0	n.a.	0	100	m.q.
honey (*Roman Meal*)	71	3.2	12.7	1.2	n.a.	0	130	.9 d
honey nut (*Roman Meal*)	72	3.3	12.1	1.6	n.a.	0	130	1.0 d
oatmeal:								
(*Pepperidge Farm*)	70	2.0	12.0	1.0	n.a.	0	160	1.0 d
(*Pepperidge Farm* 1½ lb.)	90	3.0	17.0	1.0	n.a.	0	200	1.0 d
(*Pepperidge Farm* Very Thin)	40	1.0	8.0	1.0	n.a.	0	80	0

Food and Measure	cal.	prot. (gms)	carbo. (gms)	tot. fat (gms)	sat. fat (gms)	chol. (mgs)	sod. (mgs)	fiber (gms)
BREAD, OATMEAL *(cont.)*								
and bran (*Oatmeal Goodness*)	90	4.0	15.0	2.0	m.q.	0	140	1.0 d
light (*Arnold* Bakery)	44	2.3	9.6	.6	n.a.	tr.	98	1.9 d
light (*Pepperidge Farm* Light Style)	45	2.0	9.0	0	0	0	95	1.0 d
sunflower seed (*Oatmeal* Goodness)	90	4.0	15.0	2.0	m.q.	0	140	1.0 d
orange raisin (*Brownberry*)	67	2.3	13.0	1.2	n.a.	tr.	83	.8 d
pita:								
oat bran (*Sahara*), ½ piece	66	2.4	15.3	.3	n.a.	0	163	1.8 d
wheat, whole (*Sahara*), 1 piece, approx. 2 oz.	150	6.0	28.0	2.0	m.q.	0	320	.7 c
white (*Sahara*), ½ piece	79	2.9	15.6	.5	n.a.	0	147	m.q.
white, mini (*Sahara*)	79	2.9	15.6	.5	n.a.	0	147	m.q.
pumpernickel:								
(*Arnold*)	70	2.7	14.7	.9	n.a.	0	198	1.3 d
(*Pepperidge Farm* Family)	80	3.0	15.0	1.0	0	0	230	2.0 d
small (*Pepperidge Farm* Party), 4 slices	60	2.0	12.0	1.0	0	0	160	1.0 d
raisin:								
bran (*Brownberry*)	61	2.2	12.4	1.3	n.a.	0	108	1.8 d
cinnamon (*Brownberry*)	66	2.2	12.8	1.3	n.a.	tr.	107	.9 d
w/cinnamon (*Monk's*)	70	3.0	10.0	2.0	m.q.	0	85	m.q.
w/cinnamon swirl (*Pepperidge Farm*)	90	2.0	16.0	2.0	0	0	100	1.0 d
walnut (*Brownberry*)	68	2.2	11.4	2.7	m.q.	tr.	96	2.3 d
rice bran:								
(*Roman Meal*)	70	2.8	12.4	1.5	n.a.	0	132	1.3 d
golden (*Monk's*)	70	3.0	14.0	1.0	n.a.	0	80	1.6 d
honey nut (*Roman Meal*)	71	2.6	12.8	1.6	n.a.	0	127	1.3 d
rye:								
(*Beefsteak* Hearty)	70	3.0	13.0	1.0	n.a.	n.a.	180	.7 d
(*Beefsteak* Mild)	70	3.0	13.0	1.0	n.a.	n.a.	180	.7 d
(*Beefsteak* Soft)	70	3.0	13.0	1.0	n.a.	0	170	.9 d
(*Braun's Old Allegheny*)	70	3.0	13.0	1.0	n.a.	0	160	.7 d
(*Weight Watchers*)	40	2.0	10.0	<1.0	n.a.	0	100	m.q.
(*Wonder*)	70	2.0	13.0	1.0	n.a.	n.a.	150	.7 d
caraway (*Brownberry* Natural)	73	2.8	15.4	.8	n.a.	0	185	1.2 d
Dijon (*Pepperidge Farm*)	50	2.0	9.0	1.0	0	0	170	1.0 d
Dijon (*Pepperidge Farm* Hearty) ..	70	3.0	15.0	1.0	n.a.	0	260	2.0 d
dill (*Arnold*)	71	2.8	14.4	1.0	n.a.	0	187	1.3 d
Jewish, seeded (*Levy's*)	76	2.8	15.9	.9	n.a.	0	181	1.4 d
Jewish, seedless (*Levy's*)	75	2.8	16.0	.8	n.a.	0	178	1.3 d
onion (*Beefsteak*)	70	3.0	12.0	1.0	n.a.	0	170	1.0 d
seedless (*Brownberry* Natural Thin Sliced)	45	1.7	9.8	.6	n.a.	0	118	.8 d
seedless (*Pepperidge Farm* Family)	80	3.0	16.0	1.0	0	0	210	2.0 d
w/seeds (*Pepperidge Farm* Family)	80	3.0	16.0	1.0	0	0	220	2.0 d
small (*Pepperidge Farm* Party), 4 slices	60	2.0	12.0	1.0	0	0	250	1.0 d

Food and Measure	cal.	prot. (gms)	carbo. (gms)	tot. fat (gms)	sat. fat (gms)	chol. (mgs)	sod. (mgs)	fiber (gms)
wheatberry (*Beefsteak*)	70	3.0	13.0	1.0	n.a.	0	160	1.0 d
sourdough:								
(*DiCarlo*)	70	3.0	12.0	1.0	n.a.	0	140	.7 d
French (*Boudin*), 2 oz. or 2 slices	130	5.0	27.0	1.0	n.a.	0	297	m.q.
sunflower and bran (*Monk's*)	70	3.0	12.0	1.0	n.a.	0	80	1.6 d
Vienna, light (*Pepperidge Farm* Light								
Style)	45	2.0	10.0	0	0	0	100	1.0 d
Vienna, thick-sliced (*Pepperidge Farm*								
Hearth)	70	2.0	13.0	1.0	0	0	125	0
wheat:								
(*Arnold* Brick Oven)	57	2.4	10.6	1.5	n.a.	tr.	104	1.7 d
(*Beefsteak* Hearty)	70	3.0	11.0	1.0	n.a.	0	160	1.4 d
(*Beefsteak* Soft)	70	3.0	12.0	1.0	n.a.	0	160	1.6 d
(*Brownberry* Hearth), 1 oz.	70	3.1	13.6	1.4	n.a.	0	150	2.0 d
(*Brownberry* Natural)	80	3.0	17.0	1.3	n.a.	0	183	2.3 d
(*Country Grain*)	70	3.0	12.0	1.0	n.a.	n.a.	160	1.3 d
(*Fresh & Natural*)	70	3.0	13.0	1.0	n.a.	0	140	1.8 d
(*Home Pride* Butter Top)	70	3.0	13.0	1.0	n.a.	n.a.	140	.8 d
(*Home Pride* 7 Grain)	70	3.0	12.0	1.0	n.a.	n.a.	140	.8 d
(*Home Pride* Stoneground)	70	3.0	12.0	1.0	n.a.	0	140	1.9 d
(*Pepperidge Farm* 1½ lb.)	90	3.0	18.0	2.0	m.q.	0	190	2.0 d
(*Pepperidge Farm* Family, 2 lb.) ...	70	2.0	13.0	1.0	0	0	130	2.0 d
(*Weight Watchers*)	40	2.0	9.0	<1.0	n.a.	0	100	m.q.
apple honey (*Brownberry*)	69	2.3	11.4	1.9	n.a.	0	148	1.5 d
cracked (*Pepperidge Farm*)	70	2.0	13.0	1.0	n.a.	0	140	1.0 d
cracked (*Wonder*)	70	3.0	13.0	1.0	n.a.	n.a.	180	.8 d
dark (*Arnold Bran'nola*)	83	4.1	17.6	1.0	n.a.	tr.	166	2.8 d
hearty (*Arnold Bran'nola*)	88	3.8	17.1	1.9	n.a.	tr.	197	2.7 d
hearty (*Brownberry Bran'nola*) ...	88	3.8	17.1	1.9	n.a.	tr.	197	2.7 d
honey wheatberry (*Arnold*)	77	3.1	16.5	1.2	n.a.	tr.	143	2.4 d
light (*Pepperidge Farm* Light Style)	45	2.0	9.0	0	0	0	90	1.0 d
light golden (*Arnold* Bakery)	44	2.3	9.5	.5	n.a.	tr.	86	2.0 d
multigrain (*Beefsteak*)	70	3.0	11.0	1.0	n.a.	0	130	1.6 d
oatmeal (*Oatmeal Goodness*)	90	4.0	15.0	2.0	m.q.	0	140	1.0 d
oatmeal (*Oatmeal Goodness* Light)	40	2.0	6.0	<1.0	n.a.	0	90	m.q.
sesame (*Pepperidge Farm* Hearty),								
2 slices	190	7.0	36.0	3.0	1.0	0	340	3.0 d
soft (*Brownberry*)	74	2.8	13.1	1.8	n.a.	tr.	127	1.0 d
sprouted (*Pepperidge Farm*)	70	3.0	11.0	2.0	m.q.	0	100	2.0 d
whole:								
(*Arnold* Stoneground 100%) ...	48	2.4	9.9	.7	n.a.	tr.	97	1.6 d
(*Daily*), 2 oz., approx. 1 piece	140	6.0	26.0	0	0	0	0	m.q.
(*Monk's* 100% Stone Ground)	70	3.0	13.0	1.0	n.a.	0	110	m.q.
(*Pepperidge Farm* Thin Sliced,								
1 lb.)	60	2.0	12.0	1.0	n.a.	0	110	2.0 d
(*Pepperidge Farm* Very Thin) ...	35	2.0	7.0	0	0	0	75	0
(*Wonder* 100%)	70	3.0	12.0	1.0	n.a.	n.a.	160	1.8 d
(*Wonder* Soft 100%)	70	4.0	10.0	1.0	n.a.	0	140	1.8 d
(*Wonder* High Fiber)	40	2.0	6.0	0	0	0	80	2.9 d

Food and Measure	cal.	prot. (gms)	carbo. (gms)	tot. fat (gms)	sat. fat (gms)	chol. (mgs)	sod. (mgs)	fiber (gms)
BREAD, WHEAT, WHOLE *(cont.)*								
(*Wonder* Light)	40	3.0	7.0	0	0	0	120	2.0 d
(*Wonder* Family)	70	3.0	13.0	1.0	n.a.	n.a.	140	.8 d
white:								
(*Arnold* Brick Oven)	61	2.2	11.3	1.2	n.a.	tr.	134	.8 d
(*Arnold* Country White)	98	3.4	18.6	1.8	n.a.	tr.	204	1.0 d
(*Arnold* Light Premium)	42	2.3	9.6	.5	n.a.	tr.	89	2.2 d
(*Beefsteak* Robust)	70	3.0	13.0	1.0	n.a.	n.a.	140	.7 d
(*Brownberry* Light Premium)	42	2.3	9.6	.5	n.a.	tr.	89	2.2 d
(*Brownberry* Natural)	59	2.2	11.1	1.1	n.a.	tr.	136	.6 d
(*Home Pride* Butter Top)	70	3.0	13.0	1.0	n.a.	n.a.	140	.7 d
(*Monk's*)	60	3.0	10.0	1.0	n.a.	0	95	m.q.
(*Pepperidge Farm* Hearty Country), 2 slices	190	7.0	38.0	2.0	1.0	0	340	2.0 d
(*Pepperidge Farm* Large Family 2 lb.)	70	2.0	13.0	1.0	0	0	150	0
(*Pepperidge Farm* Thin Sliced 1 lb.)	80	2.0	14.0	2.0	m.q.	0	130	0
(*Pepperidge Farm* Very Thin)	40	1.0	8.0	0	0	0	80	0
(*Weight Watchers*)	40	2.0	10.0	<1.0	n.a.	0	100	m.q.
(*Wonder*)	70	3.0	13.0	1.0	n.a.	n.a.	140	.7 d
(*Wonder* High Fiber)	40	2.0	6.0	0	0	0	80	2.9 d
(*Wonder* Light)	40	3.0	7.0	0	0	0	110	2.0 d
(*Wonder* Thin Sliced)	50	2.0	10.0	1.0	n.a.	0	120	.5 d
w/buttermilk (*Wonder*)	70	2.0	13.0	1.0	n.a.	n.a.	160	.7 d
extra fiber (*Arnold* Brick Oven) ..	55	2.2	12.1	.8	n.a.	tr.	93	2.1 d
sandwich (*Pepperidge Farm*), 2 slices	130	4.0	24.0	2.0	0	0	260	0
toasting (*Pepperidge Farm*)	90	3.0	17.0	1.0	0	0	200	1.0 d
BREAD, BROWN AND SERVE:								
(*du Jour Austrian*)	70	3.0	13.0	1.0	n.a.	0	140	.6 d
(*du Jour French*)	70	3.0	13.0	1.0	n.a.	0	140	.6 d
Italian (*Pepperidge Farm*), 1 oz.	80	2.0	14.0	1.0	n.a.	0	150	0
BREAD, BROWN, CANNED:								
(*B&M/Friends*), 1.6 oz.	94	2.0	22.0	0	0	0	320	2.0 d
(*S&W* New England), 2 slices	76	2.0	17.0	0	0	0	172	m.q.
raisin (*B&M/Friends*), 1.6 oz.	92	2.0	21.0	0	0	0	345	2.0 d
BREAD, REFRIGERATED, see "Bread dough"								
BREAD, SWEET, MIX[1]:								
banana (*Pillsbury*), 1/12 loaf	170	3.0	27.0	6.0	m.q.	n.a.	200	m.q.
blueberry nut (*Pillsbury*), 1/12 loaf ..	150	2.0	26.0	4.0	m.q.	n.a.	150	m.q.
cherry nut (*Pillsbury*), 1/12 loaf	180	3.0	29.0	5.0	m.q.	n.a.	150	m.q.
cornbread:								
(*Aunt Jemima* Easy), 1 serving ...	196	3.5	32.7	6.3	1.3	13	679	1.4 d
(*Dromedary*), 3 tbsp. dry	100	2.0	19.0	2.0	m.q.	n.a.	280	m.q.
(*Dromedary*), 2″ × 2″ square	130	3.0	20.0	3.0	m.q.	n.a.	480	m.q.
(*Martha White* Cotton Pickin'), 1/4 pan	170	3.0	31.0	3.0	m.q.	2	540	m.q.

1. *Prepared according to package directions, except as noted.*

Food and Measure	cal.	prot. (gms)	carbo. (gms)	tot. fat (gms)	sat. fat (gms)	chol. (mgs)	sod. (mgs)	fiber (gms)
(*Pillsbury/Ballard*), ⅛ recipe	140	3.0	25.0	3.0	m.q.	n.a.	570	m.q.
white (*Robin Hood/Gold Medal* Pouch Mix), ⅙ mix[1]	150	4.0	22.0	5.0	m.q.	m.q.	490	m.q.
yellow (*Martha White* Light Crust), 2 oz.	140	4.0	21.0	4.0	m.q.	26	400	m.q.
yellow (*Robin Hood/Gold Medal* Pouch Mix), ⅙ mix[1]	150	4.0	23.0	5.0	m.q.	m.q.	500	m.q.
cranberry (*Pillsbury*), 1/12 loaf	160	2.0	30.0	4.0	m.q.	n.a.	160	m.q.
date (*Pillsbury*), 1/12 loaf	160	2.0	32.0	3.0	m.q.	n.a.	150	m.q.
date nut (*Dromedary*), 1/12 pkg. dry	166	2.0	26.0	7.0	m.q.	n.a.	242	m.q.
date nut (*Dromedary*), 1/12 loaf	183	2.0	26.0	8.0	m.q.	n.a.	248	m.q.
gingerbread:								
(*Betty Crocker* Classic), ⅑ mix[2] ..	220	3.0	35.0	7.0	2.0	30	330	m.q.
(*Betty Crocker* Classic), ⅑ mix[3] ..	210	3.0	35.0	6.0	2.0	0	330	m.q.
(*Pillsbury*), 3″ square	190	2.0	36.0	4.0	m.q.	n.a.	310	m.q.
nut (*Pillsbury*), 1/12 loaf	170	3.0	28.0	6.0	m.q.	n.a.	190	m.q.
BREAD CRUMBS:								
plain (*Devonsheer*), 1 oz.	108	3.9	21.6	1.4	n.a.	0	272	.9 d
plain (*Progresso*), 2 tbsp.	60	2.0	11.0	<1.0	n.a.	0	110	m.q.
plain or Italian, dry, grated (*Tone's*), 1 tsp.	8	.3	1.5	.1	<.1	<1	15	.1 d
Italian style:								
(*Devonsheer*), 1 oz.	104	3.6	21.1	1.3	n.a.	0	408	.9 d
(*Progresso*), 2 tbsp.	60	2.0	11.0	<1.0	n.a.	0	240	m.q.
whole wheat (*Jaclyn's*), ½ oz.	28	4.0	13.0	1.0	n.a.	0	5	m.q.
BREAD DOUGH:								
frozen:								
honey walnut (*Bridgford*), 1 oz. ..	76	3.0	13.8	.9	n.a.	0	152	m.q.
white (*Bridgford*), 1 oz.	76	2.5	13.8	1.2	n.a.	0	156	m.q.
white (*Rich's*), 2 slices	120	4.0	23.0	1.0	n.a.	0	300	m.q.
refrigerated:								
(*Roman Meal*), 1-oz. slice	85	2.3	12.6	2.8	.9	0	199	.6 d
cornbread twists (*Pillsbury*), 1 twist	70	1.0	8.0	4.0	<1.0	0	150	m.q.
French, crusty (*Pillsbury*), 1″ slice	60	2.0	11.0	<1.0	0	0	120	m.q.
wheat (*Pipin' Hot*), 1″ slice	70	0	12.0	2.0	0	0	170	m.q.
white (*Pipin' Hot*), 1″ slice	70	3.0	12.0	2.0	0	0	170	m.q.
BREADFRUIT:								
untrimmed, 1 lb.	365	3.8	96.0	.8	(0)	0	6	5.2 c
trimmed:								
1 oz.	29	.3	7.7	.1	(0)	0	1	.4 c
¼ small, approx. 3.4 oz.	99	1.0	26.0	.2	(0)	0	2	1.4 c
½ cup	114	1.2	29.8	.3	(0)	0	2	1.6 c
BREADFUIT SEEDS:								
raw[4]:								
in shell, 1 lb.	590	22.8	90.2	17.2	4.7	0	n.a.	5.2 c

1. *Prepared with egg and whole milk.*
2. *Prepared with egg.*
3. *Prepared with cholesterol-free egg product or egg white.*
4. *South American cultivar.*

Food and Measure	cal.	prot. (gms)	carbo. (gms)	tot. fat (gms)	sat. fat (gms)	chol. (mgs)	sod. (mgs)	fiber (gms)
BREADFRUIT SEEDS, RAW *(cont.)*								
shelled, 1 oz.	54	2.1	8.3	1.6	.4	0	n.a.	.5 c
boiled[1]:								
in soft shell, 1 lb.	274	8.7	52.3	3.8	1.0	0	n.a.	2.9 c
shelled, 1 oz.	48	1.5	9.1	.7	.2	0	n.a.	.5 c
roasted,[2] shelled, 1 oz.	59	1.8	11.4	.8	.2	0	n.a.	.6 c
BREADNUT TREE SEEDS:								
raw, 1 oz., approx. 8–14 seeds	62	1.7	13.1	.3	.1	0	n.a.	.7 c
dried, 1 oz.	104	2.5	22.6	.5	.1	0	n.a.	1.6 c
BREADSTICKS, 1 piece, except as noted:								
plain (*Stella D'oro*)	41	1.0	6.5	1.2	m.q.	n.a.	m.q.	m.q.
plain, dietetic (*Stella D'oro*)	46	1.3	7.3	1.4	m.q.	n.a.	<10	m.q.
onion (*Stella D'oro*)	40	1.2	6.1	1.3	m.q.	n.a.	m.q.	m.q.
pizza (*Fattorie & Pandea*), 3 pieces	59	2.0	10.0	1.0	n.a.	0	100	m.q.
pizza (*Stella D'oro*)	43	1.3	6.9	1.2	m.q.	n.a.	m.q.	m.q.
refrigerated (*Roman Meal*)	117	3.1	17.4	3.9	m.q.	n.a.	274	m.q.
sesame:								
(*Fattorie & Pandea*), 3 pieces	65	2.0	10.0	2.0	m.q.	0	100	m.q.
(*Stella D'oro*)	51	1.4	6.3	2.2	m.q.	n.a.	m.q.	m.q.
dietetic (*Stella D'oro*)	49	1.3	6.1	2.1	m.q.	n.a.	<10	m.q.
soft, refrigerated (*Pillsbury*)	100	3.0	17.0	2.0	<1.0	0	230	m.q.
soft, refrigerated (*Roman Meal*)	117	3.1	17.4	3.9	1.2	0	274	.8 d
wheat (*Stella D'oro*)	42	1.3	6.1	1.4	m.q.	n.a.	m.q.	m.q.
wheat, whole (*Fattorie & Pandea*), 3 pieces	57	2.0	10.0	1.0	n.a.	0	100	m.q.
BREAKFAST, FROZEN, see specific listings								
BREAKFAST BAR, 1 bar (see also "Granola and cereal bar"):								
all varieties, except chocolate caramel (*Figurines* 100 Diet Bar)	100	2.0	11.0	5.0	m.q.	n.a.	45	m.q.
chocolate:								
caramel (*Figurines* 100 Diet Bar)	100	2.0	10.0	6.0	m.q.	n.a.	55	m.q.
crunch (*Carnation*)	190	6.0	19.0	10.0	3.0	<1	270	1.2 d
chocolate chip (*Carnation*)	200	6.0	20.0	11.0	4.2	<1	170	1.4 d
peanut butter chocolate chip (*Carnation*)	200	7.0	20.0	11.0	3.0	<1	170	1.4 d
peanut butter crunch (*Carnation*) ..	190	7.0	18.0	10.0	2.8	<1	180	1.0 d
BREAKFAST BEVERAGE, see specific flavors								
BREAKFAST SANDWICH, see "Egg breakfast sandwich" and specific listings								
BREAKFAST STRIPS, see "Bacon, substitute"								

1. *Pacific area cultivar.*
2. *South American cultivar.*

Food and Measure	cal.	prot. (gms)	carbo. (gms)	tot. fat (gms)	sat. fat (gms)	chol. (mgs)	sod. (mgs)	fiber (gms)
BRINJAL, see "Eggplant"								
BRITO, see "Burrito"								
BROAD BEAN:								
raw:								
untrimmed, 1 lb.	317	24.6	51.5	2.6	.6	0	220	9.7 c
trimmed, 1 oz.	20	1.6	3.3	.2	<.1	0	14	.6 c
trimmed, ½ cup	40	3.1	6.4	.4	.1	0	28	1.2 c
1 medium, approx. .3 oz.	6	.5	1.0	.1	<.1	0	4	.2 c
boiled, drained, 4 oz.	64	5.4	11.5	.6	.2	0	47	2.2 c
BROAD BEAN, MATURE, DRIED:								
raw, 1 oz.	97	7.4	16.5	.4	.1	0	4	4.1 d
raw, ½ cup	256	19.6	43.7	1.2	.2	0	9	10.9 d
boiled, 4 oz.	125	8.6	22.3	.5	.1	0	6	5.8 d
boiled, ½ cup	93	6.5	16.7	.3	.1	0	4	4.3 d
BROAD BEAN, MATURE, CANNED:								
w/liquid, 4 oz.	81	6.2	14.1	.2	<.1	0	514	.5 c
w/liquid, ½ cup	91	7.0	15.9	.3	<.1	0	580	.5 c
BROCCOLI:								
raw:								
untrimmed, 1 lb.	77	8.3	14.5	1.0	.2	0	73	7.7 d
trimmed, 1 oz.	8	.8	1.5	.1	<.1	0	8	.8 d
1 spear, approx. 8.7 oz.	42	4.5	7.9	.5	.1	0	40	4.2 d
chopped, ½ cup	12	1.3	2.3	.2	<.1	0	12	1.2 d
boiled, drained:								
4 oz.	32	3.4	5.7	.4	<.1	0	29	2.9 d
1 spear, approx. 6.3 oz.	51	5.4	9.1	.6	.1	0	46	4.7 d
chopped, ½ cup	22	2.3	3.9	.2	<.1	0	20	2.0 d
BROCCOLI, FROZEN:								
boiled, drained, spears or chopped,								
4 oz.	32	3.5	6.1	.1	<.1	0	27	2.5 d
boiled, drained, spears or chopped,								
½ cup	26	2.9	4.9	.1	<.1	0	22	2.0 d
(*Health Valley*), ½ cup	26	3.0	5.0	0	0	0	24	3.2 d
spears:								
10-oz. pkg.	84	8.7	15.2	1.0	.2	0	49	6.0 d
(*A&P*), 3.3 oz.	25	3.0	5.0	<1.0	(0)	0	20	m.q.
(*Bird's Eye*), 3.3 oz.	25	3.0	5.0	0	0	0	20	3.0 d
(*Frosty Acres*), 3.3 oz.	25	3.0	5.0	0	0	0	20	1.0 c
(*Green Giant Harvest Fresh*),								
½ cup	20	2.0	4.0	0	0	0	115	2.0 d
(*Seabrook*), 3.3 oz.	25	3.0	5.0	0	0	0	20	1.0 c
(*Southern*), 3.5 oz.	30	3.0	4.8	.2	(0)	0	30	m.q.
baby (*Bird's Eye* Deluxe), 3.3 oz.	30	3.0	5.0	0	0	0	15	3.0 d
baby (*Seabrook*), 3.3 oz.	30	3.0	5.0	0	0	0	14	1.0 c
mini (*Green Giant*), 4–5 spears or								
⅕ pkg.	18	2.0	5.0	0	0	0	25	3.0 d

Food and Measure	cal.	prot. (gms)	carbo. (gms)	tot. fat (gms)	sat. fat (gms)	chol. (mgs)	sod. (mgs)	fiber (gms)
BROCCOLI, FROZEN, SPEARS *(cont.)*								
whole (*Bird's Eye* Farm Fresh),								
4 oz.	30	4.0	6.0	0	0	0	25	3.0 d
florets (*Birds Eye* Deluxe), 3.3 oz.	25	3.0	5.0	0	0	0	20	3.0 d
florets (*Frosty Acres*), 3.3 oz.	30	3.0	5.0	0	0	0	14	1.0 c
cuts:								
(*A&P*), 3.3 oz.	25	3.0	5.0	<1.0	(0)	0	25	m.q.
(*Birds Eye*), 3.3 oz.	25	3.0	5.0	0	0	0	25	3.0 d
(*Birds Eye* Portion Pack), 3 oz.	20	3.0	4.0	0	0	0	20	2.0 d
(*Frosty Acres*), 3.3 oz.	25	3.0	5.0	0	0	0	50	1.0 c
(*Green Giant* Polybag), ½ cup	12	1.0	3.0	0	0	0	15	2.0 d
(*Green Giant Harvest Fresh*),								
½ cup	16	2.0	3.0	0	0	0	95	2.0 d
(*Seabrook*), 3.3 oz.	25	3.0	5.0	0	0	0	50	1.0 c
(*Stokely Singles*), 3 oz.	25	3.0	5.0	1.0	(0)	0	15	m.q.
chopped:								
10-oz. pkg.	75	8.0	13.6	.8	.1	0	68	4.8 d
(*A&P*), 3.3 oz.	25	3.0	5.0	<1.0	(0)	0	25	m.q.
(*Birds Eye*), 3.3 oz.	25	3.0	5.0	0	0	0	15	3.0 d
(*Finast*), 3.3 oz.	25	3.0	5.0	0	0	0	20	m.q.
(*Frosty Acres*), 3.3 oz.	25	3.0	5.0	0	0	0	18	1.0 c
(*Seabrook*), 3.3 oz.	25	3.0	5.0	0	0	0	18	1.0 c
(*Southern*), 3.5 oz.	28	2.9	4.4	.3	(0)	0	25	m.q.
in butter sauce:								
cuts (*Green Giant* One Serving),								
4.5 oz.	45	3.0	7.0	2.0	<1.0	5	420	3.0 d
spears (*Birds Eye* Butter Sauce								
Combinations), 3.3 oz.	45	2.0	5.0	2.0	m.q.	5	320	2.0 d
spears (*Green Giant*), ½ cup	40	2.0	6.0	2.0	<1.0	5	350	2.0 d
in cheese sauce:								
(*Birds Eye* Cheese Sauce								
Combinations), 5 oz.	130	6.0	12.0	7.0	m.q.	10	560	2.0 d
(*Freezer Queen Family Side*								
Dishes), 4.5 oz.	48	2.0	8.0	1.0	n.a.	n.a.	280	m.q.
cuts:								
(*Finast*), ⅓ cup or 3.3 oz.	45	3.0	6.0	0	0	0	310	m.q.
(*Green Giant* One Serving),								
5 oz.	70	4.0	11.0	3.0	<1.0	5	660	3.0 d
(*Stokely Singles*), 4 oz.	80	5.0	7.0	4.0	m.q.	15	200	m.q.
in cheese flavored sauce (*Green*								
Giant), ½ cup	60	3.0	9.0	2.0	<1.0	2	530	2.0 d
BROCCOLI AND CHEESE,								
frozen:								
in pastry (*Pepperidge Farm*), 1 piece	230	5.0	18.0	16.0	m.q.	m.q.	380	m.q.
BROCCOLI COMBINATIONS,								
frozen:								
and carrots:								
baby, and water chestnuts (*Birds*								
Eye Farm Fresh), 4 oz.	45	2.0	10.0	0	0	0	35	3.0 d

Food and Measure	cal.	prot. (gms)	carbo. (gms)	tot. fat (gms)	sat. fat (gms)	chol. (mgs)	sod. (mgs)	fiber (gms)
baby whole, and chestnuts (*Stokely* *Singles*), 3 oz.	30	2.0	6.0	1.0	0	0	22	m.q.
and cauliflower:								
(*A&P*), 3.2 oz.	25	2.0	4.0	<1.0	(0)	0	20	m.q.
(*Frosty Acres* Swiss Mix), 3 oz. ...	25	2.0	5.0	0	0	0	36	1.0 c
(*Stokely Singles*), 3 oz.	20	2.0	4.0	1.0	0	0	15	m.q.
medley (*Green Giant Valley* *Combinations*), ½ cup	30	2.0	10.0	1.0	(0)	0	80	3.0 d
cauliflower and carrots:								
(*Birds Eye* Farm Fresh), 4 oz.	35	2.0	7.0	0	0	0	40	3.0 d
baby (*Stokely Singles*), 3 oz.	25	2.0	5.0	1.0	(0)	0	25	m.q.
no sauce (*Green Giant* One Serving), 4 oz.	25	2.0	7.0	0	0	0	45	3.0 d
in butter sauce (*Birds Eye* Butter Sauce Combinations), 3.3 oz. ..	45	2.0	6.0	2.0	m.q.	5	290	2.0 d
in butter sauce (*Green Giant*), ½ cup	30	1.0	6.0	1.0	<1.0	5	240	3.0 d
w/cheese sauce (*Birds Eye* Cheese Sauce Combinations), 4.5 oz. ..	110	5.0	11.0	5.0	m.q.	5	410	2.0 d
in cheese sauce (*Birds Eye For One*), 5 oz.	110	6.0	11.0	5.0	m.q.	5	410	2.0 d
in cheese sauce (*Green Giant* One Serving), 5 oz.	70	3.0	12.0	3.0	<1.0	5	610	2.0 d
in cheese-flavored sauce (*Green Giant*), ½ cup	60	3.0	9.0	2.0	<1.0	2	490	2.0 d
baby, in cheese sauce (*Stokely Singles*), 4 oz.	70	4.0	8.0	3.0	m.q.	15	180	m.q.
cauliflower and red peppers (*Birds Eye* Farm Fresh), 4 oz.	30	3.0	5.0	0	0	0	25	3.0 d
corn and red peppers (*Birds Eye* Farm Fresh), 4 oz.	60	3.0	14.0	1.0	(0)	0	15	3.0 d
fanfare (*Green Giant Valley* *Combinations*), ½ cup	70	3.0	13.0	2.0	m.q.	n.a.	330	2.9 d
green beans, pearl onions and red peppers (*Birds Eye* Farm Fresh), 4 oz.	35	2.0	7.0	0	0	0	15	3.0 d
red peppers, bamboo shoots and straw mushrooms (*Birds Eye* Farm Fresh), 4 oz.	30	3.0	5.0	0	0	0	20	3.0 d
w/rotini, in cheese sauce (*Green Giant* One Serving), 5.5 oz. ...	120	4.0	20.0	3.0	<1.0	5	520	m.q.
BROTH, see "Bouillon, dehydrated" and "Soup"								
BROTWURST, see "Bratwurst"								
BROWN GRAVY:								
canned or in jars:								
(*Heinz* HomeStyle), 2 oz. or ¼ cup	25	1.0	3.0	1.0	n.a.	n.a.	320	n.a.
(*McCormick/Schilling*), ⅓ cup ...	30	.7	4.7	1.0	n.a.	n.a.	417	n.a.

Food and Measure	cal.	prot. (gms)	carbo. (gms)	tot. fat (gms)	sat. fat (gms)	chol. (mgs)	sod. (mgs)	fiber (gms)
BROWN GRAVY *(cont.)*								
w/onions *(Heinz* HomeStyle), 2 oz.								
of ¼ cup	25	10	3.0	1.0	n.a.	n.a.	330	m.q.
mix[1]:								
dry, .75-oz. pkg.	75	2.4	13.1	1.7	.8	2	1072	.1 c
prepared w/water, ¼ cup	19	.6	3.3	.4	.2	<1	269	<.1 c
(French's), ¼ cup	20	1.0	4.0	1.0	n.a.	n.a.	250	n.a.
(Hain), ¼ pkg. dry	16	1.0	3.0	0	0	0	600	n.a.
(Lawry's), 1 cup	94	3.8	16.5	1.4	n.a.	n.a.	1500	.1 c
(McCormick/Schilling), 1 pkg. dry	91	2.0	14.0	3.0	m.q.	n.a.	1251	n.a.
(McCormick/Schilling), ¼ cup ...	23	.5	3.5	.8	n.a.	n.a.	313	n.a.
(McCormick/Schilling Lite), ¼ cup	10	<1.0	2.0	1.0	n.a.	n.a.	450	n.a.
(Pillsbury), ¼ cup	15	<1.0	3.0	0	0	0	300	n.a.
(Tone's), 1 tsp. dry	10	.3	2.0	.2	.1	<1	239	<.1 d
BROWNIE (see also "Cookie"):								
Dutch chocolate *(Awrey's* Cake),								
¹⁄₁₆ cake	340	3.0	40.0	20.0	4.0	35	260	1.0 d
fudge:								
(Little Debbie), 2-oz. piece	240	3.0	39.0	8.0	m.q.	<1	140	m.q.
(Little Debbie), 3-oz. piece	350	4.0	57.0	12.0	m.q.	<1	180	m.q.
nut *(Awrey's* Sheet Cake), 1.25-oz.								
piece	150	2.0	16.0	9.0	1.0	25	115	1.0 d
nut, iced *(Awrey's* Sheet Cake),								
2.5-oz. piece	300	3.0	36.0	17.0	3.0	40	210	1.0 d
walnut *(Tastykake),* 3-oz. piece ...	335	3.9	53.4	14.2	3.3	22	222	5.4 d
BROWNIE, FROZEN:								
chocolate *(Weight Watchers),* ⅓ pkg.,								
1.25 oz.	100	3.0	16.0	3.0	<1.0	5	150	m.q.
chocolate chip, double *(Nestlé* Toll								
House Ready to Bake), 1.4 oz.	150	2.0	19.0	7.0	m.q.	n.a.	60	m.q.
hot fudge *(Pepperidge Farm*								
Newport), 1 ramekin	400	4.0	50.0	20.0	10.0	80	160	m.q.
BROWNIE MIX[2], 1 piece:								
(Duncan Hines Gourmet Truffle)	280	2.0	38.0	13.0	m.q.	n.a.	110	m.q.
(Duncan Hines Gourmet Turtle)	240	3.0	34.0	10.0	m.q.	n.a.	145	m.q.
(Estee), 2″ square	50	<1.0	8.0	2.0	<1.0	0	5	m.q.
caramel fudge chunk *(Pillsbury),*								
2″ square	170	2.0	25.0	7.0	m.q.	n.a.	105	m.q.
caramel swirl *(Betty Crocker),*								
approx. .9 oz.	120	1.0	21.0	4.0	1.0	10	115	m.q.
chocolate, German *(Betty Crocker),*								
approx. 1 oz.	160	1.0	24.0	7.0	2.0	10	110	m.q.
chocolate, milk *(Duncan Hines)*	160	1.0	22.0	7.0	m.q.	n.a.	95	m.q.
chocolate chip *(Betty Crocker),*								
approx. .9 oz.	140	1.0	20.0	6.0	2.0	10	75	m.q.
frosted *(Betty Crocker),* approx.								
1.1 oz.	160	1.0	26.0	6.0	2.0	10	120	m.q.

1. *Prepared according to package directions, except as noted.*
2. *Prepared according to package directions.*

Food and Measure	cal.	prot. (gms)	carbo. (gms)	tot. fat (gms)	sat. fat (gms)	chol. (mgs)	sod. (mgs)	fiber (gms)
frosted (*Betty Crocker MicroRave*),								
approx. 1.3 oz.	180	2.0	27.0	7.0	2.0	0	120	m.q.
fudge:								
(*Betty Crocker*), approx. .9 oz.	150	1.0	23.0	6.0	1.0	15	105	m.q.
(*Betty Crocker* Family Size),								
approx. .9 oz.	140	1.0	22.0	5.0	1.0	10	100	m.q.
(*Betty Crocker* Supreme), approx.								
1 oz.	120	1.0	21.0	3.0	1.0	10	85	m.q.
(*Betty Crocker MicroRave*),								
approx. 1 oz.	150	2.0	22.0	6.0	2.0	0	110	m.q.
(*Duncan Hines*)	160	2.0	22.0	7.0	m.q.	n.a.	105	m.q.
(*Finast* Ultra Moist), 1/16 pkg. ...	130	2.0	20.0	5.0	m.q.	n.a.	120	m.q.
(*Pillsbury* Microwave)	190	2.0	25.0	9.0	m.q.	n.a.	105	m.q.
(*Robin Hood/Gold Medal* Pouch								
Mix), 1/16 pkg.	100	1.0	16.0	4.0	m.q.	n.a.	85	m.q.
chewy (*Duncan Hines*)	130	1.0	18.0	5.0	m.q.	n.a.	90	m.q.
deluxe (*Pillsbury*), 2″ square	150	2.0	21.0	6.0	m.q.	n.a.	100	m.q.
deluxe (*Pillsbury* Family Size),								
2″ square	150	1.0	20.0	7.0	m.q.	n.a.	95	m.q.
deluxe, w/walnuts (*Pillsbury*),								
2″ square	150	2.0	19.0	8.0	m.q.	n.a.	90	m.q.
double (*Pillsbury*), 2″ square	160	2.0	24.0	6.0	m.q.	n.a.	105	m.q.
peanut butter (*Duncan Hines*) ...	150	3.0	16.0	8.0	m.q.	n.a.	105	m.q.
triple, chunky (*Pillsbury*),								
2″ square	170	2.0	25.0	7.0	m.q.	n.a.	105	m.q.
rocky road, fudge (*Pillsbury*),								
2″ square	170	2.0	24.0	8.0	m.q.	n.a.	95	m.q.
walnut:								
(*Betty Crocker*), approx. .9 oz.	140	1.0	18.0	7.0	1.0	10	80	m.q.
(*Betty Crocker MicroRave*),								
approx. 1.1 oz.	160	2.0	21.0	7.0	2.0	0	95	m.q.
(*Finast* Ultra Moist), 1/16 pkg. ...	130	1.0	19.0	6.0	m.q.	n.a.	110	m.q.
white, Vienna (*Duncan Hines*)	240	3.0	29.0	12.0	m.q.	n.a.	135	m.q.
BROWNING SAUCE:								
(*Gravymaster*), 1 tsp.	12	.5	2.4	tr.	(0)	0	<1	tr.c
BRUSSELS SPROUTS:								
raw:								
untrimmed, 1 lb.	174	13.8	36.6	1.2	.3	0	101	6.2 c
trimmed, 1 oz.	12	1.0	2.5	.1	<.1	0	7	.4 c
trimmed, ½ cup	19	1.5	3.9	.1	<.1	0	11	.7 c
1 sprout, approx. .7 oz.	8	.6	1.7	.1	<.1	0	5	.3 c
boiled, drained:								
4 oz.	44	2.9	9.8	.6	.1	0	24	4.9 d
½ cup	30	2.0	6.8	.4	.1	0	17	3.4 d
1 sprout, approx. .7 oz.	8	.5	1.8	.1	<.1	0	4	.9 d
BRUSSELS SPROUTS, FROZEN:								
10-oz. pkg.	116	10.7	22.4	1.2	.2	0	28	6.2 d
boiled, drained, 4 oz.	48	4.1	9.4	.4	.1	0	26	2.0 d
boiled, drained, ½ cup	33	2.8	6.5	.3	.1	0	18	1.4 d

Food and Measure	cal.	prot. (gms)	carbo. (gms)	tot. fat (gms)	sat. fat (gms)	chol. (mgs)	sod. (mgs)	fiber (gms)
BRUSSELS SPROUTS, FROZEN *(cont.)*								
(*A&P*), 3.3 oz.	35	3.0	7.0	<1.0	(0)	0	15	m.q.
(*Birds Eye*), 3.3 oz.	35	3.0	7.0	0	0	0	15	3.0 d
(*Frosty Acres*), 3.3 oz.	35	3.0	7.0	0	0	0	12	1.0 c
(*Green Giant* Polybag), ½ cup	25	2.0	6.0	0	0	0	10	2.0 d
(*Seabrook*), 3.3 oz.	35	3.0	7.0	0	0	0	12	1.0 c
(*Southern*), 3.5 oz.	37	3.2	7.5	0	0	0	20	m.q.
(*Stokely Singles*), 3 oz.	35	4.0	7.0	0	0	0	10	m.q.
baby (*Seabrook*), 3.3 oz.	40	4.0	7.0	0	0	0	5	1.0 c
in butter sauce (*Green Giant*), ½ cup	40	3.0	8.0	1.0	<1.0	5	280	4.0 d
in butter sauce (*Stokely Singles*), 4 oz.	50	4.0	10.0	1.0	n.a.	5	325	m.q.
w/cauliflower and carrots (*Birds Eye* Farm Fresh), 4 oz.	40	3.0	8.0	0	0	0	30	4.0 d
w/cheese sauce, baby (*Birds Eye* Cheese Sauce Combinations), 4.5 oz.	130	6.0	12.0	7.0	m.q.	5	500	2.0 d
BUCKWHEAT, whole grain:								
1 oz.	97	3.8	20.3	1.0	.2	0	<1	m.q.
1 cup	584	22.5	121.6	5.8	1.3	0	1	m.q.
BUCKWHEAT FLOUR:								
1 oz.	95	3.6	20.0	.9	.2	0	n.a.	m.q.
1 cup	402	15.1	84.7	3.7	.8	0	n.a.	m.q.
whole grain (*Arrowhead Mills*), 2 oz.	190	7.0	41.0	1.0	n.a.	0	0	7.1 d
BUCKWHEAT GROATS:								
brown or white (*Arrowhead Mills*), 2 oz.	190	7.0	41.0	1.0	n.a.	0	1	7.1 d
roasted:								
dry, 1 oz.	98	3.3	21.2	.8	.2	0	3	.5 c
dry, 1 cup	567	19.2	122.9	4.4	1.0	0	18	3.0 c
cooked, 4 oz.	104	3.8	22.6	.7	.1	0	5	.6 c
cooked, 1 cup	182	6.7	39.5	1.2	.3	0	8	1.0 c
BUFFALO, WATER, see "Water buffalo"								
BULGUR (see also "Tabbouleh mix"):								
dry, 1 oz.	97	3.5	21.5	.4	<.1	0	5	5.2 d
dry, 1 cup	479	17.2	106.2	1.9	.3	0	23	25.6 d
cooked, 4 oz.	94	3.5	21.1	.3	.1	0	6	.4 c
cooked, 1 cup	152	5.6	33.8	.4	.1	0	9	.6 c
BULLOCK'S HEART, see "Custard apple"								
BUN, see "Roll"								
BUN, SWEET, honey (see also "Roll, sweet"), 1 piece:								
glazed (*Hostess Breakfast Bake Shop*)	360	5.0	38.0	21.0	10.0	15	230	.8 d
glazed (*Tastykake*), 3.25 oz.	362	5.9	42.3	20.4	4.3	<2	219	3.6 d

Food and Measure	cal.	prot. (gms)	carbo. (gms)	tot. fat (gms)	sat. fat (gms)	chol. (mgs)	sod. (mgs)	fiber (gms)
iced (*Hostess Breakfast Bake Shop*)	430	5.0	55.0	22.0	10.0	20	240	1.7 d
iced (*Tastykake*), 3.25 oz.	348	5.0	50.0	14.9	3.3	<2	254	1.5 d
BUN, SWEET, FROZEN (see also "Roll, frozen"):								
cinnamon (*Rich's Ever Fresh*), 2.5-oz.								
piece	293	4.0	38.0	14.6	m.q.	n.a.	m.q.	m.q.
honey, mini (*Rich's Ever Fresh*),								
1.36-oz. piece	133	1.8	17.5	6.6	m.q.	n.a.	m.q.	m.q.
BURBOT, meat only, raw:								
1 lb.	407	87.6	0	3.7	.7	270	438	0
1 oz.	26	5.5	0	.2	<.1	17	27	0
1 fillet, approx. 4.1 oz., yield from								
1½-lb. whole fish	104	22.4	0	.9	.2	69	112	0
BURDOCK ROOT:								
raw:								
untrimmed, 1 lb.	245	5.2	59.0	.5	(0)	0	17	6.6 c
trimmed, 1 oz.	20	.4	4.9	<.1	(0)	0	1	.5 c
1 medium, approx. 7.3 oz.	112	1.3	13.6	.1	(0)	0	4	1.5 c
pieces, ½ cup	43	.9	10.3	.1	(0)	0	3	1.2 c
boiled, drained:								
4 oz.	100	2.4	24.0	.2	(0)	0	5	2.1 c
1 medium, approx. 5.9 oz.	146	3.5	35.1	.2	(0)	0	7	3.0 c
1" pieces, ½ cup	55	1.3	13.2	.1	(0)	0	3	1.2 c
BURGER KING:								
breakfast, 1 serving:								
bagel	272	10.0	44.0	6.0	1.0	29	438	m.q.
bagel, w/cream cheese	370	12.0	45.0	16.0	6.0	58	523	m.q.
bagel sandwich:								
w/bacon, egg, and cheese	453	21.0	46.0	20.0	7.0	252	872	m.q.
w/egg and cheese	407	19.0	46.0	16.0	5.0	247	759	m.q.
w/ham, egg, and cheese	438	25.0	46.0	17.0	6.0	266	1114	m.q.
w/sausage, egg, and cheese ...	626	27.0	49.0	36.0	12.0	293	1137	m.q.
biscuit:								
plain	332	5.0	42.0	17.0	3.0	2	754	m.q.
w/bacon	378	8.0	42.0	20.0	5.0	8	867	m.q.
w/bacon and egg	467	14.0	43.0	27.0	7.0	213	1033	m.q.
w/sausage	478	11.0	44.0	29.0	8.0	33	1007	m.q.
w/sausage and egg	568	17.0	45.0	36.0	10.0	238	1172	m.q.
croissant	180	4.0	18.0	10.0	2.0	4	285	m.q.
Croissan'wich:								
w/bacon, egg, and cheese	361	15.0	19.0	24.0	8.0	227	719	m.q.
w/egg and cheese	315	13.0	19.0	20.0	7.0	222	607	m.q.
w/ham, egg, and cheese	346	19.0	19.0	21.0	7.0	241	962	m.q.
w/sausage, egg, and cheese ...	534	21.0	22.0	40.0	13.0	268	985	m.q.
danish:								
apple cinnamon	390	6.0	62.0	13.0	3.0	19	305	m.q.
cheese	406	6.0	60.0	16.0	5.0	7	454	m.q.
cinnamon raisin	449	7.0	63.0	18.0	4.0	15	286	m.q.
french toast sticks	538	10.0	53.0	32.0	5.0	80	537	m.q.

Food and Measure	cal.	prot. (gms)	carbo. (gms)	tot. fat (gms)	sat. fat (gms)	chol. (mgs)	sod. (mgs)	fiber (gms)
BURGER KING, BREAKFAST *(cont.)*								
mini muffins:								
blueberry	292	4.0	37.0	14.0	3.0	72	244	m.q.
lemon poppyseed	318	5.0	33.0	18.0	3.0	72	253	m.q.
raisin oat bran	291	5.0	46.0	12.0	2.0	0	343	m.q.
scrambled egg platter:								
regular	549	17.0	44.0	34.0	9.0	365	893	m.q.
w/bacon	610	21.0	44.0	39.0	11.0	373	1043	m.q.
w/sausage	768	26.0	47.0	53.0	15.0	412	1271	m.q.
Tater Tenders	213	2.0	25.0	12.0	3.0	0	318	m.q.
sandwiches, 1 serving:								
bacon double cheeseburger	515	32.0	26.0	31.0	14.0	105	748	m.q.
bacon double cheeseburger deluxe	592	33.0	28.0	39.0	16.0	111	804	m.q.
barbecue bacon double								
cheeseburger	536	32.0	31.0	31.0	14.0	105	795	m.q.
Burger Buddies	349	18.0	31.0	17.0	7.0	52	717	m.q.
chicken sandwich	685	26.0	56.0	40.0	8.0	82	1417	m.q.
chicken sandwich, BK Broiler . . .	379	24.0	31.0	18.0	3.0	53	764	m.q.
cheeseburger	318	17.0	28.0	15.0	7.0	48	651	m.q.
cheeseburger, double	483	30.0	29.0	27.0	13.0	100	851	m.q.
cheeseburger deluxe	390	18.0	29.0	23.0	8.0	56	652	m.q.
hamburger	272	15.0	28.0	11.0	4.0	37	505	m.q.
hamburger deluxe	344	15.0	28.0	19.0	6.0	43	496	m.q.
mushroom Swiss double								
cheeseburger	473	31.0	27.0	27.0	12.0	95	746	m.q.
Ocean Catch fish fillet	495	20.0	49.0	25.0	4.0	57	879	m.q.
Whopper	614	27.0	45.0	36.0	12.0	90	865	m.q.
Whopper, w/cheese	706	32.0	47.0	44.0	16.0	115	1177	m.q.
Whopper, double	844	46.0	45.0	53.0	19.0	169	933	m.q.
Whopper, double, w/cheese	935	51.0	47.0	61.0	24.0	194	1245	m.q.
sandwich condiments/toppings:								
bacon bits, 1 pkt.	16	1.0	0	1.0	n.a.	5	n.a.	n.a.
BK Broiler sauce, .5 oz.	90	0	0	10.0	1.0	7	95	n.a.
Bull's-Eye barbecue sauce, .5 oz.	22	0	5.0	0	0	0	47	n.a.
cheese, American, .9 oz.	92	5.0	1.0	7.0	5.0	25	312	0
cheese, Swiss, .9 oz.	82	6.0	1.0	6.0	4.0	20	352	0
cream cheese, 1 oz.	98	2.0	1.0	10.0	5.0	28	86	0
croutons, .25 oz.	31	1.0	5.0	1.0	n.a.	n.a.	90	n.a.
lettuce, .75 oz.	3	0	0	0	0	0	2	m.q.
mayonnaise, 1 oz.	194	0	2.0	21.0	4.0	16	142	0
mushroom topping, .8 oz.	13	1.0	1.0	1.0	n.a.	0	70	n.a.
mustard, 1 pkt.	2	0	0	0	0	0	34	n.a.
onion, .25 oz.	5	0	1.0	0	0	0	0	m.q.
pickles, .5 oz.	1	0	0	0	0	0	119	m.q.
tartar sauce, 1 oz.	134	0	2.0	14.0	2.0	20	202	n.a.
tomato, 1 oz.	6	0	1.0	0	0	0	3	m.q.
Chicken Tenders, 6 pieces	236	16.0	14.0	13.0	3.0	46	541	m.q.
dipping sauces, 1 oz.:								
barbecue	36	0	9.0	0	0	0	397	n.a.

Food and Measure	cal.	prot. (gms)	carbo. (gms)	tot. fat (gms)	sat. fat (gms)	chol. (mgs)	sod. (mgs)	fiber (gms)
Burger King A.M. Express	84	0	21.0	0	0	0	18	n.a.
honey	91	0	23.0	0	0	0	12	n.a.
ranch	171	0	2.0	18.0	3.0	0	208	n.a.
sweet & sour	45	0	11.0	0	0	0	52	n.a.
salad, w/out dressing, 1 serving:								
chef salad	178	17.0	7.0	9.0	4.0	103	568	m.q.
chunky chicken salad	142	20.0	8.0	4.0	1.0	49	443	m.q.
garden salad	95	6.0	8.0	5.0	3.0	15	125	m.q.
side salad	25	1.0	5.0	0	0	0	27	m.q.
Newman's Own salad dressings, 1 pkt.:								
bleu cheese	300	3.0	2.0	32.0	7.0	58	512	0
French	290	0	23.0	22.0	3.0	0	400	n.a.
Italian, reduced calorie	170	0	3.0	18.0	3.0	0	762	n.a.
olive oil and vinegar	310	0	2.0	33.0	5.0	0	214	0
ranch	350	1.0	4.0	37.0	7.0	20	316	n.a.
Thousand Island	290	1.0	15.0	26.0	5.0	36	403	n.a.
side dishes, 1 serving:								
french fries, medium, salted	372	5.0	43.0	20.0	5.0	0	238	m.q.
onion rings	339	5.0	38.0	19.0	5.0	0	628	m.q.
dessert and shakes, 1 serving:								
apple pie	311	3.0	44.0	14.0	4.0	4	412	m.q.
chocolate shake	326	9.0	49.0	10.0	6.0	31	198	n.a.
chocolate shake, syrup added	409	10.0	68.0	11.0	6.0	33	248	n.a.
strawberry shake, syrup added ..	394	9.0	66.0	10.0	6.0	33	230	n.a.
vanilla shake	334	9.0	51.0	10.0	6.0	33	213	(0)
"BURGER," VEGETARIAN:								
canned (*Worthington Vegetarian Burger*), ½ cup	150	19.0	9.0	4.0	1.0	0	780	m.q.
canned (*Worthington Vegetarian Burger* No Salt Added), ½ cup	160	17.0	9.0	6.0	m.q.	0	500	m.q.
frozen (*Morningstar Farms Grillers*), 2.25-oz. patty	180	13.0	5.0	12.0	2.0	0	350	m.q.
frozen (*Worthington FriPats*), 2.25-oz. piece	180	13.0	5.0	12.0	2.0	0	350	m.q.
mix[1]:								
(*Love Natural Foods Loveburger*), 2 oz. mix, 4 oz. burger	245	17.0	20.0	11.0	m.q.	0	224	8.0 d
(*Nature's Burger* Original), 3-oz. burger[2]	152	7.0	21.0	4.0	m.q.	0	228	m.q.
(*Worthington Granburger*), 6 tbsp. mix	110	19.9	7.0	1.0	n.a.	0	700	m.q.
barbecue (*Nature's Burger*), 3-oz. burger[2]	117	4.0	24.0	.8	n.a.	0	423	m.q.
pizza (*Nature's Burger*), 3-oz. burger[2]	121	5.0	24.0	1.0	n.a.	0	406	m.q.

1. *Prepared according to package directions, except as noted.*
2. *Does not include value for fat from butter or oil used in cooking.*

Food and Measure	cal.	prot. (gms)	carbo. (gms)	tot. fat (gms)	sat. fat (gms)	chol. (mgs)	sod. (mgs)	fiber (gms)
"BURGER," VEGETARIAN, MIX *(cont.)*								
w/tofu (*Fantastic Foods*), 3.4-oz.								
burger[1]	133	11.0	14.0	5.0	m.q.	n.a.	320	m.q.
BURGUNDY, see "Wine"								
BURRITO, frozen:								
(*Hormel* Burrito Grande), 5½ oz.	380	14.0	45.0	16.0	m.q.	n.a.	877	m.q.
bean and cheese (*Old El Paso*),								
1 piece	330	14.0	45.0	11.0	m.q.	m.q.	740	m.q.
beef:								
(*Hormel*), 1 piece	205	9.0	31.0	8.0	m.q.	m.q.	780	m.q.
beef and bean:								
(*Patio*), 5-oz. pkg.	370	11.0	43.0	16.0	m.q.	m.q.	830	m.q.
(*Patio Britos*), 3.63 oz.	250	6.0	33.0	10.0	m.q.	15	340	m.q.
green chili (*Patio*), 5-oz. pkg.	330	12.0	43.0	12.0	m.q.	m.q.	770	m.q.
hot (*Old El Paso*), 1 piece	310	12.0	41.0	11.0	m.q.	m.q.	710	m.q.
medium (*Old El Paso*), 1 piece	330	13.0	41.0	13.0	5.0	29	630	m.q.
mild (*Old El Paso*), 1 piece	320	13.0	42.0	11.0	m.q.	m.q.	500	m.q.
and bean red chili (*Patio*), 5-oz.								
pkg.	340	11.0	44.0	13.0	m.q.	m.q.	810	m.q.
nacho (*Patio Britos*), 3.63 oz.	270	9.0	30.0	13.0	m.q.	25	420	m.q.
cheese (*Hormel*), 1 piece	210	9.0	32.0	5.0	m.q.	m.q.	792	m.q.
cheese, nacho (*Patio Britos*),								
3.63 oz.	250	7.0	32.0	10.0	m.q.	20	330	m.q.
chicken, spicy (*Patio Britos*),								
3.63 oz.	250	6.0	33.0	10.0	m.q.	25	330	m.q.
chicken and rice (*Hormel*), 1 piece	200	9.0	32.0	4.0	m.q.	m.q.	594	m.q.
chili:								
green (*Patio Britos*), 3.63 oz.	250	6.0	33.0	10.0	m.q.	15	420	m.q.
hot (*Hormel*), 1 piece	240	9.0	33.0	8.0	m.q.	m.q.	619	m.q.
red (*Patio Britos*), 3.63 oz.	240	6.0	31.0	10.0	m.q.	15	370	m.q.
red hot (*Patio*), 5-oz. pkg.	360	12.0	43.0	15.0	m.q.	m.q.	800	m.q.
BURRITO DINNER, frozen:								
(*Patio*), 12 oz.	517	18.0	74.0	16.0	m.q.	m.q.	1643	m.q.
beef and bean (*Old El Paso* Festive								
Dinners), 11 oz.	470	23.0	72.0	9.0	m.q.	m.q.	1180	m.q.
BURRITO DINNER MIX:								
(*Old El Paso*), 1 burrito[2]	299	11.0	36.0	13.0	4.0	23	430	4.0 d
(*Tio Sancho* Dinner Kit):								
seasoning mix, 3.25 oz.	265	12.3	49.3	2.1	n.a.	n.a.	5031	5.5 c
1 tortilla	125	3.3	24.0	1.9	n.a.	n.a.	569	.1 c
BURRITO ENTREE, frozen:								
bean and cheese (*Old El Paso*),								
1 pkg.	340	19.0	43.0	13.0	m.q.	m.q.	770	m.q.
beef and bean:								
hot (*Old El Paso*), 1 pkg.	340	11.0	41.0	14.0	m.q.	m.q.	950	m.q.
medium (*Old El Paso*), 1 pkg.	330	11.0	41.0	14.0	m.q.	m.q.	730	m.q.
mild (*Old El Paso*), 1 pkg.	330	12.0	40.0	13.0	m.q.	m.q.	660	m.q.
chicken (*Weight Watchers*), 7.62 oz.	310	15.0	34.0	13.0	4.0	60	790	m.q.

1. *Does not include value for fat from butter or oil used in cooking.*
2. *Prepared according to package directions, with filling.*

Food and Measure	cal.	prot. (gms)	carbo. (gms)	tot. fat (gms)	sat. fat (gms)	chol. (mgs)	sod. (mgs)	fiber (gms)
BURRITO FILLING MIX:								
beans (*Del Monte*), ½ cup	110	6.0	20.0	1.0	n.a.	n.a.	900	n.a.
BURRITO SEASONING MIX:								
(*Lawry's*), 1 pkg.	132	6.0	23.3	1.7	n.a.	0	2516	.9 c
(*Old El Paso*), ⅛ pkg.	17	1.0	3.0	0	0	0	275	1.0 d
BUSH NUT, see "Macadamia nut"								
BUTTER:								
regular:								
1 stick or 4 oz.	813	1.0	0	92.0	57.2	248	12	0
1 tbsp.	100	.1	0	11.4	7.1	31	1	0
1 tsp.	34	<.1	0	3.8	2.4	10	<1	0
(*Darigold* Quarters), 1 tsp.	35	0	0	4.0	2.5	11	<2	0
(*Land O'Lakes*), 1 tsp.	35	0	0	4.0	m.q.	10	0	0
regular, salted:								
1 stick or 4 oz.	813	1.0	0	92.0	57.2	248	937	0
1 tbsp.	100	.1	0	11.4	7.1	31	115	0
1 tsp.	34	<.1	0	3.8	2.4	10	39	0
1 pat, 90 per lb.	36	<.1	0	4.1	2.5	11	41	0
(*Darigold* Lightly Salted), 1 tsp. . . .	25	0	0	3.0	1.7	7	25	0
(*Darigold* Quarters), 1 tsp.	35	0	0	4.0	2.5	11	40	0
(*Hotel Bar/Kellers*), 1 tsp.	35	0	0	4.0	m.q.	m.q.	35	0
(*Land O'Lakes*), 1 tsp.	35	0	0	4.0	m.q.	10	40	0
whipped:								
½ cup or 1 stick	542	.6	<.1	61.3	38.2	165	8	0
1 tbsp.	67	.1	tr.	7.6	4.7	20	1	0
1 tsp.	23	tr.	tr.	2.6	1.6	7	<1	0
1 pat, 1¼″ × ⅓″, 120 per lb. . . .	27	<.1	tr.	3.1	1.9	8	1	0
(*Breakstone's*), 1 tbsp.	70	0	0	7.0	m.q.	m.q.	n.a.	0
(*Darigold*), 1 tsp.	25	0	0	3.0	1.6	7	<2	0
(*Land O'Lakes*), 1 tsp.	25	0	0	3.0	m.q.	5	0	0
whipped, salted:								
½ cup or 1 stick	542	.6	<.1	61.3	38.2	165	625	0
1 tbsp.	67	.1	tr.	7.6	4.7	20	78	0
1 tsp.	23	tr.	tr.	2.6	1.6	7	26	0
1 pat, 120 per lb.	27	<.1	tr.	3.1	1.9	8	31	0
(*Land O'Lakes*), 1 tsp.	25	0	0	3.0	m.q.	5	25	0
BUTTER OIL:								
1 oz.	248	.1	0	28.2	17.6	73	n.a.	0
1 tbsp.	112	<.1	0	12.7	7.9	33	n.a.	0
BUTTERBEAN, see "Lima bean"								
BUTTERBUR:								
raw:								
untrimmed, 1 lb.	57	1.6	14.4	.2	(0)	0	28	5.2 c
trimmed, 1 oz.	4	.1	1.0	<.1	(0)	0	2	.4 c
trimmed, ½ cup	7	.2	1.7	<.1	(0)	0	4	.6 c
1 stalk, approx. .2 oz.	1	<.1	.2	tr.	(0)	0	tr.	.1 c
boiled, drained, 4 oz.	9	.3	2.4	<.1	(0)	0	5	.9 c
BUTTERBUR, CANNED:								
4 oz.	12	.1	.4	.1	(0)	0	5	1.2 c

Food and Measure	cal.	prot. (gms)	carbo. (gms)	tot. fat (gms)	sat. fat (gms)	chol. (mgs)	sod. (mgs)	fiber (gms)
BUTTERBUR, CANNED *(cont.)*								
3 stalks, approx. 1.6 oz.	1	<.1	.2	<.1	(0)	0	2	.4 c
chopped, ½ cup	2	.1	.2	.1	(0)	0	3	.6 c
BUTTERFISH, meat only, raw:								
1 lb.	663	78.4	0	36.4	m.q.	295	401	0
1 oz.	41	4.9	0	2.3	m.q.	18	25	0
1 fillet, approx. 1.1 oz., yield from								
½-lb. whole fish	47	5.5	0	2.6	m.q.	21	28	0
BUTTERMILK, see "Milk" and								
"Milk, dry"								
BUTTERNUT, dried:								
in shell, 1 lb.	750	30.5	14.8	69.8	1.6	0	1	2.3 c
shelled, 1 oz.	174	7.1	3.4	16.2	.4	0	tr.	.5 c
BUTTERNUT SQUASH:								
raw:								
untrimmed, 1 lb.	172	3.8	44.6	.4	.1	0	15	5.3 c
trimmed, 1 oz.	13	.3	3.3	<.1	tr.	0	1	.4 c
cubed, ½ cup	32	.7	8.1	.1	<.1	0	3	1.0 c
baked, 4 oz.	45	1.0	11.9	.1	<.1	0	5	1.4 c
baked, cubed, ½ cup	41	.9	10.7	.1	<.1	0	4	1.3 c
BUTTERNUT SQUASH,								
FROZEN:								
12-oz. pkg.	192	6.0	49.0	.3	.1	0	8	4.2 c
boiled, drained, 4 oz.	44	1.4	11.4	.1	<.1	0	2	1.0 c
boiled, drained, mashed, ½ cup	47	1.5	12.1	.1	<.1	0	2	1.0 c
BUTTERSCOTCH, see "Candy"								
BUTTERSCOTCH CHIPS,								
BAKING:								
(*Nestlé* Toll House Morsels), 1 oz. ..	150	1.0	19.0	8.0	m.q.	n.a.	25	(0)
BUTTERSCOTCH TOPPING:								
(*Kraft*), 1 tbsp.	60	0	13.0	1.0	0	0	70	(0)
caramel flavor (*Smucker's* Special								
Recipe), 2 tbsp.	160	1.0	33.0	3.0	n.a.	n.a.	40	(0)
flavor (*Smucker's*), 2 tbsp.	140	0	33.0	0	0	0	75	(0)

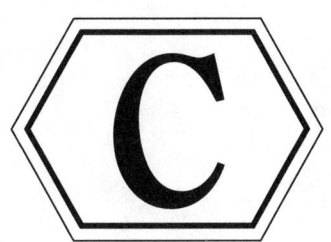

Food and Measure	cal.	prot. (gms)	carbo. (gms)	tot. fat (gms)	sat. fat (gms)	chol. (mgs)	sod. (mgs)	fiber (gms)
CABBAGE:								
raw:								
untrimmed, 1 lb.	86	4.4	19.5	.7	.1	0	65	4.0 d
trimmed, 1 oz.	7	.3	1.5	.1	tr.	0	5	.3 d
1 head, 5¾″ diam., approx.								
2.5 lb.	215	11.0	48.8	1.6	.2	0	164	10.0 d
shredded, ½ cup	8	.4	1.9	.1	tr.	0	6	.4 d
boiled, drained:								
4 oz.	24	1.1	5.4	.3	<.1	0	22	.7 c
1 head, approx. 2.8 lb.	270	12.1	60.2	3.1	.4	0	239	7.6 c
shredded, ½ cup	16	.7	3.6	.2	<.1	0	14	.5 c
CABBAGE, CHINESE:								
bok-choy:								
raw:								
untrimmed, 1 lb.	52	6.0	8.7	.8	.1	0	257	4.0 d
trimmed, 1 oz.	4	.4	.6	.1	tr.	0	19	.3 d
shredded, ½ cup	5	.5	.8	.1	tr.	0	23	.4 d
boiled, drained, 4 oz.	14	1.8	2.0	.2	<.1	0	39	1.8 d
boiled, drained, shredded, ½ cup	10	1.3	1.5	.1	<.1	0	29	1.4 d
pe-tsai:								
raw:								
untrimmed, 1 lb.	68	5.1	13.6	.8	.2	0	38	4.2 d
trimmed, 1 oz.	5	.3	.9	.1	<.1	0	3	.3 d
shredded, ½ cup	6	.5	1.2	.1	<.1	0	3	.4 d
boiled, drained:								
4 oz.	16	1.7	2.7	.2	<.1	0	10	1.8 d
1 leaf, approx. .5 oz.	2	.2	.3	<.1	tr.	0	1	.2 d
shredded, ½ cup	8	.9	1.4	.1	<.1	0	6	1.0 d

Food and Measure	cal.	prot. (gms)	carbo. (gms)	tot. fat (gms)	sat. fat (gms)	chol. (mgs)	sod. (mgs)	fiber (gms)
CABBAGE, RED:								
raw:								
untrimmed, 1 lb.	100	5.0	22.2	.9	.1	0	38	7.2 d
trimmed, 1 oz.	8	.4	1.7	.1	tr.	0	3	.6 d
shredded, ½ cup	10	.5	2.1	.1	<.1	0	4	.7 d
boiled, drained:								
4 oz.	24	1.2	5.3	.2	<.1	0	9	2.7 d
1 leaf, approx. .8 oz.	5	.2	1.0	<.1	tr.	0	2	.5 d
shredded, ½ cup	16	.8	3.5	.2	<.1	0	6	1.8 d
CABBAGE, SAVOY:								
raw:								
untrimmed, 1 lb.	100	7.3	22.1	.4	<.1	0	102	2.9 c
trimmed, 1 oz.	8	.6	1.7	<.1	tr.	0	8	.2 c
shredded, ½ cup	10	.7	2.1	<.1	tr.	0	10	.3 c
boiled, drained, 4 oz.	27	2.0	6.1	.1	<.1	0	27	.8 c
boiled, drained, shredded, ½ cup ..	18	1.3	4.0	.1	tr.	0	17	.5 c
CABBAGE, SWAMP, see "Swamp cabbage"								
CABBAGE ENTREE, frozen:								
stuffed, w/meat, in tomato sauce								
(*Lean Cuisine*), 10¾ oz.	220	14.0	19.0	10.0	2.0	55	930	m.q.
CABBAGE SALAD, see "Coleslaw"								
CADI, see "Cardoon"								
CAIMIT:								
ripe, trimmed, 1 oz.	19	.2	4.1	.5	n.a.	0	m.q.	.3 c
CAJUN SAUCE, see "Creole sauce"								
CAJUN SEASONING:								
(*Tone's*), 1 tsp.	9	.4	2.1	.2	<.1	0	215	.5 d
CAKE (see also "Cake, frozen," "Cake, snack" and "Cake mix"):								
(*Awrey's* Best Wishes), ¼ of 6" cake	150	1.0	18.0	9.0	3.0	25	170	0
(*Awrey's* Best Wishes, Miniature),								
3-oz. cake	320	5.0	33.0	22.0	9.0	0	280	0
(*Awrey's* Four-in-One Occasion),								
1.3-oz. piece	150	1.0	18.0	8.0	2.0	25	170	0
apple streusel (*Awrey's*), 2" × 2"								
piece	160	2.0	18.0	9.0	1.0	15	120	0
banana, iced (*Awrey's*), 2" × 2"								
piece	140	1.0	17.0	8.0	2.0	20	120	0
Black Forest torte (*Awrey's*), 1/14 cake	350	3.0	38.0	21.0	7.0	50	330	1.0 d
blueberry crunch (*Entenmann's*),								
1-oz. slice	70	1.0	16.0	0	0	0	85	m.q.
carrot supreme, iced (*Awrey's*), 2" ×								
2" piece	210	3.0	23.0	12.0	3.0	25	170	0
carrot, three-layer, cream cheese								
iced (*Awrey's*), 1/12 cake	390	5.0	44.0	23.0	5.0	45	310	1.0 d
chocolate:								
(*Awrey's*), .8-oz. piece	70	1.0	11.0	3.0	1.0	15	110	0

Food and Measure	cal.	prot. (gms)	carbo. (gms)	tot. fat (gms)	sat. fat (gms)	chol. (mgs)	sod. (mgs)	fiber (gms)
(*Awrey's* Happy Birthday), 1.4-oz. piece	150	1.0	18.0	8.0	3.0	25	150	1.0 d
double:								
iced (*Awrey's*), 2″ × 2″ piece ..	130	2.0	21.0	6.0	2.0	15	150	1.0 d
two-layer (*Awrey's*), 1/12 cake ..	250	3.0	38.0	11.0	3.0	35	260	1.0 d
three-layer (*Awrey's*), 1/12 cake	310	3.0	48.0	14.0	4.0	35	290	2.0 d
torte (*Awrey's*), 1/14 cake	340	3.0	51.0	15.0	4.0	35	300	2.0 d
German, iced (*Awrey's*), 2″ × 2″ piece	160	2.0	19.0	9.0	3.0	20	150	0
German, three-layer (*Awrey's*), 1/12 cake	350	3.0	46.0	18.0	6.0	40	300	1.0 d
milk, yellow, two-layer (*Awrey's*), 1/12 cake	290	3.0	33.0	17.0	5.0	50	320	0
white iced, two-layer (*Awrey's*), 1/12 cake	270	3.0	34.0	15.0	5.0	40	290	1.0 d
coconut, butter cream (*Awrey's*), 2″ × 2″ piece	160	1.0	19.0	9.0	3.0	25	180	0
coconut, yellow, three-layer (*Awrey's*), 1/12 cake	350	3.0	40.0	21.0	7.0	50	340	0
coffee:								
caramel nut (*Awrey's*), 1/12 cake ..	140	2.0	15.0	8.0	2.0	5	150	0
long john (*Awrey's*), 1/12 cake	160	2.0	19.0	8.0	2.0	10	130	0
devil's food, white iced (*Awrey's*), 2″ × 2″ piece	150	1.0	17.0	8.0	3.0	25	160	1.0 d
lemon, three-layer (*Awrey's*), 1/12 cake	320	2.0	38.0	19.0	5.0	45	310	0
lemon, yellow, two-layer (*Awrey's*), 1/12 cake	290	2.0	33.0	17.0	5.0	45	310	0
Neapolitan, torte (*Awrey's*), 1/14 cake	380	3.0	43.0	22.0	7.0	55	370	0
orange, frosty, iced (*Awrey's*), 2″ × 2″ piece	150	1.0	19.0	8.0	2.0	20	170	0
orange, three-layer (*Awrey's*), 1/12 cake	320	2.0	40.0	17.0	4.0	35	320	0
peanut butter, torte (*Awrey's*), 1/14 cake	380	7.0	44.0	22.0	5.0	40	340	1.0 d
pineapple crunch (*Entenmann's*), 1-oz. slice	70	1.0	16.0	0	0	0	85	m.q.
pistachio, torte (*Awrey's*), 1/14 cake	370	3.0	41.0	22.0	7.0	35	370	1.0 d
pound (*Drake's*), 1/10 cake, approx. 1.1 oz.	110	2.0	16.0	5.0	1.0	25	70	m.q.
pound, golden (*Awrey's*), 1/14 loaf ...	130	2.0	19.0	5.0	1.0	20	150	0
raisin spice, iced (*Awrey's*), 2″ × 2″ piece	160	1.0	21.0	8.0	2.0	20	120	0
raspberry nut (*Awrey's*), 1/16 cake ...	310	3.0	39.0	16.0	3.0	30	220	0
sponge (*Awrey's*), 2″ × 2″ piece	80	1.0	11.0	3.0	1.0	15	125	0
strawberry supreme, torte (*Awrey's*), 1/14 cake	270	3.0	38.0	12.0	3.0	45	310	1.0 d
walnut, torte (*Awrey's*), 1/14 cake ...	320	2.0	38.0	19.0	4.0	30	290	0
yellow (*Awrey's*), .9-oz. piece	80	1.0	12.0	3.0	1.0	20	135	0

Food and Measure	cal.	prot. (gms)	carbo. (gms)	tot. fat (gms)	sat. fat (gms)	chol. (mgs)	sod. (mgs)	fiber (gms)
CAKE *(cont.)*								
yellow, white iced (*Awrey's*), 2″ × 2″								
piece	150	1.0	18.0	9.0	3.0	25	180	0
CAKE, FROZEN (see also "Cake, snack, frozen"):								
banana, single layer, iced (*Sara Lee*),								
⅛ cake	170	1.0	28.0	6.0	m.q.	n.a.	160	m.q.
Black Forest, two-layer (*Sara Lee*),								
⅛ cake	190	2.0	28.0	8.0	m.q.	n.a.	100	m.q.
Boston cream (*Pepperidge Farm*								
Supreme), 2⅞ oz.	290	3.0	39.0	14.0	6.0	50	190	m.q.
Boston cream pie (*Weight Watchers*),								
½ pkg. or 3 oz.	160	3.0	34.0	4.0	1.0	5	260	m.q.
carrot:								
(*Weight Watchers*), ½ pkg. or								
3 oz.	170	4.0	27.0	5.0	<1.0	5	280	m.q.
cream cheese iced (*Pepperidge*								
Farm Old Fashioned), 1½ oz. ..	150	1.0	19.0	9.0	3.0	15	160	m.q.
single layer, iced (*Sara Lee*),								
⅛ cake	250	3.0	30.0	13.0	m.q.	25	240	m.q.
cheesecake:								
(*Weight Watchers*), ½ pkg.,								
3.9 oz.	210	10.0	29.0	7.0	2.0	20	230	m.q.
brownie (*Weight Watchers*), ½ pkg.								
or 3.5 oz.	200	9.0	34.0	5.0	1.0	10	260	m.q.
cream:								
plain (*Sara Lee*), ⅙ cake	230	5.0	27.0	11.0	m.q.	m.q.	153	m.q.
cherry (*Sara Lee*), ⅙ cake	243	4.0	35.0	8.0	m.q.	m.q.	184	m.q.
strawberry (*Sara Lee*), ⅙ cake	222	4.0	34.0	8.0	m.q.	m.q.	171	m.q.
French (*Sara Lee* Classics),								
⅛ cake	250	4.0	23.0	16.0	m.q.	20	120	m.q.
nondairy, see "cheesecake, nondairy," below								
strawberry (*Weight Watchers*),								
½ pkg. or 3.9 oz.	180	7.0	28.0	4.0	2.0	20	210	m.q.
strawberry, French (*Sara Lee*								
Classics), ⅛ cake	240	3.0	28.0	13.0	m.q.	20	125	m.q.
cheesecake, nondairy, all flavors								
(*Tofutti Better than Cheesecake*),								
⅒ cake or 2 oz.	160	2.0	16.0	10.0	m.q.	0	110	m.q.
cherries and cream (*Weight*								
Watchers), ½ pkg. or 3 oz.	190	3.0	32.0	6.0	1.0	5	200	m.q.
chocolate:								
(*Pepperidge Farm* Supreme),								
2⅞ oz.	300	3.0	37.0	16.0	7.0	25	140	m.q.
(*Sara Lee* Free & Light), ⅛ cake	110	2.0	26.0	0	0	0	140	m.q.
(*Weight Watchers*), ½ pkg.								
or 2.5 oz.	180	5.0	31.0	5.0	<1.0	5	250	m.q.

Food and Measure	cal.	prot. (gms)	carbo. (gms)	tot. fat (gms)	sat. fat (gms)	chol. (mgs)	sod. (mgs)	fiber (gms)
double, three layer (*Sara Lee*), ⅛ cake	220	3.0	26.0	11.0	m.q.	20	130	m.q.
fudge, double (*Weight Watchers*), ½ pkg. or 2.75 oz.	200	4.0	34.0	5.0	<1.0	5	190	m.q.
fudge layer (*Pepperidge Farm*), 1⅝ oz.	180	1.0	23.0	10.0	m.q.	20	140	m.q.
fudge stripe layer (*Pepperidge Farm*), 1⅝ oz.	170	2.0	20.0	9.0	3.0	20	140	m.q.
German (*Weight Watchers*), ½ pkg. or 2.5 oz.	200	4.0	31.0	7.0	<1.0	5	220	m.q.
German layer (*Pepperidge Farm*), 1⅝ oz.	180	1.0	22.0	10.0	4.0	20	170	m.q.
mousse (*Sara Lee* Classics), ⅛ cake	260	3.0	23.0	17.0	m.q.	20	100	m.q.
coconut layer (*Pepperidge Farm*), 1⅝ oz.	180	1.0	24.0	8.0	3.0	20	120	m.q.
coffee, all butter:								
cheese (*Sara Lee*), ⅛ cake	210	4.0	25.0	11.0	m.q.	m.q.	220	m.q.
pecan (*Sara Lee*), ⅛ cake	160	3.0	19.0	8.0	m.q.	m.q.	180	m.q.
streusel (*Sara Lee*), ⅛ cake	160	3.0	20.0	7.0	m.q.	m.q.	160	m.q.
devil's food layer (*Pepperidge Farm*), 1⅝ oz.	180	1.0	24.0	9.0	3.0	20	135	m.q.
golden layer (*Pepperidge Farm*), 1⅝ oz.	180	1.0	24.0	9.0	3.0	20	110	m.q.
lemon coconut (*Pepperidge Farm* Supreme), 3 oz.	280	3.0	38.0	13.0	6.0	30	220	m.q.
lemon cream (*Pepperidge Farm* Supreme), 1⅝ oz.	170	2.0	21.0	9.0	3.0	20	120	m.q.
pineapple cream (*Pepperidge Farm* Supreme), 2 oz.	190	2.0	28.0	7.0	2.0	20	130	m.q.
pound:								
(*Pepperidge Farm* Old Fashioned Cholesterol Free), 1 oz.	110	1.0	13.0	6.0	1.0	0	85	m.q.
(*Sara Lee* Free & Light), ⅒ cake	70	1.0	17.0	0	0	0	105	m.q.
all butter (*Sara Lee* Original), ⅒ cake	130	2.0	14.0	7.0	m.q.	m.q.	85	m.q.
all butter (*Sara Lee* Family Size Original), ⅟₁₅ cake	130	2.0	14.0	7.0	m.q.	m.q.	85	m.q.
strawberry cream (*Pepperidge Farm* Supreme), 2 oz.	190	1.0	30.0	7.0	3.0	20	120	m.q.
strawberry shortcake (*Sara Lee*), ⅛ cake	190	2.0	26.0	8.0	m.q.	n.a.	90	m.q.
strawberry stripe layer (*Pepperidge Farm*), 1.5 oz.	160	1.0	21.0	8.0	3.0	20	120	m.q.
vanilla layer (*Pepperidge Farm*), 1⅝ oz.	190	1.0	25.0	8.0	3.0	20	120	m.q.
CAKE, REFRIGERATED:								
cinnamon swirl (*Pillsbury*), ⅛ pkg.	180	2.0	22.0	9.0	2.0	0	170	m.q.
pecan streusel (*Pillsbury*), ⅛ pkg. ...	180	2.0	21.0	9.0	2.0	0	170	m.q.

Food and Measure	cal.	prot. (gms)	carbo. (gms)	tot. fat (gms)	sat. fat (gms)	chol. (mgs)	sod. (mgs)	fiber (gms)
CAKE, SNACK (see also "Cake, snack, frozen"), 1 piece, except as noted:								
apple:								
(*Hostess* Light)	130	2.0	29.0	1.0	<1.0	0	150	.5 d
bar, baked (*Sunbelt*), 1.31 oz. ...	130	1.0	28.0	2.0	m.q.	<1	130	m.q.
delight (*Little Debbie*), 1.25 oz. ..	140	2.0	24.0	4.0	m.q.	<1	95	m.q.
spice (*Little Debbie*), 2.2 oz.	270	2.0	41.0	11.0	m.q.	<1	180	m.q.
banana:								
(*Hostess Suzy Q's*)	240	2.0	3.8	9.0	m.q.	20	200	m.q.
(*Hostess Twinkies*)	150	2.0	26.0	5.0	2.0	20	200	.5 d
(*Tastykake* Creamie), 1.5 oz.	185	1.5	24.6	7.1	1.6	8	91	.6 d
slices (*Little Debbie*), 3 oz.	340	3.0	54.0	12.0	m.q.	<1	260	m.q.
twins (*Little Debbie*), 2.2 oz.	250	2.0	40.0	9.0	m.q.	<1	190	m.q.
brownie, see "Brownie"								
butterscotch (*Tastykake Krimpets*), 1 oz.	103	1.2	19.0	2.6	1.2	22	83	.3 d
caramel peanut filled, chocolate coated (*Little Debbie Peanut Cluster*), 1.6 oz.	230	3.0	28.0	12.0	m.q.	<1	120	m.q.
cherry cordial (*Little Debbie*), 1.3 oz.	170	1.0	23.0	8.0	m.q.	n.a.	80	m.q.
chocolate:								
(*Hostess Choco Bliss*)	200	2.0	29.0	9.0	4.0	5	210	1.2 d
(*Hostess Choco-Diles*)	240	2.0	32.0	11.0	8.0	20	180	1.5 d
(*Hostess Ding Dongs*), ...	170	2.0	21.0	9.0	6.0	5	115	1.0 d
(*Hostess Ho-Hos*)	120	1.0	16.0	6.0	4.0	10	70	.6 d
(*Hostess Suzy Q's*)	250	2.0	37.0	10.0	4.0	15	300	2.0 d
(*Little Debbie*), 2.5 oz.	320	2.0	45.0	14.0	m.q.	<1	135	m.q.
(*Little Debbie*), 3 oz.	390	2.0	53.0	19.0	m.q.	<1	140	m.q.
(*Little Debbie Choco-Cake*), 2.17 oz.	270	2.0	37.0	13.0	m.q.	<1	220	m.q.
(*Little Debbie Choco-Cake*), 2.7 oz.	330	2.0	46.0	15.0	m.q.	<1	240	m.q.
(*Little Debbie Choco-Jel*), 1.16 oz.	150	1.0	21.0	7.0	m.q.	<1	80	m.q.
(*Little Debbie Holiday Cake*), 2.4 oz.	310	2.0	42.0	14.0	m.q.	<1	130	m.q.
(*Tastykake* Creamie), 1.5 oz.	168	1.7	24.0	7.6	2.0	12	126	.9 d
(*Tastykake* Juniors), 3.3 oz.	341	4.1	57.1	12.3	3.4	60	223	3.6 d
(*Tastykake* Kandy Kakes), .7 oz.	78	1.0	12.5	3.1	2.3	0	35	.9 d
cream filled:								
(*Drake's Devil Dog*), approx. 1.5 oz.	160	2.0	24.0	6.0	1.0	0	135	m.q.
(*Drake's Ring Ding*), approx. 1.5 oz.	180	2.0	23.0	10.0	3.0	0	115	m.q.
(*Tastykake Krimpets*)	124	1.3	20.2	4.3	m.q.	6	113	.2 d
fudge crispy (*Little Debbie*), 2.08 oz.	260	2.0	48.0	7.0	m.q.	<1	90	m.q.
fudge round (*Little Debbie*), 1.19 oz.	150	1.0	23.0	6.0	m.q.	<1	70	m.q.

Food and Measure	cal.	prot. (gms)	carbo. (gms)	tot. fat (gms)	sat. fat (gms)	chol. (mgs)	sod. (mgs)	fiber (gms)
fudge round (*Little Debbie*),								
2.75 oz.	330	3.0	55.0	12.0	m.q.	<1	180	m.q.
mint, cream filled (*Drake's Ring*								
Ding), approx. 1.5 oz.	190	2.0	22.0	11.0	3.0	0	115	m.q.
roll, cream filled (*Drake's Yodel*),								
approx. 1.1 oz.	150	2.0	16.0	9.0	2.0	5	65	m.q.
roll, Swiss, cream filled (*Drake's*),								
approx. 1.4 oz.	170	2.0	22.0	8.0	2.0	15	140	m.q.
slices (*Little Debbie*), 3 oz.	320	3.0	56.0	9.0	m.q.	<1	280	m.q.
twins (*Little Debbie*), 2.2 oz.	240	2.0	41.0	7.0	m.q.	<1	200	m.q.
vanilla pudding filled *Hostess* Light)	130	2.0	28.0	1.0	<1.0	0	180	.6 d
chocolate chip (*Little Debbie*),								
2.4 oz.	320	2.0	40.0	16.0	m.q.	<1	180	m.q.
coconut:								
(*Tastykake* Juniors), 3.3 oz.	296	3.9	60.1	6.0	3.0	49	304	3.5 d
covered (*Hostess Sno Balls*)	150	1.0	26.0	4.0	2.0	2	160	1.0 d
crunch (*Little Debbie*), 2 oz.	320	2.0	35.0	19.0	m.q.	<2	80	m.q.
round (*Little Debbie*), 1.13 oz. ...	150	1.0	21.0	7.0	m.q.	<1	80	m.q.
coffee:								
(*Drake's Jr.*), approx. 1.1 oz.	140	2.0	18.0	6.0	1.0	10	90	m.q.
(*Drake's* Small), approx. 2 oz. ...	220	3.0	33.0	9.0	2.0	15	160	m.q.
(*Little Debbie*), 2.1 oz.	250	3.0	39.0	9.0	m.q.	<1	210	m.q.
(*Tastykake* Koffee Kake Juniors),								
2.5 oz.	261	3.4	43.8	8.5	2.1	40	212	.9 d
cinnamon crumb (*Drake's*),								
approx. 1.33 oz.	150	2.0	22.0	6.0	1.0	10	110	m.q.
cream filled (*Tastykake* Koffee								
Kake), 1 oz.	110	1.4	17.5	4.0	.9	16	81	.4 d
crumb cake (*Hostess*)	120	1.0	19.0	5.0	2.0	10	80	.7 d
crumb cake (*Hostess* Light)	80	1.0	19.0	1.0	<1.0	0	95	.4 d
cupcake:								
butter cream, cream filled								
(*Tastykake*), 1.1 oz.	118	1.4	19.5	4.2	1.5	6	120	.9 d
chocolate:								
(*Hostess*)	180	2.0	30.0	6.0	3.0	5	290	.9 d
(*Tastykake*), 1.1 oz.	100	1.5	18.8	2.6	1.0	4	122	1.2 d
(*Tastykake* Royale), 1.6 oz.	171	1.9	27.6	6.6	1.8	7	130	1.5 d
cream filled (*Drake's Ring*								
Ding), approx. 1 oz.	100	1.0	16.0	4.0	1.0	0	110	m.q.
cream filled (*Tastykake*), 1.1 oz.	118	1.4	19.4	4.2	1.3	4	119	1.0 d
cream filled (*Tastykake* Tastylite),								
1.1 oz.	100	1.4	21.5	1.3	.5	0	116	.8 d
creme filled (*Hostess* Light)	130	2.0	26.0	2.0	<1.0	0	190	.9 d
creme (*Tastykake* Kreme Kup),								
.9 oz.	86	1.3	14.6	2.8	1.0	4	113	.6 d
golden, cream filled (*Drake's*								
Sunny Doodle), approx. 1 oz. ..	100	1.0	16.0	3.0	1.0	10	100	m.q.
orange (*Hostess*)	160	1.0	27.0	5.0	1.0	10	150	.5 d
vanilla, cream filled (*Tastykake*								
Tastylite)	100	1.1	20.9	1.5	.6	0	121	.5 d

CAKE, SNACK *(cont.)*

Food and Measure	cal.	prot. (gms)	carbo. (gms)	tot. fat (gms)	sat. fat (gms)	chol. (mgs)	sod. (mgs)	fiber (gms)
dessert cup (*Hostess*)	90	2.0	18.0	2.0	<1.0	15	170	.4 d
dessert cup (*Little Debbie*), .79 oz.	80	1.0	4.0	1.0	n.a.	<1	170	m.q.
devil's food:								
(*Little Debbie* Devil Cremes),								
2.5 oz.	300	3.0	43.0	13.0	m.q.	<1	330	m.q.
(*Little Debbie* Devil Cremes),								
1.3 oz.	160	1.0	22.0	7.0	m.q.	<1	170	m.q.
(*Little Debbie* Devil Squares),								
2.2 oz.	270	2.0	41.0	11.0	m.q.	<1	150	m.q.
donut, see "Donut"								
(*Drake's Funny Bone*), approx.								
1.25 oz.	150	3.0	18.0	8.0	2.0	0	110	m.q.
(*Drake's Zoinks*), approx. 1.25 oz.	130	1.0	20.0	5.0	1.0	10	130	m.q.
fancy (*Little Debbie*), 2.6 oz.	340	2.0	46.0	16.0	m.q.	<1	150	m.q.
fig (*Little Debbie Figaroos*), 1.5 oz.	160	1.0	31.0	4.0	m.q.	<1	105	m.q.
fruit (*Hostess Fruit Loaf*)	400	4.0	77.0	9.0	m.q.	7	520	m.q.
golden, creme filled:								
(*Hostess Twinkies*)	150	2.0	27.0	5.0	2.0	20	200	.5 d
(*Hostess Twinkies* Light)	110	2.0	21.0	2.0	<1.0	0	160	.4 d
(*Little Debbie*), 1.4 oz.	150	1.0	23.0	6.0	m.q.	<1	150	m.q.
(*Little Debbie*), 2.5 oz.	270	3.0	41.0	11.0	m.q.	<1	270	m.q.
(*Hostess Lil' Angels*)	90	1.0	14.0	2.0	m.q.	2	95	m.q.
(*Hostess Tiger Tail*)	240	4.0	38.0	8.0	4.0	25	290	1.3 d
jelly (*Tastykake Krimpets*), 1 oz.	85	1.1	18.8	1.0	.7	21	82	.6 d
jelly roll (*Little Debbie*), 2.2 oz.	250	1.0	43.0	9.0	m.q.	<1	160	m.q.
lemon (*Tastykake* Juniors), 3.3 oz. ..	306	3.1	64.2	4.0	m.q.	m.q.	255	m.q.
lemon stix (*Little Debbie*), 1.5 oz. ..	220	2.0	29.0	10.0	m.q.	<1	55	m.q.
(*Little Debbie* Be My Valentine),								
2.5 oz.	330	2.0	44.0	17.0	m.q.	<1	125	m.q.
(*Little Debbie Caravella*), 1.2 oz. ...	200	2.0	26.0	9.0	m.q.	<1	95	m.q.
(*Little Debbie* Christmas Tree),								
1.6 oz.	220	1.0	28.0	11.0	m.q.	<1	80	m.q.
(*Little Debbie* Doodle Dandies),								
2.5 oz.	320	2.0	44.0	16.0	m.q.	<1	140	m.q.
(*Little Debbie* Easter Bunny), 2.5 oz.	320	2.0	45.0	15.0	m.q.	<1	135	m.q.
(*Little Debbie* Star Crunch), 1.08 oz.	150	1.0	22.0	6.0	m.q.	<1	95	m.q.
marshmallow supreme (*Little*								
Debbie), 1.25 oz.	150	1.0	24.0	5.0	m.q.	<1	60	m.q.
mint wafer, chocolate coated (*Little*								
Debbie Mint Sprints), 1.33 oz.	200	2.0	24.0	10.0	m.q.	<1	90	m.q.
orange (*Tastykake* Juniors), 3.3 oz.	337	3.4	61.0	9.2	2.6	51	236	.9 d
peanut butter:								
(*Tastykake* Kandy Kakes), .7 oz.	87	1.8	11.0	4.2	2.4	5	38	.6 d
bar (*Little Debbie*), 1.83 oz.	260	6.0	30.0	13.0	m.q.	<1	200	m.q.
bar (*Little Debbie*), 2.5 oz.	370	8.0	41.0	18.0	m.q.	<1	270	m.q.
wafer, chocolate coated (*Little*								
Debbie Nutty Bar), 2.5 oz.	390	5.0	41.0	23.0	m.q.	<1	150	m.q.

Food and Measure	cal.	prot. (gms)	carbo. (gms)	tot. fat (gms)	sat. fat (gms)	chol. (mgs)	sod. (mgs)	fiber (gms)
wafer, chocolate coated (*Little Debbie Nutty Bar*), 2 oz.	310	4.0	32.0	20.0	m.q.	<1	120	m.q.
peanut butter and jelly sandwich (*Little Debbie*), 1.13 oz.	150	2.0	20.0	6.0	m.q.	<1	105	m.q.
pecan twins (*Little Debbie*), 2 oz. ...	220	3.0	34.0	10.0	m.q.	<1	170	m.q.
pecan twirls (*Tastykake*), 1 oz.	109	1.0	16.8	4.9	m.q.	m.q.	74	m.q.
pie, see "Pie, snack"								
pudding cakes (*Hostess*)	170	2.0	32.0	4.0	m.q.	8	200	m.q.
pumpkin delights (*Little Debbie*), 1.1 oz.	140	1.0	21.0	6.0	m.q.	<1	105	m.q.
strawberry (*Hostess Twinkies* Fruit N Creme), 1.5 oz.	140	1.0	27.0	3.0	1.0	20	180	.5 d
strawberry (*Hostess Twinkies* Fruit N Creme), 1.75 oz.	160	2.0	32.0	3.0	1.0	20	210	.5 d
Swiss roll (*Little Debbie*), 2.17 oz. ..	270	2.0	38.0	12.0	m.q.	<1	130	m.q.
Swiss roll (*Little Debbie*), 2.25 oz. ..	280	2.0	40.0	12.0	m.q.	<1	135	m.q.
(*Tastykake* Tasty Twist)	18	.3	2.7	.6	n.a.	n.a.	m.q.	m.q.
vanilla:								
(*Little Debbie*), 2.6 oz.	330	2.0	46.0	16.0	m.q.	<1	135	m.q.
(*Little Debbie*), 3 oz.	390	1.0	53.0	19.0	m.q.	<1	130	m.q.
(*Little Debbie* Holiday Cake), 2.5 oz.	320	1.0	45.0	16.0	m.q.	<1	125	m.q.
(*Tastykake* Creamie), 1.5 oz.	184	1.4	24.9	9.0	2.2	26	117	.6 d
cream filled (*Tastykake Krimpets*), 1.1 oz.	116	1.2	19.0	4.1	1.4	19	77	.5 d
wafer, peanut butter filled (*Little Debbie* Peanut Butter Naturals), 1.25 oz.	170	5.0	19.0	10.0	m.q.	<1	90	m.q.
CAKE, SNACK, FROZEN, 1 piece:								
apple crisp (*Sara Lee* Lights), 3 oz.	150	1.0	31.0	2.0	m.q.	5	130	m.q.
apple 'N spice bake (*Pepperidge Farm* Dessert Lights), 4.25 oz.	170	2.0	37.0	2.0	0	10	105	m.q.
Black Forest (*Sara Lee* Lights), 3.6 oz.	170	3.0	34.0	5.0	m.q.	10	85	m.q.
Boston cream pie (*Pepperidge Farm* Hyannis), 1 ramekin	230	4.0	34.0	10.0	4.0	70	125	2.0 d
carrot:								
(*Pepperidge Farm* Classic), 2.5 oz.	260	2.0	32.0	16.0	6.0	50	280	m.q.
(*Sara Lee* Deluxe), 1.8-oz. cake ..	180	3.0	26.0	7.0	m.q.	n.a.	200	m.q.
(*Sara Lee* Lights), 2.5 oz.	170	4.0	30.0	4.0	m.q.	5	75	m.q.
cheesecake:								
classic (*Sara Lee*), 2 oz. cake	200	4.0	16.0	14.0	m.q.	n.a.	150	m.q.
French (*Sara Lee* Lights), 3.2 oz.	150	5.0	24.0	4.0	m.q.	15	90	m.q.
French, strawberry (*Sara Lee* Lights), 3.5 oz.	150	3.0	29.0	2.0	m.q.	5	65	m.q.
strawberry (*Pepperidge Farm* Manhattan), 1 ramekin	300	6.0	49.0	9.0	5.0	150	250	m.q.

Food and Measure	cal.	prot. (gms)	carbo. (gms)	tot. fat (gms)	sat. fat (gms)	chol. (mgs)	sod. (mgs)	fiber (gms)
CAKE, SNACK, FROZEN *(cont.)*								
cherries supreme (*Pepperidge Farm* Dessert Lights), 3.25 oz.	170	0	38.0	2.0	0	80	35	m.q.
chocolate:								
double (*Pepperidge Farm* Classic), 2.25 oz.	250	2.0	31.0	13.0	4.0	35	180	m.q.
double (*Sara Lee* Lights), 2.5 oz.	150	4.0	23.0	5.0	m.q.	10	85	m.q.
fudge (*Sara Lee*), 1.6-oz. cake ...	190	2.0	24.0	10.0	m.q.	n.a.	125	m.q.
German (*Pepperidge Farm* Classic), 2.25 oz.	250	2.0	29.0	13.0	4.0	45	230	m.q.
chocolate mousse:								
(*Pepperidge Farm* Dessert Lights), 1.5 oz.	190	3.0	25.0	9.0	3.0	5	260	m.q.
(*Sara Lee*), 3-oz. serving	180	5.0	20.0	9.0	m.q.	15	125	m.q.
(*Sara Lee* Lights), 3 oz.	170	4.0	20.0	8.0	m.q.	10	60	m.q.
coconut (*Pepperidge Farm* Classic), 2.25 oz.	230	2.0	31.0	11.0	4.0	20	160	m.q.
coffee:								
apple cinnamon (*Sara Lee* Individually Wrapped), 2.9-oz. cake	290	4.0	40.0	13.0	m.q.	n.a.	270	m.q.
butter streusel (*Sara Lee* Individually Wrapped), 2-oz. cake	230	4.0	27.0	12.0	m.q.	m.q.	270	m.q.
w/cinnamon streusel (*Weight Watchers* Microwave), ½ pkg. or 2.25 oz.	190	3.0	28.0	7.0	1.0	5	250	m.q.
pecan (*Sara Lee* Individually Wrapped), 2.2-oz. cake	280	5.0	30.0	16.0	m.q.	n.a.	270	m.q.
donut, see "Donut, frozen"								
lemon cream (*Sara Lee* Lights), 3.2 oz.	180	3.0	29.0	6.0	m.q.	10	60	m.q.
lemon supreme (*Pepperidge Farm* Dessert Lights), 2.75 oz.	170	4.0	26.0	5.0	1.0	50	100	m.q.
pound, all butter (*Sara Lee*), 1.6-oz. cake	200	2.0	23.0	11.0	m.q.	n.a.	190	m.q.
raspberry vanilla swirl (*Pepperidge Farm* Dessert Lights), 3.25 oz.	160	4.0	25.0	5.0	1.0	15	140	m.q.
shortcake, strawberry (*Pepperidge Farm* Dessert Lights), 3 oz. ...	170	2.0	30.0	5.0	1.0	70	50	1.0 d
vanilla fudge swirl (*Pepperidge Farm* Classic), 2.25 oz.	250	2.0	33.0	11.0	4.0	35	160	m.q.
CAKE FROSTING, see "Frosting"								
CAKE MIX[1], ⅟₁₂ cake, except as noted:								
angel food:								
(*Betty Crocker* Traditional), ⅟₁₂ mix, dry	130	3.0	30.0	0	0	0	170	m.q.

1. *Prepared according to basic package directions, except as noted.*

Food and Measure	cal.	prot. (gms)	carbo. (gms)	tot. fat (gms)	sat. fat (gms)	chol. (mgs)	sod. (mgs)	fiber (gms)
(*Duncan Hines*)	140	3.0	30.0	0	0	0	130	m.q.
chocolate, confetti, lemon pudding or white (*Betty Crocker*),								
¹⁄₁₂ mix, dry	150	3.0	34.0	0	0	0	300	m.q.
strawberry (*Betty Crocker*),								
¹⁄₁₂ mix, dry	150	3.0	35.0	0	0	0	260	m.q.
apple:								
cinnamon (*Betty Crocker SuperMoist*)	250	3.0	36.0	10.0	2.0	55	280	m.q.
cinnamon (*Betty Crocker SuperMoist*)[1]	210	3.0	36.0	6.0	2.0	0	280	m.q.
streusel (*Betty Crocker MicroRave*), ¹⁄₆ cake	240	2.0	33.0	11.0	3.0	45	190	m.q.
streusel (*Betty Crocker MicroRave*), ¹⁄₆ cake[1]	210	2.0	33.0	8.0	2.0	0	200	m.q.
banana (*Pillsbury Plus*)	250	3.0	36.0	11.0	m.q.	n.a.	290	m.q.
Black Forest cherry (*Pillsbury Bundt*), ¹⁄₁₆ cake	240	3.0	38.0	8.0	m.q.	n.a.	310	m.q.
Black Forest mousse (*Duncan Hines Tiarra*)	260	3.0	33.0	13.0	m.q.	n.a.	270	m.q.
Boston cream (*Betty Crocker Classic*), ¹⁄₈ cake	270	4.0	50.0	6.0	m.q.	n.a.	390	m.q.
Boston cream (*Pillsbury Bundt*) ¹⁄₁₆ cake	270	3.0	43.0	10.0	m.q.	n.a.	310	m.q.
butter:								
Brickle (*Betty Crocker SuperMoist*)	250	3.0	38.0	10.0	2.0	55	280	m.q.
Brickle (*Betty Crocker SuperMoist*)[1]	220	3.0	38.0	6.0	2.0	0	280	m.q.
chocolate (*Betty Crocker SuperMoist*)	270	3.0	35.0	13.0	7.0	75	450	m.q.
pecan (*Betty Crocker SuperMoist*)	250	3.0	35.0	11.0	3.0	55	320	m.q.
pecan (*Betty Crocker SuperMoist*)[1]	220	3.0	35.0	7.0	2.0	0	320	m.q.
recipe (*Pillsbury Plus*)	260	3.0	34.0	12.0	m.q.	n.a.	370	m.q.
recipe, golden (*Duncan Hines*) ..	270	3.0	36.0	13.0	m.q.	n.a.	270	m.q.
yellow (*Betty Crocker SuperMoist*)	260	3.0	37.0	11.0	6.0	75	350	m.q.
carrot:								
(*Betty Crocker SuperMoist*)	250	3.0	35.0	11.0	3.0	55	310	m.q.
(*Betty Crocker SuperMoist*)[1]	220	3.0	35.0	7.0	2.0	0	310	m.q.
(*Dromedary*)	232	3.0	23.0	15.0	m.q.	n.a.	292	m.q.
(*Estee*), ¹⁄₁₀ cake	100	1.0	18.0	2.0	<1.0	0	65	m.q.
'n spice (*Pillsbury Plus*)	260	3.0	36.0	11.0	m.q.	n.a.	330	m.q.
cheesecake, ¹⁄₈ cake:								
(*Jell-O* No Bake)	280	5.0	36.0	13.0	m.q.	30	350	m.q.
lemon (*Jello-O* No Bake)	270	5.0	36.0	13.0	m.q.	25	400	m.q.
lite (*Royal No-Bake*)	210	5.0	23.0	10.0	m.q.	n.a.	380	m.q.
New York style (*Jello-O* No Bake)	280	6.0	38.0	12.0	m.q.	30	420	m.q.
real (*Royal No-Bake*)	280	5.0	31.0	9.0	m.q.	n.a.	370	m.q.

1. *Prepared with cholesterol-free egg product.*

Food and Measure	cal.	prot. (gms)	carbo. (gms)	tot. fat (gms)	sat. fat (gms)	chol. (mgs)	sod. (mgs)	fiber (gms)
CAKE MIX *(cont.)*								
cherry chip (*Betty Crocker SuperMoist*)	190	3.0	37.0	3.0	1.0	0	270	m.q.
cherries and cream (*Duncan Hines Tiarra*)	250	4.0	34.0	11.0	m.q.	n.a.	265	m.q.
chocolate:								
(*Estee*), 1/10 cake	100	1.0	18.0	2.0	1.0	0	100	m.q.
(*Pillsbury* Microwave), 1/8 cake	210	2.0	23.0	13.0	m.q.	n.a.	260	m.q.
dark (*Pillsbury Plus*)	250	3.0	32.0	12.0	m.q.	n.a.	380	m.q.
double supreme (*Pillsbury* Microwave), 1/8 cake	330	3.0	39.0	19.0	m.q.	n.a.	340	m.q.
chip, see "chocolate chip," below								
fudge:								
(*Betty Crocker SuperMoist*)	260	4.0	34.0	12.0	3.0	55	470	m.q.
(*Duncan Hines* Butter Recipe)	270	4.0	34.0	13.0	m.q.	n.a.	350	m.q.
(*Pillsbury Bundt Tunnel of Fudge*), 1/16 cake	260	3.0	37.0	12.0	m.q.	n.a.	310	m.q.
(*Pillsbury Bundt Tunnel of Fudge* Microwave), 1/8 cake	290	3.0	36.0	17.0	m.q.	n.a.	320	m.q.
dark Dutch (*Duncan Hines*)	280	4.0	33.0	15.0	m.q.	n.a.	375	m.q.
marble (*Duncan Hines*)	260	3.0	36.0	11.0	m.q.	n.a.	285	m.q.
marble (*Pillsbury Plus*)	270	4.0	36.0	12.0	m.q.	n.a.	300	m.q.
w/vanilla frosting (*Betty Crocker MicroRave*), 1/6 cake	310	3.0	40.0	15.0	4.0	35	300	m.q.
German:								
(*Betty Crocker SuperMoist*)	260	3.0	35.0	12.0	3.0	55	420	m.q.
(*Betty Crocker SuperMoist*)[1]	220	3.0	35.0	8.0	2.0	0	420	m.q.
(*Pillsbury Plus*)	250	3.0	36.0	11.0	m.q.	n.a.	340	m.q.
w/coconut pecan frosting (*Betty Crocker MicroRave*), 1/6 cake	320	3.0	37.0	18.0	5.0	35	250	m.q.
milk (*Betty Crocker SuperMoist*)	260	4.0	35.0	12.0	3.0	55	340	m.q.
milk (*Betty Crocker SuperMoist*)[1]	210	3.0	35.0	7.0	2.0	0	340	m.q.
mousse (*Duncan Hines Tiarra*)	270	3.0	29.0	16.0	m.q.	n.a.	235	m.q.
mousse, Amaretto (*Duncan Hines Tiarra*)	270	3.0	29.0	16.0	m.q.	n.a.	230	m.q.
pudding (*Betty Crocker* Classic), 1/6 cake	230	3.0	44.0	5.0	m.q.	n.a.	250	m.q.
Swiss (*Duncan Hines*)	280	4.0	33.0	15.0	m.q.	n.a.	375	m.q.
w/chocolate frosting (*Pillsbury* Microwave), 1/8 cake	300	2.0	35.0	17.0	m.q.	n.a.	310	m.q.
w/vanilla frosting (*Pillsbury* Microwave), 1/8 cake	300	2.0	36.0	17.0	m.q.	n.a.	300	m.q.
chocolate chip:								
(*Betty Crocker SuperMoist*)	280	3.0	36.0	14.0	3.0	55	320	m.q.
(*Betty Crocker SuperMoist*)[1]	220	3.0	36.0	7.0	2.0	0	320	m.q.
(*Pillsbury Plus*)	270	3.0	33.0	14.0	m.q.	n.a.	290	m.q.

1. *Prepared with cholesterol-free egg product.*

Food and Measure	cal.	prot. (gms)	carbo. (gms)	tot. fat (gms)	sat. fat (gms)	chol. (mgs)	sod. (mgs)	fiber (gms)
chocolate (*Betty Crocker*								
SuperMoist)	260	4.0	34.0	12.0	3.0	55	400	m.q.
chocolate macaroon (*Pillsbury*								
Bundt), 1/16 cake	240	3.0	36.0	10.0	m.q.	n.a.	300	m.q.
cinnamon:								
(*Streusel Swirl*), 1/16 cake	260	3.0	38.0	11.0	m.q.	n.a.	200	m.q.
(*Streusel Swirl* Microwave),								
1/8 cake	240	2.0	33.0	11.0	m.q.	n.a.	180	m.q.
pecan (*Betty Crocker MicroRave*),								
1/6 cake	290	3.0	39.0	13.0	3.0	45	210	m.q.
pecan (*Betty Crocker MicroRave*),								
1/6 cake [1]	240	3.0	39.0	8.0	2.0	0	220	m.q.
coffee (*Aunt Jemima* Easy),								
1 serving	156	2.1	27.1	4.4	.8	1	279	.7 d
coffee, apple cinnamon (*Pillsbury*),								
1/8 cake	240	3.0	40.0	7.0	m.q.	n.a.	150	m.q.
devil's food:								
(*Betty Crocker SuperMoist*)	260	4.0	35.0	12.0	3.0	55	450	m.q.
(*Betty Crocker SuperMoist*) [1]	220	3.0	35.0	7.0	2.0	0	450	m.q.
(*Duncan Hines*)	280	4.0	33.0	15.0	m.q.	n.a.	375	m.q.
(*Finast* Ultra Moist)	250	3.0	33.0	11.0	m.q.	n.a.	360	m.q.
(*Pillsbury Plus*)	270	4.0	32.0	14.0	m.q.	n.a.	370	m.q.
w/chocolate frosting (*Betty Crocker*								
MicroRave), 1/6 cake	310	2.2	37.0	17.0	5.0	35	250	m.q.
w/chocolate frosting (*Betty Crocker*								
MicroRave), 1/6 cake [1]	240	2.0	37.0	9.0	3.0	0	250	m.q.
fudge, see "chocolate," above								
gingerbread (*Dromedary*), 2" × 2"								
square or 3 tbsp. dry	100	1.0	19.0	2.0	m.q.	n.a.	190	m.q.
lemon:								
(*Betty Crocker SuperMoist*)	260	3.0	36.0	11.0	3.0	55	280	m.q.
(*Betty Crocker SuperMoist*) [1]	220	3.0	36.0	7.0	2.0	0	280	m.q.
(*Duncan Hines* Supreme)	260	3.0	36.0	11.0	m.q.	n.a.	285	m.q.
(*Estee*), 1/10 cake	100	1.0	18.0	2.0	<1.0	0	68	m.q.
(*Pillsbury Bundt Tunnel of*								
Lemon), 1/16 cake	270	2.0	45.0	9.0	m.q.	n.a.	300	m.q.
(*Pillsbury* Microwave), 1/8 cake ...	220	2.0	23.0	13.0	m.q.	n.a.	180	m.q.
(*Pillsbury Plus*)	250	3.0	34.0	11.0	m.q.	n.a.	290	m.q.
(*Streusel Swirl*), 1/16 cake	270	3.0	39.0	11.0	m.q.	n.a.	340	m.q.
chiffon (*Betty Crocker* Classic) ...	200	4.0	36.0	5.0	m.q.	n.a.	200	m.q.
double supreme (*Pillsbury*								
Microwave), 1/8 cake	300	2.0	40.0	15.0	m.q.	n.a.	210	m.q.
w/lemon frosting (*Betty Crocker*								
MicroRave), 1/6 cake	300	2.0	37.0	16.0	4.0	45	250	m.q.
w/lemon frosting (*Pillsbury*								
Microwave), 1/8 cake	300	2.0	37.0	17.0	m.q.	n.a.	220	m.q.

1. *Prepared with cholesterol-free egg product.*

Food and Measure	cal.	prot. (gms)	carbo. (gms)	tot. fat (gms)	sat. fat (gms)	chol. (mgs)	sod. (mgs)	fiber (gms)
CAKE MIX, LEMON *(cont.)*								
pudding (*Betty Crocker* Classic),								
⅙ cake	230	2.0	45.0	5.0	m.q.	n.a.	270	m.q.
marble (*Betty Crocker SuperMoist*) ..	250	2.0	35.0	11.0	3.0	55	290	m.q.
marble (*Betty Crocker SuperMoist*)[1]	210	2.0	35.0	7.0	2.0	0	290	m.q.
pineapple:								
(*Duncan Hines* Supreme)	260	3.0	36.0	11.0	m.q.	n.a.	285	m.q.
cream (*Pillsbury Bundt*), 1/16 cake	260	2.0	41.0	9.0	m.q.	n.a.	300	m.q.
upside-down (*Betty Crocker*								
Classic), ⅑ cake[2]	250	2.0	39.0	10.0	4.0	40	210	m.q.
upside-down (*Betty Crocker*								
Classic), ⅑ cake[3]	240	2.0	39.0	9.0	3.0	0	220	m.q.
pound:								
(*Dromedary*), 5 tbsp. dry	130	1.0	20.0	5.0	m.q.	n.a.	140	m.q.
(*Dromedary*), ½" slice	150	2.0	21.0	6.0	m.q.	n.a.	160	m.q.
(*Estee*), 1/10 cake	100	1.0	18.0	2.0	<1.0	0	68	m.q.
(*Martha White*), 1/10 cake	120	2.0	19.0	4.0	m.q.	8	110	m.q.
golden (*Betty Crocker* Classic) ...	200	2.0	28.0	9.0	3.0	35	170	m.q.
rainbow chip (*Betty Crocker*								
SuperMoist)	250	3.0	34.0	11.0	3.0	55	320	m.q.
sour cream:								
chocolate (*Betty Crocker*								
SuperMoist)	260	3.0	35.0	12.0	3.0	55	430	m.q.
chocolate (*Betty Crocker*								
SuperMoist)[1]	220	3.0	35.0	8.0	2.0	0	430	m.q.
white (*Betty Crocker SuperMoist*)	180	3.0	36.0	3.0	1.0	0	300	m.q.
spice:								
(*Betty Crocker SuperMoist*)	260	3.0	36.0	11.0	3.0	55	320	m.q.
(*Betty Crocker SuperMoist*)[1]	220	3.0	36.0	7.0	2.0	0	320	m.q.
(*Duncan Hines*)	260	3.0	36.0	11.0	m.q.	n.a.	285	m.q.
strawberry (*Duncan Hines*								
Supreme)	260	3.0	36.0	11.0	m.q.	n.a.	285	m.q.
strawberry (*Pillsbury Plus*)	260	3.0	37.0	11.0	m.q.	n.a.	300	m.q.
vanilla:								
French (*Duncan Hines*)	260	3.0	36.0	11.0	m.q.	n.a.	285	m.q.
golden:								
(*Betty Crocker SuperMoist*)	280	3.0	36.0	14.0	3.0	55	270	m.q.
(*Betty Crocker SuperMoist*)[1] ...	220	3.0	36.0	7.0	2.0	0	270	m.q.
w/rainbow chip frosting (*Betty*								
Crocker MicroRave), ⅙ cake	320	2.0	40.0	17.0	5.0	35	230	m.q.
white:								
(*Betty Crocker SuperMoist*)[4]	240	3.0	37.0	9.0	2.0	0	250	m.q.
(*Betty Crocker SuperMoist*)[5]	220	3.0	37.0	7.0	2.0	0	250	m.q.
(*Duncan Hines*)	250	3.0	36.0	10.0	m.q.	n.a.	260	m.q.
(*Estee*), 1/10 cake	100	1.0	18.0	2.0	<1.0	0	68	m.q.
(*Pillsbury Plus*)	240	3.0	35.0	10.0	m.q.	n.a.	290	m.q.

1. *Prepared with cholesterol-free egg product.*
2. *Prepared with egg and butter.*
3. *Prepared with cholesterol-free egg product and margarine.*
4. *Prepared with 3 egg whites and ⅓ cup oil.*
5. *Prepared with 3 egg whites and 3 tbsp. oil.*

Food and Measure	cal.	prot. (gms)	carbo. (gms)	tot. fat (gms)	sat. fat (gms)	chol. (mgs)	sod. (mgs)	fiber (gms)
yellow:								
(*Betty Crocker SuperMoist*)	260	3.0	36.0	11.0	3.0	55	300	m.q.
(*Betty Crocker SuperMoist*)[1]	220	3.0	36.0	7.0	2.0	0	300	m.q.
(*Duncan Hines*)	260	3.0	36.0	11.0	m.q.	n.a.	285	m.q.
(*Finast* Ultra Moist)	240	3.0	34.0	10.0	m.q.	n.a.	280	m.q.
(*Pillsbury* Microwave), ⅛ cake ...	220	2.0	23.0	13.0	m.q.	n.a.	170	m.q.
(*Pillsbury Plus*)	260	3.0	36.0	12.0	m.q.	n.a.	300	m.q.
w/chocolate frosting:								
(*Betty Crocker MicroRave*),								
⅙ cake	300	2.0	36.0	16.0	4.0	35	210	m.q.
(*Betty Crocker MicroRave*),								
⅙ cake[1]	230	2.0	36.0	9.0	3.0	0	210	m.q.
(*Pillsbury* Microwave), ⅛ cake	300	2.0	36.0	17.0	m.q.	n.a.	220	m.q.
CALABASH GOURD, see "Gourd,								
white-flowered"								
CALALOO, see "Amaranth"								
CALAMARI, see "Squid"								
CALF, see "Veal"								
CALVE'S LIVER, see "Liver, veal"								
CANDY:								
almond, candy coated (*Brach's* Jordan								
Almonds), 1 oz.	120	2.0	23.0	2.0	m.q.	n.a.	0	m.q.
(*Baby Ruth*), 1 oz.	130	2.0	18.0	6.0	m.q.	n.a.	60	m.q.
(*Boyer Smoothie,* .275 oz.), 1 piece	38	1.3	6.3	3.8	m.q.	n.a.	n.a.	n.a.
(*Boyer Smoothie,* .5 oz.), 1 piece ...	75	2.5	12.5	7.5	m.q.	n.a.	n.a.	n.a.
(*Boyer Smoothie,* 1.6 oz.), 2 pieces	250	5.0	24.0	15.0	m.q.	n.a.	n.a.	n.a.
(*Brach Royals*), 1 oz.	100	1.0	20.0	2.0	m.q.	n.a.	60	m.q.
breath mint, see "mint," below								
bridge mix (*Brach's*), 1 oz.	130	1.0	19.0	6.0	m.q.	n.a.	40	m.q.
(*Butterfinger*), 1 oz.	130	2.0	19.0	6.0	m.q.	n.a.	60	m.q.
butterscotch:								
(*Brach's* Disks), 1 oz.	110	0	27.0	0	0	n.a.	220	(0)
(*Callard & Bowser*), 1 oz.	115	0	25.2	1.9	n.a.	n.a.	n.a.	(0)
(*Featherweight*), 1 piece	25	0	6.0	0	0	0	25	(0)
candy cane, see "seasonal or								
specialty," below								
caramel:								
(*Brach's* Milk Maid), 1 oz.	110	1.0	22.0	2.0	m.q.	n.a.	70	(0)
(*Featherweight*), 1 piece	30	0	5.0	1.0	n.a.	0	10	(0)
(*Kraft*), 1 piece	30	0	6.0	1.0	0	0	25	(0)
(*Sugar Babies* Regular/Tidbits),								
1⅝-oz. pkg.	180	1.0	40.0	2.0	m.q.	n.a.	85	(0)
(*Sugar Daddy*), 1⅜-oz. pop	150	1.0	33.0	1.0	n.a.	n.a.	85	(0)
chocolate (*Brach's* Milk Maid),								
1 oz.	110	1.0	20.0	3.0	m.q.	n.a.	55	(0)
chocolate, vanilla (*Estee*), 1 piece	20	<1.0	3.0	1.0	<1.0	0	10	(0)

1. *Prepared with cholesterol-free egg product.*

Food and Measure	cal.	prot. (gms)	carbo. (gms)	tot. fat (gms)	sat. fat (gms)	chol. (mgs)	sod. (mgs)	fiber (gms)
CANDY, CARAMEL *(cont.)*								
chocolate coated (*Pom Poms*),								
1 oz.	100	1.0	15.0	3.0	m.q.	n.a.	70	m.q.
chocolate coated, w/cookies								
(*Twix*), 2-oz. piece	140	2.0	19.0	7.0	m.q.	n.a.	60	m.q.
milk chocolate coated (*Rolo*),								
1.93 oz. or 8 pieces	270	3.0	37.0	12.0	m.q.	15	110	(0)
w/peanut, chocolate coated (*Oh*								
Henry!), 2 oz.	280	6.0	32.0	14.0	m.q.	n.a.	85	m.q.
carob milk bar (*Caroby*), 4 sections	150	4.0	13.0	9.0	m.q.	n.a.	55	m.q.
cherry:								
chocolate cream (*Brach's*), 1 oz.	110	1.0	21.0	2.0	m.q.	n.a.	20	m.q.
dark chocolate coated (*Brach's*),								
1 oz.	110	1.0	22.0	2.0	m.q.	n.a.	20	m.q.
milk chocolate coated (*Brach's*),								
1 oz.	110	0	22.0	2.0	m.q.	n.a.	20	m.q.
chocolate (see also "Chocolate,								
baking"):								
(*Brach's* Jots), 1 oz.	130	1.0	21.0	5.0	m.q.	n.a.	30	m.q.
almond (*Estee*), 2 squares	60	1.0	4.5	4.5	2.0	2	10	m.q.
almond (*Featherweight*), 1 section	90	1.0	6.0	7.0	m.q.	n.a.	20	m.q.
w/almonds (*Hershey's Golden*								
Almond), 1.6 oz. or ½ bar	260	5.0	20.0	17.0	m.q.	5	35	m.q.
w/almonds (*Hershey's Solitaires*),								
1.6 oz. or ½ bar	260	6.0	20.0	17.0	m.q.	5	25	m.q.
w/almonds, roasted (*Cadbury*),								
1 oz.	150	3.0	15.0	9.0	m.q.	n.a.	40	m.q.
assorted (*Brach's* 1 lb.), 1 oz. ...	110	0	23.0	2.0	m.q.	n.a.	25	m.q.
assorted, wrapped (*Brach's*), 1 oz.	110	0	24.0	2.0	m.q.	n.a.	20	m.q.
candy coated (*Holidays*), 1 oz. ...	140	2.0	19.0	6.0	m.q.	n.a.	40	m.q.
candy coated (*M&M's*), 1.69 oz.	250	3.0	34.0	12.0	m.q.	n.a.	70	m.q.
w/caramel (*Caramello*), 1.6 oz. ..	220	3.0	28.0	11.0	m.q.	10	60	m.q.
coconut (*Estee*), 2 squares	60	1.0	4.5	4.5	3.0	2	10	m.q.
cream (*Callard & Bowser*), 1 oz.	120	.3	22.3	3.7	(0)	n.a.	n.a.	m.q.
crunch (*Estee*), 2 squares	45	1.0	4.0	3.0	2.0	2	10	m.q.
crunch (*Featherweight*), 1 section	80	1.0	7.0	6.0	m.q.	n.a.	20	m.q.
dark, deluxe (*Estee*), 2 squares ..	60	1.0	5.0	5.0	3.0	2	0	m.q.
dark, sweet (*Hershey's Special*								
Dark), 1.45 oz.	220	3.0	25.0	12.0	m.q.	0	5	m.q.
w/fruit and nuts (*Cadbury*), 1 oz.	150	2.0	17.0	8.0	m.q.	n.a.	40	m.q.
fruit & nut (*Estee*), 2 squares	60	1.0	4.5	4.5	2.0	2	10	m.q.
w/krisps and honey (*Cadbury*),								
1 oz.	150	2.0	18.0	7.0	m.q.	n.a.	40	m.q.
milk:								
(*Brach's* Stars), 1 oz.	150	2.0	17.0	8.0	m.q.	n.a.	30	m.q.
(*Cadbury Dairy Milk*), 1 oz. ...	150	2.0	17.0	8.0	m.q.	m.q.	45	m.q.
(*Estee*), 2 squares	60	1.0	4.5	4.5	3.0	2	10	m.q.
(*Featherweight*), 1 section	80	1.0	7.0	6.0	m.q.	n.a.	20	m.q.
(*Hershey's*), 1.55 oz.	240	4.0	25.0	14.0	m.q.	10	40	m.q.

Food and Measure	cal.	prot. (gms)	carbo. (gms)	tot. fat (gms)	sat. fat (gms)	chol. (mgs)	sod. (mgs)	fiber (gms)
(*Hershey's Kisses*), 1.46 oz. or 9 pieces	220	3.0	23.0	13.0	m.q.	10	35	m.q.
(*Nabisco* Stars), 1 oz., approx. 13 pieces	160	2.0	19.0	8.0	m.q.	n.a.	35	m.q.
(*Nestlé*), 1.45 oz.	220	3.0	25.0	13.0	m.q.	n.a.	25	m.q.
w/almonds (*Hershey's*), 1.45 oz.	230	5.0	20.0	14.0	m.q.	15	55	m.q.
w/almonds (*Hershey's* Kisses), 1 oz., approx. 6 pieces	160	3.0	14.0	10.0	n.a.	n.a.	25	m.q.
w/almonds (*Nestlé*), 1.45 oz. ...	230	4.0	22.0	14.0	m.q.	n.a.	25	m.q.
creamy (*Hershey's Symphony*), 1.75 oz. or 5 sections	270	4.0	28.0	16.0	m.q.	m.q.	45	m.q.
creamy, w/almonds and toffee chips (*Hershey's Symphony*), 1.75 oz.	280	5.0	26.0	17.0	m.q.	m.q.	50	m.q.
w/crisps (*Krackel*), 1.55 oz. ...	230	3.0	27.0	13.0	m.q.	10	80	m.q.
w/crisps (*Nestlé Crunch*), 1.4 oz.	210	3.0	26.0	10.0	m.q.	n.a.	35	m.q.
w/crisps and peanuts (*Nestlé 100 Grand*), 1.5 oz.	200	2.0	31.0	8.0	m.q.	n.a.	55	m.q.
w/fruit and nuts (*Chunky*), 1.4 oz.	210	4.0	22.0	12.0	m.q.	n.a.	20	m.q.
w/peanuts (*Brach's* Peanut Clusters), 1 oz.	150	3.0	15.0	9.0	m.q.	n.a.	25	m.q.
w/peanuts (*Mr. Goodbar*), 1.75 oz.	290	7.0	23.0	19.0	m.q.	15	20	m.q.
w/pecan and caramel (*Demet's* Turtles), .6-oz. piece	90	1.0	10.0	5.0	m.q.	n.a.	15	m.q.
mint (*Estee*), 2 squares	60	1.0	5.0	5.0	3.0	2	0	n.a.
peanut (*Estee*), 2 squares	60	1.0	4.5	4.5	2.0	2	10	m.q.
w/peanuts, candy coated (*M&M's*), 1.74 oz.	250	6.0	29.0	13.0	m.q.	n.a.	55	m.q.
white, w/almonds (*Nestlé Alpine*), 1.25 oz.	210	3.0	17.0	14.0	m.q.	n.a.	35	m.q.
chocolate, tofu:								
(*Barat* Passionettes), 1 piece, approx. .4 oz.	70	1.0	6.0	5.0	m.q.	0	5	m.q.
w/almonds (*Barat* Bar), 1 oz.	170	3.0	13.0	11.0	m.q.	0	10	m.q.
w/almonds and raisins (*Barat* Bar), 1 oz.	160	3.0	14.0	11.0	m.q.	0	10	m.q.
mints (*Barat* Bits), .75 oz.	120	2.0	11.0	8.0	m.q.	0	15	m.q.
mints, after dinner (*Barat*), 1 piece	40	1.0	4.0	2.0	m.q.	0	0	m.q.
pastilles (*Barat* Bits), .75 oz.	120	2.0	11.0	8.0	m.q.	0	10	m.q.
peanuts, dipped (*Barat* Bits), 1 oz.	120	4.0	8.0	8.0	m.q.	0	15	m.q.
raisins, smothered (*Barat* Bits), 1 oz.	120	1.0	14.0	7.0	m.q.	0	10	m.q.
truffle, w/praline (*Barat* Bar), 1 oz.	170	4.0	12.0	11.0	m.q.	0	10	m.q.
cinnamon (*Brach's* Disks), 1 oz.	110	0	27.0	0	0	0	15	0

Food and Measure	cal.	prot. (gms)	carbo. (gms)	tot. fat (gms)	sat. fat (gms)	chol. (mgs)	sod. (mgs)	fiber (gms)
CANDY, CINNAMON *(cont.)*								
cinnamon (*Brach's* Imperials), 1 oz.	110	0	27.0	0	0	0	5	0
coconut:								
chocolate coated:								
(*Mounds*), 1.9-oz. piece	260	2.0	31.0	14.0	m.q.	0	85	m.q.
(*Sunbelt Macaroo*), 2 oz.	288	3.0	33.0	16.0	m.q.	<1	75	m.q.
dark or milk chocolate (*Bounty*), 1.05 oz.	150	1.0	18.0	8.0	m.q.	n.a.	50	m.q.
w/almonds (*Almond Joy*), 1.76-oz. piece	250	3.0	28.0	14.0	m.q.	0	70	m.q.
Neapolitan (*Brach's*), 1 oz.	120	1.0	24.0	2.0	m.q.	n.a.	40	m.q.
coffee flavor (*Brach's*), 1 oz.	120	0	25.0	2.0	m.q.	n.a.	35	0
corn, see "seasonal or specialty," below								
cough drops (*Beech-Nut*), 1 piece ..	10	0	3.0	0	0	0	0	0
cough drops (*Halls* Cough Tablets), 1 piece	15	tr.	3.7	tr.	(0)	0	tr.	0
creme center, chocolate coated, 1 piece:								
(*Spangler* Opera Creme Chocolate Drop)	80	<1.0	15.0	2.0	m.q.	0	40	m.q.
caramel w/nuts (*Spangler* Peanut Cluster)	100	2.0	11.0	6.0	m.q.	0	30	m.q.
cherry creme w/nuts (*Spangler* Peanut Cluster)	110	2.0	12.0	5.0	m.q.	0	20	m.q.
fudge w/nuts (*Spangler* Peanut Cluster)	140	2.0	17.0	6.0	m.q.	0	25	m.q.
fudge w/nuts (*Spangler* Pecan Cluster)	140	1.0	18.0	7.0	m.q.	0	40	m.q.
maple creme w/nuts (*Spangler* Peanut Cluster)	110	2.0	12.0	5.0	m.q.	0	15	m.q.
mint, dark chocolate coated (*Spangler Bittersweets*)	80	<1.0	14.0	2.0	m.q.	0	25	m.q.
vanilla creme w/nuts (*Spangler* Peanut Cluster)	110	2.0	13.0	5.0	m.q.	0	20	m.q.
(*Estee Estee-ets*), 5 pieces	35	1.0	4.0	2.0	1.0	<1	10	n.a.
filled, assorted (*Brach's*), 1 oz.	110	0	27.0	0	0	0	15	(0)
fruit flavored:								
all flavors:								
(*Brach's* Fruit Bunch), 1 oz. ...	90	0	23.0	0	0	0	20	0
(*Skittles*), 2.3 oz.	265	0	60.0	3.0	m.q.	0	35	0
chews:								
(*Bonkers!*), 1 piece	20	0	5.0	0	0	0	0	0
(*Rascals*), 1 piece	4	tr.	1.0	tr.	0	0	tr.	0
(*Starburst*), 2.07 oz.	240	0	48.0	5.0	m.q.	0	30	0
drops (*Featherweight*), 1/3 oz. ..	30	0	8.0	0	0	0	15	0
berry patch, orchard or tropical blend (*Featherweight*), 1 piece ..	12	0	3.0	0	0	0	0	0

Food and Measure	cal.	prot. (gms)	carbo. (gms)	tot. fat (gms)	sat. fat (gms)	chol. (mgs)	sod. (mgs)	fiber (gms)
fudge:								
(*Kraft* Fudgies), 1 piece	35	0	6.0	1.0	0	0	25	m.q.
chocolate cheese or mint, w/								
walnuts (*Woodys*), 1 oz.	120	2.0	18.0	4.0	2.0	5	25	m.q.
maple walnut (*Woodys*), 1 oz.	120	1.0	19.0	4.0	1.0	5	25	m.q.
granola bar or snack, see "Granola								
and cereal bars"								
gum, chewing, all flavors, 1 piece,								
except as noted:								
(*Beech-Nut*)	10	0	2.0	0	0	0	0	0
(*Big Red*)	10	0	2.3	0	0	0	0	0
(*Care Free*)	8	0	2.0	0	0	0	0	0
(*Chewels*)	8	tr.	2.0	tr.	0	0	tr.	0
(*Clorets* Stick)	9	tr.	2.3	tr.	0	0	tr.	0
(*Dentyne*)	6	tr.	1.5	tr.	0	0	tr.	0
(*Dentyne* Sugarless)	5	tr.	1.1	tr.	0	0	tr.	0
(*Doublemint*)	10	0	2.3	0	0	0	0	0
(*Extra*)	8	0	0	0	0	0	0	0
(*Freedent*)	10	0	2.3	0	0	0	0	0
(*Freshen-Up*)	13	tr.	3.1	tr.	0	0	tr.	0
(*Fruit Stripe*)	10	0	2.0	0	0	0	0	0
(*Juicy Fruit*)	10	0	2.3	0	0	0	0	0
(*Sticklets*)	7	tr.	1.9	tr.	0	0	tr.	0
(*Wrigley's Spearmint*)	10	0	2.3	0	0	0	0	0
balls (*Brach's Gumdinger*), 1 oz.	110	0	24.0	2.0	n.a.	0	5	0
bubble:								
(*Bubble Yum*)	25	0	7.0	0	0	0	0	0
(*Bubble Yum* Sugarless)	20	0	5.0	0	0	0	0	0
(*Bubblicious*)	25	tr.	6.2	tr.	0	0	tr.	0
(*Bubblicious* Sugarless)	5	tr.	1.3	tr.	0	0	tr.	0
(*Care Free*)	10	0	2.0	0	0	0	0	0
(*Extra*)	7	0	0	0	0	0	0	0
(*Fruit Stripe*)	10	0	2.0	0	0	0	0	0
(*Hubba Bubba* Original Sugar								
Free)	14	0	0	0	0	0	0	0
all flavors except cola (*Hubba*								
Bubba)	23	0	5.8	0	0	0	0	0
cola (*Hubba Bubba*)	23	0	5.3	0	0	0	0	0
grape (*Hubba Bubba* Sugar								
Free)	13	0	0	0	0	0	0	0
candy coated:								
(*Beechies*)	6	0	2.0	0	0	0	0	0
(*Chiclets*)	6	tr.	1.5	tr.	0	0	tr.	0
(*Chiclets* Tiny), 1 pkg.	8	tr.	<.1	tr.	0	0	tr.	0
(*Clorets*)	6	tr.	1.5	tr.	0	0	tr.	0
gum drops (*Estee*), 4 pieces	25	6.0	0	0	0	0	0	0
gummy bears (*Estee*), 4 pieces	20	1.0	4.0	0	0	0	0	0
hard, 1 piece, except as noted:								
(*Estee*), 2 pieces	25	6.0	0	0	0	0	0	0

Food and Measure	cal.	prot. (gms)	carbo. (gms)	tot. fat (gms)	sat. fat (gms)	chol. (mgs)	sod. (mgs)	fiber (gms)
CANDY, HARD *(cont.)*								
all fruit flavors (*Life Savers*)	8	0	2.0	0	0	0	0	0
butter creme mint (*Life Savers*) ..	8	0	2.0	0	0	0	5	0
butter rum (*Life Savers*)	8	0	2.0	0	0	0	10	0
butterscotch (*Life Savers*)	8	0	2.0	0	0	0	10	0
cinnamon (*Life Savers* Cin-O-Mon)	8	0	2.0	0	0	0	0	0
mint, except butter creme (*Life Savers*)	8	0	2.0	0	0	0	0	0
root beer (*Life Savers*)	8	0	2.0	0	0	0	0	0
(*Heath Bits'O Brickle*), 3 oz.	448	1.0	50.0	28.0	m.q.	n.a.	472	n.a.
(*Heath* Soft'n Crunchy Bar), 2 pieces or 1³⁄₁₆ oz.	190	1.0	19.0	12.0	m.q.	n.a.	85	n.a.
honey (*Bit-O-Honey*), 1.7 oz.	200	1.0	39.0	4.0	m.q.	n.a.	125	n.a.
(*Hot Tamales*), 1 piece	9	<.1	2.1	tr.	0	0	1	0
jellied and gummed (see also "licorice" and specific listings):								
(*Brach's* Gummi Bears/Worms), 1 oz.	100	2.0	22.0	0	0	0	15	0
(*Brach's* Jube), 1 oz.	100	0	24.0	0	0	0	10	0
beans (*Brach's*), 1 oz.	100	0	26.0	0	0	0	10	0
beans (*Just Born Teenee Beanee* Gourmet), 1 piece	4	tr.	1.1	tr.	0	0	<1	0
cherry, sour (*Brach's* Jels), 1 oz.	100	0	26.0	0	0	0	10	0
cinnamon (*Brach's* Cinnamon Bears), 1 oz.	80	0	21.0	0	0	0	10	0
eggs (*Just Born* Petite), 1 piece ..	4	tr.	1.1	tr.	0	0	<1	0
eggs (*Rodda*), 1 piece	7	<.1	1.7	tr.	0	0	1	0
juicy (*Callard & Bowser*), 1 oz. ..	90	0	22.9	0	0	0	n.a.	0
mint, assorted (*Brach's*), 1 oz. ...	100	0	26.0	0	0	0	0	0
rainbow (*Brach's* Rainbow Bears), 1 oz.	100	0	24.0	0	0	0	10	0
spearmint leaves (*Brach's*), 1 oz.	100	0	24.0	0	0	0	10	0
(*Jolly Joes*), 1 piece	9	<.1	2.1	tr.	0	0	1	0
(*Jujyfruits*), 1 oz. or 11 pieces	100	<1.0	25.0	<1.0	0	0	0	0
lemon drops (*Brach's*), 1 oz.	110	0	27.0	0	0	0	5	0
licorice, 1 oz.:								
(*Brach's* Red Laces/Twin Twists)	100	2.0	22.0	0	0	0	10	0
(*Brach's* Twists)	100	2.0	22.0	1.0	(0)	0	50	0
(*Pearson's Licorice Nip*)	120	1.0	23.0	3.0	n.a.	0	70	0
candy coated (*Good & Fruity*)	106	.6	25.7	.1	(0)	0	8	0
candy coated (*Good & Plenty*) ...	106	1.0	25.9	<.1	(0)	0	52	0
cherry (*Y&S Bites*)	100	1.0	23.0	1.0	(0)	0	85	0
cherry (*Y&S Nibs*)	100	1.0	23.0	1.0	(0)	0	80	0
strawberry (*Y&S Twizzlers*)	100	1.0	23.0	1.0	(0)	0	95	0
lollipop:								
all flavors:								
(*Brach's Pops*), 1 oz.	110	0	27.0	0	0	0	10	0
(*Estee*), 1 piece	25	0	6.0	0	0	0	0	0
(*Life Savers*), 1 piece	45	0	11.0	0	0	0	10	0

Food and Measure	cal.	prot. (gms)	carbo. (gms)	tot. fat (gms)	sat. fat (gms)	chol. (mgs)	sod. (mgs)	fiber (gms)
(*Spangler Dum Dums*), 1 piece	25	<1.0	6.0	<1.0	(0)	0	0	0
(*Spangler Saf-T-Pops*), 1 piece	45	<1.0	11.0	<1.0	(0)	0	0	0
bubble gum center (*Spangler Blo Bubble*), 1 piece	57	<1.0	14.0	<1.0	(0)	0	5	0
all flavors, except chocolate:								
(*Tootsie Pop*), 1 oz.	111	.1	26.4	.6	.1	tr.	1	(0)
chocolate (*Tootsie Pop*), 1 oz.	110	.1	26.2	.6	.2	tr.	2	(0)
lozenge (*Listerine* Throat Lozenge), 1 piece	9	tr.	2.0	tr.	(0)	0	tr.	0
malted milk balls, milk chocolate coated (*Brach's*), 1 oz.	130	1.0	21.0	5.0	m.q.	m.q.	40	m.q.
(*Mars*), 1.76-oz. bar	240	4.0	30.0	11.0	m.q.	n.a.	85	m.q.
marshmallow (see also "seasonal and specialty," below, and specific listings):								
(*Brach's* Perkys Circus Peanuts), 1 oz.	100	0	26.0	0	0	0	10	0
(*Campfire*), 2 large or 24 mini pieces	40	0	10.0	0	0	0	10	0
(*Funmallows*), 1 piece	30	0	7.0	0	0	0	15	0
(*Kraft* Jet-Puffed), 1 piece	25	0	6.0	0	0	0	5	0
(*Spangler* Circus Peanuts), 1 oz. or 4 pieces	110	<1.0	26.0	<1.0	(0)	0	5	0
coconut, toasted (*Just Born*), 1 piece	30	.3	6.1	.6	(0)	0	6	.7 d
cup:								
(*Boyer Mallow Cup*, .275 oz.), 1 piece	36	.5	7.5	2.5	m.q.	n.a.	n.a.	0
(*Boyer Mallo Cup*, .5 oz.), 1 piece	71	1.0	15.0	5.0	m.q.	n.a.	n.a.	0
(*Boyer Mallo Cup*, 1.6 oz.), 2 pieces	224	2.0	30.0	11.0	m.q.	n.a.	n.a.	0
miniature (*Funmallows*), 10 pieces	18	0	5.0	0	0	0	5	0
miniature (*Kraft*), 10 pieces	18	0	5.0	0	0	0	5	0
(*Mike & Ike*), 1 piece	9	<.1	2.1	tr.	0	0	1	0
(*Milky Way*), 2.15-oz. bar	280	3.0	42.0	11.0	m.q.	n.a.	150	m.q.
(*Milky Way* Dark), 1.76-oz.	220	1.0	36.0	8.0	m.q.	n.a.	115	m.q.
mint (see also "peppermint," "seasonal and specialty," and specific listings):								
(*Brach's* Coolers/Starlight), 1 oz.	110	0	27.0	0	0	0	15	0
(*Brach's* Creme de Menthe), 1 oz.	150	2.0	16.0	9.0	m.q.	n.a.	20	0
(*Brach's* Jots/Pearls), 1 oz.	120	0	25.0	2.0	m.q.	n.a.	10	0
(*Brach's* Kentucky Mints), 1 oz. ..	110	0	27.0	0	0	0	0	0
(*Certs* Sugar Free), 1 piece	6	tr.	1.6	tr.	0	0	tr.	0
(*Featherweight* Cool Blue), 1 piece	25	0	6.0	0	0	0	0	0
(*Mint Meltaway*), .33-oz. piece ...	50	0	5.0	3.0	m.q.	0	10	0

Food and Measure	cal.	prot. (gms)	carbo. (gms)	tot. fat (gms)	sat. fat (gms)	chol. (mgs)	sod. (mgs)	fiber (gms)
CANDY, MINT *(cont.)*								
all flavors (*Breath Savers*), 1 piece	8	0	2.0	0	0	0	0	0
assorted (*Brach's* Dessert Mints),								
1 oz.	110	0	27.0	0	0	n.a.	0	0
butter or party (*Kraft*), 1 piece ..	8	0	2.0	0	0	0	0	0
chocolate coated:								
(*Junior Mints*), 1 oz., approx.								
12 pieces	120	1.0	24.0	3.0	m.q.	n.a.	10	n.a.
(*York Peppermint Pattie*), 1.5 oz.	180	1.0	34.0	4.0	m.q.	0	20	n.a.
dark chocolate (*After Eight*),								
1 piece	35	0	6.0	1.0	n.a.	n.a.	0	n.a.
regular, creme or thin (*Brach's*),								
1 oz.	110	0	24.0	2.0	m.q.	n.a.	10	n.a.
clear (*Clorets*), 1 piece	8	tr.	2.1	tr.	0	0	tr.	0
mini (*Certs Sugar Free*), 1 piece ..	1	tr.	.4	tr.	0	0	tr.	0
parfait (*Brach's*), 1 oz.	150	2.0	16.0	9.0	m.q.	n.a.	35	(0)
pressed (*Clorets*), 1 piece	6	tr.	1.6	tr.	0	0	tr.	0
(*Munch*), 1.42-oz. bar	220	6.0	19.0	14.0	m.q.	n.a.	110	m.q.
(*Necco Sky Bar*), 1.5-oz. bar	196	1.9	31.5	7.1	m.q.	n.a.	57	0
nonpareils (*Nestlé Sno-Caps*), 1 oz.	140	1.0	21.0	6.0	m.q.	n.a.	0	m.q.
nonpareils, dark chocolate (*Brach's*),								
1 oz.	140	1.0	20.0	6.0	m.q.	n.a.	20	m.q.
nougat, chocolate coated, all flavors								
(*Charleston Chew!*), 1 oz.	120	1.0	22.0	3.0	m.q.	n.a.	40	m.q.
nougat, jelly (*Brach's*), 1 oz.	100	0	24.0	1.0	n.a.	0	35	m.q.
nut (*Brach's* Nut Goodies), 1 oz. ...	130	2.0	21.0	4.0	m.q.	n.a.	10	m.q.
orange (*Brach's* Orangettes), 1 oz.	100	0	24.0	0	0	0	20	0
orange sticks, chocolate coated								
(*Brach's*), 1 oz.	110	1.0	23.0	2.0	m.q.	n.a.	25	m.q.
peanut:								
(*Brach's* Jots), 1 oz.	140	3.0	18.0	6.0	m.q.	n.a.	25	m.q.
butter toffee (*Flavor House*), 1 oz.	150	4.0	17.0	7.0	m.q.	n.a.	90	m.q.
chocolate coated:								
(*Brach's* Small), 1 oz.	140	4.0	15.0	7.0	m.q.	n.a.	40	m.q.
(*Goobers*), 1⅜ oz.	220	6.0	19.0	13.0	m.q.	n.a.	15	m.q.
(*Nabisco*), 1 oz., approx.								
14 pieces	160	4.0	14.0	9.0	m.q.	n.a.	15	m.q.
milk chocolate (*Brach's*), 1 oz.	150	3.0	15.0	9.0	m.q.	m.q.	30	m.q.
filled (*Brach's*), 1 oz.	110	1.0	25.0	1.0	n.a.	n.a.	20	m.q.
French burnt (*Brach's*), 1 oz.	130	4.0	18.0	5.0	m.q.	0	5	m.q.
peanut brittle (*Estee*), .25 oz.	35	<1.0	5.0	1.0	<1.0	0	30	m.q.
peanut brittle (*Kraft*), 1 oz.	130	3.0	20.0	5.0	1.0	0	135	m.q.
peanut butter:								
(*PB Max*), 1.48 oz.	240	5.0	20.0	16.0	m.q.	n.a.	160	m.q.
candy coated (*Reese's Pieces*),								
1.85 oz.	260	8.0	32.0	11.0	m.q.	5	90	m.q.
chocolate coated, w/cookies								
(*Twix*), 1.77-oz. bar	130	3.0	14.0	7.0	m.q.	n.a.	70	m.q.

Food and Measure	cal.	prot. (gms)	carbo. (gms)	tot. fat (gms)	sat. fat (gms)	chol. (mgs)	sod. (mgs)	fiber (gms)
cup:								
(*Boyer*, .275 oz.), 1 piece	38	1.3	6.0	3.8	m.q.	n.a.	n.a.	m.q.
(*Boyer*, .5 oz.), 1 piece	75	2.5	12.0	7.5	m.q.	n.a.	n.a.	m.q.
(*Boyer*, 1.6 oz.), 2 pieces	250	5.0	23.0	15.0	m.q.	n.a.	n.a.	m.q.
(*Estee*), 1 piece	40	1.0	3.0	3.0	2.5	<1	20	m.q.
chocolate coated (*Reese's*),								
1.8 oz.	280	6.0	26.0	17.0	m.q.	10	180	m.q.
kisses (*Brach's*), 1 oz.	110	1.0	22.0	2.0	m.q.	n.a.	135	m.q.
peanut caramel cluster (*Brach's*),								
1 oz.	150	4.0	15.0	8.0	m.q.	n.a.	50	m.q.
peanut parfait (*Brach's*), 1 oz.	160	3.0	14.0	10.0	m.q.	n.a.	60	m.q.
peppermint kisses (*Brach's*), 1 oz. ...	100	0	24.0	1.0	n.a.	n.a.	25	n.a.
peppermint swirls (*Featherweight*),								
1 piece	20	0	5.0	0	0	0	0	0
popcorn, caramel coated:								
(*Estee*), 1-oz. bag	140	3.0	25.0	3.0	1.5	5	55	m.q.
(*Orville Redenbacher*), 2.5 cups ..	240	2.0	29.0	14.0	m.q.	0	90	m.q.
and peanuts (*Cracker Jack*), 1 oz.	120	2.0	22.0	3.0	m.q.	0	85	m.q.
raisins, chocolate coated:								
(*Brach's*), 1 oz.	130	1.0	20.0	5.0	m.q.	n.a.	30	m.q.
(*Estee*), 10 pieces	30	<1.0	5.0	1.0	1.0	<1	10	m.q.
(*Nabisco*), 1 oz., approx.								
29 pieces	130	1.0	21.0	5.0	m.q.	n.a.	15	m.q.
(*Raisinets*), 1⅜ oz.	180	2.0	28.0	6.0	m.q.	n.a.	10	m.q.
raspberry, filled (*Brach's*), 1 oz. ...	110	0	27.0	0	0	0	15	(0)
ribbon, crimp (*Brach's*), 1 oz.	110	0	27.0	0	0	0	15	0
rock (*Brach's* Cut Rock), 1 oz.	110	0	27.0	0	0	0	10	0
(*Rolaids*), 1 piece	4	tr.	1.1	tr.	0	0	n.a.	0
seasonal and specialty, 1 oz., except								
as noted:								
autumn leaves (*Brach's*)	100	0	26.0	0	0	0	15	0
Christmas:								
(*Brach's* Jots)	130	1.0	21.0	5.0	m.q.	n.a.	30	n.a.
(*Brach's* Perkys)	90	0	23.0	0	0	0	20	0
bell, chocolate, in foil (*Brach's*)	150	2.0	17.0	8.0	m.q.	n.a.	25	m.q.
candy cane (*Brach's*)	110	0	27.0	0	0	0	10	0
candy cane (*Spangler*), 1 piece	60	<1.0	14.0	<1.0	0	0	0	0
chocolate, assorted (*Brach's*) ..	110	0	23.0	2.0	m.q.	n.a.	25	m.q.
jellies (*Brach's*)	100	0	24.0	0	0	0	10	0
jellies, snowbase (*Brach's*)	100	0	24.0	0	0	0	5	0
mint (*Brach's* Pearls)	110	0	25.0	1.0	n.a.	0	5	0
mint (*Brach's* Starlight)	110	0	27.0	0	0	0	15	0
nougat (*Brach's*)	110	0	24.0	2.0	m.q.	n.a.	20	m.q.
ornaments (*Brach's*)	150	2.0	17.0	8.0	m.q.	n.a.	50	n.a.
Santa, chocolate, in foil								
(*Brach's*)	140	2.0	18.0	7.0	m.q.	n.a.	40	m.q.
Santa, marshmallow (*Brach's*) ..	120	1.0	23.0	3.0	m.q.	n.a.	35	0

Food and Measure	cal.	prot. (gms)	carbo. (gms)	tot. fat (gms)	sat. fat (gms)	chol. (mgs)	sod. (mgs)	fiber (gms)
CANDY, SEASONAL, CHRISTMAS *(cont.)*								
snowmen or trees,								
marshmallow:								
(*Just Born*), 1 large	111	.7	26.8	.1	(0)	n.a.	8	0
(*Just Born*), 1 small	37	.2	8.9	<.1	(0)	n.a.	3	0
Easter:								
assorted (*Brach's* Chicks &								
Rabbits)	100	0	26.0	0	0	0	10	0
assorted (*Brach's* Easter Fun)	100	0	26.0	0	0	0	10	0
eggs:								
(*Brach's* Hide'n Seek)	110	0	27.0	0	0	0	5	0
(*Brach's* Robin's Eggs)	140	1.0	20.0	6.0	m.q.	n.a.	30	0
chocolate, in foil (*Brach's*) ...	150	2.0	17.0	8.0	m.q.	n.a.	25	m.q.
chocolate malted milk								
(*Brach's*)	130	1.0	21.0	5.0	m.q.	n.a.	40	m.q.
jelly (*Brach's*)	100	0	24.0	0	0	0	15	0
jelly (*Brach's* Tiny)	100	0	26.0	0	0	0	10	0
jelly, speckled (*Brach's*)	110	0	27.0	0	0	0	40	0
jelly, spiced (*Brach's*)	90	0	22.0	0	0	0	10	0
marshmallow (*Brach's*)	100	0	25.0	0	0	0	5	0
pastel (*Brach's* Fiesta)	120	1.0	23.0	3.0	m.q.	n.a.	25	0
eggs, creme (*Cadbury*),								
1.37 oz.	190	2.0	26.0	8.0	m.q.	n.a.	0	n.a.
eggs, creme mini (*Cadbury*) ...	140	2.0	20.0	7.0	m.q.	n.a.	n.a.	n.a.
eggs, creme, chocolate coated:								
cherry (*Brach's*)	110	1.0	23.0	2.0	m.q.	n.a.	20	m.q.
chocolate buttercream								
(*Brach's*)	120	1.0	22.0	3.0	m.q.	n.a.	50	m.q.
coconut (*Brach's*)	110	0	22.0	3.0	m.q.	n.a.	40	m.q.
fruit and nut (*Brach's*)	110	0	23.0	2.0	m.q.	n.a.	35	m.q.
maple (*Brach's*)	110	0	23.0	2.0	m.q.	n.a.	30	m.q.
vanilla (*Brach's*)	110	0	23.0	2.0	m.q.	n.a.	25	m.q.
corn (*Brach's*)	100	0	26.0	0	0	0	66	0
mint (*Brach's* Starlight)	110	0	27.0	0	0	0	15	0
nougats (*Brach's*)	100	0	24.0	1.0	n.a.	0	25	m.q.
peeps, marshmallow (*Just Born*)								
1 piece	27	.2	6.6	<.1	(0)	0	2	0
rabbits, jel (*Brach's* Jube)	100	0	24.0	0	0	0	15	0
rabbits, marshmallow:								
(*Brach's*)	120	1.0	22.0	3.0	m.q.	0	55	0
(*Just Born*), 1 large	111	.7	26.8	.1	0	0	8	0
(*Just Born*), 1 small	28	.2	6.7	<.1	0	0	2	0
Halloween:								
(*Brach's* Mellowcremes)	100	0	26.0	0	0	0	40	0
(*Brach's* Trick or Treat Party								
Pack)	110	0	27.0	0	0	0	20	0
cats (*Brach's* Scary Cats)	100	0	26.0	0	0	0	85	0
cats, marshmallow (*Just Born*),								
1 piece	28	.2	6.7	<.1	0	0	2	0

Food and Measure	cal.	prot. (gms)	carbo. (gms)	tot. fat (gms)	sat. fat (gms)	chol. (mgs)	sod. (mgs)	fiber (gms)
corn, Indian (*Brach's*)	100	0	26.0	0	0	0	75	0
corn, three color (*Brach's*)	100	0	26.0	0	0	0	95	0
jelly beans (*Brach's*)	100	0	26.0	0	0	0	15	0
lollipops (*Brach's* Picture Pops)	110	0	27.0	0	0	0	10	0
pumpkin heads, crazy (*Brach's*)	100	0	24.0	1.0	n.a.	0	15	0
pumpkins:								
(*Brach's*)	100	0	26.0	0	0	0	65	0
marshmallow (*Just Born*),								
1 large	111	.7	26.8	.1	0	0	8	0
marshmallow (*Just Born*),								
1 small	14	.1	3.4	<.1	0	0	1	0
witches teeth (*Brach's*)	100	0	26.0	0	0	0	75	0
holiday mints (*Brach's*)	110	0	26.0	1.0	n.a.	0	0	0
holiday mix (*Brach's*)	110	0	27.0	0	0	0	10	0
Valentine's Day:								
(*Brach's* Heart Box, ½ lb.)	110	1.0	23.0	2.0	m.q.	n.a.	35	n.a.
(*Brach's* Love)	150	2.0	17.0	8.0	m.q.	n.a.	25	n.a.
(*Brach's* Mellowcremes)	100	0	26.0	0	0	0	75	0
(*Brach's* Valentine Heart, 1 lb.)	110	1.0	23.0	2.0	m.q.	n.a.	30	n.a.
(*Brach's* Valentine Heart, ⅓ lb.)	110	1.0	23.0	2.0	m.q.	n.a.	25	n.a.
chocolate (*Brach's* I Luv U) ...	150	2.0	17.0	8.0	m.q.	n.a.	25	n.a.
hearts:								
(*Brach's*, 14/28 oz.)	110	1.0	23.0	2.0	m.q.	n.a.	30	n.a.
(*Brach's* Conversation,								
Large)	110	0	27.0	0	0	0	5	0
(*Brach's* Conversation, Small)	110	0	27.0	0	0	0	0	0
(*Brach's* Sassy Hearts)	100	0	25.0	0	0	0	0	0
cherry jel (*Brach's* Jube)	100	0	26.0	0	0	0	20	0
cinnamon (*Brach's* Imperial)	110	0	27.0	0	0	0	5	0
fruity (*Brach's*)	100	0	24.0	0	0	0	5	0
jelly, red (*Brach's*)	100	0	24.0	0	0	0	10	0
kisses, nougat (*Brach's*)	110	0	24.0	2.0	m.q.	n.a.	15	n.a.
(*Snickers*), 2.07-oz. bar	280	6.0	35.0	14.0	m.q.	n.a.	160	n.a.
sour balls (*Brach's*), 1 oz.	110	0	27.0	0	0	0	15	0
spice (*Brach's* Spicettes), 1 oz.	100	0	26.0	0	0	0	15	0
straws, mint filled (*Brach's*), 1 oz. ..	110	0	26.0	1.0	n.a.	0	10	0
taffy:								
all flavors (*Brach's* Salt Water								
Taffy), 1 oz.	100	0	24.0	1.0	n.a.	0	30	0
apple flavor chews (*Beich's Laffy*								
Taffy), 1 oz., approx. 2 pieces	110	0	26.0	1.0	n.a.	0	55	0
banana flavor chews (*Beich's Laffy*								
Taffy), 1 oz., approx. 2 pieces	120	0	26.0	1.0	n.a.	0	55	0
cherry flavor chews, sweet and								
sour (*Beich's Laffy Taffy*), 1 oz.,								
approx. 2 pieces	110	0	26.0	1.0	n.a.	0	55	0
grape flavor chews (*Beich's Laffy*								
Taffy), 1 oz., approx. 2 pieces	110	0	26.0	1.0	n.a.	0	60	0

Food and Measure	cal.	prot. (gms)	carbo. (gms)	tot. fat (gms)	sat. fat (gms)	chol. (mgs)	sod. (mgs)	fiber (gms)
CANDY, TAFFY *(cont.)*								
passion punch flavor chews								
(*Beich's Laffy Taffy*), 1 oz.,								
approx. 2 pieces	120	0	26.0	1.0	n.a.	0	50	0
strawberry flavor chews (*Beich's*								
Laffy Taffy), 1 oz., approx.								
2 pieces	110	0	26.0	1.0	n.a.	0	55	0
watermelon flavor chews (*Beich's*								
Laffy Taffy), 1 oz., approx.								
2 pieces	110	0	26.0	1.0	n.a.	0	55	0
(*3 Musketeers*), 2.13-oz. bar	260	2.0	46.0	8.0	m.q.	n.a.	120	m.q.
toffee:								
(*Brach's*), 1 oz.	110	1.0	23.0	2.0	m.q.	0	80	0
(*Callard & Bowser*), 1 oz.	135	.5	19.2	6.5	n.a.	0	n.a.	0
(*Skor*), 1.4 oz.	220	2.0	22.0	14.0	m.q.	25	125	n.a.
English (*Bits 'O Heath*), 3.5 oz. ..	520	3.0	62.0	31.0	m.q.	n.a.	390	n.a.
English (*Heath* Bar), 2 pieces,								
1³⁄₁₆ oz.	180	1.0	20.0	11.0	m.q.	n.a.	130	m.q.
(*Tootsie Roll*), 1 oz.	112	.3	22.8	2.5	.6	tr.	6	(0)
wafer:								
assorted (*Necco*), 2.02-oz. roll ...	225	.3	56.5	0	0	0	5	(0)
chocolate (*Necco*), 2.02-oz. roll ..	226	.5	56.3	.1	0	0	5	(0)
bar, chocolate coated (*Kit Kat*),								
1.63 oz.	250	3.0	29.0	13.0	m.q.	10	60	m.q.
CANE SYRUP:								
1 tbsp.	52	0	13.4	0	0	0	<1	0
CANNELLINI BEAN, see "Kidney								
bean, white"								
CANNELLONI, canned:								
mini (*Chef Boyardee*), 7.5 oz.	230	9.0	33.0	7.0	m.q.	m.q.	1050	m.q.
CANNELLONI ENTREE, frozen:								
beef and pork, w/mornay sauce								
(*Lean Cuisine*), 9⅝ oz.	260	17.0	25.0	10.0	4.0	45	950	m.q.
cheese (*Dining Lite*), 9 oz.	310	19.0	38.0	9.0	m.q.	70	650	m.q.
cheese, w/tomato sauce (*Lean*								
Cuisine), 9⅛ oz.	260	21.0	22.0	10.0	5.0	35	910	m.q.
Florentine (*Celentano*), 12 oz.	350	21.0	48.0	8.0	m.q.	n.a.	620	m.q.
CANOLA OIL:								
1 oz.	251	0	0	28.4	2.0	0	0	0
½ cup	964	0	0	109.0	7.7	0	0	0
1 tbsp.	124	0	0	14.0	1.0	0	0	0
(*Hain*), 1 tbsp.	120	0	0	14.0	1.0	0	0	0
(*Nucoa Heart Beat*), 1 tbsp.	120	0	0	14.0	1.0	0	0	0
CANTALOUPE:								
untrimmed, 1 lb.	82	2.0	19.3	.6	n.a.	0	20	1.9 d
pulp, 1 oz.	10	.2	2.4	.1	(0)	0	3	.3 d
½ of 5″-diam. melon	94	2.3	22.3	.7	(0)	0	23	2.1 d
cubed, ½ cup	29	.7	6.7	.2	(0)	0	7	.6 d

Food and Measure	cal.	prot. (gms)	carbo. (gms)	tot. fat (gms)	sat. fat (gms)	chol. (mgs)	sod. (mgs)	fiber (gms)
CAPE GOOSEBERRY, see								
"Ground cherry"								
CAPOCOLLO:								
(*Hormel*), 1 oz.	80	5.0	0	6.0	m.q.	m.q.	273	0
CAPON, see "Chicken, capon"								
CAPON GIBLETS, see "Chicken								
giblets"								
CAPONATA, see "Eggplant								
appetizer"								
CARAMBOLA:								
untrimmed, 1 lb.	142	2.3	33.7	1.5	n.a.	0	7	5.0 d
trimmed, 1 oz.	9	.2	2.2	.1	(0)	0	1	.3 d
1 medium, approx. 4.7 oz.	42	.7	9.9	.4	(0)	0	2	1.5 d
cubed, ½ cup	23	.4	5.4	.2	(0)	0	1	.8 d
CARAMEL, see "Candy"								
CARAMEL TOPPING:								
(*Kraft*), 1 tbsp.	60	1.0	13.0	0	0	0	45	0
flavored (*Smucker's*), 2 tbsp.	140	1.0	33.0	0	0	0	110	0
hot (*Smucker's*), 2 tbsp.	150	1.0	28.0	4.0	m.q.	0	75	0
CARAWAY SEED:								
1 oz.	94	5.6	14.1	4.1	.2	0	5	3.6 c
1 tbsp.	22	1.3	3.3	1.0	<.1	0	1	.9 c
1 tsp.	7	.4	1.1	.3	tr.	0	tr.	.3 c
(*Spice Islands*), 1 tsp.	8	.4	.8	.4	tr.	0	<1	.2 c
(*Tone's*), 1 tsp.	7	.4	1.1	.3	<.1	0	<1	.5 d
CARDAMOM:								
ground:								
1 oz.	88	3.1	19.4	1.9	.2	0	5	3.2 c
1 tbsp.	18	.6	4.0	.4	<.1	0	1	.7 c
1 tsp.	6	.2	1.4	.1	tr.	0	tr.	.1 c
(*Tone's*), 1 tsp.	6	.2	1.3	.1	<.1	0	<1	.2 d
seed (*Spice Islands*), 1 tsp.	6	.2	1.3	.1	tr.	0	tr.	.2 c
CARDONI, see "Cardoon"								
CARDOON:								
raw:								
untrimmed, 1 lb.	44	1.6	10.9	.2	<.1	0	378	m.q.
trimmed, 1 oz.	6	.2	1.4	<.1	tr.	0	48	m.q.
shredded, ½ cup	18	.6	4.4	.1	<.1	0	151	m.q.
boiled, drained, 4 oz.	25	.9	6.0	.1	<.1	0	200	m.q.
CARIBOU, meat only:								
raw, 1 oz.	36	6.4	0	1.0	.4	24	16	0
roasted[1]:								
12 oz., yield from 1 lb. raw								
boneless	568	101.3	0	15.0	5.8	372	204	0
4 oz.	189	33.8	0	5.0	1.9	124	68	0
diced, 1 cup, approx. 4.9 oz.	234	41.7	0	6.2	2.4	153	84	0

---

1. *Without added ingredients.*

Food and Measure	cal.	prot. (gms)	carbo. (gms)	tot. fat (gms)	sat. fat (gms)	chol. (mgs)	sod. (mgs)	fiber (gms)
CARISSA:								
untrimmed, 1 lb.	240	2.0	53.2	5.1	n.a.	0	11	3.5 c
trimmed, 1 oz.	18	.1	3.9	.4	(0)	0	1	.3 c
1 medium, approx. .8 oz.	12	.1	2.7	.3	(0)	0	1	.2 c
sliced, ½ cup	46	.4	10.2	1.0	(0)	0	2	.7 c
CARL'S JR.:								
breakfast, 1 serving:								
bacon, 2 strips, .4 oz.	50	3.0	0	4.0	3.0	8	200	0
eggs, scrambled, 2.4 oz.	120	9.0	2.0	9.0	4.0	245	105	0
English muffin, w/margarine, 2 oz.	180	4.0	28.0	6.0	2.0	0	275	m.q.
French toast dips, w/out syrup,								
4.7 oz.	480	8.0	54.0	25.0	10.0	54	576	m.q.
hash brown nuggets, 3 oz.	170	2.0	20.0	9.0	4.0	10	350	m.q.
hot cakes w/margarine, w/out								
syrup, 5.5 oz.	360	7.0	59.0	12.0	3.0	15	1190	m.q.
sausage, 1 patty, .5 oz.	190	7.0	1.0	17.0	4.0	25	275	0
Sunrise Sandwich, w/bacon,								
4.5 oz.	370	17.0	32.0	19.0	8.0	120	750	m.q.
Sunrise Sandwich, w/sausage,								
6.1 oz.	500	22.0	31.0	32.0	12.0	165	990	m.q.
sandwiches, 1 serving:								
California Roast Beef 'n Swiss,								
7.4 oz.	360	31.0	43.0	8.0	4.0	130	1070	m.q.
Charbroiler BBQ Chicken								
Sandwich, 6.3 oz.	320	28.0	40.0	5.0	2.0	50	955	m.q.
Charbroiler Chicken Club								
Sandwich, 8.3 oz.	510	26.0	53.0	22.0	2.0	85	1165	m.q.
Country Fried Steak Sandwich,								
7.2 oz.	610	25.0	54.0	33.0	12.0	45	1290	m.q.
Double Western Bacon								
Cheeseburger, 7.5 oz.	890	42.0	61.0	53.0	25.0	145	1620	m.q.
Famous Star Hamburger, 8.1 oz.	590	24.0	42.0	36.0	13.0	45	890	m.q.
fish fillet, 7.9 oz.	550	22.0	58.0	26.0	11.0	90	945	m.q.
Happy Star hamburger, 3 oz.	220	12.0	26.0	8.0	4.0	45	445	m.q.
Old Time Star hamburger, 5.9 oz.	400	24.0	38.0	17.0	7.0	80	760	m.q.
Super Star hamburger, 10.6 oz. ..	770	37.0	44.0	50.0	21.0	125	990	m.q.
Western Bacon Cheeseburger,								
7.5 oz.	630	33.0	49.0	33.0	15.0	105	1415	m.q.
potatoes, 1 serving:								
bacon and cheese, 14.1 oz.	650	23.0	63.0	34.0	12.0	45	1820	m.q.
broccoli and cheese, 14 oz.	470	15.0	61.0	17.0	5.0	10	690	m.q.
cheese, 14.2 oz.	350	18.0	72.0	22.0	7.0	40	785	m.q.
Fiesta, 15.2 oz.	550	25.0	60.0	23.0	9.0	40	1230	m.q.
Lite, 9.8 oz.	250	8.0	54.0	3.0	0	0	35	m.q.
sour cream and chive, 10.4 oz. ..	350	8.0	49.0	13.0	5.0	10	140	m.q.
salad-to-go, 1 serving:								
chef, 10.7 oz.	180	19.0	11.0	7.0	3.0	63	581	m.q.
chicken, 10.9 oz.	206	23.0	12.0	8.0	3.0	83	453	m.q.
garden, 4.1 oz.	46	2.0	4.0	2.0	1.0	7	57	m.q.

Food and Measure	cal.	prot. (gms)	carbo. (gms)	tot. fat (gms)	sat. fat (gms)	chol. (mgs)	sod. (mgs)	fiber (gms)
taco, 14.3 oz.	356	29.0	18.0	19.0	6.0	99	690	m.q.
salad dressing, 1 oz.:								
blue cheese	151	1.0	0	15.0	3.0	18	255	0
French, reduced calorie	38	0	5.0	2.0	0	0	292	0
house	110	1.0	2.0	11.0	3.0	10	170	(0)
Italian	120	0	1.0	13.0	2.0	0	210	(0)
Thousand Island	110	0	4.0	11.0	3.0	5	200	(0)
side dishes, 1 serving:								
french fries, regular, 6 oz.	360	8.0	43.0	17.0	11.0	15	626	m.q.
onion rings, 3.2 oz.	310	4.0	38.0	15.0	7.0	10	260	m.q.
zucchini, 4.3 oz.	300	5.0	33.0	16.0	7.0	10	480	m.q.
soup, 6.6-oz. serving:								
Boston clam chowder	140	6.0	12.0	8.0	3.0	22	861	m.q.
broccoli, cream of	140	7.0	14.0	6.0	4.0	22	845	m.q.
chicken noodle, old fashioned	80	4.0	11.0	1.0	tr.	14	605	m.q.
Lumber Jack Mix vegetable	70	2.0	10.0	3.0	tr.	3	807	m.q.
bakery products, 1 serving:								
blueberry muffin, 3.5 oz.	256	4.0	40.0	7.0	1.0	34	360	m.q.
bran muffin, 4 oz.	220	4.0	34.0	6.0	0	50	300	m.q.
brownie, fudge, 4.5 oz.	597	8.0	88.0	27.0	7.0	tr.	295	m.q.
chocolate chip cookie, 2.5 oz. ...	327	3.0	41.0	17.0	6.0	3	170	m.q.
cinnamon roll, 4 oz.	459	7.0	70.0	16.0	1.0	tr.	226	m.q.
danish (varieties), 4 oz.	519	7.0	73.0	21.0	1.0	tr.	230	m.q.
shakes, regular, 11.6 oz.	353	11.0	61.0	7.0	4.0	17	255	(0)
CAROB FLAVOR DRINK MIX:								
powder, 1 oz.	105	.5	26.5	.1	tr.	0	29	.5 c
powder, 3 tsp.	45	.2	11.2	tr.	tr.	0	12	.2 c
beverage:								
1 cup whole milk and 3 tsp.								
powder	195	8.2	22.6	8.2	5.1	33	132	.2 c
1 cup lowfat 2% milk and 3 tsp.								
powder	166	8.3	22.9	4.7	2.9	18	134	.2 c
1 cup lowfat 1% milk and 3 tsp.								
powder	147	8.2	22.9	2.6	1.6	10	135	.2 c
1 cup skim milk and 3 tsp. powder	131	8.6	23.1	.4	.3	4	138	.2 c
CAROB FLOUR:								
1 oz.	51	1.3	25.2	.2	tr.	0	10	3.0 d
1 cup	185	4.8	91.6	.7	.1	0	36	10.9 d
1 tbsp.	14	.4	7.1	.1	tr.	0	3	.8 d
CARP, meat only:								
raw:								
1 lb.	574	80.9	0	25.4	4.9	298	223	0
1 oz.	36	5.1	0	1.6	.3	19	14	0
1 fillet, approx. 7.7 oz., yield from								
3-lb. whole fish	276	38.9	0	12.2	2.4	143	107	0
baked, broiled, or microwaved[1],								
4 oz.	184	25.9	0	8.1	1.6	95	71	0

1. *Without added ingredients.*

Food and Measure	cal.	prot. (gms)	carbo. (gms)	tot. fat (gms)	sat. fat (gms)	chol. (mgs)	sod. (mgs)	fiber (gms)
CARROT:								
raw:								
untrimmed, 1 lb.	174	4.1	41.0	.8	.1	0	139	12.9 d
trimmed, 1 oz.	12	.3	2.9	.1	tr.	0	10	.9 d
1 medium, 7½″ long × 1⅛″,								
approx. 2.8 oz.	31	.7	7.3	.1	<.1	0	25	2.3 d
shredded, ½ cup	24	.6	5.6	.1	<.1	0	19	1.8 d
boiled, drained:								
4 oz.	51	1.2	11.9	.2	<.1	0	75	2.2 d
1 medium, approx. 1.6 oz.	21	.5	4.8	.1	<.1	0	30	.9 d
sliced, ½ cup	35	.9	8.2	.1	<.1	0	52	1.5 d
CARROT, CANNED, ½ cup,								
except as noted:								
w/liquid:								
4 oz.	26	.7	5.7	.2	<.1	0	273	1.2 d
sliced	28	.8	6.2	.2	<.1	0	297	1.4 d
low-sodium, 4 oz.	26	.7	5.7	.2	<.1	0	44	1.3 d
low-sodium, sliced	28	.8	6.2	.2	<.1	0	48	1.4 d
whole, sliced or diced (*Del Monte*)	30	0	7.0	0	0	0	265	m.q.
drained:								
4 oz.	26	.7	6.3	.2	<.1	0	273	1.7 d
sliced	17	.5	4.0	.1	<.1	0	176	1.1 d
low-sodium, 4 oz.	26	.7	6.3	.2	<.1	0	48	1.7 d
low-sodium, sliced	17	.5	4.0	.1	<.1	0	31	1.1 d
(*A&P*)	30	1.0	6.0	<1.0	(0)	0	300	m.q.
(*A&P* No Salt Added)	25	<1.0	6.0	<1.0	(0)	0	40	m.q.
(*Stokely*)	35	1.0	7.0	0	0	0	300	m.q.
(*Stokely* No Salt or Sugar Added) ...	35	1.0	7.0	0	0	0	35	m.q.
whole, baby (*Allens*)	30	1.0	6.0	<1.0	(0)	0	240	m.q.
whole, tiny (*S&W* Fancy)	30	1.0	7.0	0	0	0	240	m.q.
sliced:								
(*Featherweight*)	30	1.0	6.0	0	0	0	30	m.q.
(*Finast*)	35	1.0	8.0	0	0	0	370	m.q.
(*Finast* No Salt Added)	35	1.0	8.0	0	0	0	30	m.q.
(*IGA*)	30	1.0	6.0	0	0	0	300	m.q.
(*Pathmark*)	35	1.0	7.0	0	0	0	310	m.q.
(*Pathmark* No Salt Added)	35	1.0	8.0	0	0	0	35	m.q.
(*S&W/Nutradiet*)	30	0	7.0	0	0	0	50	m.q.
diced or julienne (*S&W* Fancy) ...	30	1.0	7.0	0	0	0	240	m.q.
small, medium or large (*Allens*) ..	30	1.0	7.0	<1.0	(0)	0	250	m.q.
diced (*Allens*)	30	1.0	5.0	<1.0	(0)	0	190	m.q.
CARROT, FROZEN:								
10-oz. pkg.	112	3.1	25.5	.6	.1	0	167	4.0 d
boiled, drained, 4 oz.	41	1.3	9.4	.1	<.1	0	67	2.0 d
boiled, drained, sliced, ½ cup	26	.9	6.0	.1	<.1	0	43	1.3 d
(*A&P*), 3.3 oz.	40	1.0	9.0	<1.0	(0)	0	45	m.q.
(*Birds Eye* Deluxe Parisienne),								
2.6 oz.	30	1.0	7.0	0	0	0	35	2.0 d
(*Seabrook*), 3.3 oz.	40	1.0	9.0	0	0	0	44	1.0 c

Food and Measure	cal.	prot. (gms)	carbo. (gms)	tot. fat (gms)	sat. fat (gms)	chol. (mgs)	sod. (mgs)	fiber (gms)
whole:								
(*Southern*), 3.5 oz.	42	1.2	8.7	.2	0	0	60	m.q.
baby (*Birds Eye* Deluxe), 3.3 oz.	40	1.0	9.0	0	0	0	45	2.0 d
baby (*Green Giant Harvest Fresh*),								
½ cup	18	1.0	5.0	0	0	0	75	2.0 d
baby (*Stokely Singles*), 3 oz.	35	1.0	8.0	0	0	0	50	m.q.
sliced (*Birds Eye*), 3.2 oz.	35	1.0	8.0	0	0	0	40	1.0 d
sliced (*Frosty Acres*), 3.3 oz.	40	1.0	9.0	0	0	0	44	1.0 c
CARROT, COMBINATIONS,								
frozen:								
baby, w/sweet peas and pearl onions								
(*Birds Eye* Deluxe), 3.3 oz. ...	50	2.0	10.0	0	0	0	60	2.0 d
CARROT CAKE, see "Cake"								
CARROT CHIP:								
(*Hain*), 1 oz.	150	2.0	16.0	9.0	m.q.	0	160	m.q.
(*Hain* No Salt Added), 1 oz.	150	2.0	16.0	7.0	m.q.	0	30	m.q.
barbecue (*Hain*), 1 oz.	140	2.0	16.0	8.0	m.q.	0	160	m.q.
CARROT JUICE, canned or								
bottled:								
1 fl. oz.	12	.3	2.8	<.1	tr.	0	9	.3 c
6 fl. oz.	73	1.7	17.1	.3	.1	0	54	1.8 c
(*Biotta*), 6 fl. oz.	51	1.5	11.3	.1	(0)	0	158	m.q.
(*Hain*), 6 fl. oz.	80	1.0	17.0	0	0	0	170	m.q.
(*Hollywood*), 6 fl. oz.	80	1.0	17.0	0	0	0	170	2.0 d
CASABA:								
untrimmed, 1 lb.	71	2.5	16.9	.3	(0)	0	33	1.4 c
pulp, 1 oz.	7	.3	1.8	<.1	(0)	0	3	.1 c
⅒ of 7¾" melon, 2" slice	43	1.5	10.2	.2	(0)	0	20	.8 c
cubed, ½ cup	23	.8	5.3	.1	(0)	0	10	.4 c
CASHEW:								
(*Beer Nuts*), 1 oz.	170	5.0	8.0	13.0	m.q.	0	65	m.q.
dry-roasted:								
1 oz., approx. 14 large, 18								
medium, or 26 small kernels ..	163	4.4	9.3	13.2	2.6	0	4	1.7 d
wholes and halves, 1 cup	787	21.0	44.8	63.5	12.5	0	21	7.8 d
(*Planters* Unsalted), 1 oz.	160	5.0	9.0	13.0	3.0	0	0	m.q.
salted:								
1 oz.	163	4.4	9.3	13.2	2.6	0	181	1.7 d
wholes and halves, 1 cup	787	21.0	44.8	63.5	12.5	0	877	7.8 d
whole (*Guys*), 1 oz.	170	5.0	5.0	14.0	m.q.	0	140	m.q.
(*Pathmark*), 1 oz.	170	4.0	9.0	13.0	m.q.	0	150	m.q.
(*Pathmark* No Frills), 1 oz.	170	5.0	8.0	13.0	3.0	0	220	m.q.
(*Planters*), 1 oz.	160	5.0	9.0	13.0	3.0	0	230	m.q.
honey-roasted (*Planters*), 1 oz.	170	4.0	11.0	12.0	2.0	0	170	m.q.
honey-roasted, w/peanuts (*Planters*),								
1 oz.	170	5.0	9.0	12.0	2.0	0	170	m.q.
oil-roasted:								
1 oz., approx. 14 large or 18								
medium	163	4.6	8.1	13.7	2.7	0	5	.4 c

Food and Measure	cal.	prot. (gms)	carbo. (gms)	tot. fat (gms)	sat. fat (gms)	chol. (mgs)	sod. (mgs)	fiber (gms)
CASHEW, OIL-ROASTED *(cont.)*								
wholes and halves, 1 cup	748	21.0	37.1	62.7	12.4	0	22	1.7 c
halves (*Planters* Unsalted), 1 oz.	170	5.0	8.0	14.0	3.0	0	0	m.q.
salted:								
1 oz., approx. 14 large or 18								
medium	163	4.6	8.1	13.7	2.7	0	177	.4 c
wholes and halves, 1 cup	748	21.0	37.1	62.7	12.4	0	814	1.7 c
(*Flavor House*), 1 oz.	180	7.0	3.0	16.0	m.q.	0	125	m.q.
(*Pathmark/Pathmark* No Frills),								
1 oz.	170	5.0	8.0	14.0	m.q.	0	150	m.q.
(*Planters* Fancy), 1 oz.	170	5.0	8.0	14.0	3.0	0	135	m.q.
halves (*Planters*), 1 oz.	170	5.0	8.0	14.0	3.0	0	135	m.q.
CASHEW BUTTER:								
1 oz.	167	5.0	7.8	14.0	2.8	0	4	.2 c
1 tbsp.	94	2.8	4.4	7.9	1.6	0	2	.1 c
(*Hain* Raw), 2 tbsp.	190	6.0	8.0	15.0	3.0	0	m.q.	m.q.
(*Hain* Raw Unsalted), 2 tbsp.	210	5.0	8.0	19.0	3.0	0	10	m.q.
(*Hain* Toasted), 2 tbsp.	210	7.0	7.0	17.0	3.0	0	15	m.q.
(*Westbrae Natural*), 2 tbsp.	190	6.0	8.0	17.0	m.q.	0	0	m.q.
salted, 1 oz.	167	5.0	7.8	14.0	2.8	0	174	.2 c
salted, 1 tbsp.	94	2.8	4.4	7.9	1.6	0	98	.1 c
CASSAVA:								
trimmed, 1 lb.	544	14.1	122.1	1.8	.5	0	36	11.3 c
trimmed, 1 oz.	34	.9	7.6	.1	<.1	0	2	.7 c
CATFISH:								
channel, raw, meat only:								
1 lb.	527	82.5	0	19.3	4.5	263	286	0
1 oz.	33	5.2	0	1.2	.3	16	18	0
1 fillet, approx. 2.8 oz., yield from								
1-lb. whole fish	92	14.4	0	3.4	.8	46	50	0
channel, breaded[1], fried, meat only:								
4 oz.	260	20.5	9.1	15.1	3.7	92	318	.5 c
1 fillet, approx. 3.1 oz., yield from								
raw unbreaded fillet	199	15.7	7.0	11.6	2.9	70	244	.4 c
CATFISH, FROZEN:								
fillets (*Delta Pride*), 4 oz.	132	18.0	4.8	4.9	m.q.	62	<1	0
ocean (*Booth*), 4 oz.	115	20.0	0	20.0	m.q.	m.q.	85	0
CATJANG:								
raw, 1 oz.	97	6.8	16.9	.6	.2	0	16	1.3 c
raw, ½ cup	288	20.0	50.1	1.7	.5	0	49	3.9 c
boiled, 4 oz.	133	9.2	23.0	.8	.2	0	22	1.8 c
boiled, ½ cup	100	7.0	17.5	.6	.2	0	16	1.4 c
CATSUP:								
1 oz.	29	.4	7.7	.1	<.1	0	336	.5 d
.2-oz. pkt.	6	.1	1.6	<.1	tr.	0	71	.1 d
1 tbsp.	16	.2	4.1	.1	<.1	0	178	.2 d
(*Del Monte*), ¼ cup	60	1.0	16.0	0	0	0	675	m.q.

1. *Recipe: 84.2% fish, 9.3% cornmeal, 4.6% egg, 1.4% milk and .5% salt.*

Food and Measure	cal.	prot. (gms)	carbo. (gms)	tot. fat (gms)	sat. fat (gms)	chol. (mgs)	sod. (mgs)	fiber (gms)
(*Del Monte* No Salt Added), ¼ cup ..	60	1.0	16.0	0	0	0	25	m.q.
(*Estee*), 1 tbsp.	6	0	0	0	0	0	20	m.q.
(*Featherweight*), 1 tbsp.	6	0	1.0	0	0	0	5	m.q.
(*Hain* Natural), 1 tbsp.	16	0	4.0	0	0	0	155	m.q.
(*Hain* Natural No Salt Added),								
1 tbsp.	16	0	4.0	0	0	0	5	m.q.
(*Heinz*), 1 tbsp.	16	.2	3.8	0	0	0	213	.2 c
(*Heinz* Lite), 1 tbsp.	8	.4	1.7	0	0	0	115	.2 c
(*Hunt's*), 1 tbsp.	15	0	4.0	0	0	0	170	m.q.
(*Hunt's* No Salt Added), 1 tbsp.	20	0	5.0	0	0	0	0	m.q.
(*Life* All Natural), 1 tbsp.	17	0	4.0	0	0	0	<10	m.q.
(*Smucker's*), 1 tsp.	8	0	2.0	0	0	0	45	m.q.
(*Stokely*), 1 tbsp.	20	0	5.0	0	0	0	190	m.q.
(*Weight Watchers*), 2 tsp.	8	0	2.0	0	0	0	110	m.q.
hot (*Heinz*), 1 tbsp.	16	.3	3.7	0	0	0	195	.1 c
low sodium (see also specific								
brands):								
1 oz.	29	.4	7.7	.1	<.1	0	6	.5 d
1 pkt., approx. .2 oz.	6	.6	1.6	<.1	tr.	0	1	.1 d
1 tbsp.	16	.2	4.1	.1	<.1	0	3	.2 d
w/onions (*Heinz*), 1 tbsp.	19	4.5	.1	(0)	0	0	289	.2 c
CAULIFLOWER:								
raw:								
untrimmed, 1 lb.	42	3.5	8.7	.3	<.1	0	26	4.2 d
trimmed, 1 oz.	7	.6	1.4	.1	tr.	0	4	.7 d
3 flowerets, approx. 5 oz.	13	1.1	2.8	.1	<.1	0	8	1.3 d
1″ pieces, ½ cup	12	1.0	2.5	.1	<.1	0	7	1.2 d
boiled, drained:								
4 oz.	27	2.1	5.2	.2	<.1	0	7	2.5 d
3 flowerets, approx. 1.9 oz.	13	1.0	2.5	.1	<.1	0	3	1.2 d
1″ pieces, ½ cup	15	1.2	2.9	.1	<.1	0	4	1.4 d
CAULIFLOWER, CANNED OR								
IN JARS:								
pickled (*Vlasic* Hot & Spicy), 1 oz.	4	0	1.0	0	0	0	435	m.q.
sweet (*Vlasic*), 1 oz.	35	0	9.0	0	0	0	225	m.q.
CAULIFLOWER, FROZEN:								
10-oz. pkg.	68	5.7	13.3	.8	.1	0	68	2.8 c
boiled, drained, 4 oz.	22	1.8	4.3	.2	<.1	0	20	.9 c
boiled, drained, 1″ pieces, ½ cup ...	17	1.5	3.4	.2	<.1	0	16	.7 c
(*A&P*), 3.3 oz.	25	2.0	5.0	<1.0	(0)	0	20	m.q.
(*Birds Eye*), 3.3 oz.	25	2.0	5.0	0	0	0	20	2.0 d
(*Finast*), 3.3 oz.	25	2.0	5.0	0	0	0	15	m.q.
(*Frosty Acres*), 3.3 oz.	25	2.0	5.0	0	0	0	16	1.0 c
(*Kohl's*), 3 oz.	20	2.0	4.0	<1.0	(0)	0	15	m.q.
(*Seabrook*), 3.3 oz.	25	2.0	5.0	0	0	0	16	1.0 c
(*Southern*), 3.5 oz.	26	2.0	4.8	.2	(0)	0	30	m.q.
(*Stokely Singles*), 3 oz.	20	2.0	4.0	0	0	0	20	m.q.
cuts (*Green Giant*), ½ cup	12	1.0	3.0	0	0	0	25	1.0 d

Food and Measure	cal.	prot. (gms)	carbo. (gms)	tot. fat (gms)	sat. fat (gms)	chol. (mgs)	sod. (mgs)	fiber (gms)
CAULIFLOWER, FROZEN *(cont.)*								
in cheese sauce:								
(*Birds Eye* Cheese Sauce								
Combinations), 5 oz.	130	5.0	12.0	7.0	m.q.	10	560	2.0 d
(*Finast*), 3.3 oz.	40	2.0	5.0	0	0	0	240	m.q.
(*Green Giant* One Serving),								
5.5 oz.	80	3.0	14.0	2.0	4.0	5	690	2.0 d
(*Stokely Singles*), 4 oz.	70	4.0	7.0	3.0	m.q.	15	170	m.q.
cheddar (*The Budget Gourmet* Side								
Dish), 5 oz.	110	6.0	10.0	5.0	m.q.	25	300	m.q.
in cheese flavored sauce (*Green*								
Giant), ½ cup	60	2.0	10.0	2.0	m.q.	n.a.	500	2.4 d
CAULIFLOWER								
COMBINATIONS, frozen:								
broccoli and carrots in cheese sauce								
(*Freezer Queen* Family Side								
Dishes), 5 oz.	60	2.0	10.0	1.0	m.q.	n.a.	360	m.q.
carrots, baby, and snow pea pods								
(*Birds Eye* Farm Fresh), 4 oz. ..	40	2.0	8.0	0	0	0	35	3.0 d
zucchini, carrots, and red peppers								
(*Birds Eye* Farm Fresh), 4 oz. ..	30	2.0	6.0	0	0	0	25	2.0 d
CAVATELLI, frozen:								
(*Celentano*), 3.2 oz.	250	10.0	52.0	1.0	n.a.	n.a.	5	m.q.
CAVIAR, granular, black and red:								
1 oz.	71	6.9	1.1	5.0	m.q.	165	420	0
1 tbsp.	40	3.9	.6	2.9	m.q.	94	240	0
CAYENNE, see "Pepper, ground"								
CELERIAC:								
raw:								
untrimmed, 1 lb.	154	5.9	35.9	1.2	n.a.	0	390	5.1 c
trimmed, 1 oz.	11	.4	2.6	.1	(0)	0	28	.4 c
trimmed, ½ cup	31	1.2	7.2	.2	(0)	0	78	1.0 c
(*Frieda* of California), 3½ oz.	40	1.8	8.5	.3	(0)	0	100	m.q.
boiled, drained, 4 oz.	28	1.1	6.7	.2	(0)	0	69	.9 c
CELERY:								
raw:								
untrimmed, 1 lb.	65	3.0	14.7	.6	.1	0	352	6.5 d
trimmed, 1 oz.	5	.2	1.0	<.1	tr.	0	25	.5 d
1 stalk, 7½" long × 1¼", approx.								
1.6 oz.	6	.3	1.5	.1	<.1	0	35	.6 d
diced, ½ cup	10	.5	2.2	.1	<.1	0	52	1.0 d
boiled, drained, 4 oz.	20	.9	4.5	.1	<.1	0	103	1.0 c
boiled, drained, diced, ½ cup	13	.6	3.0	.1	<.1	0	68	.7 c
CELERY FLAKES:								
(*Tone's*), 1 tsp.	9	.4	.9	.5	<.1	0	4	.3 d
CELERY KNOB OR ROOT, see								
"Celeriac"								
CELERY ROOT JUICE, bottled:								
(*Biotta*), 6 fl. oz.	67	2.7	13.1	.2	(0)	0	195	m.q.

Food and Measure	cal.	prot. (gms)	carbo. (gms)	tot. fat (gms)	sat. fat (gms)	chol. (mgs)	sod. (mgs)	fiber (gms)
CELERY SALT:								
(*Tone's*), 1 tsp.	6	.3	.6	.4	<.1	0	1584	.2 d
CELERY SEED:								
1 oz.	111	5.1	11.7	7.2	.6	0	45	3.4 c
1 tbsp.	25	1.2	2.7	1.6	.1	0	10	.8 c
1 tsp.	8	.4	.8	.5	<.1	0	3	.2 c
(*Spice Islands*), 1 tsp.	11	.4	1.1	.5	<.1	0	4	.3 c
(*Tone's*), 1 tsp.	9	.4	.9	.5	<.1	0	4	.3 d
CELLOPHANE NOODLES, see "Noodles, Chinese"								
CELTUS:								
untrimmed, 1 lb.	76	2.9	12.4	1.0	n.a.	0	36	1.4 c
trimmed, 1 oz.	6	.2	1.0	.1	(0)	0	3	.1 c
1 leaf, approx. .4 oz.	2	.1	.3	<.1	(0)	0	1	<.1 c
CEREAL, READY-TO-EAT, dry (see also specific grain listings):								
amaranth:								
flakes (*Health Valley*), 1 oz. or ½ cup	100	3.0	20.0	3.0	m.q.	0	10	2.7 d
w/bananas (*Health Valley*), 1 oz. or ½ cup	100	4.0	20.0	2.0	m.q.	0	5	4.2 d
w/raisins (*Health Valley Amaranth Crunch*), 1 oz. or ¼ cup	110	4.0	21.0	1.0	n.a.	0	5	2.8 d
bran (see also specific bran listings, below):								
(*All Bran*), 1 oz., approx. ⅓ cup	70	4.0	22.0	1.0	n.a.	0	260	10.0 d
(*Arrowhead Mills* Bran Flakes), 1 oz.	100	4.0	20.0	1.0	n.a.	0	1	4.1 d
(*Bran Buds*), 1 oz., approx. ⅓ cup	70	3.0	22.0	1.0	n.a.	0	170	8.0 d
(*Bran Chex*), 1 oz. or ⅔ cup	90	2.0	24.0	0	0	0	200	4.0 d
(*Kellogg's 40% + Bran Flakes*), 1 oz., approx. ⅔ cup	90	3.0	23.0	0	0	0	220	5.0 d
(*Kellogg's Heartwise*), 1 oz., approx. 1 cup	90	3.0	23.0	1.0	n.a.	0	125	6.0 d
(*Nabisco 100% Bran*), 1 oz.	70	3.0	22.0	2.0	m.q.	0	190	10.0 d
(*Post* Natural Bran Flakes), 1 oz.	90	3.0	23.0	0	0	0	240	5.0 d
(*Quaker Crunchy Bran*), 1 oz., approx. ⅔ cup	89	2.0	22.6	1.3	.4	0	316	5.2 d
apple and cinnamon (*Health Valley 100% Natural*), 1 oz. or ¼ cup	70	3.0	22.0	1.0	n.a.	0	10	5.1 d
apple cinnamon (*Health Valley 10 Bran O's*), 1 oz.	90	3.0	19.0	<1.0	(0)	0	5	m.q.
apple spice or cinnamon (*Ralston Bran News*), 1 oz. or ¾ cup ...	100	2.0	23.0	0	0	0	160	3.0 d
extra fiber (*All Bran*), 1 oz., approx. ½ cup	50	3.0	22.0	1.0	n.a.	0	140	14.0 d

Food and Measure	cal.	prot. (gms)	carbo. (gms)	tot. fat (gms)	sat. fat (gms)	chol. (mgs)	sod. (mgs)	fiber (gms)
CEREAL, READY-TO-EAT, BRAN *(cont.)*								
w/fruit (*Fruitful Bran*), 1 oz.								
cereal w/.3 oz. fruit, approx.								
⅔ cup	110	3.0	29.0	0	0	0	230	5.0 d
w/fruit and nuts (*Müeslix*), 1 oz.								
cereal w/.4 oz. fruit and nuts,								
approx. ½ cup	140	3.0	32.0	2.0	m.q.	0	140	4.0 d
w/raisins:								
(*Health Valley* Flakes), 1 oz. or								
½ cup	100	3.0	21.0	1.0	n.a.	0	5	6.0 d
(*Health Valley* 100% Natural),								
1 oz. or ¼ cup	70	4.0	20.0	1.0	n.a.	0	5	4.5 d
(*Kellogg's* Raisin Bran), 1 oz.								
cereal w/.4 oz. raisins,								
approx. ¾ cup	120	3.0	31.0	1.0	n.a.	0	230	5.0 d
(*Post* Natural Raisin Bran),								
1.4 oz.	120	3.0	31.0	1.0	n.a.	0	200	6.0 d
(*Total Raisin Bran*), 1.5 oz. or								
1 cup	140	3.0	33.0	1.0	n.a.	0	190	4.0 d
and nuts (*Raisin Nut Bran*),								
1 oz. or ½ cup	110	3.0	20.0	3.0	m.q.	0	140	2.5 d
corn:								
(*Arrowhead Mills* Corn Flakes),								
1 oz.	110	2.0	25.0	1.0	n.a.	0	4	2.8 d
(*Arrowhead Mills* Puffed Corn),								
.5 oz.	50	3.0	11.0	0	0	0	<1	.4 d
(*Corn Chex*), 1 oz. or 1 cup	110	2.0	25.0	0	0	0	310	m.q.
(*Corn Pops*), 1 oz., approx. 1 cup	110	1.0	26.0	0	0	0	90	m.q.
(*Country* Corn Flakes), 1 oz. or								
1 cup	110	2.0	24.0	<1.0	n.a.	0	280	m.q.
(*Featherweight* Corn Flakes),								
1¼ cup	110	2.0	25.0	0	0	0	<10	m.q.
(*Health Valley Lites* Puffed Corn),								
.5 oz. or ½ cup	50	3.0	11.0	0	0	0	0	.3 d
(*Honeycomb*), 1 oz.	110	2.0	25.0	0	0	0	170	tr.d
(*Kellogg's Corn Flakes*), 1 oz.,								
approx. 1 cup	100	2.0	24.0	0	0	0	250	1.0 d
(*Kellogg's Frosted Flakes*), 1 oz.,								
approx. ¾ cup	110	1.0	26.0	0	0	0	200	n.a.
(*Nutri•Grain*), 1 oz., approx.								
½ cup	100	2.0	24.0	1.0	n.a.	0	170	3.0 d
(*Post Toasties*), 1 oz.	110	2.0	24.0	0	0	0	310	tr.d
(*Total Corn Flakes*), 1 oz. or								
1 cup	110	2.0	24.0	1.0	n.a.	0	280	n.a.
blue (*Health Valley* Corn Flakes),								
1 oz. or ½ cup	90	3.0	19.0	2.0	m.q.	0	11	2.8 d
chocolate flavor (*Cocoa Puffs*),								
1 oz. or 1 cup	110	1.0	25.0	1.0	n.a.	0	170	m.q.

Food and Measure	cal.	prot. (gms)	carbo. (gms)	tot. fat (gms)	sat. fat (gms)	chol. (mgs)	sod. (mgs)	fiber (gms)
w/fruit (*Health Valley Fruit Lites*),								
.5 oz. or ½ cup	45	2.0	10.0	0	0	0	2	.3 d
w/nuts and honey (*Nut & Honey*								
Crunch), 1 oz., approx. ⅔ cup	110	2.0	24.0	1.0	n.a.	0	200	m.q.
granola, see "mixed grain," below								
millet (*Arrowhead Mills* Puffed								
Millet), .5 oz.	50	2.0	11.0	0	0	0	<1	.5 d
mixed grain:								
(*Almond Delight*), 1 oz. or ¾ cup	110	2.0	23.0	2.0	m.q.	0	200	1.0 d
(*Apple Jacks*), 1 oz., approx. 1 cup	110	2.0	26.0	0	0	0	125	1.0 d
(*Arrowhead Mills* Arrowhead								
Crunch), 1 oz.	120	3.0	18.0	3.0	m.q.	0	11	3.5 d
(*Arrowhead Mills* Nature O's),								
1 oz.	110	5.0	20.0	1.0	n.a.	0	4	2.8 d
(*Booberry*), 1 oz. or 1 cup	110	1.0	24.0	1.0	n.a.	0	210	m.q.
(*Breakfast With Barbie*), 1 oz.,								
approx. 1 cup	110	1.0	25.0	1.0	n.a.	0	70	m.q.
(*Cap'n Crunch*), 1 oz., approx.								
¾ cup	113	1.5	23.8	1.7	.8	0	241	.8 d
(*Cap'n Crunch's Crunchberries*),								
1 oz., approx. ¾ cup	113	1.5	23.6	1.7	.9	0	247	.7 d
(*Cap'n Crunch's Peanut Butter*								
Crunch), 1 oz., approx. ¾ cup	119	2.1	21.6	3.0	.9	0	281	.8 d
(*Cinnamon Toast Crunch*), 1 oz.								
or ¾ cup	120	1.0	22.0	3.0	m.q.	0	220	m.q.
(*Count Chocula*), 1 oz. or 1 cup ..	110	2.0	24.0	1.0	n.a.	0	210	m.q.
(*Crispix*), 1 oz., approx. 1 cup ...	110	2.0	22.0	0	0	0	220	m.q.
(*Crunchy Nut Oh!s*), 1 oz.,								
approx. 1 cup	127	1.7	21.5	4.2	2.4	0	164	.9 d
(*Double Chex*), 1 oz. or ⅔ cup ...	100	2.0	24.0	0	0	0	190	1.0 d
(*Familia* Champion), 2 oz.,								
approx. ½ cup	200	7.0	40.0	4.0	m.q.	0	30	m.q.
(*Familia* Crunchy), 1 oz., approx.								
¼ cup	116	3.0	20.0	2.0	m.q.	0	1	m.q.
(*Familia* No Added Sugar), 2 oz.,								
approx. ½ cup	206	7.0	37.0	4.0	m.q.	0	2	m.q.
(*Fiber One*), 1 oz. or ½ cup	60	2.0	23.0	1.0	n.a.	0	140	13.0 d
(*Frankenberry*), 1 oz. or 1 cup ...	110	1.0	24.0	1.0	n.a.	0	210	m.q.
(*Froot Loops*), 1 oz., approx.								
1 cup	110	2.0	25.0	0	0	0	125	1.0 d
(*Fruit Yummy Mummy*), 1 oz. or								
1 cup	110	1.0	24.0	1.0	n.a.	0	160	m.q.
(*Golden Grahams*), 1 oz. or								
¾ cup	110	1.0	24.0	1.0	n.a.	0	280	m.q.
(*Grape Nuts*), 1 oz.	110	3.0	23.0	0	0	0	170	3.0 d
(*Grape Nuts* Flakes), 1 oz.	100	3.0	23.0	1.0	0	0	160	3.0 d
(*Health Valley Fiber 7* Flakes),								
1 oz. or ½ cup	100	4.0	21.0	0	0	0	10	2.7 d

Food and Measure	cal.	prot. (gms)	carbo. (gms)	tot. fat (gms)	sat. fat (gms)	chol. (mgs)	sod. (mgs)	fiber (gms)
CEREAL, READY-TO-EAT, MIXED GRAIN *(cont.)*								
(*Health Valley Healthy O's*), 1 oz. or ¾ cup	100	3.0	21.0	1.0	n.a.	0	1	3.4 d
(*Heartland*), 1 oz., approx. ¼ cup	130	3.0	18.0	4.0	m.q.	0	80	2.0 d
(*Honey Graham Chex*), 1 oz. or ⅔ cup	110	1.0	25.0	1.0	n.a.	0	180	m.q.
(*Honey Graham Oh!s*), 1 oz., approx. 1 cup	122	1.4	22.6	3.2	1.5	0	217	.7 d
(*Just Right*), 1 oz., approx. ⅔ cup	100	3.0	23.0	1.0	n.a.	0	190	2.0 d
(*Kaboom*), 1 oz. or 1 cup	110	2.0	23.0	1.0	n.a.	0	290	m.q.
(*King Vitaman*), 1 oz., approx. 1½ cup	110	2.0	23.0	1.0	0	0	280	1.2 d
(*Kix*), 1 oz. or 1½ cup	110	2.0	24.0	1.0	n.a.	0	260	m.q.
(*Morning Funnies*), 1 oz. or 1 cup	110	1.0	25.0	1.0	n.a.	0	70	m.q.
(*Nintendo Cereal System*), 1 oz., approx. 1 cup	110	1.0	25.0	1.0	n.a.	0	70	m.q.
(*Nutri•Grain Nuggets*), 1 oz., approx. ¼ cup	100	3.0	23.0	1.0	n.a.	0	170	3.0 d
(*Product 19*), 1 oz., approx. 1 cup	100	3.0	24.0	0	0	0	320	1.0 d
(*Quaker 100% Natural*), 1 oz., approx. ¼ cup	127	3.3	18.0	5.5	3.1	0	14	2.0 d
(*Ralston Dinersaurs*), 1 oz. or 1 cup	110	1.0	25.0	1.0	n.a.	0	70	m.q.
(*Special K*), 1 oz., approx. 1 cup	110	6.0	20.0	0	0	0	230	m.q.
(*Sunflakes Multi-Grain*), 1 oz. or 1 cup	100	2.0	24.0	1.0	n.a.	0	240	3.0 d
(*Teenage Mutant Ninja Turtles*), 1 oz. or 1 cup	110	1.0	26.0	0	0	0	190	m.q.
(*The Real Ghostbusters*), 1 oz. or 1 cup	110	1.0	26.0	1.0	n.a.	0	115	m.q.
(*Trix*), 1 oz. or 1 cup	110	1.0	25.0	1.0	n.a.	0	140	m.q.
w/almonds (*Honey Bunches of Oats*), 1 oz.	120	2.0	22.0	3.0	m.q.	0	160	1.0 d
almond date (*Health Valley Healthy Crunch*), 1 oz. or ¼ cup	100	2.0	15.0	3.0	m.q.	0	1	5.6 d
w/almonds and raisins (*Nutri•Grain*), 1 oz. cereal w/.4 oz. nuts and fruit, approx. ⅔ cup	140	3.0	31.0	2.0	m.q.	0	220	3.0 d
apple cinnamon (*Health Valley Healthy Crunch*), 1 oz. or ¼ cup	100	2.0	16.0	3.0	m.q.	0	2	5.4 d
apple and cinnamon (*Quaker 100% Natural*), 1 oz., approx. ¼ cup	126	3.0	18.9	4.9	2.7	0	13	1.6 d
w/apples and raisins (*Apple Raisin Crisp*), 1 oz. cereal w/.3 oz. fruit, approx. ⅔ cup	130	2.0	32.0	0	0	0	230	3.0 d
w/bananas and Hawaiian fruit (*Health Valley Sprouts 7*), 1 oz. or ¼ cup	90	3.0	20.0	1.0	n.a.	0	5	4.3 d

Food and Measure	cal.	prot. (gms)	carbo. (gms)	tot. fat (gms)	sat. fat (gms)	chol. (mgs)	sod. (mgs)	fiber (gms)
chocolate chip (*Cookie-Crisp*), 1 oz. or 1 cup	110	1.0	25.0	1.0	n.a.	n.a.	190	m.q.
cinnamon and raisin (*Nature Valley* 100% Natural), 1 oz. or ⅓ cup	120	2.0	20.0	4.0	m.q.	0	90	1.0 d
coconut (*Heartland*), 1 oz., approx. ¼ cup	130	3.0	18.0	5.0	m.q.	0	80	2.0 d
w/dates, raisins, walnuts, and oat clusters (*Fruit & Fibre*), 1.25 oz.	120	3.0	27.0	2.0	m.q.	0	170	5.0 d
w/fruit (*Health Valley Fruit & Fitness*), 2 oz. or 1 cup	190	8.0	33.0	3.0	m.q.	0	4	7.7 d
w/fruit and nuts:								
(*Just Right*), 1 oz. cereal w/.3 oz. fruit and nuts, approx. ¾ cup	140	3.0	30.0	1.0	n.a.	0	190	2.0 d
(*Müeslix* Five Grain), 1 oz. cereal w/.45 oz. fruit and nuts, approx. ½ cup	140	4.0	32.0	1.0	n.a.	0	55	4.0 d
(*Nature Valley* 100% Natural), 1 oz. or ⅓ cup	130	2.0	19.0	5.0	m.q.	0	75	1.0 d
w/fruit, tropical, and oat clusters (*Fruit & Fibre*), 1.25 oz.	120	3.0	27.0	3.0	m.q.	0	170	5.0 d
fruit flavor (*Body Buddies*), 1 oz. or 1 cup	110	2.0	24.0	1.0	n.a.	0	280	m.q.
granola:								
(*C.W. Post* Hearty), 1 oz.	130	2.0	21.0	4.0	m.q.	0	80	tr.d
w/almonds (*Sun Country* 100% Natural), 1 oz., approx. ¼ cup	130	3.1	18.8	5.3	.6	0	11	1.4 d
banana almond (*Sunbelt*), 1 oz.	130	3.0	20.0	4.0	m.q.	<1	25	m.q.
fruit and nut (*Sunbelt*), 1 oz. ...	120	3.0	19.0	5.0	m.q.	<1	20	m.q.
maple nut (*Arrowhead Mills*), 2 oz.	250	8.0	36.0	9.0	m.q.	0	9	11.9 d
w/raisins (*Sun Country*), 1 oz., approx. ¼ cup	125	2.7	19.4	4.8	.5	0	10	1.8 d
w/raisins and dates (*Sun Country* 100% Natural), 1 oz., approx. ¼ cup	123	2.5	19.8	4.5	.5	0	9	1.8 d
honey roasted (*Honey Bunches of Oats*), 1 oz.	110	2.0	24.0	2.0	m.q.	0	180	1.0 d
w/peaches, raisins, almonds, and oat clusters (*Fruit & Fibre*), 1.25 oz.	120	3.0	26.0	2.0	m.q.	0	170	5.0 d
w/raisins:								
(*Grape Nuts*), 1 oz.	100	3.0	23.0	0	0	0	140	2.0 d
(*Health Valley Sprouts 7*), 1 oz. or ¼ cup	90	4.0	20.0	1.0	n.a.	0	5	4.7 d
(*Heartland*), 1 oz., approx. ¼ cup	130	3.0	18.0	4.0	m.q.	0	80	2.0 d

Food and Measure	cal.	prot. (gms)	carbo. (gms)	tot. fat (gms)	sat. fat (gms)	chol. (mgs)	sod. (mgs)	fiber (gms)
CEREAL, READY-TO-EAT, MIXED GRAIN *(cont.)*								
w/raisins and almonds (*Nutrific*), 1 oz. cereal w/.5 oz. fruit and nuts, approx. 1 cup	140	4.0	31.0	2.0	m.q.	0	240	6.0 d
raisin and date (*Quaker* 100% Natural), 1 oz., approx. ¼ cup	123	3.0	18.4	5.0	2.6	0	14	1.8 d
raisin, dates, and almonds (*Ralston Muesli*), 1.45 oz. or ½ cup	140	4.0	32.0	2.0	m.q.	0	95	3.0 d
raisin, peaches, and pecans (*Ralston Muesli*), 1.45 oz. or ½ cup	150	4.0	30.0	3.0	m.q.	0	95	3.0 d
raisin, walnuts, and cranberries (*Ralston Fruit Muesli*), 1.45 oz. or ½ cup	150	4.0	30.0	3.0	m.q.	0	95	3.0 d
vanilla wafer (*Cookie-Crisp*), 1 oz. or 1 cup	110	1.0	25.0	1.0	n.a.	0	220	m.q.
oat:								
(*Alpha-Bits*), 1 oz.	110	2.0	24.0	1.0	n.a.	0	190	tr.d
(*Apple Cinnamon Cheerios*), 1 oz. or ¾ cup	110	2.0	22.0	2.0	m.q.	0	180	1.5 d
(*Cheerios*), 1 oz., approx. 1¼ cup	110	4.0	20.0	2.0	m.q.	0	290	2.0 d
(Cinnamon *Life*), 1 oz., approx. ⅔ cup	101	5.0	18.9	1.7	m.q.	0	182	2.5 d
(*General Mills* Oatmeal Crisp), 1 oz. or 1 cup	110	2.0	22.0	2.0	m.q.	0	180	1.0 d
(*General Mills* Toasted Oat), 1 oz. or ⅓ cup	130	2.0	20.0	5.0	m.q.	0	90	1.0 d
(*Honey Nut Cheerios*), 1 oz. or ¾ cup	110	3.0	23.0	1.0	n.a.	0	250	1.5 d
(*Life*), 1 oz., approx. ⅔ cup	101	5.1	18.7	1.7	m.q.	0	186	2.5 d
(*Oat Chex*), 1 oz. or ½ cup	100	3.0	22.0	1.0	n.a.	0	240	1.0 d
(*Post* Oat Flakes), 1 oz.	110	4.0	21.0	1.0	n.a.	0	130	2.0 d
(*Quaker Oat Squares*), 1 oz., approx. ½ cup	105	3.7	21.3	1.6	m.q.	0	159	2.4 d
w/marshmallow (*Lucky Charms*), 1 oz. or 1 cup	110	2.0	24.0	1.0	n.a.	0	180	m.q.
w/raisins (*General Mills* Oatmeal Raisin Crisp), 1 oz. or ½ cup ..	110	2.0	21.0	2.0	m.q.	0	140	1.0 d
oat bran:								
(*Arrowhead Mills* Oat Bran Flakes), 1 oz.	110	4.0	20.0	2.0	m.q.	0	9	3.4 d
(*Common Sense*), 1 oz., approx. ½ cup	100	4.0	22.0	1.0	n.a.	0	270	3.0 d
(*Cracklin' Oat Bran*), 1 oz., approx. ½ cup	110	3.0	20.0	0	0	0	140	4.0 d
(*Health Valley* Flakes), 1 oz. or ½ cup	100	3.0	20.0	.4	n.a.	0	2	3.7 d

Food and Measure	cal.	prot. (gms)	carbo. (gms)	tot. fat (gms)	sat. fat (gms)	chol. (mgs)	sod. (mgs)	fiber (gms)
(*Health Valley Oat Bran O's*), 1 oz. or ¾ cup	90	3.0	20.0	2.0	m.q.	0	3	2.5 d
almond crunch (*Health Valley Real*), 1 oz. or ¼ cup	110	3.0	17.0	3.0	m.q.	0	4	3.3 d
w/almonds and dates (*Health Valley Flakes*), 1 oz. or ½ cup	100	3.0	22.0	.8	n.a.	0	10	3.7 d
fruit, Hawaiian (*Health Valley Real*), 1 oz. or ¼ cup	130	5.0	22.0	3.0	m.q.	0	2	4.5 d
fruit and nut (*Health Valley Oat Bran O's*), 1 oz. or ¾ cup	90	4.0	19.0	2.0	m.q.	0	6	4.5 d
w/raisins:								
(*Common Sense*), 1 oz. cereal w/.3 oz. raisins, approx. ½ cup	120	4.0	29.0	0	0	0	250	3.0 d
(*General Mills Raisin Oat Bran*), 1.5 oz. or ¾ cup	150	4.0	31.0	2.0	m.q.	0	130	3.0 d
(*Health Valley* Flakes), 1 oz. or ½ cup	100	3.0	21.0	.8	n.a.	0	10	3.7 d
(*Raisin Oat Bran Options*), 1.45 oz., approx. 1 cup	130	4.0	32.0	1.0	n.a.	0	150	3.0 d
and nuts (*Health Valley Real*), 1 oz. or ¼ cup	110	3.0	18.0	3.0	m.q.	0	6	3.5 d
(*Popeye* Sweet Crunch), 1 oz., approx. 1 cup	113	1.3	23.6	1.8	1.0	0	254	.7 d
rice:								
(*Arrowhead Mills* Puffed Rice), .5 oz.	50	1.0	11.0	0	0	0	<1	.4 d
(*Cocoa Pebbles*), 1 oz.	110	1.0	25.0	1.0	n.a.	0	160	tr.d
(*Featherweight* Crisp Rice), 1 cup	110	2.0	26.0	0	0	0	<10	m.q.
(*Fruity Pebbles*), 1 oz.	110	1.0	25.0	1.0	n.a.	0	160	tr.d
(*Health Valley Lites* Puffed Rice), .5 oz. or ½ cup	50	1.0	12.0	0	0	0	0	.4 d
(*Kellogg's Frosted Krispies*), 1 oz., approx. ¾ cup	110	1.0	26.0	0	0	0	200	m.q.
(*Kellogg's Rice Krispies*), 1 oz., approx. 1 cup	110	2.0	25.0	0	0	0	290	m.q.
(*Quaker* Puffed Rice), .5 oz., approx. 1 cup	54	1.0	12.5	.1	0	0	1	.2 d
(*Rice Chex*), 1 oz. or 1⅛ cup	110	1.0	25.0	0	0	0	280	.5 d
chocolate flavor (*Cocoa Krispies*), 1 oz., approx. ¾ cup	110	1.0	25.0	0	0	0	190	m.q.
w/fruit (*Health Valley Fruit Lites*), .5 oz. or ½ cup	45	1.0	11.0	0	0	0	2	.3 d
w/marshmallow bits (*Fruity Marshmallow Krispies*), 1 oz. cereal w/.3 oz. marshmallows, approx. 1¼ cup	140	2.0	32.0	0	0	0	210	m.q.

Food and Measure	cal.	prot. (gms)	carbo. (gms)	tot. fat (gms)	sat. fat (gms)	chol. (mgs)	sod. (mgs)	fiber (gms)
CEREAL, READY-TO-EAT *(cont.)*								
rice bran (*Health Valley Rice Bran*								
O's), 1 oz. or ¾ cup	110	2.0	22.0	1.0	n.a.	0	7	1.8 d
rice bran w/almonds and dates								
(*Health Valley*), 1 oz. or ½ cup	110	2.0	19.0	3.0	m.q.	0	4	2.7 d
(*Smurf-Magic Berries*), 1 oz.	120	2.0	26.0	1.0	n.a.	0	60	tr.d
wheat:								
(*Arrowhead Mills* Puffed Wheat),								
.5 oz.	50	2.0	11.0	0	0	0	<1	.9 d
(*Arrowhead Mills* Wheat Flakes),								
1 oz.	110	3.0	23.0	1.0	n.a.	0	4	2.8 d
(*Clusters*), 1 oz. or ½ cup	110	3.0	20.0	3.0	m.q.	0	140	3.0 d
(*Finast* Puffed Wheat), approx.								
1 cup	50	2.0	11.0	0	0	0	0	m.q.
(*Health Valley Lites* Puffed Wheat),								
.5 oz. or ½ cup	50	2.0	11.0	0	0	0	0	1.4 d
(*Honey Smacks*), 1 oz., approx. ¾								
cup	110	2.0	25.0	1.0	n.a.	0	70	1.0 d
(*Nutri•Grain*), 1 oz., approx. ⅔								
cup	100	3.0	24.0	0	0	0	170	3.0 d
(*Quaker* Puffed Wheat), .5 oz.,								
approx. 1 cup	50	2.4	10.5	.2	0	0	1	1.0 d
(*Total*), 1 oz. or 1 cup	100	3.0	22.0	1.0	n.a.	0	140	3.0 d
(*Wheat Chex*), 1 oz. or ⅔ cup ...	100	3.0	23.0	0	0	0	230	2.0 d
(*Wheaties*), 1 oz. or 1 cup	100	3.0	23.0	1.0	n.a.	0	200	3.0 d
apple cinnamon filled (*Kellogg's*								
Apple Cinnamon Squares),								
1 oz., approx. ½ cup	90	2.0	23.0	0	0	0	5	2.0 d
blueberry filled (*Kellogg's*								
Blueberry Squares), 1 oz.,								
approx. ½ cup	90	2.0	23.0	0	0	0	5	3.0 d
brown sugar, nut and honey filled								
(*Nut & Honey Crunch* Biscuits),								
1 oz., approx. ½ cup	100	3.0	22.0	1.0	n.a.	0	5	3.0 d
w/fruit (*Health Valley Fruit Lites*),								
.5 oz. or ½ cup	45	1.0	11.0	0	0	0	2	1.5 d
honey sweetened puffs (*Super*								
Golden Crisp), 1 oz.	110	2.0	26.0	0	0	0	45	tr.d
w/raisins (*Crispy Wheats'N*								
Raisins), 1 oz. or ¾ cup	100	2.0	23.0	1.0	n.a.	0	140	2.0 d
raisin filled (*Kellogg's Raisin*								
Squares), 1 oz., approx. ½ cup	90	2.0	23.0	0	0	0	0	2.0 d
w/raisins (*Nutri•Grain*), 1 oz.								
cereal w/.4 oz. raisins, approx.								
⅔ cup	130	3.0	32.0	0	0	0	170	3.0 d
raspberry filled (*Fruit Wheats*),								
1 oz.	90	2.0	23.0	0	0	0	15	3.0 d

Food and Measure	cal.	prot. (gms)	carbo. (gms)	tot. fat (gms)	sat. fat (gms)	chol. (mgs)	sod. (mgs)	fiber (gms)
shredded:								
(*Frosted Mini-Wheats*), 1 oz.,								
approx. 4 biscuits	100	3.0	24.0	0	0	0	0	3.0 d
(*Nabisco*), 1 piece or ⅚ oz.	80	2.0	19.0	<1.0	n.a.	0	0	3.0 d
(*Nutri•Grain*), 1 oz., approx.								
½ cup	90	4.0	22.0	0	0	0	0	4.0 d
(*Quaker*), 2 biscuits or 1.4 oz.	132	3.9	31.6	.6	n.a.	0	1	3.7 d
(*S.W. Graham*), 1 oz., approx.								
½ cup	100	3.0	23.0	0	0	0	190	3.0 d
(*Sunshine*), 1 biscuit	90	2.0	19.0	1.0	n.a.	0	0	m.q.
bran (*Nabisco Shredded Wheat 'n*								
Bran), 1 oz.	90	3.0	23.0	<1.0	n.a.	0	0	4.0 d
bite size (*Frosted Mini-Wheats*),								
1 oz., approx. ½ cup	100	3.0	24.0	0	0	0	0	3.0 d
bite size (*Sunshine*), ⅔ cup	110	3.0	22.0	1.0	n.a.	0	0	m.q.
cinnamon (*S.W. Graham*), 1 oz.,								
approx. ½ cup	100	2.0	24.0	0	0	0	160	2.0 d
mini (*Nabisco* Spoon Size), 1 oz.	90	3.0	23.0	<1.0	n.a.	0	0	3.0 d
strawberry filled (*Kellogg's*								
Strawberry Squares), 1 oz.,								
approx. ½ cup	90	2.0	23.0	0	0	0	5	3.0 d
CEREAL, COOKING[1] (see also								
specific grain listings):								
bran (*H-O Brand* Super Bran),								
⅓ cup	110	4.0	18.0	2.0	0	0	0	8.0 d
bulgur, see "wheat," below								
farina, see "wheat," below								
grain, multi:								
four grain (*Arrowhead Mills*),								
1 oz.	94	4.0	18.0	1.0	n.a.	0	1	7.4 d
seven grain (*Arrowhead Mills*),								
1 oz.	100	4.0	17.0	1.0	n.a.	0	<1	4.0 d
w/apple cinnamon (*Roman Meal*),								
⅓ cup dry or ⅔ cup cooked ...	112	3.7	23.8	2.8	m.q.	<1	14	5.7 d
oat bran:								
(*Arrowhead Mills*), 1 oz.	110	6.0	17.0	1.0	n.a.	0	1	5.1 d
(*Quaker/Mother's*), ⅓ cup dry or								
⅔ cup cooked	92	5.7	16.6	2.1	.2	0	1	4.2 d
(*3-Minute Brand* Regular or								
Instant), 1 oz.	90	6.0	17.0	2.0	m.q.	0	0	4.1 d
(*Wholesome 'N Hearty*), 1 oz.	100	4.0	18.0	2.0	m.q.	0	0	5.0 d
apple and cinnamon (*Health Valley*								
Natural), 1 oz. or ¼ cup	100	3.0	19.0	1.0	n.a.	0	10	3.8 d
apple cinnamon (*Wholesome 'N*								
Hearty Instant), 1⅜-oz. pkt.	130	3.0	30.0	2.0	m.q.	0	160	5.0 d
honey (*Wholesome 'N Hearty*								
Instant), 1¼-oz. pkt.	110	3.0	26.0	2.0	m.q.	0	160	5.0 d

1. *Uncooked, except as noted. Cooked cereals prepared without salt.*

Food and Measure	cal.	prot. (gms)	carbo. (gms)	tot. fat (gms)	sat. fat (gms)	chol. (mgs)	sod. (mgs)	fiber (gms)
CEREAL, COOKING, OAT BRAN *(cont.)*								
raisins and spice *(Health Valley Natural)*, 1 oz. or ¼ cup	110	3.0	19.0	1.0	n.a.	0	10	3.8 d
oatmeal and oats:								
(Arrowhead Mills Instant), 1 oz.	100	5.8	18.0	2.0	m.q.	0	0	4.3 d
(H-O Brand Gourmet), ⅓ cup ...	100	5.0	18.0	2.0	0	0	0	3.0 d
(H-O Brand Instant), 1 pkt.	110	4.0	18.0	2.0	0	0	230	3.0 d
(H-O Brand Instant-box), ½ cup	130	5.0	22.0	2.0	0	0	<5	3.0 d
(H-O Brand Quick), ½ cup	130	5.0	23.0	2.0	0	0	<5	3.0 d
(Instant Quaker), 1 pkt.	94	3.8	18.0	2.0	.3	0	270	2.8 d
(Maypo 30 Second), 1 oz.	100	4.0	19.0	1.0	n.a.	0	0	2.0 d
(Quaker Quick/Old Fashioned), ⅓ cup dry or ⅔ cup cooked ...	99	4.4	18.6	2.0	.3	0	1	2.7 d
(Quaker Extra), 1 pkt.	95	4.4	17.6	2.0	.2	0	219	2.9 d
(3-Minute Brand Quick or Old Fashioned), 1 oz.	100	5.0	18.0	2.0	m.q.	0	0	3.0 d
(Total Instant), 1.2 oz.	110	4.0	22.0	2.0	m.q.	0	220	3.0 d
(Total Quick), 1 oz.	90	4.0	18.0	2.0	m.q.	0	0	2.5 d
apple and cinnamon:								
(H-O Brand Instant), 1 pkt. ...	130	3.0	26.0	2.0	0	0	220	3.0 d
(Instant Quaker), 1 pkt.	118	3.3	26.0	1.5	.3	0	128	3.0 d
(Oatmeal Swirlers), 1.7-oz. pkt.	160	3.0	34.0	2.0	m.q.	0	120	2.0 d
(Total Instant), 1.5 oz.	150	4.0	32.0	2.0	m.q.	0	105	3.0 d
apple, date, and almond *(Arrowhead Mills* Instant), 1 oz.	130	5.0	23.0	3.0	m.q.	0	3	3.7 d
apple spice *(Arrowhead Mills* Instant), 1 oz.	130	5.0	23.0	2.0	m.q.	0	1	3.4 d
apples and spice *(Quaker Extra)*, 1 pkt.	133	4.3	26.7	1.9	.3	0	191	3.0 d
cherry *(Oatmeal Swirlers)*, 1.7-oz. pkt.	150	3.0	33.0	2.0	m.q.	0	130	2.0 d
chocolate, milk *(Oatmeal Swirlers)*, 1.7-oz. pkt.	170	3.0	37.0	2.0	m.q.	0	100	2.0 d
cinnamon raisin *(Total* Instant), 1.8 oz.	170	4.0	38.0	2.0	m.q.	0	130	3.0 d
cinnamon, raisin, and almond *(Arrowhead Mills* Instant), 1 oz.	140	6.0	23.0	3.0	m.q.	0	3	4.3 d
cinnamon and spice *(Instant Quaker)*, 1 pkt.	164	4.5	34.9	2.1	.4	0	322	3.1 d
cinnamon spice *(Oatmeal Swirlers)*, 1.6-oz. pkt.	160	3.0	35.0	2.0	m.q.	0	100	2.0 d
w/fiber:								
(H-O Brand Instant), 1 pkt. ...	110	5.0	18.0	2.0	0	0	140	3.0 d
(H-O Brand Instant-box), ⅓ cup	100	5.0	15.0	2.0	0	0	5	3.0 d
apple and bran *(H-O Brand* Instant), 1 pkt.	130	3.0	26.0	2.0	0	0	140	3.0 d

Food and Measure	cal.	prot. (gms)	carbo. (gms)	tot. fat (gms)	sat. fat (gms)	chol. (mgs)	sod. (mgs)	fiber (gms)
raisin and bran (*H-O Brand* Instant), 1 pkt.	150	4.0	32.0	2.0	0	0	140	3.0 d
maple flavored (*Maypo* Vermont Style), 1 oz.	105	4.0	20.0	1.0	n.a.	0	0	2.0 d
maple brown sugar:								
(*H-O Brand* Instant), 1 pkt. ...	160	4.0	32.0	2.0	0	0	285	3.0 d
(*Instant Quaker*), 1 pkt.	152	4.5	31.6	2.1	.4	0	320	2.8 d
(*Oatmeal Swirlers*), 1.6-oz. pkt.	160	3.0	35.0	2.0	m.q.	0	100	2.0 d
(*Total* Instant), 1.6 oz.	160	4.0	34.0	2.0	m.q.	0	150	3.0 d
w/oat bran (*3-Minute Brand* Quick), 1 oz.	100	5.0	18.0	2.0	m.q.	0	0	3.3 d
peaches and cream (*Instant Quaker*), 1 pkt.	129	3.4	26.3	2.2	.9	0	179	2.3 d
raisins:								
(*3-Minute Brand*), 1 oz.	100	5.0	18.0	2.0	m.q.	0	0	3.0 d
and cinnamon (*Quaker Extra*), 1 pkt.	129	4.1	26.6	1.9	.3	0	119	2.7 d
date and walnut (*Instant Quaker*), 1 pkt.	141	4.0	25.1	3.8	.4	0	216	2.4 d
w/oat bran (*3-Minute Brand*), 1 oz.	100	4.0	18.0	2.0	m.q.	0	0	3.0 d
and spice (*H-O Brand* Instant), 1 pkt.	150	4.0	32.0	2.0	0	0	240	3.0 d
and spice (*Instant Quaker*), 1 pkt.	149	4.1	31.5	2.0	.3	0	266	2.8 d
strawberry (*Oatmeal Swirlers*), 1.6-oz. pkt.	150	3.0	32.0	2.0	m.q.	0	120	2.0 d
strawberries and cream (*Instant Quaker*), 1 pkt.	129	3.4	26.6	2.0	1.1	0	204	2.2 d
sweet'n mellow (*H-O Brand* Instant), 1 pkt.	150	5.0	30.0	2.0	0	0	270	3.0 d
w/wheat, dates, raisins, and almonds (*Roman Meal Premium*), 1.3 oz. or ⅓ cup ...	140	4.0	26.0	3.0	m.q.	0	0	3.0 d
w/wheat, honey, coconut, and almonds (*Roman Meal Premium*), 1.3 oz. or ⅓ cup dry	150	5.0	21.0	6.0	m.q.	0	5	3.1 d
w/wheat, rye, bran, and flax (*Roman Meal*), 1.2 oz. or ⅓ cup dry	116	5.0	25.0	1.7	m.q.	0	5	5.0 d
rice, brown (*Arrowhead Mills* Rise & Shine), 1.5 oz.	160	3.0	35.0	1.0	n.a.	0	<1	1.6 d
rye, cream of (*Roman Meal*), 1.3 oz., ⅓ cup dry	110	4.0	27.0	<1.0	n.a.	0	0	5.4 d
wheat:								
(*Arrowhead Mills* Bear Mush), 1 oz.	100	3.0	21.0	0	0	0	<1	1.3 d
(*Cream of Wheat* Instant), 1 oz. ..	100	3.0	22.0	0	0	0	0	1.0 d

Food and Measure	cal.	prot. (gms)	carbo. (gms)	tot. fat (gms)	sat. fat (gms)	chol. (mgs)	sod. (mgs)	fiber (gms)
CEREAL, COOKING, WHEAT *(cont.)*								
(Cream of Wheat Quick), 1 oz. ...	100	3.0	22.0	0	0	0	80	1.0 d
(Mix'n Eat Cream of Wheat Instant, Original), 1-oz. pkt.	100	3.0	21.0	0	0	0	180	1.0 d
(Wheat Hearts), 1 oz. dry or ¾ cup cooked	110	4.0	21.0	1.0	n.a.	0	0	m.q.
(Wheatena), 1 oz.	100	3.0	21.0	1.0	n.a.	0	0	4.0 d
apple 'n cinnamon *(Mix'n Eat Cream of Wheat* Instant), 1¼-oz. pkt.	130	2.0	30.0	0	0	0	300	1.0 d
brown sugar cinnamon *(Mix'n Eat Cream of Wheat* Instant), 1¼-oz. pkt.	130	2.0	30.0	0	0	0	180	1.0 d
bulgur *(Arrowhead Mills)*, 2 oz. ..	200	6.0	43.0	1.0	n.a.	0	0	5.4 d
cracked *(Arrowhead Mills)*, 2 oz.	180	7.0	40.0	1.0	n.a.	0	1	2.3 d
farina *(H-O Brand* Instant), 1 pkt.	110	3.0	22.0	0	0	0	235	3.0 d
farina, cream *(H-O Brand)*, 3 tbsp.	120	3.0	26.0	0	0	0	0	3.0 d
maple brown sugar *(Mix'n Eat Cream of Wheat* Instant), 1¼-oz. pkt.	130	2.0	30.0	0	0	0	180	1.0 d
w/rye, bran, and flax *(Roman Meal)*, 1 oz. or ⅓ cup dry	80	4.0	15.0	.5	n.a.	0	0	5.0 d
whole *(Quaker/Mother's* Hot Natural), ⅓ cup dry or ⅔ cup cooked	92	2.9	20.9	.6	.1	0	1	2.2 d
wheat and barley *(Maltex)*, 1 oz. ...	105	3.0	21.0	1.0	n.a.	0	0	3.0 d
CEREAL, FREEZE-DRIED:								
granola, w/blueberries and milk *(Mountain House)*, ½ cup[1]	290	8.0	44.0	8.0	m.q.	m.q.	m.q.	m.q.
CEREAL BAR, see "Granola and cereal bar"								
CEREAL BEVERAGE, see "Coffee, substitute"								
CEREAL GRAIN, see specific grain listings								
CEREAL SNACK, 1 pouch:								
(Apple Cinnamon Cheerios-to-Go) ..	110	2.0	22.0	2.0	m.q.	0	180	1.5 d
(Cheerios-to-Go)	80	3.0	15.0	2.0	m.q.	0	220	2.0 d
(Honey Nut Cheerios-to-Go)	110	3.0	23.0	1.0	n.a.	0	250	1.5 d
CERVELAT, see "Summer sausage" and "Thuringer cervelat"								
CHABLIS, see "Wine"								
CHAMPAGNE, see "Wine"								
CHARD, SWISS, see "Swiss chard"								

1. *Prepared according to package directions.*

Food and Measure	cal.	prot. (gms)	carbo. (gms)	tot. fat (gms)	sat. fat (gms)	chol. (mgs)	sod. (mgs)	fiber (gms)
CHAYOTE:								
raw:								
untrimmed, 1 lb.	108	4.0	24.3	1.4	n.a.	0	18	3.1 c
trimmed, 1 oz.	7	.3	1.5	.1	(0)	0	1	.2 c
1 medium, 5¾″ × 2⅞″ × 2⅜″,								
approx. 7.2 oz.	49	1.8	11.0	.6	(0)	0	8	1.4 c
1″ pieces, ½ cup	16	.6	3.6	.2	(0)	0	3	.5 c
boiled, drained, 4 oz.	27	.7	5.8	.5	(0)	0	1	.7 c
boiled, drained, 1″ pieces, ½ cup ...	19	.5	4.1	.4	(0)	0	1	.5 c
CHEDDARWURST:								
(*Hillshire Farm* Bun Size), 2 oz.	200	8.0	1.0	18.0	m.q.	m.q.	480	(0)
(*Hillshire Farm* Links), 2 oz.	190	8.0	1.0	17.0	m.q.	m.q.	480	(0)
CHEESE (see also "Cheese food,"								
"Cheese product," and "Cheese								
spread"), 1 oz., except as								
noted:								
American, processed:								
1 oz.	106	6.3	.5	8.9	5.6	27	406	0
1″ cube	66	3.9	.3	5.5	3.5	17	250	0
(*Borden* Loaf or Slices)	110	6.0	1.0	9.0	m.q.	m.q.	40	0
(*Dorman's*)	110	6.0	1.0	9.0	m.q.	m.q.	440	0
(*Dorman's* Loaf Low Sodium)	110	6.0	1.0	9.0	m.q.	m.q.	140	0
(*Hoffman's*)	110	6.0	1.0	9.0	m.q.	m.q.	400	0
(*Land O'Lakes*)	110	6.0	<1.0	9.0	6.0	25	405	0
(*Kraft* Deluxe Loaf)	110	6.0	1.0	9.0	5.0	25	430	0
(*Kraft* Deluxe Slices)	110	6.0	1.0	9.0	5.0	25	450	0
hot pepper (*Sargento*)	110	6.0	.5	9.0	m.q.	27	410	(0)
sharp (*Old English* Loaf)	110	6.0	1.0	9.0	5.0	30	400	0
sharp (*Old English* Slices)	110	6.0	1.0	9.0	5.0	30	440	0
asiago, wheel (*Frigo*)	110	7.0	1.0	9.0	m.q.	m.q.	400	0
babybel (*Laughing Cow*)	91	7.0	tr.	7.0	m.q.	22	227	0
babybel, mini (*Laughing Cow*),								
¾ oz.	74	4.7	tr.	6.0	m.q.	18	170	0
(*Bel Paese* Domestic Traditional) ...	101	6.0	.7	8.0	m.q.	20	145	0
(*Bel Paese* Imported)	90	5.7	.3	7.4	m.q.	22	196	0
(*Bel Paese* Lite)	76	7.0	1.0	5.0	m.q.	16	155	0
(*Bel Paese* Medallion Process)	71	3.4	1.3	5.9	m.q.	18	193	0
blue:								
1 oz.	100	6.1	.7	8.2	5.3	21	396	0
1″ cube	61	3.7	.4	5.0	3.2	13	241	0
(*Dorman's* Danablu 50%)	100	6.4	.3	8.2	5.0	23	200	0
(*Dorman's* Danablu 60%)	108	4.8	.3	9.7	6.9	31	200	0
(*Frigo*)	100	6.0	1.0	8.0	m.q.	m.q.	400	0
(*Hickory Farms* Domestic)	101	6.1	.7	8.3	m.q.	21	396	0
(*Kraft*)	100	6.0	1.0	9.0	5.0	30	330	0
(*Sargento*)	100	6.0	1.0	8.0	m.q.	21	400	0
blue castello (*Dorman's* 70%)	134	3.7	.1	12.3	9.0	29	286	0
crumbled, 1 cup not packed	477	28.9	3.2	38.8	25.2	102	1884	0

Food and Measure	cal.	prot. (gms)	carbo. (gms)	tot. fat (gms)	sat. fat (gms)	chol. (mgs)	sod. (mgs)	fiber (gms)
CHEESE, BLUE *(cont.)*								
saga *(Dorman's 70%)*	134	3.7	.1	12.3	9.0	29	286	0
bonbel *(Laughing Cow)*	100	6.0	tr.	8.0	m.q.	24	227	0
bonbel, mini *(Laughing Cow)*								
¾ oz.	74	4.7	tr.	6.0	m.q.	18	170	0
bonbino *(Laughing Cow)*	103	7.0	tr.	9.0	m.q.	27	227	0
brick:								
1 oz.	105	6.6	.8	8.4	5.3	27	159	0
1″ cube	64	4.0	.5	5.1	3.2	16	96	0
(Dorman's)	110	7.0	1.0	8.0	m.q.	m.q.	180	0
(Kraft)	110	7.0	0	9.0	5.0	30	180	0
(Land O'Lakes)	110	7.0	1.0	8.0	5.0	25	160	0
Brie:								
4½-oz. pkg.	427	26.6	.6	35.4	m.q.	128	806	0
1 oz.	95	5.9	.1	7.9	m.q.	28	178	0
(Dorman's)	81	5.1	.3	6.6	4.0	20	229	0
(Sargento)	100	6.0	.1	8.0	m.q.	28	180	0
burger cheese *(Sargento)*	110	6.0	.5	9.0	m.q.	27	410	0
Butternip *(Hickory Farms)*	110	5.2	1.1	9.4	m.q.	25	82	0
Cajun *(Sargento)*	110	7.0	.3	9.0	m.q.	28	165	0
caljack *(Churney)*	100	6.0	1.0	8.0	m.q.	m.q.	m.q.	0
Camembert:								
1⅓-oz. wedge	114	7.5	.2	9.2	5.8	27	320	0
1 oz.	85	5.6	.1	6.9	4.3	20	239	0
1″ cube	51	3.4	<.1	4.1	2.6	12	144	0
(Dorman's 45%)	82	6.0	.3	6.3	3.9	17	226	0
(Dorman's 50%)	89	5.6	.3	7.3	4.4	23	285	0
(Hickory Farms)	90	6.0	.1	7.0	m.q.	26	239	0
(Sargento)	90	6.0	.1	7.0	m.q.	20	240	0
caraway	107	7.1	.9	8.3	m.q.	m.q.	196	0
cheddar:								
1 oz.	114	7.1	.4	9.4	6.0	30	176	0
1″ cube	69	4.3	.2	5.7	3.6	18	107	0
shredded, 1 cup not packed	455	28.1	1.5	37.5	23.8	119	701	0
(Alpine Lace Cheddar Flavored) ..	100	7.0	1.0	8.0	5.0	25	95	0
(Darigold)	110	7.0	<1.0	9.0	5.9	29	170	0
(Dorman's)	110	7.0	1.0	9.0	m.q.	m.q.	200	0
(Dorman's Chedda-Delite)	90	7.0	1.0	7.0	m.q.	m.q.	100	0
(Featherweight Low Sodium)	110	7.0	1.0	9.0	m.q.	m.q.	5	0
(Frigo)	110	7.0	1.0	9.0	m.q.	m.q.	200	0
(Hickory Farms)	110	7.0	1.0	9.0	m.q.	30	176	0
(Kraft)	110	7.0	1.0	9.0	5.0	30	180	0
(Land O'Lakes)	110	7.0	<1.0	9.0	6.0	30	175	0
(Laughing Cow)	110	7.0	tr.	9.0	m.q.	28	227	0
(Sargento)	110	7.0	.4	9.0	m.q.	30	176	0
(Sargento New York)	110	7.0	.4	9.0	m.q.	30	180	0
mild:								
(Weight Watchers Natural)	80	8.0	1.0	5.0	3.0	15	150	0

Food and Measure	cal.	prot. (gms)	carbo. (gms)	tot. fat (gms)	sat. fat (gms)	chol. (mgs)	sod. (mgs)	fiber (gms)
(*Weight Watchers* Natural Low Sodium)	80	8.0	1.0	5.0	3.0	15	70	0
reduced fat (*Kraft* Light Naturals)	80	9.0	0	5.0	3.0	20	220	0
shredded (*Weight Watchers* Natural)	80	8.0	1.0	5.0	3.0	15	150	0
raw milk (*Hickory Farms Light Choice* Low Sodium)	114	6.0	0	8.0	m.q.	30	100	0
reduced fat (*Dorman's* Low Sodium)	80	8.0	1.0	5.0	3.4	20	100	0
sharp (*Weight Watchers* Natural) ..	80	8.0	1.0	5.0	3.0	15	150	0
sharp or extra sharp (*Axelrod*) ...	110	7.0	1.0	9.0	m.q.	30	200	0
sharp, reduced fat (*Kraft* Light Naturals)	80	9.0	1.0	5.0	3.0	20	220	0
sharp, slicing (*Boar's Head*)	110	7.0	1.0	9.0	m.q.	18	100	0
sharp, white, reduced fat (*Cracker Barrel Light*)	80	9.0	1.0	5.0	3.0	20	220	0
smokey sharp, processed (*Hoffman's*)	110	6.0	1.0	9.0	m.q.	m.q.	440	0
super sharp, processed (*Hoffman's*)	110	6.0	2.0	8.0	m.q.	m.q.	390	0
Vermont (*Churny*)	110	7.0	1.0	9.0	5.0	30	180	0
cheddar jack (*Dorman's* Chedda-Jack)	90	7.0	1.0	7.0	m.q.	m.q.	100	0
Cheshire	110	6.6	1.4	8.7	m.q.	29	198	0
Chutter (*Hickory Farms* Cold Pack)	87	6.0	2.6	5.8	m.q.	46	213	0
colby:								
1 oz.	112	6.7	.7	9.1	5.7	27	171	0
1″ cube	68	4.1	.4	5.5	3.5	16	104	0
(*Alpine Lace Colby-Lo*)	80	7.0	1.0	5.0	4.0	20	85	0
(*Dorman's*)	110	7.0	1.0	9.0	m.q.	m.q.	190	0
(*Hickory Farms Light Choice* Low Sodium)	100	8.0	1.0	6.0	m.q.	20	4	0
(*Hickory Farms* Longhorn)	112	6.7	.7	8.6	m.q.	27	171	0
(*Kraft*)	110	7.0	1.0	9.0	5.0	30	180	0
(*Land O'Lakes*)	110	7.0	1.0	9.0	6.0	25	170	0
(*Sargento*)	110	7.0	1.0	9.0	m.q.	27	170	0
(*Weight Watchers* Natural)	80	8.0	1.0	5.0	2.0	15	130	0
low fat, calcium enriched (*Hickory Farms Light Choice*)	100	7.0	1.0	8.0	m.q.	m.q.	180	0
reduced fat (*Kraft* Light Naturals)	80	9.0	0	5.0	3.0	20	220	0
colby jack (*Sargento*)	110	7.0	.5	9.0	m.q.	27	160	0
colby and Monterey Jack, reduced fat, shredded (*Kraft* Light Naturals)	80	8.0	1.0	5.0	3.0	20	220	0
cottage cheese, ½ cup, except as noted:								
creamed:								
4 oz.	117	14.1	3.0	5.1	3.2	17	457	0

Food and Measure	cal.	prot. (gms)	carbo. (gms)	tot. fat (gms)	sat. fat (gms)	chol. (mgs)	sod. (mgs)	fiber (gms)
CHEESE, COTTAGE CHEESE, CREAMED *(cont.)*								
1 oz.	29	3.5	.8	1.3	.8	4	115	0
small curd, ½ cup not packed ..	108	13.1	2.8	4.7	3.0	16	425	0
small curd (*Knudsen*), 4 oz. ...	120	14.0	4.0	5.0	3.0	20	370	0
large curd, ½ cup not packed ..	116	14.1	3.0	5.1	3.2	17	456	0
large curd (*Knudsen*), 4 oz. ...	120	14.0	4.0	5.0	3.0	20	340	0
(*Bison* 4% fat)	120	14.0	4.0	5.0	m.q.	20	420	0
(*Borden* 4% fat)	120	14.0	4.0	5.0	m.q.	m.q.	400	0
(*Borden* Unsalted)	120	14.0	4.0	5.0	m.q.	m.q.	40	0
(*Breakstone's*), 4 oz.	110	13.0	3.0	5.0	3.0	25	370	0
(*Crowley* 4% fat)	120	14.0	4.0	5.0	m.q.	15	390	0
(*Darigold* 4%), 4 oz.	120	14.0	4.0	4.2	3.2	17	510	0
(*Friendship* California Style 4%)	120	14.0	4.0	5.0	m.q.	17	380	0
chive (*Bison*)	120	14.0	4.0	5.0	m.q.	20	420	(0)
w/fruit, 4 oz. or ½ cup not packed	140	11.2	15.0	3.8	2.4	13	457	tr.c
w/fruit, 1 oz.	35	2.8	3.8	1.0	.6	3	115	tr.c
garden salad (*Bison*)	110	12.0	4.0	4.0	m.q.	15	420	m.q.
w/peaches (*Crowley* 4%)	140	10.0	17.0	3.0	m.q.	10	340	m.q.
w/pineapple:								
(*Bison*)	140	10.0	18.0	4.0	m.q.	15	340	m.q.
(*Crowley* 4%)	140	11.0	15.0	4.0	m.q.	15	330	m.q.
(*Friendship* 4%)	140	11.0	15.0	4.0	m.q.	17	300	m.q.
(*Knudsen* 4%), 4 oz.	140	10.0	14.0	5.0	3.0	25	260	m.q.
dry curd, unsalted:								
4 oz.	96	19.5	2.1	.5	.3	8	14	0
1 oz.	24	4.9	.5	.1	<.1	2	4	0
½ cup not packed	62	12.5	1.3	.3	.2	5	9	0
(*Borden*)	80	18.0	3.0	1.0	m.q.	m.q.	20	0
(*Breakstone's*), 4 oz.	90	16.0	6.0	0	0	10	65	0
(*Darigold*), 4 oz.	80	18.0	3.0	1.0	.4	10	15	0
lowfat:								
2%, 4 oz., approx. ½ cup not packed	101	15.5	4.1	2.2	1.4	9	459	0
2%, 1 oz.	25	3.9	1.0	.5	.3	2	115	0
2% (*Breakstone's*), 4 oz.	100	14.0	4.0	2.0	1.0	15	510	0
2% (*Darigold* Trim), 4 oz.	100	14.0	4.0	3.2	2.0	17	510	0
2% (*Knudsen*), 4 oz.	100	14.0	4.0	2.0	1.0	15	370	0
2% (*Sealtest*), 4 oz.	100	14.0	4.0	2.0	1.0	15	340	0
2% (*Weight Watchers*)	100	14.0	4.0	2.0	m.q.	m.q.	460	0
w/apple spiced, 2% (*Knudsen*), 6 oz.	180	16.0	20.0	2.0	2.0	15	280	m.q.
w/fruit cocktail, 2% (*Knudsen*), 4 oz.	130	11.0	16.0	2.0	2.0	10	330	m.q.
w/mandarin orange, 2% (*Knudsen*), 4 oz.	110	11.0	11.0	2.0	2.0	10	320	m.q.
w/peach, 2% (*Knudsen*), 6 oz.	170	16.0	19.0	2.0	2.0	15	270	m.q.
w/pear, 2% (*Knudsen*), 4 oz. ..	110	11.0	12.0	2.0	2.0	10	320	m.q.

Food and Measure	cal.	prot. (gms)	carbo. (gms)	tot. fat (gms)	sat. fat (gms)	chol. (mgs)	sod. (mgs)	fiber (gms)
w/pineapple, 2% (*Knudsen*), 6 oz.	170	16.0	18.0	2.0	2.0	15	300	m.q.
w/strawberry, 2% (*Knudsen*), 6 oz.	170	16.0	19.0	2.0	2.0	15	320	m.q.
1½% (*Lite-Line*)	90	14.0	4.0	2.0	m.q.	m.q.	400	0
1%, 4 oz., approx. ½ cup not packed	82	14.0	3.1	1.2	.7	5	459	0
1%, 1 oz.	20	3.5	.8	.3	.2	1	115	0
1% (*Bison*)	90	14.0	4.0	2.0	m.q.	5	350	0
1% (*Crowley*)	90	14.0	4.0	1.0	m.q.	5	390	0
1% (*Crowley* No Salt Added) ..	90	14.0	4.0	1.0	m.q.	5	50	0
1% (*Friendship*)	90	14.0	4.0	1.0	m.q.	5	350	0
1% (*Friendship* No Salt Added)	90	14.0	4.0	1.0	m.q.	5	31	0
1% (*Light n' Lively*), 4 oz.	80	14.0	4.0	2.0	1.0	10	370	0
1% (*Weight Watchers*)	90	14.0	4.0	1.0	m.q.	m.q.	460	0
calcium fortified, 1% (*Crowley*)	90	14.0	4.0	1.0	m.q.	5	390	0
garden salad, 1% (*Light n' Lively*), 4 oz.	80	18.0	5.0	2.0	1.0	10	350	m.q.
lactose reduced, 1% (*Friendship*)	90	14.0	4.0	1.0	m.q.	5	350	0
w/peach and pineapple, 1% (*Light n' Lively*), 4 oz.	100	11.0	12.0	1.0	1.0	10	320	m.q.
w/pineapple, 1% (*Crowley*)	110	11.0	15.0	1.0	m.q.	5	330	m.q.
w/pineapple, 1% (*Friendship*) ..	110	11.0	15.0	1.0	m.q.	5	300	m.q.
nonfat (*Knudsen*), 4 oz.	70	15.0	3.0	0	0	5	420	0
pot style, large curd, lowfat 2% (*Friendship*)	100	14.0	4.0	2.0	m.q.	9	405	0
cream cheese:								
3-oz. pkg.	297	6.4	2.3	29.6	18.7	93	251	0
1 oz.	99	2.1	.8	9.9	6.2	31	84	0
1″ cube	56	1.2	.4	5.6	3.5	18	48	0
(*Crowley*)	110	2.0	1.0	9.0	m.q.	30	100	0
(*Darigold*)	99	2.2	.8	9.9	6.2	31	84	0
(*Dorman's* 65%)	90	3.0	.6	8.4	5.1	26	200	0
(*Dorman's* 70%)	102	2.7	.6	9.9	6.1	30	200	0
(*Philadelphia Brand*)	100	2.0	1.0	10.0	6.0	30	90	0
w/chives (*Philadelphia Brand*) ...	90	2.0	1.0	9.0	5.0	30	125	(0)
w/pimiento (*Philadelphia Brand*)	90	2.0	1.0	9.0	5.0	30	150	(0)
cream cheese, soft:								
(*Friendship*)	103	1.5	.8	<10.0	m.q.	31	70	0
(*Philadelphia Brand*)	100	1.0	2.0	10.0	5.0	30	100	0
w/chives and onion (*Philadelphia Brand*)	100	2.0	2.0	9.0	5.0	30	100	(0)
w/herb and garlic (*Philadelphia Brand*)	100	1.0	2.0	9.0	5.0	25	160	(0)
w/olives and pimiento (*Philadelphia Brand*)	90	2.0	2.0	8.0	5.0	25	160	(0)
w/pineapple (*Philadelphia Brand*)	90	1.0	4.0	8.0	5.0	25	90	(0)

Food and Measure	cal.	prot. (gms)	carbo. (gms)	tot. fat (gms)	sat. fat (gms)	chol. (mgs)	sod. (mgs)	fiber (gms)
CHEESE, CREAM CHEESE, SOFT *(cont.)*								
w/smoked salmon (*Philadelphia Brand*)	90	2.0	1.0	9.0	5.0	25	180	0
w/strawberries (*Philadelphia Brand*)	90	1.0	4.0	8.0	5.0	20	75	(0)
cream cheese, whipped:								
(*Philadelphia Brand*)	100	2.0	1.0	10.0	6.0	30	85	0
w/chives (*Philadelphia Brand*)	90	2.0	1.0	8.0	5.0	30	150	(0)
w/onions (*Philadelphia Brand*)	90	2.0	2.0	8.0	5.0	25	170	(0)
w/smoked salmon (*Philadelphia Brand*)	90	2.0	2.0	8.0	5.0	30	170	0
danbo (*Dorman's 20%*)	62	8.9	.3	2.8	1.7	9	200	0
danbo (*Dorman's 45%*)	98	7.3	.3	7.5	4.6	23	200	0
(*Dorman's* Crema Dania 70%)	134	3.7	.1	12.3	9.0	29	286	0
Edam:								
7-oz. pkg.	706	49.5	2.8	55.0	34.8	177	1911	0
1 oz.	101	7.1	.4	7.9	5.0	25	274	0
(*Dorman's*)	100	7.0	1.0	8.0	m.q.	m.q.	200	0
(*Dorman's 45%*)	91	6.7	.3	7.0	4.3	21	200	0
(*Hickory Farms* Domestic)	100	6.0	.9	8.4	m.q.	24	182	0
(*Kaukauna*)	100	7.0	<1.0	8.0	m.q.	25	275	0
(*Kraft*)	90	8.0	0	7.0	4.0	20	310	0
(*Land O'Lakes*)	100	7.0	<1.0	8.0	5.0	25	275	0
(*Laughing Cow*)	100	6.0	tr.	8.0	m.q.	26	227	0
(*May-Bud*)	100	7.0	0	8.0	m.q.	m.q.	275	0
(*Sargento*)	100	7.0	.4	8.0	m.q.	25	270	0
farmer:								
(*Friendship*), ½ cup	160	16.0	4.0	12.0	m.q.	40	356	0
(*Friendship* No Salt Added), ½ cup	160	16.0	4.0	12.0	m.q.	40	8	0
(*Hickory Farms Light Choice*)	90	6.0	1.0	7.0	m.q.	20	150	0
(*Kaukauna*)	100	7.0	<1.0	8.0	m.q.	25	m.q.	0
(*May-Bud*)	90	6.0	1.0	7.0	m.q.	20	210	0
(*Sargento*)	100	7.0	1.0	8.0	m.q.	26	130	0
style (*Hickory Farms*)	90	6.0	1.0	7.0	m.q.	20	210	0
feta:								
sheep's milk	75	4.0	1.2	6.0	4.2	25	316	0
(*Churny* Natural)	75	4.7	1.2	6.5	4.2	25	316	0
(*Dorman's 45%*)	91	5.9	.4	7.3	m.q.	m.q.	m.q.	0
(*Sargento*)	80	4.0	1.0	6.0	m.q.	25	320	0
fontina:								
8-oz. pkg.	883	58.1	3.5	70.7	43.6	263	m.q.	0
1 oz.	110	7.3	.4	8.8	5.4	33	m.q.	0
(*Sargento*)	110	7.0	.4	9.0	m.q.	33	m.q.	0
gjetost:								
goat's milk, 8-oz. pkg.	1057	21.9	96.8	67.0	43.5	m.q.	1362	0
goat's milk	132	2.7	12.1	8.4	5.4	m.q.	170	0
(*Sargento*)	130	3.0	12.0	8.0	m.q.	m.q.	170	0

Food and Measure	cal.	prot. (gms)	carbo. (gms)	tot. fat (gms)	sat. fat (gms)	chol. (mgs)	sod. (mgs)	fiber (gms)
goat's milk, fresh	82	4.5	.9	6.8	m.q.	20	180	0
Gouda:								
7-oz. pkg.	705	49.4	4.4	54.3	34.9	226	1622	0
1 oz.	101	7.1	.6	7.8	5.0	32	232	0
(Dorman's)	100	7.0	1.0	8.0	m.q.	m.q.	210	0
(Kaukauna)	100	7.0	1.0	8.0	m.q.	30	230	0
(Kraft)	110	7.0	0	9.0	5.0	30	200	0
(Land O'Lakes)	100	7.0	1.0	8.0	5.0	30	230	0
(Laughing Cow)	110	7.0	tr.	9.0	m.q.	28	227	0
(May-Bud)	100	7.0	1.0	8.0	m.q.	m.q.	230	0
(Sargento)	100	7.0	1.0	8.0	m.q.	32	230	0
w/caraway seed (Kaukauna)	100	7.0	<1.0	8.0	m.q.	30	230	(0)
w/hickory smoke flavor								
(Kaukauna)	100	7.0	<1.0	8.0	m.q.	25	230	0
mini (Laughing Cow), ¾ oz.	80	5.3	tr.	6.4	m.q.	21	170	0
grated (Polly-O)	130	11.0	1.0	10.0	m.q.	25	530	0
Gruyère, 6-oz. pkg.	702	50.7	.6	55.0	32.2	187	571	0
Gruyère	117	8.5	.1	9.2	5.4	31	95	0
havarti:								
(Casino)	120	6.0	0	11.0	7.0	35	140	0
(Dorman's 45%)	91	6.7	.3	7.0	4.3	21	200	0
(Dorman's 60%)	118	5.4	.3	10.6	6.5	31	200	0
(Hickory Farms Danish Special) ..	117	5.1	.3	10.5	m.q.	31	198	0
(Sargento)	120	5.0	.3	11.0	m.q.	31	200	0
hot pepper (Hickory Farms)	106	6.3	.5	8.9	m.q.	27	406	(0)
Italian style, grated (Sargento)	110	8.0	1.0	8.0	m.q.	26	105	0
Jarlsberg (Hickory Farms)	100	7.0	1	7.0	m.q.	16	130	0
Jarlsberg (Norseland Jarlsberg)	97	7.0	1.0	7.0	4.2	18	135	0
(Laughing Cow Reduced mini), ¾ oz.	45	6.0	tr.	2.5	m.q.	8	170	0
Limburger:								
8-oz. pkg.	742	45.5	1.1	61.9	38.0	204	1816	0
1 oz.	93	5.7	.1	7.7	4.8	26	227	0
(Sargento)	90	6.0	.1	8.0	m.q.	26	230	0
natural (Mohawk Valley Little								
Gem)	90	6.0	0	8.0	5.0	25	250	0
mascarpone (Galbani Imported)	128	1.5	1.2	13.1	m.q.	39	17	0
Monterey Jack:								
6-oz. pkg.	635	41.6	1.2	51.5	m.q.	m.q.	912	0
1 oz.	106	6.9	.2	8.6	m.q.	m.q.	152	0
(Alpine Lace Monti-Jack-Lo)	80	7.0	1.0	5.0	4.0	15	75	0
(Axelrod)	100	6.0	1.0	8.0	m.q.	30	150	0
(Darigold)	110	7.0	<1.0	8.0	m.q.	25	150	0
(Dorman's)	100	6.0	1.0	8.0	m.q.	m.q.	180	0
(Hickory Farms Light Choice Low								
Sodium)	110	6.0	0	8.0	m.q.	30	100	0
(Kaukauna)	110	7.0	<1.0	9.0	m.q.	25	150	0
(Kraft)	110	6.0	0	9.0	5.0	30	190	0
(Land O'Lakes)	110	7.0	<1.0	9.0	5.0	20	150	0

Food and Measure	cal.	prot. (gms)	carbo. (gms)	tot. fat (gms)	sat. fat (gms)	chol. (mgs)	sod. (mgs)	fiber (gms)
CHEESE, MONTEREY JACK *(cont.)*								
(May-Bud)	110	7.0	0	9.0	m.q.	m.q.	150	0
(Sargento)	110	7.0	.2	9.0	m.q.	25	150	0
(Weight Watchers Natural)	80	8.0	1.0	5.0	2.0	15	120	0
w/caraway *(Kraft)*	100	7.0	1.0	8.0	5.0	30	180	(0)
w/jalapeño pepper *(Axelrod)*	100	6.0	1.0	8.0	m.q.	30	220	(0)
w/jalapeño pepper *(Kraft)*	110	7.0	1.0	9.0	5.0	30	190	(0)
w/peppers, reduced fat *(Kraft* Light Naturals)	80	8.0	1.0	5.0	3.0	20	220	(0)
reduced fat *(Dorman's* Low Sodium)	80	8.0	1.0	5.0	3.1	18	90	0
reduced fat *(Kraft* Light Naturals)	80	9.0	0	5.0	3.0	20	220	0
mozzarella:								
(Dorman's)	90	7.0	1.0	6.0	m.q.	m.q.	190	0
(Hickory Farms)	72	6.9	.8	4.5	m.q.	16	132	0
(Hickory Farms Light Choice Low Sodium)	80	8.0	1.0	5.0	m.q.	15	90	0
(Polly-O Lite)	70	7.0	1.0	4.0	m.q.	15	200	0
(Weight Watchers Natural)	70	8.0	1.0	4.0	2.0	15	150	0
fresh *(Polly-O Fior di Latte)*	80	5.0	1.0	6.0	m.q.	20	20	0
shredded *(Weight Watchers* Natural)	80	8.0	1.0	4.0	2.0	15	150	0
whole milk:								
1 oz.	80	5.5	.6	6.1	3.7	22	106	0
(Crowley)	90	5.0	1.0	7.0	m.q.	25	240	0
(Polly-O)	90	5.0	1.0	6.0	m.q.	20	280	0
(Sargento)	90	6.0	1.0	7.0	m.q.	25	120	0
low moisture *(Frigo)*	90	6.0	1.0	7.0	4.0	15	190	0
part skim milk:								
1 oz.	72	6.9	.8	4.5	2.9	16	132	0
(Crowley)	70	8.0	1.0	4.0	m.q.	15	240	0
(Polly-O)	80	6.0	1.0	5.0	m.q.	15	280	0
low moisture:								
1 oz.	79	7.8	.9	4.9	3.1	15	150	0
1″ cube	49	4.8	.6	3.0	1.9	10	93	0
(Alpine Lace)	70	7.0	1.0	5.0	3.0	15	75	0
(Dorman's Low Sodium)	80	8.0	1.0	5.0	2.6	15	90	0
(Frigo)	80	7.0	1.0	5.0	m.q.	10	190	0
(Kraft)	80	8.0	1.0	5.0	3.0	15	200	0
(Land O'Lakes)	80	8.0	1.0	5.0	3.0	15	150	0
(Sargento)	80	8.0	1.0	5.0	m.q.	15	150	0
reduced fat *(Frigo)*	60	8.0	1.0	3.0	2.0	10	150	0
w/jalapeño pepper *(Kraft)*	80	8.0	1.0	5.0	3.0	20	230	(0)
low moisture:								
1 oz.	90	6.1	.7	7.0	4.4	25	118	0
1″ cube	56	3.8	.4	4.3	2.7	16	73	0
(Kraft)	90	6.0	1.0	7.0	4.0	20	190	0
reduced fat *(Dorman's* Low Sodium)	80	9.0	1.0	4.0	2.5	17	90	0

Food and Measure	cal.	prot. (gms)	carbo. (gms)	tot. fat (gms)	sat. fat (gms)	chol. (mgs)	sod. (mgs)	fiber (gms)
reduced fat (*Kraft* Light Naturals)	80	8.0	1.0	4.0	3.0	15	200	0
Muenster:								
6-oz. pkg.	626	3.8	1.9	51.1	32.5	163	1067	0
1 oz.	104	6.6	.3	8.5	5.4	27	178	0
(*Alpine Lace*)	100	7.0	1.0	8.0	5.0	30	85	0
(*Dorman's*)	110	7.0	0	9.0	m.q.	m.q.	190	0
(*Dorman's 50%*)	100	6.4	.3	8.2	5.0	24	200	0
(*Dorman's* Low Sodium)	110	7.0	0	9.0	m.q.	m.q.	95	0
(*Hickory Farms*)	100	6.6	.3	8.5	m.q.	25	180	0
(*Hickory Farms Light Choice* Low								
Sodium)	110	7.0	0	9.0	m.q.	27	95	0
(*Kaukauna*)	110	7.0	<1.0	9.0	m.q.	25	180	0
(*Land O'Lakes*)	100	7.0	<1.0	9.0	5.0	25	180	0
red rind (*Sargento*)	100	7.0	.3	9.0	m.q.	27	180	0
reduced fat (*Dorman's* Low								
Sodium)	80	8.0	0	5.0	3.1	18	140	0
Neufchâtel:								
3-oz. pkg.	221	8.5	2.5	19.9	12.6	65	339	0
1 oz.	74	2.8	.8	6.6	4.2	22	113	0
(*Philadelphia Brand* Light)	80	3.0	1.0	7.0	4.0	25	115	0
chocolate (*Hickory Farms*)	110	2.0	8.0	8.0	m.q.	33	90	(0)
date, nut, rum (*Hickory Farms*) ..	100	2.0	4.0	8.0	m.q.	31	80	(0)
garlic and herbs (*Kaukauna*)	80	3.0	1.0	7.0	m.q.	25	150	(0)
orange (*Hickory Farms*)	100	2.0	4.0	8.0	m.q.	45	75	(0)
peach (*Hickory Farms*)	90	2.0	3.0	8.0	m.q.	39	85	(0)
pineapple (*Hickory Farms*)	90	2.0	2.0	8.0	m.q.	33	60	(0)
strawberry (*Hickory Farms*)	90	2.0	3.0	8.0	m.q.	32	70	(0)
vegetable, garden (*Kaukauna*) ...	80	3.0	1.0	7.0	m.q.	25	200	(0)
New Holland, w/herbs (*Hickory*								
Farms Light Choice)	90	7.0	1.0	8.0	m.q.	27	100	(0)
Parmesan:								
(*Hickory Farms*)	110	10.0	1.0	7.0	m.q.	m.q.	350	0
(*Kraft*)	100	9.0	1.0	7.0	4.0	20	290	0
fresh (*Sargento*)	110	10.0	1.0	7.0	m.q.	19	450	0
hard, 5-oz. pkg.	557	50.8	4.6	36.7	23.3	96	2274	0
hard	111	10.1	.9	7.3	4.7	19	454	0
grated:								
1 oz.	129	11.8	1.1	8.5	5.4	22	528	0
1 tbsp.	23	2.1	.2	1.5	1.0	4	93	0
(*Frigo*)	130	12.0	1.0	9.0	m.q.	m.q.	510	0
(*Kraft*)	130	12.0	1.0	9.0	5.0	30	430	0
(*Polly-O*)	130	11.0	1.0	9.0	m.q.	20	530	0
(*Progresso*), 1 tbsp.	23	2.0	<1.0	2.0	1.0	4	95	0
(*Sargento*)	130	12.0	2.0	9.0	m.q.	22	530	0
Reggiano (*Galbani* Imported)	105	10.1	n.a.	7.1	m.q.	21	188	0
wheel or fresh grated (*Frigo*)	110	10.0	1.0	7.0	m.q.	m.q.	350	0
Parmesan and Romano, grated								
(*Frigo*)	130	12.0	1.0	9.0	m.q.	m.q.	510	0

Food and Measure	cal.	prot. (gms)	carbo. (gms)	tot. fat (gms)	sat. fat (gms)	chol. (mgs)	sod. (mgs)	fiber (gms)
CHEESE *(cont.)*								
Parmesan and Romano, grated								
(*Sargento*)	110	10.0	1.0	7.0	m.q.	24	400	0
pasta, Italian, grated (*Frigo*								
Parmazest)	120	7.0	5.0	8.0	m.q.	m.q.	430	0
pimiento, processed:								
1 oz.	106	6.3	.5	8.9	5.6	27	405	tr.c
1″ cube	66	3.9	.3	5.5	3.4	16	250	tr.c
(*Kraft* Deluxe)	100	6.0	1.0	8.0	5.0	25	440	(0)
pizza, shredded (*Frigo*)	90	6.0	1.0	7.0	m.q.	20	190	0
pizza, shredded, low fat (*Frigo*)	65	9.0	1.0	3.0	m.q.	10	150	0
Port du Salut, 6-oz. pkg.	598	40.4	1.0	47.9	28.4	209	908	0
Port du Salut	100	6.7	.2	8.0	4.7	35	151	0
port wine (*Hickory Farms*)	97	5.6	2.4	6.9	m.q.	18	262	0
pot cheese (*Sargento*)	25	5.0	1.0	.2	m.q.	m.q.	1	0
primavera (*Bel Paese* Lite)	68	6.0	2.0	4.0	m.q.	14	165	(0)
provolone:								
6-oz. pkg.	598	43.5	3.6	45.3	29.0	117	1488	0
1 oz.	100	7.3	.6	7.6	4.8	20	248	0
(*Alpine Lace Provo-Lo*)	70	7.0	1.0	5.0	5.0	15	85	0
(*Dorman's*)	90	7.0	1.0	7.0	m.q.	m.q.	290	0
(*Dorman's* Low Sodium)	90	7.0	1.0	m.q.	m.q.	m.q.	140	0
(*Frigo*)	100	7.0	1.0	7.0	m.q.	m.q.	230	0
(*Hickory Farms Light Choice* Low								
Sodium)	90	7.0	1.0	7.0	m.q.	20	140	0
(*Kraft*)	100	7.0	1.0	7.0	4.0	25	260	0
(*Land O'Lakes*)	100	7.0	1.0	8.0	5.0	20	250	0
(*Sargento*)	100	7.0	1.0	8.0	m.q.	20	250	0
smoked (*Frigo*)	100	7.0	1.0	7.0	m.q.	m.q.	230	0
pub (*Hickory Farms*)	94	5.6	2.4	6.9	m.q.	18	237	0
queso blanco (*Sargento*)	100	7.0	.3	9.0	m.q.	27	180	0
queso de papa (*Sargento*)	110	7.0	.4	9.0	m.q.	30	180	0
queso de taco (*Hickory Farms*)	106	6.3	.5	8.9	m.q.	27	450	0
ricotta:								
(*Polly-O* Lite), 2 oz.	80	7.0	3.0	4.0	m.q.	15	65	0
(*Sargento*)	40	3.0	1.0	3.0	m.q.	13	25	0
(*Sargento* Lite)	23	3.0	1.0	1.0	m.q.	4	20	0
whole milk:								
4 oz.	197	12.8	3.4	14.7	9.4	58	95	0
1 oz.	49	3.2	.9	3.7	2.4	14	24	0
½ cup	216	14.0	3.8	16.1	10.3	63	104	0
(*Crowley*), 2 oz.	100	6.0	3.0	7.0	m.q.	25	50	0
(*Frigo*)	50	3.0	1.0	4.0	m.q.	15	100	0
(*Polly-O*), 2 oz.	100	7.0	2.0	7.0	m.q.	20	45	0
part skim milk:								
4 oz.	156	12.9	5.8	9.0	5.6	35	142	0
1 oz.	39	3.2	1.5	2.2	1.4	9	35	0
½ cup	171	14.1	6.4	9.8	6.1	38	155	0
(*Crowley*), 2 oz.	80	7.0	3.0	4.0	m.q.	15	50	0

Food and Measure	cal.	prot. (gms)	carbo. (gms)	tot. fat (gms)	sat. fat (gms)	chol. (mgs)	sod. (mgs)	fiber (gms)
(*Frigo*)	45	3.0	1.0	3.0	m.q.	10	100	0
(*Polly-O*), 2 oz.	90	7.0	2.0	6.0	m.q.	20	45	0
(*Sargento*)	30	3.0	1.0	2.0	m.q.	10	30	0
low fat (*Frigo*)	20	3.0	1.0	1.0	m.q.	5	20	0
Romano:								
5-oz. pkg.	549	45.2	5.2	38.3	m.q.	148	1704	0
1 oz.	110	9.0	1.0	7.6	m.q.	29	340	0
(*Kraft* Natural)	100	8.0	1.0	7.0	4.0	20	250	0
(*Sargento*)	110	9.0	1.0	8.0	m.q.	29	340	0
grated:								
(*Frigo*)	130	12.0	1.0	9.0	m.q.	m.q.	510	0
(*Kraft*)	130	11.0	1.0	9.0	6.0	30	350	0
(*Polly-O*)	130	11.0	1.0	10.0	m.q.	30	530	0
(*Progresso*), 1 tbsp.	23	2.0	<1.0	2.0	1.0	6	70	0
loaf (*Hickory Farms*)	110	9.0	1.0	8.0	m.q.	m.q.	350	0
wedge (*Frigo*)	110	9.0	1.0	8.0	m.q.	m.q.	350	0
Roquefort, sheep's milk, 3-oz. pkg.	314	18.3	1.7	26.0	16.4	76	1538	0
Roquefort, sheep's milk	105	6.1	.6	8.7	5.5	26	513	0
Slim Jack (*Dorman's*)	90	6.0	1.0	7.0	m.q.	m.q.	90	0
smoked (*Hickory Farms Light Choice*								
Smoky Lyte)	80	7.0	1.0	6.0	m.q.	5	449	0
smoked (*Sargento* Smokestick)	100	7.0	1.0	7.0	m.q.	24	390	0
string:								
(*Frigo*)	80	7.0	1.0	5.0	m.q.	m.q.	190	0
(*Polly-O*), 1-oz. stick	90	7.0	2.0	6.0	m.q.	15	200	0
(*Sargento*)	80	8.0	1.0	5.0	m.q.	15	150	0
low moisture (*Kraft*)	80	8.0	1.0	5.0	3.0	20	230	0
smoked (*Sargento*)	80	8.0	1.0	5.0	m.q.	15	150	0
Swiss:								
(*Alpine Lace Swiss-Lo*)	100	8.0	1.0	7.0	4.0	20	35	0
(*Boar's Head* Domestic)	110	7.0	1.0	8.0	m.q.	25	75	0
(*Boar's Head* No Salt Added)	100	8.0	<1.0	8.0	m.q.	26	12	0
(*Casino*)	110	8.0	1.0	8.0	5.0	30	35	0
(*Dorman's*)	100	8.0	0	8.0	m.q.	m.q.	80	0
(*Dorman's* No Salt Added)	100	8.0	0	8.0	m.q.	m.q.	8	0
(*Dorman's* Reduced Fat)	90	10.0	0	5.0	2.8	17	80	0
(*Hickory Farms* Domestic)	110	8.1	1.0	7.8	m.q.	25	75	0
(*Hickory Farms Light Choice*								
Lorraine)	100	8.0	0	7.8	m.q.	25	35	0
(*Hickory Farms Light Choice* Low								
Sodium)	100	8.0	0	8.0	m.q.	26	8	0
(*Kraft*)	110	8.0	1.0	8.0	5.0	25	40	0
(*Kraft* Light Naturals)	90	10.0	1.0	5.0	3.0	20	45	0
(*Kraft* 75% Very Low Sodium) ...	110	8.0	1.0	8.0	5.0	25	10	0
(*Land O'Lakes*)	110	8.0	1.0	8.0	5.0	25	75	0
(*Sargento*)	110	8.0	1.0	8.0	m.q.	26	75	0
(*Sargento* Finland)	110	8.0	1.0	8.0	m.q.	26	75	0
(*Weight Watchers* Natural)	90	9.0	1.0	5.0	3.0	15	50	0
aged (*Kraft*)	110	8.0	1.0	8.0	5.0	25	45	0

Food and Measure	cal.	prot. (gms)	carbo. (gms)	tot. fat (gms)	sat. fat (gms)	chol. (mgs)	sod. (mgs)	fiber (gms)
CHEESE, SWISS *(cont.)*								
baby (*Cracker Barrel* Natural) ...	110	7.0	0	9.0	5.0	25	65	0
creamy (*Hickory Farms* Cold Pack)	92	5.6	2.5	7.2	m.q.	24	237	0
natural	107	8.1	1.0	7.8	5.0	26	74	0
natural, 1″ cube	56	4.3	.5	4.1	2.7	14	39	0
processed:								
1 oz.	95	7.0	.6	7.1	4.6	24	388	0
1″ cube	60	4.4	.4	4.5	2.9	15	245	0
(*Borden*)	100	7.0	1.0	8.0	m.q.	m.q.	380	0
(*Kraft* Deluxe)	90	7.0	1.0	7.0	4.0	25	420	0
reduced fat (*Kraft* Light Naturals)	90	10.0	1.0	5.0	3.0	20	70	0
smoked (*Dorman's*)	100	7.0	1.0	7.0	m.q.	m.q.	390	0
Swiss and cheddar, smokey (*Hoffman's*)	110	7.0	1.0	8.0	m.q.	m.q.	410	0
taco:								
(*Sargento*)	110	7.0	.5	9.0	m.q.	27	160	0
shredded (*Frigo*)	110	7.0	1.0	9.0	m.q.	m.q.	200	0
shredded (*Kraft*)	110	7.0	1.0	9.0	5.0	30	190	0
taleggio (*Tal-Fino* Brand Imported)	89	5.4	.2	7.4	m.q.	m.q.	176	0
Tilsit:								
(*Sargento*)	100	7.0	1.0	7.0	m.q.	29	210	0
whole milk, 6-oz. pkg.	578	41.5	3.2	44.2	28.5	173	1280	0
whole milk	96	6.9	.5	7.4	4.8	29	213	0
Tybo (*Dorman's* 45%)	98	7.3	.3	7.5	4.7	23	200	0
Tybo, red wax (*Sargento*)	100	7.0	.3	7.0	m.q.	23	200	0
CHEESE, SUBSTITUTE AND IMITATION, 1 oz.:								
American:								
(*Churny* Delicia)	80	6.0	1.0	6.0	m.q.	3	300	0
(*Golden Image*)	90	7.0	2.0	6.0	2.0	5	360	0
(*Weight Watchers* Slices)	50	6.0	2.0	2.0	1.0	5	400	0
(*Weight Watchers* Low Sodium Slices)	50	7.0	2.0	2.0	1.0	5	120	0
and caraway (*Churny* Delicia)	80	6.0	1.0	6.0	m.q.	3	275	(0)
hickory smoke (*Churny* Delicia) ..	80	6.0	0	6.0	m.q.	1	470	0
and hot pepper (*Churny* Delicia)	80	6.0	1.0	6.0	m.q.	3	300	(0)
and salami (*Churny* Delicia)	80	6.0	1.0	6.0	m.q.	3	370	(0)
cheddar:								
imitation (*Frigo*)	90	5.0	1.0	7.0	1.0	0	280	0
imitation (*Sargento*)	90	7.0	<1.0	6.0	m.q.	2	350	0
mild, imitation (*Golden Image*) ...	110	7.0	0	9.0	2.0	5	190	0
sharp (*Weight Watchers* Slices) ...	50	6.0	2.0	2.0	1.0	5	400	0
shredded (*Fisher Ched-O-Mate*) ..	90	6.0	1.0	7.0	m.q.	n.a.	330	0
cheese food:								
(*Cheeztwin*)	90	5.0	3.0	6.0	m.q.	n.a.	400	0
(*Fisher Sandwich-Mate*)	90	5.0	3.0	6.0	m.q.	n.a.	400	0
(*Lite-Line* Low Cholesterol)	90	5.0	2.0	7.0	m.q.	n.a.	430	0

Food and Measure	cal.	prot. (gms)	carbo. (gms)	tot. fat (gms)	sat. fat (gms)	chol. (mgs)	sod. (mgs)	fiber (gms)
colby:								
(*Dorman's* LoChol)	90	7.0	1.0	6.0	1.1	1	140	0
imitation (*Golden Image*)	110	7.0	1.0	9.0	2.0	5	190	0
longhorn style (*Churny* Delicia) ..	80	6.0	1.0	6.0	m.q.	3	550	0
cream cheese, imitation, all flavors								
(*Tofutti Better than Cream*								
Cheese)	80	1.0	1.0	8.0	3.0	0	200	m.q.
creamed cheese (*Weight Watchers*) ..	35	3.0	1.0	2.0	m.q.	n.a.	40	0
mozzarella:								
imitation (*Frigo*)	90	6.0	1.0	7.0	1.0	0	240	0
imitation (*Sargento*)	80	7.0	<1.0	6.0	m.q.	2	310	0
shredded (*Fisher Pizza-Mate*)	90	6.0	1.0	7.0	m.q.	n.a.	310	0
muenster (*Dorman's* LoChol)	100	7.0	1.0	7.0	1.1	1	140	0
(*Nucoa Heart Beat*), 1 oz. or								
1½ slices	50	7.0	2.0	2.0	1.0	0	280	0
Swiss (*Dorman's* LoChol)	100	7.0	1.0	7.0	1.1	1	140	0
Swiss (*Weight Watchers* Slices)	50	6.0	2.0	2.0	1.0	15	400	0
CHEESE BLINTZ, frozen:								
(*King Kold*), 2.5-oz. piece	113	6.0	18.9	1.6	m.q.	m.q.	272	m.q.
(*King Kold* No Salt Added), 2.5-oz.								
piece	96	6.4	18.6	.5	m.q.	m.q.	78	m.q.
CHEESE CURLS, see "Corn								
chips, puffs, and similar snacks"								
CHEESE DANISH, see "Danish								
pastry"								
CHEESE DIP:								
blue (*Kraft* Premium), 2 tbsp.	50	1.0	2.0	4.0	2.0	10	210	0
nacho (*Kraft* Premium), 2 tbsp.	55	2.0	2.0	4.0	2.0	10	200	0
CHEESE ENCHILADA, see								
"Enchilada"								
CHEESE FOOD, 1 oz.								
American:								
cold pack	94	5.6	2.4	6.9	4.4	18	274	0
processed	93	5.6	2.1	7.0	4.4	18	337	0
(*Borden* Singles)	90	5.0	3.0	7.0	m.q.	m.q.	350	0
(*Borden* Slices)	100	6.0	2.0	7.0	m.q.	m.q.	420	0
(*Darigold*)	80	5.0	2.0	6.0	3.8	16	381	0
(*Kraft* Singles)	90	5.0	2.0	7.0	4.0	25	390	0
colored (*Hoffman's*)	100	5.0	3.0	7.0	m.q.	m.q.	490	0
grated (*Kraft*)	130	8.0	8.0	7.0	4.0	25	740	0
sharp (*Borden* Singles)	90	5.0	2.0	7.0	m.q.	m.q.	470	0
white (*Kraft* Singles)	90	5.0	2.0	7.0	4.0	20	400	0
w/bacon:								
(*Cracker Barrel*)	90	5.0	3.0	7.0	4.0	20	280	0
(*Hoffman's* Chees'N Bacon)	90	6.0	3.0	6.0	m.q.	m.q.	540	0
(*Kraft* Cheez'N Bacon)	90	6.0	2.0	7.0	4.0	25	400	0
w/caraway (*Hoffman's* Swisson Rye)	90	6.0	2.0	7.0	m.q.	m.q.	400	(0)
cheddar:								
(*Land O'Lakes* La Chedda)	90	6.0	2.0	7.0	4.0	20	335	0

Food and Measure	cal.	prot. (gms)	carbo. (gms)	tot. fat (gms)	sat. fat (gms)	chol. (mgs)	sod. (mgs)	fiber (gms)
CHEESE FOOD, CHEDDAR *(cont.)*								
bacon w/horseradish, cold pack								
(*Kaukauna* Cup)	100	6.0	3.0	7.0	m.q.	25	250	(0)
extra sharp (*Cracker Barrel*)	90	5.0	3.0	7.0	4.0	20	240	0
nacho, cold pack (*Kaukauna* Cup)	100	6.0	3.0	7.0	m.q.	25	250	0
port wine (*Cracker Barrel*)	100	4.0	3.0	7.0	4.0	20	230	0
sharp (*Cracker Barrel*)	100	4.0	4.0	7.0	4.0	20	230	0
sharp or smokey (*Kaukauna* Lite)	70	5.0	5.0	4.0	m.q.	15	230	0
sharp, extra sharp, or smokey,								
cold pack (*Kaukauna* Cup)	100	6.0	3.0	7.0	m.q.	25	250	0
sharp, cold pack (*Wispride*)	100	5.0	2.0	7.0	m.q.	25	210	0
w/garlic (*Kraft*)	90	5.0	2.0	7.0	4.0	20	370	(0)
horseradish, hearty, cold pack								
(*Kaukauna* Cup)	100	6.0	3.0	7.0	m.q.	25	250	(0)
w/jalapeño pepper:								
(*Hoffman's*)	90	5.0	2.0	7.0	m.q.	m.q.	580	(0)
(*Kraft*)	90	5.0	2.0	7.0	4.0	20	390	(0)
(*Kraft* Singles)	90	5.0	2.0	7.0	4.0	25	450	(0)
(*Land O'Lakes*)	90	6.0	2.0	7.0	4.0	20	360	(0)
hot (*Velveeta* Mexican)	100	6.0	3.0	7.0	4.0	25	430	(0)
mild (*Velveeta* Mexican)	100	6.0	3.0	7.0	4.0	25	420	(0)
Mexican, hot, shredded (*Velveeta*) ..	100	6.0	3.0	7.0	4.0	25	430	(0)
Mexican, mild, shredded (*Velveeta*)	100	6.0	3.0	7.0	4.0	25	420	(0)
Monterey Jack (*Kraft* Singles)	90	5.0	2.0	7.0	4.0	25	390	0
(*Nippy*)	90	5.0	2.0	7.0	4.0	20	380	0
w/onion (*Hoffman's* Chees'N Onion)	100	5.0	3.0	7.0	m.q.	m.q.	490	(0)
onion (*Land O'Lakes*)	90	6.0	2.0	7.0	4.0	15	330	(0)
pepperoni (*Land O'Lakes*)	90	6.0	1.0	7.0	4.0	20	395	0
pimiento (*Kraft* Singles)	90	5.0	2.0	7.0	4.0	25	390	(0)
port wine, cold pack (*Kaukauna*								
Cup)	100	6.0	3.0	7.0	m.q.	25	250	0
port wine, cold pack (*Wispride*)	100	5.0	3.0	7.0	m.q.	25	210	0
salami (*Hoffman's* Chees'N Salami)	90	5.0	3.0	6.0	m.q.	m.q.	560	0
salami (*Land O'Lakes*)	100	5.0	2.0	8.0	5.0	20	400	0
sharp (*Kraft* Singles)	100	6.0	1.0	8.0	5.0	25	400	0
shredded (*Velveeta*)	100	6.0	3.0	7.0	4.0	20	410	0
Swiss:								
processed	92	6.2	1.3	6.8	m.q.	23	440	0
(*Kraft* Singles)	90	6.0	2.0	7.0	4.0	25	440	0
country (*Kaukauna* Lite)	70	6.0	5.0	4.0	m.q.	15	200	0
country, cold pack (*Kaukauna*								
Cup)	100	6.0	3.0	7.0	m.q.	25	250	0
(*Velveeta*)	100	6.0	3.0	7.0	4.0	20	410	0
CHEESE NUGGETS, frozen:								
mozzarella, breaded (*Banquet Cheese*								
Hot Bites), 2.63 oz.	240	14.0	16.0	13.0	m.q.	m.q.	530	m.q.

Food and Measure	cal.	prot. (gms)	carbo. (gms)	tot. fat (gms)	sat. fat (gms)	chol. (mgs)	sod. (mgs)	fiber (gms)
CHEESE-NUT BALL OR LOG,								
1 oz.:								
ball, cheddar, w/almonds								
and bacon (*Kaukauna*)	100	6.0	3.0	7.0	m.q.	25	250	m.q.
port wine (*Cracker Barrel*)	90	5.0	4.0	6.0	3.0	15	260	m.q.
sharp (*Cracker Barrel*)	100	5.0	4.0	7.0	3.0	20	250	m.q.
sharp, w/bell and jalapeño peppers								
(*Kaukauna*)	100	6.0	3.0	7.0	m.q.	25	250	m.q.
ball, green onion flavor w/almonds								
(*Kaukauna*)	100	6.0	3.0	7.0	m.q.	25	250	m.q.
ball or log, port wine w/almonds								
(*Kaukauna*)	100	6.0	3.0	7.0	m.q.	25	250	m.q.
ball or log, sharp cheddar w/almonds								
(*Kaukauna*)	100	6.0	3.0	7.0	m.q.	25	250	m.q.
log:								
cheddar, sharp or smokey,								
w/almonds (*Cracker Barrel*) ...	90	5.0	4.0	6.0	3.0	15	410	m.q.
cheddar, sharp or port wine								
(*Sargento*)	100	6.0	3.0	7.0	m.q.	18	250	m.q.
double, hickory smoke/white sharp								
cheddar (*Kaukauna*)	100	6.0	3.0	7.0	m.q.	25	250	m.q.
double, white sharp cheddar/green								
onion (*Kaukauna*)	100	6.0	3.0	7.0	m.q.	25	250	m.q.
Swiss almond (*Sargento*)	90	6.0	2.0	7.0	m.q.	21	350	m.q.
Swiss almond w/almonds								
(*Kaukauna*)	100	6.0	3.0	7.0	m.q.	25	250	m.q.
CHEESE OMELET, see "Egg								
breakfast"								
CHEESE PASTRY POCKET:								
(*Tastykake*), 3 oz.	325	4.4	40.8	16.7	3.9	11	231	1.3 d
CHEESE PRODUCT, processed,								
1 oz.:								
American flavor:								
(*Alpine Lace*)	90	6.0	2.0	7.0	4.0	20	200	0
(*Borden* Light)	70	6.0	1.0	5.0	m.q.	m.q.	420	0
(*Harvest Moon*)	70	6.0	2.0	4.0	2.0	15	420	0
(*Kraft Light* Singles)	70	6.0	2.0	4.0	3.0	15	420	0
(*Light N' Lively* Singles)	70	6.0	2.0	4.0	3.0	15	420	0
(*Lite-Line*)	50	7.0	1.0	2.0	m.q.	m.q.	410	0
(*Lite-Line* Reduced Sodium)	70	6.0	2.0	4.0	m.q.	m.q.	90	0
(*Lite-Line* Sodium Lite)	70	6.0	2.0	4.0	m.q.	m.q.	200	0
white (*Kraft Light* Singles)	70	6.0	2.0	4.0	2.0	15	410	0
white (*Light n' Lively* Singles) ...	70	6.0	2.0	4.0	2.0	15	410	0
cheddar flavor:								
medium (*Spreadery*)	70	5.0	3.0	4.0	2.0	15	250	0
mild (*Lite-Line*)	50	7.0	1.0	2.0	m.q.	m.q.	380	0
sharp (*Kraft Light*)	70	6.0	2.0	4.0	2.0	15	380	0
sharp (*Light N' Lively* Singles) ...	70	6.0	2.0	4.0	2.0	15	380	0

Food and Measure	cal.	prot. (gms)	carbo. (gms)	tot. fat (gms)	sat. fat (gms)	chol. (mgs)	sod. (mgs)	fiber (gms)
CHEESE PRODUCT, CHEDDAR FLAVOR *(cont.)*								
sharp *(Lite-Line)*	50	7.0	1.0	2.0	m.q.	m.q.	440	0
sharp *(Spreadery)*	70	5.0	3.0	4.0	2.0	15	240	0
Vermont white *(Spreadery)*	70	5.0	3.0	4.0	2.0	15	230	0
cream cheese *(Philadelphia Brand*								
Light)	60	3.0	2.0	5.0	3.0	10	160	0
(Kraft Free Singles)	45	7.0	4.0	0	0	5	420	0
Mexican, mild, w/jalapeños								
(Spreadery)	70	5.0	3.0	4.0	3.0	15	260	(0)
mozzarella flavor *(Lite-Line)*	50	7.0	1.0	2.0	m.q.	m.q.	340	0
Muenster flavor *(Lite-Line)*	50	7.0	1.0	2.0	m.q.	m.q.	450	0
nacho *(Spreadery)*	70	5.0	3.0	4.0	2.0	15	240	0
Neufchatel:								
garlic and herb *(Spreadery)*	70	2.0	1.0	6.0	4.0	20	140	(0)
onion, French *(Spreadery)*	70	2.0	2.0	6.0	4.0	20	135	(0)
ranch, classic *(Spreadery)*	70	2.0	1.0	7.0	4.0	20	190	(0)
w/strawberries *(Spreadery)*	70	2.0	m.q.	5.0	3.0	15	270	(0)
vegetable, garden *(Spreadery)* ...	70	2.0	2.0	6.0	3.0	20	220	(0)
port wine *(Spreadery)*	70	5.0	3.0	4.0	2.0	15	250	0
sandwich slices *(Lunch Wagon)*	90	5.0	2.0	7.0	2.0	5	370	0
Swiss flavor:								
(Kraft Light)	70	6.0	2.0	3.0	2.0	15	350	0
(Light N' Lively Singles)	70	6.0	2.0	3.0	2.0	15	350	0
(Lite-Line)	50	7.0	1.0	2.0	m.q.	m.q.	380	0
(Velveeta Light)	70	6.0	3.0	4.0	2.0	15	470	0
CHEESE PUFFS, see "Corn chips,								
puffs, and similar snacks"								
CHEESE SAUCE (see also "Welsh								
rarebit"):								
aged *(White House)*, 3.5 oz.	213	4.0	10.0	18.0	m.q.	m.q.	810	0
cheddar:								
(Lucky Leaf/Musselman's), 4 oz.	220	3.0	12.0	18.0	m.q.	m.q.	1000	0
aged *(Lucky Leaf/Musselman's)*,								
4 oz.	240	5.0	11.0	20.0	m.q.	m.q.	920	0
aged, mild *(Lucky Leaf/*								
Musselman's), 4 oz.	200	5.0	9.0	18.0	m.q.	m.q.	790	0
aged, sharp *(Lucky Leaf/*								
Musselman's), 4 oz.	230	9.0	6.0	17.0	m.q.	m.q.	850	0
four cheese, refrigerated *(Contadina*								
Fresh), 6 oz.	470	12.0	8.0	45.0	m.q.	147	500	0
jalapeño *(White House)*, 3.5 oz.	193	3.0	10.0	16.0	m.q.	m.q.	890	(0)
nacho:								
(Kaukauna), 1 oz.	80	3.0	4.0	6.0	m.q.	8	330	0
(Lucky Leaf/Musselman's), 4 oz.	220	4.0	11.0	18.0	m.q.	m.q.	1010	0
(White House), 3.5 oz.	193	3.0	10.0	16.0	m.q.	m.q.	890	0

Food and Measure	cal.	prot. (gms)	carbo. (gms)	tot. fat (gms)	sat. fat (gms)	chol. (mgs)	sod. (mgs)	fiber (gms)
CHEESE SAUCE MIX:								
1.2-oz. pkt.	158	8.0	11.9	9.0	4.2	18	1447	<.1 c
½ cup[1]	154	8.0	11.6	8.6	4.7	27	783	<.1 c
(French's), ¼ cup[1]	80	3.0	7.0	4.0	m.q.	m.q.	430	n.a.
(McCormick/Schilling), ¼ pkg.	35	2.0	3.5	1.5	n.a.	n.a.	477	n.a.
(Tone's), 1 tsp.	9	.4	1.9	.3	n.a.	n.a.	228	n.a.
nacho (McCormick/Schilling), ¼ pkg.	42	3.0	4.5	1.5	n.a.	n.a.	409	n.a.
CHEESE SPREAD, 1 oz., except as noted:								
American, processed:								
5-oz. jar	412	23.3	12.4	30.2	18.9	78	1910	0
1 oz.	82	4.7	2.5	6.0	3.8	16	381	0
1″ cube	51	2.9	1.5	3.7	2.3	10	235	0
(Kraft)	80	4.0	2.0	6.0	3.0	15	470	0
w/pimiento (Sargento Cracker Snacks)	110	6.0	.5	9.0	m.q.	27	410	(0)
sharp (Sargento Cracker Snacks)	110	6.0	.5	9.0	m.q.	27	410	0
w/bacon (Kraft)	80	5.0	1.0	7.0	4.0	20	560	0
w/bacon (Squeez-A-Snak)	80	5.0	1.0	7.0	4.0	20	500	0
blue (Roka)	70	3.0	2.0	6.0	4.0	20	270	0
brick (Sargento Cracker Snacks) . . .	100	6.0	1.0	9.0	m.q.	25	430	0
cheddar, sharp (Weight Watchers Cup), 1 oz. or 2 tbsp.	70	4.0	7.0	3.0	2.0	10	190	0
(Cheez Whiz)	80	4.0	2.0	6.0	3.0	20	470	0
cream cheese, see "Cheese"								
garlic flavor (Squeez-A-Snak)	80	5.0	1.0	7.0	4.0	20	430	(0)
hickory smoke flavor (Squeez-A-Snak)	80	5.0	1.0	7.0	4.0	20	440	0
w/jalapeño pepper:								
(Cheez Whiz)	80	4.0	2.0	6.0	4.0	20	430	(0)
(Kraft)	70	2.0	3.0	5.0	3.0	15	95	(0)
(Squeez-A-Snak)	80	5.0	1.0	6.0	4.0	20	510	(0)
loaf (Kraft)	80	5.0	2.0	6.0	4.0	20	470	(0)
(Land O'Lakes Golden Velvet)	80	5.0	2.0	6.0	4.0	15	380	0
(Laughing Cow Cheezbits), ⅙ oz. . . .	13	.8	.1	1.0	m.q.	3	55	0
Limburger (Mohawk Valley)	70	4.0	0	6.0	3.0	20	420	0
Mexican:								
hot (Velveeta)	80	5.0	3.0	6.0	3.0	20	520	(0)
mild (Cheez Whiz)	80	4.0	2.0	6.0	4.0	20	430	(0)
mild (Velveeta)	80	5.0	3.0	6.0	3.0	20	440	(0)
(Micro Melt)	80	4.0	2.0	6.0	m.q.	15	380	0
Neufchâtel, see "Cheese"								
olives and pimiento (Kraft)	60	2.0	2.0	5.0	3.0	15	160	(0)
pimiento (Kraft)	70	2.0	3.0	5.0	3.0	15	120	(0)
pimiento (Velveeta)	80	5.0	3.0	6.0	3.0	20	400	(0)
pineapple (Kraft)	70	2.0	4.0	5.0	3.0	15	75	(0)

1. *Prepared with whole milk.*

Food and Measure	cal.	prot. (gms)	carbo. (gms)	tot. fat (gms)	sat. fat (gms)	chol. (mgs)	sod. (mgs)	fiber (gms)
CHEESE SPREAD *(cont.)*								
port wine (*Weight Watchers* Cup),								
1 oz. or 2 tbsp.	70	4.0	7.0	3.0	2.0	10	190	0
sharp (*Old English*)	80	5.0	1.0	7.0	4.0	20	480	0
sharp (*Squeez-A-Snak*)	80	5.0	1.0	7.0	4.0	20	440	0
Swiss (*Sargento* Cracker Snacks) ...	100	7.0	1.0	7.0	m.q.	24	390	0
(*Velveeta*)	80	5.0	3.0	6.0	4.0	20	430	0
(*Velveeta* Slices)	90	5.0	3.0	6.0	4.0	20	400	0
CHEESE SNACK STICKS:								
cheddar (*Flavor Tree*), ¼ cup	129	2.7	11.9	8.1	m.q.	n.a.	335	.1 c
CHEESE STICKS, breaded, frozen:								
cheddar (*Farm Rich*), 3 oz.	300	10.9	19.0	21.0	m.q.	m.q.	740	m.q.
hot pepper (*Farm Rich*), 3 oz.	260	8.0	20.0	17.0	m.q.	m.q.	700	m.q.
mozzarella (*Farm Rich*), 3 oz.	240	10.0	19.0	13.0	m.q.	m.q.	570	m.q.
provolone (*Farm Rich*), 3 oz.	270	10.0	22.0	16.0 ·	m.q.	m.q.	820	m.q.
CHEESE TOPPING (see also "Cheese sauce"):								
cheddar, w/bacon (*Tone's*), 1 tsp. ...	10	.5	.7	1.0	.5	1	81	0
CHEESEBURGER, see "Beef entree, frozen"								
CHEESECAKE, see "Cake"								
CHEESEFURTER, see "Frankfurter, cheese"								
CHERIMOYA:								
untrimmed, 1 lb.	277	3.8	70.8	1.2	n.a.	0	n.a.	6.5 c
trimmed, 1 oz.	27	.4	6.8	.1	(0)	0	n.a.	.6 c
1 medium, approx. 1.9 lb.	515	7.1	131.3	2.2	n.a.	0	n.a.	12.0 c
CHERRY:								
sour, red:								
untrimmed, 1 lb.	203	4.1	49.7	1.2	.3	0	13	.8 c
trimmed:								
1 oz.	14	.3	3.5	.1	<.1	0	1	.2 c
½ cup	39	.8	9.4	.2	.1	0	3	.2 c
w/pits, ½ cup	26	.5	6.3	.2	<.1	0	2	.1 c
sweet:								
untrimmed, 1 lb.	293	4.9	67.6	3.9	1.0	0	2	6.3 d
trimmed, 1 oz.	20	.3	4.7	.3	.1	0	tr.	.4 d
trimmed, ½ cup	52	.9	12.0	.7	.2	0	1	1.1 d
10 medium, approx. 2.6 oz.	49	.8	11.3	.7	.1	0	tr.	1.0 d
CHERRY, CANNED:								
sour, red:								
(*A&P*), ½ cup	50	<1.0	12.0	<1.0	(0)	0	5	m.q.
pitted:								
(*White House*), 3.5 oz.	43	0	11.0	0	0	0	5	m.q.
tart (*Lucky Leaf/Musselman's*), 4 oz.	50	1.0	11.0	0	0	0	0	m.q.
in water (*Stokely*), ½ cup	45	1.0	10.0	0	0	0	15	m.q.

Food and Measure	cal.	prot. (gms)	carbo. (gms)	tot. fat (gms)	sat. fat (gms)	chol. (mgs)	sod. (mgs)	fiber (gms)
in water, 4 oz.	41	.9	10.0	.1	<.1	0	8	.1 c
in water, ½ cup	43	.9	10.9	.1	<.1	0	9	.1 c
in light syrup, 4 oz.	85	.8	21.9	.1	<.1	0	8	.1 c
in light syrup, ½ cup	94	.9	24.3	.1	<.1	0	9	.1 c
in heavy syrup, 4 oz.	103	.8	26.4	.1	<.1	0	8	.1 c
in heavy syrup, ½ cup	116	.9	29.8	.1	<.1	0	9	.1 c
in extra heavy syrup, 4 oz.	129	.8	33.1	.1	<.1	0	8	.1 c
in extra heavy syrup, ½ cup	148	.9	38.0	.1	<.1	0	9	.1 c
sweet:								
in water, 4 oz.	52	.9	13.3	.1	<.1	0	1	.2 c
in water, ½ cup	57	1.0	14.6	.2	<.1	0	2	.3 c
in juice, 4 oz.	61	1.0	15.7	<.1	tr.	0	3	.3 d
in juice, ½ cup	68	1.1	17.3	<.1	tr.	0	3	.3 d
in light syrup, 4 oz.	76	.7	19.6	.2	<.1	0	3	.4 c
in light syrup, ½ cup	85	.8	21.8	.2	<.1	0	3	.4 c
in heavy syrup, 4 oz.	94	.7	24.1	.2	<.1	0	3	.4 c
in heavy syrup, ½ cup	107	.8	27.4	.2	<.1	0	3	.4 c
in extra heavy syrup, 4 oz.	116	.7	29.7	.2	<.1	0	3	.4 c
in extra heavy syrup, ½ cup	133	.8	34.1	.2	<.1	0	3	.4 c
dark, w/pits (*Del Monte*), ½ cup ..	90	0	23.0	0	0	0	<10	m.q.
dark, pitted (*Del Monte*), ½ cup ..	90	0	24.0	0	0	0	<10	m.q.
light, w/pits (*Del Monte*), ½ cup ..	100	0	26.0	0	0	0	<10	m.q.
packaged (*Mott's* Cherry Fruit								
Pak), 3.75 oz.	72	0	17.0	0	0	0	8	m.q.
CHERRY, FROZEN:								
sour, red, unsweetened:								
18-oz. pkg.	237	4.7	56.2	2.2	.5	0	4	1.5 c
4 oz.	52	1.0	12.5	.5	.1	0	1	.3 c
½ cup	36	.7	8.5	.3	.1	0	1	.2 c
sweet, sweetened:								
10-oz. pkg.	254	3.3	63.5	.4	.1	0	3	1.1 c
4 oz.	101	1.3	25.4	.1	<.1	0	1	.5 c
½ cup	116	1.5	29.0	.2	<.1	0	2	.5 c
(*Lucky Leaf*), 4 oz.	130	1.0	31.0	0	0	0	150	m.q.
CHERRY, MARASCHINO, in jars:								
w/liquid, 1 oz.	33	.1	8.3	.1	0	0	n.a.	.1 c
CHERRY COBBLER, see								
"Cobbler"								
CHERRY DRINK MIX[1], 8 fl. oz.,								
except as noted:								
(*Finast*)	80	0	21.0	0	0	0	15	(0)
(*Kool-Aid* Presweetened)	80	0	20.0	0	0	0	0	(0)
(*Kool-Aid* Sugar Free)	4	0	0	0	0	0	0	(0)
(*Pathmark* No Frills)	90	0	22.0	0	0	0	65	(0)
(*Wylers* Fruit Slush), 4 fl. oz.	157	0	39.3	0	0	0	10	(0)
regular or black (*Kool-Aid*)	100	0	25.0	0	0	0	0	(0)

1. *Prepared according to package directions.*

Food and Measure	cal.	prot. (gms)	carbo. (gms)	tot. fat (gms)	sat. fat (gms)	chol. (mgs)	sod. (mgs)	fiber (gms)
CHERRY FRUIT CONCENTRATE:								
black (*Hain*), 1 oz. or 2 tbsp.	70	0	18.0	0	0	0	30	n.a.
CHERRY FRUIT ROLL, see "Fruit snack"								
CHERRY JUICE:								
black (*Smucker's* Naturally 100%), 8 fl. oz.	130	0	31.0	0	0	0	10	m.q.
blend (*Dole Pure & Light* Mountain Cherry), 6 fl. oz.	87	.2	22.0	.1	(0)	0	8	m.q.
blend (*Libby's Juicy Juice*), 6 fl. oz. ..	90	0	22.0	0	0	0	5	m.q.
CHERRY JUICE COCKTAIL:								
(*Welch's Orchard*), 6 fl. oz.	180	0	45.0	0	0	0	10	(0)
CHERRY JUICE DRINK:								
(*Hi-C*), 8.45 fl. oz.	141	.2	34.8	.1	(0)	0	24	(0)
(*Hi-C*), 6 fl. oz.	100	.1	24.7	.1	(0)	0	17	(0)
(*Kool-Aid Koolers*), 8.45 fl. oz.	140	0	38.0	0	0	0	10	(0)
(*Tang* Fruit Box), 8.45 fl. oz.	120	0	32.0	0	0	0	10	(0)
CHERRY PASTRY POCKET:								
(*Tastykake*), 3 oz.	325	4.4	40.8	16.7	3.9	11	231	1.3 d
CHERRY PIE, see "Pie"								
CHERRY PIE FILLING, see "Pie filling"								
CHERVIL, dried:								
1 oz.	67	6.6	13.9	1.1	n.a.	0	24	3.2 c
1 tbsp.	4	.4	.9	.1	(0)	0	2	.2 c
1 tsp.	1	.1	.3	<.1	(0)	0	tr.	.1 c
(*Tone's*), 1 tsp.	1	.1	.3	<.1	(0)	0	2	.1 d
CHESTNUT, CHINESE[1]:								
raw, in shell, 1 lb.	852	16.0	187.0	4.2	.6	0	13	6.2 c
raw, 1 oz.	64	1.2	13.9	.3	<.1	0	1	.5 c
boiled or steamed, 1 oz.	44	.8	9.6	.2	<.1	0	1	.3 c
dried, 1 oz.	103	1.9	22.7	.5	.1	0	2	.8 c
roasted, 1 oz.	68	1.3	14.9	.3	.1	0	1	.5 c
CHESTNUT, EUROPEAN[1]:								
raw:								
in shell, 1 lb.	714	8.1	152.8	7.6	1.4	0	9	33.3 d
unpeeled, 1 oz.	60	.7	12.9	.6	.1	0	1	2.8 d
unpeeled, 1 cup, approx. 13 kernels	308	3.5	66.0	3.3	.6	0	4	14.5 d
peeled, 1 oz.	56	.5	12.5	.4	.1	0	1	.3 c
boiled or steamed, 1 oz.	37	.8	7.9	.4	.1	0	8	.2 c
dried:								
in shell, 1 lb.	1357	23.2	280.5	16.1	3.0	0	135	19.8 c
unpeeled, 1 oz.	106	1.8	22.0	1.3	.2	0	11	1.6 c
peeled, 1 oz.	105	1.4	22.3	1.1	.2	0	11	1.4 c

1. *Shelled, except as noted.*

Food and Measure	cal.	prot. (gms)	carbo. (gms)	tot. fat (gms)	sat. fat (gms)	chol. (mgs)	sod. (mgs)	fiber (gms)
roasted:								
in shell, 1 lb.	700	9.1	151.3	6.3	1.2	0	6	33.4 d
peeled, 1 oz.	70	.9	15.0	.6	.1	0	1	3.3 d
peeled, 1 cup, approx. 17 kernels	350	4.3	75.7	3.2	.6	0	3	16.7 d
CHESTNUT, ITALIAN, see								
"Chestnut, European"								
CHESTNUT, JAPANESE[1]:								
raw, in shell, 1 lb.	462	6.7	104.5	1.6	.2	0	43	2.9 c
raw, 1 oz.	44	.6	9.9	.2	<.1	0	4	.3 c
boiled or steamed, 1 oz.	16	.2	3.6	.1	<.1	0	1	.1 c
dried:								
in shell, 1 lb.	1078	15.7	243.7	3.7	.5	0	101	6.8 c
1 oz.	102	1.5	23.1	.4	.1	0	10	.6 c
1 cup	558	8.1	126.2	1.9	.3	0	52	3.5 c
roasted, 1 oz.	57	.8	12.8	.2	<.1	0	m.q.	.3 c
CHESTNUT, SWEET, see								
"Chestnut, European"								
CHEWING GUM, see "Candy"								
CHIA SEEDS, dried:								
1 oz.	134	4.7	13.6	7.5	3.0	0	m.q.	7.2 c
CHIANTI, see "Wine"								
CHICKEN, BROILER OR								
FRYER[2]:								
raw:								
meat w/skin, ½ chicken, 1 lb.,								
yield from 1.5 lbs. w/bone	990	85.6	0	69.3	19.2	347	321	0
meat w/skin, 1 oz.	61	5.3	0	4.3	1.2	21	20	0
meat only, 1 oz.	34	6.1	0	.9	.2	20	22	0
dark meat w/skin, 1 oz.	67	4.7	0	5.2	1.5	23	21	0
dark meat only, 1 oz.	35	5.7	0	1.2	.3	23	24	0
light meat w/skin, 1 oz.	53	5.7	0	3.1	.9	19	18	0
light meat only, 1 oz.	32	6.6	0	.5	.1	16	19	0
back, meat w/skin, 1 oz.	90	4.0	0	8.1	2.4	22	18	0
back, meat only, 1 oz.	39	5.5	0	1.7	.4	23	23	0
breast, meat w/skin, 1 oz.	49	5.9	0	2.6	.8	18	18	0
breast, meat only, 1 oz.	31	6.5	0	.4	.1	16	18	0
drumstick, meat w/skin, 1 oz. ...	46	5.5	0	2.5	.7	23	24	0
drumstick, meat only, 1 oz.	34	5.8	0	1.0	.2	22	25	0
leg, meat w/skin, 1 oz.	53	5.1	0	3.4	1.0	24	22	0
leg, meat only, 1 oz.	34	5.7	0	1.1	.3	23	24	0
neck, meat w/skin, 1 oz.	84	4.0	0	7.4	2.1	28	18	0
neck, meat only, 1 oz.	44	5.0	0	2.5	.6	24	23	0
thigh, meat w/skin, 1 oz.	60	4.9	0	4.3	1.2	24	22	0
thigh, meat only, 1 oz.	34	5.6	0	1.1	.3	24	24	0
wing, meat w/skin, 1 oz.	63	5.2	0	4.5	1.3	22	21	0
wing, meat only, 1 oz.	36	6.2	0	1.0	.3	16	23	0

1. *Shelled, except as noted.*
2. *Cooked poultry is prepared without added ingredients, except as noted.*

Food and Measure	cal.	prot. (gms)	carbo. (gms)	tot. fat (gms)	sat. fat (gms)	chol. (mgs)	sod. (mgs)	fiber (gms)
CHICKEN, BROILER OR FRYER *(cont.)*								
fried, batter dipped[1], meat w/skin:								
4 oz.	328	25.6	10.7	19.7	5.2	99	331	<.1 c
dark meat, 4 oz.	338	24.8	10.6	21.1	5.6	101	335	<.1 c
light meat, 4 oz.	312	26.6	10.7	17.4	4.7	94	324	<.1 c
back, 4 oz.	375	24.9	11.6	24.8	6.6	100	359	<.1 c
breast, 4 oz.	295	28.2	10.2	15.0	4.0	96	312	<.1 c
breast, 4.9 oz., yield from								
½ breast, 11.3 oz. w/bone	364	34.8	12.6	18.5	4.9	119	385	.1 c
drumstick, 4 oz.	304	24.9	9.4	17.9	4.7	98	305	<.1 c
drumstick, 2.5 oz., yield from								
3.4 oz.-drumstick w/bone	193	15.8	6.0	11.3	3.0	62	194	<.1 c
leg, 4 oz.	310	24.7	9.9	18.3	4.9	102	316	<.1 c
leg, 5.6 oz., yield from 7.2-oz. leg								
w/bone	431	34.4	13.8	25.6	6.8	142	442	.1 c
neck, 4 oz.	374	22.5	9.9	26.7	7.1	103	313	<.1 c
neck, 1.8 oz., yield from 2.5-oz.								
neck w/bone	172	10.3	4.5	12.2	3.2	47	143	<.1 c
thigh, 4 oz.	314	24.5	10.3	18.7	5.0	105	327	<.1 c
thigh, 3 oz., yield from 3.7-oz.								
thigh w/bone	238	18.6	7.8	14.2	3.8	80	248	<.1 c
wing, 4 oz.	367	22.5	12.4	24.7	6.6	90	363	<.1 c
wing, 1.7 oz., yield from 2.8-oz.								
wing w/bone	159	9.7	5.4	10.7	2.9	39	157	<.1 c
fried, batter dipped[1], skin only,								
1 oz.	112	2.9	6.6	8.2	2.2	21	165	<.1 c
fried, flour coated, meat w/skin:								
½ chicken, 11.1 oz., yield from								
15.6 oz. w/bone	844	89.7	9.9	46.8	12.7	283	264	<.1 c
4 oz.	305	32.4	3.6	16.9	4.6	102	95	<.1 c
dark meat, 4 oz.	323	30.9	4.6	19.2	5.2	104	101	<.1 c
light meat, 4 oz.	279	34.5	2.1	13.7	3.8	99	87	<.1 c
back, 4 oz.	375	31.5	7.4	23.5	6.4	101	102	<.1 c
breast, 4 oz.	252	36.1	1.9	10.1	2.8	101	86	<.1 c
breast, 3.5 oz., yield from								
½ breast, 8.3 oz. w/bone	218	31.2	1.6	8.7	2.4	88	75	<.1 c
drumstick, 4 oz.	278	30.6	1.8	15.6	4.2	102	101	<.1 c
drumstick, 1.7 oz., yield from								
2.6-oz. drumstick, w/bone	120	13.2	.8	6.7	1.8	44	44	0
leg, approx. 4 oz., yield from								
5.5-oz. leg w/bone	285	30.1	2.8	16.2	4.4	105	99	<.1 c
neck, 4 oz.	376	27.2	4.8	26.8	7.2	107	93	<.1 c
neck, 1.3 oz., yield from 1.8-oz.								
neck w/bone	119	8.6	1.5	8.5	2.3	34	29	<.1 c
thigh, 4 oz.	297	30.3	3.6	17.0	4.6	110	100	<.1 c
thigh, 2.2 oz., yield from 2.9-oz.								
thigh w/bone	162	16.6	2.0	9.3	2.5	60	55	<.1 c

1. *Batter made from enriched wheat flour, egg yolk, nonfat dry milk, salt, and water.*

Food and Measure	cal.	prot. (gms)	carbo. (gms)	tot. fat (gms)	sat. fat (gms)	chol. (mgs)	sod. (mgs)	fiber (gms)
wing, 4 oz.	364	29.6	2.7	25.1	6.9	92	87	<.1 c
wing, 1.1 oz., yield from 2.2-oz.								
wing w/bone	103	8.4	.8	7.1	1.9	26	25	0
fried, flour coated, skin only, 1 oz.	142	5.4	2.6	12.1	3.3	21	15	<.1 c
roasted:								
meat w/skin, ½ chicken, 10.5 oz.,								
yield from 15.8 oz. w/bone	715	81.6	0	40.7	11.3	263	244	0
meat, w/skin, 4 oz.	271	31.0	0	15.4	4.3	100	93	0
meat only, 4 oz.	215	32.8	0	8.4	2.3	101	98	0
meat only, chopped or diced,								
1 cup not packed	266	40.5	0	10.4	2.9	125	120	0
skin only, 1 oz.	129	5.8	0	11.5	3.2	24	18	0
dark meat:								
w/skin, 4 oz.	287	29.4	0	17.9	5.0	103	99	0
meat only, 4 oz.	232	31.0	0	11.0	3.0	105	105	0
meat only, chopped or diced,								
1 cup not packed	286	38.3	0	13.6	3.7	130	130	0
light meat:								
w/skin, 4 oz.	252	32.9	0	12.3	3.5	95	85	0
meat only, 4 oz.	196	35.1	0	5.1	1.4	96	87	0
meat only, chopped or diced,								
1 cup not packed	242	43.3	0	6.3	1.8	118	108	0
back, meat w/skin, 4 oz.	340	29.4	0	23.8	6.6	100	99	0
back, meat only, 4 oz.	271	32.0	0	14.9	4.1	102	109	0
breast:								
meat w/skin, ½ breast, 3.5 oz.,								
yield from 8.5 oz. w/bone ...	193	29.2	0	7.6	2.2	83	69	0
meat w/skin, 4 oz.	223	33.8	0	8.8	2.5	95	81	0
meat only, ½ breast, 3 oz.,								
yield from 8.5 oz. w/bone								
and skin	142	26.7	0	3.1	.9	73	63	0
meat only, 4 oz.	187	35.2	0	4.0	1.1	96	84	0
drumstick:								
meat w/skin, 1 drumstick,								
1.8 oz., yield from 2.9 oz.								
w/bone	112	14.1	0	5.8	1.6	48	47	0
meat w/skin, 4 oz.	245	30.7	0	12.6	3.5	103	102	0
meat only, 1 drumstick, 1.6 oz.,								
yield from 2.9 oz. w/bone								
and skin	76	12.5	0	2.5	.7	41	42	0
meat only, 4 oz.	195	32.1	0	6.4	1.7	105	108	0
leg:								
meat w/skin, 1 leg, 4 oz., yield								
from 5.7 oz. w/bone	265	29.6	0	15.4	4.2	105	99	0
meat only, 1 leg, 3.4 oz., yield								
from 5.7 oz. w/bone and								
skin	182	25.7	0	8.0	2.2	89	87	0

Food and Measure	cal.	prot. (gms)	carbo. (gms)	tot. fat (gms)	sat. fat (gms)	chol. (mgs)	sod. (mgs)	fiber (gms)
CHICKEN, BROILER OR FRYER, ROASTED, LEG *(cont.)*								
meat only, 4 oz.	217	30.7	0	9.6	2.6	107	103	0
thigh:								
meat w/skin, 1 thigh, 2.2 oz.,								
yield from 2.9 oz. w/bone ...	153	15.5	0	9.6	2.7	58	52	0
meat w/skin, 4 oz.	280	28.4	0	17.6	4.9	105	95	0
meat only, 1 thigh, 1.8 oz.,								
yield from 2.9 oz. w/bone								
and skin	109	13.5	0	5.7	1.6	49	46	0
meat only, 4 oz.	237	29.4	0	12.3	3.4	108	100	0
wing:								
meat w/skin, 1 wing, 1.2 oz.,								
yield from 2.3 oz. w/bone ...	99	9.1	0	6.6	1.9	29	28	0
meat w/skin, 4 oz.	329	30.5	0	22.1	6.2	95	93	0
meat only, 1 wing, .7 oz., yield								
from 2.3 oz. w/bone and								
skin	43	6.4	0	1.7	.5	18	19	0
meat only, 4 oz.	230	34.5	0	9.2	2.6	96	104	0
simmered, neck:								
meat w/skin, 1 neck, 1.3 oz., yield								
from 2 oz. w/bone	94	7.5	0	6.9	1.9	27	20	0
meat w/skin, 4 oz.	280	22.2	0	20.5	5.7	79	59	0
meat only, 1 neck, .6 oz., yield								
from 2 oz. w/bone and skin	32	4.4	0	1.5	.4	14	12	0
meat only, 4 oz.	203	27.9	0	9.3	2.4	90	73	0
stewed:								
meat with skin, ½ chicken,								
11.8 oz., yield from 1.1 lbs.								
w/bone	730	82.4	0	42.0	11.7	262	224	0
meat w/skin, 4 oz.	248	28.0	0	14.2	4.0	88	76	0
meat only, 4 oz.	201	30.9	0	7.6	2.1	94	79	0
meat only, chopped or diced,								
1 cup not packed	248	38.2	0	9.4	2.6	116	98	0
skin only, 1 oz.	103	4.3	0	9.4	2.6	18	16	0
dark meat:								
w/skin, 4 oz.	264	26.6	0	16.6	4.6	93	79	0
meat only, 4 oz.	218	29.4	0	10.2	2.8	100	84	0
meat only, chopped or diced,								
1 cup not packed	269	36.4	0	12.6	3.4	123	104	0
light meat:								
w/skin, 4 oz.	228	29.6	0	11.3	3.2	84	71	0
meat only, 4 oz.	180	32.7	0	4.5	1.3	87	74	0
meat only, chopped or diced,								
1 cup not packed	223	40.4	0	5.6	1.6	107	91	0
back, meat w/skin, 4 oz.	293	25.2	0	20.6	5.7	88	73	0
back, meat only, 4 oz.	237	28.7	0	12.7	3.4	96	76	0
breast:								
meat w/skin, ½ breast, 3.9 oz.,								
yield from 9.5 oz. w/bone ...	202	30.1	0	8.2	2.3	83	68	0

Food and Measure	cal.	prot. (gms)	carbo. (gms)	tot. fat (gms)	sat. fat (gms)	chol. (mgs)	sod. (mgs)	fiber (gms)
meat w/skin, 4 oz.	209	31.1	0	8.4	2.4	85	70	0
meat only, ½ breast, 3.4 oz., yield from 9.5 oz. w/bone and skin	144	27.5	0	2.9	.8	73	59	0
meat only, 4 oz.	171	32.9	0	3.4	1.0	87	71	0
drumstick:								
meat w/skin, 1 drumstick, 2 oz., yield from 3.1 oz. w/bone ...	116	14.4	0	6.1	1.7	48	43	0
meat w/skin, 4 oz.	231	28.7	0	12.1	3.3	94	86	0
meat only, 1.6 oz., yield from 3.1-oz. whole drumstick	78	12.7	0	2.6	.7	40	37	0
meat only, 4 oz.	192	31.2	0	6.5	1.7	100	91	0
leg:								
meat w/skin, 1 leg, 4.4 oz., yield from 6.3 oz. w/bone ...	275	30.2	0	16.2	4.5	105	92	0
meat w/skin, 4 oz.	249	27.4	0	14.7	4.0	95	83	0
meat, 1 leg, 3.6 oz., yield from 6.3 oz. w/bone and skin	187	26.5	0	8.1	2.2	90	78	0
meat only, 4 oz.	210	29.8	0	9.1	2.5	101	88	0
thigh:								
meat w/skin, 1 thigh, 2.4 oz., yield from 3.2 oz. w/bone ...	158	15.8	0	10.0	2.8	57	49	0
meat w/skin, 4 oz.	263	26.4	0	16.7	4.7	95	81	0
meat only, 1 thigh, 1.9 oz., yield from 3.2 oz. w/bone and skin	107	13.8	0	5.4	1.5	49	41	0
meat only, 4 oz.	221	28.4	0	11.1	3.1	102	85	0
wing:								
meat w/skin, 1 wing, 1.4 oz., yield from 2.7 oz. w/bone ...	100	9.1	0	6.7	1.9	28	27	0
meat w/skin, 4 oz.	282	25.8	0	19.1	5.3	79	76	0
meat only, 1 wing, .8 oz., yield from 2.7 oz. w/bone and skin	43	6.5	0	1.7	.5	18	18	0
meat only, 4 oz.	205	30.8	0	8.1	2.3	84	83	0
CHICKEN, CAPON[1]:								
raw:								
meat w/skin:								
½ capon, 2.1 lbs., yield from 2.9 lbs. w/bone	2257	180.9	0	164.6	47.7	720	431	0
1 lb.	1061	85.1	0	77.4	22.5	340	204	0
1 oz.	66	5.3	0	4.8	1.4	21	13	0
roasted, meat w/skin, ½ capon, 1.4 lbs., yield from 2 lbs. w/bone ..	1457	184.5	0	74.2	20.8	549	313	0
roasted, meat w/skin, 4 oz.	260	32.8	0	13.2	3.7	98	56	0

1. *Cooked poultry is prepared without added ingredients.*

Food and Measure	cal.	prot. (gms)	carbo. (gms)	tot. fat (gms)	sat. fat (gms)	chol. (mgs)	sod. (mgs)	fiber (gms)
CHICKEN, ROASTER[1]:								
raw:								
meat w/skin:								
½ chicken, 1.5 lbs., yield from								
2 lbs. w/bone	1444	114.5	0	105.9	30.2	484	457	0
1 lb.	980	77.7	0	71.9	20.5	331	308	0
1 oz.	61	4.9	0	4.5	1.3	21	19	0
meat only, 1 lb.	503	92.2	0	12.2	3.0	295	340	0
meat only, 1 oz.	31	5.8	0	.8	.2	18	21	0
dark meat only, 1 lb.	513	85.0	0	16.4	4.2	327	431	0
dark meat only, 1 oz.	32	5.3	0	1.0	.3	20	27	0
light meat only, 1 lb.	494	100.7	0	7.4	1.7	259	231	0
light meat only, 1 oz.	31	6.3	0	.5	.1	16	14	0
roasted:								
meat w/skin, ½ chicken, 1 lb.,								
yield from 1.5 lbs. w/bone	1071	115.0	0	64.3	17.9	365	349	0
meat w/skin, 4 oz.	253	27.2	0	15.2	4.2	86	83	0
meat only, 4 oz.	189	28.4	0	7.5	2.1	85	85	0
meat only, chopped or diced,								
1 cup not packed	233	35.0	0	9.3	2.5	104	105	0
dark meat only, 4 oz.	202	26.4	0	9.9	2.8	85	108	0
dark meat only, chopped or diced,								
1 cup not packed	250	32.6	0	12.3	3.4	104	133	0
light meat only, 4 oz.	174	30.8	0	4.6	1.2	85	58	0
light meat only, chopped or diced,								
1 cup not packed	214	38.0	0	5.7	1.5	105	71	0
CHICKEN, STEWING[1]:								
raw:								
meat w/skin:								
½ chicken, 14 oz., yield from								
1.25 lbs. w/bone	1028	69.9	0	80.9	22.7	282	283	0
1 lb.	1170	79.6	0	92.2	25.9	322	322	0
1 oz.	73	5.0	0	5.8	1.6	20	20	0
meat only, 1 lb.	671	96.4	0	28.7	7.1	286	358	0
meat only, 1 oz.	42	6.0	0	1.8	.4	18	22	0
dark meat only, 1 lb.	712	89.4	0	36.8	9.4	349	458	0
dark meat only, 1 oz.	45	5.6	0	2.3	.6	22	29	0
light meat only, 1 lb.	621	104.8	0	19.1	4.4	213	240	0
light meat only, 1 oz.	39	6.5	0	1.2	.3	13	15	0
stewed:								
meat w/skin, ½ chicken, 9.2 oz.,								
yield from 13.5 oz. w/bone	744	70.2	0	49.2	13.3	205	190	0
meat w/skin, 4 oz.	323	30.5	0	21.4	5.8	90	83	0
meat only, 4 oz.	269	34.5	0	13.5	3.5	94	88	0
meat only, chopped or diced,								
1 cup not packed	332	42.6	0	16.6	4.3	117	109	0
dark meat only, 4 oz.	293	31.9	0	17.3	4.6	108	108	0

1. *Cooked poultry is prepared without added ingredients.*

Food and Measure	cal.	prot. (gms)	carbo. (gms)	tot. fat (gms)	sat. fat (gms)	chol. (mgs)	sod. (mgs)	fiber (gms)
dark meat only, chopped or diced,								
1 cup not packed	361	39.4	0	21.4	5.7	132	133	0
light meat only, 4 oz.	242	37.5	0	9.0	2.2	79	66	0
light meat only, chopped or diced,								
1 cup not packed	298	46.3	0	11.2	2.8	98	81	0
CHICKEN, BONELESS AND								
LUNCHEON MEAT:								
breast, 1 oz.:								
(*Longacre* Premium)	45	4.0	1.0	3.0	m.q.	20	280	0
(*Mr. Turkey*)	32	4.8	.6	1.1	m.q.	9	242	0
hickory smoked (*Louis Rich*)	30	5.1	.6	.8	.3	14	356	0
oven-roasted:								
(*Louis Rich* Deluxe)	30	4.9	.6	.8	.3	14	332	0
(*Louis Rich* Thin Sliced), .4-oz.								
slice	12	1.9	.2	.3	.1	6	130	0
(*Oscar Mayer*)	29	5.2	.6	.7	.2	15	414	0
roast (*Oscar Mayer* Thin Sliced),								
.4-oz. slice	13	2.1	.3	.4	.1	5	151	0
smoked (*Hillshire Farm* Deli								
Select)	31	6.0	<1.0	.2	m.q.	m.q.	290	0
smoked (*Oscar Mayer*)	25	5.3	.2	.4	.1	15	397	0
ham, see "Chicken ham"								
roll:								
(*Pilgrim's Pride*), 1-oz. slice	35	5.2	.4	1.2	m.q.	15	260	0
light meat, 6-oz. pkg.	271	33.2	4.2	12.5	3.4	85	992	0
light meat, 1-oz. slice	45	5.5	.7	2.1	.6	14	166	0
sliced (*Longacre*), 1 oz.	60	4.0	1.0	5.0	m.q.	25	210	0
white meat, oven-roasted (*Louis*								
Rich), 1-oz. slice	35	4.9	.1	1.7	.5	16	301	0
CHICKEN, CANNED (see also								
"Chicken entree, canned"):								
boned, w/broth, 5-oz. can	234	30.9	0	11.3	3.1	m.q.	714	0
boned, w/broth, 1 oz.	47	6.2	0	2.3	.6	m.q.	143	0
chunk:								
(*Featherweight*), 3 oz.	90	16.0	0	3.0	m.q.	65	60	0
breast (*Hormel*), 6¾ oz.	350	41.0	0	20.0	m.q.	m.q.	855	0
dark (*Hormel*), 6¾ oz.	327	42.0	0	18.0	m.q.	m.q.	933	0
style (*Swanson* Mixin' Chicken),								
2½ oz.	130	13.0	1.0	8.0	m.q.	m.q.	230	0
white and dark (*Hormel*), 6¾ oz.	340	39.0	0	20.0	m.q.	m.q.	857	0
white and dark, unsalted (*Hormel*),								
6¾ oz.	330	42.0	0	18.0	m.q.	m.q.	75	0
loaf (*Hormel*), 2 oz.	130	7.0	0	10.0	m.q.	m.q.	608	0
white (*Swanson*), 2½ oz.	100	15.0	0	4.0	m.q.	35	235	0
white and dark (*Swanson*), 2½ oz. ..	100	16.0	0	4.0	m.q.	40	240	0
"CHICKEN," VEGETARIAN:								
canned:								
(*Worthington FriChik*), 2 pieces,								
approx. 3.2 oz.	180	11.0	4.0	13.0	m.q.	0	610	m.q.

Food and Measure	cal.	prot. (gms)	carbo. (gms)	tot. fat (gms)	sat. fat (gms)	chol. (mgs)	sod. (mgs)	fiber (gms)
"CHICKEN," VEGETARIAN, CANNED *(cont.)*								
sliced, drained *(Worthington)*,								
2 slices, approx. 2.1 oz.	90	4.0	2.0	8.0	m.q.	0	330	m.q.
diced, drained *(Worthington)*,								
¼ cup	90	4.0	2.0	8.0	m.q.	0	330	m.q.
frozen:								
(Worthington Crispy Chik), 3 oz.	280	10.0	17.0	19.0	m.q.	0	500	m.q.
diced *(Worthington* Meatless								
Chicken), ½ cup	190	13.0	5.0	13.0	2.0	0	680	m.q.
nuggets, homestyle *(Morningstar								
Farms Country Crisps)*, 3 oz. ..	250	8.0	18.0	16.0	m.q.	0	480	m.q.
nuggets, zesty *(Morningstar								
Farms Country Crisps)*, 3 oz. ..	280	9.0	17.0	19.0	3.0	0	740	m.q.
patty *(Morningstar Farms Country								
Crisps)*, 2.5-oz. patty	220	8.0	13.0	15.0	2.0	0	620	m.q.
patty *(Worthington Crispy Chik)*,								
2.5-oz. patty	220	8.0	13.0	15.0	2.0	0	620	m.q.
pie *(Worthington)*, 8-oz. pie	380	7.0	43.0	20.0	3.0	0	1200	m.q.
roll *(Worthington Chic-ketts)*,								
½ cup	160	19.0	6.0	7.0	1.0	0	640	m.q.
roll *(Worthington* Meatless								
Chicken), 2½ oz.	150	11.0	4.0	10.0	1.0	0	570	m.q.
slices *(Worthington* Meatless								
Chicken), 2 slices, 2 oz.	130	9.0	3.0	9.0	1.0	0	460	m.q.
sticks *(Worthington Chik Stiks)*,								
1 piece, approx. 1.7 oz.	110	9.0	4.0	7.0	1.0	0	390	m.q.
CHICKEN BOLOGNA:								
(Health Valley), 1 slice	85	4.0	1.0	8.0	m.q.	13	329	0
CHICKEN COATING MIX, see								
"Chicken seasoning and coating								
mix"								
CHICKEN DINNER, frozen:								
a la king *(Armour Classics Lite)*,								
11.25 oz.	290	19.0	38.0	7.0	m.q.	55	630	m.q.
a la king *(Le Menu)*, 10.25 oz.	330	23.0	29.0	13.0	m.q.	m.q.	830	m.q.
barbecue-style *(Stouffer's Dinner								
Supreme)*, 10.5 oz.	390	22.0	24.0	23.0	m.q.	m.q.	1250	m.q.
boneless *(Swanson Hungry Man)*,								
17.75 oz.	700	48.0	65.0	28.0	m.q.	m.q.	1530	m.q.
breast:								
baked, w/gravy *(Stouffer's Dinner								
Supreme)*, 10 oz.	300	30.0	20.0	11.0	m.q.	m.q.	830	m.q.
glazed *(Le Menu* LightStyle),								
10 oz.	230	25.0	25.0	3.0	m.q.	55	430	m.q.
Marsala *(Armour Classics Lite)*,								
10.5 oz.	250	2.0	27.0	7.0	m.q.	80	930	m.q.
Burgundy *(Armour Classics Lite)*,								
10 oz.	210	23.0	25.0	2.0	m.q.	45	780	m.q.

Food and Measure	cal.	prot. (gms)	carbo. (gms)	tot. fat (gms)	sat. fat (gms)	chol. (mgs)	sod. (mgs)	fiber (gms)
cacciatore (*The Budget Gourmet*),								
11 oz.	300	20.0	27.0	13.0	m.q.	60	810	m.q.
casserole (*Pillsbury Microwave*								
Classic), 1 pkg.	400	21.0	30.0	22.0	m.q.	m.q.	890	m.q.
and cheese, casserole (*Pillsbury*								
Microwave Classic), 1 pkg.	480	21.0	33.0	29.0	m.q.	m.q.	940	m.q.
Cordon Bleu (*Le Menu*), 11 oz.	460	23.0	47.0	20.0	m.q.	m.q.	850	m.q.
and dumplings (*Banquet*), 10 oz. ...	430	17.0	34.0	24.0	m.q.	45	940	m.q.
fettuccine (*Armour Classics*), 11 oz.	260	17.0	28.0	9.0	m.q.	50	660	m.q.
Florentine (*Stouffer's Dinner*								
Supreme), 11 oz.	430	33.0	32.0	18.0	m.q.	m.q.	930	m.q.
fried:								
(*Banquet*), 10 oz.	400	15.0	45.0	22.0	m.q.	m.q.	1100	m.q.
(*Banquet Extra Helping*), 16 oz. ...	570	20.0	70.0	28.0	m.q.	m.q.	1470	m.q.
(*Kid Cuisine*), 7.25 oz.	420	15.0	41.0	22.0	m.q.	m.q.	1050	m.q.
(*Stouffer's Dinner Supreme*),								
10⅝ oz.	450	25.0	35.0	23.0	m.q.	m.q.	990	m.q.
barbecue flavored (*Swanson*),								
10 oz.	540	25.0	61.0	22.0	m.q.	m.q.	1160	m.q.
dark meat (*Swanson*), 9.75 oz.	560	22.0	55.0	28.0	m.q.	m.q.	1130	m.q.
dark meat (*Swanson Hungry Man*),								
1 pkg.	860	36.0	77.0	45.0	m.q.	m.q.	1660	m.q.
white meat:								
(*Banquet Extra Helping*), 16 oz.	570	20.0	70.0	28.0	m.q.	m.q.	1470	m.q.
(*Swanson*), 10.25 oz.	550	22.0	60.0	25.0	m.q.	m.q.	1460	m.q.
(*Swanson Hungry Man*), 1 pkg.	870	35.0	80.0	46.0	m.q.	m.q.	2150	m.q.
glazed (*Armour Classics*), 10.75 oz.	300	15.0	24.0	16.0	m.q.	60	960	m.q.
herb roasted (*Healthy Choice*),								
11 oz.	260	20.0	38.0	3.0	1.0	40	300	m.q.
herb roasted (*Le Menu* LightStyle),								
10 oz.	240	27.0	18.0	7.0	m.q.	70	400	m.q.
mesquite (*Armour Classics*), 9.5 oz.	370	15.0	42.0	16.0	m.q.	55	660	m.q.
mesquite (*Healthy Choice*), 10.5 oz.	310	21.0	52.0	2.0	<1.0	45	270	m.q.
Mexicana (*The Budget Gourmet*),								
12.8 oz.	510	23.0	70.0	15.0	m.q.	40	1210	m.q.
and noodles (*Armour Classics*),								
11 oz.	230	19.0	23.0	7.0	m.q.	50	660	m.q.
nuggets:								
(*Kid Cuisine*), 6.25 oz.	400	11.0	46.0	19.0	m.q.	60	610	m.q.
(*Swanson*), 8.75 oz.	470	19.0	47.0	23.0	m.q.	m.q.	650	m.q.
w/barbecue sauce (*Banquet Extra*								
Helping), 10 oz.	640	29.0	56.0	36.0	m.q.	m.q.	1390	m.q.
platter (*Freezer Queen*), 6 oz.	410	14.0	36.0	23.0	m.q.	m.q.	950	m.q.
w/sweet and sour sauce (*Banquet*								
Extra Helping), 10 oz.	650	28.1	64.0	34.0	m.q.	m.q.	m.q.	m.q.
Oriental (*Armour Classics Lite*),								
10 oz.	180	18.0	24.0	1.0	m.q.	35	660	m.q.
Oriental (*Healthy Choice*), 11.25 oz.	220	21.0	31.0	2.0	<1.0	55	460	m.q.

Food and Measure	cal.	prot. (gms)	carbo. (gms)	tot. fat (gms)	sat. fat (gms)	chol. (mgs)	sod. (mgs)	fiber (gms)
CHICKEN DINNER *(cont.)*								
parmigiana:								
(Armour Classics), 11.5 oz.	370	22.0	27.0	19.0	m.q.	75	1060	m.q.
(Healthy Choice), 11.5 oz.	280	23.0	38.0	3.0	2.0	60	310	m.q.
(Le Menu), 11.75 oz.	410	26.0	31.0	20.0	m.q.	m.q.	1030	m.q.
(Stouffer's Dinner Supreme), 11.5 oz.	360	31.0	25.0	15.0	m.q.	m.q.	1150	m.q.
and pasta divan *(Healthy Choice)*, 11.5 oz.	310	23.0	45.0	4.0	2.0	60	510	m.q.
pattie platter *(Freezer Queen)*, 7.5 oz.	360	17.0	33.0	17.0	m.q.	m.q.	1160	m.q.
roast *(The Budget Gourmet)*, 11.2 oz.	280	19.0	34.0	7.0	m.q.	40	1110	m.q.
w/supreme sauce *(Stouffer's Dinner Supreme)*, 11⅜ oz.	360	33.0	29.0	12.0	m.q.	m.q.	990	m.q.
sweet and sour:								
(Armour Classics Lite), 11 oz. ...	240	18.0	39.0	2.0	m.q.	35	820	m.q.
(Healthy Choice), 11.5 oz.	280	22.0	44.0	2.0	<1.0	50	260	m.q.
(Le Menu), 11.25 oz.	400	19.0	41.0	18.0	m.q.	m.q.	1020	m.q.
(Le Menu LightStyle), 10 oz.	250	18.0	29.0	7.0	m.q.	2	530	m.q.
teriyaki *(The Budget Gourmet)*, 12 oz.	360	20.0	44.0	12.0	m.q.	55	610	m.q.
w/wine and mushroom sauce *(Armour Classics)*, 10.75 oz. ..	280	22.0	24.0	11.0	m.q.	50	900	m.q.
in wine sauce *(Le Menu)*, 10 oz. ...	280	26.0	27.0	7.0	m.q.	m.q.	680	m.q.
CHICKEN ENTREE, CANNED:								
a la king *(Swanson)*, 5¼ oz.	190	10.0	9.0	12.0	m.q.	m.q.	690	m.q.
chow mein *(La Choy Bi-Pack)*, ¾ cup	80	7.0	8.0	3.0	m.q.	18	980	1.0 d
and dumplings:								
(Featherweight), 7½ oz.	160	12.0	18.0	5.0	m.q.	m.q.	115	m.q.
(Luck's), 7¼ oz.	240	16.0	18.0	11.0	m.q.	m.q.	605	m.q.
(Swanson), 7½ oz.	220	11.0	19.0	11.0	m.q.	m.q.	980	m.q.
Oriental *(La Choy Bi-Pack)*, ¾ cup	240	9.0	47.0	2.0	m.q.	m.q.	1400	1.0 d
stew:								
(Swanson), 7⅝ oz.	160	9.0	15.0	7.0	m.q.	m.q.	990	m.q.
w/dumplings *(Heinz)*, 7½ oz.	210	9.0	22.0	9.0	m.q.	m.q.	850	m.q.
w/wild rice *(Featherweight)*, 7½ oz.	140	10.0	23.0	1.0	m.q.	20	400	m.q.
CHICKEN ENTREE, FREEZE-DRIED:								
stew *(Mountain House)*, 1 cup[1]	230	9.0	30.0	8.0	m.q.	m.q.	209	m.q.
CHICKEN ENTREE, FROZEN (see also "Chicken sandwich"):								
a la gratin *(Myers)*, 3.5 oz.	129	9.0	9.0	7.0	m.q.	m.q.	276	m.q.
a la king:								
(Banquet Cookin' Bags), 4 oz. ...	110	8.0	9.0	5.0	m.q.	m.q.	n.a.	n.a.
(Dining Lite), 9 oz.	240	14.0	30.0	7.0	m.q.	40	780	m.q.

1. *Prepared according to package directions.*

Food and Measure	cal.	prot. (gms)	carbo. (gms)	tot. fat (gms)	sat. fat (gms)	chol. (mgs)	sod. (mgs)	fiber (gms)
(*Freezer Queen Cook-In-Pouch*),								
4 oz.	70	9.0	6.0	1.0	m.q.	m.q.	460	n.a.
(*Myers*), 3.5 oz.	137	9.0	6.0	9.0	m.q.	m.q.	357	n.a.
(*Weight Watchers*), 9 oz.	240	17.0	28.0	6.0	3.0	20	490	n.a.
w/rice (*Freezer Queen* Single								
Serve), 9 oz.	270	20.0	37.0	5.0	m.q.	m.q.	520	m.q.
w/rice (*Stouffer's*), 9.5 oz.	290	19.0	34.0	9.0	m.q.	m.q.	890	m.q.
w/seasoned rice (*Le Menu*								
LightStyle), 8.25 oz.	240	19.0	29.0	5.0	1.0	30	670	m.q.
almond, w/rice and vegetables (*La*								
Choy Fresh & Lite), 9.75 oz.	270	14.0	40.1	8.0	m.q.	42	1092	3.0 d
a l'orange:								
(*Healthy Choice*), 9 oz.	260	22.0	39.0	2.0	<1.0	45	90	m.q.
(*Tyson Gourmet Selection*), 9.5 oz.	300	21.0	36.0	8.0	m.q.	m.q.	670	m.q.
w/almond rice (*Lean Cuisine*),								
8 oz.	260	24.0	30.0	5.0	1.0	55	430	m.q.
au gratin (*The Budget Gourmet* Slim								
Selects), 9.1 oz.	260	20.0	21.0	11.0	m.q.	70	820	m.q.
and beef luau (*Tyson Gourmet*								
Selection), 10.5 oz.	330	18.0	42.0	10.0	m.q.	m.q.	1030	m.q.
breast, boneless:								
barbecue marinated (*Tyson*),								
3.75 oz.	120	22.0	5.0	3.0	m.q.	m.q.	400	n.a.
butter garlic marinated (*Tyson*),								
3.75 oz.	160	21.0	3.0	7.0	m.q.	m.q.	320	n.a.
chunks (*Tyson*), 3 oz.	240	13.0	10.0	17.0	m.q.	30	430	m.q.
fillets (*Pilgrim's Pride*), 3 oz.	195	15.1	10.8	10.2	m.q.	26	450	m.q.
fillets (*Tyson*), 3 oz.	190	13.0	15.0	9.0	m.q.	25	400	m.q.
in herb cream sauce (*Lean*								
Cuisine), 9.5 oz.	260	26.0	17.0	10.0	3.0	80	840	m.q.
herb roasted, w/rice and								
vegetables (*Le Menu*								
LightStyle), 7.75 oz.	260	22.0	29.0	6.0	2.0	45	500	m.q.
Italian marinated (*Tyson*),								
3.75 oz.	130	22.0	6.0	2.0	m.q.	m.q.	320	n.a.
lemon pepper marinated (*Tyson*),								
3.75 oz.	120	22.0	4.0	2.0	m.q.	m.q.	210	n.a.
Marsala w/vegetables (*Lean*								
Cuisine), 8⅛ oz.	190	25.0	11.0	5.0	1.0	80	400	m.q.
Parmesan (*Lean Cuisine*), 10 oz.	260	27.0	19.0	8.0	2.0	80	870	m.q.
patties, see "patties," below								
tenders:								
(*Banquet* Chicken Hot Bites),								
2.25 oz.	150	11.0	12.0	6.0	m.q.	m.q.	280	m.q.
(*Banquet* Chicken Hot Bites								
Microwave), 4 oz.	260	19.0	24.0	10.0	m.q.	m.q.	560	m.q.
(*Pilgrim's Pride*), 3 oz.	181	12.7	11.1	9.5	m.q.	26	430	m.q.
Southern fried (*Banquet*								
Chicken Hot Bites), 2.25 oz.	160	10.0	13.0	7.0	m.q.	m.q.	340	m.q.

Food and Measure	cal.	prot. (gms)	carbo. (gms)	tot. fat (gms)	sat. fat (gms)	chol. (mgs)	sod. (mgs)	fiber (gms)
CHICKEN ENTREE, FROZEN, BREAST, TENDERS *(cont.)*								
Southern fried (*Tyson*), 3 oz. . .	220	14.0	15.0	11.0	m.q.	25	630	m.q.
teriyaki marinated (*Tyson*),								
3.75 oz.	130	22.0	6.0	2.0	m.q.	m.q.	290	n.a.
and broccoli (*Green Giant* Entrees),								
9.5 oz.	340	23.0	28.0	15.0	m.q.	m.q.	890	m.q.
cacciatore:								
(*Freezer Queen* Single Serve),								
9 oz.	270	20.0	33.0	6.0	m.q.	m.q.	710	m.q.
(*Swanson* Homestyle Recipe),								
10.95 oz.	260	15.0	33.0	8.0	m.q.	m.q.	1030	m.q.
w/vermicelli (*Lean Cuisine*),								
10⅞ oz.	250	21.0	26.0	7.0	1.0	45	860	m.q.
Cajun style (*Pilgrim's Pride*), 3 oz.[1]	241	13.3	8.6	17.0	m.q.	51	480	m.q.
cannelloni, see "Cannelloni entree"								
cashew, in sauce, w/rice (*Stouffer's*),								
9.5 oz.	380	31.0	29.0	16.0	m.q.	m.q.	1140	m.q.
w/cheddar, boneless (*Tyson* Chick'n								
Cheddar), 2.6 oz.	220	11.0	11.0	15.0	m.q.	40	310	m.q.
chow mein:								
(*Chun King*), 13 oz.	370	25.0	53.0	6.0	m.q.	m.q.	1560	m.q.
(*Dining Lite*), 9 oz.	180	10.0	31.0	2.0	m.q.	30	650	m.q.
(*Healthy Choice*), 8.5 oz.	220	16.0	31.0	3.0	1.0	45	440	m.q.
w/out noodles (*Stouffer's*), 8 oz. . .	130	13.0	11.0	4.0	m.q.	m.q.	1080	m.q.
w/rice (*Lean Cuisine*), 11.25 oz.	250	14.0	36.0	5.0	1.0	35	980	m.q.
chunks:								
(*Country Pride*), 3 oz.	240	10.0	15.0	15.0	m.q.	m.q.	560	m.q.
(*Tyson* Chick'n Chunks), 2.6 oz.	220	10.0	11.0	15.0	m.q.	35	500	m.q.
Southern fried (*Country Pride*),								
3 oz.	280	10.0	14.0	20.0	m.q.	m.q.	690	m.q.
Southern fried (*Tyson* Chick'n								
Chunks), 2.6 oz.	220	10.0	11.0	15.0	m.q.	35	540	m.q.
Cordon Bleu (*Swift International*),								
6 oz.	360	30.0	23.0	17.0	m.q.	m.q.	1010	m.q.
Cordon Bleu, breaded (*Weight*								
Watchers), 8 oz.	220	19.0	14.0	9.0	5.0	50	630	m.q.
creamed (*Myers*), 3.5 oz.	151	12.0	5.0	10.0	m.q.	m.q.	372	n.a.
creamed (*Stouffer's*), 6.5 oz.	300	19.0	8.0	21.0	m.q.	m.q.	670	n.a.
croquettes (*Myers*), 3.5 oz.	168	16.0	10.0	7.0	m.q.	m.q.	364	n.a.
croquettes, breaded, gravy and								
(*Freezer Queen Family Suppers*),								
7 oz.	240	12.0	20.0	12.0	m.q.	m.q.	1000	m.q.
diced (*Tyson*), 3 oz.	150	26.0	0	5.0	m.q.	70	50	0
Dijon (*Tyson Gourmet Selection*),								
8.5 oz.	310	17.0	22.0	17.0	m.q.	m.q.	840	m.q.
Dijon, w/pasta and vegetables (*Le*								
Menu LightStyle), 8.5 oz.	240	22.0	21.0	7.0	2.0	40	500	m.q.

1. *Edible portion.*

Food and Measure	cal.	prot. (gms)	carbo. (gms)	tot. fat (gms)	sat. fat (gms)	chol. (mgs)	sod. (mgs)	fiber (gms)
divan (*Stouffer's*), 8.5 oz.	320	24.0	11.0	20.0	m.q.	m.q.	780	m.q.
drumsnackers (*Banquet* Chicken Hot Bites), 2.63 oz.	220	10.0	13.0	15.0	m.q.	m.q.	530	m.q.
drumsnackers (*Banquet* Platters), 7 oz.	430	20.0	49.0	19.0	m.q.	m.q.	690	m.q.
drumsters (*Pilgrim's Pride*), 3 oz. ...	200	11.5	10.5	12.5	m.q.	38	320	m.q.
and dumplings (*Banquet Family Entrees*), 7 oz.	280	12.0	28.0	14.0	m.q.	m.q.	m.q.	m.q.
and egg noodles, w/broccoli (*The Budget Gourmet*), 10 oz.	450	23.0	31.0	26.0	m.q.	130	1110	m.q.
empress, w/seasoned rice (*Le Menu LightStyle*), 8.25 oz.	210	16.0	26.0	5.0	1.0	30	690	m.q.
enchilada, see "Enchilada entree"								
escalloped, and noodles (*Stouffer's*), 10 oz.	420	21.0	27.0	25.0	m.q.	m.q.	1230	m.q.
fajita, see "Fajita entree"								
w/fettuccine (*The Budget Gourmet*), 10 oz.	400	23.0	29.0	21.0	m.q.	100	740	m.q.
fettuccini (*Weight Watchers*), 8.25 oz.	280	22.0	25.0	9.0	3.0	40	590	m.q.
fiesta (*Healthy Choice*), 8.5 oz.	250	21.0	29.0	6.0	1.0	45	880	m.q.
Francais (*Tyson Gourmet Selection*), 9.5 oz.	280	19.0	20.0	14.0	m.q.	m.q.	1130	m.q.
French recipe (*The Budget Gourmet Slim Selects*), 10 oz.	260	21.0	21.0	10.0	m.q.	60	790	m.q.
fried:								
(*Banquet/Banquet* Hot'n Spicy), 6.4 oz.	330	18.0	29.0	19.0	m.q.	m.q.	1210	m.q.
(*Pilgrim's Pride*), 3 oz.[1]	255	12.0	11.9	17.7	m.q.	38	480	m.q.
(*Swanson* Homestyle Recipe), 7 oz.[1]	390	18.0	33.0	21.0	m.q.	m.q.	1100	m.q.
(*Swanson* 1 lb. Take-Out Pre-Fried), 3.25 oz.[1]	270	15.0	16.0	16.0	m.q.	m.q.	650	m.q.
breast portions (*Banquet*), 5.75 oz.	220	16.0	13.0	11.0	m.q.	m.q.	710	m.q.
breast portions (*Swanson* Plump & Juicy), 4.5 oz.[1]	360	23.0	21.0	20.0	m.q.	m.q.	800	m.q.
thighs and drumsticks (*Banquet*), 6.25 oz.	250	14.0	14.0	14.0	m.q.	m.q.	790	m.q.
white meat (*Banquet* Platter), 9 oz.	430	38.0	21.0	22.0	m.q.	105	m.q.	m.q.
white meat, hot'n spicy (*Banquet* Platter), 9 oz.	430	38.0	21.0	22.0	m.q.	105	m.q.	m.q.
glazed:								
(*Dining Lite*), 9 oz.	220	17.0	30.0	4.0	m.q.	45	680	m.q.
(*Healthy Choice*), 8.5 oz.	220	21.0	27.0	3.0	1.0	50	390	m.q.
w/vegetable rice (*Lean Cuisine*), 8.5 oz.	270	26.0	23.0	8.0	1.0	55	810	m.q.

1. *Edible portion.*

Food and Measure	cal.	prot. (gms)	carbo. (gms)	tot. fat (gms)	sat. fat (gms)	chol. (mgs)	sod. (mgs)	fiber (gms)
CHICKEN ENTREE, FROZEN *(cont.)*								
hot'n spicy (*Banquet* Snack'n),								
3.75 oz.	140	6.0	8.0	9.0	m.q.	m.q.	480	m.q.
Imperial:								
(*Chun King*), 13 oz.	300	17.0	54.0	1.0	m.q.	m.q.	1540	m.q.
(*Weight Watchers*), 9.25 oz.	240	21.0	32.0	3.0	1.0	35	640	m.q.
w/rice (*La Choy Fresh & Lite*),								
11 oz.	260	13.0	45.0	6.0	m.q.	46	1269	3.1 d
Italiano, w/fettuccini and vegetables								
(*Right Course*), 9⅝ oz.	280	24.0	29.0	8.0	2.0	45	560	m.q.
Kiev:								
(*Le Menu*), 8 oz.	530	20.0	24.0	39.0	m.q.	m.q.	780	m.q.
(*Swift International*), 6 oz.	420	27.0	22.0	24.0	m.q.	m.q.	1030	m.q.
(*Tyson Gourmet Selection*),								
9.25 oz.	520	16.0	40.0	33.0	m.q.	m.q.	1200	m.q.
(*Weight Watchers*), 7 oz.	230	13.0	23.0	9.0	3.0	30	610	m.q.
Mandarin (*The Budget Gourmet* Slim								
Selects), 10 oz.	290	19.0	40.0	6.0	m.q.	25	690	m.q.
Marsala (*The Budget Gourmet*),								
10 oz.	250	15.0	37.0	5.0	m.q.	65	660	m.q.
Marsala (*Tyson Gourmet Selection*),								
10.5 oz.	300	19.0	26.0	13.0	m.q.	m.q.	900	m.q.
mesquite (*Tyson Gourmet Selection*),								
9.5 oz.	320	23.0	35.0	10.0	m.q.	m.q.	700	m.q.
nibbles (*Swanson* Homestyle Recipe),								
4.25 oz.[1]	340	10.0	29.0	20.0	m.q.	m.q.	730	m.q.
nibbles (*Swanson* Plump & Juicy),								
3.25 oz.[1]	300	12.0	19.0	19.0	m.q.	m.q.	690	m.q.
and noodles:								
(*Dining Lite*), 9 oz.	240	17.0	28.0	7.0	m.q.	50	570	m.q.
(*Myers*), 3.5 oz.	136	8.0	9.0	8.0	m.q.	m.q.	399	m.q.
homestyle (*Stouffer's*), 10 oz.	310	23.0	21.0	15.0	m.q.	m.q.	1020	m.q.
homestyle (*Weight Watchers*), 9 oz.	240	19.0	25.0	7.0	2.0	30	450	m.q.
nuggets:								
(*Banquet* Chicken Hot Bites),								
2.63 oz.	210	11.0	11.0	14.0	m.q.	m.q.	550	m.q.
(*Banquet* Platters), 6.4 oz.	430	17.0	46.0	21.0	m.q.	m.q.	630	m.q.
(*Country Pride*), 3 oz.	250	11.0	14.0	16.0	m.q.	m.q.	460	m.q.
(*Freezer Queen Deluxe Family								
Suppers*), 3 oz.	270	14.0	15.0	17.0	m.q.	m.q.	770	m.q.
(*Pilgrim's Pride*), 3 oz.	202	12.4	10.4	12.3	m.q.	31	370	m.q.
(*Swanson* Plump & Juicy), 3 oz.[1]	230	13.0	14.0	14.0	m.q.	m.q.	360	m.q.
(*Tyson* Microwave), 3.5 oz.	220	10.0	11.0	15.0	m.q.	m.q.	m.q.	m.q.
(*Weight Watchers*), 5.9 oz.	270	15.0	24.0	12.0	4.0	50	540	m.q.
breast, Southern fried w/barbecue								
sauce (*Banquet* Microwave								
Chicken Hot Bites), 4.5 oz.	370	19.0	20.0	23.0	m.q.	m.q.	930	m.q.

1. *Edible portion.*

Food and Measure	cal.	prot. (gms)	carbo. (gms)	tot. fat (gms)	sat. fat (gms)	chol. (mgs)	sod. (mgs)	fiber (gms)
w/cheddar (*Banquet* Chicken Hot Bites), 2.63 oz.	250	11.0	11.0	18.0	m.q.	m.q.	560	m.q.
hot'n spicy (*Banquet* Chicken Hot Bites), 2.63 oz.	250	10.0	10.0	19.0	m.q.	m.q.	380	m.q.
hot'n spicy, w/barbecue sauce (*Banquet* Microwave Chicken Hot Bites), 4.5 oz.	360	20.0	23.0	21.0	m.q.	m.q.	820	m.q.
Southern fried (*Banquet* Chicken Hot Bites), 2.63 oz.	220	10.0	13.0	14.0	m.q.	m.q.	530	m.q.
Southern fried, w/barbecue sauce (*Banquet* Microwave Chicken Hot Bites), 4.5 oz.	370	19.0	20.0	23.0	m.q.	m.q.	930	m.q.
w/sweet and sour sauce (*Banquet* Microwave Chicken Hot Bites), 4.5 oz.	360	20.0	22.0	21.0	m.q.	m.q.	770	m.q.
Oriental:								
(*Lean Cuisine*), 9⅜ oz.	230	22.0	23.0	6.0	1.0	100	790	m.q.
(*Tyson Gourmet Selection*), 10.25 oz.	270	20.0	32.0	7.0	m.q.	m.q.	1140	m.q.
spicy (*La Choy Fresh & Lite*), 9.75 oz.	270	11.0	52.0	4.0	m.q.	42	560	4.0 d
parmigiana (*Celentano*), 9 oz.	330	32.0	15.0	20.0	m.q.	m.q.	560	m.q.
parmigiana (*Tyson Gourmet Selection*), 11.25 oz.	380	19.0	37.0	17.0	m.q.	m.q.	1100	m.q.
patties:								
(*Banquet* Platters), 7.5 oz.	380	15.0	34.0	21.0	m.q.	m.q.	760	m.q.
(*Country Pride*), 3 oz.	250	12.0	14.0	16.0	m.q.	m.q.	570	m.q.
(*Pilgrim's Pride*), 3 oz.	205	12.0	11.4	12.4	m.q.	28	340	m.q.
(*Tyson*), 2.6 oz.	220	10.0	11.0	15.0	m.q.	35	640	m.q.
(*Tyson* Thick & Crispy), 2.6 oz.	220	11.0	13.0	14.0	m.q.	40	490	m.q.
breast:								
(*Banquet* Chicken Hot Bites), 2.63 oz.	210	11.0	13.0	13.0	m.q.	m.q.	460	m.q.
and bun (*Banquet* Microwave Chicken Hot Bites), 4-oz. pkg.	310	16.0	31.0	14.0	m.q.	m.q.	664	m.q.
Southern fried:								
(*Banquet* Chicken Hot Bites), 2.63 oz.	210	11.0	13.0	12.0	m.q.	m.q.	620	m.q.
(*Country Pride*), 3 oz.	240	11.0	13.0	16.0	m.q.	m.q.	630	m.q.
(*Tyson*), 2.6 oz.	220	11.0	9.0	15.0	m.q.	35	460	m.q.
Southern fried, and biscuit (*Banquet* Microwave Chicken Hot Bites), 4 oz.	320	12.0	37.0	14.0	m.q.	m.q.	980	m.q.
Southern fried (*Weight Watchers*), 6.5 oz.	320	17.0	27.0	16.0	7.0	65	690	m.q.

Food and Measure	cal.	prot. (gms)	carbo. (gms)	tot. fat (gms)	sat. fat (gms)	chol. (mgs)	sod. (mgs)	fiber (gms)
CHICKEN ENTREE, FROZEN *(cont.)*								
picatta (*Tyson Gourmet Selection*),								
9 oz.	240	19.0	19.0	10.0	m.q.	m.q.	680	m.q.
pie:								
(*Banquet*), 7 oz.	550	15.0	39.0	36.0	m.q.	35	860	m.q.
(*Banquet* Supreme Microwave),								
7 oz.	430	15.0	30.0	28.0	m.q.	40	740	m.q.
(*Morton*), 7 oz.	420	14.0	27.0	28.0	m.q.	35	740	m.q.
(*Myers*), 3.5 oz.	129	7.0	10.0	7.0	m.q.	m.q.	253	m.q.
(*Stouffer's*), 10 oz.	530	22.0	35.0	33.0	m.q.	m.q.	1260	m.q.
(*Swanson* Homestyle Recipe),								
8 oz.	410	15.0	41.0	21.0	m.q.	m.q.	1030	m.q.
(*Swanson* Pot Pie), 7 oz.	380	11.0	35.0	22.0	m.q.	m.q.	760	m.q.
(*Swanson Hungry Man*), 16 oz. ..	630	22.0	57.0	35.0	m.q.	m.q.	1600	m.q.
primavera:								
(*Celentano*), 11.5 oz.	270	25.0	18.0	10.0	m.q.	m.q.	580	m.q.
and vegetable (*Banquet Cookin'*								
Bags), 4 oz.	100	6.0	14.0	2.0	m.q.	m.q.	m.q.	m.q.
and vegetable (*Banquet Family*								
Entrees), 7 oz.	140	9.0	18.0	3.0	m.q.	m.q.	m.q.	m.q.
sesame (*Right Course*), 10 oz.	320	25.0	34.0	9.0	2.0	50	590	m.q.
sliced, gravy and (*Freezer Queen*								
Cook-In-Pouch), 5 oz.	80	7.0	6.0	3.0	m.q.	m.q.	820	n.a.
steaks, chicken fried (*Pilgrim's*								
Pride), 3 oz.	183	13.9	8.3	10.4	m.q.	21	640	m.q.
sticks (*Banquet* Chicken Hot Bites),								
2.63 oz.	220	10.0	11.0	15.0	m.q.	m.q.	350	m.q.
sticks (*Country Pride*), 3 oz.	240	10.0	16.0	15.0	m.q.	m.q.	400	m.q.
sweet and sour:								
(*Banquet Cookin' Bags*), 4 oz. ...	130	5.0	22.0	2.0	m.q.	m.q.	n.a.	n.a.
(*Tyson Gourmet Selection*), 11 oz.	420	22.0	50.0	15.0	m.q.	m.q.	850	n.a.
w/rice (*The Budget Gourmet*),								
10 oz.	350	18.0	53.0	7.0	m.q.	40	640	m.q.
w/rice (*Freezer Queen* Single								
Serve), 9 oz.	300	20.0	48.0	4.0	m.q.	m.q.	700	m.q.
w/rice and vegetables (*La Choy*								
Fresh & Lite), 10 oz.	260	13.0	50.1	3.0	m.q.	53	601	3.7 d
tenders (*Weight Watchers*),								
10.19 oz.	240	16.0	43.0	1.0	<1.0	40	600	m.q.
tenderloins, in barbecue sauce (*Right*								
Course), 8.75 oz.	270	20.0	35.0	6.0	1.0	40	590	m.q.
tenderloins, in peanut sauce (*Right*								
Course), 9.25 oz.	330	27.0	32.0	10.0	2.0	50	570	m.q.
tenders (*Tyson* Microwave), 3.5 oz.	230	16.0	19.0	11.0	m.q.	m.q.	m.q.	m.q.
thighs and drumsticks (*Swanson*								
Plump & Juicy, 3.25 oz.[1]	290	15.0	17.0	18.0	m.q.	m.q.	610	m.q.
and vegetables, w/vermicelli (*Lean*								
Cuisine), 11.75 oz.	270	20.0	29.0	7.0	1.0	45	980	m.q.

1. *Edible portion.*

Food and Measure	cal.	prot. (gms)	carbo. (gms)	tot. fat (gms)	sat. fat (gms)	chol. (mgs)	sod. (mgs)	fiber (gms)
walnut, crunchy (*Chun King*),								
13 oz.	310	16.0	49.0	5.0	m.q.	m.q.	1700	m.q.
wings:								
(*Pilgrim's Pride* Wing Zappers),								
3 oz.[1]	187	16.1	1.8	12.8	m.q.	90	340	n.a.
all varieties (*Tyson Flyers*), 3.5 oz.								
or 6–7 wings	220	23.0	0	14.0	m.q.	m.q.	400	0
Southern fried (*Pilgrim's Pride*),								
3 oz.[1]	228	13.3	5.1	17.2	m.q.	51	480	m.q.
CHICKEN ENTREE,								
PACKAGED, 1 serving:								
Acapulco (*Hormel Top Shelf*)	390	28.0	41.0	13.0	m.q.	55	1320	m.q.
breast of, glazed (*Hormel Top Shelf*)	210	22.0	22.0	3.0	m.q.	75	1150	m.q.
sweet and sour (*Hormel Top Shelf*) . .	270	24.0	41.0	1.0	m.q.	60	280	m.q.
CHICKEN ENTREE,								
REFRIGERATED, 5 oz.:								
bleu cheese, Italian (*Chicken By*								
George)	190	29.0	1.0	8.0	m.q.	80	650	n.a.
Cajun (*Chicken By George*)	200	29.0	1.0	9.0	m.q.	80	450	n.a.
lemon herb (*Chicken By George*) . . .	150	27.0	2.0	4.0	m.q.	70	480	n.a.
mesquite barbecue (*Chicken By*								
George)	170	29.0	5.0	4.0	m.q.	70	680	n.a.
mustard, country, and dill (*Chicken*								
By George)	180	29.0	1.0	7.0	m.q.	80	530	n.a.
teriyaki (*Chicken By George*)	180	30.0	6.0	4.0	m.q.	65	340	n.a.
tomato herb and basil (*Chicken By*								
George)	190	28.0	4.0	7.0	m.q.	90	430	n.a.
CHICKEN ENTREE MIX:								
barbecue style (*Lipton Microeasy*),								
¼ pkg. dry	110	2.0	24.0	<1.0	m.q.	n.a.	980	m.q.
barbecue style (*Lipton Microeasy*),								
¼ pkg.[2]	220	16.0	24.0	6.0	m.q.	m.q.	1020	m.q.
country style (*Lipton Microeasy*),								
¼ pkg. dry	80	3.0	15.0	<1.0	m.q.	n.a.	840	m.q.
country style (*Lipton Microeasy*),								
¼ pkg.[2]	190	18.0	15.0	6.0	m.q.	m.q.	880	m.q.
CHICKEN FAT:								
1 oz.	178	1.1	0	19.3	5.7	16	9	0
CHICKEN FRANKFURTER:								
1 oz.	73	3.7	1.9	5.5	1.6	28	388	0
1 link, approx. 1.6 oz.	116	5.8	3.1	8.8	2.5	45	617	0
(*Health Valley* Weiners), 1 link	96	5.0	1.0	8.0	m.q.	49	90	0
(*Longacre*), 1 oz.	63	4.0	1.0	5.0	m.q.	30	230	0
batter-wrapped (*Tyson* Corn Dogs),								
3.5 oz.	280	9.0	28.0	14.0	m.q.	75	70	m.q.

1. *Edible portion.*
2. *Prepared according to package directions, with chicken.*

Food and Measure	cal.	prot. (gms)	carbo. (gms)	tot. fat (gms)	sat. fat (gms)	chol. (mgs)	sod. (mgs)	fiber (gms)
CHICKEN GIBLETS[1]:								
broiler-fryer:								
raw, 1 oz.	35	5.1	.5	1.3	.4	74	22	0
raw, 2.6 oz.[2]	93	13.4	1.4	3.4	1.0	196	58	0
fried, flour coated:								
4 oz.	314	36.9	4.9	15.3	4.3	506	128	<.1 c
1.6 oz.[3]	122	14.3	1.9	5.9	1.7	196	50	tr.c
chopped or diced, 1 cup	402	47.2	6.3	19.5	5.5	647	164	<.1 c
simmered:								
4 oz.	178	29.3	1.1	5.4	1.7	446	66	0
1.6 oz.[4]	71	11.6	.4	2.1	.7	177	26	0
chopped or diced, 1 cup	228	37.5	1.4	6.9	2.2	570	85	0
roaster:								
raw, 1 oz.	36	5.1	.3	1.4	.4	67	22	0
raw, 4 oz.[5]	144	20.5	1.3	5.7	1.7	267	87	0
simmered, 4 oz.	187	30.4	1.0	5.9	1.9	405	68	0
simmered, chopped or diced,								
1 cup	239	38.8	1.2	7.6	2.4	517	86	0
capon:								
raw, 1 oz.	37	5.2	.4	1.5	.5	83	22	0
raw, 4.1 oz.[6]	150	21.0	1.6	6.0	1.9	335	89	0
simmered, 4 oz.	186	29.9	.9	6.1	20.0	492	62	0
simmered, chopped or diced,								
1 cup	238	38.3	1.1	7.8	2.6	629	80	0
CHICKEN GIZZARD, broiler-fryer:								
raw, 1 medium, approx. 1.3 oz.	44	6.7	.2	1.6	.4	48	28	0
simmered, 1 oz.	43	7.7	.3	1.0	.3	55	19	0
simmered, 1 medium, approx. .8 oz.	34	6.0	.3	.8	.2	43	15	0
CHICKEN GRAVY:								
canned:								
1 oz.	22	.5	1.5	1.6	.4	<1	164	n.a.
¼ cup	47	1.1	3.2	3.4	.8	1	344	n.a.
(Franco-American), 2 oz.	45	0	3.0	4.0	m.q.	n.a.	240	n.a.
(Heinz HomeStyle), 2 oz. or ¼ cup	35	1.0	3.0	2.0	m.q.	m.q.	350	n.a.
w/chunky chicken (Hormel Great								
Beginnings), 5 oz.	147	14.0	5.0	8.0	m.q.	m.q.	567	n.a.
giblet (Franco-American), 2 oz. ..	30	1.0	3.0	2.0	m.q.	n.a.	310	n.a.
mix[7]:								
1 oz. dry[8]	102	3.2	17.6	2.4	.6	2	1390	.1 c
¼ cup[8]	21	.7	3.6	.5	.1	1	283	<.1 c

1. *Cooked giblets are prepared without added ingredients, except as noted.*
2. *Includes 1 gizzard, 1 heart, and 1 liver from 3.3-lb. raw broiler-fryer.*
3. *Includes 1 gizzard, 1 heart, and 1 liver from 2.2-lb. fried broiler-fryer.*
4. *Includes 1 gizzard, 1 heart, and 1 liver from 2.5-lb. stewed chicken.*
5. *Includes 1 gizzard, 1 heart, and 1 liver from 4.6-lb. raw chicken.*
6. *Includes 1 gizzard, 1 heart, and 1 liver from 6.5-lb. raw capon.*
7. *Prepared according to package directions, with water, except as noted.*
8. *Contains chicken fat, soybeans, and cottonseed oil.*

Food and Measure	cal.	prot. (gms)	carbo. (gms)	tot. fat (gms)	sat. fat (gms)	chol. (mgs)	sod. (mgs)	fiber (gms)
(French's Gravy for Chicken),								
¼ cup	25	1.0	4.0	1.0	n.a.	n.a.	270	n.a.
(Lawry's), 1 cup	99	2.5	15.5	2.8	m.q.	n.a.	980	.1 c
(McCormick/Schilling), ¼ cup ...	22	.8	3.7	.4	n.a.	n.a.	300	n.a.
(Pillsbury), ¼ cup [1]	25	<1.0	4.0	1.0	n.a.	m.q.	230	n.a.
(Tone's), 1 tsp. dry	11	.3	1.9	.2	.2	<1	157	(0)
CHICKEN HAM:								
(Pilgrim's Pride), 1-oz. slice	35	4.0	.8	1.8	m.q.	18	430	0
CHICKEN HEART, see "Heart"								
CHICKEN LIVER, see "Liver"								
CHICKEN LIVER PATE, see "Pâté"								
CHICKEN LUNCHEON MEAT, see "Chicken, boneless and luncheon meat"								
CHICKEN NUGGETS, see "Chicken entree, frozen"								
CHICKEN PIE, see "Chicken entree, frozen"								
CHICKEN SALAD:								
(Longacre), 1 oz.	64	3.0	3.0	5.0	m.q.	15	110	n.a.
(Longacre Saladfest), 1 oz.	47	4.0	1.0	3.0	m.q.	15	150	n.a.
CHICKEN SANDWICH, frozen:								
(MicroMagic), 4.5 oz.	390	13.0	42.0	16.0	m.q.	35	650	m.q.
barbecue *(Tyson* Microwave), 4 oz.	230	16.0	27.0	6.0	m.q.	m.q.	510	m.q.
breast *(Tyson* Microwave), 3.5 oz. ...	275	14.0	27.0	12.0	m.q.	m.q.	m.q.	m.q.
mini *(Tyson* Microwave), 3.5 oz. ...	230	12.0	39.0	5.0	m.q.	m.q.	m.q.	m.q.
pocket:								
(Lean Pockets Supreme), 1 pkg. ...	280	14.0	34.0	9.0	m.q.	m.q.	500	m.q.
n' cheddar *(Hot Pockets)*, 5 oz. ...	310	16.0	38.0	11.0	m.q.	m.q.	720	m.q.
Oriental *(Lean Pockets)*, 1 pkg. ...	250	14.0	35.0	6.0	m.q.	m.q.	840	m.q.
Parmesan *(Lean Pockets)*, 1 pkg.	270	19.0	35.0	6.0	m.q.	m.q.	750	m.q.
CHICKEN SAUCE MIX (see also "Chicken gravy"), 1 pkg.:								
cacciatore *(McCormick/Schilling* Sauce Blends)	132	3.6	28.0	4.8	m.q.	n.a.	1092	m.q.
creole *(McCormick/Schilling* Sauce Blends)	140	2.0	24.0	4.8	m.q.	n.a.	1084	m.q.
curry *(McCormick/Schilling* Sauce Blends)	152	2.4	24.0	5.6	m.q.	n.a.	1288	m.q.
Dijon *(McCormick/Schilling* Sauce Blends)	156	3.2	20.0	6.8	m.q.	n.a.	1414	m.q.
mesquite marinade *(McCormick/ Schilling* Sauce Blends)	132	1.6	24.0	3.0	m.q.	n.a.	2068	m.q.

1. *Prepared with milk and water.*

Food and Measure	cal.	prot. (gms)	carbo. (gms)	tot. fat (gms)	sat. fat (gms)	chol. (mgs)	sod. (mgs)	fiber (gms)
CHICKEN SAUCE MIX *(cont.)*								
teriyaki (*McCormick/Schilling* Sauce Blends)	172	6.8	28.0	3.6	m.q.	n.a.	1380	m.q.
CHICKEN SEASONING AND COATING MIX:								
(*Featherweight*), ¼ pkg.	18	1.0	8.0	0	0	0	30	m.q.
(*Golden Dipt*), 1 oz.	90	2.0	20.0	0	0	0	1430	m.q.
(*McCormick/Schilling* Bag'n Season), 1 pkg.	177	3.7	22.6	1.4	n.a.	n.a.	2564	m.q.
(*Shake'n Bake*), ¼ pouch	80	2.0	14.0	2.0	m.q.	0	450	m.q.
(*Shake'n Bake Oven Fry* Extra Crispy), ¼ pouch	110	3.0	20.0	2.0	m.q.	0	810	m.q.
barbecue (*Shake'n Bake*), ¼ pouch	90	1.0	18.0	2.0	m.q.	0	840	m.q.
batter, Cajun (*Tone's*), 1 tsp.	12	.3	2.6	.1	<.1	0	75	.1 d
fried (*McCormick/Schilling*), ¼ tsp.	1	.1	.2	<.1	(0)	n.a.	132	n.a.
homestyle (*Shake'n Bake Oven Fry*), ¼ pouch	80	1.0	15.0	2.0	m.q.	0	970	m.q.
CHICKEN SIDE DISH MIX:								
meatless style (*Hain* 3-Grain Side Dish), ½ cup	100	4.0	17.0	1.0	n.a.	0	390	m.q.
CHICKEN SPREAD, canned:								
1 oz.	55	4.4	1.5	3.3	m.q.	m.q.	m.q.	n.a.
1 tbsp.	25	2.0	.7	1.5	m.q.	m.q.	m.q.	n.a.
(*Hormel*), ½ oz.	30	2.0	0	2.0	m.q.	m.q.	m.q.	0
(*Underwood* Light), 2⅛ oz.	80	11.0	2.0	3.0	1.0	30	330	n.a.
chunky (*Underwood*), 2⅛ oz.	150	10.0	2.0	9.0	3.0	40	440	n.a.
smoky (*Underwood*), 2⅛ oz.	150	10.0	10.0	8.0	2.0	40	290	n.a.
CHICK-PEA:								
raw:								
1 oz.	103	5.5	17.2	1.7	.2	0	7	1.8 d
½ cup	364	19.3	60.7	6.0	.6	0	24	6.4 d
(*Arrowhead Mills*), 2 oz.	200	12.0	35.0	3.0	m.q.	0	9	7.0 d
boiled, 4 oz.	186	10.0	31.1	2.9	.3	0	8	4.0 d
boiled, ½ cup	134	7.3	22.5	2.1	.2	0	6	2.9 d
CHICK-PEA, CANNED:								
w/liquid, 4 oz.	135	5.6	25.7	1.3	.1	0	339	1.5 c
w/liquid, ½ cup	143	5.9	27.1	1.4	.1	0	359	1.6 c
(*A&P*), ½ cup	100	6.0	17.0	1.0	n.a.	0	270	m.q.
(*Allens*), ½ cup	110	5.0	18.0	<1.0	n.a.	0	320	m.q.
(*Finast*), 8 oz.	210	10.0	35.0	3.0	m.q.	0	250	m.q.
(*Green Giant*), ½ cup	90	6.0	18.0	2.0	n.a.	0	320	5.0 d
(*Old El Paso*), ½ cup	190	5.0	16.0	<1.0	n.a.	0	250	m.q.
(*Progresso*), ½ cup	110	9.0	22.0	1.0	n.a.	0	200	6.0 d
(*S&W/Nutradiet*), ½ cup	100	5.0	19.0	1.0	n.a.	0	5	m.q.
large (*S&W* Lite 50% Less Salt), ½ cup	110	6.0	21.0	1.0	n.a.	0	295	m.q.
CHICK-PEA FLOUR:								
(*Arrowhead Mills*), 2 oz.	200	12.0	35.0	3.0	m.q.	0	9	7.4 d

Food and Measure	cal.	prot. (gms)	carbo. (gms)	tot. fat (gms)	sat. fat (gms)	chol. (mgs)	sod. (mgs)	fiber (gms)
CHICORY, WITLOOF:								
untrimmed, 1 lb.	61	4.0	12.9	.4	.1	0	28	m.q.
trimmed, 1 oz.	4	.3	.9	<.1	tr.	0	2	m.q.
trimmed, ½ cup	7	.5	1.7	.1	<.1	0	3	m.q.
1 head, 5–7″ long, approx. 2.1 oz. ...	8	.5	1.7	.1	<.1	0	4	m.q.
CHICORY GREENS:								
untrimmed, 1 lb.	87	6.3	17.5	1.1	.3	0	167	3.0 c
trimmed, 1 oz.	7	.5	1.3	.1	<.1	0	13	.2 c
trimmed, chopped, ½ cup	21	1.5	4.2	.3	.1	0	41	.7 c
CHICORY ROOT:								
untrimmed, 1 lb.	272	5.2	65.1	.7	.2	0	186	7.3 c
trimmed, 1 oz.	21	.4	5.0	.1	<.1	0	14	.6 c
1 medium, approx. 2.6 oz.	44	.8	10.5	.1	<.1	0	30	1.2 c
1″ pieces, ½ cup	33	.6	7.9	.1	<.1	0	23	.9 c
CHIKUWA, see "Fish paste cake"								
CHILI, canned:								
(*Chef Boyardee* Chili Mac), 7.5 oz. ...	230	8.0	26.0	11.0	m.q.	m.q.	1410	m.q.
(*Heinz* Chili Con Carne), 7.75 oz. ...	350	15.0	27.0	21.0	m.q.	m.q.	1000	m.q.
(*Heinz* Chili Mac), 7.5 oz.	250	10.0	26.0	12.0	m.q.	m.q.	860	m.q.
w/beans:								
4 oz.	127	6.5	13.5	6.2	2.7	19	592	2.4 c
½ cup	144	7.3	15.3	7.0	3.0	22	668	2.8 c
(*Dennison's*, 40 oz.), 8 oz.	340	17.0	29.0	17.0	m.q.	m.q.	1050	8.0 d
(*Dennison's*, 30 oz.), 7.5 oz.	310	16.0	28.0	15.0	m.q.	m.q.	840	8.0 d
(*Dennison's*, 15 oz.), 7.5 oz.	310	16.0	27.0	15.0	m.q.	m.q.	875	8.0 d
(*Dennison's* Cook-Off), 7.5 oz. ..	340	17.0	25.0	19.0	m.q.	m.q.	915	8.0 d
(*Estee*), 7.5 oz.	370	16.0	27.0	20.0	10.0	60	125	m.q.
(*Featherweight*), 7.5 oz.	280	19.0	29.0	10.0	m.q.	30	440	m.q.
(*Hormel*, 40 oz.), 8 oz.	320	17.0	25.0	17.0	m.q.	m.q.	1135	m.q.
(*Hormel*, 25 oz.), 8⅓ oz.	350	18.0	26.0	20.0	m.q.	m.q.	1202	m.q.
(*Hormel*, 15 oz.), 7.5 oz.	310	17.0	23.0	17.0	m.q.	m.q.	1127	m.q.
(*Hormel Micro-Cup*), 7.5 oz.	250	15.0	23.0	11.0	m.q.	65	980	m.q.
(*Libby's*, 24 oz.), 8 oz.	290	14.0	27.0	14.0	m.q.	m.q.	860	m.q.
(*Libby's*, 15 oz.), 7.5 oz.	270	13.0	25.0	13.0	m.q.	m.q.	810	m.q.
(*Nalley's*), 7.5 oz.	260	17.0	27.0	9.0	m.q.	m.q.	880	m.q.
(*Nalley's* Thick), 7.5 oz.	260	16.0	29.0	9.0	m.q.	m.q.	840	m.q.
(*Van Camp's*), 1 cup	352	14.9	20.9	23.2	m.q.	m.q.	1215	2.3 c
(*Wolf* Brand), 8 oz.	345	15.0	21.8	22.0	m.q.	m.q.	1013	2.3 c
beef (*Chef Boyardee*), 7.5 oz.	330	15.0	30.0	17.0	m.q.	m.q.	1005	m.q.
chunky (*Dennison's*), 7.5 oz.	310	16.0	28.0	14.0	m.q.	m.q.	780	10.0 d
extra spicy (*Wolf* Brand),								
7.75 oz.	324	14.1	20.6	20.6	m.q.	m.q.	926	2.2 c
hot:								
(*Dennison's*, 40 oz.), 8 oz.	350	17.0	29.0	19.0	m.q.	m.q.	950	7.0 d
(*Dennison's*, 15 oz.), 7.5 oz. ..	310	16.0	26.0	16.0	m.q.	m.q.	910	7.0 d
(*Gebhardt*), 4 oz.	189	7.1	9.2	14.2	.2	17	497	2.1 d
(*Heinz*), 7.75 oz.	330	15.0	30.0	16.0	m.q.	m.q.	1140	m.q.
(*Hormel*, 15 oz.), 7.5 oz.	310	16.0	24.0	16.0	m.q.	m.q.	1121	m.q.

Food and Measure	cal.	prot. (gms)	carbo. (gms)	tot. fat (gms)	sat. fat (gms)	chol. (mgs)	sod. (mgs)	fiber (gms)
CHILI, WITH BEANS, HOT *(cont.)*								
(*Nalley's*), 7.5 oz.	280	17.0	30.0	10.0	m.q.	m.q.	810	m.q.
jalapeño (*Nalley's*), 7.5 oz.	260	14.0	29.0	10.0	m.q.	m.q.	920	m.q.
vegetarian:								
mild (*Health Valley*), 4 oz.	130	8.0	16.0	3.0	m.q.	0	730	8.2 d
mild (*Health Valley* No Salt								
Added), 4 oz.	130	8.0	16.0	3.0	m.q.	0	25	8.2 d
spicy (*Health Valley*), 4 oz.	130	8.0	16.0	3.0	m.q.	0	430	8.2 d
spicy (*Health Valley* No Salt								
Added), 4 oz.	130	8.0	16.0	3.0	m.q.	0	25	8.2 d
w/out beans:								
(*Dennison's*, 19 oz.), 9.5 oz.	380	22.0	18.0	24.0	m.q.	m.q.	1335	m.q.
(*Dennison's*, 15 oz.), 7.5 oz.	300	17.0	15.0	19.0	m.q.	m.q.	1380	m.q.
(*Hormel*, 25 oz.), 8⅓ oz.	430	20.0	13.0	33.0	m.q.	m.q.	1070	m.q.
(*Hormel*, 15 oz.), 7.5 oz.	370	17.0	12.0	28.0	m.q.	m.q.	1012	m.q.
(*Hormel*), 10.5-oz. can	540	24.0	19.0	41.0	m.q.	m.q.	1384	m.q.
(*Libby's*), 7.5 oz.	390	18.0	11.0	30.0	m.q.	m.q.	800	m.q.
(*Nalley's* Big Chunk), 7.5 oz.	270	17.0	14.0	16.0	m.q.	m.q.	810	m.q.
(*Van Camp's*), 1 cup	412	15.4	12.1	33.5	m.q.	m.q.	1499	1.6 c
(*Wolf* Brand), 8 oz.	387	20.7	16.2	26.6	m.q.	m.q.	1042	2.0 c
(*Wolf* Brand Chili-Mac), 7.75 oz.	317	11.5	22.9	19.9	m.q.	m.q.	854	1.1 c
extra spicy (*Wolf* Brand), 7.5 oz.	363	19.4	15.3	24.9	m.q.	m.q.	962	1.9 c
w/franks (*Van Camp's Chilee*								
Weenee), 1 cup	309	14.4	27.6	15.7	m.q.	m.q.	1057	2.2 c
hot (*Hormel*, 15 oz.), 7.5 oz.	370	17.0	12.0	28.0	m.q.	m.q.	985	m.q.
w/chicken, spicy (*Hain*), 7.5 oz. . . .	130	11.0	19.0	2.0	m.q.	40	1030	m.q.
vegetarian:								
(*Gebhardt*), 4 oz.	219	9.6	6.9	17.1	m.q.	0	555	m.q.
(*Worthington*), ⅔ cup	190	10.0	15.0	10.0	1.0	0	550	m.q.
w/lentils, mild (*Health Valley*),								
4 oz.	130	8.0	16.0	3.0	m.q.	0	200	8.2 d
w/lentils, mild (*Health Valley* No								
Salt Added), 4 oz.	130	8.0	16.0	3.0	m.q.	0	50	8.2 d
spicy:								
(*Hain*), 7.5 oz.	160	7.0	29.0	1.0	m.q.	0	1060	m.q.
(*Hain* Reduced Sodium),								
7.5 oz.	170	7.0	31.0	1.0	m.q.	0	200	m.q.
(*Natural Touch*), ⅔ cup	230	12.0	19.0	12.0	1.0	0	890	m.q.
tempeh, spicy (*Hain*), 7.5 oz. . . .	160	7.0	24.0	4.0	m.q.	0	1350	m.q.
CHILI BEAN, canned:								
(*Hunt's*), 4 oz.	102	5.7	18.1	0	0	0	488	m.q.
(*S&W*), ½ cup	130	7.0	23.0	1.0	n.a.	n.a.	520	m.q.
baked style, hot (*Campbell's*),								
7.75 oz.	180	10.0	38.0	4.0	m.q.	n.a.	870	m.q.
Caliente style (*Green Giant/Joan of*								
Arc), ½ cup	100	6.0	20.0	1.0	n.a.	0	700	7.0 d
in chili gravy (*Dennison's*), 7.5 oz. . .	180	12.0	30.0	1.0	n.a.	n.a.	770	12.0 d
hot (*A&P*), ½ cup	140	8.0	24.0	1.0	n.a.	n.a.	440	m.q.

Food and Measure	cal.	prot. (gms)	carbo. (gms)	tot. fat (gms)	sat. fat (gms)	chol. (mgs)	sod. (mgs)	fiber (gms)
hot (*Allens*), ½ cup	90	5.0	17.0	<1.0	n.a.	n.a.	420	m.q.
Mexican style (*Allens*), ½ cup	135	8.0	24.0	<1.0	n.a.	n.a.	430	m.q.
Mexican style (*Van Camp's*), 1 cup	210	11.4	39.0	2.4	m.q.	n.a.	730	m.q.
in sauce (*Hormel*), 5 oz.	130	6.0	19.0	3.0	m.q.	n.a.	453	m.q.
spiced (*Gebhardt*), 4 oz.	113	7.5	19.7	1.1	.1	0	590	6.7 d
CHILI DIP:								
(*La Victoria*), 1 tbsp.	6	<1.0	1.0	<1.0	n.a.	n.a.	90	n.a.
CHILI ENTREE, CANNED, see "Chili, canned"								
CHILI ENTREE, FREEZE-DRIED[1]:								
w/beans (*Mountain House*), 1 cup ..	390	20.0	38.0	16.0	m.q.	m.q.	153	m.q.
w/beef (*Mountain House* Chili Mac), 1 cup	250	12.0	31.0	8.0	m.q.	m.q.	115	m.q.
CHILI ENTREE, FROZEN:								
con carne (*Swanson* Homestyle Recipe), 8¼ oz.	270	20.0	26.0	10.0	m.q.	m.q.	740	m.q.
con carne, w/beans (*Stouffer's*), 8¾ oz.	260	19.0	24.0	10.0	m.q.	m.q.	1270	m.q.
vegetarian (*Right Course*), 9¾ oz. ...	280	9.0	45.0	7.0	1.0	0	590	m.q.
CHILI ENTREE, PACKAGED:								
con carne suprema (*Hormel Top Shelf*), 1 serving	320	24.0	30.0	12.0	m.q.	65	1140	m.q.
CHILI MIX[2]:								
(*Gebhardt Chili Quik*), 1.5-oz. pkt. dry	82	2.5	16.8	1.1	.1	0	2784	3.0 d
(*Old El Paso* Chili con Carne), 1 cup	162	19.0	8.0	7.0	m.q.	47	510	1.5 d
w/beans (*Old El Paso*), 1 cup	217	15.0	17.0	10.0	m.q.	32	480	6.0 d
w/beans, vegetarian (*Fantastic Foods*), ½ cup	104	8.0	19.0	.8	n.a.	0	180	m.q.
CHILI PEPPER, HOT, see "Pepper, chili, hot"								
CHILI POWDER (see also "Chili seasoning"):								
1 oz.	89	3.5	15.5	4.8	m.q.	0	286	6.3 c
1 tbsp.	24	.9	4.1	1.3	m.q.	0	76	1.7 c
1 tsp.	8	.3	1.4	.4	n.a.	0	26	.6 c
(*Gebhardt*), 1 tsp.	6	0	1.0	0	0	0	30	m.q.
hot or mild (*Tone's*), 1 tsp.	8	.3	1.4	.4	.1	0	25	.6 d
CHILI SAUCE:								
(*Featherweight*), 1 tbsp.	8	0	2.0	0	0	0	10	m.q.
(*Heinz*), 1 tbsp.	16	.2	3.6	0	0	0	225	.2 c
(*S&W Chili Makin's*), ½ cup	100	5.0	20.0	1.0	n.a.	0	782	m.q.
green, mild (*El Molino*), 2 tbsp. ...	10	0	2.0	0	0	0	210	m.q.
hot dog:								
(*Gebhardt*), 2 tbsp.	20	1.0	2.0	1.0	n.a.	n.a.	150	m.q.

1. *Prepared according to package directions.*
2. *Prepared according to package directions, except as noted.*

Food and Measure	cal.	prot. (gms)	carbo. (gms)	tot. fat (gms)	sat. fat (gms)	chol. (mgs)	sod. (mgs)	fiber (gms)
CHILI SAUCE, HOT DOG *(cont.)*								
(*Wolf* Brand), 1.25 oz., approx.								
⅙ cup	44	1.5	4.4	2.3	m.q.	n.a.	199	.4 c
w/beef (*Chef Boyardee*), 1 oz.	30	1.0	4.0	1.0	n.a.	n.a.	140	m.q.
tomato (*Del Monte*), ¼ cup	70	1.0	17.0	0	0	0	835	m.q.
CHILI SEASONING (see also								
"Chili powder"):								
(*Lawry's* Seasoning Blends),								
1 pkg.	143	4.9	26.6	1.8	n.a.	0	2291	2.1 c
(*Tone's*), 1 tsp.	12	.3	2.4	.3	.1	0	231	.4 d
mix:								
(*McCormick/Schilling*), ¼ pkg.	27	1.0	4.5	.5	n.a.	n.a.	290	m.q.
(*Old El Paso*), ⅕ pkg.	21	1.0	4.0	1.0	n.a.	0	717	1.0 d
(*Tio Sancho*), 1.23 oz.	109	4.1	60.9	2.2	m.q.	n.a.	832	4.2 c
hot (*Hain*), ¼ pkg.	30	1.0	5.0	1.0	n.a.	0	370	m.q.
medium (*Hain*), ¼ pkg.	30	1.0	5.0	1.0	n.a.	0	300	m.q.
mild (*Hain*), ¼ pkg.	30	1.0	5.0	1.0	n.a.	0	330	m.q.
CHIMICHANGA, frozen:								
beef (*Old El Paso*), 1 piece	370	12.0	34.0	21.0	m.q.	m.q.	470	m.q.
chicken (*Old El Paso*), 1 piece	360	13.0	33.0	20.0	m.q.	m.q.	470	m.q.
CHIMICHANGA DINNER, frozen:								
beef (*Old El Paso* Festive								
Dinners), 11 oz.	540	23.0	65.0	21.0	m.q.	m.q.	1200	m.q.
beef and cheese (*Old El Paso* Festive								
Dinners), 11 oz.	510	22.0	53.0	23.0	m.q.	m.q.	1400	m.q.
CHIMICHANGA ENTREE,								
frozen, 1 pkg.:								
bean and cheese (*Old El Paso*)	380	12.0	40.0	19.0	m.q.	20	610	m.q.
beef (*Old El Paso*)	380	10.0	35.0	23.0	m.q.	m.q.	470	m.q.
beef and pork (*Old El Paso*)	340	13.0	35.0	16.0	m.q.	m.q.	700	m.q.
chicken (*Old El Paso*)	370	10.0	35.0	21.0	m.q.	m.q.	460	m.q.
CHINESE GOOSEBERRY, see								
"Kiwifruit"								
CHINESE PARSLEY, see								
"Coriander"								
CHINESE PRESERVING								
MELON, see "Waxgourd"								
CHINESE RADISH, see "Radish,								
Oriental"								
CHINESE WATERCHESTNUT,								
see "Waterchestnut"								
CHINESE YAM, see "Yam bean								
tuber"								
CHITTERLINGS, pork:								
raw, 1 oz.	71	2.9	0	6.5	2.3	45	10	0
simmered, 6 oz., yield from 1 lb. raw								
untrimmed	518	17.5	0	49.2	17.3	245	66	0
simmered, 4 oz.	344	11.6	0	32.6	11.5	162	44	0

Food and Measure	cal.	prot. (gms)	carbo. (gms)	tot. fat (gms)	sat. fat (gms)	chol. (mgs)	sod. (mgs)	fiber (gms)
CHIVES:								
1 lb.	115	12.7	17.2	2.7	.5	0	27	14.5 d
1 oz.	7	.8	1.1	.2	<.1	0	2	.9 d
chopped, 1 tbsp.	1	.1	.1	<.1	tr.	0	tr.	.1 d
CHIVES, FREEZE-DRIED:								
¼ cup	2	.2	.5	<.1	tr.	0	24	.1 c
1 tbsp.	1	<.1	.1	<.1	tr.	0	6	<.1 c
(*Tone's*), 1 tsp.	<1	<.1	<.1	tr.	0	0	m.q.	tr.d
CHOCOLATE, see "Candy"								
CHOCOLATE, BAKING, 1 oz.,								
except as noted:								
bars:								
semi-sweet:								
(*Baker's*)	140	1.0	17.0	9.0	m.q.	n.a.	0	m.q.
(*Hershey's* Premium)	140	1.0	16.0	8.0	m.q.	n.a.	0	m.q.
(*Nestlé*)	160	2.0	16.0	9.0	m.q.	n.a.	0	m.q.
sweet (*Baker's German*)	140	1.0	17.0	10.0	m.q.	n.a.	0	m.q.
unsweetened:								
(*Baker's*)	140	3.0	9.0	15.0	m.q.	n.a.	0	m.q.
(*Hershey's*)	190	4.0	7.0	16.0	m.q.	0	5	m.q.
(*Nestlé*)	180	4.0	9.0	14.0	m.q.	n.a.	0	m.q.
white (*Nestlé* Premier), ½ oz. ...	80	1.0	8.0	5.0	m.q.	n.a.	15	m.q.
chips:								
milk:								
(*Baker's*)	140	2.0	18.0	8.0	m.q.	5	25	m.q.
(*Baker's* Big Chip), ¼ cup	240	3.0	30.0	13.0	m.q.	10	40	m.q.
(*Hershey's*)	150	2.0	27.0	12.0	m.q.	10	55	m.q.
(*Nestlé* Toll House Morsels) ...	150	1.0	19.0	7.0	m.q.	n.a.	15	m.q.
mint (*Hershey's*), 1.5 oz. or ¼ cup	230	2.0	28.0	12.0	m.q.	n.a.	<1	m.q.
mint (*Nestlé* Toll House Morsels)	150	2.0	18.0	8.0	m.q.	n.a.	0	m.q.
semi-sweet:								
(*Baker's*), ¼ cup	200	2.0	28.0	11.0	m.q.	n.a.	0	m.q.
(*Baker's* Big Chip), ¼ cup	220	2.0	31.0	13.0	m.q.	n.a.	0	m.q.
(*Nestlé* Toll House Morsels) ...	150	2.0	18.0	8.0	m.q.	n.a.	0	m.q.
chocolate flavor (*Baker's*),								
¼ cup	200	2.0	30.0	9.0	m.q.	0	30	m.q.
regular or mini (*Hershey's*),								
1.5 oz. or ¼ cup	220	2.0	26.0	12.0	m.q.	0	5	m.q.
vanilla (white), milk (*Hershey's*),								
1.5 oz. or ¼ cup	240	3.0	25.0	14.0	m.q.	n.a.	65	m.q.
chunks or pieces:								
milk (*Hershey's* Chunks)	160	2.0	16.0	9.0	m.q.	n.a.	25	m.q.
milk (*Nestlé* Toll House *Treasures*)	150	2.0	17.0	9.0	m.q.	n.a.	20	m.q.
semi-sweet (*Hershey's* Chunks) ..	140	1.0	15.0	8.0	m.q.	n.a.	n.a.	m.q.
semi-sweet (*Nestlé* Toll House								
Treasures)	150	2.0	18.0	8.0	m.q.	n.a.	0	m.q.
white (*Nestlé* Toll House Premier								
Treasures)	160	2.0	15.0	10.0	m.q.	n.a.	25	m.q.

Food and Measure	cal.	prot. (gms)	carbo. (gms)	tot. fat (gms)	sat. fat (gms)	chol. (mgs)	sod. (mgs)	fiber (gms)
CHOCOLATE, BAKING *(cont.)*								
premelted, unsweetened (*Nestlé*								
Choco Bake)	190	4.0	7.0	16.0	m.q.	n.a.	0	m.q.
shreds (*Tone's*), 1 tsp.	21	.1	2.2	1.4	.8	0	1	.1 d
CHOCOLATE CAKE, see "Cake"								
CHOCOLATE FLAVOR DRINK,								
canned:								
(*Frostee*), 8 fl. oz.	200	2.0	30.0	8.0	m.q.	n.a.	160	(0)
plain or Dutch (*Sego* Lite), 10 fl. oz.	150	11.0	20.0	3.0	m.q.	5	480	(0)
plain or malt (*Sego* Very Chocolate),								
10 fl. oz.	225	11.0	43.0	1.0	n.a.	5	450	(0)
CHOCOLATE FLAVOR DRINK								
MIX (see also "Carob flavor								
mix" and "Cocoa"):								
powder:								
1 oz.	99	.9	25.6	.9	.5	0	60	.2 c
2–3 heaping tsp. or .8 oz.	75	.7	19.5	.7	.4	0	45	.2 c
(*Carnation* Instant Breakfast),								
1 pouch	130	6.0	25.0	1.0	.5	2	135	.2 d
(*Carnation* Instant Breakfast No								
Sugar Added), 1 pouch	70	6.0	10.0	1.0	.5	2	115	.2 d
(*Hershey's*), .8 oz. or 3 tsp.	90	1.0	22.0	4.0	m.q.	0	40	m.q.
(*Nestlé Quik*), ¾ oz., approx. 2½								
heaping tsp.	90	1.0	20.0	1.0	m.q.	0	25	m.q.
(*Nestlé Quik* Sugar Free), .2 oz.,								
approx. 1 heaping tsp.	18	1.0	3.0	<1.0	n.a.	n.a.	35	m.q.
(*Pillsbury* Instant Breakfast),								
1 pouch	130	6.0	26.0	0	0	0	190	m.q.
malt:								
(*Carnation* Instant Breakfast),								
1 pouch	130	6.0	24.0	2.0	.7	3	160	.2 d
(*Carnation* Instant Breakfast No								
Sugar Added), 1 pouch	70	6.0	8.0	2.0	.8	2	135	.2 d
(*Pillsbury* Instant Breakfast),								
1 pouch	130	6.0	26.0	0	0	0	190	m.q.
beverage:								
w/whole milk:								
1 cup milk and 2–3 heaping tsp.								
powder	226	8.8	30.9	8.8	5.5	33	165	.2 c
(*Nestlé Quik*), 1 cup milk and								
approx. 2½ heaping tsp.								
powder	230	9.0	31.0	9.0	m.q.	m.q.	150	m.q.
(*Pillsbury* Instant Breakfast),								
1 cup	290	14.0	38.0	9.0	m.q.	m.q.	310	m.q.
malt (*Pillsbury* Instant								
Breakfast), 1 cup	290	14.0	38.0	9.0	m.q.	m.q.	310	m.q.
w/lowfat 2% milk:								
1 cup milk and 2–3 heaping tsp.								
powder	196	8.8	31.2	5.4	3.3	18	167	.2 c

Food and Measure	cal.	prot. (gms)	carbo. (gms)	tot. fat (gms)	sat. fat (gms)	chol. (mgs)	sod. (mgs)	fiber (gms)
(*Nestlé Quik*), 1 cup milk and approx. 2½ heaping tsp. powder	210	9.0	31.0	5.0	m.q.	m.q.	150	m.q.
sugar free (*Nestlé Quik*), 1 cup milk and approx. 1 heaping tsp. powder	140	9.0	15.0	5.0	m.q.	m.q.	150	m.q.
1 cup lowfat 1% milk and 2–3 heaping tsp. powder	177	8.7	31.2	3.3	2.0	10	168	.2 c
w/skim milk:								
1 cup milk and 2–3 heaping tsp. powder	161	9.1	31.4	1.1	.7	4	171	.2 c
(*Nestlé Quik*), 1 cup milk and approx. 2½ heaping tsp. powder	170	9.0	31.0	1.0	m.q.	m.q.	150	m.q.
CHOCOLATE MILK, 1 cup, except as noted:								
1 fl. oz.	26	1.0	3.2	1.1	.7	4	19	<.1 c
1 cup	208	7.9	25.9	8.5	5.3	30	149	.2 c
(*Hershey's*)	210	7.0	28.0	9.0	m.q.	m.q.	120	m.q.
(*Meadow Gold*)	210	8.0	25.0	8.0	m.q.	m.q.	240	m.q.
lowfat:								
2% (*Borden* Dutch Brand)	180	8.0	25.0	5.0	m.q.	m.q.	180	m.q.
2% (*Darigold*)	190	8.0	28.0	5.0	3.1	17	210	m.q.
2% (*Hershey's*)	190	8.0	29.0	5.0	m.q.	20	130	m.q.
1% (*Knudsen*)	190	10.0	32.0	3.0	m.q.	m.q.	370	m.q.
mix, see "Chocolate flavor drink mix" and "Chocolate syrup"								
CHOCOLATE MOUSSE, see "Mousse"								
CHOCOLATE SYRUP (see also "Chocolate topping"):								
1 fl. oz. or 2 tbsp.	82	.7	22.1	.3	.2	0	36	.1 c
1 cup whole milk and 2 tbsp. syrup	232	8.8	33.5	8.5	5.3	33	156	.1 c
1 cup lowfat 2% milk and 2 tbsp. syrup	203	8.8	33.8	5.0	3.1	18	158	.1 c
1 cup lowfat 1% milk and 2 tbsp. syrup	184	8.7	33.8	2.9	1.8	10	159	.1 c
1 cup skim milk and 2 tbsp. syrup ..	168	9.1	34.0	.7	.5	4	162	.1 c
w/added nutrients:								
1 fl. oz.	92	.7	24.7	.5	.3	0	57	.2 c
1 tbsp.	46	.3	12.4	.2	.1	0	29	.1 c
1 cup whole milk and 1 tbsp. syrup	196	8.4	23.8	8.4	5.2	33	148	.1 c
1 cup lowfat 2% milk and 1 tbsp. syrup	167	8.4	24.1	4.9	3.1	18	151	.1 c
1 cup lowfat 1% milk and 1 tbsp. syrup	148	8.3	24.1	2.8	2.0	10	152	.1 c
1 cup skim milk and 1 tbsp. syrup	132	8.7	24.3	.6	.4	4	155	.1 c
(*Estee*), 1 tbsp.	20	<1.0	5.0	<1.0	<1.0	0	5	m.q.

Food and Measure	cal.	prot. (gms)	carbo. (gms)	tot. fat (gms)	sat. fat (gms)	chol. (mgs)	sod. (mgs)	fiber (gms)
CHOCOLATE SYRUP *(cont.)*								
(*Hershey's*), 1 oz. or 2 tbsp.	80	1.0	17.0	1.0	n.a.	0	20	m.q.
(*Nestlé Quik*), 1.22 oz., approx.								
2 tbsp.	100	1.0	22.0	1.0	n.a.	0	45	m.q.
(*Nestlé Quik*), 1 cup whole milk and								
1.22 oz. syrup	240	9.0	33.0	8.0	n.a.	n.a.	160	n.a.
(*Nestlé Quik*), 1 cup 2% lowfat milk								
and 1.22 oz. syrup	220	9.0	34.0	5.0	n.a.	n.a.	160	n.a.
(*Nestlé Quik*), 1 cup skim milk and								
1.22 oz. syrup	180	9.0	34.0	1.0	n.a.	n.a.	170	n.a.
CHOCOLATE TOPPING (see also								
"Chocolate syrup") 2 tbsp.,								
except as noted:								
(*Kraft*), 1 tbsp.	50	1.0	11.0	0	0	0	15	m.q.
(*Smucker's Magic Shell*)	190	1.0	16.0	15.0	m.q.	n.a.	25	m.q.
dark, flavored (*Smucker's* Special								
Recipe)	130	1.0	31.0	1.0	n.a.	n.a.	45	m.q.
flavored syrup (*Smucker's*)	130	1.0	27.0	2.0	m.q.	n.a.	40	m.q.
fudge:								
(*Hershey's*)	100	1.0	14.0	4.0	m.q.	5	30	m.q.
(*Smucker's*)	130	1.0	31.0	1.0	n.a.	n.a.	45	m.q.
(*Smucker's Magic Shell*)	190	1.0	16.0	15.0	m.q.	n.a.	50	m.q.
hot:								
(*Kraft*), 1 tbsp.	70	1.0	11.0	2.0	1.0	0	50	m.q.
(*Smucker's*)	110	1.0	18.0	4.0	m.q.	n.a.	55	m.q.
(*Smucker's* Special Recipe)	150	2.0	23.0	5.0	m.q.	n.a.	60	m.q.
Swiss milk chocolate (*Smucker's*)	140	3.0	31.0	1.0	n.a.	n.a.	70	m.q.
milk, w/almonds (*Nestlé Candytops*),								
1.25 oz.	230	2.0	14.0	18.0	m.q.	m.q.	15	m.q.
milk, w/crisps (*Nestlé Crunch*								
Candytops), 1.25 oz.	220	2.0	16.0	17.0	m.q.	m.q.	40	m.q.
nut (*Smucker's Magic Shell*)	200	2.0	15.0	16.0	m.q.	n.a.	40	m.q.
white, w/almonds (*Nestlé Candytops*),								
1.25 oz.	230	3.0	12.0	19.0	m.q.	n.a.	20	m.q.
CHOPS, VEGETARIAN, canned:								
(*Worthington Choplets*), 2 slices,								
3.25 oz.	100	17.0	5.0	2.0	m.q.	0	350	m.q.
CHORIZO, beef and pork:								
1 oz.	125	6.8	(0)	10.9	4.1	m.q.	m.q.	0
CHOW MEIN, see specific entree								
listings								
CHOW MEIN, VEGETARIAN,								
mix:								
Mandarin (*Tofu Classics*), ½ cup[1] ...	110	8.0	14.0	6.0	m.q.	0	390	m.q.
Mandarin (*Tofu Classics*), ½ cup[2] ...	134	8.0	14.0	9.0	m.q.	0	390	m.q.
CHOW MEIN NOODLES, see								
"Noodles, Chinese"								

1. *Prepared according to package directions, with tofu.*
2. *Prepared according to package directions, with tofu and 1 tbsp. oil.*

Food and Measure	cal.	prot. (gms)	carbo. (gms)	tot. fat (gms)	sat. fat (gms)	chol. (mgs)	sod. (mgs)	fiber (gms)
CHOWDER, see "Soup"								
CHRYSANTHEMUM GARLAND:								
raw:								
untrimmed, 1 lb.	76	6.8	19.0	.8	n.a.	0	225	3.9 c
trimmed, 1 oz.	5	.4	1.2	<.1	(0)	0	15	.3 c
1 stem, 8¾" long, .5 oz.	2	.2	.6	<.1	(0)	0	7	.1 c
1" pieces, ½ cup	2	.2	.5	<.1	(0)	0	7	.1 c
boiled, drained, 4 oz.	23	1.9	4.9	.1	(0)	0	60	1.3 c
boiled, drained, 1" pieces, ½ cup ...	10	.8	2.2	.1	(0)	0	27	.6 c
CHUB, see "Cisco, smoked"								
CIDER, see "Apple cider"								
CILANTRO, see "Coriander"								
CINNAMON, ground:								
1 oz.	74	1.1	22.6	.9	.2	0	7	6.9 c
1 tbsp.	18	.3	5.4	.2	<.1	0	2	1.7 c
1 tsp.	6	.1	1.8	.1	tr.	0	1	.6 c
(*Spice Islands*), 1 tsp.	6	.1	1.4	<.1	(0)	0	<1	.3 c
(*Tone's*), 1 tsp.	6	.1	1.8	.1	<.1	0	1	.6 d
CINNAMON DANISH, see "Danish pastry"								
CISCO, meat only:								
raw:								
1 lb.	446	86.1	0	8.7	1.9	m.q.	249	0
1 oz.	28	5.4	0	.5	.1	m.q.	16	0
1 fillet, approx. 2.8 oz., yield from 1-lb. whole fish	78	15.0	0	1.5	.3	m.q.	47	0
smoked, 4 oz.	201	18.6	0	13.5	2.0	36	545	0
smoked, 1 oz.	50	4.6	0	3.3	.5	9	135	0
CITRUS DRINK MIX[1]:								
blend (*Crystal Light* Sugar Free), 8 fl. oz.	4	0	0	0	0	0	0	0
CITRUS FRUIT JUICE DRINK:								
(*Hi-C* Citrus Cooler), 6 fl. oz.	95	.1	23.3	<.1	(0)	0	17	(0)
aseptic box (*Five Alive*), 8.45 fl. oz.	123	.8	30.7	0	0	0	32	(0)
chilled or frozen[2]:								
(*Five Alive*), 6 fl. oz.	87	.6	21.8	0	0	0	23	(0)
berry (*Five Alive*), 6 fl. oz.	88	.2	22.1	.1	(0)	0	21	(0)
tropical (*Five Alive*), 6 fl. oz.	85	.4	21.3	.1	(0)	0	19	(0)
frozen[3]:								
undiluted, 12-fl.-oz. can	684	4.9	170.5	.3	<.1	0	12	.8 d
1 fl. oz.	14	.1	3.6	tr.	tr.	0	1	<.1 d
8 fl. oz.	114	.8	28.4	tr.	tr.	0	7	.2 d
CITRUS PUNCH:								
chilled or frozen[2] (*Minute Maid*), 6 fl. oz.	93	.1	23.1	<.1	0	0	18	(0)

1. *Prepared according to package directions.*
2. *Diluted according to package directions.*
3. *Diluted according to package directions, except as noted.*

Food and Measure	cal.	prot. (gms)	carbo. (gms)	tot. fat (gms)	sat. fat (gms)	chol. (mgs)	sod. (mgs)	fiber (gms)
CITRUS SALAD:								
(*Florigold*), 8 oz.	120	2.7	27.2	0	0	0	3	m.q.
CLAM, mixed species, meat only:								
raw:								
1 lb.	335	57.9	11.6	4.4	.4	152	253	0
1 oz.	21	3.6	.7	.3	<.1	10	16	0
9 large or 20 small, approx.								
6.3 oz.	133	23.0	4.6	1.8	.2	60	100	0
boiled, poached, or steamed[1], 4 oz.	168	29.0	5.8	2.2	2.1	76	127	0
breaded[2], fried:								
4 oz.	229	16.1	11.7	12.6	3.0	69	413	.2 c
20 small, approx. 6.6 oz.	379	26.8	19.2	21.0	5.0	115	684	.3 c
CLAM, CANNED:								
mixed species:								
drained, 4 oz.	168	29.0	5.8	2.2	.2	76	127	0
drained, 1 cup	236	40.9	8.2	3.1	.3	107	179	0
liquid only, 4 oz.	2	.5	.1	<.1	m.q.	n.a.	244	0
liquid only, 1 cup	6	1.0	.2	.1	m.q.	n.a.	516	0
chopped or minced:								
(*Gorton's*), ½ can	70	12.0	4.0	1.0	m.q.	m.q.	640	0
(*Progresso*), ½ cup	70	12.0	2.0	<1.0	m.q.	31	140	0
w/liquid (*Doxsee*), 6.5 oz.	100	14.0	8.0	<1.0	m.q.	m.q.	1160	0
w/liquid (*Orleans*), 6.5 oz.	100	14.0	8.0	<1.0	m.q.	m.q.	1160	0
CLAM CHOWDER, see "Soup"								
CLAM DIP:								
(*Breakstone's*), 2 tbsp.	50	1.0	2.0	4.0	3.0	15	220	n.a.
(*Breakstone's* Gourmet Chesapeake),								
2 tbsp.	50	1.0	2.0	4.0	3.0	20	200	n.a.
(*Kraft*), 2 tbsp.	60	1.0	3.0	4.0	1.0	10	240	n.a.
(*Kraft* Premium), 2 tbsp.	45	1.0	2.0	4.0	2.0	20	210	n.a.
(*Sealtest*), 2 tbsp.	50	1.0	2.0	4.0	3.0	15	220	n.a.
CLAM ENTREE, frozen:								
battered, fried (*Mrs. Paul's*), 2.5 oz.	200	10.0	21.0	9.0	m.q.	15	450	m.q.
strips, crunchy (*Gorton's* Microwave								
Specialty), 3.5 oz.	330	10.0	24.0	22.0	6.0	30	430	m.q.
CLAM JUICE:								
(*Doxsee*), 3 fl. oz.	4	<1.0	0	0	0	n.a.	110	0
(*Snow's*), 3 fl. oz.	4	<1.0	0	0	0	n.a.	110	0
CLAM SAUCE, CANNED:								
red:								
(*Buitoni*), approx. 5 oz.	190	8.0	28.0	6.0	1.0	20	560	m.q.
(*Ferrara*), 4 oz.	70	5.0	8.0	2.0	0	10	320	m.q.
(*Progresso*), ½ cup	70	5.0	7.0	3.0	m.q.	m.q.	560	m.q.
white:								
(*Ferrara*), 4 oz.	80	5.0	4.0	5.0	1.0	10	570	m.q.
(*Progresso*), ½ cup	110	9.0	1.0	8.0	m.q.	m.q.	280	m.q.

1. *Without added ingredients.*
2. *Recipe: 84.2% clams, 9.3% bread crumbs, 4.6% egg, 1.4% milk, and .5% salt.*

Food and Measure	cal.	prot. (gms)	carbo. (gms)	tot. fat (gms)	sat. fat (gms)	chol. (mgs)	sod. (mgs)	fiber (gms)
(*Progresso* Authentic Pasta Sauces), ½ cup	130	8.0	4.0	9.0	1.0	19	460	<1.0 d
CLAM SAUCE, REFRIGERATED:								
red (*Contadina Fresh*), 7.5 oz.	120	7.0	15.0	4.0	m.q.	35	800	m.q.
white (*Contadina Fresh*), 6 oz.	290	8.0	13.0	23.0	m.q.	94	800	m.q.
CLAM AND TOMATO JUICE, see "Tomato–clam juice cocktail"								
CLOVES, ground:								
1 oz.	92	1.7	17.4	5.7	1.2	0	69	2.7 c
1 tbsp.	21	.4	4.0	1.3	.3	0	16	.6 c
1 tsp.	7	.1	1.3	.4	.1	0	5	.2 c
(*Tone's*), 1 tsp.	7	.1	1.4	.4	.1	0	5	.2 d
(*Spice Islands*), 1 tsp.	7	.1	1.2	.2	n.a.	0	4	.2 c
COATING MIX, see "Seasoning and coating mix" and specific listings								
COBBLER, ⅛ pie:								
apple, deep dish (*Awrey's*)	320	2.0	48.0	14.0	3.0	0	300	1.0 d
blueberry, deep dish (*Awrey's*)	310	2.0	45.0	14.0	3.0	0	360	2.0 d
COBBLER, FROZEN:								
apple (*Pet-Ritz*), ⅙ pkg., 4.33 oz. ..	290	1.0	50.0	9.0	m.q.	n.a.	m.q.	m.q.
apple (*Stilwell*), 4 oz.	200	2.0	4.0	4.0	m.q.	n.a.	225	m.q.
blackberry (*Pet-Ritz*), ⅙ pkg., 4.33 oz.	250	2.0	39.0	10.0	m.q.	n.a.	m.q.	m.q.
blackberry (*Stilwell*), 4 oz.	280	3.0	50.0	8.0	m.q.	n.a.	220	m.q.
blueberry (*Pet-Ritz*), ⅙ pkg., 4.33 oz.	370	3.0	50.0	12.0	m.q.	n.a.	m.q.	m.q.
cherry (*Pet-Ritz*), ⅙ pkg., 4.33 oz.	280	2.0	46.0	10.0	m.q.	n.a.	m.q.	m.q.
cherry (*Stilwell*), 4 oz.	250	3.0	46.0	6.0	m.q.	n.a.	205	m.q.
peach (*Pet-Ritz*), ⅙ pkg., 4.33 oz. ..	260	2.0	46.0	10.0	m.q.	n.a.	m.q.	m.q.
peach (*Stilwell*), 4 oz.	270	2.0	55.0	5.0	m.q.	n.a.	200	m.q.
strawberry (*Pet-Ritz*), ⅙ pkg., 4.33 oz.	290	1.0	50.0	9.0	m.q.	n.a.	m.q.	m.q.
COCKTAIL SAUCE (see also "Seafood sauce"), 1 tbsp., except as noted:								
(*Del Monte*), ¼ cup	70	1.0	17.0	0	0	0	765	n.a.
(*Estee*)	10	<1.0	2.0	<1.0	<1.0	0	35	n.a.
(*Great Impressions*)	21	.2	4.7	.1	(0)	0	182	n.a.
(*Great Impressions* Brandy Glow) ...	68	.2	1.6	6.7	m.q.	10	106	n.a.
(*Great Impressions* Low Salt)	21	.2	4.8	.1	(0)	0	6	n.a.
(*Heinz*)	17	.2	3.8	.1	(0)	0	180	n.a.
(*Sauceworks*)	14	0	3.0	0	0	0	170	n.a.
(*Stokely*)	18	0	5.0	0	0	0	90	n.a.
regular or extra hot (*Golden Dipt*) ..	20	0	5.0	0	0	0	210	n.a.
COCOA, powder:								
(*Bensdorp*), 1 oz.	130	6.0	8.0	7.0	m.q.	<1.0	5	m.q.
(*Hershey's*), 1 oz. or ⅓ cup	120	7.0	13.0	4.0	m.q.	0	10	m.q.

Food and Measure	cal.	prot. (gms)	carbo. (gms)	tot. fat (gms)	sat. fat (gms)	chol. (mgs)	sod. (mgs)	fiber (gms)
COCOA *(cont.)*								
(Hershey's European), 1 oz.	90	7.0	8.0	3.0	m.q.	0	15	m.q.
(Nestlé), 1.5 oz. or ½ cup	180	11.0	21.0	6.0	m.q.	n.a.	6	m.q.
COCOA BUTTER OIL:								
1 oz.	251	0	0	28.4	16.9	0	0	0
½ cup	964	0	0	109.0	65.1	0	0	0
1 tbsp.	120	0	0	13.6	8.1	0	0	0
COCOA MIX:								
powder, 1-oz. pkt. or 3–4 heaping								
tsp.	102	3.1	22.5	1.1	.7	n.a.	143	.2 c
6 fl. oz. water and 3–4 heaping tsp.								
powder	103	3.1	22.5	1.1	.7	n.a.	149	.2 c
w/added nutrients[1]:								
powder, 1.1-oz. pkt.	120	1.9	24.0	3.0	1.8	n.a.	201	m.q.
1 fl. oz.	20	.3	4.0	.5	.3	n.a.	35	m.q.
6 fl. oz. water and 1.1-oz. pkt.								
powder	120	1.9	24.1	3.0	1.8	n.a.	207	m.q.
reduced calorie, Aspartame								
sweetened:								
powder, .5-oz. pkt.	48	3.8	8.5	.4	.3	n.a.	m.q.	m.q.
1 fl. oz.	8	.6	1.4	.1	<.1	n.a.	m.q.	m.q.
6 fl. oz. water and .5-oz. pkt. ..	48	3.8	8.5	.4	.3	n.a.	m.q.	m.q.
regular or w/mini marshmallows								
(Finast), 6 fl. oz.	110	2.0	24.0	1.0	m.q.	n.a.	150	m.q.
chocolate *(Pathmark* No Frills),								
1 oz. dry	110	2.0	24.0	1.0	m.q.	n.a.	110	m.q.
(Carnation 70-Calorie), 1 pkt.	70	3.0	16.0	.3	.2	1	135	.2 c
(Featherweight), .44 oz.	50	2.0	8.0	1.0	m.q.	0	110	m.q.
(Hills Bros), 2 tbsp. dry, or 6 fl. oz.[2]	110	3.0	23.0	1.0	m.q.	n.a.	55	m.q.
(Hills Bros Sugar Free), 3 tsp. dry,								
or 6 fl. oz.[2]	60	2.0	9.0	2.0	m.q.	n.a.	145	m.q.
(Pathmark), 1 oz. or 4 heaping tsp.	110	2.0	24.0	1.0	m.q.	n.a.	160	m.q.
(Swiss Miss Lite), .76-oz. pkt.	70	1.0	17.0	.8	.2	n.a.	160	m.q.
Amaretto creme *(Swiss Miss)*,								
1.25 oz.	150	2.0	29.0	3.0	m.q.	n.a.	220	m.q.
chocolate:								
(Swiss Miss), 1 oz.	110	1.0	24.0	1.0	n.a.	n.a.	125	m.q.
(Swiss Miss Sugar Free), .5 oz. ..	50	2.0	9.0	1.0	.2	<1	130	m.q.
double rich *(Swiss Miss)*, 1 oz. ...	110	2.0	24.0	1.0	n.a.	0	125	m.q.
fudge *(Carnation)*, 1-oz. pkt.	110	1.0	24.0	1.3	1.1	1	135	.3 d
milk:								
(Carnation), 1-oz. pkt. or								
4 heaping tsp.	110	2.0	24.0	1.1	1.0	1	130	.2 d
(Swiss Miss), 1-oz. pkt.	110	1.0	20.0	3.0	1.3	<1	170	m.q.
(Swiss Miss Sugar Free), .5 oz. ..	60	3.0	10.0	0	0	n.a.	125	m.q.
milk and marshmallow *(Weight*								
Watchers), 1 pkt.	60	6.0	10.0	0	0	0	160	m.q.

1. *Prepared according to package directions, except as noted.*
2. *Prepared according to package directions.*

Food and Measure	cal.	prot. (gms)	carbo. (gms)	tot. fat (gms)	sat. fat (gms)	chol. (mgs)	sod. (mgs)	fiber (gms)
rich (*Carnation*), 1-oz. pkt. or								
4 heaping tsp.	110	1.0	24.0	1.1	1.0	1	120	.2 d
rich (*Carnation* Sugar Free),								
1 pkt.	50	4.0	8.0	.4	.2	3	160	.1 d
w/marshmallows:								
(*Carnation*), 1-oz. pkt. or								
4 heaping tsp.	110	1.0	24.0	1.0	.9	1	120	.2 d
chocolate (*Carnation*), 1-oz. pkt.	110	1.0	24.0	1.2	1.1	2	120	.2 d
mini:								
(*Pathmark*), 1 oz.	110	2.0	24.0	1.0	m.q.	n.a.	140	m.q.
(*Swiss Miss*), 1 oz.	110	1.0	23.0	1.0	n.a.	n.a.	140	m.q.
Swiss Miss Sugar Free), .5-oz.								
pkg.	50	3.0	9.0	<1.0	n.a.	n.a.	120	m.q.
mint (*Featherweight*), .44 oz.	50	2.0	8.0	1.0	m.q.	0	110	m.q.
mocha (*Carnation* Sugar Free),								
1 pkt.	50	3.0	9.0	.3	.2	2	140	.1 d
COCONUT, mature kernel:								
in shell, 1 lb.	834	7.9	35.9	79.0	70.0	0	47	21.2 d
shelled:								
1 oz.	100	.9	4.3	9.5	8.4	0	6	2.6 d
1 piece, 2″ × 2″ × ½″, approx.								
1.6 oz.	159	1.5	6.9	15.1	13.4	0	9	4.1 d
shredded or grated, 1 cup	283	2.7	12.2	26.8	23.8	0	16	7.2 d
shredded or grated, 1 cup packed	460	4.3	19.8	43.5	38.6	0	26	11.7 d
COCONUT, CANNED OR								
PACKAGED, see "Coconut,								
dried"								
COCONUT, DRIED (desiccated):								
creamed, 1 oz.	194	1.5	6.1	19.6	17.4	0	11	1.1 c
unsweetened, 1 oz.	187	2.0	6.7	18.3	16.3	0	11	1.5 c
sweetened, flaked:								
canned:								
4 oz.	505	3.8	46.6	36.1	32.0	0	23	2.4 c
1 oz.	126	.9	11.6	9.0	8.0	0	6	.6 c
1 cup	341	2.6	31.5	24.4	21.6	0	15	1.7 c
(*Baker's Angel Flake*), ⅓ cup ..	110	1.0	10.0	9.0	m.q.	0	5	m.q.
packaged:								
7-oz. pkg.	944	6.5	94.7	64.0	56.7	0	509	4.2 c
1 oz.	134	.9	13.5	9.1	8.1	0	73	.6 c
1 cup	351	2.4	35.2	23.8	21.1	0	189	1.6 c
(*Baker's Angel Flake*), ⅓ cup ..	120	1.0	10.0	8.0	m.q.	0	75	m.q.
(*Finast* Snowflake), 1 oz.	137	1.0	12.0	9.0	m.q.	0	<1	m.q.
toasted (*Baker's Angel Flake*),								
⅓ cup	200	2.0	17.0	17.0	m.q.	0	85	m.q.
sweetened, shredded:								
7-oz. pkg.	997	5.7	94.9	70.6	62.6	0	522	4.3 c
1 oz.	142	.8	13.5	10.1	8.9	0	74	.6 c
cookie shred, 1 cup	466	2.7	44.3	33.0	29.3	0	244	2.0 c
(*Baker's* Premium Shred), ⅓ cup	140	1.0	12.0	9.0	m.q.	0	85	m.q.

Food and Measure	cal.	prot. (gms)	carbo. (gms)	tot. fat (gms)	sat. fat (gms)	chol. (mgs)	sod. (mgs)	fiber (gms)
COCONUT, DRIED *(cont.)*								
toasted, 1 oz.	168	1.5	12.6	13.4	11.8	0	11	.7 c
COCONUT CREAM[1]:								
raw:								
1 oz.	94	1.0	1.9	9.8	8.7	0	1	m.q.
1 cup	792	8.7	16.0	83.2	73.8	0	10	m.q.
1 tbsp.	49	.5	1.0	5.2	4.6	0	1	m.q.
canned, sweetened:								
1 oz.	54	.8	2.4	5.0	4.5	0	14	m.q.
1 cup	568	8.0	24.7	52.5	46.5	0	149	m.q.
1 tbsp.	36	.5	1.6	3.4	3.0	0	10	m.q.
(*Coco Lopez*), 2 tbsp.	120	0	20.0	5.0	m.q.	0	10	m.q.
(*Holland House*), 1 fl. oz.	81	0	18.0	m.q.	m.q.	0	21	m.q.
COCONUT MILK[2]:								
raw:								
1 oz.	65	.6	1.6	6.8	6.0	0	4	m.q.
1 cup	552	5.5	13.3	57.2	50.7	0	37	m.q.
1 tbsp.	35	.3	.8	3.6	3.2	0	2	m.q.
canned:								
1 oz.	56	.6	.8	6.0	5.4	0	4	m.q.
1 cup	445	4.6	6.3	48.2	42.7	0	29	m.q.
1 tbsp.	30	.3	.4	3.2	2.8	0	2	m.q.
frozen:								
1 oz.	57	.5	1.6	5.9	5.2	0	3	m.q.
1 cup	486	3.9	13.4	49.9	44.3	0	29	m.q.
1 tbsp.	30	.2	.8	3.1	2.8	0	2	m.q.
COCONUT OIL:								
1 oz.	251	0	0	28.4	24.5	0	0	0
½ cup	964	0	0	109.0	94.3	0	0	0
1 tbsp.	120	0	0	13.6	11.8	0	0	0
(*Hain*), 1 tbsp.	120	0	0	14.0	12.0	0	0	0
COCONUT WATER[3]:								
1 oz.	5	.2	1.1	.1	<.1	0	30	<.1 c
1 cup	46	1.7	8.9	.5	.4	0	252	.1 c
1 tbsp.	3	.1	.6	<.1	<.1	0	16	tr.c
COD, ATLANTIC, meat only:								
raw:								
1 lb.	372	80.8	0	3.1	.6	195	246	0
1 oz.	23	5.0	0	.2	<.1	12	15	0
1 fillet, approx. 8.1 oz., yield from								
3-lb. whole fish	190	41.1	0	1.6	.3	99	125	0
baked, broiled, or microwaved[4],								
4 oz.	119	25.9	0	1.0	.2	62	88	0
dried, salted, 1 oz.	81	17.6	0	.7	.1	42	1968	0

1. *Liquid expressed from grated coconut meat.*
2. *Liquid expressed from mixture of grated coconut meat and water.*
3. *Liquid from coconuts.*
4. *Without added ingredients.*

Food and Measure	cal.	prot. (gms)	carbo. (gms)	tot. fat (gms)	sat. fat (gms)	chol. (mgs)	sod. (mgs)	fiber (gms)
COD, ATLANTIC, CANNED, w/liquid:								
11-oz. can	327	71.0	0	2.7	.5	171	680	0
4 oz.	119	25.8	0	1.0	.2	62	247	0
COD, FROZEN, fillet:								
(*Booth*), 4 oz.	89	20.0	0	1.0	m.q.	m.q.	350	0
(*Booth* Individually Wrapped),								
4 oz.	90	20.0	0	1.0	m.q.	m.q.	80	0
(*Gorton's Fishmarket Fresh*), 5 oz. ...	110	26.0	0	1.0	m.q.	m.q.	90	0
(*SeaPak*), 4 oz.	90	20.0	0	1.0	m.q.	m.q.	135	0
(*Van de Kamp's* Natural), 4 oz.	90	20.0	0	1.0	0	25	90	0
skinless (*Finast*), 4 oz.	80	18.0	0	1.0	m.q.	m.q.	200	0
COD, PACIFIC, meat only, raw:								
1 lb.	372	81.2	0	2.9	.4	168	322	0
1 oz.	23	5.1	0	.2	<.1	10	20	0
1 fillet, approx. 4.1 oz., yield from								
1½-lb. whole fish	95	20.8	0	.7	.1	43	82	0
COD ENTREE, frozen:								
fillet:								
au gratin (*Booth*), 9.5 oz.	280	27.0	18.0	11.0	m.q.	m.q.	1160	m.q.
breaded (*Van de Kamp's* Light),								
1 piece	250	17.0	20.0	11.0	2.0	35	510	m.q.
breaded (*Mrs. Paul's* Light),								
1 piece	240	15.0	22.0	11.0	m.q.	m.q.	430	m.q.
Florentine (*Booth*), 9.5 oz.	244	20.0	29.0	6.0	m.q.	m.q.	880	m.q.
w/lemon butter sauce and rice								
(*Booth*), 9.5 oz.	567	22.0	27.0	38.0	m.q.	m.q.	1330	m.q.
w/mushroom sauce and rice								
(*Booth*), 9.5 oz.	280	27.0	19.0	11.0	m.q.	m.q.	1010	m.q.
minced, nuggets, crunchy (*Frionor*								
Bunch O'Crunch), 8 pieces or								
4 oz.	320	14.0	19.0	21.0	3.0	m.q.	411	<.1 d
COD LIVER OIL:								
regular or mint (*Hain*), 1 tbsp.	120	0	0	14.0	m.q.	85	0	0
cherry (*Hain*), 1 tbsp.	120	0	0	14.0	m.q.	75	0	0
COFFEE:								
brewed, 6 fl. oz.	4	.1	.8	0	0	0	4	0
(*Chock Full O'Nuts* Regular/								
Decaffeinated), 6 fl. oz.	2	m.q.	m.q.	0	0	0	0	0
instant:								
regular, 1 oz. powder	68	3.5	11.7	.1	<.1	0	10	0
regular, 1 rounded tsp. powder ..	4	.2	.7	tr.	tr.	0	1	0
(*Kava*), 1 tsp. powder	2	0	1.0	0	0	0	<5	0
(*Nescafé/Nescafé Decaf*), 8 fl. oz.								
prepared	4	<1.0	1.0	<1.0	(0)	0	0	0
(*Nescafé* Classic/Brava/Silka),								
8 fl. oz. prepared	4	<1.0	1.0	<1.0	(0)	0	0	0

Food and Measure	cal.	prot. (gms)	carbo. (gms)	tot. fat (gms)	sat. fat (gms)	chol. (mgs)	sod. (mgs)	fiber (gms)
COFFEE, INSTANT *(cont.)*								
w/chicory (*Nescafé* Mountain Blend/Mountain Blend Decaffeinated), 8 fl. oz. prepared	6	<1.0	1.0	<1.0	(0)	0	0	0
w/chicory (*Sunrise*), 8 fl. oz. prepared	6	<1.0	1.0	<1.0	(0)	0	0	0
freeze-dried, prepared:								
(*Taster's Choice* Original/Original Decaffeinated), 8 fl. oz.	4	<1.0	1.0	<1.0	(0)	0	0	0
Colombian (*Taster's Choice* Colombian Select), 8 fl. oz.	4	<1.0	1.0	<1.0	(0)	0	0	0
dark roast (*Taster's Choice* Maragor/Maragor Decaffeinated), 8 fl. oz.	4	<1.0	1.0	<1.0	(0)	0	0	0
COFFEE, FLAVORED[1], 6 fl. oz.:								
café Amaretto (*General Foods International*)	50	0	7.0	2.0	m.q.	0	20	(0)
café Francais (*General Foods International*)	60	0	6.0	3.0	m.q.	0	15	(0)
café Francais (*General Foods International Sugar Free*)	35	0	3.0	2.0	m.q.	0	30	(0)
café Irish creme (*General Foods International*)	50	0	8.0	2.0	m.q.	0	15	(0)
café Vienna:								
(*General Foods* International)	60	0	10.0	2.0	m.q.	0	110	(0)
(*General Foods* International Sugar Free)	30	0	3.0	2.0	m.q.	0	80	(0)
(*Hills Bros* Cafe Coffees)	60	1.0	9.0	2.0	m.q.	n.a.	35	(0)
chocolate, double Dutch (*General Foods* International)	50	0	8.0	2.0	m.q.	0	15	(0)
chocolate mint, Dutch (*General Foods International*)	50	0	8.0	2.0	m.q.	0	80	(0)
mocha:								
(*General Foods* International Suisse)	50	0	7.0	3.0	m.q.	0	15	(0)
(*General Foods* International Suisse Sugar Free)	30	0	3.0	2.0	m.q.	0	15	(0)
(*MJB*)	52	.6	9.5	1.3	m.q.	n.a.	54	(0)
banana nut (*MJB* Sugar Free)	39	.8	4.9	1.8	m.q.	n.a.	60	(0)
cherry (*MJB*)	53	.5	9.7	1.4	m.q.	n.a.	17	(0)
fudge (*MJB* Sugar Free)	39	1.2	4.5	1.8	m.q.	n.a.	88	(0)
mint (*MJB*)	53	.4	9.9	1.3	m.q.	n.a.	16	(0)
mint (*MJB* Sugar Free)	37	.7	5.6	1.3	m.q.	n.a.	43	(0)
Swiss (*Hills Bros* Cafe Coffees)	60	1.0	8.0	2.0	m.q.	n.a.	10	(0)
Swiss (*Hills Bros* Cafe Coffees Sugar Free)	40	1.0	5.0	2.0	m.q.	n.a.	25	(0)
vanilla (*MJB* Sugar Free)	39	.7	5.2	1.7	m.q.	n.a.	50	(0)

1. *Prepared according to package directions.*

Food and Measure	cal.	prot. (gms)	carbo. (gms)	tot. fat (gms)	sat. fat (gms)	chol. (mgs)	sod. (mgs)	fiber (gms)
orange:								
cappuccino (*General Foods* International)	60	0	10.0	2.0	m.q.	0	100	(0)
cappuccino (*General Foods* International Sugar Free)	30	0	3.0	2.0	m.q.	0	60	(0)
Capri (*Hills Bros* Cafe Coffees) ..	60	1.0	9.0	2.0	m.q.	n.a.	30	(0)
COFFEE, SUBSTITUTE, cereal grain beverage:								
powder:								
1 tsp.	9	.1	1.9	.1	<.1	0	2	tr.c
(*Pero*), 1 serving	4	<1.0	<1.0	0	0	0	<2	(0)
(*Pionier*), 1 serving	6	0	1.4	0	0	0	0	(0)
beverage:								
6 fl. oz. water and 1 tsp. powder	9	.1	1.9	.1	<.1	0	7	tr.c
6 fl. oz. whole milk and 1 tsp. powder	121	6.1	10.4	6.2	3.8	25	91	tr.c
6 fl. oz. lowfat 2% milk and 1 tsp. powder	100	6.2	10.7	3.6	2.2	14	94	tr.c
6 fl. oz. lowfat 1% milk and 1 tsp. powder	86	6.1	10.6	2.0	1.2	8	94	tr.c
6 fl. oz. skim milk and 1 tsp. powder	74	6.4	10.8	.4	.2	3	97	tr.c
(*Kaffree Roma*), 8 fl. oz.[1]	6	0	1.0	0	0	0	m.q.	n.a.
regular or coffee flavor (*Postum* Instant), 6 fl. oz.[1]	12	0	3.0	0	0	0	0	n.a.
COFFEE CAKE, see "Cake"								
COFFEE-FLAVORED DRINK MIX:								
(*Carnation* Instant Breakfast), 1 pouch	130	6.0	25.0	.2	.1	3	150	.1 d
COFFEE LIQUEUR:								
53 proof, 1 fl. oz.	117	tr.	16.3	.1	<.1	0	3	0
cream, 34 proof, 1 fl. oz.	102	.9	6.5	4.9	3.0	n.a.	29	0
COFFEE WHITENER, see "Creamer, nondairy"								
COGNAC, see "Liquor"								
COLA, see "Soft drinks and mixers"								
COLD CUTS, see "Luncheon meat" and specific listings								
COLESLAW[2]:								
4 oz.	78	1.5	14.1	3.0	.4	9	26	.7 c
½ cup	42	.8	7.5	1.6	.2	5	14	.4 c
1 tbsp.	6	.1	1.0	.2	<.1	1	2	.1 c
COLLARDS:								
raw:								
untrimmed, 1 lb.	80	4.1	18.4	.6	n.a.	0	51	1.5 c
trimmed, 1 oz.	9	.4	2.0	.1	(0)	0	6	.2 c

1. *Prepared according to package directions.*
2. *Recipe: 41% cabbage, 12% celery, 12% table cream, 10% sugar, 7% green pepper, 6% lemon juice, 4% onion, 3% pimiento, 3% vinegar, 2% salt, dry mustard, and white pepper.*

Food and Measure	cal.	prot. (gms)	carbo. (gms)	tot. fat (gms)	sat. fat (gms)	chol. (mgs)	sod. (mgs)	fiber (gms)
COLLARDS, RAW *(cont.)*								
chopped, ½ cup	6	.3	1.3	<.1	(0)	0	4	.1 c
boiled, drained, 4 oz.	31	1.5	7.0	.2	(0)	0	18	.6 c
boiled, drained, chopped, ½ cup ...	17	.9	3.9	.1	(0)	0	10	.3 c
COLLARDS, CANNED:								
chopped (*Allens*), ½ cup	20	2.0	2.0	<1.0	(0)	0	15	m.q.
chopped, w/pork (*Luck's*), 7.5 oz. ...	90	2.0	7.0	7.0	m.q.	m.q.	420	m.q.
COLLARDS, FROZEN:								
10-oz. pkg.	93	7.7	18.3	1.1	n.a.	0	136	2.8 c
boiled, drained, 4 oz.	41	3.4	8.1	.5	(0)	0	57	1.2 c
boiled, drained, chopped, ½ cup ...	31	2.5	6.1	.4	(0)	0	42	.9 c
chopped (*Seabrook*), 3.3 oz.	25	3.0	4.0	0	0	0	45	1.0 c
chopped (*Southern*), 3.5 oz.	30	2.7	4.6	.4	(0)	0	60	m.q.
COLORADO PINYON PINE, see "Pine nut, piñon"								
COOKIE:								
almond, 1 piece:								
(*Stella D'oro* Breakfast Treats)	101	1.6	15.4	3.6	m.q.	n.a.	m.q.	m.q.
(*Stella D'oro* Chinese Dessert)	169	2.4	19.5	8.9	m.q.	n.a.	m.q.	m.q.
toast (*Stella D'oro* Mandel)	58	1.3	10.2	1.4	n.a.	n.a.	m.q.	m.q.
almond-date (*Health Valley Fruit Jumbos*), 1 piece	70	2.0	10.0	3.0	m.q.	0	30	1.1 d
amaranth (*Health Valley Amaranth Cookies*), 1 piece	90	2.0	12.0	3.0	m.q.	0	30	2.3 d
animal crackers:								
(*Barnum's*), 5 pieces, ½ oz.	60	1.0	11.0	2.0	<1.0	0	70	m.q.
(*FFV*), 1.25-oz. pkg.	160	2.0	26.0	6.0	1.0	0	150	m.q.
(*Finast*), 1 oz., approx. 15 pieces	120	2.0	22.0	3.0	m.q.	n.a.	110	m.q.
(*Keebler*), 5 pieces, approx. ½ oz.	70	1.0	11.0	2.0	<1.0	0	75	m.q.
(*Sunshine*), 13 pieces	130	2.0	21.0	4.0	1.0	0	160	m.q.
anise:								
(*Stella D'oro* Anisette Sponge), 1 piece	51	1.1	9.9	.8	n.a.	n.a.	m.q.	m.q.
(*Stella D'oro* Anisette Toast), 1 piece	46	.8	9.3	.6	n.a.	n.a.	m.q.	m.q.
(*Stella D'oro* Anisette Toast Jumbo), 1 piece	109	2.0	23.0	1.0	n.a.	n.a.	m.q.	m.q.
apple:								
bar (*Apple Newtons*), ¾-oz. piece	70	1.0	15.0	2.0	<1.0	0	70	m.q.
bar, Dutch (*Stella D'oro*), 1 piece	112	1.4	18.9	3.3	m.q.	n.a.	m.q.	m.q.
pastry, dietetic (*Stella D'oro*), 1 piece	86	1.0	13.0	3.3	m.q.	n.a.	<10	m.q.
apple n' raisin (*Archway*), 1 piece ...	120	2.0	20.0	3.0	m.q.	10	169	1.0 d
apple-raisin bar (*Weight Watchers*), 1 piece	100	1.0	18.0	3.0	m.q.	n.a.	115	m.q.
apricot-almond (*Health Valley Fancy Fruit Chunks*), 2 pieces	90	2.0	14.0	4.0	m.q.	0	45	1.8 d
apricot-raspberry (*Pepperidge Farm Fruit Cookies*), 2 pieces	100	1.0	15.0	4.0	2.0	10	50	m.q.

Food and Measure	cal.	prot. (gms)	carbo. (gms)	tot. fat (gms)	sat. fat (gms)	chol. (mgs)	sod. (mgs)	fiber (gms)
apricot-raspberry (*Pepperidge Farm* Zurich), 1 piece	60	1.0	10.0	2.0	1.0	0	30	m.q.
arrowroot biscuit (*National*), ¼-oz. piece	20	0	3.0	1.0	<1.0	<2	15	m.q.
assorted:								
(*Archway* Select Assortment), 1 piece	50	1.0	7.0	2.0	m.q.	5	40	m.q.
(*Stella D'oro* Hostess), 1 piece ...	42	.5	5.5	2.0	m.q.	n.a.	m.q.	m.q.
(*Stella D'oro* Lady Stella), 1 piece	42	.6	5.5	2.0	m.q.	n.a.	m.q.	m.q.
fig, apple, strawberry (*Newtons*), 1¼-oz. piece	120	1.0	24.0	3.0	1.0	0	110	m.q.
brownie (see also "Brownie"):								
chocolate nut (*Pepperidge Farm* Old Fashioned), 2 pieces	110	1.0	11.0	7.0	2.0	<5	45	m.q.
cream sandwich (*Pepperidge Farm* Capri), 1 piece	80	0	10.0	5.0	1.0	0	45	m.q.
butter flavor:								
(*Pepperidge Farm* Chessmen), 2 pieces	90	1.0	12.0	4.0	2.0	10	60	m.q.
chocolate coated (*Keebler* Baby Bear), 3 pieces, approx. ½ oz.	70	1.0	10.0	2.0	<1.0	0	55	m.q.
chocolate coated (*Keebler E.L. Fudge*), 2 pieces, approx. ½ oz.	80	<1.0	10.0	4.0	1.0	<5	40	m.q.
caramel patties (*FFV*), 2 pieces, approx. 1 oz.	150	1.0	20.0	7.0	m.q.	n.a.	125	m.q.
carrot walnut (*Pepperidge Farm* Wholesome Choice), 1 piece ...	60	1.0	11.0	1.0	<1.0	0	45	m.q.
(*Carr's Hob-Nobs*), 1 piece	72	1.1	9.6	3.2	m.q.	n.a.	78	m.q.
(*Carr's Muesli*), 1 piece	84	1.1	10.8	4.1	m.q.	n.a.	30	m.q.
chocolate:								
(*Stella D'oro* Castelets), 1 piece ..	64	.8	9.0	2.8	m.q.	n.a.	m.q.	m.q.
(*Stella D'oro* Margherite), 1 piece	72	.9	10.2	3.1	m.q.	n.a.	m.q.	m.q.
(*Weight Watchers*), 3 pieces	80	1.0	13.0	3.0	m.q.	n.a.	70	m.q.
creme wafer (*Featherweight*), 1 piece	20	0	3.0	1.0	n.a.	0	0	m.q.
fudge:								
(*Estee*), 1 piece	30	<1.0	4.0	1.0	<1.0	0	0	m.q.
(*Stella D'oro* Swiss), 1 piece ...	68	.8	8.5	3.4	m.q.	n.a.	m.q.	m.q.
bar (*Tastykake*), 1.8 oz.	205	2.3	35.0	6.8	2.1	6	155	1.4 d
mint (*Keebler Grasshopper*), 2 pieces, approx. ½ oz.	70	<1.0	10.0	3.0	1.0	0	35	m.q.
middles (*Nabisco*), ½-oz. piece ..	80	1.0	9.0	5.0	2.0	<5	35	m.q.
snaps (*Nabisco*), 4 pieces or ½ oz.	70	1.0	11.0	2.0	1.0	<2	75	m.q.
wafer (*Nabisco* Famous Wafers), ½ oz., approx. 2½ pieces	70	1.0	11.0	2.0	<1.0	<2	110	m.q.

Food and Measure	cal.	prot. (gms)	carbo. (gms)	tot. fat (gms)	sat. fat (gms)	chol. (mgs)	sod. (mgs)	fiber (gms)
COOKIE *(cont.)*								
chocolate chip:								
(*Almost Home* Real Chocolate								
Chip), ½-oz. piece	60	1.0	7.0	3.0	1.0	<2	45	m.q.
(*Archway*), 1 piece	50	1.0	7.0	3.0	m.q.	5	40	m.q.
(*Chips Ahoy!* Pure Chocolate								
Chip), ½-oz. piece	50	1.0	7.0	2.0	<1.0	0	40	m.q.
(*Drake's*), 2 pieces, approx. 1 oz.	140	1.0	18.0	6.0	2.0	0	110	m.q.
(*Duncan Hines*), 2 pieces	110	1.0	15.0	5.0	m.q.	n.a.	90	m.q.
(*Featherweight*), 1 piece	45	1.0	6.0	2.0	m.q.	0	0	m.q.
(*Finast*), 1 oz.	90	1.0	18.0	7.0	m.q.	0	60	m.q.
(*Grandma's* Big Cookies),								
2 pieces, approx. 2.75 oz.	370	4.0	50.0	17.0	m.q.	5	270	m.q.
(*Keebler Chips Deluxe*), 1 piece,								
approx. ½ oz.	80	<1.0	10.0	4.0	1.0	<5	75	m.q.
(*Keebler Soft Batch*), 1 piece,								
approx. ½ oz.	80	<1.0	10.0	4.0	1.0	0	70	m.q.
(*Mini Chips Ahoy!*), 6 pieces	70	1.0	9.0	3.0	1.0	0	45	m.q.
(*Pepperidge Farm* Old Fashioned),								
2 pieces	100	1.0	12.0	5.0	2.0	5	45	m.q.
(*Tastykake* Soft'n Chewy), 1.4 oz.	174	2.3	25.5	7.3	2.1	10	168	.9 d
bar (*Tastykake*), 1 piece, 1.5 oz. ..	193	3.0	28.3	8.4	1.5	4	97	1.0 d
w/candy coated chocolate (*Keebler*								
Rainbow Chips Deluxe), 1 piece,								
approx. ½ oz.	80	1.0	11.0	3.0	1.0	<5	45	m.q.
chewy (*Chips Ahoy!*), ½-oz. piece	60	1.0	7.0	3.0	1.0	<2	40	m.q.
chocolate:								
(*Drake's*), 2 pieces, approx.								
1 oz.	130	2.0	19.0	5.0	1.0	0	85	m.q.
(*Tastykake* Soft'n Chewy),								
1.4 oz.	171	2.1	26.2	7.0	2.1	3	111	1.1 d
chunk (*Chips Ahoy!* Selections),								
½-oz. piece	90	1.0	10.0	5.0	2.0	10	65	m.q.
walnut (*Chips Ahoy!* Selections),								
½-oz. piece	95	1.0	9.0	6.0	2.0	5	70	m.q.
walnut (*Pepperidge Farm* Beacon								
Hill), 1 piece	120	2.0	14.0	7.0	2.0	5	65	1.0 d
w/chocolate middle (*Keebler Magic*								
Middles), 1 piece, approx.								
½ oz.	80	1.0	9.0	5.0	1.0	<5	25	m.q.
chunk:								
(*Pepperidge Farm* Nantucket),								
1 piece	120	1.0	15.0	6.0	2.0	5	60	1.0 d
pecan (*Chips Ahoy!* Selections),								
½-oz. piece	100	1.0	10.0	6.0	2.0	10	65	m.q.
pecan (*Pepperidge Farm*								
Chesapeake), 1 piece	120	1.0	14.0	7.0	2.0	5	60	1.0 d
pecan (*Pepperidge Farm* Special								
Collection), 1 piece	70	0	8.0	4.0	1.0	10	25	m.q.

Food and Measure	cal.	prot. (gms)	carbo. (gms)	tot. fat (gms)	sat. fat (gms)	chol. (mgs)	sod. (mgs)	fiber (gms)
chunky (*Chips Ahoy!* Selections),								
½-oz. piece	90	1.0	11.0	5.0	2.0	10	90	m.q.
double (*Featherweight*), 1 piece ...	45	1.0	6.0	2.0	m.q.	0	0	m.q.
fudge (*Almost Home*), ½-oz. piece	70	1.0	9.0	3.0	<1.0	<2	50	m.q.
fudge (*Grandma's* Big Cookies),								
2 pieces, 2.75 oz.	350	4.0	54.0	13.0	m.q.	5	380	m.q.
milk:								
(*Duncan Hines*), 2 pieces	110	1.0	15.0	5.0	m.q.	n.a.	95	m.q.
macadamia (*Pepperidge Farm*								
Sausalito), 1 piece	120	1.0	14.0	7.0	2.0	5	65	m.q.
macadamia (*Pepperidge Farm*								
Special Collection), 1 piece ..	70	1.0	8.0	4.0	1.0	<5	35	m.q.
mint (*Keebler Soft Batch*), 1 piece	80	1.0	10.0	4.0	1.0	0	70	m.q.
snaps (*Nabisco*), 3 pieces or ½ oz.	70	1.0	11.0	2.0	1.0	0	50	m.q.
sprinkled (*Chips Ahoy!*), 1 piece ..	50	1.0	7.0	2.0	<1.0	0	40	m.q.
striped (*Chips Ahoy!*), ½-oz.								
piece	90	1.0	10.0	5.0	2.0	0	45	m.q.
toffee (*Pepperidge Farm* Old								
Fashioned), 2 pieces	100	1.0	12.0	5.0	2.0	5	75	m.q.
walnut (*Keebler Soft Batch*),								
1 piece, approx. ½ oz.	80	1.0	10.0	4.0	1.0	0	70	m.q.
chocolate sandwich:								
(*Estee*), 1 piece	50	<1.0	7.0	2.0	1.0	0	15	m.q.
(*Little Debbie*), 1.8 oz.	250	3.0	35.0	12.0	m.q.	<1	260	m.q.
(*Oreo*), ½-oz. piece	50	1.0	8.0	2.0	<1.0	<2	75	m.q.
(*Oreo Big Stuf*), 1¾-oz. piece	250	2.0	33.0	12.0	4.0	<5	220	m.q.
(*Oreo Double Stuf*), ½-oz. piece ..	70	1.0	9.0	4.0	1.0	<2	75	m.q.
fudge covered (*Oreo*), ¾-oz.								
piece	110	1.0	13.0	6.0	4.0	<2	80	m.q.
fudge creme filled (*Keebler*								
Chocolate Creme Sandwich),								
1 piece, approx. ½ oz.	80	1.0	12.0	4.0	1.0	0	70	m.q.
fudge w/fudge creme filling								
(*Keebler E.L. Fudge*), 1 piece	70	<1.0	9.0	3.0	<1.0	0	50	m.q.
fudge w/peanut butter creme filling								
(*Keebler E.L. Fudge*), 1 piece	50	1.0	7.0	3.0	<1.0	0	50	m.q.
white fudge covered (*Oreo*), ¾-oz.								
piece	110	1.0	14.0	6.0	4.0	<2	75	m.q.
chocolate-filled sandwich:								
(*Pepperidge Farm* Brussels),								
2 pieces	110	1.0	13.0	5.0	2.0	0	65	m.q.
(*Pepperidge Farm* Lido), 1 piece ..	90	1.0	10.0	5.0	1.0	<5	30	m.q.
(*Pepperidge Farm* Milano),								
2 pieces	120	1.0	15.0	6.0	2.0	5	45	m.q.
(*Pepperidge Farm* Orleans),								
2 pieces	120	1.0	14.0	8.0	2.0	0	40	m.q.
fudge creme (*Keebler E.L. Fudge*),								
1 piece	60	<1.0	8.0	3.0	<1.0	<5	35	m.q.

Food and Measure	cal.	prot. (gms)	carbo. (gms)	tot. fat (gms)	sat. fat (gms)	chol. (mgs)	sod. (mgs)	fiber (gms)
COOKIE, CHOCOLATE-FILLED SANDWICH *(cont.)*								
mint (*Pepperidge Farm* Brussels Mint), 2 pieces	130	1.0	17.0	7.0	2.0	0	40	m.q.
mint (*Pepperidge Farm* Mint Milano), 2 pieces	150	1.0	17.0	7.0	2.0	5	60	m.q.
orange (*Pepperidge Farm* Orange Milano), 2 pieces	150	1.0	17.0	7.0	2.0	5	60	m.q.
chocolate peanut bar (*Ideal*), ¾-oz. piece	90	2.0	11.0	5.0	2.0	0	80	m.q.
(*Cinnamon Raisin Nut Newtons*), ½-oz. piece	60	1.0	11.0	2.0	<1.0	0	50	m.q.
coconut:								
(*Drake's*), 2 pieces, approx. 1 oz.	130	2.0	20.0	5.0	2.0	0	95	m.q.
chocolate-filled (*Pepperidge Farm* Tahiti), 1 piece	90	0	9.0	6.0	2.0	5	25	m.q.
dietetic (*Stella D'oro*), 1 piece ...	52	.8	6.8	2.4	m.q.	n.a.	<10	m.q.
macaroon (*Stella D'oro*), 1 piece	60	.7	6.6	3.4	m.q.	n.a.	m.q.	m.q.
coffee, chocolate praline-filled (*Pepperidge Farm* Cappucino), 1 piece	50	0	6.0	3.0	1.0	<5	20	m.q.
creme sandwich, see specific listings								
date pecan (*Health Valley Fancy Fruit Chunks*), 2 pieces	90	2.0	15.0	4.0	m.q.	0	45	1.7 d
date pecan (*Pepperidge Farm* Kitchen Hearth), 2 pieces	110	1.0	15.0	5.0	2.0	10	40	m.q.
devil's food (*FFV* Trolley Cakes), 2 pieces or 2 oz.	120	2.0	25.0	2.0	m.q.	n.a.	80	m.q.
devil's food cakes (*Nabisco*), 1 piece	70	1.0	15.0	1.0	<1.0	0	40	m.q.
egg biscuit:								
(*Stella D'oro*), 1 piece	43	1.6	6.7	1.1	n.a.	n.a.	m.q.	m.q.
(*Stella D'oro Anginetti*), 1 piece ..	31	.5	4.9	1.0	n.a.	n.a.	m.q.	m.q.
(*Stella D'oro* Jumbo), 1 piece	47	1.0	9.1	.7	n.a.	n.a.	m.q.	m.q.
dietetic (*Stella D'oro*), 1 piece ...	43	1.7	6.5	1.1	n.a.	n.a.	<10	m.q.
dietetic (*Stella D'oro* Kitchel), 1 piece	8	.2	.7	.5	n.a.	n.a.	<10	m.q.
Roman (*Stella D'oro*), 1 piece	137	2.7	20.4	5.0	m.q.	n.a.	m.q.	m.q.
sugared (*Stella D'oro*), 1 piece ...	75	1.6	14.3	1.4	n.a.	n.a.	m.q.	m.q.
(*Estee*), all varieties, except fudge, sandwich and wafer, 1 piece ...	30	<1.0	4.0	1.0	<1.0	0	0	m.q.
(*Estee* Original Sandwich), 1 piece ..	45	<1.0	6.0	2.0	<1.0	0	5	m.q.
(*FFV* Kreem Pilot Bread), 1 piece ..	60	1.0	9.0	2.0	m.q.	n.a.	60	m.q.
(*FFV* Royal Dainty), 2 pieces, approx. .7 oz.	120	1.0	14.0	6.0	m.q.	n.a.	90	m.q.
(*FFV* T.C. Rounds), 2 pieces, approx. 1 oz.	160	1.0	20.0	8.0	m.q.	n.a.	65	m.q.
(*FFV* Tango), 2 pieces, approx. 1.2 oz.	160	1.0	26.0	5.0	m.q.	n.a.	50	m.q.
fig:								
bar (*Fig Newtons*), ½-oz. piece ..	60	1.0	11.0	1.0	<1.0	0	6	m.q.

Food and Measure	cal.	prot. (gms)	carbo. (gms)	tot. fat (gms)	sat. fat (gms)	chol. (mgs)	sod. (mgs)	fiber (gms)
bar (*Keebler*), 1 piece	60	1.0	11.0	2.0	<1.0	0	70	m.q.
bar, vanilla (*FFV*), 1 piece	70	1.0	12.0	1.0	<1.0	0	55	m.q.
bar, whole wheat (*FFV*), 1 piece	70	1.0	11.0	2.0	<1.0	0	50	m.q.
pastry, dietetic (*Stella D'oro*), 1 piece	89	1.0	13.0	3.7	m.q.	n.a.	<10	m.q.
fruit:								
(*Health Valley Fruit & Fitness*), 5 pieces	200	4.0	40.0	6.0	m.q.	0	249	4.0 d
slices (*Stella D'oro*), 1 piece	60	1.1	8.7	2.2	m.q.	n.a.	m.q.	m.q.
tropical (*Health Valley Fancy Fruit Chunks*), 2 pieces	80	2.0	13.0	3.0	m.q.	0	45	1.7 d
tropical (*Health Valley Fruit Jumbos*), 1 piece	70	1.0	10.0	2.0	m.q.	0	26	1.5 d
fudge bar, caramel and peanut (*Heyday*), ¾-oz. piece	110	2.0	12.0	6.0	2.0	0	40	m.q.
ginger (*Pepperidge Farm* Gingerman), 2 pieces	70	1.0	10.0	3.0	0	5	50	m.q.
ginger boys (*FFV*), 1.25-oz. pkg. ..	150	2.0	26.0	5.0	1.0	0	210	m.q.
gingersnaps:								
(*Archway*, 80/pkg.), 1 piece	25	1.0	4.0	<1.0	n.a.	0	20	m.q.
(*Archway*, 54/pkg.), 1 piece	35	0	6.0	1.0	n.a.	0	30	m.q.
(*FFV*), 5 pieces, approx. 1 oz. ...	130	2.0	22.0	4.0	1.0	0	140	m.q.
(*Nabisco* Old Fashioned), ¼-oz. piece	30	<1.0	6.0	1.0	<1.0	0	45	m.q.
(*Sunshine*), 5 pieces	100	1.0	16.0	3.0	1.0	0	120	m.q.
graham cracker:								
(*Bugs Bunny*), 5 pieces or ½ oz.	60	1.0	11.0	2.0	<1.0	0	70	m.q.
(*Keebler*), 4 pieces, approx. ½ oz.	70	1.0	12.0	2.0	<1.0	0	85	m.q.
(*Nabisco*), 2 pieces or ½ oz.	60	1.0	11.0	1.0	<1.0	0	90	m.q.
(*Regal*), 2 pieces, approx. 1 oz. ..	140	1.0	19.0	7.0	m.q.	n.a.	120	m.q.
(*Rokeach*), 8 pieces or 1 oz.	120	2.0	21.0	3.0	m.q.	n.a.	m.q.	m.q.
(*Sunshine Grahamy Bears*), 9 pieces	130	2.0	21.0	5.0	1.0	0	160	m.q.
amaranth (*Health Valley Amaranth Graham Crackers*), 7 pieces ...	110	3.0	25.0	3.0	m.q.	0	110	3.1 d
apple cinnamon (*Honey Maid Graham Bites*), 11 pieces or ½ oz.	60	1.0	11.0	2.0	<1.0	0	80	m.q.
brown sugar'n spice (*Honey Maid Graham Bites*), 11 pieces or ½ oz.	60	1.0	11.0	2.0	<1.0	0	80	m.q.
chocolate:								
(*Keebler Thin Bits*), 12 pieces, approx. ½ oz.	70	1.0	9.0	3.0	<1.0	0	75	m.q.
(*Nabisco*), ½-oz. piece	60	1.0	7.0	3.0	2.0	0	30	m.q.
(*Teddy Grahams*), 11 pieces or ½ oz.	60	1.0	10.0	2.0	<1.0	0	90	m.q.

Food and Measure	cal.	prot. (gms)	carbo. (gms)	tot. fat (gms)	sat. fat (gms)	chol. (mgs)	sod. (mgs)	fiber (gms)
COOKIE, GRAHAM CRACKER, CHOCOLATE *(cont.)*								
vanilla creme filled (*Teddy Grahams Bearwich's*),								
4 pieces	70	1.0	10.0	3.0	<1.0	0	60	m.q.
cinnamon:								
(*Honey Maid*), 2 pieces or ½ oz.	60	1.0	12.0	1.0	<1.0	0	85	m.q.
(*Keebler* Alpha Grahams),								
6 pieces	70	1.0	10.0	2.0	<1.0	0	55	m.q.
(*Keebler* Cinnamon Crisp),								
4 pieces, approx. ½ oz.	70	1.0	11.0	2.0	<1.0	0	85	m.q.
(*Keebler Thin Bits*), 12 pieces,								
approx. ½ oz.	70	1.0	10.0	3.0	<1.0	0	50	m.q.
(*Sunshine*), 1 piece	70	1.0	11.0	3.0	1.0	0	95	m.q.
(*Teddy Grahams*),								
11 pieces, ½ oz.	60	1.0	11.0	2.0	<1.0	0	90	m.q.
vanilla creme filled (*Teddy Grahams Bearwich's*),								
4 pieces	70	1.0	10.0	3.0	<1.0	0	60	m.q.
fudge covered (*Keebler* Deluxe),								
2 pieces, approx. ½ oz.	90	<1.0	11.0	4.0	1.0	0	60	m.q.
w/fudge (*Nabisco Cookies'N Fudge*), 1 piece..............	45	<1.0	6.0	2.0	1.0	0	35	m.q.
honey:								
(*Health Valley* Fancy), 7 pieces	130	3.0	21.0	5.0	m.q.	0	89	3.5 d
(*Honey Maid*), 2 pieces, ½ oz.	60	1.0	11.0	1.0	<1.0	0	90	m.q.
(*Keebler* Honey Grahams),								
4 pieces, approx. ½ oz.	70	1.0	12.0	2.0	<1.0	0	85	m.q.
(*Sunshine*), 1 piece	60	1.0	10.0	2.0	<1.0	0	90	m.q.
(*Teddy Grahams*),								
11 pieces or ½ oz.	60	1.0	11.0	2.0	<1.0	0	90	m.q.
honey'n oat bran (*Honey Maid* Graham Bites), 11 pieces or ½ oz.	60	1.0	11.0	2.0	<1.0	0	55	m.q.
oat bran (*Health Valley*), 7 pieces	130	3.0	25.0	2.0	m.q.	0	47	3.4 d
vanilla (*Teddy Grahams*), 11 pieces or ½ oz.	60	1.0	10.0	2.0	<1.0	0	75	m.q.
vanilla, chocolate creme filled (*Teddy Grahams Bearwich's*),								
4 pieces or ½ oz.	70	1.0	10.0	3.0	<1.0	0	65	m.q.
wheat (*Carr's* Home Wheat Graham), 1 piece	74	1.0	10.9	3.3	m.q.	n.a.	<1	m.q.
hazelnut (*Pepperidge Farm* Old Fashioned), 2 pieces	110	1.0	15.0	6.0	2.0	0	75	m.q.
honey:								
cinnamon, crisp (*Health Valley Honey Jumbos*), 1 piece	70	1.0	10.0	2.0	m.q.	0	35	2.6 d
oat bran, fancy (*Health Valley Honey Jumbos*), 1 piece	70	1.0	10.0	2.0	m.q.	0	22	1.6 d
peanut butter, crisp (*Health Valley Honey Jumbos*), 1 piece	70	2.0	10.0	2.0	m.q.	0	24	1.5 d

Food and Measure	cal.	prot. (gms)	carbo. (gms)	tot. fat (gms)	sat. fat (gms)	chol. (mgs)	sod. (mgs)	fiber (gms)
jelly tarts (*FFV*), 1 piece	60	<1.0	11.0	2.0	<1.0	0	55	m.q.
lemon (*Featherweight*), 1 piece	45	1.0	6.0	2.0	m.q.	0	0	m.q.
lemon nut crunch (*Pepperidge Farm* Old Fashioned), 2 pieces	110	1.0	13.0	7.0	2.0	<5	50	m.q.
marshmallow:								
chocolate cake (*Mallomars*), ½-oz. piece	60	1.0	9.0	3.0	1.0	0	20	m.q.
chocolate cake (*Pinwheels*), 1-oz. piece	130	1.0	20.0	5.0	2.0	0	40	m.q.
fudge cake (*Nabisco* Puffs), ¾-oz. piece	90	1.0	14.0	4.0	3.0	0	45	m.q.
fudge cake (*Nabisco* Twirls), 1-oz. piece	140	1.0	20.0	6.0	4.0	0	70	m.q.
mint sandwich (*FFV*), 2 pieces, approx. 1.1 oz.	160	2.0	22.0	7.0	m.q.	n.a.	50	m.q.
mint sandwich (*Mystic Mint*), ½-oz. piece	90	1.0	11.0	5.0	3.0	<2	65	m.q.
molasses:								
(*Archway*), 1 piece	100	1.0	18.0	2.0	m.q.	10	155	2.0 d
(*Grandma's* Old Time Big Cookies), 2 pieces or 2.75 oz.	320	4.0	58.0	9.0	m.q.	5	520	m.q.
(*Nabisco Pantry*), ½-oz. piece	80	1.0	13.0	3.0	<1.0	0	75	m.q.
crisps (*Pepperidge Farm* Old Fashioned), 2 pieces	70	1.0	8.0	3.0	0	0	50	m.q.
oat bran:								
animal cookies (*Health Valley*), 7 pieces	110	3.0	20.0	4.0	m.q.	0	50	3.0 d
fruit (*Health Valley Oat Bran Fruit Jumbos*), 1 piece	70	1.0	10.0	2.0	m.q.	0	22	1.5 d
fruit and nut (*Health Valley*), 2 pieces	110	3.0	17.0	4.0	m.q.	0	70	2.8 d
raisin (*Awrey's*), 1 piece	100	1.0	14.0	4.0	1.0	0	115	1.0 d
raisin (*Health Valley Fancy Fruit Chunks*), 2 pieces	90	2.0	15.0	3.0	m.q.	0	95	1.6 d
oatmeal:								
(*Archway*), 1 piece	110	2.0	19.0	3.0	m.q.	5	90	1.0 d
(*Archway* Ruth's Golden), 1 piece	120	2.0	20.0	4.0	m.q.	5	122	1.2 d
(*Baker's Bonus*), ½-oz. piece ...	80	1.0	12.0	3.0	1.0	0	65	m.q.
(*Drake's*), 2 pieces, approx. 1 oz.	120	2.0	19.0	4.0	1.0	0	50	m.q.
(*FFV*), 5 pieces, approx. 1 oz. ...	130	2.0	20.0	4.0	1.0	0	150	m.q.
(*Keebler* Old Fashion), 1 piece, approx. ½ oz.	80	1.0	12.0	3.0	1.0	0	110	m.q.
(*Little Debbie*), 2.75-oz. serving ..	340	5.0	52.0	12.0	m.q.	<2	440	m.q.
apple filled (*Archway*), 1 piece ...	90	1.0	18.0	1.0	n.a.	5	115	1.0 d
apple spice (*Grandma's* Big Cookies), 2 pieces or 2.75 oz.	330	5.0	51.0	12.0	m.q.	10	570	m.q.
chocolate chunk (*Chips Ahoy!* Selections), ½-oz. piece	95	1.0	10.0	5.0	2.0	<5	50	m.q.
chocolate chunk (*Pepperidge Farm* Dakota), 1 piece	110	1.0	15.0	6.0	2.0	5	70	1.0 d

Food and Measure	cal.	prot. (gms)	carbo. (gms)	tot. fat (gms)	sat. fat (gms)	chol. (mgs)	sod. (mgs)	fiber (gms)
COOKIE, OATMEAL *(cont.)*								
w/chocolate middle (*Keebler Magic Middles*), 1 piece, approx. ½ oz.	80	1.0	8.0	5.0	1.0	0	30	m.q.
date filled (*Archway*), 1 piece	100	1.0	18.0	2.0	m.q.	5	105	1.0 d
iced (*Archway*), 1 piece	140	2.0	22.0	5.0	m.q.	5	107	1.7 d
Irish (*Pepperidge Farm* Old Fashioned), 2 pieces	90	1.0	13.0	5.0	1.0	5	80	m.q.
raisin:								
(*Almost Home*), ½-oz. piece ...	70	1.0	10.0	3.0	<1.0	<2	40	m.q.
(*Archway*), 1 piece	100	2.0	18.0	3.0	m.q.	5	107	.9 d
(*Duncan Hines*), 2 pieces	110	1.0	15.0	5.0	m.q.	n.a.	75	m.q.
(*Entenmann's*), 2 pieces	80	1.0	17.0	0	0	0	120	m.q.
(*Featherweight*), 1 piece	45	1.0	6.0	2.0	m.q.	0	0	m.q.
(*Keebler Soft Batch*), 1 piece, approx. ½ oz.	70	1.0	10.0	3.0	<1.0	0	65	m.q.
(*Pepperidge Farm* Old Fashioned), 2 pieces	110	1.0	15.0	5.0	2.0	10	115	m.q.
(*Pepperidge Farm* Santa Fe), 1 piece	100	1.0	16.0	4.0	1.0	<5	70	1.0 d
(*Sunshine*), 2 pieces	110	1.0	16.0	5.0	1.0	0	125	m.q.
(*Tastykake* Soft'n Chewy), 1.4 oz.	161	3.4	26.8	5.4	1.0	3	158	1.0 d
bar (*Tastykake*), 1.8 oz.	212	3.2	31.8	8.3	2.2	17	255	1.2 d
raisin bran (*Archway*), 1 piece ...	100	2.0	18.0	3.0	m.q.	5	95	1.0 d
spice (*Weight Watchers*), 3 pieces	80	1.0	13.0	2.0	m.q.	n.a.	75	m.q.
peach-apricot:								
bar, vanilla (*FFV*), 1 piece	70	<1.0	14.0	1.0	<1.0	0	50	m.q.
bar, whole wheat (*FFV*), 1 piece	70	<1.0	11.0	2.0	<1.0	0	50	m.q.
pastry (*Stella D'oro*), 1 piece	93	1.2	13.6	3.8	m.q.	n.a.	m.q.	m.q.
pastry, dietetic (*Stella D'oro*), 1 piece	87	1.2	12.3	3.7	m.q.	n.a.	<10	m.q.
peanut (*Health Valley Fancy Peanut Chunks*), 2 pieces	100	2.0	14.0	3.0	m.q.	0	585	2.3 d
peanut butter:								
(*Featherweight*), 1 piece	40	1.0	5.0	2.0	m.q.	0	10	m.q.
(*Grandma's* Big Cookies), 2 pieces or 2.75 oz.	410	7.0	43.0	30.0	m.q.	10	410	m.q.
chocolate chip (*Keebler Soft Batch*), 1 piece, approx. ½ oz.	80	1.0	9.0	5.0	1.0	0	55	m.q.
chocolate chunk (*Pepperidge Farm* Cheyenne), 1 piece	110	2.0	13.0	6.0	2.0	5	80	1.0 d
chocolate filled (*Pepperidge Farm* Nassau), 1 piece	80	1.0	9.0	5.0	1.0	<5	45	m.q.
cream filled (*Pitter Patter*), 1 piece, approx. ½ oz.	90	2.0	12.0	4.0	<1.0	0	115	m.q.
creme wafer (*Featherweight*), 1 piece	25	1.0	3.0	1.0	n.a.	0	0	m.q.

Food and Measure	cal.	prot. (gms)	carbo. (gms)	tot. fat (gms)	sat. fat (gms)	chol. (mgs)	sod. (mgs)	fiber (gms)
nut (*Keebler Soft Batch*), 1 piece, approx. ½ oz.	80	1.0	9.0	4.0	1.0	0	60	m.q.
sandwich:								
(*Estee*), 1 piece	50	1.0	5.0	3.0	1.0	0	35	m.q.
(*FFV*), 2 pieces, approx. 1.1 oz.	170	2.0	21.0	8.0	m.q.	n.a.	110	m.q.
(*Nutter Butter*), ½-oz. piece ...	70	1.0	9.0	3.0	<1.0	<2	50	m.q.
peanut creme patties (*Nutter Butter*), 2 pieces or ½ oz.	80	2.0	8.0	4.0	<1.0	0	45	m.q.
pecan crunch (*Archway*), 1 piece ...	60	1.0	8.0	3.0	m.q.	5	45	m.q.
praline pecan (*FFV*), 1 piece	40	<1.0	10.0	2.0	1.0	<5	40	m.q.
prune pastry, dietetic (*Stella D'oro*), 1 piece	95	1.2	15.0	3.4	m.q.	n.a.	<10	m.q.
raisin:								
(*Stella D'oro* Golden Bars), 1 piece	109	1.6	16.0	4.3	m.q.	n.a.	m.q.	m.q.
bar, iced (*Keebler*), 1 piece	80	1.0	11.0	4.0	1.0	0	85	m.q.
soft (*Grandma's* Big Cookies), 2 pieces, or 2.75 oz.	320	3.0	54.0	10.0	m.q.	10	280	m.q.
raisin bran (*Pepperidge Farm* Kitchen Hearth), 2 pieces	110	1.0	13.0	5.0	2.0	<5	55	m.q.
raisin nut (*Health Valley Fruit Jumbos*), 1 piece	70	2.0	10.0	3.0	m.q.	0	35	.9 d
raisin oatmeal (*Archway*), 1 piece ...	50	1.0	7.0	2.0	m.q.	0	20	m.q.
raspberry bar (*Raspberry Newtons*), ¾-oz. piece	70	1.0	15.0	2.0	<1.0	0	70	m.q.
raspberry filled:								
(*Pepperidge Farm* Chantilly), 1 piece	80	1.0	14.0	2.0	1.0	<5	35	m.q.
(*Pepperidge Farm* Linzer), 1 piece	120	2.0	20.0	4.0	1.0	<5	55	m.q.
chocolate (*Pepperidge Farm* Chantilly), 1 piece	90	1.0	14.0	3.0	1.0	<5	35	m.q.
sandwich, see specific listings								
sesame (*Stella D'oro* Regina), 1 piece	48	.9	6.1	2.2	m.q.	n.a.	m.q.	m.q.
sesame, dietetic (*Stella D'oro* Regina), 1 piece	41	.8	5.1	2.0	m.q.	n.a.	<10	m.q.
shortbread:								
(*Lorna Doone*), 3 pieces or ½ oz.	70	1.0	9.0	4.0	<1.0	<5	65	m.q.
(*Pepperidge Farm* Old Fashioned), 2 pieces	150	1.0	17.0	8.0	2.0	<5	85	m.q.
(*Weight Watchers*), 3 pieces	80	1.0	13.0	2.0	m.q.	n.a.	95	m.q.
w/chocolate cream center (*Keebler Magic Middles*), 1 piece, approx. ½ oz.	80	1.0	9.0	5.0	1.0	<5	25	m.q.
country (*FFV*), 1 piece	70	1.0	9.0	4.0	1.0	<5	45	m.q.
fudge striped (*Keebler* Fudge Stripes), 1 piece, approx. ½ oz.	50	<1.0	7.0	3.0	<1.0	0	55	m.q.

Food and Measure	cal.	prot. (gms)	carbo. (gms)	tot. fat (gms)	sat. fat (gms)	chol. (mgs)	sod. (mgs)	fiber (gms)
COOKIE, SHORTBREAD *(cont.)*								
fudge striped (*Nabisco Cookies 'n Fudge*), ½-oz. piece	60	1.0	7.0	3.0	1.0	0	50	m.q.
pecan (*Nabisco*), ½-oz. piece	80	1.0	8.0	5.0	1.0	<2	40	m.q.
pecan (*Pecan Sandies*), 1 piece, approx. ½ oz.	80	<1.0	9.0	5.0	1.0	<5	75	m.q.
pecan (*Pepperidge Farm* Old Fashioned), 1 piece	70	1.0	7.0	5.0	2.0	0	15	m.q.
spice drops (*Stella D'oro* Pfeffernusse), 1 piece	35	.5	6.7	.8	n.a.	n.a.	m.q.	m.q.
(*Stella D'oro Angel Bars*), 1 piece ..	76	1.0	7.3	4.7	m.q.	n.a.	m.q.	m.q.
(*Stella D'oro Angel Wings*), 1 piece	74	1.1	7.0	4.7	m.q.	n.a.	m.q.	m.q.
(*Stella D'oro Angelica Goodies*), 1 piece	106	1.7	15.7	4.0	m.q.	n.a.	m.q.	m.q.
(*Stella D'oro Como Delight*), 1 piece	145	2.1	17.9	7.2	m.q.	n.a.	m.q.	m.q.
(*Stella D'oro Holiday Trinkets*), 1 piece	38	.6	4.6	1.9	m.q.	n.a.	m.q.	m.q.
(*Stella D'oro Love Cookies*), 1 piece	106	1.3	13.4	5.2	m.q.	n.a.	m.q.	m.q.
(*Stella D'oro Royal Nuggets*), 1 piece	2	.1	.1	.1	n.a.	n.a.	n.a.	n.a.
strawberry:								
(*Pepperidge Farm* Fruit Cookies), 2 pieces	100	1.0	15.0	5.0	2.0	10	50	m.q.
bar (*Strawberry Newtons*), ¾-oz. piece	70	1.0	15.0	2.0	<1.0	0	70	m.q.
creme wafer (*Featherweight*), 1 piece	20	0	3.0	1.0	n.a.	0	0	m.q.
(*Suddenly S'Mores*), ¾-oz. piece ...	100	1.0	15.0	4.0	2.0	0	90	m.q.
sugar:								
(*Almost Home* Old Fashioned), ½-oz. piece	70	1.0	10.0	3.0	<1.0	<2	80	m.q.
(*Pepperidge Farm* Old Fashioned), 2 pieces	100	1.0	13.0	5.0	2.0	10	55	m.q.
wafer (*Biscos*), 4 pieces or ½ oz.	70	<1.0	10.0	3.0	<1.0	0	20	m.q.
wafer, vanilla (*Tastykake*), 10 pieces	34	.3	4.1	1.9	.5	0	11	<.1 d
tea biscuit (*Social Tea*), ⅙-oz. piece	20	<1.0	4.0	1.0	<1.0	<2	20	m.q.
tofu (*Health Valley The Great Tofu Cookie*), 2 pieces	90	2.0	16.0	3.0	m.q.	0	29	1.4 d
vanilla:								
(*Featherweight*), 1 piece	45	1.0	6.0	2.0	m.q.	0	0	m.q.
(*Pepperidge Farm* Bordeaux), 2 pieces	70	1.0	11.0	3.0	1.0	0	40	m.q.
(*Pepperidge Farm* Pirouettes), 2 pieces	70	0	9.0	4.0	1.0	<5	35	m.q.
(*Stella D'oro Castelets*), 1 piece ..	72	1.0	10.0	3.1	m.q.	n.a.	m.q.	m.q.
(*Stella D'oro Margherite*), 1 piece	72	1.0	10.8	2.8	m.q.	n.a.	m.q.	m.q.
chocolate coated (*Pepperidge Farm* Orleans), 3 pieces	90	0	11.0	6.0	2.0	0	30	m.q.

Food and Measure	cal.	prot. (gms)	carbo. (gms)	tot. fat (gms)	sat. fat (gms)	chol. (mgs)	sod. (mgs)	fiber (gms)
chocolate laced (*Pepperidge Farm* Pirouettes), 2 pieces	70	1.0	8.0	4.0	1.0	<5	20	m.q.
chocolate nut coated (*Pepperidge Farm* Geneva), 2 pieces	130	1.0	14.0	6.0	2.0	0	50	m.q.
creme sandwich:								
(*Cameo*), ½-oz. piece	70	1.0	10.0	3.0	1.0	0	50	m.q.
(*Keebler* French Vanilla Creme), 1 piece, approx. ½ oz.	80	<1.0	12.0	4.0	<1.0	0	80	m.q.
(*Nabisco Cookie Break*), ½-oz. piece	50	1.0	7.0	2.0	<1.0	0	35	m.q.
(*Nabisco Giggles*), ½-oz. piece	60	1.0	8.0	3.0	<1.0	<2	20	m.q.
shortbread (*Tastykake*), .4 oz. ...	55	.7	6.4	3.0	.7	0	31	.1 d
wafer:								
(*Archway*), 1 piece	30	0	6.0	<1.0	n.a.	0	30	m.q.
(*FFV*), 1 oz., approx. 8 pieces	130	1.0	19.0	5.0	1.0	<5	100	m.q.
(*Nabisco Nilla* Wafers), ½ oz., approx. 3½ pieces	60	1.0	11.0	2.0	<1.0	<5	45	m.q.
cinnamon (*Nabisco Nilla* Wafers), ½ oz., approx. 3½ pieces	60	1.0	11.0	2.0	<1.0	<5	45	m.q.
creme (*Featherweight*), 1 piece	20	0	3.0	1.0	n.a.	0	0	m.q.
golden (*Keebler*), 4 pieces	80	<1.0	10.0	3.0	1.0	0	60	m.q.
wafer (see also specific listings):								
brown edged (*Nabisco*), ½ oz., approx. 2½ pieces	70	1.0	10.0	3.0	<1.0	<2	45	m.q.
creme, fudge covered (*Keebler Fudge Sticks*), 2 pieces, approx. ½ oz.	100	<1.0	13.0	5.0	1.0	0	35	m.q.
creme filled, assorted (*Estee*), 1 piece	30	<1.0	4.0	2.0	<1.0	0	5	m.q.
creme filled, chocolate, vanilla (*Estee*), 1 piece	20	<1.0	3.0	1.0	<1.0	0	5	m.q.
fudge striped (*Nabisco Cookies 'n Fudge*), ½-oz. piece	70	1.0	9.0	4.0	2.0	0	30	m.q.
snack, chocolate, strawberry, vanilla (*Estee*), 1 piece	80	<1.0	11.0	4.0	<1.0	0	<5	m.q.
snack, chocolate coated (*Estee*), 1 piece	130	2.0	14.0	7.0	3.0	0	10	m.q.
waffle cremes (*Biscos*), 2 pieces or ½ oz.	70	<1.0	10.0	4.0	<1.0	0	20	m.q.
wheat free (*Health Valley The Great Wheat-Free Cookie*), 4 pieces	130	2.0	25.0	3.0	m.q.	0	35	3.3 d
COOKIE, FROZEN, 1.2 oz., approx. 2 pieces:								
chocolate chip:								
(*Nestlé* Toll House Ready To Bake)	150	1.0	20.0	7.0	m.q.	n.a.	115	m.q.
double (*Nestlé* Toll House Ready To Bake)	150	2.0	19.0	7.0	m.q.	n.a.	60	m.q.

Food and Measure	cal.	prot. (gms)	carbo. (gms)	tot. fat (gms)	sat. fat (gms)	chol. (mgs)	sod. (mgs)	fiber (gms)
COOKIE, FROZEN, CHOCOLATE CHIP *(cont.)*								
w/nuts (*Nestlé* Toll House Ready To Bake)	160	2.0	19.0	8.0	m.q.	n.a.	90	m.q.
oatmeal raisin (*Nestlé* Toll House Ready To Bake)	130	2.0	21.0	5.0	m.q.	n.a.	55	m.q.
COOKIE, REFRIGERATED,								
1 piece:								
chocolate chip (*Pillsbury*)	70	1.0	9.0	3.0	<1.0	5	55	m.q.
oatmeal raisin (*Pillsbury*)	60	1.0	9.0	3.0	<1.0	0	55	m.q.
peanut butter (*Pillsbury*)	70	1.0	9.0	3.0	<1.0	5	75	m.q.
sugar (*Pillsbury*)	70	1.0	9.0	3.0	<1.0	5	70	m.q.
COOKIE MIX[1], 2 pieces:								
chocolate chip:								
(*Betty Crocker Big Batch*)[2]	120	1.0	16.0	6.0	m.q.	m.q.	100	m.q.
(*Duncan Hines*)	130	1.0	20.0	5.0	m.q.	n.a.	85	m.q.
(*Finast*)	110	1.0	16.0	5.0	m.q.	n.a.	290	m.q.
oatmeal raisin (*Duncan Hines*)	130	2.0	18.0	6.0	m.q.	n.a.	70	m.q.
peanut butter (*Duncan Hines*)	140	3.0	15.0	7.0	m.q.	n.a.	120	m.q.
sugar, golden (*Duncan Hines*)	130	1.0	17.0	6.0	m.q.	n.a.	70	m.q.
CORIANDER:								
untrimmed, 1 lb.	77	9.1	10.0	2.3	n.a.	0	108	3.1 c
trimmed, 1 oz.	6	.7	.7	.2	(0)	0	8	.2 c
trimmed, ¼ cup	1	.1	.1	<.1	(0)	0	1	<.1 c
9 plants, approx. .8 oz.	4	.5	.5	.1	(0)	0	6	.2 c
CORIANDER LEAF, DRIED:								
1 oz.	79	6.2	14.8	1.3	n.a.	0	60	2.9 c
1 tbsp.	5	.4	.9	.1	(0)	0	4	.2 c
1 tsp.	2	.1	.3	<.1	(0)	0	1	.1 c
(*Tone's*), 1 tsp.	2	.1	.3	<.1	(0)	0	1	.1 d
CORIANDER SEED:								
1 oz.	84	3.5	15.6	5.0	.3	0	10	8.3 c
1 tbsp.	15	.6	2.8	.9	.1	0	2	1.5 c
1 tsp.	5	.2	1.0	.3	<.1	0	1	.5 c
(*Spice Islands*), 1 tsp.	6	.2	.8	.3	<.1	0	<1	.4 c
CORN, sweet, fresh:								
raw:								
untrimmed, 1 lb.	140	5.3	31.1	1.9	.3	0	25	5.2 d
trimmed, 1 oz.	24	.9	5.4	.3	.1	0	4	.9 d
kernels from 1 ear, approx. 3.2 oz.	77	2.9	17.1	1.1	.2	0	14	2.9 d
cut, ½ cup	66	2.5	14.6	.9	.1	0	12	2.5 d
boiled, drained:								
4 oz.	122	3.8	28.5	1.5	.2	0	19	4.2 d
kernels from 1 ear, approx. 2.7 oz.	83	2.6	19.3	1.0	.2	0	13	2.8 d
cut, ½ cup	89	2.7	20.6	1.1	.2	0	14	3.0 d

1. *Prepared according to package directions.*
2. *Prepared with eggs and margarine.*

Food and Measure	cal.	prot. (gms)	carbo. (gms)	tot. fat (gms)	sat. fat (gms)	chol. (mgs)	sod. (mgs)	fiber (gms)
CORN, CANNED, ½ cup, except as noted:								
(*Green Giant* Delicorn)	80	2.0	19.0	<1.0	n.a.	0	350	2.0 d
in brine, w/liquid (*Green Giant*)	70	2.0	18.0	0	0	0	350	2.0 d
kernel:								
w/liquid:								
4 oz.	69	2.2	16.8	.5	.1	0	287	.9 d
½ cup	79	2.5	19.0	.6	.1	0	324	1.0 d
low-sodium, 4 oz.	69	2.2	16.8	.5	.1	0	3	.9 d
low-sodium	79	2.5	19.0	.6	.1	0	4	1.0 d
drained, 4 oz.	92	3.0	21.1	1.1	.2	0	m.q.	1.5 d
drained	66	2.2	15.2	.8	.1	0	m.q.	1.1 d
(*A&P*)	80	2.0	20.0	1.0	m.q.	0	350	m.q.
(*A&P* No Salt Added)	80	2.0	18.0	<1.0	n.a.	0	10	m.q.
(*Featherweight*)	80	2.0	16.0	1.0	n.a.	0	10	m.q.
(*Finast*)	90	2.0	20.0	1.0	n.a.	0	390	m.q.
(*Finast* No Salt Added)	80	3.0	19.0	1.0	n.a.	0	<10	m.q.
(*Green Giant*)	80	2.0	18.0	0	0	0	280	2.7 d
(*Green Giant* 50% Less Salt, No Sugar)	50	2.0	11.0	1.0	n.a.	0	140	2.0 d
(*Pathmark* No Frills), 1 cup	160	5.0	38.0	1.0	n.a.	0	550	m.q.
(*Pathmark* No Salt Added)	70	2.0	16.0	1.0	n.a.	0	10	m.q.
(*S&W/Nutradiet*)	80	2.0	15.0	1.0	n.a.	0	0	m.q.
golden:								
w/liquid (*Del Monte*)	70	2.0	17.0	1.0	n.a.	0	355	m.q.
(*Del Monte* No Salt Added)	80	2.0	18.0	1.0	n.a.	0	<10	m.q.
(*Green Giant* 50% Less Salt) ..	70	2.0	16.0	<1.0	n.a.	0	175	2.0 d
(*Green Giant* No Salt or Sugar Added)	80	3.0	18.0	<1.0	n.a.	0	0	2.0 d
(*Green Giant Pantry Express*)	80	2.0	18.0	<1.0	0	0	210	1.0 d
(*Pathmark*)	90	2.0	19.0	1.0	n.a.	0	330	m.q.
(*Stokely*)	90	2.0	20.0	0	0	0	300	m.q.
(*Stokely* No Salt or Sugar Added)	80	2.0	16.0	0	0	0	5	m.q.
sweet (*IGA*)	70	2.0	16.0	1.0	n.a.	0	<10	m.q.
vacuum-pack (*Green Giant*) ...	80	2.0	20.0	0	0	0	330	2.0 d
vacuum-pack (*Stokely*)	90	3.0	22.0	0	0	0	300	m.q.
no salt added, see specific brands								
sweet (*Green Giant* Sweet Select)	60	2.0	12.0	1.0	n.a.	0	280	2.0 d
white:								
(*Stokely*)	90	3.0	21.0	0	0	0	290	m.q.
w/liquid (*Del Monte*)	70	2.0	16.0	0	0	0	355	m.q.
vacuum pack (*Green Giant*) ...	80	2.0	20.0	0	0	0	290	2.0 d
young tender (*S&W* Premium) ...	90	2.0	20.0	1.0	n.a.	0	295	m.q.
vacuum-pack:								
4 oz.	90	2.7	22.0	.6	.1	0	308	.9 c
½ cup	83	2.5	20.4	.5	.1	0	286	.8 c
(*A&P*)	100	2.0	25.0	1.0	n.a.	0	300	m.q.
(*Finast*), 4 oz.	90	5.0	20.0	1.0	n.a.	0	150	m.q.
(*Green Giant Niblets*)	80	3.0	16.0	1.0	n.a.	0	280	1.7 d

Food and Measure	cal.	prot. (gms)	carbo. (gms)	tot. fat (gms)	sat. fat (gms)	chol. (mgs)	sod. (mgs)	fiber (gms)
CORN, CANNED, KERNEL, VACUUM-PACK *(cont.)*								
(Pathmark)	120	3.0	25.0	1.0	n.a.	0	350	m.q.
low-sodium	83	2.5	20.4	.5	.1	0	3	.8 c
cream style:								
4 oz.	82	2.0	20.6	.5	.1	0	323	1.1 d
½ cup	93	2.2	23.2	.5	.1	0	365	1.3 d
(A&P)	100	2.0	25.0	1.0	n.a.	0	330	m.q.
(Finast)	105	2.0	25.0	1.0	n.a.	0	350	m.q.
(Green Giant)	100	2.0	24.0	<1.0	n.a.	0	390	2.0 d
(Pathmark No Frills), 1 cup	210	5.0	51.0	1.0	n.a.	0	700	m.q.
(S&W Premium Homestyle No Starch Added)	120	3.0	24.0	1.0	n.a.	0	285	m.q.
(S&W Premium Homestyle Starch Added)	105	2.0	25.0	1.0	n.a.	0	435	m.q.
(S&W/Nutradiet)	100	3.0	21.0	1.0	n.a.	0	0	m.q.
golden:								
(Del Monte)	80	2.0	18.0	1.0	n.a.	0	355	m.q.
(Del Monte No Salt Added)	80	2.0	20.0	1.0	n.a.	0	<10	m.q.
(Pathmark)	100	2.0	25.0	1.0	n.a.	0	350	m.q.
(Stokely)	100	2.0	23.0	0	0	0	380	m.q.
low-sodium, 4 oz.	82	2.0	20.6	.5	.1	0	3	.6 c
low-sodium	93	2.2	23.2	.5	.1	0	4	.6 c
white *(Del Monte)*	90	2.0	21.0	0	0	0	355	m.q.
white *(Stokely)*	100	2.0	23.0	0	0	0	380	m.q.
vacuum pack, w/liquid *(Del Monte)* ..	90	3.0	22.0	1.0	n.a.	0	355	m.q.
vacuum pack, w/liquid *(Del Monte* No Salt Added)	90	3.0	22.0	1.0	n.a.	0	<10	m.q.
w/peppers *(Green Giant Mexicorn)*	80	2.0	19.0	<1.0	n.a.	0	450	2.0 d
w/red and green peppers, w/liquid, 4 oz. or ½ cup	86	2.7	20.7	.6	.1	0	396	.7 c
w/beans, carrots, and pasta, in tomato sauce *(Green Giant Pantry Express)*	80	2.0	17.0	2.0	0	0	330	3.0 d
CORN, DRIED:								
(John Cope's), 1 oz. dry or 4 oz. prepared	101	3.0	20.5	1.2	n.a.	0	0	m.q.
CORN, FREEZE-DRIED:								
(Mountain House), ½ cup[1]	90	2.0	18.0	1.0	n.a.	0	<1	m.q.
CORN, FROZEN:								
(Health Valley), ½ cup	76	2.0	17.0	0	0	0	4	1.7 d
on the cob:								
kernels from 8-oz. ear	123	4.1	29.4	1.0	.2	0	6	.9 c
boiled, drained, kernels from 4-oz. ear	59	2.0	14.1	.5	.1	0	3	.4 c
boiled, drained, kernels, ½ cup ..	77	2.6	18.3	.6	.1	0	3	.5 c
(A&P), 1 ear	120	4.0	28.0	1.0	n.a.	0	0	m.q.
(A&P Cob Treats), 2 ears	130	5.0	28.0	1.0	n.a.	0	5	m.q.

1. *Prepared according to package directions.*

Food and Measure	cal.	prot. (gms)	carbo. (gms)	tot. fat (gms)	sat. fat (gms)	chol. (mgs)	sod. (mgs)	fiber (gms)
(*Birds Eye*), 1 ear	120	4.0	29.0	1.0	n.a.	0	0	m.q.
(*Birds Eye Big Ears*), 1 ear	160	5.0	37.0	1.0	n.a.	0	0	m.q.
(*Birds Eye Little Ears*), 2 ears ...	130	4.0	30.0	1.0	n.a.	0	0	m.q.
(*Frosty Acres*), 1 ear	120	4.0	29.0	1.0	n.a.	0	0	m.q.
(*Green Giant* One Serving), 2 half ears	120	4.0	26.0	1.0	<1.0	0	10	2.0 d
(*Green Giant Nibblers*, 6 ears), 2 ears	120	4.0	27.0	1.0	n.a.	0	10	2.0 d
(*Green Giant Nibblers* Supersweet), 2 ears	90	3.0	19.0	2.0	m.q.	0	10	2.0 d
(*Green Giant Niblet Ears*), 1 ear	120	4.0	27.0	1.0	n.a.	0	10	2.0 d
(*Green Giant Niblet Ears* Supersweet), 1 ear	90	3.0	19.0	2.0	m.q.	0	10	2.0 d
(*Ore-Ida*), 1 ear[1]	180	5.0	39.0	2.0	m.q.	0	40	m.q.
(*Seabrook*), 5″ ear	120	4.0	29.0	1.0	n.a.	0	4	1.0 c
(*Southern*), 5″ ear	140	5.0	30.0	1.0	n.a.	0	n.a.	m.q.
baby (*Birds Eye* Deluxe), 2.6 oz.	25	2.0	4.0	0	0	0	10	2.0 d
miniature (*Ore-Ida Mini-Gold*), 2 ears	180	5.0	39.0	2.0	m.q.	0	40	m.q.
kernel:								
kernels cut off cob, 10-oz. pkg. ..	250	8.6	59.1	2.2	.3	0	9	6.0 d
kernels cut off cob, boiled, drained, ½ cup	67	2.5	16.8	.1	tr.	0	4	1.7 d
(*A&P*), 3.3 oz.	80	3.0	18.0	<1.0	n.a.	0	0	m.q.
(*Birds Eye* Sweet), 3.3 oz.	80	3.0	20.0	1.0	n.a.	0	0	2.0 d
(*Birds Eye* Tender Sweet Deluxe), 3.3 oz.	80	3.0	20.0	1.0	n.a.	0	0	2.0 d
(*Finast*), 3.3 oz.	80	3.0	20.0	1.0	n.a.	0	5	m.q.
(*Green Giant Harvest Fresh Niblets*), ½ cup	80	2.0	17.0	1.0	n.a.	0	40	2.0 d
(*Green Giant* Niblets), ½ cup	90	2.0	19.0	<1.0	n.a.	0	5	2.0 d
(*Green Giant Niblets* Supersweet), ½ cup	60	2.0	13.0	1.0	n.a.	0	5	2.0 d
cut:								
(*Birds Eye* Portion Pack), 3 oz.	70	3.0	18.0	1.0	n.a.	0	0	2.0 d
(*Frosty Acres*), 3.3 oz.	80	3.0	20.0	1.0	n.a.	0	3	1.0 c
(*Seabrook*), 3.3 oz.	80	3.0	20.0	1.0	n.a.	0	3	1.0 c
(*Southern*), 3.5 oz.	98	3.1	21.3	.7	n.a.	0	20	m.q.
(*Stokely Singles*), 3 oz.	75	3.0	18.0	1.0	n.a.	0	5	m.q.
petite (*Birds Eye* Deluxe), 2.6 oz.	70	2.0	16.0	1.0	n.a.	0	0	2.0 d
white:								
(*Green Giant*), ½ cup	90	2.0	19.0	1.0	n.a.	0	5	2.0 d
(*Seabrook*), 3.3 oz.	80	3.0	19.0	1.0	n.a.	0	3	1.0 c
shoepeg (*Green Giant Harvest Fresh*), ½ cup	90	3.0	19.0	1.0	n.a.	0	60	2.0 d
cream style (*Green Giant*), ½ cup ..	110	3.0	25.0	1.0	0	0	370	2.5 d

1. *5.3-oz. edible portion.*

Food and Measure	cal.	prot. (gms)	carbo. (gms)	tot. fat (gms)	sat. fat (gms)	chol. (mgs)	sod. (mgs)	fiber (gms)
CORN, FROZEN *(cont.)*								
in butter sauce:								
(The Budget Gourmet Side Dish),								
5.5 oz.	190	4.0	31.0	6.0	m.q.	15	310	m.q.
(Finast), ½ cup	170	4.0	30.0	4.0	m.q.	n.a.	390	m.q.
(Green Giant Niblets), ½ cup	100	2.0	18.0	2.0	m.q.	n.a.	280	2.0 d
(Green Giant Niblets One Serving),								
4.5 oz.	120	3.0	24.0	2.0	<1.0	5	350	3.0 d
(Stokely Singles), 4 oz.	110	3.0	23.0	1.0	m.q.	5	230	m.q.
on cob *(Stokely Singles)*, 1 ear ...	70	2.0	16.0	1.0	m.q.	5	200	m.q.
golden *(Green Giant)*, ½ cup	100	3.0	19.0	2.0	1.0	5	310	2.0 d
tender sweet *(Birds Eye* Butter								
Sauce Combinations), 3.3 oz. ..	90	2.0	17.0	2.0	m.q.	5	250	2.0 d
white *(Green Giant)*, ½ cup	100	2.0	20.0	2.0	<1.0	5	280	2.3 d
in sauce, country style *(The Budget*								
Gourmet Side Dish), 5.75 oz. ..	140	4.0	19.0	5.0	m.q.	15	290	n.a.
CORN, TOASTED, 1 oz.:								
original *(Cornnuts)*	120	2.0	19.0	4.0	m.q.	0	200	2.7 d
barbecue *(Cornnuts)*	110	3.0	16.0	4.0	m.q.	0	290	2.5 d
nacho cheese *(Cornnuts)*	110	3.0	16.0	4.0	m.q.	0	200	2.4 d
unsalted *(Cornnuts)*	120	2.0	19.0	4.0	m.q.	0	30	2.7 d
CORN, WHOLE GRAIN:								
1 oz.	103	2.7	21.1	1.3	.2	0	10	.8 c
1 cup	605	15.6	123.3	7.9	1.1	0	58	4.8 c
blue *(Arrowhead Mills)*, 2 oz.	210	6.0	41.0	3.0	m.q.	0	1	5.6 d
yellow *(Arrowhead Mills)*, 2 oz.	210	4.0	43.0	2.0	m.q.	0	1	6.8 d
CORN BRAN, crude:								
1 oz.	64	2.4	24.3	.3	<.1	0	2	24.0 d
1 cup	170	6.4	65.1	.7	.1	0	5	64.3 d
CORN CAKE:								
(Quaker Grain Cakes), .32-oz. piece	35	.7	7.4	.2	(0)	0	53	.1 d
CORN CHIPS, PUFFS, AND								
SIMILAR SNACKS, 1 oz.,								
except as noted:								
(Azteca Unsalted)	140	2.0	18.0	7.0	m.q.	0	110	m.q.
(Bachman)	160	2.0	15.0	10.0	m.q.	0	160	m.q.
(Bugles)	150	2.0	18.0	8.0	m.q.	0	290	m.q.
(Corn Snackers), .5-oz. pkg.	60	1.0	10.0	2.0	m.q.	0	190	m.q.
(Dipsy Doodles Rippled Corn Chips)	160	2.0	15.0	10.0	m.q.	0	180	m.q.
(Featherweight Low Salt)	170	2.0	15.0	11.0	m.q.	0	3	m.q.
(Fritos), approx. 34 pieces	150	1.0	16.0	9.0	m.q.	0	230	m.q.
(Fritos Dip Size), approx. 13 pieces	150	2.0	17.0	9.0	m.q.	0	210	m.q.
(Fritos Crisp 'n Thin)	160	1.0	16.0	10.0	m.q.	0	210	m.q.
(Health Valley)	160	1.0	13.0	11.0	m.q.	0	90	1.0 d
(Health Valley No Salt Added)	160	1.0	13.0	11.0	m.q.	0	1	1.0 d
(Planters)	160	2.0	15.0	10.0	2.0	0	160	m.q.
(Snyder's)	160	2.0	14.0	11.0	2.0	0	150	m.q.
(Wise Corn Chips or Crunchies)	160	2.0	15.0	10.0	m.q.	0	180	m.q.
(Wise Corn Ridgies)	160	2.0	15.0	10.0	m.q.	0	180	m.q.

Food and Measure	cal.	prot. (gms)	carbo. (gms)	tot. fat (gms)	sat. fat (gms)	chol. (mgs)	sod. (mgs)	fiber (gms)
(*Wise Toasted Corn Spirals*)	160	2.0	15.0	10.0	m.q.	0	125	m.q.
barbecue flavor (*Bachman* BBQ) ...	150	<1.0	17.0	9.0	m.q.	0	230	m.q.
barbecue flavor (*Fritos* Bar-B-Q),								
approx. 34 pieces	150	2.0	16.0	9.0	m.q.	0	320	m.q.
blue (*Arrowhead Mills* Corn Curls)	120	3.0	22.0	2.0	m.q.	0	54	4.0 d
blue (*Arrowhead Mills* Corn Curls								
Unsalted)	120	3.0	22.0	2.0	m.q.	0	1	4.0 d
cheese:								
(*Chee•tos* Puffed Balls), approx.								
38 pieces	160	2.0	15.0	10.0	m.q.	tr.	360	m.q.
(*Chee•tos* Puffs), approx.								
33 pieces	160	1.0	16.0	10.0	m.q.	tr.	330	m.q.
(*Cheez Doodles* Baked Corn Puffs)	150	2.0	17.0	8.0	m.q.	n.a.	360	m.q.
(*Cheez Doodles* Fried Corn Puffs)	160	2.0	15.0	10.0	m.q.	n.a.	220	m.q.
(*Featherweight* Cheese Curls Low								
Salt)	150	2.0	16.0	9.0	m.q.	0	81	m.q.
(*Jax* Baked)	140	2.0	17.0	7.0	m.q.	n.a.	290	m.q.
(*Jax* Crunchy)	160	2.0	14.0	11.0	m.q.	n.a.	250	m.q.
(*Planters* Cheez Balls)	160	2.0	14.0	11.0	2.0	5	270	m.q.
(*Planters* Cheez Curls)	160	2.0	14.0	11.0	2.0	5	290	m.q.
(*Wise Cheez Waffies*)	140	3.0	14.0	8.0	m.q.	n.a.	420	m.q.
cheddar (*Health Valley*)	160	3.0	15.0	10.0	m.q.	2	120	1.0 d
crunchy (*Chee•tos*), approx.								
26 pieces	150	2.0	15.0	10.0	m.q.	tr.	280	m.q.
crunchy (*Chee•tos* Light)	140	2.0	19.0	6.0	m.q.	0	360	m.q.
nacho (*Bugles*)	160	2.0	17.0	9.0	m.q.	n.a.	250	m.q.
nacho (*Corn Snackers*),								
.5-oz. pkg.	60	1.0	10.0	2.0	m.q.	n.a.	240	m.q.
nacho (*Wise Corn Spirals*)	160	2.0	16.0	10.0	m.q.	n.a.	190	m.q.
chili cheese (*Fritos*), approx.								
34 pieces	160	2.0	16.0	10.0	m.q.	0	310	m.q.
ranch (*Fritos Wild 'n Mild*), approx.								
32 pieces	150	2.0	16.0	9.0	m.q.	0	230	m.q.
tortilla:								
(*Bachman*)	140	2.0	19.0	6.0	m.q.	0	140	m.q.
(*Bachman* No Salt)	140	2.0	19.0	6.0	m.q.	0	0	m.q.
(*Buenitos Tortilla Chips*)	150	2.0	18.0	8.0	m.q.	0	80	3.6 d
(*Buenitos Tortilla Chips* No Salt								
Added)	150	2.0	18.0	8.0	m.q.	0	1	3.6 d
(*Doritos*), approx. 18 pieces	140	2.0	19.0	6.0	m.q.	0	230	m.q.
(*Doritos Cool Ranch*), approx.								
16 pieces	140	2.0	18.0	7.0	m.q.	0	190	m.q.
(*Doritos Cool Ranch* Light)	120	2.0	21.0	4.0	m.q.	0	240	m.q.
(*Featherweight* Round Low Salt) ..	150	2.0	18.0	8.0	m.q.	0	10	m.q.
(*La Famous*)	140	2.0	18.0	7.0	m.q.	0	180	m.q.
(*La Famous* No Salt Added)	140	2.0	18.0	7.0	m.q.	0	5	m.q.
(*Laura Scudder's* Restaurant Style								
Lightly Salted)	140	2.0	18.0	7.0	m.q.	0	90	m.q.

Food and Measure	cal.	prot. (gms)	carbo. (gms)	tot. fat (gms)	sat. fat (gms)	chol. (mgs)	sod. (mgs)	fiber (gms)
CORN CHIPS, TORTILLA *(cont.)*								
(Old El Paso Nachips), approx.								
9 pieces	150	2.0	18.0	7.0	m.q.	0	80	1.5 d
(Tostitos), approx. 11 pieces	140	2.0	18.0	8.0	m.q.	0	170	m.q.
blue *(Bearitos* Organic)	146	2.9	17.4	7.0	m.q.	0	29	.6 d
blue *(Bearitos* Organic No Salt) ..	137	2.6	17.1	6.5	m.q.	0	3	1.0 d
crispy *(Old El Paso)*, approx.								
16 pieces	150	2.0	17.0	8.0	m.q.	0	105	.5 d
nacho:								
(Bachman)	140	2.0	18.0	6.0	m.q.	n.a.	210	m.q.
(Bravos Strips)	140	2.0	18.0	7.0	m.q.	0	220	m.q.
(Bravos Rounds)	150	2.0	18.0	8.0	m.q.	n.a.	180	m.q.
(Doritos), approx. 15 pieces ...	140	2.0	18.0	7.0	m.q.	0	240	m.q.
(Doritos Light)	120	2.0	21.0	4.0	m.q.	0	290	m.q.
(Featherweight Low Salt)	150	2.0	18.0	8.0	m.q.	0	45	m.q.
(Laura Scudder's Triangles) ...	140	2.0	18.0	7.0	m.q.	0	220	m.q.
(Tio Sancho), .5 oz.	70	4.1	.7	5.7	m.q.	n.a.	282	.1 c
jalapeño flavor *(Bravos)*	150	2.0	19.0	7.0	m.q.	0	170	m.q.
jalapeño flavor *(Laura Scudder's*								
Strips)	150	2.0	19.0	7.0	m.q.	0	170	m.q.
sharp *(Tostitos)*, approx.								
11 pieces	150	2.0	17.0	8.0	m.q.	0	200	m.q.
picante flavor, savory and mild								
(Laura Scudder's Restaurant								
Style Strips)	150	2.0	19.0	7.0	m.q.	0	190	m.q.
ranch *(Eagle)*	140	2.0	17.0	8.0	m.q.	1	190	m.q.
salsa *(Doritos Salsa Rio)*, approx.								
15 pieces	140	1.0	19.0	7.0	m.q.	0	170	m.q.
sesame:								
(Hain)	140	2.0	19.0	7.0	m.q.	0	190	m.q.
(Hain No Salt Added)	140	2.0	19.0	7.0	m.q.	0	<5	m.q.
cheese *(Hain)*	160	2.0	20.0	8.0	m.q.	<5	270	m.q.
taco flavor *(Doritos)*	140	2.0	18.0	7.0	m.q.	0	220	m.q.
taco style *(Hain)*	160	2.0	15.0	11.0	m.q.	<5	320	m.q.
yellow *(Bearitos* Organic)	143	2.1	18.1	6.4	m.q.	0	58	1.1 d
yellow *(Bearitos* Organic No Salt)	148	2.2	17.2	7.2	m.q.	0	2	1.4 d
yellow *(Arrowhead Mills* Corn								
Chips), .75 oz.	90	2.0	18.0	1.0	n.a.	0	31	3.0 d
yellow, w/cheese *(Arrowhead Mills*								
Corn Chips), .75 oz.	90	2.0	15.0	2.0	m.q.	n.a.	30	3.0 d
CORN DOG, see "Frankfurter,								
batter-wrapped"								
CORN DOG BATTER MIX:								
(Golden Dipt Corny Dog), 1 oz.	100	3.0	22.0	0	0	0	490	m.q.
CORN FLAKE CRUMBS:								
(Kellogg's), 1 oz.	100	2.0	24.0	0	0	0	290	1.0 d
CORN FLOUR:								
whole-grain, 1 oz.	102	2.0	21.8	1.1	.2	0	1	3.8 d
whole-grain, 1 cup	422	8.1	89.9	4.5	.6	0	6	15.7 d

Food and Measure	cal.	prot. (gms)	carbo. (gms)	tot. fat (gms)	sat. fat (gms)	chol. (mgs)	sod. (mgs)	fiber (gms)
masa, 1 oz.	103	2.6	21.6	1.1	.2	0	1	.5 c
masa, 1 cup	416	10.7	87.0	4.3	.6	0	6	1.9 c
(*Quaker Masa Harina* De Maiz), 1.3								
oz., approx. ⅓ cup	137	3.5	27.4	1.5	n.a.	0	2	2.7 d
(*Quaker Masa Trigo*), 1.3 oz.,								
approx. ⅓ cup	149	3.5	24.7	4.0	m.q.	0	794	1.0 d
white (*Tone's* Masa Harina), 1 tsp. ...	8	.2	1.7	.1	<.1	0	<1	.2 d
CORN FRITTER, frozen:								
(*Mrs. Paul's*), 2 pieces	240	5.0	35.0	9.0	m.q.	10	560	m.q.
CORN GRITS:								
dry:								
1 oz.	105	2.5	22.6	.3	<.1	0	<1	.3 c
1 cup	579	13.7	124.2	1.8	.3	0	1	.8 c
1 tbsp.	36	.9	7.7	.1	<.1	0	tr.	tr.c
white (*Arrowhead Mills*), 2 oz. ...	200	5.0	43.0	1.0	n.a.	0	1	1.5 d
white, enriched (*Quaker/Aunt*								
Jemima Regular/Quick), 3 tbsp.	101	2.4	22.4	.2	n.a.	0	1	1.4 d
yellow:								
(*Arrowhead Mills*), 2 oz.	200	5.0	44.0	1.0	n.a.	0	1	1.5 d
enriched (*Quaker* Quick),								
3 tbsp.	101	2.4	22.4	.2	n.a.	0	1	1.2 d
enriched (*Tone's*), 1 tsp.	12	.3	2.6	<.1	tr.	0	tr.	.1 d
cooked:								
4 oz.	68	1.6	14.7	.2	<.1	0	tr.	.1 c
1 cup	146	3.5	31.4	.5	.1	0	tr.	.2 c
salted, 4 oz.	68	1.6	14.7	.2	<.1	0	253	.1 c
salted, 1 cup	146	3.5	31.4	.5	.1	0	540	.2 c
instant, dry:								
(*Albers* Hominy Quick Grits),								
½ cup	150	4.0	33.0	0	0	0	0	m.q.
w/imitation bacon bits (*Quaker*),								
1-oz. pkt.	101	2.7	21.6	.4	n.a.	0	544	1.5 d
w/real cheddar cheese flavor								
(*Quaker*), 1-oz. pkt.	104	2.2	21.6	1.0	n.a.	n.a.	497	1.3 d
w/imitation ham bits (*Quaker*),								
1-oz. pkt.	99	2.7	21.3	.3	n.a.	0	665	1.7 d
white hominy product (*Quaker*),								
.8-oz. pkt.	79	1.9	17.7	.1	n.a.	0	385	1.2 d
CORN NUGGETS, frozen:								
breaded, fried (*Stilwell Quickkrisp*),								
3 oz.	210	3.0	30.0	8.0	m.q.	1	420	m.q.
CORN OIL, 1 tbsp., except as								
noted:								
1 oz.	251	0	0	28.4	3.6	0	0	0
½ cup	964	0	0	109.0	13.9	0	0	0
1 tbsp.	120	0	0	13.6	1.7	0	0	0
(*Crisco*)	120	0	0	14.0	2.0	0	0	0
(*Hain*)	120	0	0	14.0	2.0	0	0	0

Food and Measure	cal.	prot. (gms)	carbo. (gms)	tot. fat (gms)	sat. fat (gms)	chol. (mgs)	sod. (mgs)	fiber (gms)
CORN OIL *(cont.)*								
(*Mazola*)	120	0	0	14.0	2.0	0	0	0
(*Pathmark*)	130	0	0	14.0	2.0	0	0	0
(*Pathmark* No Frills)	130	0	0	14.0	2.0	0	0	0
(*Wesson*)	120	0	0	14.0	2.0	0	0	0
spray (*Mazola* No Stick), 2.5-second								
spray	6	0	0	1.0	.1	0	0	0
CORN OIL SPREAD, see "Margarine"								
CORN PASTA, see "Pasta"								
CORN PUDDING[1]:								
4 oz.	124	5.0	14.5	6.0	2.9	84	62	.4 c
½ cup	136	5.5	16.0	6.6	3.2	93	69	.5 c
CORN SALAD:								
raw, 1 oz. or ½ cup	6	.6	1.0	.1	(0)	0	n.a.	.2 c
CORN SOUFFLE, frozen:								
(*Stouffer's*), ⅓ of 12-oz. pkg.	160	5.0	18.0	7.0	m.q.	n.a.	560	m.q.
CORN SYRUP (see also "Pancake syrup"):								
dark (*Karo*), 1 tbsp.	60	0	15.0	0	0	0	40	0
light (*Karo*), 1 tbsp.	60	0	15.0	0	0	0	30	0
CORNBREAD, see "Bread, sweet, mix" and "Bread dough"								
CORNED BEEF, see "Beef, corned"								
CORNISH GAME HEN, frozen:								
(*Tyson*), 3.5 oz.	240	28.0	0	14.0	m.q.	75	70	0
CORNMEAL (see also "Corn flour" and "Polenta"):								
degermed, 1 oz.	104	8.5	22.0	.5	.1	0	1	1.5 d
degermed, 1 cup	506	11.7	107.2	2.3	.3	0	5	7.2 d
self-rising:								
bolted:								
1 oz.	95	2.3	19.9	1.0	.1	0	353	.3 c
1 cup	408	10.1	85.7	4.2	.6	0	1521	1.3 c
w/wheat flour, 1 oz.	99	2.4	20.8	.8	.1	0	374	.2 c
w/wheat flour, 1 cup	592	14.3	124.8	4.8	.7	0	2242	1.3 c
degermed, 1 oz.	101	2.4	21.2	.5	.1	0	382	.2 c
degermed, 1 cup	489	11.6	103.2	2.4	.3	0	1860	.7 c
white (*Aunt Jemima*), 1 oz., approx. ⅙ cup	98	2.3	21.1	.5	n.a.	0	381	.2 c
white, enriched, bolted (*Aunt Jemima*), 1 oz., approx. 3 tbsp.	99	2.3	20.4	.9	n.a.	0	382	m.q.
white or yellow (*Albers*), 1 oz.	100	2.0	22.0	1.0	n.a.	0	0	1.5 d
white or yellow, enriched (*Quaker/ Aunt Jemima*), 1 oz., approx. 3 tbsp.	102	2.4	22.2	.5	n.a.	0	1	1.2 d

1. *Recipe: 55% yellow corn, 23% whole milk, 14% egg, 4% sugar, 3% butter, 1% salt, and pepper.*

Food and Measure	cal.	prot. (gms)	carbo. (gms)	tot. fat (gms)	sat. fat (gms)	chol. (mgs)	sod. (mgs)	fiber (gms)
whole grain:								
1 oz.	103	2.3	21.8	1.0	.1	0	10	3.1 d
1 cup	442	9.9	93.8	4.4	.6	0	43	13.4 d
blue (*Arrowhead Mills*), 2 oz.	210	6.0	41.0	3.0	m.q.	0	1	5.6 d
yellow or hi-lysine (*Arrowhead*								
Mills), 2 oz.	210	4.0	43.0	2.0	m.q.	0	1	6.8 d
yellow, bolted (*Tone's*), 1 tsp.	9	.2	1.9	.1	<.1	0	tr.	.2 d
CORNMEAL MIX:								
buttermilk, self-rising, white (*Aunt*								
Jemima), 3 tbsp.	101	2.5	20.2	1.1	n.a.	0	439	m.q.
white, bolted (*Aunt Jemima*), 1 oz.,								
approx. 1/6 cup	99	2.4	20.8	.7	n.a.	0	337	m.q.
yellow, self-rising (*Aunt Jemima*),								
1 oz. or 3 tbsp.	100	2.0	21.0	1.0	n.a.	0	490	m.q.
CORNSTARCH:								
1 oz.	108	.1	25.9	<.1	tr.	0	3	.3 d
1 cup	488	.3	116.8	.1	<.1	0	11	1.2 d
1 tbsp.	30	<.1	7.3	tr.	tr.	0	1	.1 d
(*Argo/Kingsford*), 1 tbsp.	30	0	7.0	0	0	0	0	tr.d
(*Tone's*), 1 tsp.	10	tr.	2.3	<.1	tr.	0	0	<.1 d
COTTONSEED FLOUR:								
partially defatted:								
1 oz.	102	11.6	11.5	1.8	.5	0	10	.6 c
1 cup	337	38.5	38.1	5.8	1.5	0	33	1.9 c
1 tbsp.	18	2.1	2.0	.3	.1	0	2	.1 c
low-fat, 1 oz.	94	14.2	10.3	.4	.1	0	10	.7 c
COTTONSEED KERNELS,								
roasted:								
1 oz.	143	9.2	6.2	10.3	2.7	0	7	.6 c
1 cup	754	48.6	32.6	54.1	14.5	0	37	3.0 c
1 tbsp.	51	3.3	2.2	3.6	1.0	0	3	.2 c
COTTONSEED MEAL:								
partially defatted, 1 oz.	104	13.9	10.9	1.4	.3	0	10	.7 c
COTTONSEED OIL:								
1 oz.	251	0	0	28.4	7.3	0	0	0
1/2 cup	964	0	0	109.0	28.2	0	0	0
1 tbsp.	120	0	0	13.6	3.5	0	0	0
COUGH DROP, see "Candy"								
COUNTRY COATING MIX, see								
"Seasoning and coating mix"								
COUSCOUS:								
dry, 1 oz.	107	3.6	22.0	.2	<.1	0	3	.2 c
dry, 1 cup	692	23.5	142.5	1.2	.2	0	18	1.1 c
cooked, 4 oz.	127	4.3	26.3	.2	<.1	0	6	.2 c
cooked, 1 cup	201	6.8	41.6	.3	.1	0	9	.2 c
mix[1]:								
(*Fantastic Foods*), 1/2 cup[1]	105	3.0	22.0	0	0	0	1	m.q.

1. *Prepared according to package directions, without added ingredients.*

Food and Measure	cal.	prot. (gms)	carbo. (gms)	tot. fat (gms)	sat. fat (gms)	chol. (mgs)	sod. (mgs)	fiber (gms)
COUSCOUS, MIX *(cont.)*								
(Fantastic Foods), ½ cup [1]	122	3.0	22.0	3.0	m.q.	m.q.	35	m.q.
(Near East), 1¼ oz. dry	120	4.0	26.0	0	0	0	5	m.q.
whole wheat *(Fantastic Foods)*,								
½ cup [2]	94	3.5	20.0	0	0	0	0	m.q.
whole wheat *(Fantastic Foods)*,								
½ cup [3]	111	3.5	20.0	2.0	m.q.	m.q.	23	m.q.
COUSCOUS PILAF MIX [4]:								
(Casbah), 1 oz. dry or ½ cup								
cooked	100	4.0	20.0	0	0	0	n.a.	m.q.
savory *(Quick Pilaf)*, ½ cup	94	4.0	19.0	0	0	0	215	m.q.
savory *(Quick Pilaf)*, ½ cup [1]	124	4.0	19.0	3.0	m.q.	m.q.	254	m.q.
COWPEA:								
raw:								
in pods, 1 lb.	208	6.8	43.7	.8	.2	0	9	4.2 c
trimmed, 1 oz.	26	.8	5.4	.1	<.1	0	1	.5 c
trimmed, ½ cup	65	2.1	13.6	.3	.1	0	3	1.3 c
boiled, drained, 4 oz.	110	3.6	23.1	.4	.1	0	5	2.2 c
boiled, drained, ½ cup	79	2.6	16.7	.3	.1	0	3	1.6 c
leafy tips:								
raw:								
untrimmed, 1 lb.	68	9.7	11.4	.6	.2	0	16	3.1 c
trimmed, 1 oz.	8	1.2	1.4	.1	<.1	0	2	.4 c
chopped, ½ cup	5	.7	.9	<.1	<.1	0	1	.2 c
boiled, drained, 4 oz.	25	5.3	3.2	.1	<.1	0	7	3.0 c
young pods, w/seeds:								
raw:								
untrimmed, 1 lb.	182	13.6	39.2	1.2	.3	0	17	7.0 c
trimmed, 1 oz.	12	.9	2.7	.1	<.1	0	1	.5 c
trimmed, ½ cup	21	1.6	4.5	.1	<.1	0	2	.8 c
1 pod, 11⅞″ × ⁵⁄₁₆″, approx.								
.5 oz.	5	.4	1.1	<.1	tr.	0	tr.	.2 c
boiled, drained, 4 oz.	39	2.9	7.9	.3	.1	0	3	1.9 c
boiled, drained, ½ cup	16	1.2	3.3	.1	<.1	0	1	.8 c
COWPEA, CANNED (see "Black-								
eyed peas" and "Cowpea,								
mature, canned")								
COWPEA, CATJANG, see								
"Catjang"								
COWPEA, FROZEN (see also								
"Black-eyed peas, frozen"):								
10-oz. pkg.	396	25.5	71.4	2.0	.5	0	17	4.6 c
boiled, drained, 4 oz.	150	9.6	26.9	.7	.2	0	6	1.7 c
boiled, drained, ½ cup	112	7.2	20.2	.6	.1	0	5	1.3 c
COWPEA, MATURE, dried:								
raw, 1 oz.	95	6.7	17.0	.4	.1	0	5	7.7 d

1. *Prepared with 2 tbsp. salted butter.*
2. *If adding ¼ tsp. salt to basic recipe, increase value listed for sodium by 75 mg.*
3. *Prepared with 2 tbsp. salted butter; if adding ¼ tsp. salt to basic recipe, increase value listed for sodium by 75 mg.*
4. *Prepared according to package directions, without added ingredients, except as noted.*

Food and Measure	cal.	prot. (gms)	carbo. (gms)	tot. fat (gms)	sat. fat (gms)	chol. (mgs)	sod. (mgs)	fiber (gms)
raw, ½ cup	283	19.8	50.4	1.1	.3	0	14	22.7 d
boiled:								
4 oz.	132	8.8	23.6	.6	.2	0	5	10.9 d
½ cup	100	6.7	17.9	.5	.1	0	3	8.3 d
(A&P), 1 cup	230	15.0	41.0	1.0	m.q.	0	15	m.q.
COWPEA, MATURE, CANNED								
(see also "Black-eyed peas, canned"):								
plain, w/liquid, 4 oz.	87	5.4	15.5	.6	.2	0	339	.8 c
plain, w/liquid, ½ cup	92	5.7	16.4	.7	.2	0	359	.8 c
w/pork, 4 oz.	94	3.1	18.7	1.8	.7	8	397	.8 c
w/pork, ½ cup	99	3.3	19.8	1.9	.7	8	420	.8 c
CRAB, ALASKA KING, meat only:								
raw:								
1 lb.	379	83.0	0	2.7	m.q.	189	3792	0
1 oz.	24	5.2	0	.2	m.q.	12	237	0
1 leg, approx. 6.1 oz., yield from 1-lb. whole leg	144	31.5	0	1.0	m.q.	72	1438	0
boiled, poached, or steamed[1]:								
4 oz.	110	21.9	0	1.7	.2	60	1216	0
1 leg, approx. 4.7 oz., yield from raw leg	129	25.9	0	m.q.	.2	72	1436	0
CRAB, BLUE, meat only:								
raw:								
1 lb.	395	81.9	.2	4.9	1.0	355	1329	0
1 oz.	25	5.1	<.1	.3	.1	22	83	0
1 crab, approx. .7 oz., yield from ⅓-lb. whole crab	18	3.8	<.1	.2	<.1	16	62	0
boiled, poached, or steamed[1]:								
4 oz.	116	22.9	0	2.0	.3	113	316	0
1 cup, approx. 4.75 oz.	138	27.3	0	2.4	.3	135	376	0
cake, fried :								
4 oz.	176	22.9	.5	8.5	1.7	170	374	.6 c
1 medium, approx. 2.1 oz.	93	12.1	.3	4.5	.9	90	198	<.1 c
CRAB, CANNED, meat only:								
blue, 4 oz.	112	23.3	0	1.4	.3	101	378	0
blue, 1 cup, approx. 4.75 oz.	133	27.7	0	1.7	.3	120	450	0
dungeness (S&W), 3.25 oz.	81	18.0	1.0	2.0	m.q.	m.q.	920	0
CRAB, DEVILED, breaded, frozen:								
(Mrs. Paul's), 3-oz. cake	180	8.0	18.0	9.0	m.q.	20	480	m.q.
miniature (Mrs. Paul's), 3½ oz.	240	9.0	25.0	12.0	m.q.	20	540	m.q.
CRAB, DUNGENESS, meat only, raw:								
1 lb.	391	79.0	3.3	4.4	.6	269	1340	0
1 oz.	24	4.9	.2	.3	<.1	17	84	0

1. *Without added ingredients.*
2. *Recipe: 82.2% cooked crab meat, 9.1% egg, 3.6% onion, and 5.1% margarine for frying.*

Food and Measure	cal.	prot. (gms)	carbo. (gms)	tot. fat (gms)	sat. fat (gms)	chol. (mgs)	sod. (mgs)	fiber (gms)
CRAB, DUNGENESS *(cont.)*								
1 crab, approx. 5.75 oz., yield from								
1½-lb. whole crab	140	1.6	1.2	1.6	.2	97	481	0
CRAB, FROZEN:								
snow (*Wakefield*), 3 oz.	60	13.0	0	1.0	m.q.	m.q.	270	0
CRAB, IMITATION[1]:								
1 lb.	463	54.5	46.4	5.9	m.q.	89	3815	0
1 oz.	29	3.4	3.0	.4	m.q.	6	238	0
(*Icicle Brand*), 3.5 oz.	99	12.0	11.0	.1	tr.	10	900	0
CRAB, QUEEN, meat only, raw:								
1 lb.	407	83.9	0	5.4	.6	248	2445	0
1 oz.	26	5.2	0	.3	<.1	16	153	0
CRAB AND SHRIMP, frozen:								
(*Wakefield*), 3 oz.	60	13.0	0	1.0	m.q.	m.q.	210	0
CRABAPPLE:								
untrimmed, 1 lb.	316	1.7	83.2	1.3	.2	0	4	2.5 c
trimmed, w/skin, 1 oz.	22	.1	5.7	.1	<.1	0	<1	.2 c
trimmed, w/skin, sliced, ½ cup	42	.2	11.0	.2	.1	0	1	.3 c
CRABAPPLE, SPICED, canned:								
(*Lucky Leaf/Musselman's*), 4 oz. ...	110	0	28.0	0	0	0	m.q.	m.q.
CRACKER:								
bacon flavor (*Keebler* Toasteds),								
4 pieces, approx. ½ oz.	60	1.0	8.0	3.0	<1.0	0	125	m.q.
bacon flavor (*Nabisco Bacon Flavor*								
Thins), 7 pieces or ½ oz.	70	1.0	9.0	4.0	1.0	0	210	m.q.
w/bacon and cheese (*Handi-Snacks*),								
1 pkg.	130	4.0	8.0	9.0	4.0	20	410	m.q.
bran (*FiberRich*), 1 piece	18	1.0	6.0	<1.0	n.a.	0	10	2.8 d
bran, toasted (*Bran Thins*), 7 pieces								
or ½ oz.	60	1.0	9.0	3.0	<1.0	0	70	m.q.
butter flavor:								
(*Escort*), 3 pieces, ½ oz.	70	1.0	9.0	4.0	<1.0	0	115	m.q.
(*Keebler Club* Low Salt), 4 pieces,								
approx. ½ oz.	60	1.0	9.0	3.0	<1.0	0	75	m.q.
(*Keebler* Toasteds Buttercrisp),								
4 pieces, approx. ½ oz.	60	1.0	8.0	3.0	<1.0	0	125	m.q.
(*Keebler Town House*), 4 pieces,								
approx. ½ oz.	70	1.0	8.0	4.0	<1.0	0	120	m.q.
(*Keebler Town House* Low Salt),								
4 pieces, approx. ½ oz.	70	1.0	8.0	4.0	<1.0	0	60	m.q.
(*Pepperidge Farm Flutters*), ¾ oz.	100	2.0	15.0	4.0	1.0	5	150	m.q.
(*Ritz*), 4 pieces or ½ oz.	70	1.0	9.0	4.0	<1.0	0	120	m.q.
(*Ritz* Low Salt), 4 pieces or ½ oz.	70	1.0	9.0	4.0	<1.0	0	60	m.q.
(*Ritz Bits*), 22 pieces or ½ oz. ...	70	1.0	9.0	4.0	<1.0	0	120	m.q.
(*Ritz Bits* Low Salt), 22 pieces or								
½ oz.	70	1.0	9.0	4.0	<1.0	0	60	m.q.
dairy (*Nabisco American Classic*),								
4 pieces or ½ oz.	70	1.0	9.0	3.0	<1.0	<2	140	m.q.

1. *Made from surimi (see "Surimi").*

Food and Measure	cal.	prot. (gms)	carbo. (gms)	tot. fat (gms)	sat. fat (gms)	chol. (mgs)	sod. (mgs)	fiber (gms)
thins (*Pepperidge Farm* Distinctive), 4 pieces	70	1.0	10.0	3.0	1.0	<5	115	m.q.
cheese or cheese flavor:								
(*Cheez-It*), 12 pieces	70	2.0	7.0	4.0	1.0	<2	135	m.q.
(*Cheez-It* Low Salt), 12 pieces ...	70	2.0	7.0	4.0	1.0	<2	65	m.q.
(*Cheese Nips*), 13 pieces or ½ oz.	70	1.0	9.0	3.0	<1.0	<2	130	m.q.
(*Combos*), 1.8 oz.	240	5.0	34.0	10.0	m.q.	n.a.	580	m.q.
(*Hain*), 1 oz.	130	3.0	17.0	6.0	m.q.	n.a.	180	m.q.
(*Ritz Bits*), 22 pieces or ½ oz. ...	70	1.0	8.0	4.0	<1.0	<2	130	m.q.
(*Rokeach*), 25 pieces or 1 oz.	140	3.0	16.0	8.0	m.q.	n.a.	m.q.	m.q.
(*Tid Bit*), 16 pieces or ½ oz.	70	1.0	8.0	4.0	1.0	<2	200	m.q.
cheddar:								
(*Better Cheddars*), 10 pieces or ½ oz.	70	2.0	8.0	4.0	<1.0	<2	130	m.q.
(*Better Cheddars* Low Salt), 10 pieces or ½ oz.	70	2.0	8.0	4.0	<1.0	<2	65	m.q.
(*Cheddar Wedges*), 31 pieces or ½ oz.	70	1.0	9.0	3.0	<1.0	<2	240	m.q.
(*Guppies*), ½ oz., approx. 12 pieces	40	1.0	5.0	2.0	m.q.	n.a.	95	m.q.
(*Keebler Town House Jrs.*), 8 pieces, approx. ½ oz.	80	1.0	8.0	4.0	<1.0	<5	95	m.q.
(*Pepperidge Farm* Goldfish), 1 oz.	120	4.0	19.0	4.0	1.0	5	230	1.0 d
Parmesan (*Pepperidge Farm* Goldfish), 1 oz.	120	4.0	19.0	4.0	1.0	<5	330	1.0 d
snacks (*Finast*), ½ oz., approx. 12 pieces	70	1.0	9.0	3.0	m.q.	n.a.	135	m.q.
sticks (*Pepperidge Farm* Snack Sticks), 8 pieces	130	4.0	19.0	5.0	2.0	0	400	1.0 d
Swiss (*Nabisco Swiss Cheese*), 7 pieces or ½ oz.	70	1.0	11.0	3.0	<1.0	<2	170	m.q.
thins (*Pepperidge Farm* Goldfish Thins), 4 pieces	50	1.0	8.0	2.0	0	0	160	m.q.
cheese sandwich:								
(*Ritz Bits*), 6 pieces or ½ oz. ..	80	1.0	7.0	5.0	1.0	<2	135	m.q.
cheddar (*Keebler Town House*), 1 piece, approx. ½ oz.	70	1.0	6.0	4.0	1.0	<5	105	m.q.
and peanut butter (*Keebler*), 2 pieces, approx. ½ oz.	70	2.0	9.0	3.0	<1.0	0	150	m.q.
wheat and American cheese (*Keebler*), 1 piece, approx. ½ oz.	70	1.0	7.0	4.0	1.0	<5	85	m.q.
and cheese (*Handi-Snacks*), 1 pkg.	120	4.0	9.0	8.0	5.0	20	360	m.q.
chicken flavored (*Chicken in a Biskit*), 7 pieces or ½ oz.	80	1.0	8.0	5.0	1.0	0	130	m.q.

Food and Measure	cal.	prot. (gms)	carbo. (gms)	tot. fat (gms)	sat. fat (gms)	chol. (mgs)	sod. (mgs)	fiber (gms)
CRACKER *(cont.)*								
chowder, see "soup and oyster," below								
(*Crisp & Light* Crackerbread), 1 slice	17	1.0	3.0	<1.0	n.a.	0	25	m.q.
(*Crisp & Light* Crackerbread Salt Free), 1 slice	17	1.0	3.0	<1.0	n.a.	0	<1	m.q.
crispbread (see also specific grains):								
(*Dar-Vida*), 1 piece	20	1.0	4.0	<1.0	n.a.	0	40	m.q.
(*Kavli* Norwegian), 1 thick piece	35	1.0	7.5	.3	n.a.	0	31	1.9 d
(*Kavli* Norwegian), 2 thin pieces	40	1.0	8.0	.3	n.a.	0	32	6 d
(*Wasa* Breakfast), 1 piece	50	2.0	8.0	1.0	n.a.	0	65	.7 d
(*Wasa* Extra Crisp), 1 piece	25	1.0	5.0	0	0	0	40	m.q.
(*Wasa* Fiber Plus), 1 piece	35	1.0	5.0	1.0	n.a.	0	65	2.8 d
dark, regular or w/caraway (*Finn Crisp*), 2 pieces	38	1.0	9.0	<1.0	n.a.	0	130	1.6 d
garlic flavor (*Weight Watchers*), 2 pieces	30	<1.0	7.0	0	0	0	55	m.q.
high fiber (*Ryvita* Crisp Bread), 1 piece	23	.9	4.0	<1.0	n.a.	0	10	2.0 d
high fiber (*Ryvita* Snackbread), 1 piece	14	.6	3.0	<1.0	n.a.	0	25	1.0 d
croissant (*Carr's*), 1 piece	25	n.a.	3.0	1.3	n.a.	n.a.	19	m.q.
(*Estee* Unsalted), 4 pieces	60	1.0	9.0	2.0	<1.0	0	0	m.q.
(*FFV* Schooners), 33 pieces, approx. ½ oz.	60	1.0	10.0	2.0	<1.0	0	130	m.q.
(*Featherweight* Low Salt), 2 pieces . .	30	0	5.0	1.0	n.a.	0	1	m.q.
garlic (*Manischewitz Garlic Tams*), 10 pieces	153	2.0	19.0	8.0	6.0	0	165	m.q.
graham, see "Cookie"								
grain, mixed (*Harvest Crisps* 5 Grain), 6 pieces or ½ oz. . . .	60	1.0	10.0	2.0	<1.0	0	135	m.q.
(*Hain* Rich), 1 oz.	130	3.0	18.0	5.0	m.q.	n.a.	160	m.q.
(*Hain* Rich No Salt Added), 1 oz. . . .	130	3.0	18.0	5.0	m.q.	n.a.	15	m.q.
herb, garden (*Pepperidge Farm Flutters*), ¾ oz.	100	2.0	14.0	4.0	1.0	0	190	m.q.
(*Hickory Farms Old Fashioned*), 10 pieces	90	2.0	16.0	3.0	m.q.	n.a.	170	m.q.
high fiber, see specific listings								
(*Manischewitz Tam Tams*), 10 pieces	147	2.0	17.0	8.0	6.0	0	171	m.q.
(*Manischewitz Tam Tams* No Salt), 10 pieces	138	2.0	18.0	7.0	5.0	0	<10	m.q.
matzo:								
(*Manischewitz* Daily Unsalted), 1-oz. board	110	3.0	24.0	.3	0	0	1	.1 d
(*Manischewitz* Passover), 1.1-oz. board	129	3.3	27.0	.4	0	0	<5	m.q.
American (*Manischewitz*), 1-oz. board	115	2.9	22.0	1.9	m.q.	0	n.a.	m.q.

Food and Measure	cal.	prot. (gms)	carbo. (gms)	tot. fat (gms)	sat. fat (gms)	chol. (mgs)	sod. (mgs)	fiber (gms)
dietetic, thin (*Manischewitz*),								
.8-oz. board	91	2.6	19.0	.4	0	0	<1	.1 d
egg (*Manischewitz* Passover),								
1.2-oz. board	132	4.0	27.0	2.0	m.q.	25	<5	m.q.
egg, miniature (*Manischewitz*								
Passover), 10 pieces, approx.								
1 oz.	108	3.0	20.0	2.0	m.q.	20	<10	m.q.
egg n' onion (*Manischewitz*), 1-oz.								
board	112	3.1	23.0	1.0	.2	15	180	m.q.
miniature (*Manischewitz*),								
10 pieces	90	2.0	20.0	<1.0	n.a.	0	<10	m.q.
tea, thin (*Manischewitz* Daily),								
.9-oz. board	103	3.0	22.0	.3	0	0	1	.1 d
thin (*Manischewitz*), .9-oz. board	100	3.0	21.0	.3	0	0	n.a.	.1 d
whole wheat w/bran								
(*Manischewitz*), 1-oz. board ...	110	4.0	21.0	.6	0	0	1	.6 d
melba toast, ½ oz., except as noted:								
plain:								
(*Devonsheer*), 1 piece	16	1.0	3.0	.4	.1	0	30	.2 d
(*Devonsheer* Rounds)	53	2.0	11.0	.6	n.a.	0	111	.8 d
(*Devonsheer* Unsalted), 1 piece	16	1.0	3.0	.4	.1	0	5	.2 d
(*Devonsheer* Unsalted Rounds)	52	1.8	10.9	.6	n.a.	0	<5	.8 d
bacon (*Old London* Rounds)	53	2.1	10.1	1.0	n.a.	0	126	.9 d
garlic (*Devonsheer* Rounds)	56	2.1	10.0	1.2	n.a.	0	132	.6 d
garlic (*Old London* Rounds)	56	2.1	9.9	1.2	n.a.	0	132	.6 d
honey bran (*Devonsheer*), 1 piece	16	1.0	3.0	.4	.1	0	25	.2 d
honey bran (*Devonsheer* Rounds)	52	2.1	10.2	.9	n.a.	0	98	.9 d
oat (*Harvest Crisps*), 6 pieces or								
½ oz.	60	1.0	10.0	2.0	<1.0	0	135	m.q.
onion (*Devonsheer* Rounds)	51	1.9	10.7	.6	n.a.	0	120	.8 d
onion (*Old London* Rounds)	52	2.0	10.2	.8	n.a.	0	121	.7 d
pumpernickel (*Old London*)	54	1.6	11.0	.6	n.a.	0	156	.8 d
rye:								
(*Devonsheer*), 1 piece	16	1.0	3.0	.4	.1	0	30	.2 d
(*Devonsheer* Rounds)	53	1.8	10.7	.6	n.a.	0	130	.9 d
(*Devonsheer* Unsalted), 1 piece	16	1.0	3.0	.4	.1	0	5	.2 d
(*Old London*)	52	1.8	10.9	.7	n.a.	0	132	.8 d
(*Old London* Rounds)	52	1.7	10.8	.7	n.a.	0	132	.9 d
sesame:								
(*Devonsheer*), 1 piece	16	1.0	3.0	.5	.1	0	25	.2 d
(*Devonsheer* Rounds)	57	2.3	9.0	1.8	m.q.	0	131	.9 d
(*Old London*)	55	2.3	8.9	1.8	m.q.	0	148	.9 d
(*Old London* Rounds)	56	2.3	8.9	1.8	m.q.	0	149	.9 d
(*Old London* Unsalted)	55	2.3	8.9	1.8	m.q.	0	5	1.0 d
vegetable (*Devonsheer*), 1 piece ..	16	1.0	3.0	.4	.1	0	25	.2 d
wheat:								
(*Estee* 6 calorie), 1 piece	6	<1.0	1.0	<1.0	<1.0	0	<5	m.q.
(*Estee* Snax), 1 oz.	100	4.0	22.0	<1.0	<1.0	0	15	m.q.
(*Old London*)	51	2.1	10.5	.7	n.a.	0	121	.9 d

Food and Measure	cal.	prot. (gms)	carbo. (gms)	tot. fat (gms)	sat. fat (gms)	chol. (mgs)	sod. (mgs)	fiber (gms)
CRACKER, MELBA TOAST, WHEAT *(cont.)*								
whole (*Devonsheer*), 1 piece ...	16	1.0	3.0	.4	.1	0	30	.2 d
whole (*Devonsheer* Unsalted),								
1 piece	16	1.0	3.0	.4	.1	0	5	.2 d
white:								
(*Old London*)	51	2.0	10.4	.6	n.a.	0	111	.8 d
(*Old London* Rounds)	48	2.0	9.8	.6	n.a.	0	111	.8 d
(*Old London* Unsalted)	51	1.8	10.7	.6	n.a.	0	4	.8 d
whole grain:								
(*Old London*)	52	2.1	10.1	.9	n.a.	0	116	.8 d
(*Old London* Rounds)	54	2.1	9.9	1.2	n.a.	0	102	.9 d
(*Old London* Unsalted)	53	2.1	10.0	1.0	n.a.	0	4	.9 d
oat (*Oat Thins*), 8 pieces or ½ oz.	70	1.0	10.0	3.0	<1.0	0	90	m.q.
oat bran (*Oat Bran Krisp*), ½ oz.,								
approx. 2 triple pieces	60	1.0	9.0	3.0	m.q.	0	140	3.2 d
onion:								
(*Hain*), 1 oz.	130	3.0	17.0	6.0	m.q.	n.a.	160	m.q.
(*Hain* No Salt Added), 1 oz.	130	3.0	17.0	6.0	m.q.	n.a.	5	m.q.
(*Keebler* Toasteds), 4 pieces,								
approx. ½ oz.	60	1.0	9.0	3.0	<1.0	0	140	m.q.
(*Manischewitz Onion Tams*),								
10 pieces	150	2.0	18.0	8.0	6.0	0	157	m.q.
minced (*Nabisco American*								
Classics), 4 pieces or ½ oz. ...	70	1.0	10.0	3.0	<1.0	0	120	m.q.
oyster, see "soup and oyster," below								
peanut butter:								
(*Combos*), 1.8 oz.	240	6.0	30.0	10.0	m.q.	n.a.	360	m.q.
cheese (*Little Debbie*), .93 oz. ...	130	4.0	14.0	6.0	m.q.	<1	260	m.q.
cheese (*Little Debbie*), 1.4 oz. ...	190	6.0	23.0	9.0	m.q.	<1	390	m.q.
cheese sandwich (*Handi-Snacks*),								
1 pkg.	190	6.0	11.0	14.0	4.0	0	180	m.q.
sandwich (*Ritz Bits*), 6 pieces or								
½ oz.	80	2.0	8.0	4.0	<1.0	0	80	m.q.
toast and (*Keebler*), 2 pieces,								
approx. ½ oz.	70	2.0	9.0	3.0	<1.0	0	120	m.q.
toasty (*Little Debbie*), .93 oz.	140	4.0	14.0	7.0	m.q.	<1	250	m.q.
toasty (*Little Debbie*), 1.4 oz.	200	6.0	21.0	12.0	m.q.	<1	380	m.q.
(*Pepperidge Farm* Original Goldfish),								
1 oz.	130	3.0	18.0	5.0	1.0	0	190	1.0 d
pizza (*Pepperidge Farm* Goldfish),								
1 oz.	130	4.0	19.0	5.0	1.0	<5	220	1.0 d
poppy, toasted (*Nabisco American*								
Classic), 4 pieces or ½ oz.	70	1.0	9.0	3.0	<1.0	0	140	m.q.
pretzel (*Pepperidge Farm* Goldfish),								
1 oz.	110	3.0	20.0	3.0	0	0	160	1.0 d
pretzel (*Pepperidge Farm* Snack								
Sticks), 8 pieces	120	3.0	23.0	3.0	0	0	430	1.0 d
pumpernickel (*Pepperidge Farm* Snack								
Sticks), 8 pieces	140	3.0	20.0	6.0	1.0	0	330	1.0 d

Food and Measure	cal.	prot. (gms)	carbo. (gms)	tot. fat (gms)	sat. fat (gms)	chol. (mgs)	sod. (mgs)	fiber (gms)
rice, harvest (*Weight Watchers* Crispbread), 2 pieces	30	<1.0	7.0	0	0	0	55	m.q.
rice bran (*Health Valley*), 7 pieces ..	130	4.0	19.0	4.0	m.q.	0	64	1.5 d
rye:								
(*Hain*), 1 oz.	120	3.0	19.0	4.0	m.q.	0	200	m.q.
(*Hain* No Salt Added), 1 oz.	120	3.0	19.0	4.0	m.q.	0	10	m.q.
(*Hickory Farms* Salt Free), 8 pieces	90	2.0	18.0	1.0	n.a.	n.a.	0	m.q.
(*Hickory Farms Wafers*), 8 pieces	90	2.0	17.0	2.0	m.q.	n.a.	250	m.q.
(*Keebler* Toasteds), 4 pieces, approx. ½ oz.	60	1.0	8.0	3.0	<1.0	0	140	m.q.
(*Rykrisp*), ½ oz.	40	1.0	11.0	0	0	0	75	3.6 d
BBQ (*Hickory Farms Rounds O' Rye*), 1 oz.	153	2.7	13.0	10.6	m.q.	n.a.	60	m.q.
dark (*Ryvita* Crisp Bread), 1 piece	26	.7	6.0	<1.0	n.a.	0	35	1.3 d
garlic (*Hickory Farms Rounds O' Rye*), 1 oz.	147	2.7	14.5	8.9	m.q.	n.a.	126	m.q.
golden (*Wasa* Crispbread), 1 piece	35	1.0	7.0	0	0	0	55	1.4 d
hearty (*Wasa* Crispbread), 1 piece	45	2.0	9.0	0	0	0	70	2.6 d
light (*Finn Crisp* Hi-Fiber), 1 piece	35	1.0	8.0	1.0	n.a.	0	60	m.q.
light (*Ryvita* Crisp Bread), 1 piece	26	.7	6.0	<1.0	n.a.	0	20	1.3 d
light (*Wasa* Crispbread Lite), 1 piece	25	1.0	5.0	0	0	0	40	1.2 d
natural (*Hickory Farms Rounds O' Rye*), 1 oz.	156	3.1	12.2	10.9	m.q.	n.a.	93	m.q.
original (*Finn Crisp* Hi-Fiber), 1 piece	40	1.0	10.0	0	0	0	95	m.q.
seasoned (*Rykrisp*), ½ oz.	45	1.0	11.0	1.0	n.a.	0	105	3.0 d
seasoned (*Rykrisp* Twindividuals), ½ oz., approx. 2 triple pieces	45	1.0	11.0	1.0	n.a.	0	105	3.0 d
sesame (*Rykrisp*), ½ oz., approx. 2 triple pieces	50	1.0	10.0	2.0	m.q.	0	105	3.0 d
sesame, toasted (*Ryvita* Crisp Bread), 1 piece	31	1.1	5.0	<1.0	n.a.	0	10	1.4 d
sour cream (*Hickory Farms Rounds O' Rye*), 1 oz.	155	2.7	12.6	10.7	m.q.	n.a.	130	m.q.
saltine:								
(*Krispy*), 5 pieces	60	1.0	11.0	1.0	<1.0	0	210	m.q.
(*Krispy* Unsalted Tops), 5 pieces	60	1.0	11.0	1.0	<1.0	0	120	m.q.
(*Premium*), 5 pieces or ½ oz. ...	60	1.0	10.0	2.0	<1.0	0	180	m.q.
(*Premium* Fat Free), 5 pieces or ½ oz.	50	1.0	12.0	0	0	0	115	m.q.
(*Premium* Low Salt), 5 pieces or ½ oz.	60	1.0	10.0	2.0	<1.0	0	115	m.q.
(*Premium* Unsalted Tops), 5 pieces or ½ oz.	60	1.0	10.0	2.0	<1.0	0	135	m.q.
(*Premium Bits*), 16 pieces or ½ oz.	70	1.0	9.0	3.0	<1.0	0	160	m.q.

Food and Measure	cal.	prot. (gms)	carbo. (gms)	tot. fat (gms)	sat. fat (gms)	chol. (mgs)	sod. (mgs)	fiber (gms)
CRACKER, SALTINE *(cont.)*								
(Rokeach), 10 pieces or 1 oz.	120	2.0	20.0	3.0	m.q.	0	n.a.	m.q.
(Zesta), 5 pieces, approx. ½ oz.	60	1.0	10.0	2.0	<1.0	0	190	m.q.
(Zesta Low Salt), 5 pieces, approx. ½ oz.	60	1.0	10.0	2.0	<1.0	0	95	m.q.
(Zesta Unsalted Tops), 5 pieces, approx. ½ oz.	60	1.0	10.0	2.0	<1.0	0	85	m.q.
wheat *(Zesta)*, 5 pieces, approx. ½ oz.	60	1.0	10.0	2.0	<1.0	0	190	m.q.
wheat, whole *(Premium Plus)*, 5 pieces or ½ oz.	60	1.0	10.0	2.0	<1.0	0	130	m.q.
sandwich, see specific cracker listings								
sesame:								
(Dar-Vida Crispbread), 1 piece ..	22	1.0	4.0	1.0	n.a.	0	40	m.q.
(FFV Crisp), 1 piece	60	1.0	10.0	2.0	<1.0	0	120	m.q.
(Hain), 1 oz.	140	3.0	16.0	7.0	m.q.	n.a.	210	m.q.
(Hain No Salt Added), 1 oz.	140	3.0	16.0	7.0	m.q.	n.a.	5	m.q.
(Keebler Toasteds), 4 pieces, approx. ½ oz.	60	1.0	8.0	3.0	<1.0	0	130	m.q.
(Pepperidge Farm Distinctive), 4 pieces	80	2.0	12.0	4.0	1.0	0	140	2.0 d
(Pepperidge Farm Snack Sticks), 8 pieces	140	4.0	19.0	5.0	1.0	0	280	1.0 d
bread wafer *(Meal Mates)*, 3 pieces or ½ oz.	70	1.0	9.0	3.0	<1.0	0	160	m.q.
golden *(Nabisco American Classic)*, 4 pieces or ½ oz.	70	1.0	9.0	3.0	<1.0	0	120	m.q.
golden *(Pepperidge Farm Flutters)*, ¾ oz.	110	2.0	13.0	5.0	1.0	0	150	m.q.
savory *(Wasa* Crispbread), 1 piece	30	2.0	4.0	1.0	n.a.	0	40	2.4 d
wafer *(FFV* Crisp), 4 pieces, approx. ½ oz.	60	2.0	9.0	2.0	<1.0	0	140	m.q.
sesame and cheese *(Twigs* Snack Sticks), 5 pieces or ½ oz.	70	1.0	8.0	4.0	<1.0	<2	140	m.q.
sesame wheat *(Wasa* Crispbread), 1 piece	50	2.0	8.0	2.0	m.q.	0	65	.6 d
snack *(Rokeach)*, 9 pieces or 1 oz. ..	130	2.0	19.0	5.0	m.q.	n.a.	m.q.	m.q.
soda or water:								
(Carr's Table Water, Bite Size), 2 pieces	25	1.0	5.0	1.0	n.a.	n.a.	15	m.q.
(Crown Pilot), ½-oz. piece	70	1.0	11.0	2.0	<1.0	0	70	m.q.
(FFV Ocean Crisps), 1 piece	60	1.0	10.0	2.0	<1.0	0	120	m.q.
(North Castles English), 1 piece ..	10	0	3.0	0	0	0	14	m.q.
(Pepperidge Farm Distinctive English Water Biscuit), 4 pieces	70	2.0	13.0	1.0	0	0	100	m.q.
(Royal Lunch), ½-oz. piece	60	1.0	10.0	2.0	<1.0	<2	80	m.q.
(Sailor Boy Pilot), 1 piece	100	2.0	17.0	3.0	<1.0	0	125	m.q.

Food and Measure	cal.	prot. (gms)	carbo. (gms)	tot. fat (gms)	sat. fat (gms)	chol. (mgs)	sod. (mgs)	fiber (gms)
soup and oyster:								
(*Dandy*), 20 pieces or ½ oz.	60	1.0	10.0	2.0	<1.0	0	220	m.q.
(*OTC*), 1 piece	25	1.0	4.0	1.0	<1.0	0	65	m.q.
(*Oysterettes*), 18 pieces or ½ oz.	60	1.0	10.0	1.0	<1.0	0	140	m.q.
(*Sunshine*), 16 pieces	60	1.0	11.0	1.0	<1.0	0	190	m.q.
sour cream and chive (*Hain*), 1 oz.	130	3.0	15.0	6.0	m.q.	n.a.	150	m.q.
sour cream and chive (*Hain* No Salt								
Added), 1 oz.	130	3.0	15.0	6.0	m.q.	n.a.	25	m.q.
sourdough (*Hain*), ½ oz.	65	2.0	9.0	3.0	m.q.	0	100	m.q.
sourdough (*Hain* Low Salt), 1 oz. . .	130	3.0	18.0	5.0	m.q.	0	10	m.q.
toast (*Uneeda* Biscuits Unsalted								
Tops), 3 pieces or ½ oz.	60	1.0	10.0	2.0	<1.0	0	100	m.q.
vegetable:								
(*Hain*), 1 oz.	130	3.0	10.0	5.0	m.q.	0	180	m.q.
(*Hain* No Salt Added), 1 oz.	130	3.0	10.0	5.0	m.q.	0	50	m.q.
(*Vegetable Thins*), 7 pieces or								
½ oz.	70	1.0	8.0	4.0	<1.0	0	140	m.q.
water, see "soda or water," above								
(*Waverly*), 4 pieces or ½ oz.	70	1.0	10.0	3.0	<1.0	0	160	m.q.
(*Waverly* Low Salt), 4 pieces or								
½ oz.	70	1.0	10.0	3.0	<1.0	0	80	m.q.
wheat:								
(*FFV* Crispy Wafer), 6 pieces,								
approx. ½ oz.	70	1.0	9.0	3.0	m.q.	n.a.	80	m.q.
(*FFV* Stoned Wheat Wafer),								
4 pieces, approx. ½ oz.	60	1.0	10.0	2.0	<1.0	0	170	m.q.
(*Finast* Snacks), ½ oz., approx.								
7 pieces	70	1.0	9.0	3.0	m.q.	n.a.	85	m.q.
(*Health Valley* Stoned Wheat),								
13 pieces	120	3.0	17.0	6.0	m.q.	0	85	3.9 d
(*Health Valley* Stoned Wheat No								
Salt Added), 13 pieces	120	3.0	17.0	6.0	m.q.	0	10	3.9 d
(*Hickory Farms Stoned Wheat*								
Wafers Salt Free), 8 pieces	100	2.0	18.0	2.0	m.q.	n.a.	0	m.q.
(*Hickory Farms Wheat Mill Wafers*								
Salt Free), 4 pieces	50	1.0	9.0	1.0	n.a.	n.a.	0	m.q.
(*Manischewitz Wheat Tams*),								
10 pieces	150	2.0	18.0	8.0	6.0	0	180	m.q.
(*Ryvita* Original Snackbread),								
1 piece	20	.5	4.0	<1.0	n.a.	0	20	.2 d
(*Sociables*), 6 pieces or ½ oz.	70	1.0	9.0	3.0	<1.0	0	135	m.q.
(*Sunshine* Wheats), 8 pieces	70	1.0	9.0	4.0	1.0	0	170	m.q.
(*Triscuit*), 3 pieces or ½ oz.	60	1.0	10.0	2.0	<1.0	0	75	m.q.
(*Triscuit* Low Salt), 3 pieces or								
½ oz.	60	1.0	10.0	2.0	<1.0	0	35	m.q.
(*Triscuit Bits*), 8 pieces or ½ oz.	60	1.0	10.0	2.0	<1.0	0	75	m.q.
(*Wheat Thins*), 8 pieces or ½ oz.	70	1.0	9.0	3.0	<1.0	0	120	m.q.
(*Wheat Thins* Low Salt), 8 pieces								
or ½ oz.	70	1.0	9.0	3.0	<1.0	0	60	m.q.

Food and Measure	cal.	prot. (gms)	carbo. (gms)	tot. fat (gms)	sat. fat (gms)	chol. (mgs)	sod. (mgs)	fiber (gms)
CRACKER, WHEAT *(cont.)*								
(Wheatsworth Stone Ground),								
4 pieces or ½ oz.	70	1.0	9.0	3.0	<1.0	0	135	m.q.
cracked:								
(Hickory Farms Wafers),								
8 pieces	100	2.0	17.0	3.0	m.q.	n.a.	290	m.q.
(Nabisco American Classic),								
4 pieces or ½ oz.	70	1.0	8.0	4.0	<1.0	0	140	m.q.
(Pepperidge Farm Distinctive),								
3 pieces	100	2.0	14.0	4.0	1.0	0	180	1.0 d
hearty *(Pepperidge Farm*								
Distinctive), 4 pieces	100	2.0	13.0	5.0	1.0	0	140	1.0 d
herb *(Health Valley* Stoned Wheat),								
13 pieces	120	3.0	17.0	6.0	m.q.	0	160	3.5 d
herb *(Health Valley* Stoned Wheat								
No Salt Added), 13 pieces	120	3.0	17.0	6.0	m.q.	0	30	3.5 d
nutty *(Wheat Thins),* 7 pieces or								
½ oz.	70	1.0	9.0	4.0	<1.0	0	170	m.q.
sesame *(Health Valley* Stoned								
Wheat), 13 pieces	130	3.0	16.0	6.0	m.q.	0	150	2.6 d
sesame *(Health Valley* Stoned								
Wheat No Salt Added),								
13 pieces	130	3.0	17.0	6.0	m.q.	0	20	2.6 d
toasted *(Pepperidge Farm*								
Distinctive), 4 pieces	80	2.0	12.0	3.0	1.0	0	140	m.q.
toasted *(Pepperidge Farm Flutters),*								
¾ oz.	110	2.0	13.0	5.0	1.0	0	170	m.q.
vegetable, seven grain *(Health*								
Valley Stoned Wheat), 13 pieces	120	3.0	17.0	5.0	m.q.	0	125	2.8 d
vegetable, seven grain *(Health*								
Valley Stoned Wheat No Salt								
Added), 13 pieces	120	3.0	17.0	5.0	m.q.	0	20	2.8 d
whole:								
(Carr's), 2 pieces	70	1.0	12.0	1.0	m.q.	m.q.	15	m.q.
(Keebler Wheatables), 12 pieces,								
approx. ½ oz.	70	1.0	9.0	3.0	<1.0	0	140	m.q.
(Manischewitz), 10 pieces	90	3.0	18.0	1.0	m.q.	0	<10	m.q.
whole grain *(Keebler Harvest*								
Wheats), 4 pieces, approx.								
½ oz.	60	1.0	8.0	3.0	<1.0	0	95	m.q.
whole grain *(Wasa* Crispbread),								
1 slice, approx. .35 oz.	30	2.0	4.0	1.0	m.q.	0	40	2.4 d
wheat'n bran *(Triscuit),* 3 pieces or								
½ oz.	60	1.0	10.0	2.0	<1.0	0	75	m.q.
zwieback toast *(Nabisco),* 2 pieces or								
½ oz.	60	2.0	10.0	1.0	<1.0	<2	20	m.q.

Food and Measure	cal.	prot. (gms)	carbo. (gms)	tot. fat (gms)	sat. fat (gms)	chol. (mgs)	sod. (mgs)	fiber (gms)
CRACKER CRUMBS AND								
MEAL:								
(*Golden Dipt*), 1 oz.	100	3.0	22.0	0	0	0	0	m.q.
matzo (*Manischewitz Farfel*), 1 cup ..	280	6.8	60.0	.8	0	0	2	.2 d
matzo meal (*Manischewitz* Daily),								
1 cup	514	13.0	109.0	1.4	0	0	3	.5 d
CRANBERRY:								
w/stems, 1 lb.	210	1.7	54.6	.9	n.a.	0	5	5.2 c
trimmed:								
1 oz.	14	.1	3.6	.1	(0)	0	<1	.3 c
whole, ½ cup	23	.2	6.0	.1	(0)	0	1	.6 c
chopped, ½ cup	27	.2	7.0	.1	(0)	0	1	.7 c
(*Ocean Spray*), 2 oz. or ½ cup	25	0	6.0	0	0	0	0	m.q.
CRANBERRY, CANNED, see								
"Cranberry sauce"								
CRANBERRY BEAN:								
raw, 1 oz.	95	6.5	17.0	.3	.1	0	2	2.6 d
raw, ½ cup	328	22.6	58.9	1.2	.3	0	6	9.1 d
boiled, 4 oz.	154	10.6	27.7	.5	.1	0	1	3.9 d
boiled, ½ cup	120	8.2	21.5	.4	.1	0	1	3.0 d
CRANBERRY BEAN, CANNED:								
w/liquid, 4 oz.	94	6.3	17.1	.3	.1	0	376	1.0 c
w/liquid, ½ cup	108	7.2	19.7	.4	.1	0	431	1.2 c
CRANBERRY FRUIT								
CONCENTRATE:								
(*Hain*), 1 oz. or 2 tbsp.	40	0	10.0	0	0	0	20	n.a.
CRANBERRY JUICE:								
(*Lucky Leaf*), 6 fl. oz.	110	0	26.0	0	0	0	10	(0)
(*Smucker's* Naturally 100%), 8 fl. oz.	130	0	30.0	0	0	0	10	(0)
CRANBERRY JUICE COCKTAIL,								
6 fl. oz., except as noted:								
bottled:								
1 fl. oz.	18	0	4.3	tr.	tr.	0	1	(0)
low-calorie, 1 fl. oz.	5	0	1.4	0	0	0	1	(0)
(*A&P*)	100	<1.0	26.0	<1.0	(0)	0	0	(0)
(*Ocean Spray*)	110	0	26.0	0	0	0	10	(0)
(*Ocean Spray* Low Calorie)	40	0	10.0	0	0	0	10	(0)
(*P&Q*)	100	<1.0	24.0	<1.0	(0)	0	0	(0)
(*Pathmark/Pathmark* No Frills) ...	100	0	26.0	0	0	0	<10	(0)
(*Sunkist*)	110	.1	28.2	.1	(0)	0	8	(0)
(*Veryfine*), 8 fl. oz.	160	<1.0	40.0	0	0	0	<10	(0)
frozen[1]:								
undiluted, 12-fl.-oz. cont.	821	.3	210.2	0	0	0	13	(0)
1 fl. oz.	17	tr.	4.4	0	0	0	1	(0)
(*Sunkist*)	110	.1	28.2	.1	0	0	0	(0)
(*Welch's*)	100	0	26.0	0	0	0	0	0
(*Welch's* No Sugar Added)	40	0	10.0	0	0	0	5	0

1. *Diluted according to package directions, except as noted.*

Food and Measure	cal.	prot. (gms)	carbo. (gms)	tot. fat (gms)	sat. fat (gms)	chol. (mgs)	sod. (mgs)	fiber (gms)
CRANBERRY JUICE DRINK:								
(*Tropicana* Cranberry Orchard Juice Sparkler), 8 fl. oz.	120	(0)	30.0	0	0	0	20	(0)
blend (*Ocean Spray Cran•tastic*), 6 fl. oz.	110	0	27.0	0	0	0	15	(0)
CRANBERRY-APPLE JUICE COCKTAIL:								
frozen[1] (*Welch's*), 6 fl. oz.	120	0	30.0	0	0	0	0	0
CRANBERRY-APPLE JUICE DRINK:								
1 fl. oz.	20	tr.	5.2	0	0	0	1	(0)
(*A&P*), 6 fl. oz.	130	<1.0	32.0	(0)	(0)	0	<1	(0)
(*Ocean Spray Cran•Apple*), 6 fl. oz.	130	0	32.0	0	0	0	10	(0)
(*Ocean Spray Cran•Apple* Low Calorie), 6 fl. oz.	40	0	10.0	0	0	0	10	(0)
(*P&Q*), 6 fl. oz.	130	<1.0	32.0	(0)	(0)	0	<1	(0)
(*Pathmark*), 6 fl. oz.	130	0	32.0	0	0	0	10	(0)
CRANBERRY-APRICOT JUICE DRINK:								
1 fl. oz.	20	.1	5.0	0	0	0	1	(0)
(*Ocean Spray Cranicot*), 6 fl. oz. ...	110	0	26.0	0	0	0	5	(0)
CRANBERRY-BLUEBERRY DRINK:								
(*Ocean Spray Cran•Blueberry*), 6 fl. oz.	120	0	30.0	0	0	0	10	(0)
CRANBERRY-BLUEBERRY JUICE COCKTAIL:								
frozen[1] (*Welch's*), 6 fl. oz.	110	0	27.0	0	0	0	0	0
CRANBERRY-GRAPE JUICE COCKTAIL:								
frozen[1] (*Welch's*), 6 fl. oz.	110	0	27.0	0	0	0	0	0
CRANBERRY-GRAPE JUICE DRINK:								
1 fl. oz.	17	tr.	4.3	tr.	tr.	0	1	(0)
(*Finast*), 6 fl. oz.	103	0	26.0	0	0	0	5	(0)
(*Ocean Spray Cran•Grape*), 6 fl. oz.	130	0	32.0	0	0	0	5	(0)
(*Pathmark*), 6 fl. oz.	103	0	26.0	0	0	0	5	(0)
CRANBERRY-ORANGE RELISH, canned:								
4 oz.	202	.3	52.4	.1	(0)	0	36	.7 c
½ cup	246	.4	63.8	.1	(0)	0	44	.8 c
CRANBERRY-RASPBERRY DRINK:								
(*Ocean Spray Cran•Raspberry*), 6 fl. oz.	110	0	27.0	0	0	0	10	(0)
(*Ocean Spray Cran•Raspberry* Low Calorie), 6 fl. oz.	40	0	10.0	0	0	0	10	(0)

1. *Diluted according to package directions.*

Food and Measure	cal.	prot. (gms)	carbo. (gms)	tot. fat (gms)	sat. fat (gms)	chol. (mgs)	sod. (mgs)	fiber (gms)
CRANBERRY-RASPBERRY JUICE COCKTAIL:								
frozen[1] (*Welch's*), 6 fl. oz.	110	0	28.0	0	0	0	0	0
CRANBERRY SAUCE, canned:								
sweetened, 4 oz.	171	.2	44.1	.2	(0)	0	33	.3 c
sweetened, ½ cup	209	.3	53.7	.2	(0)	0	40	.4 c
(*A&P*), 2 oz.	100	<1.0	25.0	<1.0	(0)	0	15	m.q.
whole or jellied:								
(*Finast*), 2 oz.	90	0	22.0	0	0	0	10	m.q.
(*Ocean Spray*), 2 oz.	90	0	22.0	0	0	0	15	m.q.
(*S&W* Old Fashioned), ½ cup	90	0	22.0	0	0	0	20	m.q.
jellied (*Pathmark*), 2 oz.	90	0	22.0	0	0	0	10	m.q.
CRANBERRY-APPLESAUCE:								
(*Ocean Spray Cran•Fruit*), 2 oz.	100	0	24.0	0	0	0	20	m.q.
CRANBERRY-ORANGE SAUCE:								
(*Ocean Spray Cran•Fruit*), 2 oz.	100	0	23.0	0	0	0	10	m.q.
CRANBERRY-RASPBERRY SAUCE:								
(*Ocean Spray Cran•Fruit*), 2 oz.	100	0	23.0	0	0	0	10	m.q.
CRANBERRY-STRAWBERRY SAUCE:								
(*Ocean Spray Cran•Fruit*), 2 oz.	100	0	23.0	0	0	0	10	m.q.
CRAWFISH ENTREE, frozen:								
etouffee (*Cajun Cookin'*), 12 oz. ...	390	23.0	51.0	10.0	m.q.	m.q.	1110	n.a.
CRAYFISH, mixed species, meat only:								
raw, 1 lb.	405	84.6	0	4.8	.8	628	241	0
raw, 1 oz., approx. 8 medium	25	5.3	0	.3	<.1	39	15	0
boiled or steamed[2], 4 oz.	129	27.1	0	1.5	.3	202	77	0
CREAM, fluid:								
half and half:								
1 oz.	37	.8	1.2	3.3	2.0	10	12	0
1 cup	315	7.2	10.4	27.8	17.3	89	98	0
1 tbsp.	20	.4	.6	1.7	1.1	6	6	0
(*Crowley*), 1 fl. oz.	35	1.0	1.0	3.0	m.q.	15	10	0
(*Darigold*), 8 fl. oz.	310	8.0	11.0	27.0	17.3	89	120	0
(*Knudsen*), 4 fl. oz.	150	4.0	5.0	13.0	m.q.	m.q.	60	0
light, coffee or table:								
1 oz.	55	.8	1.0	5.5	3.4	19	11	0
1 cup	469	6.5	8.8	46.3	28.9	159	95	0
1 tbsp.	29	.4	.6	2.9	1.8	10	6	0
medium, 25% fat:								
1 oz.	69	.7	1.0	7.1	4.4	25	10	0
1 cup	583	5.9	8.3	59.8	37.2	209	88	0
1 tbsp.	37	.4	.5	3.8	2.3	13	6	0
sour, see "Cream, sour"								

1. *Diluted according to package directions.*
2. *Without added ingredients.*

Food and Measure	cal.	prot. (gms)	carbo. (gms)	tot. fat (gms)	sat. fat (gms)	chol. (mgs)	sod. (mgs)	fiber (gms)
CREAM *(cont.)*								
whipping, light:								
1 oz.	83	.6	.8	8.8	5.5	31	10	0
1 cup, approx. 2 cups whipped ...	699	5.2	7.1	73.9	46.2	265	82	0
1 tbsp., approx. 2 tbsp. whipped	44	.3	.4	4.6	2.9	17	5	0
whipping, heavy:								
1 oz.	98	.6	.8	10.5	6.5	39	11	0
1 cup, approx. 2 cups whipped ...	821	4.9	6.6	88.1	54.8	326	89	0
1 tbsp., approx. 2 tbsp. whipped	52	.3	.4	5.6	3.5	21	6	0
(*Crowley*), 1 fl. oz.	110	1.0	1.0	11.0	m.q.	40	10	0
(*Darigold/Darigold UHT*), 1 cup	790	6.0	8.0	81.0	50.8	290	90	0
(*Darigold* Classic), 1 cup	858	5.1	6.9	90.0	23.7	334	77	0
whipped topping, frozen:								
(*Kraft* Real Cream), ¼ cup	30	0	2.0	2.0	2.0	10	5	0
(*La Creme*), 1 tbsp.	16	0	1.0	1.0	n.a.	<1	5	0
whipped topping, pressurized:								
1 oz.	73	.9	3.5	6.3	3.9	22	37	0
1 cup	154	1.9	7.5	13.3	8.3	46	78	0
1 tbsp.	8	.1	.4	.7	.4	2	4	0
(*Crowley*), 1 tbsp.	20	<1.0	<1.0	1.0	m.q.	5	10	0
whipped topping, nondairy, see "Cream topping, nondairy"								
CREAM, SOUR:								
1 oz.	61	.9	1.2	5.9	3.7	13	15	0
1 cup	493	7.3	9.8	48.2	30.0	102	123	0
1 tbsp.	26	.4	.5	2.5	1.6	5	6	0
(*Bison*), 1 oz.	50	1.0	1.0	5.0	m.q.	20	15	0
(*Breakstone's*), 1 tbsp.	30	0	1.0	3.0	2.0	10	5	0
(*Crowley*), 1 oz.	50	1.0	1.0	5.0	m.q.	20	15	0
(*Darigold*), 1 tbsp.	23	.9	1.1	2.8	1.8	5	5	0
(*Friendship*), 1 oz., 2 tbsp.	55	1.0	1.0	5.0	m.q.	42	15	0
(*Knudsen Hampshire*), 1 oz.	60	1.0	1.0	6.0	3.0	20	10	0
(*Sealtest*), 1 tbsp.	30	0	1.0	3.0	2.0	10	5	0
French onion (*Crowley*), 1 oz.	50	1.0	1.0	5.0	m.q.	20	130	0
half and half:								
1 oz.	38	.8	1.2	3.4	2.1	11	11	0
1 tbsp.	20	.4	.6	1.8	1.1	6	6	0
(*Breakstone's Light Choice*), 1 tbsp.	25	1.0	1.0	2.0	1.0	5	10	0
(*Sealtest Light*), 1 tbsp.	25	1.0	1.0	2.0	1.0	5	10	0
imitation (*Pet*), 1 tbsp.	25	<1.0	<1.0	2.0	m.q.	<1	25	0
light:								
(*Crowley*), 1 oz.	30	1.0	2.0	2.0	m.q.	5	25	0
(*Knudsen*), 1 oz.	40	1.0	2.0	3.0	2.0	10	20	0
(*Weight Watchers*), 1 oz. or 2 tbsp.	35	2.0	2.0	2.0	m.q.	m.q.	40	0
lowfat (*Friendship Lite Delite*), 1 oz. or 2 tbsp.	35	1.0	2.0	2.0	m.q.	8	25	0

Food and Measure	cal.	prot. (gms)	carbo. (gms)	tot. fat (gms)	sat. fat (gms)	chol. (mgs)	sod. (mgs)	fiber (gms)
CREAM, SOUR, NONDAIRY:								
1 oz.	59	.7	1.9	5.5	5.0	0	29	0
1 cup	479	5.5	15.3	44.9	40.9	0	235	0
dressing (*Crowley*), 1 oz.	40	1.0	1.0	4.0	m.q.	0	5	0
CREAM GRAVY, canned:								
(*Franco-American*), 2 oz.	35	0	4.0	2.0	m.q.	n.a.	220	n.a.
CREAM NUT, see "Brazil nut"								
CREAM PUFF, frozen:								
Bavarian (*Rich's*), 1 piece	150	2.0	17.0	8.0	m.q.	25	70	m.q.
CREAM OF TARTAR:								
(*Tone's*), 1 tsp.	2	0	.6	0	0	0	n.a.	0
CREAM TOPPING, DAIRY, see								
"Cream"								
CREAM TOPPING, NONDAIRY:								
frozen, semisolid:								
1 oz.	90	.4	6.5	7.2	6.2	0	7	0
1 cup	239	.9	17.3	19.0	16.3	0	19	0
1 tbsp.	13	.1	.9	1.0	.9	0	1	0
(*Birds Eye Cool Whip*), 1 tbsp.	12	0	1.0	1.0	m.q.	0	0	0
(*Birds Eye Cool Whip Lite*),								
1 tbsp.	8	0	1.0	<1.0	m.q.	0	0	0
(*Kraft* Whipped Topping), ¼ cup	35	0	2.0	3.0	3.0	0	10	0
(*Pet Whip*), 1 tbsp.	14	0	1.0	1.0	m.q.	0	0	0
extra creamy (*Birds Eye Cool*								
Whip Dairy Recipe), 1 tbsp.	14	0	1.0	1.0	m.q.	0	0	0
mix[1]:								
1.5 oz. dry	245	2.1	22.3	17.0	15.6	0	52	0
(*D-Zerta*), 1 tbsp.	8	0	0	1.0	(0)	0	5	0
(*Dream Whip*), 1 tbsp.	10	0	1.0	0	0	0	0	0
(*Featherweight*), 1 tbsp.	4	0	0	0	0	0	5	0
pressurized:								
1 oz.	75	.3	4.6	6.3	5.4	0	18	0
1 cup	184	.7	11.3	15.6	13.2	0	43	0
1 tbsp.	11	<.1	.6	.9	.8	0	2	0
(*Rich's Richwhip*), ¼ oz.	20	0	1.0	2.0	m.q.	0	5	0
prewhipped (*Estee*), 1 tbsp.	4	<1.0	<1.0	<1.0	<1.0	0	0	0
prewhipped (*Rich's Richwhip*),								
1 tbsp.	12	0	1.0	1.0	m.q.	0	0	0
unwhipped (*Rich's Richwhip*), ¼ oz.	20	0	1.0	2.0	m.q.	0	10	0
CREAMER, NONDAIRY:								
(*Crowley*), ½ oz.	16	<1.0	1.0	1.0	n.a.	5	5	0
(*Diehl*), 1 tsp.	10	0	1.0	<1.0	0	0	0	0
(*IGA*), 1 tsp.	10	0	2.0	<1.0	n.a.	0	5	0
(*N-Rich*), 1 tsp.	10	.1	2.0	.6	.3	0	2	0
(*Pathmark* No Frills), 1 tsp.	10	0	1.0	0	0	0	5	0
liquid (*Coffee-mate*), 1 tbsp.	16	0	2.0	1.0	.3	0	5	0

1. *Prepared according to package directions, except as noted.*

Food and Measure	cal.	prot. (gms)	carbo. (gms)	tot. fat (gms)	sat. fat (gms)	chol. (mgs)	sod. (mgs)	fiber (gms)
CREAMER, NONDAIRY *(cont.)*								
liquid, frozen:								
1 oz.[1]	39	.3	3.2	2.8	.5	0	22	0
½ cup[1]	163	1.2	13.7	12.0	2.3	0	95	0
1 tbsp.[1]	20	.2	1.7	1.5	.3	0	12	0
1 oz.[2]	39	.3	3.2	2.8	2.6	0	22	0
½ cup[2]	164	1.2	13.7	12.0	11.2	0	95	0
1 tbsp.[2]	20	.2	1.7	1.5	1.4	0	12	0
(*Finast*), ½ oz.	20	0	2.0	2.0	<1.0	0	10	0
(*Rich's Coffee Rich*), ½ oz.	20	0	2.0	2.0	<1.0	0	10	0
(*Rich's Farm Rich*), ½ oz.	20	0	2.0	2.0	<1.0	0	5	0
(*Rich's Poly Rich*), ½ oz.	20	0	1.0	2.0	0	0	5	0
(*Rich's Poly Rich*), ½ oz.	20	0	2.0	1.0	<1.0	0	5	0
powdered:								
1 oz.[1]	155	1.4	15.6	10.1	9.2	0	51	0
½ cup[1]	257	2.3	16.7	25.8	15.3	0	85	0
1 tsp.[1]	11	.1	1.1	.7	.7	0	4	0
(*Coffee-mate*), 1 tsp.	10	<1.0	1.0	<1.0	.7	0	<5	0
(*Coffee-mate Lite*), 1 tsp.	8	<1.0	2.0	<1.0	.3	0	0	0
(*Cremora*), 1 tsp.	10	0	1.0	<1.0	n.a.	0	5	0
CREME DE MENTHE:								
72 proof, 1 fl. oz.	125	0	14.0	.1	tr.	0	2	0
CREOLE SAUCE:								
Cajun (*Enrico's* Light), 4 oz.	76	2.0	9.0	2.8	m.q.	0	284	n.a.
CRESS, GARDEN:								
raw:								
untrimmed, 1 lb.	103	8.4	17.7	2.3	.1	0	45	3.5 c
trimmed, 1 oz.	9	.7	1.6	.2	tr.	0	4	.3 c
trimmed, ½ cup	8	.7	1.4	.2	tr.	0	4	.3 c
boiled, drained, 4 oz.	26	2.2	4.3	.7	<.1	0	9	1.0 c
boiled, drained, ½ cup	16	1.3	2.6	.4	<.1	0	5	.6 c
CRESS, WATER, see "Watercress"								
CRISPBREAD, see "Cracker"								
CROAKER, Atlantic, meat only:								
raw:								
1 lb.	474	80.7	0	14.4	4.9	277	252	0
1 oz.	29	5.0	0	.9	.3	17	16	0
1 fillet, approx. 2.8 oz., yield from 1-lb. whole fish	83	14.1	0	2.5	.9	48	44	0
breaded[3], fried:								
4 oz.	251	20.6	8.6	14.4	3.9	95	395	.2 c
1 fillet, approx. 3.1 oz., yield from raw unbreaded fillet	192	15.8	6.6	11.0	3.0	73	303	.1 c
CROISSANT, 1 piece:								
(*Pepperidge Farm* Sandwich Quartet)	170	4.0	22.0	7.0	m.q.	0	250	tr.d
butter:								
(*Awrey's*), 3 oz.	300	5.0	32.0	17.0	8.0	45	280	1.0 d

1. *Containing hydrogenated vegetable oil and soy protein.*
2. *Containing lauric acid oil (lauric oils include modified coconut oil, hydrogenated coconut oil and/or palm kernel oil) and sodium caseinate.*
3. *Recipe: 84.2% fish, 9.3% bread crumbs, 4.6% egg, 1.4% milk, and .5% salt.*

Food and Measure	cal.	prot. (gms)	carbo. (gms)	tot. fat (gms)	sat. fat (gms)	chol. (mgs)	sod. (mgs)	fiber (gms)
(*Awrey's*), 2 oz.	200	3.0	21.0	11.0	5.0	30	190	1.0 d
(*Awrey's*), 1 oz.	100	2.0	10.0	6.0	3.0	15	90	0
margarine (*Awrey's*), 2.5 oz.	250	4.0	26.0	14.0	3.0	5	360	1.0 d
margarine (*Awrey's*), 1.25 oz.	120	2.0	13.0	7.0	2.0	5	180	0
wheat (*Awrey's*), 2.5 oz.	240	4.0	24.0	14.0	3.0	5	390	1.0 d
CROISSANT, FROZEN, butter, 1 piece:								
(*Sara Lee*), 1.5 oz.	170	4.0	19.0	9.0	m.q.	m.q.	250	m.q.
petite (*Pepperidge Farm*)	140	3.0	13.0	7.0	m.q.	m.q.	160	m.q.
petite (*Sara Lee*), 1 oz.	120	3.0	13.0	6.0	m.q.	m.q.	160	m.q.
CROOKNECK SQUASH:								
raw:								
untrimmed, 1 lb.	84	4.2	18.2	1.1	.2	0	7	4.9 d
ends trimmed, 1 oz.	5	.3	1.1	.1	<.1	0	1	.3 d
ends trimmed, sliced, ½ cup	12	.6	2.6	.2	<.1	0	1	.7 d
boiled, drained, 4 oz.	23	1.0	4.9	.4	.1	0	1	1.2 d
boiled, drained, sliced, ½ cup	18	.8	3.9	.3	.1	0	1	1.0 d
CROOKNECK SQUASH, CANNED:								
drained, no salt added, 4 oz.	15	.7	3.4	.1	<.1	0	6	1.1 d
drained, sliced, no salt added, ½ cup	14	.7	3.2	.1	<.1	0	5	1.1 d
yellow, cut (*Allens*), ½ cup	16	1.0	3.0	<1.0	(0)	0	230	m.q.
CROOKNECK SQUASH, FROZEN:								
10 oz.	57	2.4	13.6	.4	.1	0	14	3.4 d
boiled, drained, 4 oz.	28	1.5	6.3	.2	<.1	0	7	1.4 d
boiled, drained, sliced, ½ cup	24	1.2	5.3	.2	<.1	0	6	1.2 d
(*Kohl's*), cooked, 4 oz.	45	1.0	11.0	<1.0	(0)	0	0	m.q.
yellow (*Seabrook*), 3.3 oz.	18	1.0	4.0	0	0	0	1	1.0 c
yellow (*Southern*), 3.5 oz.	21	1.5	4.1	.1	(0)	0	20	m.q.
CROUTON, ½ oz., except as noted:								
Caesar salad (*Brownberry*)	62	1.8	8.0	2.6	m.q.	<1	165	.5 d
cheddar cheese (*Brownberry*)	63	1.8	8.3	2.8	m.q.	3	155	.3 d
cheddar and Romano cheese (*Pepperidge Farm*)	60	2.0	10.0	2.0	0	0	200	m.q.
cheese and garlic (*Pepperidge Farm*)	70	2.0	9.0	3.0	1.0	0	180	m.q.
onion and garlic (*Brownberry*)	60	1.6	8.8	2.2	m.q.	1	190	.4 d
onion and garlic (*Pepperidge Farm*) ..	70	2.0	9.0	3.0	0	0	160	m.q.
seasoned:								
(*Brownberry*)	59	1.6	8.5	2.2	m.q.	<1	155	.5 d
(*Pepperidge Farm*)	70	2.0	9.0	3.0	1.0	0	180	m.q.
(*Weight Watchers*), 1 pouch	30	1.0	5.0	0	0	n.a.	120	m.q.
sour cream and chive (*Pepperidge Farm*)	70	2.0	9.0	3.0	1.0	0	170	m.q.
toasted (*Brownberry*)	56	1.7	9.7	1.4	n.a.	0	145	.4 d
CROWDER PEA, see "Peas, crowder"								

Food and Measure	cal.	prot. (gms)	carbo. (gms)	tot. fat (gms)	sat. fat (gms)	chol. (mgs)	sod. (mgs)	fiber (gms)
CUCUMBER, w/peel:								
untrimmed, 1 lb.	56	2.4	12.8	.6	.1	0	9	4.4 d
ends trimmed, 1 oz.	4	.2	.8	<.1	tr.	0	1	.3 d
1 medium, 8¼" long × 2⅛", approx.								
10.9 oz. untrimmed	39	1.6	8.8	.4	.1	0	6	3.0 d
sliced, ½ cup	7	.3	1.5	.1	<.1	0	1	.5 d
CUCUMBER, PICKLED, see "Pickle"								
CUCUMBER DIP:								
creamy (*Kraft* Premium), 2 tbsp.	50	1.0	2.0	4.0	3.0	10	130	(0)
CUCUMBER AND ONION DIP:								
(*Breakstone's*), 2 tbsp.	50	1.0	2.0	4.0	3.0	15	160	n.a.
(*Sealtest*), 2 tbsp.	50	1.0	2.0	4.0	3.0	15	160	n.a.
CUMIN SEED:								
1 oz.	106	5.0	12.5	6.3	m.q.	0	48	3.0 c
1 tbsp.	22	1.1	2.7	1.3	n.a.	0	10	.6 c
1 tsp.	8	.4	.9	.5	(0)	0	4	.2 c
(*Spice Islands*), 1 tsp.	7	.3	.7	.4	(0)	0	3	.1 c
(*Tone's*), 1 tsp.	7	.4	.9	.4	(0)	0	3	.2 d
CUPCAKE, see "Cake, snack"								
CUPU ASSU OIL:								
1 oz.	251	0	0	28.4	15.1	0	0	0
½ cup	964	0	0	109.0	58.0	0	0	0
1 tbsp.	120	0	0	13.6	7.2	0	0	0
CURRANT, BLACK, European:								
w/stems, 1 lb.	282	6.2	68.4	1.8	.2	0	8	24.1 d
trimmed, 1 oz.	18	.4	4.4	.1	tr.	0	1	1.5 d
trimmed, ½ cup	36	.8	8.6	.2	<.1	0	1	3.0 d
CURRANT, RED OR WHITE:								
w/stems, 1 lb.	249	6.2	61.3	.9	.1	0	5	15.1 c
trimmed, 1 oz.	16	.4	3.9	.1	tr.	0	<1	1.0 c
trimmed, ½ cup	31	.8	7.7	.1	<.1	0	1	1.9 c
CURRANT, ZANTE, dried:								
1 lb.	1282	18.5	336.0	1.2	.1	0	35	7.1 c
1 oz.	80	1.2	21.0	.1	tr.	0	2	.4 c
½ cup	204	2.9	53.3	.2	<.1	0	6	1.1 c
(*Del Monte*), ½ cup	200	2.0	53.0	0	0	0	<10	m.q.
CURRY POWDER:								
1 oz.	92	3.6	16.5	3.9	m.q.	0	15	4.6 c
1 tbsp.	20	.8	3.7	.9	m.q.	0	3	1.0 c
1 tsp.	6	.3	1.2	.3	m.q.	0	1	.3 c
(*Tone's*), 1 tsp.	6	.3	1.2	.3	<.1	0	1000	.3 d
CURRY SAUCE MIX:								
1.25-oz. pkt.	151	3.3	17.9	8.2	1.2	tr.	1444	.5 c
½ cup[1]	135	5.3	12.9	7.4	3.0	18	638	.2 c
CUSK, meat only, raw:								
1 lb.	396	86.2	0	3.1	m.q.	186	143	0

1. *Prepared according to package directions, with whole milk.*

Food and Measure	cal.	prot. (gms)	carbo. (gms)	tot. fat (gms)	sat. fat (gms)	chol. (mgs)	sod. (mgs)	fiber (gms)
1 oz.	25	5.4	0	.2	m.q.	12	9	0
1 fillet, approx. 4.3 oz., yield from 2-lb. whole fish	106	23.2	0	.8	m.q.	50	38	0
CUSTARD, see "Pudding mix"								
CUSTARD APPLE:								
untrimmed, 1 lb.	267	4.5	66.3	1.6	n.a.	0	11	9.0 c
trimmed, 1 oz.	29	.5	7.1	.2	(0)	0	1	1.0 c
CUTLET, VEGETARIAN, canned:								
(*Worthington*), 1½ slices or 3.25 oz.	100	16.0	4.0	2.0	m.q.	0	270	m.q.
(*Worthington* Multigrain), 2 slices or 3.25 oz.	90	14.0	6.0	1.0	m.q.	0	260	m.q.
CUTTLEFISH, mixed species, meat only, raw:								
1 lb.	359	73.7	3.7	3.2	.5	507	1686	0
1 oz.	22	4.6	.2	.2	<.1	32	105	0

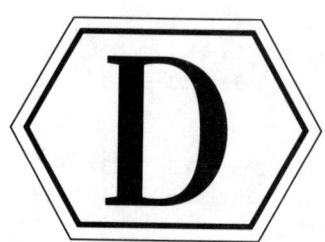

Food and Measure	cal.	prot. (gms)	carbo. (gms)	tot. fat (gms)	sat. fat (gms)	chol. (mgs)	sod. (mgs)	fiber (gms)
DAIKON, see "Radish, Oriental"								
DAIQUIRI[1]:								
1 fl. oz.	56	tr.	2.0	tr.	tr.	0	1	(0)
DAIQUIRI MIX:								
bottled:								
(*Holland House*), 1 fl. oz.	36	0	9.0	0	0	0	111	(0)
raspberry (*Holland House*),								
1 fl. oz.	30	0	7.0	0	0	0	4	(0)
strawberry (*Holland House*),								
1 fl. oz.	31	0	7.0	0	0	0	3	(0)
instant (*Bar-Tender's*), 3½ fl. oz.[2]	177	0	18.0	0	0	0	50	0
instant (*Holland House*), .56 oz. dry	65	0	16.0	0	0	0	21	(0)
DAIRY QUEEN/BRAZIER:								
sandwiches:								
BBQ beef, 4.5 oz.	225	12.0	34.0	4.0	1.0	20	700	m.q.
chicken fillet:								
breaded, 6.7 oz.	430	24.0	37.0	20.0	4.0	55	760	m.q.
breaded, w/cheese, 7.2 oz.	480	27.0	38.0	25.0	7.0	70	980	m.q.
grilled, 6.5 oz.	300	25.0	33.0	8.0	2.0	50	800	m.q.
fish fillet, 6 oz.	370	16.0	39.0	16.0	3.0	45	630	m.q.
fish fillet, w/cheese, 6.5 oz.	420	19.0	40.0	21.0	6.0	60	850	m.q.
hamburger:								
single, 5 oz.	310	17.0	29.0	13.0	6.0	45	580	m.q.
single, w/cheese, 5.5 oz.	365	20.0	30.0	18.0	9.0	60	800	m.q.
double, 7 oz.	460	31.0	29.0	25.0	12.0	95	630	m.q.
double, w/cheese, 8 oz.	570	37.0	31.0	34.0	18.0	120	1070	m.q.
DQ Homestyle Ultimate Burger,								
9.7 oz.	700	43.0	30.0	47.0	21.0	140	1110	m.q.

1. *Recipe: 69.4% rum, 25.5% lime juice, 5.1% sugar.*
2. *Prepared according to package directions, with liquor.*

Food and Measure	cal.	prot. (gms)	carbo. (gms)	tot. fat (gms)	sat. fat (gms)	chol. (mgs)	sod. (mgs)	fiber (gms)
hot dog:								
3.5 oz.	280	9.0	23.0	16.0	6.0	25	700	m.q.
w/cheese, 4 oz.	330	12.0	24.0	21.0	9.0	35	920	m.q.
w/chili, 4.5 oz.	320	11.0	26.0	19.0	7.0	30	720	m.q.
¼ lb. *Super Dog*, 7 oz.	590	20.0	41.0	38.0	16.0	60	1360	m.q.
side dishes and dressings:								
dressing, french, reduced calorie,								
2 oz.	90	<1.0	11.0	5.0	1.0	0	450	0
dressing, Thousand Island, 2 oz.	225	<1.0	10.0	21.0	3.0	25	570	0
french fries, 3.5 oz.	300	4.0	40.0	14.0	3.0	0	160	m.q.
french fries, large, 4.5 oz.	390	5.0	52.0	18.0	4.0	0	200	m.q.
onion rings, 3 oz.	240	4.0	29.0	12.0	3.0	0	135	m.q.
salad, garden, w/out dressing,								
10 oz.	200	13.0	7.0	13.0	7.0	185	240	m.q.
salad, side, w/out dressing,								
4.8 oz.	25	1.0	4.0	0	0	0	15	m.q.
desserts and shakes:								
banana split, 13 oz.	510	9.0	93.0	11.0	8.0	30	250	m.q.
Blizzard:								
Heath, small, 10.3 oz.	560	11.0	79.0	23.0	11.0	40	280	n.a.
Heath, regular, 14.3 oz.	820	16.0	114.0	36.0	17.0	60	410	n.a.
strawberry, small, 9.4 oz.	500	9.0	64.0	12.0	8.0	35	160	n.a.
strawberry, regular, 13.5 oz. ...	740	13.0	92.0	16.0	11.0	50	230	n.a.
Breeze:								
Heath, small, 9.6 oz.	450	11.0	78.0	12.0	3.0	10	230	n.a.
Heath, regular, 13.4 oz.	680	15.0	113.0	21.0	6.0	15	360	n.a.
strawberry, small, 8.7 oz.	400	9.0	63.0	<1.0	<1.0	5	115	n.a.
strawberry, regular, 12.5 oz. ...	590	12.0	90.0	1.0	<1.0	5	170	n.a.
Buster Bar, 5.3 oz.	450	11.0	40.0	29.0	9.0	15	220	n.a.
Brownie Delight, hot fudge,								
10.8 oz.	710	11.0	102.0	29.0	14.0	35	340	n.a.
cone:								
chocolate, regular, 5 oz.	230	6.0	36.0	7.0	5.0	20	115	m.q.
chocolate, large, 7.5 oz.	350	8.0	54.0	11.0	8.0	30	170	m.q.
chocolate dipped, regular,								
5.5 oz.	330	6.0	40.0	16.0	8.0	20	100	m.q.
vanilla, small, 3 oz.	140	4.0	22.0	4.0	3.0	15	60	m.q.
vanilla, regular, 5 oz.	230	6.0	36.0	7.0	5.0	20	95	m.q.
vanilla, large, 7.5 oz.	340	9.0	53.0	10.0	7.0	30	140	m.q.
Dilly Bar, 3 oz.	210	3.0	21.0	13.0	6.0	10	50	n.a.
DQ frozen cake slice,								
undecorated, 5.8 oz.	380	6.0	50.0	18.0	8.0	20	210	n.a.
DQ Sandwich, 2.2 oz.	140	3.0	24.0	4.0	2.0	5	135	m.q.
malt, vanilla, regular, 14.7 oz. ...	610	13.0	106.0	14.0	8.0	45	230	n.a.
Mr. Misty, regular, 11.6 oz.	250	0	63.0	0	0	0	0	n.a.
Nutty Double Fudge, 9.7 oz.	580	10.0	85.0	22.0	10.0	35	170	m.q.
Peanut Buster parfait, 10.8 oz. ...	710	16.0	94.0	32.0	10.0	30	410	m.q.
QC Big Scoop:								
chocolate, 4.5 oz.	310	5.0	40.0	14.0	10.0	35	100	n.a.

Food and Measure	cal.	prot. (gms)	carbo. (gms)	tot. fat (gms)	sat. fat (gms)	chol. (mgs)	sod. (mgs)	fiber (gms)
DAIRY QUEEN/BRAZIER, QC BIG SCOOP (cont.)								
vanilla, 4.5 oz.	300	5.0	39.0	14.0	9.0	35	100	n.a.
shake:								
chocolate, regular, 14 oz.	540	12.0	94.0	14.0	8.0	45	290	n.a.
vanilla, regular, 14 oz.	520	12.0	88.0	14.0	8.0	45	230	n.a.
vanilla, large, 16.3 oz.	600	13.0	101.0	16.0	10.0	50	260	n.a.
sundae, chocolate, regular, 6.2 oz.	300	6.0	54.0	7.0	5.0	20	100	n.a.
Waffle Cone Sundae, strawberry,								
6.1 oz.	350	8.0	56.0	12.0	5.0	20	220	n.a.
yogurt:								
cone, regular, 5 oz.	180	6.0	38.0	<1.0	<1.0	<5	80	0
cone, large, 7.5 oz.	260	9.0	56.0	<1.0	<1.0	5	115	0
cup, regular, 5 oz.	170	6.0	35.0	<1.0	<1.0	<5	70	0
cup, large, 7 oz.	230	8.0	49.0	<1.0	<1.0	<5	100	0
strawberry sundae, regular,								
12.5 oz.	200	6.0	43.0	<1.0	<1.0	<5	80	n.a.
DANDELION GREENS:								
raw, trimmed, 1 lb.	204	12.3	41.7	3.2	n.a.	0	345	7.3 c
raw, 1 oz. or ½ cup chopped	13	.8	2.6	.2	(0)	0	22	.5 c
boiled, drained, 4 oz.	37	2.3	7.3	.7	(0)	0	50	1.5 c
boiled, drained, chopped, ½ cup ...	17	1.0	3.3	.3	(0)	0	23	.7 c
DANISH PASTRY, 1 piece:								
apple filled:								
(*Awrey's* Round), 4.5 oz.	390	4.0	50.0	20.0	4.0	10	390	1.0 d
(*Awrey's* Round), 2.75 oz.	270	3.0	34.0	14.0	3.0	5	310	1.0 d
(*Awrey's* Square), 3 oz.	220	3.0	34.0	8.0	2.0	10	230	1.0 d
fried (*Hostess Breakfast Bake Shop*)	400	4.0	46.0	22.0	10.0	20	340	1.7 d
miniature (*Awrey's*), 1.7 oz.	160	2.0	21.0	8.0	2.0	5	170	0
cheese filled:								
(*Awrey's* Round), 4.5 oz.	420	5.0	52.0	22.0	5.0	15	530	1.0 d
(*Awrey's* Round), 2.75 oz.	280	3.0	34.0	15.0	3.0	10	350	1.0 d
(*Awrey's* Square), 2.5 oz.	210	4.0	25.0	11.0	3.0	15	300	1.0 d
miniature (*Awrey's*), 1.7 oz.	170	2.0	21.0	9.0	2.0	5	200	4.0 d
cinnamon-raisin filled:								
(*Awrey's* Square), 3 oz.	290	3.0	41.0	12.0	3.0	15	280	1.0 d
miniature (*Awrey's*), 1.5 oz.	160	2.0	21.0	8.0	2.0	5	150	1.0 d
cinnamon-walnut (*Awrey's* Round),								
2.75 oz.	300	4.0	31.0	18.0	3.0	5	290	1.0 d
pineapple filled, miniature (*Awrey's*),								
1.7 oz.	157	2.0	21.0	8.0	2.0	5	180	1.0 d
raspberry filled:								
Awrey's Square), 3 oz.	260	3.0	45.0	8.0	2.0	10	210	1.0 d
fried (*Hostess Breakfast Bake Shop*)	390	4.0	49.0	20.0	10.0	20	290	1.7 d
strawberry filled:								
(*Awrey's* Round), 4.5 oz.	400	4.0	53.0	20.0	4.0	10	410	1.0 d
(*Awrey's* Round), 2.75 oz.	270	3.0	34.0	14.0	3.0	5	320	1.0 d
miniature (*Awrey's*), 1.7 oz.	160	2.0	21.0	8.0	2.0	5	180	0

Food and Measure	cal.	prot. (gms)	carbo. (gms)	tot. fat (gms)	sat. fat (gms)	chol. (mgs)	sod. (mgs)	fiber (gms)
DANISH PASTRY, FROZEN,								
1 piece:								
apple:								
(*Pepperidge Farm*), 2¼ oz.	220	2.0	35.0	8.0	m.q.	n.a.	130	m.q.
(*Sara Lee Free & Light*), ⅛ pkg. ...	130	2.0	30.0	0	0	0	120	m.q.
(*Sara Lee* Individual), 1.3 oz.	120	2.0	15.0	6.0	m.q.	n.a.	120	m.q.
twist (*Sara Lee*), ⅛ pkg.	190	3.0	22.0	10.0	m.q.	10	200	m.q.
cheese:								
(*Pepperidge Farm*), 2¼ oz.	240	3.0	25.0	14.0	m.q.	m.q.	230	m.q.
(*Sara Lee* Individual), 1.3 oz.	130	2.0	13.0	8.0	m.q.	n.a.	130	m.q.
twist (*Sara Lee*), ⅛ pkg.	200	3.0	21.0	12.0	m.q.	15	270	m.q.
cinnamon-raisin (*Pepperidge Farm*),								
2¼ oz.	250	3.0	35.0	11.0	m.q.	n.a.	170	m.q.
cinnamon-raisin (*Sara Lee* Individual),								
1.3 oz.	150	2.0	17.0	8.0	m.q.	n.a.	140	m.q.
raspberry (*Pepperidge Farm*), 2¼ oz.	220	3.0	31.0	9.0	m.q.	n.a.	140	m.q.
raspberry twist (*Sara Lee*), ⅛ pkg.	200	3.0	25.0	9.0	m.q.	15	220	m.q.
DANISH PASTRY,								
REFRIGERATED, 1 piece:								
caramel, w/nuts (*Pillsbury*)	160	2.0	19.0	8.0	2.0	0	240	m.q.
cinnamon-raisin, w/icing (*Pillsbury*)	150	2.0	20.0	7.0	2.0	0	230	m.q.
orange, w/icing (*Pillsbury*)	150	2.0	19.0	7.0	2.0	0	250	m.q.
DASHEEN, see "Taro"								
DATE:								
pitted:								
(*Bordo*), 2 oz.	204	1.2	47.2	1.2	n.a.	0	5	1.5 c
(*Dole*), ½ cup	280	5.0	62.0	0	0	0	0	m.q.
(*Dromedary*), 1 oz. or 5 dates ...	100	1.0	23.0	0	0	0	0	m.q.
chopped (*Dromedary*), ¼ cup	130	1.0	31.0	0	0	0	0	m.q.
diced (*Bordo*), 2 oz.	203	1.0	47.5	1.1	n.a.	0	5	1.2 c
domestic, natural and dry:								
w/pits, 1 lb.	1123	8.0	300.1	1.8	n.a.	0	10	20.8 d
pitted:								
1 oz.	78	.6	20.8	.1	n.a.	0	1	1.4 d
10 dates, 2.9 oz.	228	1.6	61.0	.4	n.a.	0	2	4.2 d
chopped, ½ cup	245	1.8	65.4	.4	n.a.	0	3	4.5 d
DATE BAR, mix[1]:								
(*Betty Crocker* Classic), 1 bar,								
approx. .4 oz.	60	1.0	9.0	2.0	1.0	0	35	m.q.
DATE NUT PASTRY:								
(*Awrey's*), 1.6-oz. piece	230	2.0	35.0	10.0	2.0	15	150	1.0 d
DEER, see "Venison"								
DIABLE SAUCE:								
(*Escoffier*), 1 tbsp.	20	0	4.0	0	0	0	160	n.a.
DIET BAR, see "Breakfast bar"								
DILL DIP:								
creamy (*Nasoya Vegi-Dip*), 1 oz.	60	2.0	4.0	4.0	m.q.	0	100	n.a.

1. *Prepared according to package directions.*

Food and Measure	cal.	prot. (gms)	carbo. (gms)	tot. fat (gms)	sat. fat (gms)	chol. (mgs)	sod. (mgs)	fiber (gms)
DILL SEASONING:								
(McCormick/Schilling Parsley Patch								
It's a Dilly), 1 tsp.	11	.4	2.0	.4	n.a.	0	5	(0)
DILL SEED:								
1 oz.	86	4.5	15.6	4.1	.2	0	6	6.0 c
1 tbsp.	20	1.1	3.6	1.0	.1	0	1	1.4 c
1 tsp.	6	.3	1.2	.3	<.1	0	tr.	.4 c
(Spice Islands), 1 tsp.	9	.3	1.2	.4	n.a.	0	<1	.4 c
(Tone's), 1 tsp.	6	.3	1.2	.3	<.1	0	2	.4 d
DILL WEED, dried:								
1 oz.	72	5.7	15.8	1.2	n.a.	0	79	3.4 c
1 tbsp.	8	.6	1.7	.1	(0)	0	6	.4 c
1 tsp.	3	.2	.6	<.1	(0)	0	2	.1 c
(Tone's), 1 tsp.	3	.2	.6	<.1	(0)	0	2	.1 d
DIP, see specific listings								
DISHCLOTH GOURD, see								
"Gourd, dishcloth"								
DOCK:								
raw:								
untrimmed, 1 lb.	70	6.4	10.2	2.2	n.a.	0	13	2.5 c
trimmed, 1 oz.	6	.6	.9	.2	(0)	0	1	.2 c
trimmed, chopped, ½ cup	15	1.3	2.1	.5	(0)	0	3	.5 c
boiled, drained, 4 oz.	23	2.1	3.3	.7	(0)	0	3	.8 c
DOGFISH, see "Shark"								
DOLPHIN FISH, meat only, raw:								
1 lb.	387	83.9	0	3.2	.9	331	397	0
1 oz.	24	5.2	0	.2	.1	21	25	0
1 fillet, approx. 7.2 oz., yield from								
3-lb. whole fish	174	37.7	0	1.4	.4	149	179	0
DOMINO'S PIZZA:								
cheese, 2 slices	376	21.6	56.3	10.1	5.5	19	483	6.4 d
deluxe, 2 slices	498	26.7	59.2	20.4	9.3	40	954	7.0 d
double cheese/pepperoni, 2 slices . .	545	32.1	55.2	25.3	13.3	48	1042	8.0 d
ham, 2 slices	417	23.2	58.0	11.0	5.9	26	805	2.1 d
pepperoni, 2 slices	460	24.1	55.6	17.5	8.4	28	825	4.5 d
sausage/mushroom, 2 slices	430	24.2	55.3	15.8	7.7	28	552	7.6 d
veggie, 2 slices	498	31.0	60.0	18.5	10.2	36	1035	8.1 d
DONUT, 1 piece:								
plain:								
(Awrey's)	490	6.0	48.0	30.0	7.0	35	650	1.0 d
(Hostess Breakfast Bake Shop								
Family Pack)	120	2.0	13.0	6.0	3.0	5	160	.6 d
(Hostess Breakfast Bake Shop								
Pantry)	190	3.0	21.0	11.0	5.0	10	270	.9 d
(Tastykake Assorted), 1.6 oz.	185	3.0	21.6	10.1	2.5	12	171	.9 d
mini *(Hostess Breakfast Bake Shop*								
Donette Gems)	60	1.0	6.0	3.0	2.0	5	80	.3 d

Food and Measure	cal.	prot. (gms)	carbo. (gms)	tot. fat (gms)	sat. fat (gms)	chol. (mgs)	sod. (mgs)	fiber (gms)
cinnamon:								
(*Hostess Breakfast Bake Shop* Family Pack)	120	2.0	14.0	6.0	3.0	5	140	.5 d
(*Hostess Breakfast Bake Shop* Pantry)	190	3.0	24.0	10.0	5.0	10	240	.9 d
(*Tastykake* Assorted), 1.6 oz.	179	2.6	24.5	8.2	2.1	11	211	.8 d
mini (*Hostess Breakfast Bake Shop* Donette Gems)	60	1.0	7.0	3.0	2.0	5	70	.3 d
mini (*Tastykake*)	48	.7	6.4	2.4	.6	4	54	.3 d
apple-filled, mini (*Hostess Breakfast Bake Shop Donette Gems*)	70	1.0	10.0	3.0	1.0	5	70	.3 d
crumb (*Hostess Breakfast Bake Shop*)	160	1.0	16.0	10.0	5.0	10	140	.9 d
crumb, mini (*Hostess Breakfast Bake Shop Donette Gems*)	80	1.0	8.0	5.0	2.0	5	70	.4 d
crunch (*Awrey's*)	600	7.0	65.0	34.0	8.0	40	730	2.0 d
crunch (*Hostess* Krunch)	110	1.0	16.0	4.0	m.q.	4	130	m.q.
frosted:								
(*Hostess Breakfast Bake Shop*), 1.5 oz.	190	2.0	20.0	12.0	7.0	5	180	1.1 d
(*Hostess O's*)	260	3.0	32.0	14.0	9.0	5	240	1.7 d
mini (*Hostess Breakfast Bake Shop* Donette Gems)	80	1.0	8.0	5.0	3.0	<5	70	.4 d
rich (*Tastykake*), 2 oz.	258	3.6	28.2	16.0	7.6	9	196	3.3 d
rich, mini (*Tastykake*)	61	.9	7.7	3.2	1.9	4	59	.5 d
strawberry filled, mini (*Hostess Breakfast Bake Shop Donette Gems*)	80	1.0	10.0	4.0	3.0	<5	70	.5 d
glazed (*Hostess Breakfast Bake Shop* Old Fashioned)	250	3.0	33.0	12.0	5.0	15	230	1.4 d
glazed whirl (*Hostess Breakfast Bake Shop*)	190	3.0	27.0	7.0	3.0	5	230	.9 d
honey wheat:								
(*Hostess Breakfast Bake Shop*) ...	250	3.0	32.0	12.0	6.0	25	280	1.2 d
(*Tastykake*), 2 oz.	209	2.3	33.3	7.5	m.q.	15	190	.9 d
mini (*Tastykake*)	40	.6	7.2	1.2	.3	3	48	.2 d
(*Hostess Breakfast Bake Shop* Old Fashioned)	170	3.0	21.0	9.0	4.0	10	230	.9 d
(*Hostess O's*)	230	3.0	34.0	10.0	4.0	5	230	1.0 d
orange glazed (*Tastykake*), 2 oz.	219	2.7	32.1	9.1	2.5	10	178	.8 d
powdered sugar:								
(*Hostess Breakfast Bake Shop* Family Pack)	120	1.0	14.0	6.0	3.0	5	135	.5 d
(*Hostess Breakfast Bake Shop* Pantry)	190	2.0	24.0	10.0	5.0	10	230	.8 d
(*Tastykake* Assorted), 1.6 oz.	188	2.6	24.4	8.6	2.2	10	221	.8 d
mini:								
(*Hostess Breakfast Bake Shop* Donette Gems)	60	1.0	7.0	3.0	2.0	5	70	.2 d
(*Tastykake*)	42	.6	6.9	1.3	.3	4	71	.2 d

Food and Measure	cal.	prot. (gms)	carbo. (gms)	tot. fat (gms)	sat. fat (gms)	chol. (mgs)	sod. (mgs)	fiber (gms)
DONUT, POWDERED SUGAR, MINI *(cont.)*								
strawberry filled (*Hostess*								
Breakfast Bake Shop								
Donette Gems)	70	1.0	10.0	3.0	1.0	5	70	.3 d
stick (*Little Debbie*), 1.67 oz.	230	2.0	26.0	13.0	m.q.	<1	180	m.q.
sugared (*Awrey's*)	610	7.0	68.0	35.0	8.0	40	735	2.0 d
DONUT, FROZEN:								
glazed (*Rich's Ever Fresh*), 1.2-oz.								
piece	141	2.4	17.2	7.0	m.q.	n.a.	m.q.	m.q.
jelly (*Rich's Ever Fresh*), 2.17-oz.								
piece	213	3.6	26.0	9.5	m.q.	n.a.	m.q.	m.q.
DRUM, freshwater, meat only, raw:								
1 lb.	541	79.5	0	22.4	5.1	290	340	0
1 oz.	34	5.0	0	1.4	.3	18	21	0
1 fillet, approx. 7 oz., yield from								
2½-lb. whole fish	236	34.7	0	9.8	2.2	127	149	0
DRUTHER'S[1]:								
breakfast, 1 serving:								
bacon and egg:								
biscuit, 3.1 oz.	258	11.8	15.2	16.3	m.q.	253	653	.6 d
plate, fried egg, 10 oz.	721	24.9	62.2	41.9	m.q.	500	1224	1.7 d
plate, scrambled egg, 11.1 oz.	742	25.9	63.9	43.0	m.q.	501	1243	1.7 d
ham and egg:								
biscuit, 3.5 oz.	217	13.0	15.1	11.2	m.q.	256	796	.6 d
plate, fried egg, 10.9 oz.	681	29.4	62.1	35.3	m.q.	511	1622	1.7 d
plate, scrambled egg, 12.1 oz.	762	27.0	64.1	44.6	m.q.	515	1408	1.7 d
sausage and egg:								
biscuit, 3.3 oz.	246	11.2	15.3	15.1	m.q.	257	674	.6 d
plate, fried egg, 10.6 oz.	741	26.0	62.5	43.4	m.q.	515	1390	1.7 d
plate, scrambled egg, 10 oz. ..	762	27.0	64.1	44.6	m.q.	515	1408	1.7 d
1 sausage, 1 biscuit, 1.7 oz.	179	5.9	13.1	11.1	m.q.	17	447	.6 d
2 sausages, 2 biscuits, 3.4 oz. ...	358	11.9	26.2	22.3	m.q.	34	894	1.1 d
biscuits and gravy, 8.1 oz.	331	5.6	418	14.7	m.q.	3	1233	1.2 d
cheeseburger, 1 serving:								
4.7 oz.	380	18.7	35.1	17.8	m.q.	69	585	.3 d
deluxe quarter, 8.7 oz.	660	32.9	45.5	37.6	m.q.	127	768	.6 d
double, 6.4 oz.	500	29.3	35.1	26.1	m.q.	105	618	.3 d
chicken:								
8 pieces, 2.6 lbs.	3664	212.9	424.6	114.1	m.q.	601	8558	10.9 d
12 pieces, 3.9 lbs.	5496	319.4	636.8	171.2	m.q.	902	12,904	16.3 d
dinner or snack:								
2-piece, breast and wing, w/								
potatoes and coleslaw, 14 oz.	970	53.7	76.0	49.9	m.q.	159	1899	2.2 d
2-piece, breast and wing,								
7.5 oz.	595	48.0	28.0	30.7	m.q.	154	1607	.6 d
2-piece, leg and thigh, w/								
potatoes and coleslaw,								
13.4 oz.	925	44.0	77.3	49.0	m.q.	157	1530	2.2 d

1. *Values for all dishes and dinners are complete as served, including accompanying biscuits, potatoes, coleslaw, and hush puppies.*

Food and Measure	cal.	prot. (gms)	carbo. (gms)	tot. fat (gms)	sat. fat (gms)	chol. (mgs)	sod. (mgs)	fiber (gms)
2-piece, leg and thigh, 7 oz. ...	549	38.2	29.4	29.8	m.q.	152	1205	.6 d
3-piece, breast, thigh, and leg, 1.1 lb.	1281	78.0	89.6	66.9	m.q.	273	2566	2.3 d
3-piece, breast, thigh, and wing, 1.1 lb.	1309	80.2	86.5	70.3	m.q.	271	2465	2.2 d
fish and chips, 11.2 oz.	729	42.3	71.2	29.8	m.q.	112	1292	3.5 d
fish dinner, 13.3 oz.	770	43.1	78.7	31.3	m.q.	117	1306	3.9 d
fish sandwich, 4.8 oz.	349	22.1	33.0	14.4	m.q.	56	821	2.3 d
hamburger, 4.4 oz.	327	15.6	34.9	13.4	m.q.	55	382	.3 d
DUCK, DOMESTICATED:								
raw:								
meat w/skin:								
½ duck, 1.4 lbs., yield from 1.9 lbs. w/bone	2561	72.8	0	249.4	83.8	481	401	0
1 lb.	1833	52.1	0	178.4	60.0	345	286	0
1 oz.	115	3.3	0	11.2	3.7	22	18	0
meat only, 1 lb.	599	82.9	0	27.0	10.5	349	336	0
meat only, 1 oz.	37	5.2	0	1.7	.7	22	21	0
roasted[1]:								
meat w/skin:								
½ duck, 13.5 oz., yield from 1.3 lbs. w/bone	1287	72.6	0	108.3	36.9	320	227	0
4 oz.	382	21.5	0	32.1	11.0	95	67	0
meat only, ½ duck, 7.8 oz., yield from 1.3 lbs. w/bone and skin w/separable fat	445	51.9	0	24.8	9.2	198	143	0
meat only, 4 oz.	228	26.6	0	12.7	4.7	101	74	0
DUCK, WILD, raw:								
meat w/skin:								
½ duck, 9.5 oz., yield from 1 lb. w/bone	571	47.0	0	41.0	13.6	216	152	0
1 lb.	957	79.0	0	68.9	22.9	363	254	0
1 oz.	60	4.9	0	4.3	1.4	23	16	0
breast meat only, ½ breast, 2.9 oz., yield from 5.4 oz. w/bone and skin w/separable fat	102	16.5	0	3.5	1.1	m.q.	47	0
breast meat only, 1 oz.	35	5.6	0	1.2	.4	m.q.	16	0
DUCK FAT:								
1 oz.	255	0	0	28.3	9.4	28	0	0
½ cup	923	0	0	102.3	34.0	103	0	0
1 tbsp.	115	0	0	12.8	4.3	13	0	0
DUCK LIVER, see "Liver"								
DUCK SAUCE, see "Sweet and sour sauce"								
DULCITA, frozen:								
apple (*Hormel*), 4 oz.	290	5.0	44.0	10.0	m.q.	n.a.	350	m.q.
cherry (*Hormel*), 4 oz.	300	5.0	48.0	9.0	m.q.	n.a.	345	m.q.

1. *Without added ingredients.*

Food and Measure	cal.	prot. (gms)	carbo. (gms)	tot. fat (gms)	sat. fat (gms)	chol. (mgs)	sod. (mgs)	fiber (gms)
DUNKIN' DONUTS, 1 piece:								
apple filled, w/cinnamon sugar,								
2.8 oz.	250	5.0	33.0	11.0	m.q.	0	280	1.0 d
Bavarian filled, w/chocolate frosting,								
2.8 oz.	240	5.0	32.0	11.0	m.q.	0	260	2.0 d
blueberry filled, 2.4 oz.	210	4.0	29.0	8.0	m.q.	0	240	2.0 d
buttermilk ring, glazed, 2.6 oz.	290	4.0	37.0	14.0	m.q.	10	370	1.0 d
cake ring, plain, 2.2 oz.	270	4.0	25.0	17.0	m.q.	10	330	1.0 d
cake ring, chocolate, w/glaze,								
2.5 oz.	324	3.5	34.0	21.0	m.q.	2	383	1.9 d
chocolate chunk cookie, 1.5 oz.	200	3.0	25.0	10.0	m.q.	30	110	1.0 d
chocolate chunk cookie, w/nuts,								
1.5 oz.	210	3.0	23.0	11.0	m.q.	30	100	2.0 d
coffee roll, glazed, 2.9 oz.	280	5.0	37.0	12.0	m.q.	0	310	2.0 d
croissant:								
plain, 2.5 oz.	310	7.0	27.0	19.0	m.q.	0	240	2.0 d
almond, 3.7 oz.	420	8.0	38.0	27.0	m.q.	0	280	3.0 d
chocolate, 3.3 oz.	440	7.0	38.0	29.0	m.q.	0	220	3.0 d
cruller, French, w/glaze, 1.3 oz. ...	140	2.0	16.0	8.0	m.q.	30	130	0
jelly filled, 2.4 oz.	220	4.0	31.0	9.0	m.q.	0	230	1.0 d
lemon filled, 2.8 oz.	260	4.0	33.0	12.0	m.q.	0	280	1.0 d
muffin:								
apple spice, 3.5 oz.	300	6.0	52.0	8.0	m.q.	25	360	2.0 d
banana nut, 3.6 oz.	310	7.0	49.0	10.0	m.q.	30	410	3.0 d
blueberry, 3.6 oz.	280	6.0	46.0	8.0	m.q.	30	340	2.0 d
bran w/raisins, 3.7 oz.	310	6.0	51.0	9.0	m.q.	15	560	4.0 d
corn, 3.4 oz.	340	7.0	51.0	12.0	m.q.	40	560	1.0 d
cranberry nut, 3.5 oz.	290	6.0	44.0	9.0	m.q.	25	360	2.0 d
oat bran, 3.4 oz.	330	7.0	50.0	11.0	m.q.	0	450	3.0 d
oatmeal pecan raisin cookie, 1.6 oz.	200	3.0	28.0	9.0	m.q.	25	100	1.0 d
whole wheat ring, glazed, 2.9 oz. ..	330	4.0	39.0	18.0	m.q.	5	380	2.0 d
yeast ring, chocolate frosted,								
1.9 oz.	200	4.0	25.0	100	m.q.	0	190	1.0 d
yeast ring, glazed, 1.9 oz.	200	4.0	26.0	9.0	m.q.	0	230	1.0 d
DUTCH BRAND LOAF, 1-oz. slice,								
except as noted:								
(*Eckrich*)	70	3.0	2.0	6.0	m.q.	m.q.	300	0
(*Eckrich* Lean Supreme)	60	4.0	2.0	4.0	m.q.	m.q.	250	0
(*Eckrich Smorgas Pac*)	70	3.0	2.0	6.0	m.q.	m.q.	300	0
(*Kahn's*), 1 slice	80	3.0	1.0	7.0	m.q.	m.q.	280	0
pork and beef, 4″ × 4″ × ³⁄₃₂″ slice	68	3.8	1.6	5.1	1.8	13	354	0

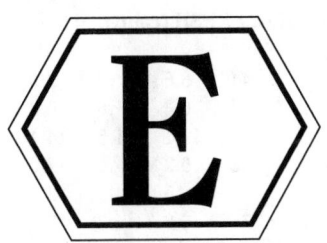

Food and Measure	cal.	prot. (gms)	carbo. (gms)	tot. fat (gms)	sat. fat (gms)	chol. (mgs)	sod. (mgs)	fiber (gms)
EAR, PORK, see "Pork ear"								
ECLAIR, frozen:								
chocolate (*Rich's*), 1 piece, 2 oz. ...	210	2.0	27.0	10.0	m.q.	35	110	m.q.
EEL, mixed species, meat only:								
raw:								
1 lb.	834	83.7	0	52.9	10.7	571	231	0
1 oz.	52	5.2	0	3.3	.7	36	14	0
1 fillet, approx. 7.2 oz., yield from								
2-lb. whole fish	375	37.6	0	23.8	4.8	257	104	0
baked, broiled, or microwaved[1],								
4 oz.	268	26.8	0	17.0	3.4	183	74	0
EGG, CHICKEN:								
raw, whole, fresh or frozen:								
1 oz.	42	3.5	.3	2.8	.9	120	36	0
1 large egg, approx. 1.75 oz.	75	6.3	.6	5.0	1.6	213	63	0
1 cup	363	30.4	3.0	24.3	7.5	1033	307	0
raw, white, fresh or frozen:								
1 oz.	14	3.0	.3	0	0	0	46	0
white from 1 large egg	17	3.5	.3	0	0	0	55	0
1 cup	121	25.6	2.5	0	0	0	399	0
raw, yolk:								
fresh:								
1 oz.	101	4.8	.5	8.8	2.7	363	12	0
yolk from 1 large egg[2]	59	2.8	.3	5.1	1.6	213	7	0
1 cup	870	40.7	4.3	75.0	23.2	3112	104	0
frozen, yolk[3], 1 oz.	88	4.5	.5	7.4	2.3	306	18	0
frozen, yolk, sugared, 1 oz.	92	3.7	2.7	7.2	2.2	328	16	0
cooked, whole, fresh:								
fried[4], 1 large egg	91	6.2	.6	6.9	1.9	211	162	0

1. *Without added ingredients.*
2. *Includes a small portion of white.*
3. *Includes approximately 17% white.*
4. *Recipe: 95% whole egg, 5% margarine, and salt.*

Food and Measure	cal.	prot. (gms)	carbo. (gms)	tot. fat (gms)	sat. fat (gms)	chol. (mgs)	sod. (mgs)	fiber (gms)
EGG, CHICKEN, COOKED, WHOLE, FRESH *(cont.)*								
hard-boiled in shell:								
1 oz.	44	3.6	.3	3.0	.9	120	35	0
1 large egg	77	6.3	.6	5.3	1.6	213	62	0
chopped, 1 cup	210	17.1	1.5	14.4	4.4	578	169	0
omelet[1], 1 large egg	92	6.3	.6	7.0	1.9	214	165	0
poached, 1 oz.	42	3.5	.3	2.8	.9	120	79	0
poached, 1 large egg	74	6.2	.6	5.0	1.5	212	140	0
scrambled[2], 1 large egg	101	6.8	1.3	7.5	2.2	215	171	0
dried, whole:								
1 oz.	168	13.0	1.4	11.9	3.6	544	148	0
1 cup, sifted	505	39.0	4.1	35.5	10.7	1631	443	0
1 tbsp.	30	2.3	.2	2.1	.6	96	26	0
stabilized (glucose reduced):								
1 oz.	174	13.7	.7	12.5	3.7	572	155	0
1 cup, sifted	523	40.9	2.0	37.4	11.2	1714	466	0
1 tbsp.	31	2.4	.1	2.2	.7	101	27	0
dried, white, stabilized (glucose reduced):								
flakes, 1 oz.	100	21.8	1.2	<.1	0	0	328	0
powder, 1 oz.	107	23.4	1.3	<.1	0	0	351	0
powder, 1 cup, sifted	402	88.2	4.8	<.1	0	0	1325	0
dried, yolk:								
1 oz.	195	8.7	.1	17.4	5.2	830	26	0
1 cup, sifted	460	20.5	.3	41.1	12.3	1962	61	0
1 tbsp.	27	1.2	<.1	2.5	.7	117	4	0
EGG, CHICKEN, SUBSTITUTE OR IMITATION:								
(Featherweight), 2 eggs	120	9.0	2.0	8.0	m.q.	15	250	0
(Fleischmann's Egg Beaters), ¼ cup	25	5.0	1.0	0	0	0	80	0
w/cheese *(Fleischmann's Egg Beaters Cheez)*, ½ cup	130	14.0	3.0	6.0	m.q.	5	440	0
frozen:								
1 oz.[3]	45	3.2	.9	3.1	.5	<1	56	0
1 cup[3]	384	27.1	7.7	26.7	4.6	5	479	0
(Morningstar Farms Scramblers), ¼ cup	60	6.0	3.0	3.0	m.q.	0	m.q.	0
(Tofutti Egg Watchers), 2 oz.	50	7.0	2.0	2.0	m.q.	0	100	n.a.
liquid[4]:								
1 oz.	24	3.4	.2	.9	.2	<1	50	0
1 cup	211	30.1	1.6	8.3	1.7	3	444	0
1½ fl. oz.	40	5.6	.3	1.6	.3	tr.	83	0
powder[5], 1 oz.	126	15.7	6.2	3.7	1.1	162	227	0
mix, tofu *(Tofu Scrambler)*, ½ cup[6]	98	11.0	7.0	5.0	m.q.	0	252	m.q.
mix, tofu *(Tofu Scrambler)*, ½ cup[7]	158	11.0	7.0	12.0	m.q.	m.q.	335	m.q.

1. *Recipe: 74% whole egg, 22% water, 4% margarine, and salt.*
2. *Recipe: 74% whole egg, 22% whole milk, 4% margarine, and salt.*
3. *Containing egg white, corn oil, and nonfat dry milk.*
4. *Containing egg white, hydrogenated soybean oil, and soy protein.*
5. *Containing egg white solids, whole egg solids, sweet whey solids, nonfat dry milk solids, and soy protein.*
6. *Prepared according to package directions, with tofu.*
7. *Prepared according to package directions, with tofu and 3 tbsp. salted butter.*

Food and Measure	cal.	prot. (gms)	carbo. (gms)	tot. fat (gms)	sat. fat (gms)	chol. (mgs)	sod. (mgs)	fiber (gms)
EGG, DUCK, fresh:								
whole, raw, 1 oz.	52	3.6	.4	3.9	1.0	251	41	0
whole, raw, 1 egg, approx. 2.5 oz.	130	9.0	1.0	9.6	2.6	619	102	0
EGG, GOOSE, fresh:								
whole, raw, 1 oz.	52	3.9	.4	3.8	1.0	m.q.	n.a.	0
whole, raw, 1 egg, approx. 5.1 oz.	267	20.0	1.9	19.1	5.2	m.q.	n.a.	0
EGG, PICKLED:								
(*Penrose*), 1 egg, approx. 2 oz.	80	8.0	1.0	5.0	m.q.	m.q.	230	0
EGG, QUAIL, fresh:								
whole, raw, 1 oz.	45	3.7	.1	3.1	1.0	239	n.a.	0
whole, raw, 1 egg, approx. .3 oz. . .	14	1.2	<.1	1.0	.3	76	n.a.	0
EGG, TURKEY, fresh:								
whole, raw, 1 oz.	48	3.9	.3	3.4	1.0	265	n.a.	0
whole, raw, 1 egg, approx. 2.8 oz.	135	10.8	.9	9.4	2.9	737	n.a.	0
EGG BREAKFAST, FREEZE-								
DRIED, ½ pkg.[1]:								
w/bacon (*Mountain House*)	170	12.0	7.0	10.0	m.q.	m.q.	165	n.a.
w/butter (*Mountain House*)	160	11.0	8.0	8.0	m.q.	m.q.	174	n.a.
omelet, cheese (*Mountain House*) . .	180	13.0	8.0	9.0	m.q.	m.q.	207	n.a.
precooked, w/bacon (*Mountain*								
House)	180	12.0	3.0	12.0	m.q.	m.q.	m.q.	n.a.
EGG BREAKFAST, FROZEN (see								
also "Egg breakfast sandwich"):								
omelet, w/cheese sauce and ham								
(*Swanson Great Starts*), 7 oz. . . .	390	19.0	15.0	29.0	m.q.	m.q.	1220	m.q.
reduced cholesterol, w/mini oat bran								
muffins (*Swanson Great Starts*),								
4.75 oz.	250	10.0	27.0	12.0	m.q.	m.q.	400	m.q.
scrambled:								
and bacon, w/home fries (*Swanson*								
Great Starts), 5.6 oz.	340	11.0	16.0	26.0	m.q.	m.q.	690	m.q.
w/cheddar cheese and fried								
potatoes (*Aunt Jemima*								
Homestyle), 5.9 oz.	250	11.0	22.0	13.0	m.q.	m.q.	910	m.q.
w/cheese and cinnamon pancakes								
(*Swanson Great Starts*), 3.4 oz.	290	7.0	14.0	23.0	m.q.	m.q.	380	m.q.
w/ham and hash browns								
(*Downyflake*), 6.25 oz.	360	13.0	17.0	26.0	m.q.	m.q.	730	m.q.
w/ham and pecan twirl								
(*Downyflake*), 6.25 oz.	470	15.0	40.0	28.0	m.q.	m.q.	670	m.q.
w/hash browns and sausage								
(*Downyflake*), 6.25 oz.	420	12.0	17.0	34.0	m.q.	m.q.	790	m.q.
and home fries (*Swanson Great*								
Starts), 4.6 oz.	260	7.0	14.0	19.0	m.q.	m.q.	380	m.q.
and sausages:								
w/hash browns (*Aunt Jemima*								
Homestyle), 5.7 oz.	290	12.0	14.0	20.0	m.q.	m.q.	810	m.q.

1. *Prepared according to package directions.*

Food and Measure	cal.	prot. (gms)	carbo. (gms)	tot. fat (gms)	sat. fat (gms)	chol. (mgs)	sod. (mgs)	fiber (gms)
EGG BREAKFAST, FROZEN, SCRAMBLED, W/SAUSAGES *(cont.)*								
w/hash browns *(Swanson Great Starts)*, 6.5 oz.	430	13.0	19.0	34.0	m.q.	m.q.	760	m.q.
w/pancakes *(Aunt Jemima Homestyle)*, 5.2 oz.	270	13.0	21.0	14.0	m.q.	m.q.	880	m.q.
w/pecan twirl *(Downyflake)*, 6.25 oz.	510	16.0	39.0	33.0	m.q.	m.q.	710	m.q.
"EGG" BREAKFAST, VEGETARIAN, frozen:								
Scramblers, hash browns and links *(Morningstar Farms* Country Breakfast), 7 oz.	360	16.0	22.0	23.0	m.q.	0	660	m.q.
Scramblers, pancakes and links *(Morningstar Farms* Country Breakfast), 6.8 oz.	380	18.0	33.0	19.0	m.q.	0	900	m.q.
EGG BREAKFAST SANDWICH, frozen:								
beefsteak and cheese *(Swanson Great Starts* Breakfast on a Muffin), 4.9 oz.	360	17.0	27.0	20.0	m.q.	m.q.	730	m.q.
Canadian bacon and cheese *(Swanson Great Starts* Breakfast on a Biscuit), 5.2 oz.	420	16.0	37.0	22.0	m.q.	m.q.	1845	m.q.
Canadian bacon and cheese *(Swanson Great Starts* Breakfast on a Muffin), 4.1 oz.	290	15.0	25.0	15.0	m.q.	m.q.	770	m.q.
English muffin *(Weight Watchers* Microwave), 4 oz.	230	13.0	25.0	8.0	3.0	160	590	m.q.
sausage and cheese *(Swanson Great Starts* Breakfast on a Biscuit), 5.5 oz.	460	18.0	35.0	28.0	m.q.	m.q.	1310	m.q.
EGG FOO YOUNG MIX[1]:								
(La Choy), 8.8 oz.	164	8.2	19.2	7.0	m.q.	n.a.	1250	m.q.
EGG ROLL, frozen:								
chicken *(Chun King)*, 3.6 oz.	220	5.0	32.0	8.0	m.q.	m.q.	600	m.q.
chicken *(Jeno's* Snacks), 3 oz., approx. 6 rolls	190	5.0	21.0	9.0	m.q.	m.q.	350	m.q.
meat and shrimp *(Chun King)*, 3.6 oz.	220	6.0	31.0	8.0	m.q.	m.q.	680	m.q.
meat and shrimp *(Jeno's* Snacks), 3 oz., approx. 6 rolls	200	5.0	21.0	11.0	m.q.	m.q.	420	m.q.
pork *(Chun King* Restaurant Style), 3 oz.	180	6.0	23.0	6.0	m.q.	m.q.	450	m.q.
shrimp *(Chun King)*, 3.6 oz.	200	4.0	31.0	6.0	m.q.	m.q.	480	m.q.
shrimp and cheese *(Jeno's* Snacks), 3 oz., approx. 6 rolls	190	7.0	22.0	8.0	m.q.	m.q.	290	m.q.
vegetarian *(Worthington)*, 3-oz. roll	160	6.0	20.0	6.0	1.0	0	530	m.q.

1. *Prepared according to package directions.*

Food and Measure	cal.	prot. (gms)	carbo. (gms)	tot. fat (gms)	sat. fat (gms)	chol. (mgs)	sod. (mgs)	fiber (gms)
EGG ROLL WRAPPER:								
(*Nasoya*), 1 piece	23	1.0	4.5	0	0	0	19	m.q.
EGG WHITE STABILIZER:								
(*Tone's*), 1 tsp.	12	<.1	3.0	tr.	0	0	1	.1 d
EGG NOG, nonalcoholic:								
canned (*Borden*), ½ cup	160	3.0	16.0	9.0	m.q.	m.q.	80	0
chilled:								
1 fl. oz.	43	1.2	4.3	2.4	1.4	19	17	0
1 quart	1368	38.7	137.6	76.0	45.1	596	553	0
1 cup	342	9.7	34.4	19.0	11.3	149	138	0
(*Crowley*), 6 fl. oz.	270	6.0	34.0	13.0	m.q.	100	200	0
(*Darigold*), 8 fl. oz.	350	6.0	43.0	17.0	m.q.	m.q.	120	0
(*Darigold* Classic), 8 fl. oz.	390	10.0	48.0	17.0	m.q.	m.q.	170	0
EGGNOG FLAVOR BEVERAGE MIX:								
powder, 1 oz.	111	.1	27.7	.3	.1	n.a.	44	tr.c
beverage[1]:								
1 cup whole milk and 1 oz.								
powder	260	8.1	39.0	8.4	5.1	33	163	0
1 cup lowfat 2% milk and 1 oz.								
powder	232	8.2	39.4	5.0	3.0	18	166	0
1 cup lowfat 1% milk and 1 oz.								
powder	213	8.1	39.4	2.9	1.7	10	167	0
1 cup skim milk and 1 oz. powder	197	8.5	39.6	.7	.4	4	170	0
EGGPLANT:								
raw:								
untrimmed, 1 lb.	95	4.0	23.0	.4	.1	0	13	5.5 d
trimmed, 1 oz.	7	.3	1.8	<.1	tr.	0	1	.4 d
1 medium, 8½" × 1⅜", approx.								
4.5 oz.	27	1.1	6.4	.1	<.1	0	4	1.5 d
1" pieces, ½ cup	11	.5	2.6	<.1	tr.	0	1	.6 d
boiled, drained, 4 oz.	32	.9	7.5	.3	<.1	0	3	1.1 c
boiled, drained, 1" cubes, ½ cup ...	13	.4	3.2	.1	<.1	0	2	.5 c
EGGPLANT APPETIZER:								
(*Progresso* Caponata), ½ can	70	2.0	4.0	4.0	m.q.	0	260	m.q.
EGGPLANT ENTREE, frozen:								
parmigiana:								
(*Celentano*), 6.25 oz.	260	9.0	36.0	10.0	m.q.	m.q.	220	m.q.
(*Celentano*), 8 oz.	280	14.0	23.0	15.0	m.q.	m.q.	400	m.q.
(*Celentano*), 10 oz.	350	18.0	29.0	19.0	m.q.	m.q.	500	m.q.
(*Mrs. Paul's*), 5 oz.	240	6.0	18.0	16.0	4.0	15	600	m.q.
rollettes (*Celentano*), 11 oz.	320	14.0	36.0	14.0	m.q.	n.a.	210	m.q.
ELDERBERRY:								
1 lb.	329	3.0	83.5	2.3	n.a.	0	n.a.	31.8 c
1 oz.	21	.2	5.2	.1	(0)	0	n.a.	2.0 c
½ cup	53	.5	13.3	.4	(0)	0	n.a.	5.1 c

1. *Cholesterol contribution from milk only.*

Food and Measure	cal.	prot. (gms)	carbo. (gms)	tot. fat (gms)	sat. fat (gms)	chol. (mgs)	sod. (mgs)	fiber (gms)
ELK, meat only:								
raw, 1 oz.	32	6.5	0	.4	.2	16	16	0
roasted[1]:								
12 oz., yield from 1 lb. raw	497	102.7	0	6.5	2.4	247	208	0
4 oz.	166	34.2	0	2.2	.8	83	69	0
diced, 1 cup, approx. 4.9 oz.	204	42.3	0	2.7	1.0	102	85	0
ENCHANADA ENTREE, see "Enchilada entree, frozen"								
ENCHILADA DINNER, FROZEN:								
beef:								
(*Banquet*), 12 oz.	500	19.0	72.0	15.0	m.q.	m.q.	1810	m.q.
(*Old El Paso* Festive Dinners),								
11 oz.	390	24.0	56.0	8.0	m.q.	m.q.	1200	m.q.
(*Patio*), 13.25 oz.	520	16.0	59.0	24.0	m.q.	40	1810	m.q.
(*Swanson*), 13.75 oz.	480	17.0	55.0	21.0	m.q.	m.q.	1350	m.q.
(*Van de Kamp's* Mexican Dinner),								
½ pkg.	200	8.0	27.0	7.0	m.q.	m.q.	740	m.q.
cheese:								
(*Banquet*), 12 oz.	550	22.0	71.0	19.0	m.q.	m.q.	2170	m.q.
(*Old El Paso* Festive Dinners),								
11 oz.	590	24.0	51.0	31.0	m.q.	m.q.	1200	m.q.
(*Patio*), 12.25 oz.	380	14.0	59.0	10.0	m.q.	20	2010	m.q.
(*Van de Kamp's* Mexican Dinner),								
½ pkg.	220	8.0	26.0	9.0	m.q.	m.q.	620	m.q.
chicken (*Old El Paso* Festive Dinners), 11 oz.	460	21.0	54.0	18.0	m.q.	m.q.	770	m.q.
ENCHILADA DINNER MIX:								
(*Old El Paso*), 1 enchilada[2]	145	7.0	11.0	8.0	3.0	21	325	2.0 d
(*Tio Sancho* Dinner Kit):								
sauce mix, 3 oz.	278	4.5	62.0	1.5	m.q.	n.a.	4058	1.8 c
1 shell	80	1.3	10.8	3.5	m.q.	n.a.	2	.6 c
ENCHILADA ENTREE, frozen:								
beef:								
(*Hormel*), 1 piece	140	6.0	17.0	5.0	m.q.	m.q.	573	m.q.
(*Old El Paso*), 1 pkg.	210	8.0	16.0	13.0	m.q.	10	720	m.q.
(*Van de Kamp's* Mexican Entrees), 1 pkg.	270	11.0	30.0	12.0	m.q.	m.q.	1040	m.q.
(*Van de Kamp's* Mexican Entrees Family Pack), ¼ pkg.	150	7.0	19.0	5.0	m.q.	m.q.	530	m.q.
and bean (*Lean Cuisine* Enchanadas), 9.25 oz.	280	15.0	32.0	10.0	2.0	60	890	m.q.
chili gravy and (*Banquet Family Entrees*), 7 oz.	270	10.0	28.0	13.0	m.q.	m.q.	m.q.	m.q.
ranchero (*Weight Watchers*), 9.12 oz.	230	20.0	17.0	10.0	3.0	40	720	m.q.
shredded (*Van de Kamp's* Mexican Entrees), 1 pkg.	360	20.0	40.0	14.0	m.q.	m.q.	1010	m.q.

1. *Without added ingredients.*
2. *Prepared according to package directions.*

Food and Measure	cal.	prot. (gms)	carbo. (gms)	tot. fat (gms)	sat. fat (gms)	chol. (mgs)	sod. (mgs)	fiber (gms)
sirloin ranchero (*The Budget Gourmet* Slim Selects), 9 oz.	290	19.0	20.0	15.0	m.q.	35	770	m.q.
cheese:								
(*Hormel*), 1 piece	151	6.0	18.0	6.0	m.q.	m.q.	676	m.q.
(*Old El Paso*), 1 pkg.	250	10.0	24.0	12.0	m.q.	m.q.	830	m.q.
(*Stouffer's*), 10⅛ oz.	590	23.0	34.0	40.0	m.q.	m.q.	880	m.q.
(*Van de Kamp's* Mexican Entrees), 1 pkg.	300	11.0	31.0	15.0	m.q.	m.q.	980	m.q.
(*Van de Kamp's* Mexican Entrees Family Pack), ¼ pkg.	200	7.0	19.0	10.0	m.q.	m.q.	460	m.q.
ranchero (*Van de Kamp's* Mexican Entrees), ½ pkg.	260	11.0	26.0	12.0	m.q.	m.q.	630	m.q.
ranchero (*Weight Watchers*), 8.87 oz.	360	18.0	30.0	18.0	5.0	60	900	m.q.
chicken:								
(*Le Menu* LightStyle), 8 oz.	280	21.0	32.0	8.0	m.q.	35	530	m.q.
(*Lean Cuisine* Enchanadas), 9⅞ oz.	270	17.0	31.0	9.0	2.0	65	850	m.q.
(*Old El Paso*), 1 pkg.	220	8.0	20.0	12.0	m.q.	m.q.	740	m.q.
(*Stouffer's*), 10 oz.	490	22.0	34.0	29.0	m.q.	m.q.	910	m.q.
(*Van de Kamp's* Mexican Entrees), 1 pkg.	260	13.0	27.0	11.0	m.q.	m.q.	1010	m.q.
w/sour cream sauce (*Old El Paso*), 1 pkg.	280	10.0	18.0	19.0	m.q.	m.q.	520	m.q.
Suiza:								
(*The Budget Gourmet* Slim Selects), 9 oz.	270	17.0	30.0	9.0	m.q.	50	1080	m.q.
(*Van de Kamp's* Mexican Entrees), 1 pkg.	230	12.0	23.0	10.0	m.q.	m.q.	390	m.q.
(*Weight Watchers*), 9 oz.	280	19.0	28.0	11.0	2.0	30	600	m.q.
vegetable, w/tofu and sauce (*Legume* Mexican), 11 oz.	270	14.0	36.0	8.0	3.0	0	390	10.3 d
ENCHILADA SAUCE:								
(*La Victoria*), 1 cup	80	1.0	10.0	5.0	m.q.	0	1520	(0)
(*Rosarita*), 3 oz.	20	0	4.0	0	0	0	430	(0)
green (*Old El Paso*), 2 tbsp.	11	<1.0	3.0	0	0	0	200	(0)
hot:								
(*Del Monte*), ½ cup	45	1.0	11.0	0	0	0	1090	(0)
(*El Molino*), 2 tbsp.	16	0	2.0	1.0	n.a.	0	100	(0)
(*Old El Paso*), ¼ cup	30	<1.0	4.0	1.0	n.a.	0	250	(0)
hot or mild (*Ortega*), 1 oz.	12	0	3.0	0	0	0	280	(0)
mild (*Del Monte*), ½ cup	45	1.0	11.0	0	0	0	1150	(0)
mild (*Old El Paso*), ¼ cup	25	<1.0	4.0	1.0	n.a.	0	250	(0)
ENCHILADA SEASONING MIX:								
(*Lawry's*), 1 pkg.	152	5.3	29.9	1.2	n.a.	n.a.	1723	1.2 c
(*Old El Paso*), 1/18 pkg.	6	0	1.0	0	0	0	80	0
ENDIVE:								
untrimmed, 1 lb.	65	4.9	13.1	.8	.2	0	87	3.5 c
trimmed, 1 oz.	5	.4	.9	.1	<.1	0	6	.3 c

Food and Measure	cal.	prot. (gms)	carbo. (gms)	tot. fat (gms)	sat. fat (gms)	chol. (mgs)	sod. (mgs)	fiber (gms)
ENDIVE *(cont.)*								
1 head, approx. 1.3 lb.	86	6.4	17.2	1.0	.2	0	115	4.6 c
chopped, ½ cup	4	.3	.8	.1	<.1	0	6	.2 c
ENDIVE, BELGIAN, see								
"Chickory, witloof"								
ENGLISH MUFFIN, see "Muffin"								
EPPAW, trimmed:								
1 lb.	680	20.9	143.7	8.2	n.a.	0	54	m.q.
1 oz.	43	1.3	9.0	.5	(0)	0	3	m.q.
½ cup	75	2.3	15.8	.9	(0)	0	6	m.q.
ESCAROLE, see "Endive"								
EXTRACT, see specific listings								

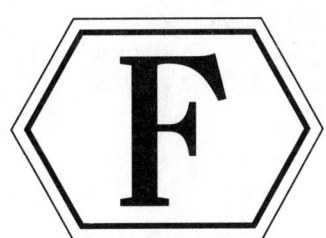

Food and Measure	cal.	prot. (gms)	carbo. (gms)	tot. fat (gms)	sat. fat (gms)	chol. (mgs)	sod. (mgs)	fiber (gms)
FAJITA ENTREE, FROZEN:								
beef (*Weight Watchers*), 6.75 oz.	250	15.0	32.0	7.0	2.0	20	630	m.q.
chicken (*Weight Watchers*), 6.75 oz.	230	17.0	30.0	5.0	2.0	30	590	m.q.
FAJITA ENTREE, REFRIGERATED:								
chicken (*Chicken By George*), 5 oz.	170	28.0	2.0	6.0	m.q.	85	370	n.a.
FAJITA MARINADE:								
(*Old El Paso*), ⅛ jar	14	0	3.0	0	0	0	450	0
(*Tone's*), 1 tsp.	9	.3	1.9	.1	(0)	0	963	n.a.
FAJITA SAUCE:								
(*Tio Sancho* Skillet Sauce), 1 oz. ...	14	.5	1.8	.5	(0)	0	590	.1 c
FAJITA SEASONING BLEND:								
(*Lawry's*), 1 pkg.	63	2.0	14.0	.4	n.a.	n.a.	2118	.5 c
FALAFEL:								
1 oz.	94	3.8	9.0	5.0	.8	0	83	.3 c
1 patty, 2¼″ diam.	57	2.3	5.4	3.0	.4	0	50	.2 c
mix:								
(*Casbah*), 1 oz. dry	103	7.0	15.0	2.0	n.a.	0	n.a.	m.q.
(*Fantastic Foods Falafil*), 6 balls or 3 oz.[1]	129	8.0	20.0	2.0	n.a.	0	188	m.q.
(*Near East*), 3 patties[2]	270	13.0	22.0	15.0	m.q.	n.a.	680	m.q.
FARINA, WHOLE GRAIN (see also "Cereal"):								
dry:								
1 oz.	105	3.0	22.1	.1	<.1	0	1	.8 d
1 cup	649	18.6	137.2	.9	.1	0	5	4.8 d
1 tbsp.	40	1.2	8.5	.1	<.1	0	tr.	.3 d
cooked:								
4 oz.	57	1.6	12.0	.1	<.1	0	tr.	1.6 d
1 cup	116	3.4	24.6	.2	<.1	0	1	3.3 d

1. *Prepared according to package directions; does not include value for fat from butter or oil used in cooking.*
2. *Prepared according to package directions.*

Food and Measure	cal.	prot. (gms)	carbo. (gms)	tot. fat (gms)	sat. fat (gms)	chol. (mgs)	sod. (mgs)	fiber (gms)
FARINA, WHOLE GRAIN, COOKED *(cont.)*								
salted, 4 oz.	57	1.6	12.0	.1	<.1	0	373	1.6 d
salted, 1 cup	116	3.4	24.6	.2	<.1	0	767	3.3 d
FAST-FOOD RESTAURANTS, see specific listings								
FAST FOODS, unspecified:								
breakfast:								
biscuit:								
plain, 2.6 oz.	276	4.3	34.4	13.4	8.7	5	584	.3 c
w/egg:								
4.8 oz.	315	11.1	24.2	20.2	6.2	232	655	.1 c
and bacon, 5.3 oz.	457	17.0	28.6	31.1	9.9	353	999	.1 c
and ham, 6.8 oz.	442	20.4	30.3	27.0	8.4	299	1381	.1 c
and sausage, 6.3 oz.	582	19.2	41.2	38.7	15.0	302	1142	.2 c
and steak, 5.2 oz.	474	17.9	37.4	28.4	8.6	272	888	.1 c
cheese and bacon, 5.1 oz. ..	477	16.3	33.4	31.4	11.4	261	1261	.3 c
w/ham, 4 oz.	387	13.4	43.8	18.4	11.4	25	1433	.3 c
w/sausage, 4.4 oz.	485	12.1	40.0	31.8	14.2	34	1071	.3 c
w/steak, 5 oz.	456	13.1	44.4	26.0	6.9	26	795	.2 c
croissant, w/egg and cheese:								
4.5 oz.	369	12.8	24.3	24.7	14.1	216	551	.2 c
and bacon, 4.6 oz.	413	16.2	23.7	28.4	15.4	215	889	.2 c
and ham, 5.4 oz.	475	18.9	24.2	33.6	17.5	213	1080	.2 c
and sausage, 5.6 oz.	524	20.3	24.7	38.2	18.2	216	1115	.2 c
Danish pastry:								
cheese, 3.2 oz.	353	5.8	28.7	24.6	5.1	20	320	.2 c
cinnamon, 3.1 oz.	349	4.8	46.9	16.7	3.5	28	326	.7 c
fruit, 3.3 oz.	335	4.8	45.1	15.9	3.3	19	333	.4 c
eggs, scrambled, 2 eggs	200	13.0	2.0	15.2	5.8	400	211	.2 c
English muffin:								
w/butter, 2.2 oz.	189	4.9	30.4	5.8	2.4	13	386	.1 c
w/cheese and sausage, 4.1 oz.	394	15.3	29.2	24.3	9.9	58	1036	.5 c
w/egg, cheese, and Canadian bacon, 5.1 oz.	383	19.8	31.5	19.8	9.1	234	785	.3 c
w/egg, cheese, and sausage, 5.8 oz.	487	21.7	31.0	30.9	12.4	274	1135	.5 c
French toast w/butter, 2 slices, 4.8 oz.	356	10.3	36.0	18.8	7.7	117	513	.1 c
French toast sticks, 5 sticks, 5 oz.	479	8.3	49.1	29.1	4.7	74	499	.2 c
pancakes, w/butter and syrup, 3 cakes, 8.2 oz.	519	8.3	90.9	14.0	5.9	57	1103	.2 c
potatoes, hashed brown, ½ cup ..	151	1.9	16.2	9.2	4.3	9	290	.4 c
sausage, 1-oz. patty	100	5.3	.3	8.4	2.9	22	349	0
sausage, .5-oz. link	48	2.5	.1	4.1	1.4	11	168	0
entrees:								
chicken, breaded and fried:								
dark meat, 1 thigh and 1 drumstick, 5.2 oz.	430	30.1	15.7	26.7	7.0	165	756	0

Food and Measure	cal.	prot. (gms)	carbo. (gms)	tot. fat (gms)	sat. fat (gms)	chol. (mgs)	sod. (mgs)	fiber (gms)
light meat, combination of								
2 pieces[1], 5.7 oz.	494	35.7	19.6	29.5	7.8	149	975	0
chicken nuggets, breaded, fried,								
6 pieces:								
plain, 3.6 oz.	290	16.9	15.5	17.7	5.5	62	542	.2 c
w/barbecue sauce, 4.6 oz.	330	17.1	25.0	18.0	5.6	61	830	.3 c
w/honey, 4.1 oz.	329	16.8	26.9	17.5	5.5	61	537	.2 c
w/mustard sauce, 4.6 oz.	323	17.4	20.9	18.9	5.7	62	791	.2 c
w/sweet and sour sauce,								
4.6 oz.	346	17.0	29.0	18.0	5.5	61	677	.3 c
chili con carne w/beans, 1 cup ...	254	24.6	21.9	8.3	3.4	133	1008	1.9 c
clams, breaded, fried, ¾ cup	451	12.8	38.8	26.4	6.6	87	833	.2 c
crab, baked[2], 2.1-oz. cake	88	15.7	2.3	1.3	.2	101	303	<.1 c
crab, soft shell, breaded, fried,								
4.4-oz. crab	334	11.0	31.2	17.9	4.4	45	1118	.2 c
crab cakes[3], 3.8-oz. cake	290	20.4	9.3	18.8	4.1	149	893	<.1 c
fish fillet, battered or breaded,								
fried, 3.2-oz. piece	211	13.3	15.5	11.2	2.6	31	484	<.1 c
oysters, battered or breaded,								
fried, 6 pieces or 4.9 oz.	368	12.5	39.9	17.9	4.6	109	677	.1 c
pizza, ⅛ of 12″ pie:								
w/cheese	109	6.0	15.9	2.5	1.2	7	261	.2 c
w/cheese, meat, and vegetables	152	10.7	17.5	4.4	1.3	17	315	.6 c
w/pepperoni	135	7.6	14.8	5.2	1.7	11	199	.5 c
scallops, breaded, fried, 6 pieces,								
5.1 oz.	386	15.8	38.5	19.4	4.9	107	919	.2 c
shrimp, breaded, fried, 6–8								
pieces, 5.8 oz.	454	18.9	40.0	24.9	5.4	201	1447	.1 c
Mexican foods:								
burrito, 2 pieces except as noted:								
w/apple or cherry, 1 small,								
2.6 oz.	231	2.5	35.0	9.5	4.6	3	211	.4 c
w/apple or cherry, 1 large,								
5.5 oz.	484	5.2	73.3	19.9	9.6	7	443	.8 c
w/beans:								
7.7 oz.	448	14.1	71.4	13.5	6.9	5	986	4.7 c
and cheese, 6.6 oz.	377	15.1	55.0	11.7	6.8	27	1166	2.0 c
and chili peppers, 7.2 oz. ...	413	16.4	58.1	14.7	7.6	33	1043	3.1 c
and meat, 8.1 oz.	508	22.5	66.0	17.8	8.3	48	1335	3.7 c
cheese and beef, 7.2 oz.	331	14.6	39.7	13.3	7.2	125	990	2.4 c
cheese and chili peppers,								
11.9 oz.	663	33.3	85.2	23.0	11.2	158	2060	5.1 c
w/beef:								
7.8 oz.	523	26.6	58.5	20.8	10.5	65	1492	1.7 c
and chili peppers, 7.1 oz. ...	426	21.5	49.5	16.5	8.0	54	1116	1.3 c

1. *Wing and breast, side or center cut.*
2. *Recipe: 94% crab, 4% flour, and 2% egg.*
3. *Recipe: 72% crab, 9% margarine, 8% egg, 8% bread crumbs, and 3% onion.*

Food and Measure	cal.	prot. (gms)	carbo. (gms)	tot. fat (gms)	sat. fat (gms)	chol. (mgs)	sod. (mgs)	fiber (gms)
FAST FOODS, MEXICAN, BURRITO, W/BEEF *(cont.)*								
cheese and chili peppers,								
10.7 oz.	634	40.9	63.7	24.8	10.4	170	2091	1.8 c
chimichanga, w/beef, 1 piece:								
6.1 oz.	425	19.6	42.8	19.7	8.5	9	910	2.3 c
and cheese, 6.5 oz.	443	20.1	39.3	23.5	11.2	51	956	2.1 c
and red chili peppers, 6.7 oz. . .	424	18.1	45.8	19.1	8.3	9	1169	1.5 c
cheese and red chili peppers,								
6.3 oz.	364	14.7	38.3	17.6	8.4	50	895	1.1 c
enchilada, w/cheese, 1 piece or								
5.7 oz.	320	9.6	28.5	18.9	10.6	44	784	2.7 c
enchilada, w/cheese and beef,								
1 piece or 6.8 oz.	324	11.9	30.5	17.6	9.0	40	1320	3.0 c
enchirito, w/cheese, beef and								
beans, 1 piece or 6.8 oz.	344	17.9	33.8	16.1	7.9	49	1251	2.0 c
frijoles, w/cheese, 1 cup	226	11.4	28.7	7.8	4.1	36	882	3.9 c
nachos, 6–8 pieces:								
w/cheese:								
4 oz.	345	9.1	36.3	19.0	7.8	18	816	2.0 c
and jalapeño peppers, 7.2 oz.	607	16.8	60.1	34.2	14.0	83	1736	4.7 c
beans, ground beef, and								
peppers, 9 oz.	568	19.8	55.8	30.7	12.5	21	1800	4.3 c
w/cinnamon and sugar, 3.8 oz.	592	7.2	63.4	36.0	18.2	39	439	1.4 c
taco, 1 small or 6 oz.	370	20.7	26.7	20.6	11.4	57	802	2.1 c
taco, 1 large or 9.3 oz.	569	31.8	41.1	31.6	17.5	87	1234	3.2 c
taco salad[1], 1½ cup	279	13.2	23.6	14.8	6.8	44	763	2.5 c
taco salad, w/chili[2], 1½ cup	288	17.4	26.6	13.1	6.0	4	886	5.2 c
tostada, 1 piece except as noted:								
w/beans and cheese, 5.1 oz. . .	223	9.6	26.5	9.9	5.4	30	543	3.8 c
w/beans, beef, and cheese,								
7.9 oz.	334	16.1	29.7	16.9	11.5	75	870	3.6 c
w/beef and cheese, 5.7 oz.	315	19.0	22.8	16.4	10.4	41	896	2.5 c
w/guacamole, 2 pieces or								
9.2 oz.	360	12.5	32.0	23.3	9.9	39	798	4.1 c
sandwiches, 1 piece:								
cheeseburger, regular:								
single meat patty:								
plain, 3.6 oz.	320	14.8	31.8	15.2	6.5	50	500	.1 c
w/condiments[3], 4 oz.	295	16.0	26.5	14.1	6.3	37	616	.3 c
w/condiments and								
vegetables[4], 5.4 oz.	359	17.8	28.1	19.8	9.2	52	976	.6 c
double meat patty:								
plain, 5.5 oz.	457	27.7	22.1	28.5	13.0	110	635	.1 c
w/condiments and								
vegetables[4], 5.9 oz.	416	21.2	35.2	21.1	8.7	60	1051	.5 c
double-decker bun, 5.6 oz. . .	461	22.1	44.3	21.6	9.5	80	892	.2 c

1. *Recipe: 41% lettuce, 17% tomato, 13% chili sauce, 12% ground beef, 9% cheese, and 7% taco shell.*
2. *Recipe: 44% chili con carne, 24% lettuce, 15% tomato, 9% cheese, and 8% taco shell.*
3. *Condiments include catsup, mustard, pickles, and onions.*
4. *Condiments and vegetables include catsup, mustard, mayonnaise-style dressing, pickles, onions, lettuce, and tomatoes.*

Food and Measure	cal.	prot. (gms)	carbo. (gms)	tot. fat (gms)	sat. fat (gms)	chol. (mgs)	sod. (mgs)	fiber (gms)
double-decker bun, w/ condiments and vegetables[1], 8 oz.	649	29.7	53.1	35.3	12.8	94	920	1.2 c
cheeseburger, large:								
single meat patty:								
plain, 6.5 oz.	608	30.1	47.4	33.0	14.8	96	1589	.2 c
w/bacon and condiments[2], 6.9 oz.	609	32.0	37.1	36.8	16.2	112	1044	.8 c
w/condiments and vegetables[1], 7.7 oz.	564	28.2	38.4	32.9	15.0	88	1107	.8 c
w/ham, condiments, and vegetables[1], 9 oz.	745	39.5	37.7	48.2	21.1	122	1713	.6 c
double meat patty, w/ condiments and vegetables[1], 9.1 oz.	706	38.0	39.7	43.7	17.7	141	1149	1.0 c
triple meat patty, plain, 10.7 oz.	796	56.1	26.7	51.0	21.7	161	1211	1.2 c
chicken fillet, 6.4 oz.	515	24.1	38.7	29.5	8.5	60	957	.4 c
chicken fillet, w/cheese, 8 oz. ...	632	29.4	41.6	38.8	12.4	76	1238	.3 c
egg and cheese, 5.1 oz.	340	15.6	25.9	19.4	6.6	291	804	.2 c
fish fillet, w/tartar sauce, 5.6 oz.	431	16.9	41.0	22.8	5.2	55	615	.6 c
fish fillet, w/tartar sauce and cheese, 6.5 oz.	524	20.6	47.6	28.6	8.1	68	939	.4 c
hamburger, small, single meat patty, w/condiments[2], 1.7 oz.	121	6.0	14.4	4.5	1.5	19	248	.2 c
hamburger, regular:								
single meat patty:								
plain, 3.2 oz.	275	12.3	30.5	11.8	4.1	36	387	.1 c
w/condiments[2], 3.8 oz.	275	13.6	32.7	10.2	3.5	43	564	.3 c
w/condiments and vegetables[1], 3.9 oz.	279	12.9	27.3	13.5	4.1	26	504	.3 c
double meat patty, plain, 6.2 oz.	544	29.9	42.9	27.9	10.4	99	554	.2 c
double meat patty, w/ condiments[2], 7.6 oz.	576	31.8	38.7	32.5	12.0	102	742	.3 c
hamburger, large:								
single meat patty, plain, 4.8 oz.	400	22.5	25.5	22.9	8.4	71	474	.1 c
single meat patty, w/condiments and vegetables[1], 7.7 oz.	511	25.7	40.1	27.4	10.4	86	825	1.0 c
double meat patty, w/ condiments and vegetables[1], 8 oz.	540	34.3	40.3	26.6	10.5	122	791	.7 c
triple meat patty, w/ condiments[2], 9.1 oz.	693	50.0	28.6	41.5	15.9	142	713	.8 c
ham and cheese, 5.1 oz.	353	20.7	33.3	15.5	6.4	58	772	.1 c
ham, egg, and cheese, 5 oz.	348	19.3	31.0	16.3	7.4	245	1005	.1 c

1. *Condiments and vegetables include catsup, mustard, mayonnaise-style dressing, pickles, onions, lettuce, and tomatoes.*
2. *Condiments include catsup, mustard, pickles, and onions.*

Food and Measure	cal.	prot. (gms)	carbo. (gms)	tot. fat (gms)	sat. fat (gms)	chol. (mgs)	sod. (mgs)	fiber (gms)
FAST FOODS *(cont.)*								
hot dog:								
plain, 3.5 oz.	242	10.4	18.0	14.5	5.1	44	671	.3 c
w/chili, 4 oz.	297	13.5	31.3	13.4	4.9	51	480	.2 c
corn flour coated (corn dog),								
6.2 oz.	460	16.8	55.8	18.9	5.2	79	972	.3 c
roast beef sandwich, plain, 4.9 oz.	346	21.5	33.5	13.8	3.6	52	792	.7 c
roast beef sandwich, w/cheese,								
6.2 oz.	402	32.2	27.1	18.0	9.0	77	1634	.2 c
steak sandwich, 7.2 oz.	459	30.3	52.0	14.1	3.8	73	798	.4 c
submarine sandwich:								
w/cold cuts, 8 oz.	456	21.9	51.0	18.6	6.8	35	1650	.7 c
w/roast beef, 7.6 oz.	411	28.6	44.3	13.0	7.1	73	845	.7 c
w/tuna salad, 9 oz.	584	29.7	55.4	28.0	5.3	47	1294	.6 c
salad, w/out dressing, 1½ cup:								
vegetable[1]	32	2.6	6.7	.2	<.1	0	53	1.4 c
w/cheese and egg[2]	102	8.8	4.8	5.8	3.0	98	119	1.0 c
w/chicken[3]	105	17.4	3.7	2.2	.6	72	209	1.0 c
w/pasta and seafood[4]	380	16.4	32.0	20.9	2.6	50	1572	1.6 c
w/shrimp[5]	107	14.5	6.6	2.5	.7	180	487	1.4 c
chef style[6]	267	26.0	4.7	16.1	8.2	139	744	1.1 c
side dishes:								
coleslaw, ¾ cup	147	1.5	12.8	11.0	1.6	5	267	.6 c
corn on cob, w/butter, 1 ear,								
5.1 oz.	155	4.5	32.0	3.4	1.6	6	30	.9 c
hush puppies, 5 pieces, 2.8 oz. . .	256	4.9	34.9	11.6	2.7	135	965	.4 c
onion rings, breaded, fried, 8–9								
rings, 2.9 oz.	275	3.7	31.3	15.5	7.0	14	430	.3 c
potato, baked, 1 potato:								
topped w/cheese sauce:								
10.4 oz.	475	14.6	46.5	28.7	10.6	19	381	1.3 c
and bacon, 10.5 oz.	451	18.4	44.4	25.9	10.1	30	973	1.3 c
and broccoli, 12 oz.	402	13.7	46.6	21.4	8.5	20	484	2.0 c
and chili, 13.9 oz.	481	23.2	55.9	21.9	13.0	31	701	3.2 c
topped w/sour cream and								
chives, 10.1 oz.	394	6.7	50.0	22.3	10.0	23	182	1.5 c
potato, french-fried:								
in beef tallow, 1 regular order,								
2.7 oz.	237	3.0	29.3	12.2	5.6	13	124	.6 c
in beef tallow, 1 large order,								
4.1 oz.	358	4.6	44.4	18.5	8.5	20	187	.9 c
in beef tallow and vegetable oil,								
1 regular order, 2.7 oz.	237	3.0	29.3	12.2	5.0	11	124	.6 c

1. *Recipe: lettuce, cabbage, cucumber, green pepper, tomato, radish, and carrot.*
2. *Recipe: lettuce, tomato, egg, cheese, celery, cucumber, and radish.*
3. *Recipe: lettuce, chicken, celery, tomato, green pepper, and carrot.*
4. *Recipe: lettuce, macaroni, salad dressing, pollock, sweet pepper, carrot, celery, carp, turbot, olives, and onion.*
5. *Recipe: lettuce, shrimp, celery, tomato, green pepper, and carrot.*
6. *Recipe: lettuce, tomato, turkey, ham, cheese, egg, celery, cucumber, radish, and carrot.*

Food and Measure	cal.	prot. (gms)	carbo. (gms)	tot. fat (gms)	sat. fat (gms)	chol. (mgs)	sod. (mgs)	fiber (gms)
in beef tallow and vegetable oil,								
1 large order, 4.1 oz.	358	4.6	44.4	18.5	7.6	16	187	.9 c
in vegetable oil, 1 regular order,								
2.7 oz.	235	3.0	29.3	12.2	3.8	0	124	.6 c
in vegetable oil, 1 large order,								
4.1 oz.	355	4.6	44.4	18.5	5.7	0	187	.9 c
potato, mashed, ⅓ cup	66	1.9	12.9	1.0	.4	2	182	.7 c
potato chips, 1 oz.	148	1.8	14.7	10.1	2.6	0	133	.4 c
potato salad, ⅓ cup	108	1.5	12.9	5.7	1.0	57	312	.3 c
desserts:								
brownie, 1 piece, 2.1 oz.	243	2.7	39.0	10.1	3.1	9	153	.5 c
cookies, animal crackers,								
2.4-oz. box	299	4.1	50.5	9.0	3.5	11	274	.2 c
cookies, chocolate chip,								
1.9-oz. box	233	2.9	36.2	12.2	5.3	12	188	.3 c
fruit pie (apple, cherry or lemon),								
fried, 3-oz. pie	266	2.4	33.1	14.4	6.5	13	325	.3 c
ice milk cone, vanilla, soft-serve,								
1 cone, 3.6 oz.	164	3.9	24.1	6.1	3.5	28	92	.1 c
sundae:								
caramel, 5.5 oz.	303	7.3	49.3	9.3	4.5	25	195	.2 c
hot fudge, 5.6 oz.	284	5.6	47.7	8.6	5.0	21	182	.2 c
strawberry, 5.4 oz.	269	6.3	44.7	7.9	3.7	21	92	.2 c
beverages:								
beer, regular, 12-fl.-oz. can	146	.9	13.2	0	0	0	19	0
beer, light, 12-fl.-oz. can	100	.7	4.8	0	0	0	10	0
coffee, brewed, 6 fl. oz.	4	.1	.8	tr.	tr.	0	4	0
coffee, instant, decaffeinated,								
6 fl. oz.	4	.2	.8	tr.	tr.	0	6	0
hot chocolate, 6 fl. oz.	103	3.1	22.5	1.1	.7	n.a.	149	.2 c
juice, 6 fl. oz.:								
grapefruit	78	1.0	18.1	.2	<.1	0	tr.	n.a.
orange	84	1.3	20.1	.1	<.1	0	tr.	.1 c
tomato	32	1.4	7.7	.1	<.1	0	658	.7 c
lemonade, 8 fl. oz.	100	.1	26.0	.1	<.1	0	8	.1 c
milk, whole, 8 fl. oz.	150	8.0	11.4	8.2	5.1	33	120	0
milk, lowfat 2%, 8 fl. oz.	121	8.1	11.7	4.7	2.9	18	122	0
orange drink, 6 fl. oz.	94	0	24.0	tr.	tr.	0	31	(0)
shake, 10 fl. oz.:								
chocolate	360	9.6	57.9	10.5	6.5	37	273	.2 c
strawberry	319	9.5	53.4	8.0	n.a.	31	234	.2 c
vanilla	314	9.8	50.8	8.4	5.3	32	232	.3 c
soda, 12-fl.-oz. can:								
cola	151	.1	38.5	.1	0	0	14	0
cola, Aspartame-sweetened ...	2	.2	.3	0	0	0	21	0
ginger ale	124	.1	31.9	0	0	0	25	0
lemon-lime	149	0	38.4	0	0	0	41	0
orange	177	0	45.8	0	0	0	46	0
pepper type	151	0	38.2	.4	n.a.	0	38	0

Food and Measure	cal.	prot. (gms)	carbo. (gms)	tot. fat (gms)	sat. fat (gms)	chol. (mgs)	sod. (mgs)	fiber (gms)
FAST FOODS, BEVERAGES, SODA *(cont.)*								
root beer	152	.1	39.2	0	0	0	49	0
tea, brewed, 6 fl. oz.	2	0	.4	tr.	tr.	0	5	0
tea, iced, instant, sugar-								
sweetened, lemon flavor,								
prepared w/water, 12 fl. oz. ...	132	.4	33.1	.2	<.1	0	n.a.	0
FAT, see specific listings								
FAT, IMITATION:								
(*Rokeach Neutral Nyafat*), 1 tbsp. ...	99	0	0	11.0	m.q.	0	0	0
FAVA BEAN, canned:								
(*Progresso*), ½ cup	90	7.0	15.0	<1.0	n.a.	0	420	12.0 d
FEET, PORK, see "Pig's feet"								
FENNEL:								
(*Frieda* of California), 1 lb.	68	5.0	11.8	.5	n.a.	0	408	m.q.
(*Frieda* of California), 1 oz.	4	.3	.7	<.1	(0)	0	26	m.q.
FENNEL SEED:								
1 oz.	98	4.8	14.8	4.2	.1	0	25	4.4 c
1 tbsp.	20	.9	3.0	.9	<.1	0	5	.9 c
1 tsp.	7	.3	1.1	.3	tr.	0	2	.3 c
(*Spice Islands*), 1 tsp.	8	.2	1.3	.2	(0)	0	2	.4 c
(*Tone's*), 1 tsp.	7	.3	1.1	.3	<.1	0	2	.3 d
FENUGREEK SEED:								
1 oz.	92	6.5	16.5	1.8	n.a.	0	19	2.9 c
1 tbsp.	36	2.6	6.5	.7	n.a.	0	7	1.1 c
1 tsp.	12	.9	2.2	.9	n.a.	0	2	.4 c
FETTUCCINI, see "Pasta"								
FETTUCCINI ENTREE, FROZEN:								
Alfredo:								
(*Healthy Choice*), 8 oz.	240	10.0	36.0	7.0	2.0	45	370	m.q.
(*Stouffer's*), ½ of 10-oz. pkg.	270	8.0	17.0	19.0	m.q.	n.a.	560	m.q.
(*Weight Watchers*), 9 oz.	210	17.0	18.0	8.0	3.0	35	600	m.q.
w/broccoli (*Dining Lite*), 9 oz.	290	12.0	33.0	12.0	m.q.	35	1020	m.q.
w/meat sauce (*The Budget Gourmet*), 10 oz.	290	16.0	34.0	10.0	m.q.	25	980	m.q.
primavera (*Green Giant*), 1 pkg. ...	230	13.0	26.0	8.0	3.0	25	610	6.0 d
primavera (*Green Giant* Microwave Garden Gourmet), 1 pkg.	260	17.0	25.0	13.0	m.q.	n.a.	640	6.0 d
FETTUCCINI ENTREE MIX:								
Alfredo (*Hain* Pasta & Sauce), ¼ pkg.	180	5.0	27.0	4.0	m.q.	n.a.	420	m.q.
Alfredo (*Kraft* Pasta & Cheese), ½ cup[1]	180	7.0	19.0	9.0	3.0	30	590	m.q.
FIELD CRESS, see "Garden cress"								
FIG:								
w/stems, 1 lb.	333	3.4	86.1	1.4	.3	0	5	5.4 c

1. *Prepared according to package directions.*

Food and Measure	cal.	prot. (gms)	carbo. (gms)	tot. fat (gms)	sat. fat (gms)	chol. (mgs)	sod. (mgs)	fiber (gms)
trimmed, 1 oz.	21	.2	5.4	.1	<.1	0	<1	.3 c
1 large, approx. 2.3 oz.	47	.5	12.3	.2	<.1	0	1	.8 c
1 medium, approx. 1.8 oz.	37	.4	9.6	.2	<.1	0	1	.6 c
FIG, CANNED:								
in water:								
4 oz.	60	.5	15.9	.1	<.1	0	1	.6 c
½ cup	65	.5	17.3	.1	<.1	0	2	.7 c
3 figs and 1¾ tbsp. liquid	42	.3	11.2	.1	<.1	0	1	.5 c
in light syrup:								
4 oz.	78	.4	20.4	.1	<.1	0	1	.6 c
½ cup	87	.5	22.6	.1	<.1	0	2	.7 c
3 figs and 1¾ tbsp. liquid	58	.3	15.3	.1	<.1	0	1	.5 c
in heavy syrup:								
4 oz.	100	.4	26.0	.1	<.1	0	1	.6 c
½ cup	114	.5	29.7	.1	<.1	0	2	.7 c
3 figs and 1¾ tbsp. liquid	75	.3	19.5	.1	<.1	0	1	.5 c
whole (*Del Monte*), ½ cup	100	0	28.0	0	0	0	<10	m.q.
whole kadota (*S&W* Fancy), ½ cup	100	0	28.0	0	0	0	<10	m.q.
in extra heavy syrup:								
4 oz.	121	.4	31.6	.1	<.1	0	1	.6 c
½ cup	140	.5	36.4	.1	<.1	0	2	.7 c
3 figs and 1¾ tbsp. liquid	91	.3	23.7	.1	<.1	0	1	.5 c
FIG, DRIED:								
uncooked:								
4 oz.	289	3.5	74.1	1.3	.3	0	15	10.5 d
½ cup	254	3.0	65.0	1.2	.2	0	11	9.3 d
10 figs, approx. 6.6 oz.	477	5.7	122.2	2.2	.4	0	20	17.4 d
Calimyrna (*Blue Ribbon/ Sun•Maid*), ½ cup	250	3.0	58.0	2.0	m.q.	0	<10	m.q.
Mission (*Blue Ribbon/Sun•Maid*), ½ cup	210	3.0	1.0	m.q.	m.q.	0	<20	m.q.
cooked, 4 oz.	122	1.5	31.3	.6	.1	0	6	2.3 c
cooked, ½ cup	140	1.7	35.9	.6	.1	0	6	2.6 c
FILBERT, shelled:								
dried, unblanched:								
1 oz.	179	3.7	4.4	17.8	1.3	0	1	1.1 c
whole, 1 cup	853	17.6	20.7	84.6	6.2	0	4	5.1 c
chopped, 1 cup	727	15.0	17.6	72.0	5.3	0	3	4.4 c
ground, 1 cup	474	9.8	11.5	47.0	3.5	0	2	2.9 c
dried, blanched, 1 oz.	191	3.6	4.5	19.1	1.4	0	1	.5 c
dry-roasted, unblanched, 1 oz.	188	2.8	5.1	18.8	1.4	0	1	1.1 c
dry-roasted, unblanched, salted, 1 oz.	188	2.8	5.1	18.8	1.4	0	221	1.1 c
oil-roasted, unblanched, 1 oz.	187	4.1	5.4	18.1	1.3	0	1	1.8 d
oil-roasted, unblanched, salted, 1 oz.	187	4.1	5.4	18.1	1.3	0	223	1.8 d

FILE POWDER, see "Gumbo file powder"

Food and Measure	cal.	prot. (gms)	carbo. (gms)	tot. fat (gms)	sat. fat (gms)	chol. (mgs)	sod. (mgs)	fiber (gms)
FINNAN HADDIE, see "Haddock, smoked"								
FINNISH POTATO, see "Potato, Finnish"								
FINOCCHIO, see "Fennel"								
FISH, see specific fish listings								
FISH BATTER MIX, see "Fish seasoning and coating mix"								
FISH CAKE, see "Fish entree"								
FISH COATING MIX, see "Fish seasoning and coating mix"								
FISH DINNER, frozen (see also specific fish listings):								
(*Morton*), 9.75 oz.	370	18.0	46.0	13.0	m.q.	65	910	m.q.
'n' chips (*Swanson*), 10 oz.	500	20.0	60.0	21.0	m.q.	m.q.	960	m.q.
nuggets (*Kid Cuisine*), 7 oz.	320	13.0	33.0	15.0	m.q.	45	750	m.q.
FISH ENTREE, FROZEN (see also specific fish listings):								
(*Banquet* Platters), 8.75 oz.	450	31.0	33.0	22.0	m.q.	95	m.q.	m.q.
au gratin (*Weight Watchers*), 9.25 oz.	200	25.0	11.0	6.0	1.0	60	700	m.q.
battered fillets:								
(*Gorton's* Crispy Batter), 2 pieces	290	11.0	18.0	19.0	8.0	35	550	m.q.
(*Gorton's* Crispy Batter, Large), 1 piece	320	12.0	20.0	21.0	m.q.	m.q.	680	m.q.
(*Gorton's* Crunchy), 2 pieces	230	13.0	16.0	13.0	3.0	40	420	m.q.
(*Gorton's* Crunchy Microwave), 2 pieces	340	10.0	17.0	26.0	12.0	30	400	m.q.
(*Gorton's* Crunchy Microwave, Large), 1 piece	320	11.0	20.0	22.0	10.0	35	500	m.q.
(*Gorton's* Potato Crisp), 2 pieces	300	12.0	18.0	20.0	6.0	30	360	m.q.
(*Gorton's* Value Pack Portions), 1 piece	180	7.0	13.0	11.0	m.q.	m.q.	490	m.q.
(*Mrs. Paul's*), 2 pieces	330	16.0	28.0	17.0	m.q.	60	650	m.q.
(*Mrs. Paul's* Crunchy), 2 pieces	280	12.0	26.0	14.0	3.0	22	730	m.q.
(*Van de Kamp's*), 1 piece	170	7.0	13.0	10.0	2.0	20	350	m.q.
minced (*Mrs. Paul's* Portions), 2 pieces	300	11.0	21.0	19.0	3.0	33	540	m.q.
tempura (*Gorton's Light Recipe*), 1 piece	200	10.0	8.0	14.0	4.0	30	400	m.q.
breaded fillets:								
reheated, 1 piece[1], 4″ × 2″ × ½″, approx. 2 oz.	155	8.9	13.5	7.0	1.8	64	332	.2 c
(*Gorton's Light Recipe*), 1 piece	180	11.0	16.0	8.0	3.0	30	380	m.q.
(*Mrs. Paul's* Crispy Crunchy), 2 pieces	220	13.0	23.0	9.0	2.0	22	380	m.q.
(*Van de Kamp's*), 2 pieces	280	11.0	18.0	18.0	3.0	35	280	m.q.

1. *Recipe: 53.1% walleye pollock, 29.2% bread crumbs, 11.7% egg, 5.4% milk, and .6% salt.*

Food and Measure	cal.	prot. (gms)	carbo. (gms)	tot. fat (gms)	sat. fat (gms)	chol. (mgs)	sod. (mgs)	fiber (gms)
crispy (*Van de Kamp's* Microwave), 1 piece	140	6.0	9.0	9.0	2.0	15	210	m.q.
crispy (*Van de Kamp's* Microwave, Large), 1 piece	290	12.0	21.0	17.0	3.0	25	640	m.q.
minced (*Mrs. Paul's* Crispy Crunchy Portions), 2 pieces ...	230	10.0	14.0	15.0	2.0	25	300	m.q.
cakes (*Mrs. Paul's*), 2 pieces	190	9.0	24.0	7.0	m.q.	20	690	m.q.
coated, fillets, ranch (*Gorton's* Specialty Microwave, Large), 1 piece	330	12.0	24.0	21.0	m.q.	m.q.	520	m.q.
Dijon (*Mrs. Paul's* Light), 8¾ oz. ..	200	21.0	17.0	5.0	2.0	60	650	m.q.
fillet of:								
Divan (*Lean Cuisine*), 12⅜ oz. ..	260	31.0	17.0	7.0	2.0	85	750	m.q.
Florentine (*Lean Cuisine*), 9 oz.	230	26.0	13.0	8.0	2.0	100	700	m.q.
Florentine (*Mrs. Paul's* Light), 8 oz.	220	25.0	10.0	8.0	4.0	95	820	m.q.
in herb sauce (*Gorton's*), 1 pkg. ...	190	26.0	3.0	8.0	5.0	90	450	m.q.
jardiniere, w/souffléed potatoes (*Lean Cuisine*), 11¼ oz.	290	31.0	18.0	10.0	4.0	110	840	m.q.
fillets, in butter sauce (*Mrs. Paul's* Light), 1 piece	140	20.0	1.0	6.0	m.q.	40	520	n.a.
'n' fries (*Swanson* Homestyle Recipe), 6½ oz.	340	11.0	37.0	16.0	m.q.	m.q.	670	m.q.
gems, fancy style (*Wakefield*), 4 oz.	80	11.0	11.0	1.0	n.a.	m.q.	m.q.	m.q.
gems, salad style (*Wakefield*), 3 oz.	70	10.0	8.0	1.0	n.a.	m.q.	m.q.	n.a.
oven-fried (*Weight Watchers*), 7.08 oz.	240	20.0	23.0	7.0	<1.0	15	380	m.q.
Mornay (*Mrs. Paul's* Light), 9 oz. ...	230	24.0	12.0	10.0	4.0	80	670	m.q.
sticks, battered:								
(*Gorton's* Crispy Batter), 4 pieces	260	9.0	16.0	18.0	6.0	25	480	m.q.
(*Gorton's* Crunchy), 4 pieces	210	7.0	15.0	13.0	4.0	25	240	m.q.
(*Gorton's* Crunchy Microwave), 6 pieces	340	11.0	24.0	22.0	7.0	35	420	m.q.
(*Gorton's* Potato Crisp), 4 pieces	260	8.0	21.0	16.0	5.0	25	390	m.q.
(*Gorton's* Value Pack), 4 pieces ..	190	9.0	17.0	9.0	m.q.	m.q.	420	m.q.
(*Mrs. Paul's*), 4 pieces	210	7.0	15.0	12.0	m.q.	25	590	m.q.
(*Van de Kamp's*), 4 pieces	160	8.0	12.0	9.0	2.0	20	350	m.q.
minced (*Mrs. Paul's*), 4 pieces ...	220	8.0	20.0	13.0	2.0	20	630	m.q.
sticks, breaded:								
reheated, 1 piece[1], 4″ × 1″ × ½″, approx. 1 oz.	76	4.4	6.7	3.4	.9	31	163	.1 c
(*Frionor Bunch o' Crunch*), 4 pieces or 2.7 oz.	210	9.0	13.0	14.0	2.0	m.q.	267	<.1 d
(*Mrs. Paul's* Crispy Crunchy), 4 pieces	140	7.0	14.0	6.0	m.q.	20	340	m.q.
(*Van de Kamp's*), 4 pieces	200	9.0	15.0	12.0	2.0	20	290	m.q.
(*Van de Kamp's* Value Pack), 4 pieces	170	8.0	13.0	10.0	2.0	20	270	m.q.

1. *Recipe: 53.1% walleye pollock, 29.2% bread crumbs, 11.7% egg, 5.4% milk, and .6% salt.*

Food and Measure	cal.	prot. (gms)	carbo. (gms)	tot. fat (gms)	sat. fat (gms)	chol. (mgs)	sod. (mgs)	fiber (gms)
FISH ENTREE, FROZEN, STICKS, BREADED *(cont.)*								
crispy (*Van de Kamp's* Microwave),								
3 pieces	130	7.0	11.0	7.0	1.0	15	280	m.q.
minced (*Mrs. Paul's* Crispy								
Crunchy), 4 pieces	190	9.0	18.0	8.0	m.q.	25	560	m.q.
whole wheat (*Booth* Microwave),								
2 oz.	150	6.0	14.0	8.0	m.q.	m.q.	210	m.q.
"FISH" ENTREE,								
VEGETARIAN, frozen:								
(*Worthington Fillets*), 2 pieces, 3 oz.	180	15.0	9.0	9.0	2.0	0	910	m.q.
FISH PASTE CAKE, Japanese:								
block (kamaboko), steamed, 4 oz. ..	111	13.6	11.0	1.0	m.q.	m.q.	1134	n.a.
stick (chikuwa), grilled, 4 oz.	143	13.8	15.3	2.4	m.q.	m.q.	1134	n.a.
FISH ROE, see "Caviar" and "Roe"								
FISH SEASONING AND								
COATING MIX:								
(*Featherweight*), ¼ pkg.	18	1.0	8.0	0	0	0	10	m.q.
(*Shake'n Bake*), ¼ pouch	70	1.0	14.0	1.0	n.a.	0	410	m.q.
batter, Cajun (*Tone's*), 1 tsp.	12	.3	2.6	.1	<.1	0	49	.1 d
batter, fish & chips (*Golden Dipt*),								
1¼ oz.	120	2.0	27.0	0	0	0	910	m.q.
blackened redfish (*Golden Dipt*),								
¼ tsp.	2	0	0	0	0	0	140	n.a.
broiled (*Golden Dipt*), ¼ tsp.	2	0	0	0	0	0	125	n.a.
fish fry (*Golden Dipt*), ⅔ oz.	60	2.0	14.0	0	0	0	430	m.q.
fish fry, Cajun style (*Golden Dipt*),								
⅔ oz.	60	2.0	14.0	0	0	0	470	m.q.
seafood:								
(*Golden Dipt*), ⅔ oz.	60	1.0	14.0	0	0	0	600	m.q.
(*Tone's*), 1 tsp.	10	.5	.9	.7	<.1	0	1	.3 d
all purpose (*Golden Dipt*), ¼ tsp.	2	0	0	0	0	0	85	n.a.
Chesapeake (*Tone's*), 1 tsp.	8	.4	.9	.3	<.1	0	1032	.3 d
Chesapeake Bay (*McCormick/*								
Schilling), ¼ tsp.	2	.1	.2	.1	n.a.	0	202	n.a.
lemon pepper (*Golden Dipt*),								
¼ tsp.	8	1	1	0	0	0	115	n.a.
shrimp and crab, Cajun style (*Golden*								
Dipt), ¼ tsp.	2	0	0	0	0	0	200	n.a.
FISH STICKS, see "Fish entree"								
5-SPICE, see "Oriental spice"								
FLAN, see "Pudding mix"								
FLATFISH, meat only:								
raw:								
1 lb.	414	85.5	0	5.4	1.3	217	367	0
1 oz.	26	5.3	0	.3	.1	14	23	0
1 fillet, approx. 5.7 oz., yield from								
2-lb. whole fish	149	30.7	0	1.9	.5	78	132	0

Food and Measure	cal.	prot. (gms)	carbo. (gms)	tot. fat (gms)	sat. fat (gms)	chol. (mgs)	sod. (mgs)	fiber (gms)
baked, broiled, or microwaved[1], 4 oz.	133	27.4	0	1.7	.4	77	119	0
FLAVOR ENHANCER:								
(*Ac'cent*), ½ tsp.	5	0	0	0	0	0	300	0
FLAX SEED:								
(*Arrowhead Mills*), 1 oz.	140	5.0	11.0	10.0	m.q.	0	<1	6.0 d
FLORENCE FENNEL, see "Fennel"								
FLOUNDER, fresh, see "Flatfish"								
FLOUNDER, FROZEN:								
(*Booth* Individually Wrapped), 4 oz.	90	19.0	0	0	0	m.q.	90	0
(*Finast*), 4 oz.	90	19.0	0	1.0	m.q.	m.q.	150	0
(*Gorton's Fishmarket Fresh*), 5 oz. ...	110	23.0	1.0	1.0	m.q.	m.q.	170	0
(*SeaPak*), 4 oz.	90	20.0	0	1.0	m.q.	m.q.	120	0
(*Van de Kamp's* Natural), 4 oz.	100	22.0	0	2.0	0	35	100	0
Atlantic (*Booth*), 4 oz.	90	19.0	0	1.0	m.q.	m.q.	180	0
FLOUNDER ENTREE, frozen:								
battered fillets (*Mrs. Paul's* Crunchy), 2 pieces	220	12.0	23.0	9.0	m.q.	40	560	m.q.
breaded fillets:								
(*Mrs. Paul's* Light), 1 piece	240	16.0	20.0	10.0	m.q.	50	450	m.q.
(*Van de Kamp's* Light), 1 piece ...	260	18.0	21.0	12.0	2.0	45	480	m.q.
stuffed (*Gorton's Microwave Entrees*), 1 pkg.	350	25.0	21.0	18.0	7.0	120	850	m.q.
FLOUR, see "Wheat flour" and specific grain listings								
FLYING FISH, meat only, raw:								
1 lb.	413	95.3	0	.9	m.q.	m.q.	m.q.	0
1 oz.	26	6.0	0	<.1	m.q.	m.q.	m.q.	0
FON GOOT, see "Yam bean tuber"								
FORESTIERA SAUCE, refrigerated:								
(*Contadina Fresh*), 7.5 oz.	270	6.0	15.0	9.0	m.q.	15	830	n.a.
FRANKFURTER:								
(*Eckrich*, 12 oz.), 1 link	110	4.0	2.0	10.0	m.q.	m.q.	300	0
(*Eckrich*, 1 lb.), 1 link	160	5.0	2.0	14.0	m.q.	m.q.	420	0
(*Eckrich* Bunsize), 1 link	190	6.0	2.0	17.0	m.q.	m.q.	500	0
(*Eckrich* Jumbo), 1 link	190	6.0	2.0	17.0	m.q.	m.q.	500	0
(*Eckrich* Jumbo Lean Supreme), 1 link	140	7.0	2.0	12.0	m.q.	m.q.	490	0
(*Hillshire Farm* Bun Size Wieners), 2 oz.	180	7.0	2.0	16.0	m.q.	m.q.	550	0
(*JM*), 1.2-oz. link	110	4.0	1.0	10.0	m.q.	16	370	0
(*JM*, 10/lb.), 1.6-oz. link	140	5.0	1.0	13.0	m.q.	22	490	0
(*JM* German Brand), 2-oz. link	160	7.0	1.0	14.0	m.q.	m.q.	620	0
(*JM* Jumbo), 2-oz. link	190	6.0	2.0	17.0	m.q.	27	620	0
(*Kahn's* Bun Size), 1 link	190	6.0	2.0	17.0	m.q.	m.q.	600	0

1. *Without added ingredients.*

Food and Measure	cal.	prot. (gms)	carbo. (gms)	tot. fat (gms)	sat. fat (gms)	chol. (mgs)	sod. (mgs)	fiber (gms)
FRANKFURTER *(cont.)*								
(*Kahn's* Bun Size Frank or Jumbo),								
1 link	190	6.0	2.0	17.0	m.q.	m.q.	560	0
(*Kahn's* Wieners), 1 link	140	5.0	1.0	13.0	m.q.	m.q.	500	0
(*OHSE* Wieners), 1 oz.	90	3.0	1.0	8.0	m.q.	m.q.	300	0
(*Oscar Mayer Bun-Length* Wieners),								
2-oz. link	184	6.3	1.4	16.9	6.2	34	571	0
(*Oscar Mayer* Light Wieners), 2-oz.								
link	127	7.3	.3	10.8	3.8	30	623	0
(*Oscar Mayer* Wieners), 1.6-oz. link	144	5.0	1.1	13.3	5.0	29	455	0
(*Oscar Mayer* Wieners), 2-oz. link ..	181	6.3	1.4	16.9	6.4	36	576	0
(*Pilgrim's Pride*, 1 lb.), 2-oz. link ..	118	7.8	1.1	8.8	m.q.	31	456	0
(*Pilgrim's Pride*, 12 oz.), 1.5-oz.								
link	88	5.8	.8	6.6	m.q.	24	342	0
bacon and cheddar cheese (*Oscar*								
Mayer Hot Dogs), 1.6-oz. link	137	6.3	1.0	12.0	5.0	29	501	0
batter-wrapped, frozen (*Hormel* Corn								
Dogs), 1 piece	220	7.0	21.0	12.0	m.q.	m.q.	656	m.q.
batter-wrapped, frozen (*Hormel*								
Tater Dogs), 1 piece	210	6.0	15.0	14.0	m.q.	m.q.	170	m.q.
beef:								
1 oz.	91	3.2	.7	8.3	3.4	14	290	0
1 link, 5″ long × ⅞″, approx.								
2 oz.	184	6.4	1.4	16.8	6.8	27	584	0
1 link, 5″ long × ¾″, approx.								
1.6 oz.	145	5.1	1.1	13.2	5.4	22	461	0
(*Boar's Head*), 1 oz.	80	4.0	<1.0	7.0	m.q.	15	m.q.	0
(*Eckrich*, 12 oz.), 1 link	110	4.0	2.0	10.0	m.q.	m.q.	310	0
(*Eckrich*, 1 lb.), 1 link	150	5.0	2.0	14.0	m.q.	m.q.	400	0
(*Eckrich* Bunsize), 1 link	190	6.0	2.0	17.0	m.q.	m.q.	520	0
(*Eckrich* Jumbo), 1 link	190	6.0	2.0	17.0	m.q.	m.q.	520	0
(*Hebrew National*), 1.7-oz. link ...	149	5.8	<1.0	14.0	m.q.	15	497	0
(*Hillshire Farm* Bun Size								
Wieners), 2 oz.	180	7.0	2.0	16.0	m.q.	m.q.	560	0
(*Hormel* 12 oz.), 1 link	100	4.0	1.0	10.0	m.q.	m.q.	362	0
(*Hormel* 1 lb.), 1 link	140	5.0	1.0	13.0	m.q.	m.q.	463	0
(*JM*), 1.2-oz. link	100	4.0	1.0	9.0	m.q.	20	350	0
(*JM*, 10/lb.), 1.6-oz. link	140	5.0	1.0	13.0	m.q.	26	480	0
(*JM* Jumbo), 2-oz. link	180	6.0	2.0	16.0	m.q.	33	600	0
(*Kahn's*), 1 link	140	5.0	2.0	13.0	m.q.	m.q.	500	0
(*Kahn's* Bun Size), 1 link	190	6.0	2.0	17.0	m.q.	m.q.	560	0
(*Kahn's* Bun Size Franks), 1 link	190	6.0	3.0	17.0	m.q.	m.q.	560	0
(*Kahn's* Jumbo), 1 link	190	6.0	3.0	18.0	m.q.	m.q.	560	0
(*King Kold*), 2 oz.	173	9.0	1.0	16.3	m.q.	m.q.	815	0
(*OHSE*), 1 oz.	85	3.0	1.0	8.0	m.q.	m.q.	280	0
(*Oscar Mayer Bun-Length* Franks),								
2-oz. link	182	6.3	1.4	16.8	7.3	34	568	0
(*Oscar Mayer* Franks), 1.6-oz. link	143	5.0	1.1	13.2	5.6	28	460	0
(*Oscar Mayer* Franks), 2-oz. link	181	6.3	1.4	16.7	7.0	35	583	0

Food and Measure	cal.	prot. (gms)	carbo. (gms)	tot. fat (gms)	sat. fat (gms)	chol. (mgs)	sod. (mgs)	fiber (gms)
(*Oscar Mayer* Light Franks), 2-oz. link	131	6.8	.9	11.1	4.6	23	594	0
w/cheddar:								
(*Kahn's* Beef n'Cheddar), 1 link	180	7.0	2.0	16.0	m.q.	m.q.	640	0
(*Oscar Mayer* Franks), 1.6-oz. link	136	5.6	1.2	12.2	5.1	27	492	0
(*Oscar Mayer* Franks), 2-oz. link	163	7.5	1.1	14.3	6.4	36	655	0
beef and pork:								
1 oz.	91	3.2	.7	8.3	3.1	14	318	0
1 link, 5" long × ⅞", approx. 2 oz.	183	6.4	1.5	16.6	6.1	29	639	0
1 link, 5" long × ¾", approx. 1.6 oz.	144	5.1	1.2	13.1	4.8	22	504	0
cheese (cheesefurter or cheese smokie):								
1 oz.	93	4.0	.4	8.2	3.0	19	307	0
1 link, approx. 1.5 oz., 8 links per 12-oz. pkg.	141	6.0	.6	12.5	4.5	29	465	0
(*Eckrich*), 1 link	180	7.0	2.0	16.0	m.q.	m.q.	530	0
(*Hillshire Farm* Bun Size Wieners), 2 oz.	180	7.0	2.0	16.0	m.q.	m.q.	530	0
(*JM* Cheese Franks), 1.6-oz. link	140	5.0	2.0	13.0	m.q.	m.q.	540	0
(*Kahn's* Cheese Wiener), 1 link ..	150	6.0	1.0	13.0	m.q.	m.q.	490	0
(*Oscar Mayer* Hot Dogs), 1.6-oz. link	143	5.4	1.1	12.9	5.3	30	480	0
w/cheese (*JM* German Brand), 2-oz. link	160	8.0	2.0	14.0	m.q.	37	620	0
chicken, see "Chicken frankfurter"								
chicken, beef, and pork (*OHSE*), 1 oz.	85	3.0	1.0	8.0	m.q.	m.q.	260	0
chili (*Hormel* Frank 'n Stuff), 1 link	165	7.0	2.0	15.0	m.q.	m.q.	517	n.a.
cocktail (*Oscar Mayer* Little Wieners), .3-oz. link	28	1.1	.2	2.6	1.0	5	92	0
hot (*Hillshire Farm* Hot Links), 2 oz.	190	8.0	2.0	16.0	m.q.	m.q.	530	0
hot, beef (*Hillshire Farm* Hot Links), 2 oz.	190	8.0	1.0	17.0	m.q.	m.q.	560	0
meat (*Hormel*, 12 oz.), 1 link	110	4.0	1.0	10.0	m.q.	m.q.	378	0
meat (*Hormel*, 1 lb.), 1 link	140	5.0	1.0	13.0	m.q.	m.q.	486	0
Mexacali (*Hormel* Mexacali Dogs), 5 oz.	400	14.0	41.0	21.0	m.q.	m.q.	952	n.a.
natural casing (*Hillshire Farm* Wieners), 2 oz.	180	6.0	2.0	17.0	m.q.	m.q.	470	0
pork and beef (*Boar's Head*), 1 oz.	80	4.0	<1.0	7.0	m.q.	15	250	0
smoked, 1 link:								
(*Hormel Range Brand Wranglers*)	170	7.0	1.0	16.0	m.q.	m.q.	600	0
(*Kahn's* Big Red Smokey)	170	8.0	2.0	14.0	m.q.	m.q.	550	0
(*Kahn's* Bun Size Smokey)	180	8.0	2.0	15.0	m.q.	m.q.	550	0
beef (*Hormel Wranglers*)	170	7.0	2.0	15.0	m.q.	m.q.	619	0

Food and Measure	cal.	prot. (gms)	carbo. (gms)	tot. fat (gms)	sat. fat (gms)	chol. (mgs)	sod. (mgs)	fiber (gms)
FRANKFURTER, SMOKED *(cont.)*								
beef *(Kahn's* Bun Size Beef								
Smokey)	190	7.0	2.0	17.0	m.q.	m.q.	530	0
w/cheese *(Hormel Wranglers)*	180	8.0	1.0	16.0	m.q.	m.q.	546	0
turkey, see "Turkey frankfurter"								
"FRANKFURTER,"								
VEGETARIAN:								
canned *(Worthington Super-Links),*								
1.7-oz. link	100	7.0	3.0	7.0	1.0	0	440	m.q.
canned *(Worthington Veja-Links),*								
2 links, approx. 2.2 oz.	140	8.0	4.0	10.0	m.q.	0	330	m.q.
frozen *(Worthington Leanies),* 1.4-oz.								
link	100	8.0	2.0	6.0	1.0	0	440	m.q.
frozen, on a stick *(Worthington* Dixie								
Dogs), 2.5-oz. piece	200	8.0	21.0	10.0	m.q.	0	640	m.q.
FRANKFURTER WRAP,								
refrigerated:								
(Weiner Wrap), 1 piece	60	1.0	10.0	2.0	m.q.	n.a.	430	m.q.
FRENCH BEAN, dried:								
raw, 1 oz.	97	5.3	18.2	.6	.1	0	5	1.1 c
raw, ½ cup	316	17.3	59.0	1.9	.2	0	16	3.4 c
boiled, 4 oz.	146	8.0	27.2	.9	.1	0	7	1.6 c
boiled, ½ cup	111	6.1	20.7	.7	.1	0	5	1.2 c
FRENCH-CUT BEAN, see "Green								
bean"								
FRENCH-FRY SEASONING:								
(Tone's), 1 tsp.	5	.2	1.0	.1	<.1	0	1551	.2 d
FRENCH TOAST, frozen, 3 oz.,								
except as noted:								
(Aunt Jemima Original)	166	6.7	26.5	4.4	1.0	46	554	1.3 d
(Downyflake), 2 slices	270	6.0	34.0	12.0	m.q.	73	380	m.q.
(Downyflake Extra Thick), 1 slice ..	150	5.0	11.0	9.0	m.q.	m.q.	340	m.q.
cinnamon swirl *(Aunt Jemima)*	171	6.7	27.5	4.3	1.0	41	516	1.3 d
w/cinnamon *(Weight Watchers*								
Microwave) ½ pkg. or 3 oz. ...	160	8.0	24.0	4.0	<1.0	5	280	m.q.
sticks:								
apple cinnamon *(Farm Rich)*	310	6.0	39.0	15.0	m.q.	n.a.	300	m.q.
blueberry *(Farm Rich)*	310	6.0	37.0	14.0	m.q.	n.a.	280	m.q.
original *(Farm Rich)*	300	5.0	37.0	15.0	m.q.	n.a.	280	m.q.
FRENCH TOAST BREAKFAST,								
frozen:								
cinnamon swirl, w/sausages								
(Swanson Great Starts), 5.5 oz.	390	12.0	37.0	21.0	m.q.	m.q.	530	m.q.
w/links *(Weight Watchers* Microwave),								
4.5 oz.	270	15.0	24.0	11.0	3.0	15	550	m.q.
mini, w/sausage *(Swanson Great*								
Starts), 2.5 oz.	190	6.0	22.0	9.0	m.q.	m.q.	320	m.q.
oatmeal, w/lite links *(Swanson Great*								
Starts), 4.65 oz.	310	13.0	35.0	13.0	m.q.	m.q.	500	m.q.

Food and Measure	cal.	prot. (gms)	carbo. (gms)	tot. fat (gms)	sat. fat (gms)	chol. (mgs)	sod. (mgs)	fiber (gms)
w/sausages (*Swanson Great Starts*), 5.5 oz.	380	12.0	35.0	21.0	m.q.	m.q.	550	m.q.
sticks, and syrup (*Aunt Jemima* Homestyle), 5.2 oz.	400	7.0	48.0	20.0	m.q.	m.q.	640	m.q.
Texas style, and sausage (*Downyflake*), 4.25 oz.	400	10.0	37.0	24.0	m.q.	m.q.	550	m.q.
vegetarian, cinnamon swirl, w/patties (*Morningstar Farms* Country Breakfast), 6.5 oz.	380	24.0	37.0	15.0	m.q.	0	1220	4.0 d
wedges, and sausages (*Aunt Jemima* Homestyle), 5.3 oz.	360	13.0	40.0	17.0	m.q.	m.q.	780	m.q.
FROG'S LEGS, meat only, raw:								
1 oz.	21	4.6	0	<1.0	m.q.	m.q.	m.q.	0
FROSTING, READY-TO-USE,								
¹⁄₁₂ can, except as noted:								
Amaretto almond (*Betty Crocker Creamy Deluxe*)	160	0	27.0	6.0	2.0	0	50	(0)
butter pecan (*Betty Crocker Creamy Deluxe*)	170	0	26.0	7.0	2.0	0	50	(0)
caramel pecan (*Pillsbury Frosting Supreme*)	160	0	21.0	8.0	m.q.	n.a.	70	(0)
cherry (*Betty Crocker Creamy Deluxe*)	160	0	27.0	6.0	2.0	0	50	(0)
chocolate:								
(*Betty Crocker Creamy Deluxe*) ...	160	<1.0	24.0	7.0	2.0	0	60	(0)
(*Duncan Hines*)	160	0	24.0	7.0	m.q.	n.a.	90	(0)
(*Pillsbury* Frost It Hot), ⅛ cake ..	50	0	12.0	0	0	0	50	(0)
creamy (*Pathmark*)	160	0	25.0	6.0	m.q.	n.a.	95	(0)
w/dinosaurs (*Betty Crocker Creamy Deluxe* Party)	160	<1.0	24.0	7.0	2.0	0	60	(0)
double Dutch (*Pillsbury Frosting Supreme*)	140	1.0	22.0	6.0	m.q.	n.a.	45	(0)
fudge:								
(*Pillsbury*), ⅛ cake	110	0	17.0	5.0	m.q.	n.a.	65	(0)
(*Pillsbury Frosting Supreme*) ...	150	<1.0	24.0	6.0	m.q.	n.a.	80	(0)
(*Pillsbury Funfetti*)	140	<1.0	22.0	6.0	m.q.	n.a.	80	(0)
creamy (*Pathmark*)	160	0	25.0	7.0	m.q.	n.a.	100	(0)
dark Dutch (*Betty Crocker Creamy Deluxe*)	160	1.0	22.0	7.0	2.0	0	70	(0)
dark Dutch (*Duncan Hines*) ...	160	0	24.0	7.0	m.q.	n.a.	95	(0)
milk:								
(*Betty Crocker Creamy Deluxe*)	160	<1.0	25.0	6.0	2.0	0	55	(0)
(*Duncan Hines*)	160	0	24.0	7.0	m.q.	n.a.	85	(0)
(*Finast*)	160	0	25.0	6.0	m.q.	n.a.	105	(0)
(*Pillsbury Frosting Supreme*) ...	150	0	23.0	6.0	m.q.	n.a.	60	(0)
mint (*Pillsbury Frosting Supreme*)	150	<1.0	24.0	7.0	m.q.	n.a.	80	(0)
mocha (*Pillsbury Frosting Supreme*)	150	<1.0	24.0	6.0	m.q.	n.a.	60	(0)

Food and Measure	cal.	prot. (gms)	carbo. (gms)	tot. fat (gms)	sat. fat (gms)	chol. (mgs)	sod. (mgs)	fiber (gms)
FROSTING, READY-TO-USE *(cont.)*								
chocolate chip:								
(*Betty Crocker Creamy Deluxe*) ...	170	<1.0	27.0	7.0	3.0	0	30	(0)
(*Pillsbury Frosting Supreme*)	150	0	27.0	5.0	m.q.	n.a.	70	(0)
double (*Betty Crocker Creamy Deluxe*)	170	<1.0	24.0	8.0	3.0	0	60	(0)
chocolate, candy coated (*Betty Crocker Creamy Deluxe* Party)	160	<1.0	24.0	7.0	2.0	0	60	(0)
chocolate coconut almond (*Betty Crocker Creamy Deluxe*)	160	1.0	21.0	8.0	3.0	0	55	(0)
coconut almond (*Pillsbury*)	160	1.0	16.0	10.0	m.q.	n.a.	85	(0)
coconut almond (*Pillsbury Frosting Supreme*)	150	1.0	17.0	9.0	m.q.	n.a.	60	(0)
coconut pecan:								
(*Betty Crocker Creamy Deluxe*) ...	160	<1.0	20.0	9.0	3.0	0	80	(0)
(*Pillsbury*)	150	1.0	20.0	7.0	m.q.	n.a.	105	(0)
(*Pillsbury Frosting Supreme*)	160	0	17.0	10.0	m.q.	n.a.	60	(0)
cream cheese (*Betty Crocker Creamy Deluxe*)	160	0	27.0	6.0	2.0	0	75	(0)
cream cheese (*Pillsbury Frosting Supreme*)	160	0	26.0	6.0	m.q.	n.a.	115	(0)
decorator, all flavors, except chocolate (*Pillsbury*), 1 tbsp. ..	70	0	12.0	2.0	m.q.	n.a.	0	(0)
decorator, chocolate (*Pillsbury*), 1 tbsp.	60	0	11.0	2.0	m.q.	n.a.	0	(0)
fudge, see "chocolate," above								
lemon (*Betty Crocker Creamy Deluxe*)	170	0	28.0	6.0	2.0	0	70	(0)
lemon (*Pillsbury Frosting Supreme*)	160	0	26.0	6.0	m.q.	n.a.	80	(0)
rainbow chip (*Betty Crocker Creamy Deluxe*)	170	<1.0	27.0	7.0	3.0	0	30	(0)
rocky road (*Betty Crocker Creamy Deluxe*)	150	<1.0	20.0	8.0	2.0	0	50	(0)
sour cream:								
chocolate (*Betty Crocker Creamy Deluxe*)	160	<1.0	23.0	7.0	2.0	0	110	(0)
vanilla (*Pillsbury Frosting Supreme*)	160	0	27.0	6.0	m.q.	n.a.	80	(0)
white (*Betty Crocker Creamy Deluxe*)	160	0	27.0	6.0	2.0	0	50	(0)
strawberry (*Pillsbury Frosting Supreme*)	160	0	26.0	6.0	m.q.	n.a.	75	(0)
vanilla:								
(*Betty Crocker Creamy Deluxe*) ...	160	0	27.0	6.0	2.0	0	30	(0)
(*Duncan Hines*)	160	0	24.0	7.0	m.q.	n.a.	80	(0)
(*Pillsbury*), 1/8 cake	120	0	19.0	5.0	m.q.	n.a.	60	(0)
(*Pillsbury Frosting Supreme*)	160	0	26.0	6.0	m.q.	n.a.	75	(0)
(*Pillsbury* Funfetti, pink and white)	150	0	24.0	6.0	m.q.	n.a.	70	(0)

Food and Measure	cal.	prot. (gms)	carbo. (gms)	tot. fat (gms)	sat. fat (gms)	chol. (mgs)	sod. (mgs)	fiber (gms)
w/teddy bears (*Betty Crocker*								
Creamy Deluxe Party)	160	0	27.0	6.0	2.0	0	25	(0)
white:								
creamy (*Pathmark*)	160	0	25.0	6.0	m.q.	n.a.	95	(0)
fluffy (*Pillsbury*)	60	0	15.0	0	0	0	65	(0)
fluffy (*Pillsbury* Frost It Hot),								
⅛ cake	50	0	12.0	0	0	0	50	(0)
FROSTING MIX, ¹⁄₁₂ pkg., except								
as noted[1]:								
(*Estee*), 1½ tbsp.	50	1.0	10.0	1.0	<1.0	0	0	(0)
cherry (*Betty Crocker* Creamy)	180	0	31.0	6.0	2.0	0	100	(0)
cherry (*Betty Crocker* Creamy)[2]	180	0	31.0	6.0	3.0	10	100	(0)
chocolate:								
fudge (*Betty Crocker* Creamy) ...	180	<1.0	30.0	6.0	2.0	0	70	(0)
fudge (*Betty Crocker* Creamy)[2] ...	180	<1.0	30.0	6.0	3.0	10	70	(0)
milk (*Betty Crocker* Creamy)	170	1.0	29.0	5.0	1.0	0	40	(0)
milk (*Betty Crocker* Creamy)[2]	170	1.0	29.0	5.0	3.0	10	40	(0)
coconut pecan (*Betty Crocker*								
Creamy)[3]	150	<1.0	19.0	8.0	3.0	0	50	(0)
coconut pecan (*Betty Crocker*								
Creamy)[4]	150	<1.0	19.0	8.0	4.0	10	50	(0)
rainbow chip (*Betty Crocker* Creamy)	190	<1.0	32.0	7.0	2.0	0	50	(0)
rainbow chip (*Betty Crocker*								
Creamy)[2]	190	<1.0	32.0	7.0	4.0	10	50	(0)
sour cream:								
chocolate fudge (*Betty Crocker*								
Creamy)	180	1.0	30.0	6.0	2.0	0	75	(0)
chocolate fudge (*Betty Crocker*								
Creamy)[2]	180	1.0	30.0	6.0	3.0	10	75	(0)
white (*Betty Crocker* Creamy) ...	170	0	31.0	5.0	1.0	0	100	(0)
white (*Betty Crocker* Creamy)[2] ...	170	0	31.0	5.0	3.0	10	100	(0)
vanilla (*Betty Crocker* Creamy)	170	0	32.0	5.0	1.0	0	50	(0)
vanilla (*Betty Crocker* Creamy)[2] ...	170	0	32.0	5.0	3.0	10	50	(0)
white (*Betty Crocker* Fluffy), ¹⁄₁₂ pkg.								
dry	70	<1.0	16.0	0	0	0	40	(0)
FROZEN DESSERT, see "Ice								
cream, substitute and								
imitation," and specific listings								
FRUCTOSE:								
(*Estee*), 1 tsp.	12	0	3.0	0	0	0	0	0
(*Featherweight*), 1 pkt. or 1 tsp.	12	0	3.0	0	0	0	0	0
FRUIT, see specific listings								
FRUIT, MIXED, CANNED,								
½ cup, except as noted:								
(*Del Monte* Fruit Cup), 5 oz.	100	0	27.0	0	0	0	<10	m.q.

1. *Prepared according to package directions, with margarine, except as noted.*
2. *Prepared with unsalted butter.*
3. *Prepared with margarine and skim milk.*
4. *Prepared with unsalted butter and 2% lowfat milk.*

Food and Measure	cal.	prot. (gms)	carbo. (gms)	tot. fat (gms)	sat. fat (gms)	chol. (mgs)	sod. (mgs)	fiber (gms)
FRUIT, MIXED, CANNED *(cont.)*								
chunky *(Del Monte)*	80	0	23.0	0	0	0	<10	m.q.
chunky *(Del Monte Lite)*	50	0	14.0	0	0	0	<10	m.q.
chunky *(S&W/Nutradiet)*	40	0	10.0	0	0	0	5	m.q.
in juice, chunky:								
(Libby Lite)	50	1.0	14.0	0	0	0	5	m.q.
(Pathmark)	50	1.0	14.0	0	0	0	15	m.q.
sweetened clarified *(S&W)*	90	1.0	21.0	0	0	0	5	m.q.
in light syrup *(A&P)*	75	<1.0	20.0	<1.0	(0)	0	10	m.q.
in light syrup *(Pathmark* No Frills),								
1 cup	150	1.0	39.0	0	0	0	20	m.q.
in heavy syrup:								
4 oz.[1]	82	.4	21.3	.1	<.1	0	5	.5 c
½ cup[1]	92	.5	24.0	.1	<.1	0	5	.5 c
chunky *(Finast)*	70	0	18.0	0	0	0	10	m.q.
fruit cocktail:								
(Del Monte)	80	0	23.0	0	0	0	<10	m.q.
(Del Monte Lite)	50	0	15.0	0	0	0	<10	m.q.
(Finast No Sugar Added)	50	1.0	14.0	0	0	0	10	m.q.
(S&W/Nutradiet Regular/								
Unsweetened)	40	0	10.0	0	0	0	5	m.q.
in water, 4 oz.	36	.5	9.7	.1	tr.	0	5	.5 c
in water	40	.5	10.4	.1	tr.	0	5	.6 c
in juice:								
4 oz.	52	.5	13.4	<.1	tr.	0	5	.7 d
½ cup	56	.6	14.7	<.1	tr.	0	4	.8 d
(Featherweight)	50	1.0	14.0	0	0	0	<10	m.q.
(IGA)	60	0	15.0	0	0	0	10	m.q.
(Libby Lite)	50	0	13.0	0	0	0	10	m.q.
pear juice *(A&P)*	50	1.0	14.0	<1.0	(0)	0	15	m.q.
sweetened clarified juice								
(S&W)	90	1.0	21.0	0	0	0	5	m.q.
in extra light syrup, 4 oz.	51	.5	13.2	.1	<.1	0	5	.5 c
in extra light syrup	55	.5	14.3	.1	<.1	0	5	.6 c
in light syrup, 4 oz.	65	.5	16.9	.1	<.1	0	7	.5 c
in light syrup	72	.5	18.8	.1	<.1	0	7	.6 c
in heavy syrup:								
4 oz.	83	.4	21.4	.1	<.1	0	7	.5 c
½ cup	93	.5	24.2	.1	<.1	0	7	.6 c
(A&P)	90	<1.0	24.0	<1.0	(0)	0	15	m.q.
(Finast)	90	0	24.0	0	0	0	9	m.q.
(Pathmark), 1 cup	180	1.0	48.0	0	0	0	35	m.q.
(S&W)	90	0	24.0	0	0	0	15	m.q.
in extra heavy syrup, 4 oz.	98	.4	26.0	.1	<.1	0	7	.5 c
in extra heavy syrup	115	.5	29.8	.1	<.1	0	7	.6 c
in fruit concentrates *(Pathmark* No								
Sugar Added)	50	1.0	14.0	0	0	0	15	m.q.

1. *Includes peaches, pears, and pineapple.*

Food and Measure	cal.	prot. (gms)	carbo. (gms)	tot. fat (gms)	sat. fat (gms)	chol. (mgs)	sod. (mgs)	fiber (gms)
fruit for salad (*Del Monte*)	90	0	22.0	0	0	0	<10	m.q.
fruit salad:								
in water, 4 oz.	34	.4	8.9	.1	<.1	0	3	.7 c
in water	37	.4	9.6	.1	<.1	0	4	.8 c
in juice, 4 oz.	57	.6	14.8	<.1	tr.	0	6	.7 d
in juice, ½ cup	62	.6	16.2	<.1	tr.	0	7	.8 d
in light syrup, 4 oz.	66	.4	17.2	.1	<.1	0	7	.7 c
in light syrup	73	.4	19.1	.1	<.1	0	7	.8 c
in heavy syrup, 4 oz.	83	.4	21.7	.1	<.1	0	7	.7 c
in heavy syrup	94	.4	24.5	.1	<.1	0	7	.8 c
in extra heavy syrup, 4 oz.	100	.4	25.8	.1	<.1	0	6	.7 c
in extra heavy syrup	114	.4	29.6	.1	<.1	0	7	.8 c
tropical:								
(*Del Monte*)	90	0	26.0	0	0	0	<10	m.q.
in heavy syrup, 4 oz.	98	.5	25.4	.1	(0)	0	2	.5 c
in heavy syrup	110	.5	28.6	.1	(0)	0	3	.6 c
FRUIT, MIXED, CHILLED:								
salad (*Kraft* Pure), ½ cup	80	1.0	18.0	0	0	0	10	m.q.
FRUIT, MIXED, DRIED:								
11-oz. pkg.[1]	712	7.2	187.7	1.4	.1	0	52	8.5 c
pitted, 1 oz.[1]	69	.7	18.2	.1	<.1	0	5	.8 c
(*Del Monte*), 2 oz.	130	1.0	34.0	0	0	0	10	m.q.
(*Sun•Maid/Sunsweet*) 2 oz.	150	1.0	39.0	0	0	0	<20	m.q.
bits (*Sun•Maid/Sunsweet*), 2 oz.	150	2.0	40.0	<1.0	(0)	0	<50	m.q.
FRUIT, MIXED, FROZEN:								
in syrup (*Birds Eye* Quick Thaw								
Pouch), 5 oz.	120	1.0	31.0	0	0	0	5	1.0 d
sweetened:								
10-oz. pkg.	278	4.0	68.8	.5	.1	0	9	m.q.
4 oz.	111	1.6	27.5	.2	<.1	0	3	m.q.
½ cup	123	1.8	30.3	.2	<.1	0	4	m.q.
FRUIT BAR, see "Snack bar"								
FRUIT BAR, FROZEN, (see also								
"Ice bar" and "Gelatin bar"),								
1 bar:								
all flavors (Minute Maid Fruit Juicee)	60	0	14.0	0	0	0	0	n.a.
cherry (*Dole Fresh Lites*)	25	<1.0	6.0	<1.0	n.a.	0	6	n.a.
coconut (*Sunkist*) 4 fl. oz.	170	3.0	15.0	10.0	m.q.	0	70	m.q.
grape (*Dole SunTops*)	40	<1.0	9.0	<1.0	n.a.	0	5	n.a.
lemon (*Dole Fresh Lites*)	25	<1.0	6.0	<1.0	n.a.	0	16	n.a.
lemonade (*Dole SunTops*)	40	<1.0	9.0	<1.0	n.a.	0	5	n.a.
lemonade (*Sunkist*), 4 fl. oz.	90	0	24	0	0	0	5	n.a.
orange (*Sunkist* Juice Bar), 4 fl. oz.	100	0	25	0	0	0	0	n.a.
orange, tropical (*Dole SunTops*)	40	<1.0	9.0	<1.0	n.a.	0	5	n.a.
pina colada (*Dole Fruit'n Juice*)	90	n.a.	16.0	3.0	m.q.	0	2	n.a.
pineapple (*Dole Fruit'n Juice*)	70	.3	17.0	<.1	n.a.	0	4	n.a.
pineapple-orange (*Dole Fresh Lites*)	25	<1.0	6.0	<1.0	n.a.	0	7	n.a.
punch (*Dole SunTops*)	40	<1.0	9.0	<1.0	n.a.	0	5	n.a.

1. *Includes prunes, apricots, apples, and pears.*

Food and Measure	cal.	prot. (gms)	carbo. (gms)	tot. fat (gms)	sat. fat (gms)	chol. (mgs)	sod. (mgs)	fiber (gms)
FRUIT BAR, FROZEN *(cont.)*								
raspberry (*Dole Fresh Lites*)	25	<1.0	6.0	<1.0	n.a.	0	6	n.a.
raspberry (*Dole Fruit'n Juice*)	70	.2	16.0	<.1	n.a.	0	14	n.a.
strawberry (*Dole Fruit'n Juice*)	70	.2	16.0	<.1	n.a.	0	6	n.a.
wildberry (*Sunkist*), 4 fl. oz.	140	0	33.0	0	0	0	15	n.a.
and cream:								
blueberry (*Dole* Fruit & Cream) ..	90	1.0	19.4	1.4	n.a.	5	20	n.a.
chocolate/banana (*Dole* Fruit & Cream)	175	2.0	22.0	9.0	m.q.	n.a.	20	n.a.
chocolate/strawberry (*Dole* Fruit & Cream)	140	2.0	23.0	8.0	m.q.	n.a.	20	n.a.
peach (*Dole* Fruit & Cream)	90	1.0	19.4	1.4	n.a.	5	19	n.a.
raspberry (*Dole* Fruit & Cream) ..	90	1.0	20.0	1.4	n.a.	5	23	n.a.
strawberry (*Dole* Fruit & Cream)	90	1.0	19.3	1.4	n.a.	5	22	n.a.
strawberry (*Sunkist*), 4 fl. oz. ...	90	0	19.0	1.0	n.a.	n.a.	30	n.a.
and yogurt:								
cherry (*Dole* Fruit & Yogurt)	80	2.0	17.0	<1.0	m.q.	m.q.	22	n.a.
raspberry (*Dole* Fruit & Yogurt) ..	70	1.0	17.0	<1.0	m.q.	m.q.	18	n.a.
strawberry (*Dole* Fruit & Yogurt)	70	1.0	17.0	<1.0	m.q.	m.q.	16	n.a.
FRUIT COCKTAIL, see "Fruit, mixed, canned"								
FRUIT COMPOTE:								
(*Rokeach*), 4 oz.	120	1.0	31.0	1.0	n.a.	0	4	m.q.
FRUIT DRINK (see also specfic fruit listings):								
(*Finast*), 8 fl. oz.	80	0	21.0	0	0	0	15	(0)
(*Hi-C* Double Fruit Cooler), 8.45 fl. oz.	131	<.1	32.3	<.1	(0)	0	25	(0)
(*Hi-C* Double Fruit Cooler), 6 fl. oz.	93	<.1	22.9	<.1	(0)	0	18	(0)
(*Hi-C* Ecto Cooler), 8.45 fl. oz.	134	.2	32.8	<.1	(0)	0	24	(0)
(*Hi-C* Ecto Cooler), 6 fl. oz.	95	.1	23.3	<.1	(0)	0	17	(0)
(*Hi-C* Hula Cooler), 6 fl. oz.	97	.1	23.9	<.1	(0)	0	17	(0)
FRUIT JUICE (see also specific fruit listings):								
tropical (*Libby's Juicy Juice*), 6 fl. oz.	100	1.0	24.0	0	0	0	5	(0)
FRUIT JUICE COCKTAIL (see also specific fruit listings):								
(*Welch's Orchard* Harvest Blend), 6 fl. oz.	110	0	27.0	0	0	0	20	0
(*Welch's Orchard* Harvest Blend Cocktails-In-A-Box), 8.45 fl. oz.	150	0	38.0	0	0	0	20	0
frozen[1] (*Welch's Orchard* Harvest Blend), 6 fl. oz.	110	0	27.0	0	0	0	10	0
FRUIT JUICE DRINK:								
mixed (*Tang* Fruit Box), 8.45 fl. oz.	140	0	36.0	0	0	0	10	(0)
FRUIT AND NUT MIX:								
(*Estee*), 4 pieces	35	1.0	3.0	2.0	2.0	<1	0	m.q.
(*Planters* Fruit'n Nut), 1 oz.	150	5.0	13.0	9.0	2.0	0	90	m.q.

1. *Diluted according to package directions.*

Food and Measure	cal.	prot. (gms)	carbo. (gms)	tot. fat (gms)	sat. fat (gms)	chol. (mgs)	sod. (mgs)	fiber (gms)
FRUIT PUNCH:								
canned, bottled, or boxed:								
(*Minute Maid*), 8.45 fl. oz.	128	.1	32.0	.1	(0)	0	24	(0)
(*Minute Maid* Juices to Go),								
11.5 fl. oz.	174	.1	43.6	.1	(0)	0	33	(0)
(*Minute Maid* Juices to Go),								
9.6 fl. oz.	145	.1	36.8	.1	(0)	0	28	(0)
(*Minute Maid On The Go*),								
10 fl. oz.	152	.1	37.9	.1	(0)	0	29	(0)
(*Pathmark*), 6 fl. oz.	90	0	22.0	0	0	0	0	(0)
(*Veryfine* 100% Juice Punch),								
8 fl. oz.	122	<1.0	30.0	0	0	0	<10	(0)
blend (*Libby's Juicy Juice*),								
8.45 fl. oz.	140	1.0	33.0	0	0	0	10	(0)
blend (*Libby's Juicy Juice*), 6 fl. oz.	100	1.0	23.0	0	0	0	10	(0)
Concord:								
(*Minute Maid*), 8.45 fl. oz.	131	.2	32.7	.1	(0)	0	25	(0)
(*Minute Maid* Juices to Go),								
11.5 fl. oz.	178	.3	44.5	.1	(0)	0	74	(0)
(*Minute Maid* Juices to Go),								
9.6 fl. oz.	148	.2	37.1	.1	(0)	0	28	(0)
(*Minute Maid On The Go*),								
10 fl. oz.	155	.2	38.7	.1	(0)	0	29	(0)
tropical:								
(*Minute Maid*), 8.45 fl. oz.	130	.1	32.0	<.1	(0)	0	24	(0)
(*Minute Maid* Juices to Go),								
11.5 fl. oz.	176	.1	43.6	<.1	(0)	0	33	(0)
(*Minute Maid* Juices to Go),								
9.6 fl. oz.	147	.1	36.4	<.1	(0)	0	28	(0)
chilled or frozen[1] (*Minute Maid*),								
6 fl. oz.	91	.1	22.7	.1	(0)	0	17	(0)
FRUIT PUNCH COCKTAIL,								
canned, bottled, or boxed:								
(*Welch's Orchard* Fruit Harvest								
Punch), 10 fl. oz.	180	0	45.0	0	0	0	0	0
(*Welch's Orchard* Fruit Harvest Punch								
Cocktails-In-A-Box),								
8.45 fl. oz.	150	0	38.0	0	0	0	20	0
island fruit (*Hawaiian Punch*),								
6 fl. oz.	90	0	22.0	0	0	0	30	(0)
FRUIT PUNCH DRINK:								
canned, bottled, or boxed:								
(*Bama*), 8.45 fl. oz.	130	0	32.0	0	0	0	15	(0)
(*Hi-C*), 8.45 fl. oz.	135	.2	33.4	<.1	(0)	0	24	(0)
(*Hi-C*), 6 fl. oz.	96	.1	23.7	<.1	(0)	0	17	(0)
(*Hi-C* Hula Punch), 8.45 fl. oz. ..	122	.1	30.2	<.1	(0)	0	24	(0)
(*Hi-C* Hula Punch), 6 fl. oz.	87	.1	21.4	<.1	(0)	0	17	(0)
(*Mott's*), 10-fl.-oz. bottle	170	0	42.0	0	0	0	4	(0)

1. *Diluted according to package directions.*

Food and Measure	cal.	prot. (gms)	carbo. (gms)	tot. fat (gms)	sat. fat (gms)	chol. (mgs)	sod. (mgs)	fiber (gms)
FRUIT PUNCH DRINK, CANNED *(cont.)*								
(*Mott's*), 9.5-fl.-oz. can	161	0	40.0	0	0	0	4	(0)
(*Tropicana* Single Serve), 10 fl. oz.	148	(0)	37.0	0	0	0	<3	(0)
(*Wyler's*), 6 fl. oz.	84	0	21.3	.1	(0)	0	8	(0)
mountain berry (*Kool-Aid Koolers*), 8.45 fl. oz.	140	0	37.0	0	0	0	10	(0)
rainbow (*Kool-Aid Koolers*), 8.45 fl. oz.	130	0	36.0	0	0	0	10	(0)
red (*Hawaiian Punch* Fruit Juicy), 6 fl. oz.	90	0	22.0	0	0	0	20	(0)
red (*Hawaiian Punch* Fruit Juicy Lite), 6 fl. oz.	60	0	15.0	0	0	0	30	(0)
tropical:								
(*Hawaiian Punch*), 6 fl. oz. ...	90	0	22.0	0	0	0	30	(0)
(*Kool-Aid Koolers*), 8.45 fl. oz.	130	0	35.0	0	0	0	10	(0)
(*Wylers*), 6 fl. oz.	157	0	39.3	0	0	0	10	0
(*Wylers* Fruit Slush), 4 fl. oz. ..	157	0	39.3	0	0	0	10	(0)
wild fruit (*Hawaiian Punch*), 6 fl. oz.	90	0	23.0	0	0	0	35	(0)
chilled (*Crowley*), 8 fl. oz.	130	0	32.0	0	0	0	15	(0)
chilled (*Minute Maid* Light'N Juicy), 6 fl. oz.	14	.1	2.9	.1	(0)	0	17	(0)
frozen[1]:								
undiluted, 12-fl.-oz. cont.	678	.7	173.1	.1	<.1	0	34	.4 d
1 fl. oz.	14	tr.	3.6	tr.	tr.	0	1	(0)
8 fl. oz.	113	.1	28.8	tr.	tr.	0	11	(0)
mix[2], 8 fl. oz., except as noted:								
2 rounded tbsp. or .9 oz. dry[3] ...	97	tr.	24.8	tr.	<.1	0	30	<.1 d
8 fl. oz. water and 2 rounded tbsp. powder[3]	97	tr.	24.8	tr.	<.1	0	38	(0)
(*Crystal Light* Sugar Free)	4	0	0	0	0	0	0	0
(*Kool-Aid* Surfin' Berry)	100	0	25.0	0	0	0	25	(0)
(*Kool-Aid* Surfin' Berry Sugar Free)	4	0	0	0	0	0	25	0
(*Pathmark* No Frills)	90	0	22.0	0	0	0	85	(0)
mountain berry:								
(*Kool-Aid*)	100	0	25.0	0	0	0	15	(0)
(*Kool-Aid* Presweetened)	80	0	20.0	0	0	0	15	(0)
(*Kool-Aid* Sugar Free)	4	0	0	0	0	0	35	(0)
no salt added:								
2 rounded tsp. or .9 oz. dry ...	97	tr.	24.8	tr.	<.1	0	11	<.1 d
8 fl. oz. water and 2 rounded tbsp. powder	97	tr.	24.8	tr.	<.1	0	10	(0)
rainbow (*Kool-Aid*)	100	0	25.0	0	0	0	0	(0)
rainbow (*Kool-Aid* Presweetened)	80	0	21.0	0	0	0	20	(0)

1. *Diluted according to package directions, except as noted.*
2. *Prepared according to package directions, except as noted.*
3. *Value for product with added sodium.*

Food and Measure	cal.	prot. (gms)	carbo. (gms)	tot. fat (gms)	sat. fat (gms)	chol. (mgs)	sod. (mgs)	fiber (gms)
tropical:								
(*Kool-Aid*)	100	0	25.0	0	0	0	0	(0)
(*Kool-Aid* Presweetened)	80	0	21.0	0	0	0	0	(0)
(*Kool-Aid* Sugar Free)	4	0	0	0	0	0	10	0
(*Wylers* Crystals)	85	0	21.1	.1	(0)	0	18	(0)
FRUIT PUNCH JUICE DRINK,								
frozen[1]:								
undiluted, 12-fl.-oz. cont.	739	1.2	182.1	3.0	.4	0	41	(0)
1 fl. oz.	15	tr.	3.8	.1	tr.	0	2	(0)
8 fl. oz.	123	.2	30.4	.5	.1	0	12	(0)
FRUIT ROLL, see "Fruit snack"								
FRUIT FOR SALAD, see "Fruit, mixed, canned"								
FRUIT SALAD, see "Fruit, mixed, canned"								
FRUIT SNACK (see also specific fruit listings):								
all flavors:								
(*Berry Bears*), 1 pouch	100	<1.0	22.0	<1.0	(0)	0	20	n.a.
(*Fruit Corners/Fruit Roll-Ups* Peel-Outs), 1 roll	50	<1.0	12.0	<1.0	(0)	0	40	m.q.
(*Fruit Wrinkles*), 1 pouch	100	<1.0	22.0	1.0	(0)	0	55	n.a.
(*Shark Bites*), 1 pouch	100	<1.0	22.0	<1.0	(0)	0	20	n.a.
(*Thunder Jets*), 1 pouch	100	<1.0	22.0	1.0	(0)	0	30	n.a.
assorted (*Flavor Tree* Fruit Circus/Fruit Bears), 1.05 oz.	117	.1	25.4	1.6	n.a.	0	12	n.a.
assorted, all shapes (*Sunkist Fun Fruits*), 1 pouch	100	.1	21.8	1.4	n.a.	0	10	n.a.
apple:								
(*Squeezit*), 6.75 oz.	110	<1.0	27.0	<1.0	(0)	0	5	n.a.
(*Weight Watchers*), 1 pouch	50	<1.0	13.0	<1.0	(0)	0	75	n.a.
roll (*Flavor Tree*), 1 piece	75	.2	18.5	0	0	0	17	m.q.
apricot roll (*Flavor Tree*), 1 piece ...	76	.3	17.7	.5	(0)	0	17	m.q.
berry (*Sunkist Fun Fruits* Berry Bunch), 1 pouch	100	.1	21.8	1.4	n.a.	0	10	n.a.
berry, wild (*Squeezit*), 6.75 oz.	110	<1.0	27.0	<1.0	(0)	0	5	n.a.
blueberry (*Garfield and Friends* Wild Blue), 1 roll	50	<1.0	12.0	<1.0	(0)	0	20	m.q.
cherry:								
(*Squeezit*), 6.75 oz.	110	<1.0	27.0	<1.0	(0)	0	30	n.a.
(*Sunkist Fun Fruits*), 1 pouch ...	100	.1	21.8	1.4	n.a.	0	10	n.a.
roll (*Flavor Tree*), 1 piece	75	.3	18.3	.1	(0)	0	18	m.q.
cinnamon flavor (*Weight Watchers*), 1 pouch	50	<1.0	13.0	<1.0	(0)	0	75	n.a.
fruit (*Garfield and Friends* Fruity Party), 1 roll	50	<1.0	12.0	<1.0	(0)	0	40	m.q.

1. *Diluted according to package directions, except as noted.*

Food and Measure	cal.	prot. (gms)	carbo. (gms)	tot. fat (gms)	sat. fat (gms)	chol. (mgs)	sod. (mgs)	fiber (gms)
FRUIT SNACK *(cont.)*								
fruit punch:								
(Garfield and Friends 1-2 Punch),								
1 pouch	100	<1.0	21.0	2.0	n.a.	0	70	n.a.
(Sunkist Fun Fruits Fantastic								
Fruit), 1 pouch	100	.1	21.8	1.4	n.a.	0	10	n.a.
roll *(Flavor Tree),* 1 piece	74	.2	18.2	0	0	0	12	m.q.
grape:								
(Squeezit), 6.75 oz.	110	<1.0	27.0	<1.0	(0)	0	30	n.a.
(Sunkist Fun Fruits), 1 pouch . . .	100	.1	21.8	1.4	n.a.	0	10	n.a.
roll *(Flavor Tree),* 1 piece	76	.2	18.5	.1	(0)	0	13	m.q.
orange *(Squeezit),* 6.75 oz.	110	<1.0	27.0	<1.0	(0)	0	5	n.a.
orange *(Sunkist Fun Fruits),*								
1 pouch	100	.1	21.8	1.4	n.a.	0	10	n.a.
punch, red *(Squeezit),* 6.75 oz.	110	<1.0	27.0	<1.0	(0)	0	5	n.a.
raspberry, roll *(Flavor Tree),* 1 piece	75	.2	18.3	.1	(0)	0	20	m.q.
strawberry:								
(Garfield and Friends), 1 pouch . .	90	<1.0	21.0	1.0	n.a.	0	60	n.a.
(Sunkist Fun Fruits), 1 pouch . . .	100	.1	21.8	1.4	n.a.	0	10	n.a.
(Weight Watchers), 1 pouch	50	<1.0	13.0	<1.0	(0)	0	75	n.a.
roll *(Flavor Tree),* 1 piece	74	.2	18.0	.1	(0)	0	11	m.q.
yogurt coated *(Sunkist Fun Fruits*								
Creme Supremes), 1 pouch . . .	114	.2	20.1	3.6	m.q.	n.a.	19	n.a.
FRUIT SPREAD (see also "Jam and								
preserves"):								
all flavors:								
(Polaner All Fruit Spreadable								
Fruit), 1 tsp.	14	0	4.0	0	0	0	0	m.q.
(Smucker's Simply Fruit), 1 tsp. . .	16	0	4.0	0	0	0	0	m.q.
(Weight Watchers), 2 tsp.	16	0	4.0	0	0	0	0	m.q.
low sugar *(Smucker's),* 1 tsp.	8	0	2.0	0	0	0	<10	m.q.
FRUIT SYRUP:								
all flavors *(Smucker's),* 2 tbsp.	100	0	26.0	0	0	0	0	n.a.
FUDGE, see "Candy"								
FUDGE TOPPING, see "Chocolate								
topping"								
FUKI, see "Butterbur"								
FUYU, see "Tofu"								

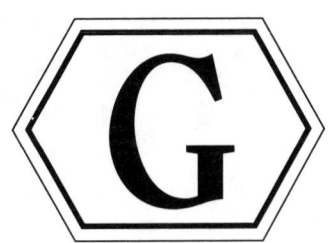

Food and Measure	cal.	prot. (gms)	carbo. (gms)	tot. fat (gms)	sat. fat (gms)	chol. (mgs)	sod. (mgs)	fiber (gms)
GARBANZO, see "Chick-pea"								
GARDEN CRESS, see "Cress, garden"								
GARDEN SALAD, canned:								
(*Joan of Arc/Read*), ½ cup	70	2.0	17.0	0	0	0	500	2.4 d
marinated (*S&W*), ½ cup	60	2.0	11.0	0	0	0	670	m.q.
GARLIC:								
untrimmed, 1 lb.	587	25.1	130.5	2.0	.4	0	67	5.9 c
trimmed, 1 oz.	42	1.8	9.4	.1	<.1	0	5	.4 c
1 clove, 1¼" × ⅝" × ⅜", approx.								
.1 oz.	4	.2	1.0	<.1	tr.	0	1	.1 c
GARLIC BREAD SEASONING:								
(*McCormick/Schilling* Garlic Bread Sprinkle), ¼ tsp.	5	<.1	.1	.4	n.a.	n.a.	25	n.a.
(*Tone's* Garlic Bread Sprinkle), 1 tsp.	17	.3	.6	1.6	.4	<1	167	<.1 d
GARLIC BREAD SPREAD:								
(*Lawry's*), ½ tbsp.	47	.2	1.0	4.6	m.q.	n.a.	15	<.1 c
GARLIC DRESSING AND DIP:								
w/tofu (*Life* All Natural), 1 tbsp. . . .	70	<1.0	1.4	7.1	m.q.	0	75	m.q.
GARLIC AND HERB DIP:								
(*Nasoya Vegi-Dip*), 1 oz.	50	2.0	6.0	2.0	m.q.	0	100	m.q.
GARLIC AND OIL:								
(*Hain*), 1 tbsp.	120	0	0	14.0	3.0	0	0	0
GARLIC POWDER:								
1 oz.	94	4.8	20.6	.2	(0)	0	7	.5 c
1 tbsp.	28	1.4	6.1	.1	(0)	0	2	.2 c
1 tsp.	9	.5	2.0	<.1	(0)	0	1	.1 c
(*Spice Islands*), 1 tsp.	5	.3	1.1	tr.	(0)	0	<1	<.1 c
(*Tone's*), 1 tsp.	9	.5	2.0	<.1	tr.	0	1	.1 d
w/parsley (*Lawry's*), 1 tsp.	12	.5	2.3	.9	n.a.	0	5	.1 c

Food and Measure	cal.	prot. (gms)	carbo. (gms)	tot. fat (gms)	sat. fat (gms)	chol. (mgs)	sod. (mgs)	fiber (gms)
GARLIC SALT:								
(*Lawry's*), 1 tsp.	4	.1	.8	<.1	(0)	0	968	<.1 c
(*Morton*), 1 tsp.	3	<1.0	<1.0	<.1	(0)	0	1300	m.q.
(*Tone's*), 1 tsp.	2	.1	.4	tr.	tr.	0	1706	<.1 d
GARLIC SEASONING:								
(*McCormick/Schilling* Season All),								
¼ tsp.	2	<.1	.1	(0)	(0)	0	163	n.a.
(*McCormick/Schilling Parsley Patch*),								
1 tsp.	13	.5	2.0	.5	n.a.	0	1	m.q.
GARLIC SPREAD:								
concentrate (*Lawry's*), 1 tbsp.	15	0	.2	1.6	m.q.	0	21	0
GEFILTE FISH, 1 ball, except as noted:								
hors d'oeuvres (*Rokeach*), 8 balls ...	60	8.0	4.0	1.0	m.q.	m.q.	m.q.	m.q.
in jelled broth:								
(*Mother's* Old Fashioned, 12 oz.)	54	7.0	4.0	.8	m.q.	m.q.	m.q.	m.q.
(*Mother's* Old Fashioned, 24 oz.)	70	9.0	5.0	1.0	m.q.	m.q.	m.q.	m.q.
(*Mother's* Old World)	70	8.0	7.0	1.0	m.q.	m.q.	m.q.	m.q.
(*Mother's* Unsalted)	45	5.0	2.0	1.0	m.q.	m.q.	m.q.	m.q.
(*Rokeach* Old Vienna, 12 oz.),								
2 oz.	54	6.0	6.0	1.0	m.q.	m.q.	m.q.	m.q.
(*Rokeach* Old Vienna, 24 oz.),								
2.6 oz.	70	8.0	8.0	1.0	m.q.	m.q.	m.q.	m.q.
(*Rokeach* Old Vienna, 31 oz.),								
3 oz.	81	9.0	9.0	1.0	m.q.	m.q.	m.q.	m.q.
(*Rokeach Redi-Jelled*), 2 oz.	46	6.0	3.0	1.0	m.q.	m.q.	222	m.q.
(*Rokeach Redi-Jelled*), 3 oz.	65	9.0	5.0	1.0	m.q.	m.q.	333	m.q.
(*Rokeach Redi-Jelled*), 4 oz.	92	12.0	6.0	2.0	m.q.	m.q.	444	m.q.
in liquid:								
(*Mother's* Old Fashioned, 12 oz.)	54	7.0	5.0	.8	m.q.	m.q.	m.q.	m.q.
(*Mother's* Old Fashioned, 24/31 oz.)	70	9.0	7.0	1.0	m.q.	m.q.	m.q.	m.q.
in natural broth (*Rokeach*, 24 oz.),								
4 oz.	60	8.0	4.0	1.0	m.q.	m.q.	835	m.q.
in natural broth (*Rokeach*, 24 oz.),								
2.6 oz.	50	7.0	4.0	1.0	m.q.	m.q.	m.q.	m.q.
sweet:								
w/broth, 1 lb.	381	41.4	33.6	7.9	1.9	135	2377	.2 c
w/broth, 1 oz.	24	2.6	2.1	.5	.1	9	149	<.1 c
w/broth, approx. 1.5 oz.	35	3.8	3.1	.7	.2	12	220	<.1 c
(*Mother's* Old World)	54	6.0	5.0	.8	m.q.	m.q.	m.q.	m.q.
whitefish, in jelled broth:								
(*Mother's*, 12 oz.)	46	7.0	3.0	.8	m.q.	m.q.	m.q.	m.q.
(*Mother's*, 24/31 oz.)	60	9.0	4.0	1.0	m.q.	m.q.	m.q.	m.q.
whitefish, in liquid:								
(*Mother's*, 12 oz.)	54	7.0	5.0	.8	m.q.	m.q.	m.q.	m.q.
(*Mother's*, 24/31 oz.)	70	9.0	7.0	1.0	m.q.	m.q.	m.q.	m.q.
whitefish and pike, in jelled broth:								
(*Mother's*, 12 oz.)	46	7.0	3.0	.8	m.q.	m.q.	m.q.	m.q.

Food and Measure	cal.	prot. (gms)	carbo. (gms)	tot. fat (gms)	sat. fat (gms)	chol. (mgs)	sod. (mgs)	fiber (gms)
(*Mother's*, 24/31 oz.)	60	9.0	4.0	1.0	m.q.	m.q.	m.q.	m.q.
(*Mother's* Old World, 12 oz.)	54	6.0	5.0	.8	m.q.	m.q.	m.q.	m.q.
(*Mother's* Old World, 24 oz.)	70	8.0	7.0	1.0	m.q.	m.q.	m.q.	m.q.
(*Rokeach*, 24/31 oz.), 2.6 oz.	60	9.0	4.0	1.0	m.q.	m.q.	m.q.	m.q.
(*Rokeach*, 12 oz.), 2 oz.	46	7.0	3.0	1.0	m.q.	m.q.	m.q.	m.q.
whitefish and pike, in liquid								
(*Mother's*)	70	9.0	7.0	1.0	m.q.	m.q.	m.q.	m.q.
GELATIN, unflavored:								
(*Knox*), 1 pkt.	25	6.0	0	0	0	0	10	0
GELATIN BAR, frozen:								
all flavors (*Jell-O Gelatin Pops*), 1 bar	35	1.0	8.0	0	0	0	5	(0)
GELATIN DESSERT:								
(*Estee*), ½ cup	8	1.0	<1.0	0	0	0	0	(0)
GELATIN DESSERT MIX[1] (see also "Pudding"), ½ cup:								
all flavors:								
(*D-Zerta*)	8	2.0	0	0	0	0	0	0
(*Jell-O*)	80	2.0	19.0	0	0	0	—[2]	(0)
except lemon (*Featherweight*)	10	2.0	1.0	0	0	0	5	0
except lemon, lime, peach, pineapple, and strawberry								
(*Royal*)	80	2.0	19.0	0	0	0	95	0
except lime (*Royal* Sugar Free) ...	6	1.0	0	0	0	0	70	0
lemon (*Featherweight*)	10	2.0	1.0	0	0	0	4	0
lemon (*Royal*)	80	2.0	19.0	0	0	0	100	0
lime (*Royal*)	80	2.0	19.0	0	0	0	90	0
lime (*Royal* Sugar Free)	6	1.0	0	0	0	0	75	0
peach (*Royal*)	80	2.0	19.0	0	0	0	100	0
pineapple (*Royal*)	80	2.0	19.0	0	0	0	90	0
strawberry (*Royal*)	80	2.0	19.0	0	0	0	100	0
GELATIN DRINK MIX, orange flavor:								
powder:								
1 oz.	108	10.0	17.1	.3	<.1	n.a.	47	<.1 c
.6-oz. pkt.	67	6.1	10.5	.2	<.1	n.a.	29	tr.c
(*Knox*), 1 envelope	39	5.7	4.0	.1	(0)	0	17	(0)
beverage, 4 fl. oz. water and								
.6-oz. pkt.	67	6.2	10.5	.2	<.1	n.a.	32	0
GERMAN SAUSAGE:								
(*Hickory Farms*), 1 oz.	100	5.0	1.0	8.0	m.q.	20	385	0
GHEE:								
1 oz.	249	0	0	28.4	m.q.	m.q.	n.a.	0
GHERKIN, see "Pickle"								
GIN, see "Liquor"								
GIN AND TONIC[3]:								
1 fl. oz.	23	tr.	2.1	tr.	tr.	0	1	(0)

1. *Prepared according to package directions.*
2. *Sodium values per serving vary according to flavor: black raspberry and concord grape, 35 mg.; lemon and wild strawberry, 75 mg.; lime 55 mg.; orange-pineapple, 65 mg.; cherry, 70 mg.; all other flavors, 50 mg.*
3. *Recipe: 74.5% tonic water, 18.7% gin, 6.8% lime juice.*

Food and Measure	cal.	prot. (gms)	carbo. (gms)	tot. fat (gms)	sat. fat (gms)	chol. (mgs)	sod. (mgs)	fiber (gms)
GINGELEY, see "Sesame seed"								
GINGER, root:								
untrimmed, 1 lb.	291	7.4	63.6	3.1	.9	0	53	4.3 c
trimmed:								
1 oz.	20	.5	4.3	.2	.1	0	4	.3 c
5 slices, ⅛" thick, 1" diam.	8	.2	1.7	.1	<.1	0	1	.1 c
sliced, ¼ cup	17	.4	3.6	.2	<.1	0	3	.3 c
GINGER, GROUND:								
1 oz.	98	2.6	20.1	1.7	.5	0	9	1.7 c
1 tbsp.	19	.5	3.8	.3	.1	0	2	.3 c
1 tsp.	6	.2	1.3	.1	<.1	0	1	.1 c
(*Spice Islands*), 1 tsp.	6	.1	1.2	.1	m.q.	0	1	.1 c
(*Tone's*), 1 tsp.	6	.2	1.3	.1	<.1	0	1	.1 d
GINGER, PICKLED, Japanese:								
1 oz.	10	.1	2.1	<.1	tr.	0	105	m.q.
GINGERBREAD, see "Bread, sweet, mix"								
GINKGO NUT:								
raw, in shell, 1 lb.	628	14.9	129.6	5.8	1.1	0	24	1.7 c
raw, shelled, 1 oz.	52	1.2	10.7	.5	.1	0	2	.1 c
dried, in shell, 1 lb.	1198	35.7	249.8	6.9	1.3	0	46	3.4 c
dried, shelled, 1 oz.	99	2.9	20.6	.8	.1	0	4	.3 c
GINKGO NUT, CANNED, drained:								
1 oz., approx. 22 small, 14 medium or 9 large	32	.6	6.3	.5	.1	0	87	.5 c
1 cup	173	3.6	34.3	2.5	.5	0	476	2.5 c
GLUTEN, see "Wheat gluten"								
GOA BEAN, see "Winged bean"								
GOAT, meat only:								
raw, 1 oz.	31	5.9	0	.7	.2	16	23	0
roasted[1]:								
12 oz., yield from 1 lb. boneless	487	92.2	0	10.3	3.2	255	294	0
4 oz.	162	30.7	0	3.4	1.1	85	98	0
diced, 1 cup, approx. 4.9 oz.	200	37.9	0	4.2	1.3	105	120	0
GOATFISH, meat only, raw:								
1 lb.	435	92.5	0	4.5	m.q.	m.q.	m.q.	0
1 oz.	27	5.8	0	.3	m.q.	m.q.	m.q.	0
GOBO ROOT, see "Burdock"								
GODFATHER'S PIZZA:								
original:								
cheese:								
mini, ¼ pie, 2.8 oz.	190	8.0	31.0	4.0	m.q.	8	260	m.q.
small, ⅙ pie, 3.6 oz.	240	12.0	32.0	7.0	m.q.	15	400	m.q.
medium, ⅛ pie, 4 oz.	270	13.0	36.0	8.0	m.q.	15	430	m.q.
large, ⅒ pie, 4.4 oz.	297	15.0	39.0	9.0	m.q.	20	494	m.q.
large, hot slice, ⅛ pie, 5.5 oz.	370	18.0	48.0	11.0	m.q.	25	620	m.q.
combo:								
mini, ¼ pie, 3.8 oz.	240	10.0	32.0	7.0	m.q.	10	450	m.q.

1. *Without added ingredients.*

Food and Measure	cal.	prot. (gms)	carbo. (gms)	tot. fat (gms)	sat. fat (gms)	chol. (mgs)	sod. (mgs)	fiber (gms)
small, ⅙ pie, 5.6 oz.	360	18.0	35.0	15.0	m.q.	30	830	m.q.
medium, ⅛ pie, 6.2 oz.	400	20.0	39.0	17.0	m.q.	35	930	m.q.
large, ⅒ pie, 6.8 oz.	437	22.0	42.0	19.0	m.q.	36	1019	m.q.
large, hot slice, ⅛ pie, 8.5 oz.	550	27.0	52.0	24.0	m.q.	45	1270	m.q.
thin crust:								
cheese:								
small, ⅙ pie, 2.6 oz.	180	9.0	21.0	6.0	m.q.	10	370	m.q.
medium, ⅛ pie, 3 oz.	210	10.0	26.0	7.0	m.q.	14	410	m.q.
large, ⅒ pie, 3.4 oz.	228	11.0	28.0	7.0	m.q.	16	464	m.q.
combo:								
small, ⅙ pie, 4.3 oz.	270	13.0	23.0	13.0	m.q.	25	710	m.q.
medium, ⅛ pie, 4.9 oz.	310	15.0	29.0	14.0	m.q.	25	790	m.q.
large, ⅒ pie, 5.4 oz.	336	17.0	31.0	16.0	m.q.	27	870	m.q.
stuffed pie:								
cheese:								
small, ⅙ pie, 4.4 oz.	310	13.0	38.0	11.0	m.q.	25	560	m.q.
medium, ⅛ pie, 4.8 oz.	350	14.0	42.0	13.0	m.q.	25	610	m.q.
large, ⅒ pie, 5.2 oz.	381	16.0	44.0	16.0	m.q.	32	677	m.q.
combo:								
small, ⅙ pie, 6.3 oz.	430	19.0	41.0	20.0	m.q.	40	1000	m.q.
medium, ⅛ pie, 7 oz.	480	21.0	45.0	23.0	m.q.	43	1105	m.q.
large, ⅒, 7.6 oz.	521	23.0	47.0	26.0	m.q.	48	1204	m.q.
GOOBER PEA, see "Peanut"								
GOOSE, domesticated:								
raw:								
meat w/skin:								
½ goose, 2.9 lbs., yield from								
3.6 lbs. w/bone	4893	209.2	0	443.5	129.0	1055	964	0
1 lb.	1683	71.9	0	152.5	44.4	363	331	0
1 oz.	105	4.5	0	9.5	2.8	23	21	0
meat only, 1 lb.	730	103.2	0	32.3	12.7	381	395	0
meat only, 1 oz.	46	6.4	0	2.0	.8	24	25	0
roasted[1]:								
meat w/skin, ½ goose, 1.7 lbs.,								
yield from 2.4 lbs. w/bone	2362	194.7	0	169.7	53.2	708	543	0
meat w/skin, 4 oz.	346	28.5	0	24.9	7.8	103	79	0
meat only, ½ goose, 1.3 lbs.,								
yield from 2.4 lbs. w/bone and								
skin w/separable fat	1406	171.2	0	74.9	26.9	569	447	0
meat only, 4 oz.	270	32.9	0	14.4	5.2	109	86	0
GOOSE FAT:								
1 oz.	255	0	0	28.3	7.9	28	0	0
½ cup	923	0	0	102.3	28.4	103	0	0
1 tbsp.	115	0	0	12.8	3.5	13	0	0
GOOSE LIVER, see "Liver"								
GOOSE LIVER PATE, see "Pâté"								
GOOSEBERRY:								
1 lb.	202	4.0	46.2	2.6	.2	0	4	8.6 c

1. *Without added ingredients.*

Food and Measure	cal.	prot. (gms)	carbo. (gms)	tot. fat (gms)	sat. fat (gms)	chol. (mgs)	sod. (mgs)	fiber (gms)
GOOSEBERRY *(cont.)*								
1 oz.	12	.2	2.9	.2	<.1	0	<1	.5 c
½ cup	34	.7	7.6	.4	<.1	0	1	1.4 c
GOOSEBERRY, CANNED:								
in light syrup, 4 oz.	83	.7	21.3	.2	<.1	0	2	1.4 c
in light syrup, ½ cup	93	.8	23.6	.3	<.1	0	3	1.5 c
GOOSEFISH, see "Monkfish"								
GOURD, DISHCLOTH:								
raw:								
untrimmed, 1 lb.	67	4.0	14.4	.7	.1	0	11	1.7 c
trimmed, 1 oz.	6	.3	1.2	.1	tr.	0	1	.1 c
1 medium, 13¼″ × 1¾″, approx.								
8.6 oz.	36	2.1	7.8	.4	<.1	0	6	.9 c
1″ slices, ½ cup	10	.6	2.1	.1	tr.	0	2	.2 c
boiled, drained, 4 oz.	64	.7	16.3	.4	<.1	0	24	.5 d
boiled, drained, 1″ slices, ½ cup ...	50	.6	12.8	.3	<.1	0	18	.4 d
GOURD, WHITE-FLOWERED:								
raw:								
untrimmed, 1 lb.	44	2.0	10.8	.1	tr.	0	8	3.5 d
trimmed, 1 oz.	4	.2	1.0	tr.	tr.	0	1	.3 d
1 medium, 17″ × 3⅛″, approx.								
2.4 lb.	106	5.0	26.1	.2	<.1	0	19	8.5 d
1″ cubes, ½ cup	8	.4	2.0	<.1	tr.	0	1	.6 d
boiled, drained, 4 oz.	17	.7	4.2	<.1	tr.	0	2	.7 c
boiled, drained, 1″ cubes, ½ cup ...	11	.4	2.7	<.1	tr.	0	1	.5 c
GOURD STRIPS, see "Kanpyo"								
GOURMET LOAF:								
(*Eckrich*), 1-oz. slice	30	4.0	1.0	1.0	m.q.	m.q.	340	(0)
GOVERNOR PLUM:								
trimmed, 1 oz.	31	.1	8.4	0	0	0	n.a.	.1 c
GRAIN, see specific listings								
GRANADILLA, see "Passion fruit"								
GRANOLA, see "Cereal"								
GRANOLA AND CEREAL BAR								
(see also "Breakfast bar" and								
"Snack bar"), 1 bar:								
w/almonds, chewy (*Sunbelt*), 1 oz. ...	120	3.0	18.0	6.0	m.q.	<1	65	m.q.
caramel nut (*Quaker Granola Dipps*),								
1 oz.	148	1.9	20.9	6.4	2.8	2	81	.7 d
chocolate chip:								
(*Kudos*)	180	3.0	21.0	9.0	n.a.	n.a.	60	m.q.
(*Quaker Chewy*), 1 oz.	128	2.0	19.3	4.7	1.5	<1	90	1.4 d
(*Quaker Granola Dipps*), 1 oz. ...	139	1.8	18.7	6.3	2.8	1	78	1.0 d
chewy (*Sunbelt*), 1.25 oz.	150	3.0	23.0	7.0	m.q.	<1	75	m.q.
chocolate coated (*Hershey's*),								
1.2 oz.	170	2.0	22.0	8.0	m.q.	n.a.	50	m.q.
fudge dipped, chewy (*Sunbelt*),								
1.63 oz.	220	2.0	29.0	11.0	m.q.	<1	60	m.q.

Food and Measure	cal.	prot. (gms)	carbo. (gms)	tot. fat (gms)	sat. fat (gms)	chol. (mgs)	sod. (mgs)	fiber (gms)
w/chocolate chips, chewy (*Sunbelt*), 1.75 oz.	220	4.0	32.0	9.0	m.q.	<1	105	m.q.
chocolate fudge (*Quaker Granola Dipps*), 1 oz.	160	2.1	20.0	7.9	m.q.	n.a.	74	m.q.
cinnamon (*Nature Valley*), .8 oz.	120	2.0	17.0	5.0	1.0	0	70	1.0 d
cocoa creme, chocolate coated (*Hershey's*), 1.2 oz.	180	2.0	22.0	9.0	m.q.	5	50	m.q.
Common Sense, raspberry filled (*Kellogg's Smart Start*), 1.5 oz.	170	2.0	28.0	6.0	m.q.	0	160	1.0 d
cookies and creme, chocolate coated (*Hershey's*), 1.2 oz.	170	2.0	22.0	8.0	m.q.	n.a.	50	m.q.
corn flakes, mixed berry filled (*Kellogg's Smart Start*), 1.5 oz.	170	2.0	27.0	7.0	m.q.	0	160	1.0 d
fudge, nutty (*Kudos*)	190	4.0	19.0	11.0	n.a.	n.a.	60	m.q.
honey and oats (*Quaker Chewy*), 1 oz.	125	2.3	19.1	4.4	1.1	<1	95	1.3 d
nut and raisin, chunky (*Quaker Chewy*), 1 oz.	131	2.5	17.2	5.8	1.3	<1	86	1.6 d
Nutri•Grain, blueberry or strawberry (*Kellogg's Smart Start*), 1.5 oz.	180	2.0	26.0	8.0	m.q.	0	170	1.0 d
oat bran-honey graham (*Nature Valley*), .8 oz.	110	2.0	16.0	4.0	<1.0	0	90	1.0 d
oats and honey:								
(*Nature Valley*), .8 oz.	120	2.0	17.0	5.0	1.0	0	65	1.0 d
chewy (*Sunbelt*), 1 oz.	130	2.0	18.0	5.0	m.q.	<1	35	m.q.
fudge dipped, chewy (*Sunbelt*), 1.38 oz.	190	2.0	24.0	10.0	m.q.	<1	55	m.q.
peanut butter:								
(*Nature Valley*), .8 oz.	120	2.0	15.0	6.0	1.0	0	70	1.0 d
(*Quaker Chewy*), 1 oz.	128	3.1	17.8	4.9	1.3	<1	116	1.2 d
(*Quaker Granola Dipps*), 1 oz. . . .	170	3.6	18.5	9.1	3.1	2	74	1.0 d
and chocolate chip (*Quaker Chewy*), 1 oz.	131	3.1	17.0	5.7	1.5	<1	112	1.2 d
chocolate chip (*Quaker Granola Dipps*), 1 oz.	174	3.6	17.4	10.0	m.q.	n.a.	102	m.q.
chocolate coated (*Hershey's*), 1.2 oz.	180	4.0	19.0	10.0	m.q.	5	65	m.q.
chocolate coated (*Kudos*), 1.3 oz.	190	4.0	18.0	12.0	m.q.	n.a.	70	m.q.
w/peanuts, fudge dipped, chewy (*Sunbelt*), 1.38 oz.	190	2.0	24.0	10.0	m.q.	<1	55	m.q.
w/peanuts, fudge dipped, chewy (*Sunbelt*), 2.25 oz.	300	6.0	36.0	18.0	m.q.	<1	90	m.q.
raisin bran (*Kellogg's Smart Start*), 1.5 oz.	160	2.0	28.0	5.0	m.q.	0	170	2.0 d
w/raisins, chewy (*Sunbelt*), 1.25 oz.	150	2.0	24.0	6.0	m.q.	<1	65	m.q.
w/raisins, fudge dipped, chewy (*Sunbelt*), 1.5 oz.	200	4.0	24.0	12.0	m.q.	<1	60	m.q.

Food and Measure	cal.	prot. (gms)	carbo. (gms)	tot. fat (gms)	sat. fat (gms)	chol. (mgs)	sod. (mgs)	fiber (gms)
GRANOLA AND CEREAL BAR *(cont.)*								
raisin and cinnamon (*Quaker Chewy*),								
1 oz.	128	2.2	18.6	5.0	1.1	<1	92	1.2 d
Rice Krispies, w/almonds (*Kellogg's*								
Smart Start), 1 oz.	130	2.0	18.0	6.0	m.q.	0	65	1.0 d
S'mores (*Quaker Chewy*), 1 oz.	126	1.9	19.7	4.4	1.4	<1	108	1.1 d
GRAPE:								
American type (slipskin: Concord,								
Delaware, Niagara):								
untrimmed, 1 lb.	165	1.7	45.1	.9	.3	0	4	2.0 c
peeled and seeded, 1 oz.	18	.2	4.9	.1	<.1	0	<1	.2 c
peeled and seeded, ½ cup	29	.3	7.9	.2	.1	0	1	.4 c
10 medium, approx. 1.4 oz.	15	.2	4.1	.1	<.1	0	tr.	.2 c
European type (adherent skin:								
Thompson seedless, Tokay,								
Muscat):								
seeded, untrimmed, 1 lb.	287	2.7	72.0	2.3	.8	0	7	2.8 d
seedless:								
untrimmed, 1 lb.	309	2.9	77.4	2.5	.8	0	7	3.0 d
or seeded, 1 oz.	20	.2	5.0	.2	.1	0	1	.2 d
or seeded, ½ cup	57	.5	14.2	.5	.2	0	2	.6 d
10 medium, ⅝″ × ⅞″, approx.								
1.75 oz.	36	.3	8.9	.3	.1	0	1	.4 d
GRAPE, CANNED, Thompson								
seedless:								
in water, 4 oz.	45	.6	11.7	.1	<.1	0	7	.2 c
in water, ½ cup	48	.6	12.6	.1	<.1	0	7	.3 c
in heavy syrup:								
4 oz.	83	.5	22.3	.1	<.1	0	6	.2 c
½ cup	94	.6	25.2	.1	<.1	0	7	.3 c
(*S&W* Premium Thompson),								
½ cup	100	0	25.0	0	0	0	5	m.q.
GRAPE DRINK (see also "Grape								
juice drink" and "Grapeade"):								
canned, bottled, boxed, or chilled:								
1 fl. oz.	14	0	3.6	tr.	tr.	0	2	0
(*A&P*), 6 fl. oz.	100	<1.0	25.0	<1.0	(0)	0	0	0
(*Bama*), 8.45 fl. oz.	120	0	29.0	0	0	0	25	0
(*Crowley*), 8 fl. oz.	130	0	32.0	0	0	0	15	0
(*Minute Maid* Light'N Juicy),								
6 fl. oz.	13	.2	2.7	<.1	(0)	0	18	0
(*Pathmark*), 6 fl. oz.	90	0	22.0	0	0	0	0	0
(*Veryfine*), 8 fl. oz.	130	.1	34.0	0	0	0	<10	0
(*Wylers* Fruit Slush), 4 fl. oz.	157	0	39.3	0	0	0	10	0
mix[1], 8 fl. oz., except as noted:								
(*Finast*)	80	0	21.0	0	0	0	15	0
(*Kool-Aid*)	100	0	25.0	0	0	0	0	0

1. *Prepared according to package directions.*

Food and Measure	cal.	prot. (gms)	carbo. (gms)	tot. fat (gms)	sat. fat (gms)	chol. (mgs)	sod. (mgs)	fiber (gms)
(*Kool-Aid* Presweetened)	80	0	20.0	0	0	0	25	0
(*Kool-Aid* Sugar Free)	4	0	0	0	0	0	0	0
(*Pathmark* No Frills)	90	0	22.0	0	0	0	20	0
(*Pathmark* No Frills Sodium Free),								
6 fl. oz.	80	0	22.0	0	0	0	0	0
GRAPE FRUIT ROLL, see "Fruit								
snack"								
GRAPE JUICE, 6 fl. oz., except as								
noted:								
canned, bottled, or boxed:								
1 fl. oz.	19	.2	4.7	<.1	tr.	0	1	0
6 fl. oz.	116	1.1	28.4	.1	<.1	0	5	0
(*IGA* Unsweetened)	120	0	30.0	0	0	0	5	0
(*Kraft* Pure 100% Unsweetened)	104	1.0	25.0	0	0	0	0	0
(*Lucky Leaf*)	130	0	32.0	0	0	0	0	0
(*Minute Maid*), 8.45 fl. oz.	150	.6	37.4	.3	(0)	0	30	0
(*Pathmark* No Frills)	113	0	27.0	0	0	0	<10	0
(*Pathmark* Unsweetened)	120	0	30.0	0	0	0	10	0
(*Sippin' Pak*), 8.45 fl. oz.	130	1.0	32.0	0	0	0	25	0
(*Veryfine* 100%), 8 fl. oz.	153	1.0	37.0	0	0	0	<20	0
(*Welch's* USDA)	120	0	30.0	0	0	0	10	0
blend (*Libby's Juicy Juice*)	100	0	25.0	0	0	0	5	0
Concord (*S&W* Unsweetened) ...	100	1.0	25.0	0	0	0	9	0
purple (*Welch's*)	120	0	30.0	0	0	0	10	0
red (*Welch's*), 8.45 fl. oz.	170	0	43.0	0	0	0	20	0
red or white (*Welch's*)	120	0	30.0	0	0	0	15	0
sparkling, red (*Welch's*)	128	0	30.0	0	0	0	30	0
sparkling, white (*Welch's*)	120	0	30.0	0	0	0	30	0
white (*Welch's*), 8.45 fl. oz.	160	0	39.0	0	0	0	20	0
chilled or frozen[1] (*Minute Maid*) ...	100	.4	25.0	.2	(0)	0	21	0
frozen[2]:								
(*Sunkist*)	69	.3	17.1	.1	(0)	0	3	0
purple or white (*Welch's*)	100	0	25.0	0	0	0	0	0
sweetened:								
undiluted	386	1.4	95.8	.7	.2	0	15	0
1 fl. oz.	16	.1	4.0	<.1	tr.	0	1	0
6 fl. oz.	96	.4	23.9	.2	.1	0	4	0
GRAPE JUICE COCKTAIL:								
canned, bottled, or boxed:								
(*Welch's Orchard*), 10 fl. oz.	170	0	43.0	0	0	0	10	0
(*Welch's Orchard*), 6 fl. oz.	110	0	27.0	0	0	0	20	0
(*Welch's Orchard* Cocktails-In-A-								
Box), 8.45 fl. oz.	150	0	38.0	0	0	0	20	0
frozen[1] (*Welch's* No Sugar Added),								
6 fl. oz.	40	0	10.0	0	0	0	5	0

1. *Diluted according to package directions.*
2. *Diluted according to package directions, except as noted.*

Food and Measure	cal.	prot. (gms)	carbo. (gms)	tot. fat (gms)	sat. fat (gms)	chol. (mgs)	sod. (mgs)	fiber (gms)
GRAPE JUICE DRINK:								
canned, bottled, or boxed:								
1 fl. oz.	16	tr.	4.0	0	0	0	tr.	0
(*Hi-C*), 8.45 fl. oz.	136	.1	33.4	.1	(0)	0	24	0
(*Hi-C*), 6 fl. oz.	96	.1	23.7	.1	(0)	0	17	0
(*Kool-Aid Koolers*), 8.45 fl. oz. ...	140	0	35.0	0	0	0	10	0
(*Tang* Fruit Box), 8.45 fl. oz.	130	0	34.0	0	0	0	10	0
frozen[1] (*Sunkist*), 6 fl. oz.	69	.3	17.0	.1	(0)	0	3	0
GRAPE-APPLE DRINK:								
(*Mott's*), 10-fl.-oz. bottle	167	0	42.0	0	0	0	<1	0
(*Mott's*), 9.5-fl.-oz. can	158	0	40.0	0	0	0	<1	0
GRAPEADE:								
chilled or frozen[1] (*Minute Maid*),								
6 fl. oz.	94	.1	23.4	<.1	0	0	18	0
GRAPEFRUIT:								
pink and red, California and Arizona:								
untrimmed, 1 lb.	86	1.2	22.4	.2	<.1	0	1	.5 c
trimmed, 1 oz.	11	.1	2.7	<.1	tr.	0	<1	.1 c
½ of 3¾"-diam. fruit, approx.								
8.5 oz.	46	.6	11.9	.1	<.1	0	<1	.3 c
sections w/juice, ½ cup	43	.6	11.1	.1	<.1	0	<1	.2 c
pink and red, Florida:								
untrimmed, 1 lb.	69	1.3	17.4	.2	<.1	0	1	.5 c
trimmed, 1 oz.	9	.2	2.1	<.1	tr.	0	tr.	.1 c
½ of 3¾"-diam. fruit, approx.								
8.5 oz.	37	.7	9.2	.1	<.1	0	<1	.3 c
sections w/juice, ½ cup	34	.6	8.6	.1	<.1	0	<1	.2 c
pink (*Ocean Spray*), ½ medium	50	1.0	13.0	0	0	0	0	m.q.
white, California:								
untrimmed, 1 lb.	81	2.0	20.2	.2	<.1	0	1	.4 c
trimmed, 1 oz.	10	.2	2.6	<.1	tr.	0	tr.	.1 c
½ of 3¾"-diam. fruit, approx.								
8.5 oz.	43	1.0	10.7	.1	<.1	0	tr.	.2 c
sections w/juice, ½ cup	42	1.0	10.5	.1	<.1	0	tr.	.2 c
white, Florida:								
untrimmed, 1 lb.	72	1.4	18.2	.2	<.1	0	1	.4 d
trimmed, 1 oz.	9	.2	2.3	<.1	tr.	0	tr.	<.1 d
½ of 3¾"-diam. fruit, approx.								
8.5 oz.	38	.7	9.7	.1	<.1	0	tr.	.2 d
sections w/juice, ½ cup	38	.7	9.4	.1	<.1	0	tr.	.2 d
white (*Ocean Spray*), ½ medium ...	45	1.0	12.0	0	0	0	0	m.q.
GRAPEFRUIT, CANNED, ½ cup,								
except as noted:								
(*S&W* Unsweetened)	40	0	9.0	0	0	0	<10	m.q.
(*S&W*/*Nutradiet*)	40	0	9.0	0	0	0	0	m.q.
in water, 4 oz.	41	.7	10.4	.1	<.1	0	2	.4 c
in water	44	.7	11.2	.1	<.1	0	2	.4 c

1. *Diluted according to package directions.*

Food and Measure	cal.	prot. (gms)	carbo. (gms)	tot. fat (gms)	sat. fat (gms)	chol. (mgs)	sod. (mgs)	fiber (gms)
in juice:								
4 oz.	42	.8	10.4	.1	<.1	0	8	.2 d
½ cup	46	.9	11.4	.1	<.1	0	9	.3 d
(Featherweight)	40	0	9.0	0	0	0	<10	m.q.
in light syrup:								
4 oz.	68	.6	17.5	.1	<.1	0	2	.4 c
½ cup	76	.7	19.6	.1	<.1	0	2	.4 c
(Finast)	80	0	20.0	<.1	(0)	0	<10	m.q.
(S&W)	80	<1.0	24.0	0	0	0	0	m.q.
(Stokely)	90	1.0	23.0	1.0	(0)	0	5	m.q.
GRAPEFRUIT, CHILLED:								
(Kraft Pure), ½ cup	50	1.0	12.0	0	0	0	0	m.q.
GRAPEFRUIT JUICE, 6 fl. oz.,								
except as noted:								
fresh:								
1 fl. oz.	12	.2	2.8	<.1	tr.	0	<1	m.q.
6 fl. oz.	72	.9	17.0	l2	<.1	0	2	m.q.
juice from 3¾"-diam. fruit	76	1.0	18.0	.2	<.1	0	2	m.q.
canned, bottled, boxed, or chilled:								
1 fl. oz.	12	.2	2.8	<.1	tr.	0	tr.	tr.
6 fl. oz.	70	1.0	16.6	.2	<.1	0	2	tr.
(Del Monte)	70	1.0	17.0	0	0	0	<10	tr.
(Kraft Pure 100%)	70	1.0	16.0	0	0	0	0	tr.
(Minute Maid)	78	1.0	18.4	.3	0	0	19	tr.
(Minute Maid On The Go),								
10 fl. oz.	130	1.7	30.7	.4	0	0	31	tr.
(Mott's), 10-fl.-oz. bottle	124	1.0	30.0	0	0	0	5	tr.
(Mott's), 9.5-fl.-oz. can.	118	1.0	29.0	0	0	0	10	tr.
(Ocean Spray)	70	1.0	16.0	0	0	0	10	tr.
(S&W)	80	1.0	18.0	0	0	0	<10	tr.
(Stokely)	76	1.0	18.0	1.0	(0)	0	5	tr.
(Sunkist Fresh Squeezed),								
8 fl. oz.	96	1.2	22.7	.2	(0)	0	3	tr.
(Tree Top)	80	1.0	19.0	0	0	0	0	tr.
(Veryfine 100%), 8 fl. oz.	101	1.4	23.0	0	0	0	<10	tr.
pink (Ocean Spray Pink Premium)	60	1.0	15.0	0	0	0	10	tr.
regular or pink (TreeSweet)	72	0	17.0	0	0	0	15	tr.
regular or ruby red (Tropicana								
100% Pure), 8 fl. oz.	101	m.q.	24.0	0	0	0	3	m.q.
sweetened, 1 fl. oz.	14	.2	3.5	<.1	tr.	0	tr.	tr.
sweetened, 6 fl. oz.	87	1.1	20.9	.2	<.1	0	3	tr.
chilled or frozen[1], pink (Minute								
Maid)	78	1.0	18.4	.3	(0)	0	19	tr.
frozen[2]:								
undiluted	302	4.1	71.5	1.0	.1	0	6	tr.
1 fl. oz.	13	.2	3.0	<.1	tr.	0	tr.	tr.

1. *Diluted according to package directions.*
2. *Diluted according to package directions, except as noted.*

Food and Measure	cal.	prot. (gms)	carbo. (gms)	tot. fat (gms)	sat. fat (gms)	chol. (mgs)	sod. (mgs)	fiber (gms)
GRAPEFRUIT JUICE, FROZEN *(cont.)*								
6 fl. oz.	51	.7	12.0	.2	<.1	0	1	tr.
(A&P)	80	<1.0	18.0	<1.0	(0)	0	0	tr.
(Minute Maid)	83	1.1	19.7	.3	(0)	0	19	tr.
(Sunkist)	56	.8	13.3	.2	(0)	0	1	tr.
(TreeSweet)	78	1.0	18.0	0	0	0	15	tr.
GRAPEFRUIT JUICE COCKTAIL, pink, 6 fl. oz., except as noted:								
canned, bottled, or boxed:								
(IGA)	80	0	20.0	0	0	0	15	(0)
(Minute Maid Juices to Go), 11.5 fl. oz.	163	.9	40.1	.2	(0)	0	34	(0)
(Minute Maid Juices to Go), 9.6 fl. oz.	136	.7	33.5	.1	(0)	0	29	(0)
(Ocean Spray)	80	0	20.0	0	0	0	15	(0)
(Pathmark)	80	0	20.0	0	0	0	15	(0)
(TreeSweet Lite)	40	1.0	10.0	0	0	0	15	(0)
(Tropicana Twister), 8 fl. oz.	110	(0)	28.0	0	0	0	1	(0)
(Veryfine), 8 fl. oz.	120	<1.0	29.0	0	0	0	<15	(0)
chilled or frozen[1] *(Minute Maid)* ...	85	.5	20.9	.1	(0)	0	18	(0)
GRAPEFRUIT JUICE DRINK:								
(Citrus Hill Plus Calcium), 6 fl. oz.	70	<1.0	19.0	<1.0	(0)	0	10	(0)
(Tropicana Juice Sparkler), 8 fl. oz.	110	(0)	26.0	0	0	0	50	(0)
(Wyler's Fruit Slush), 4 fl. oz.	157	0	39.3	0	0	0	10	(0)
GRAPESEED OIL:								
1 oz.	251	0	0	28.4	2.70	0	0	0
½ cup	964	0	0	109.0	10.50	0	0	0
1 tbsp.	120	0	0	13.6	1.3	0	0	0
GRAVY, see specific listings								
GRAVY MIX[2] (see also specific listings)								
country *(Tone's),* 1 tsp. dry	12	.2	1.5	.5	n.a.	<1	114	<.1 d
homestyle:								
(French's), ¼ cup	20	1.0	4.0	1.0	n.a.	n.a.	250	n.a.
(McCormick/Schilling), ¼ cup ...	24	.5	3.8	.8	n.a.	n.a.	295	n.a.
(Pillsbury), ¼ cup	15	<1.0	3.0	0	0	n.a.	300	n.a.
GREAT NORTHERN BEAN:								
raw, 1 oz.	96	6.2	17.7	.3	.1	0	4	11.3 d
raw, ½ cup	309	20.0	58.6	1.0	.3	0	12	36.4 d
boiled, 4 oz.	134	9.4	23.9	.5	.2	0	2	6.1 d
boiled, ½ cup	104	7.3	18.6	.4	.1	0	2	4.7 d
GREAT NORTHERN BEAN, CANNED:								
w/liquid, 4 oz.	129	8.4	23.8	.4	.1	0	5	2.6 c
w/liquid, ½ cup	150	9.7	27.6	.5	.2	0	6	3.0 c
(A&P), 1 cup	210	14.0	38.0	1.0	m.q.	0	0	m.q.

1. *Diluted according to package directions.*
2. *Prepared according to package directions, except as noted.*

Food and Measure	cal.	prot. (gms)	carbo. (gms)	tot. fat (gms)	sat. fat (gms)	chol. (mgs)	sod. (mgs)	fiber (gms)
(*Allens*), ½ cup	105	5.0	17.0	<1.0	m.q.	0	440	m.q.
(*Green Giant/Joan of Arc*), ½ cup ...	80	6.0	18.0	1.0	m.q.	0	290	5.0 d
w/pork (*Allens*), ½ cup	100	5.0	19.0	1.0	m.q.	m.q.	320	m.q.
w/pork (*Luck's*), 7.25 oz.	220	12.0	32.0	5.0	m.q.	m.q.	645	13.0 d
GREEN BEAN:								
raw:								
untrimmed, 1 lb.	123	7.3	28.5	.5	.1	0	23	8.4 d
trimmed, 1 oz.	9	.5	2.0	<.1	tr.	0	2	.6 d
trimmed, ½ cup	17	1.0	3.9	.1	<.1	0	3	1.2 d
boiled, drained, 4 oz.	40	2.1	8.9	.3	.1	0	3	2.0 d
boiled, drained, ½ cup	22	1.2	4.9	.2	<.1	0	2	1.1 d
GREEN BEAN, CANNED, ½ cup,								
except as noted:								
w/liquid, 4 oz.	17	1.0	4.0	.1	<.1	0	417	.7 d
w/liquid	18	1.0	4.2	.1	<.1	0	442	.7 d
drained, 4 oz.	23	1.3	5.1	.1	<.1	0	285	1.5 d
drained	13	.8	3.1	.1	<.1	0	170	.9 d
(*Green Giant* 50% Less Salt)	18	1.0	4.0	0	0	0	150	1.0 d
(*Pathmark*)	20	1.0	5.0	0	0	0	350	m.q.
(*Stokely*)	20	1.0	4.0	0	0	0	360	m.q.
(*Stokely* No Salt or Sugar)	20	1.0	4.0	0	0	0	5	m.q.
whole:								
(*Finast*)	25	1.0	4.0	0	0	0	400	m.q.
(*IGA*), 1 cup	45	2.0	8.0	0	0	0	640	m.q.
(*S&W* Vertical Pack)	20	1.0	4.0	0	0	0	385	m.q.
whole or cut (*A&P*)	20	1.0	4.0	<1.0	(0)	0	350	m.q.
whole or cut (*Pathmark*)	20	1.0	4.0	0	0	0	430	m.q.
whole, cut, or French style, w/liquid:								
(*Del Monte*)	20	1.0	4.0	0	0	0	355	m.q.
stringless (*S&W*)	20	1.0	4.0	0	0	0	3850	m.q.
cut:								
(*A&P*)	20	1.0	5.0	<1.0	(0)	0	340	m.q.
(*Featherweight*)	25	1.0	5.0	0	0	0	<10	m.q.
(*Finast*)	25	1.0	4.0	0	0	0	400	m.q.
(*Finast* No Salt Added)	20	1.0	4.0	0	0	0	10	m.q.
(*Finast* Veri-Green)	20	1.0	4.0	0	0	0	320	m.q.
(*Green Giant*)	16	1.0	4.0	0	0	0	300	1.0 d
(*Green Giant Pantry Express*)	12	<1.0	3.0	0	0	0	20	1.0 d
(*IGA*)	20	1.0	5.0	0	0	0	10	m.q.
(*S&W* Premium Golden)	20	1.0	5.0	0	0	0	385	m.q.
(*S&W/Nutradiet*)	20	1.0	4.0	0	0	0	5	m.q.
w/liquid (*Del Monte* No Salt								
Added)	20	1.0	4.0	0	0	0	<10	m.q.
cut or French style (*Allens*)	20	1.0	4.0	<1.0	(0)	0	350	m.q.
almondine (*Green Giant*)	45	2.0	5.0	3.0	0	0	300	2.0 d
dilled (*S&W*)	60	1.0	15.0	0	0	0	3850	m.q.
French style:								
(*A&P*)	20	1.0	4.0	<1.0	(0)	0	350	m.q.
(*Green Giant*)	16	1.0	4.0	0	0	0	330	1.0 d

Food and Measure	cal.	prot. (gms)	carbo. (gms)	tot. fat (gms)	sat. fat (gms)	chol. (mgs)	sod. (mgs)	fiber (gms)
GREEN BEAN, CANNED, FRENCH STYLE *(cont.)*								
or cut:								
(*Finast*)	20	1.0	4.0	0	0	0	400	m.q.
(*Pathmark* Blue Lake)	20	1.0	4.0	0	0	0	430	m.q.
(*Pathmark* No Frills), 1 cup	35	2.0	8.0	0	0	0	640	m.q.
(*S&W* Premium Blue Lake) ...	20	1.0	4.0	0	0	0	385	m.q.
or regular (*A&P* No Salt Added)	20	1.0	4.0	<1.0	(0)	0	10	m.q.
or regular (*Pathmark* No Salt Added)	20	1.0	5.0	0	0	0	10	m.q.
Italian (*Allens*)	18	1.0	3.0	<1.0	(0)	0	260	m.q.
Italian, cut (*Del Monte*)	25	1.0	6.0	0	0	0	355	m.q.
kitchen sliced (*Green Giant*)	16	1.0	4.0	0	0	0	280	1.0 d
low-sodium (see also specific brands):								
w/liquid, 4 oz.	17	1.0	4.0	.1	<.1	0	2	.7 d
w/liquid	18	1.0	4.2	.1	<.1	0	2	.7 d
drained, 4 oz.	23	1.3	5.1	.1	<.1	0	2	1.5 d
drained	13	.8	3.1	.1	<.1	0	1	.9 d
w/potatoes and mushrooms, in sauce								
(*Green Giant Pantry Express*) ..	50	1.0	9.0	2.0	<1.0	0	430	2.0 d
seasoned, w/liquid:								
4 oz.	18	.9	4.0	.2	.1	0	423	1.0 c
½ cup	18	1.0	4.0	.2	.1	0	425	1.0 c
French style (*Del Monte*)	20	1.0	4.0	0	0	0	355	m.q.
w/shelled beans and pork (*Luck's*),								
8 oz.	200	9.0	24.0	8.0	m.q.	m.q.	840	9.0 d
shelly beans (*Allens*)	35	2.0	6.0	<1.0	(0)	0	395	m.q.
GREEN BEAN, FREEZE-DRIED:								
(*Mountain House*), ½ cup[1]	35	1.0	6.0	0	0	0	tr.	m.q.
GREEN BEAN, FROZEN:								
10-oz. pkg.	94	5.1	21.5	.6	.1	0	8	5.1 d
boiled, drained, 4 oz.	29	1.5	6.9	.2	<.1	0	15	1.8 d
boiled, drained, ½ cup	18	.9	4.2	.1	<.1	0	9	1.1 d
(*Green Giant*), ½ cup	14	1.0	4.0	0	0	0	10	1.5 d
whole:								
(*Birds Eye* Deluxe), 3 oz.	25	1.0	5.0	0	0	0	0	2.0 d
(*Birds Eye* Farm Fresh), 4 oz.	30	2.0	7.0	0	0	0	0	2.0 d
(*Seabrook*), 3 oz.	25	1.0	5.0	0	0	0	1	1.0 c
(*Southern*), 3.5 oz.	33	1.6	6.8	.1	(0)	0	20	m.q.
cut:								
(*A&P*), 3 oz.	25	1.0	6.0	<1.0	(0)	0	140	m.q.
(*Birds Eye* Portion Pack), 3 oz. ...	25	1.0	6.0	0	0	0	0	2.0 d
(*Finast*), 3 oz.	25	1.0	6.0	0	0	0	5	m.q.
(*Frosty Acres*), 3 oz.	25	1.0	6.0	0	0	0	3	1.0 c
(*Green Giant Harvest Fresh*), ½ cup	16	1.0	4.0	0	0	0	95	1.0 d

1. *Prepared according to package directions.*

Food and Measure	cal.	prot. (gms)	carbo. (gms)	tot. fat (gms)	sat. fat (gms)	chol. (mgs)	sod. (mgs)	fiber (gms)
(*Seabrook*), 3 oz.	25	1.0	6.0	0	0	0	3	1.0 c
(*Stokely Singles*), 3 oz.	30	2.0	6.0	1.0	(0)	0	5	m.q.
cut or French style (*Birds Eye*),								
3 oz.	25	1.0	6.0	0	0	0	0	2.0 d
French style:								
(*A&P*), 3 oz.	25	1.0	6.0	<1.0	(0)	0	0	m.q.
(*Finast*), 3 oz.	25	1.0	6.0	0	0	0	5	m.q.
(*Frosty Acres*), 3 oz.	25	1.0	6.0	0	0	0	3	1.0 c
(*Seabrook*), 3 oz.	25	1.0	6.0	0	0	0	3	1.0 c
(*Southern*), 3.5 oz.	34	1.6	6.9	.1	(0)	0	20	m.q.
Italian:								
(*Birds Eye*), 3 oz.	30	2.0	7.0	0	0	0	0	3.0 d
(*Seabrook*), 3 oz.	30	2.0	7.0	0	0	0	3	1.0 c
cut (*Finast*), 3 oz.	30	2.0	7.0	0	0	0	5	m.q.
style (*Frosty Acres*), 3 oz.	30	2.0	7.0	0	0	0	3	1.0 c
petite (*Birds Eye* Deluxe), 2.6 oz. ..	20	1.0	5.0	0	0	0	0	2.0 d
in butter sauce (*Green Giant* One								
Serving), 5.5 oz.	60	2.0	8.0	2.0	1.0	5	370	3.0 d
in butter sauce, cut (*Green Giant*),								
½ cup	30	1.0	4.0	1.0	<1.0	5	230	1.5 d
GREEN BEAN COMBINATIONS,								
frozen:								
Bavarian style recipe, w/spaetzle, in								
sauce (*Birds Eye* International),								
3.3 oz.	100	2.0	11.0	5.0	m.q.	10	350	2.0 d
French, w/toasted almonds (*Birds								
Eye* Combinations), 3 oz.	50	3.0	8.0	2.0	m.q.	0	340	2.0 d
and mushroom, creamy (*Green Giant*								
Garden Gourmet*), 1 pkg.	220	6.0	29.0	11.0	6.0	25	860	4.0 d
mushroom casserole (*Stouffer's*),								
4.75 oz.	160	3.0	13.0	11.0	m.q.	n.a.	680	m.q.
GREEN BEAN SALAD, see "Bean								
salad"								
GREEN PEPPER, see "Pepper,								
sweet"								
GRENADINE:								
(*Rose's*), 1 fl. oz.	65	0	16.0	0	0	0	27	(0)
GRITS, see "Corn grits"								
GROUND CHERRY:								
in husk, 1 lb.	226	8.1	47.8	3.0	m.q.	0	m.q.	11.9 c
trimmed, 1 oz.	15	.5	3.2	.2	tr.	0	m.q.	.8 c
trimmed, ½ cup	37	1.3	7.8	.5	tr.	0	m.q.	2.0 c
GROUND HUSK TOMATO, see								
"Tomatillo"								
GROUND NUT, see "Peanut"								
GROUPER, mixed species, meat								
only:								
raw:								
1 lb.	417	87.9	0	4.6	1.1	166	239	0

Food and Measure	cal.	prot. (gms)	carbo. (gms)	tot. fat (gms)	sat. fat (gms)	chol. (mgs)	sod. (mgs)	fiber (gms)
GROUPER, RAW *(cont.)*								
1 oz.	26	5.5	0	.3	.1	10	15	0
1 fillet, approx. 9.1 oz., yield from								
3-lb. whole fish	238	50.2	0	2.6	.6	95	136	0
baked, broiled, or microwaved[1],								
4 oz.	134	28.2	0	1.5	.3	53	60	0
GUACAMOLE, see "Avocado dip"								
GUACAMOLE SEASONING:								
blend (*Lawry's*), 1 pkg.	60	1.7	12.6	.4	(0)	0	1495	.8 c
mix (*Old El Paso*), ⅐ pkg.	7	0	2.0	0	0	0	240	0
GUAVA, COMMON:								
untrimmed, 1 lb.	183	3.0	43.1	2.2	.6	0	9	20.3 c
trimmed, 1 oz.	15	.2	3.4	.2	<.1	0	1	1.6 c
trimmed, ½ cup	42	.7	9.8	.5	.1	0	2	4.6 c
1 medium, approx. 4 oz.	45	.7	10.7	.5	.2	0	2	5.0 c
GUAVA, STRAWBERRY:								
untrimmed, 1 lb.	268	2.2	66.9	2.3	.7	0	141	24.7 c
trimmed, 1 oz.	20	.2	4.9	.2	<.1	0	11	1.8 c
trimmed, ½ cup	85	.7	21.2	.7	.2	0	45	7.8 c
1 medium, approx. .2 oz.	4	<.1	1.0	<.1	<.1	0	2	.4 c
GUAVA FRUIT DRINK, Hawaiian:								
(*Ocean Spray Mauna La'i*), 6 fl. oz.	100	0	25.0	0	0	0	10	(0)
GUAVA JUICE:								
bottled or frozen[2] (*Welch's Orchard*								
Tropicals), 6 fl. oz.	100	0	25.0	0	0	0	20	0
GUAVA NECTAR:								
(*Libby's*), 6 fl. oz.	110	0	26.0	0	0	0	15	m.q.
GUAVA SAUCE, cooked:								
4 oz.	41	.4	10.8	.2	<.1	0	4	2.3 c
½ cup	43	.4	11.3	.2	<.1	0	4	2.4 c
GUAVA-PASSION FRUIT DRINK,								
Hawaiian:								
(*Ocean Spray Mauna La'i*), 6 fl. oz.	100	0	25.0	0	0	0	10	(0)
(*Pathmark* Hawaii), 6 fl. oz.	100	0	25.0	0	0	0	10	(0)
GUAVA-STRAWBERRY								
TROPICAL REFRESHER:								
(*Veryfine*), 8 fl. oz.	120	.3	30.0	0	0	0	<25	(0)
GUINEA HEN, fresh, raw:								
meat w/skin:								
1 lb.	717	106.1	0	29.3	m.q.	m.q.	m.q.	0
1 oz.	45	6.6	0	1.8	m.q.	m.q.	m.q.	0
½ hen, 12.2 oz., yield from								
14.6 oz. w/bone	545	80.7	0	22.3	m.q.	m.q.	m.q.	0
meat only:								
1 lb.	499	93.6	0	11.2	m.q.	286	m.q.	0
1 oz.	31	5.9	0	.7	m.q.	18	m.q.	0

1. *Without added ingredients.*
2. *Diluted according to package directions.*

Food and Measure	cal.	prot. (gms)	carbo. (gms)	tot. fat (gms)	sat. fat (gms)	chol. (mgs)	sod. (mgs)	fiber (gms)
½ hen, 9.3 oz., yield from 14.6 oz. w/bone and skin w/ separable fat	292	54.5	0	6.5	m.q.	166	m.q.	0
GUMBO, see "Okra"								
GUMBO FILE POWDER:								
(*Tone's*), 1 tsp.	8	.2	1.7	.2	<.1	0	<1	.6 d

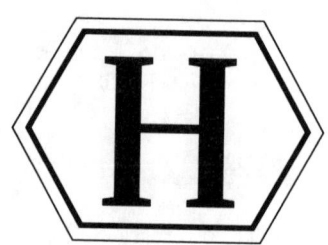

Food and Measure	cal.	prot. (gms)	carbo. (gms)	tot. fat (gms)	sat. fat (gms)	chol. (mgs)	sod. (mgs)	fiber (gms)
HÄAGEN-DAZS ICE CREAM								
SHOP (see also "Ice cream"):								
sorbet:								
lemon, 4 fl. oz.	140	1.0	34.0	0	0	n.a.	5	n.a.
orange, 4 oz.	113	1.0	30.0	0	0	n.a.	7	n.a.
raspberry, 4 oz.	93	0	22.0	0	0	n.a.	7	n.a.
yogurt, frozen, soft-serve, 1 fl. oz.:								
banana, nonfat	25	1.0	5.0	0	0	0	15	n.a.
chocolate	30	1.0	4.0	1.0	n.a.	3	13	(0)
chocolate, nonfat	30	1.0	6.0	0	0	0	20	(0)
coffee	28	1.0	4.0	1.0	n.a.	3	13	0
raspberry	30	1.0	5.0	1.0	n.a.	3	15	n.a.
strawberry, nonfat	25	1.0	5.0	0	0	0	10	n.a.
vanilla	28	1.0	4.0	1.0	n.a.	3	13	0
HADDOCK, meat only:								
raw:								
1 lb.	396	85.8	0	3.3	.6	261	310	0
1 oz.	25	5.4	0	.2	<.1	16	19	0
1 fillet, approx. 6.8 oz., yield from								
2½-lb. whole fish	168	36.5	0	1.4	.3	111	132	0
baked, broiled, or microwaved[1], 4 oz.	127	27.5	0	1.1	.2	84	99	0
smoked, 4 oz.	132	28.6	0	1.1	.2	87	865	0
smoked, 1 oz.	33	7.2	0	.3	<.1	22	216	0
HADDOCK, FROZEN, fillet:								
(*Booth* Individually Wrapped), 4 oz.	90	21.0	0	0	0	m.q.	70	0
(*Gorton's Fishmarket Fresh*), 5 oz. ..	110	25.0	0	1.0	m.q.	m.q.	120	0
(*SeaPak*), 4 oz.	90	18.0	0	1.0	m.q.	m.q.	120	0
(*Van de Kamp's* Natural), 4 oz.	90	21.0	0	1.0	0	20	125	0
HADDOCK ENTREE, frozen:								
battered fillets (*Mrs. Paul's*								
Crunchy), 2 pieces	190	14.0	22.0	5.0	m.q.	25	580	m.q.

1. *Without added ingredients.*

Food and Measure	cal.	prot. (gms)	carbo. (gms)	tot. fat (gms)	sat. fat (gms)	chol. (mgs)	sod. (mgs)	fiber (gms)
battered fillets (*Van de Kamp's*), 2 pieces	250	12.0	19.0	15.0	3.0	30	580	m.q.
breaded fillets:								
(*Mrs. Paul's* Light), 1 piece	220	17.0	15.0	9.0	m.q.	45	350	m.q.
(*Van de Kamp's*), 2 pieces	270	12.0	19.0	16.0	3.0	25	290	m.q.
(*Van de Kamp's* Light), 1 piece	240	15.0	21.0	11.0	2.0	35	380	m.q.
in lemon butter (*Gorton's Microwave Entrees*), 1 pkg.	360	23.0	19.0	21.0	10.0	100	730	m.q.
HAKE, see "Whiting"								
HALIBUT, ATLANTIC AND PACIFIC, meat only:								
raw:								
1 lb.	497	94.4	0	10.4	1.5	146	245	0
1 oz.	31	5.9	0	.6	.1	9	15	0
½ fillet, approx. 7.2 oz., yield from 5-lb. whole fish	223	42.5	0	4.7	.7	65	110	0
baked, broiled, or microwaved[1], 4 oz.	159	30.3	0	3.3	.5	46	78	0
HALIBUT, FROZEN:								
steaks, w/out seasoning mix (*SeaPak*), 6-oz. pkg.	160	36.0	0	1.0	m.q.	m.q.	120	0
HALIBUT, GREENLAND, meat only, raw:								
1 lb.	845	65.2	0	62.8	11.0	209	363	0
1 oz.	53	4.1	0	3.9	.7	13	23	0
½ fillet, approx. 7.2 oz., yield from 5-lb. whole fish	380	29.3	0	28.2	4.9	94	163	0
HALIBUT ENTREE, frozen:								
battered fillets (*Van de Kamp's*), 2 pieces	150	8.0	16.0	6.0	1.0	10	400	m.q.
HALVAH:								
(*Fantastic Foods*), 1.5-oz. bar	232	8.0	17.0	10.0	m.q.	0	0	m.q.
HAM[2], fresh (see also "Ham, cured"), boneless:								
whole leg, separable lean and fat:								
raw, 1 oz.	74	4.8	0	5.9	2.1	21	13	0
roasted:								
4 oz.	333	28.4	0	23.5	8.5	105	67	0
1.5-oz. slice, 4⅛″ × 2¼″ × ¼″	125	10.6	0	8.8	3.2	40	25	0
chopped or diced, 1 cup not packed	411	35.0	0	29.0	10.5	131	83	0
whole leg, separable lean only:								
raw, 1 oz.	39	5.8	0	1.5	.5	19	16	0
roasted:								
4 oz.	249	32.1	0	12.5	4.3	107	73	0
1.5-oz. slice, 4⅛″ × 2¼″ × ¼″	94	12.0	0	4.7	1.6	40	27	0

1. *Without added ingredients.*
2. *Cooked meats are prepared without added ingredients.*

Food and Measure	cal.	prot. (gms)	carbo. (gms)	tot. fat (gms)	sat. fat (gms)	chol. (mgs)	sod. (mgs)	fiber (gms)
HAM, WHOLE LEG, LEAN ONLY *(cont.)*								
chopped or diced, 1 cup not packed	309	39.7	0	15.4	5.3	131	90	0
rump half, separable lean and fat:								
raw, 1 oz.	66	5.2	0	4.9	1.8	19	17	0
roasted:								
4 oz.	311	30.2	0	20.2	7.3	108	69	0
1.5-oz. slice, 4⅛″ × 2¼″ × ¼″	117	11.3	0	7.6	2.7	40	26	0
chopped or diced, 1 cup not packed	384	37.3	0	24.9	9.1	133	85	0
rump half, separable lean only:								
raw, 1 oz.	39	6.0	0	1.5	.5	17	19	0
roasted:								
4 oz.	251	33.0	0	12.1	4.2	109	74	0
1.5-oz. slice, 4⅛″ × 2¼″ × ¼″	94	12.4	0	4.5	1.6	41	28	0
chopped or diced, 1 cup not packed	309	40.8	0	14.9	5.1	134	90	0
shank half, separable lean and fat:								
raw, 1 oz.	80	4.7	0	6.6	2.4	19	16	0
roasted:								
4 oz.	344	27.6	0	25.1	9.1	104	66	0
1.5-oz. slice, 4⅛″ × 2¼″ × ¼″	129	10.3	0	9.4	3.4	39	25	0
chopped or diced, 1 cup not packed	425	34.0	0	31.0	11.3	129	82	0
shank half, separable lean only:								
raw, 1 oz.	39	5.9	0	1.6	.6	17	19	0
roasted:								
4 oz.	244	32.0	0	11.9	4.1	104	73	0
1.5-oz. slice, 4⅛″ × 2¼″ × ¼″	91	12.0	0	4.5	1.5	39	27	0
chopped or diced, 1 cup not packed	301	39.5	0	14.7	5.1	129	90	0
HAM[1], CANNED:								
regular (approx. 13% fat):								
unheated, 1 oz.	54	4.8	<.1	3.7	1.2	11	352	0
unheated, chopped or diced, 1 cup not packed	266	23.8	<.1	18.2	6.0	55	1736	0
roasted, 4 oz.	256	23.3	.5	17.2	5.7	70	1067	0
roasted, chopped or diced, 1 cup not packed	317	28.7	.6	21.3	7.1	86	1317	0
extra lean and regular:								
unheated, 1 oz.	41	5.1	0	2.1	.7	11	362	0
unheated, chopped or diced, 1 cup not packed	201	25.2	0	10.4	3.4	54	1787	0
roasted, 4 oz.	189	23.7	.6	9.6	3.2	46	1211	0
roasted, chopped or diced, 1 cup not packed	234	29.3	.7	11.8	3.9	57	1495	0
extra lean (approx. 4% fat):								
unheated, 1 oz.	34	5.2	0	1.3	.4	11	356	0

1. *Cooked meats are prepared without added ingredients.*

Food and Measure	cal.	prot. (gms)	carbo. (gms)	tot. fat (gms)	sat. fat (gms)	chol. (mgs)	sod. (mgs)	fiber (gms)
unheated, chopped or diced, 1 cup								
not packed	168	25.9	0	6.4	2.1	53	1757	0
roasted, 4 oz.	154	24.0	.6	5.5	1.8	34	1287	0
roasted, chopped or diced, 1 cup								
not packed	191	29.6	.7	6.8	2.3	41	1589	0
(*Black Label*, 5 lb.), 4 oz.	140	20.0	0	7.0	m.q.	m.q.	1245	0
(*Black Label*, 3 lb.), 4 oz.	140	20.0	0	7.0	m.q.	m.q.	1315	0
(*Black Label*, 1½ lb.), 4 oz.	150	21.0	0	7.0	m.q.	m.q.	1324	0
(*EXL*), 4 oz.	120	22.0	0	4.0	m.q.	m.q.	1382	0
(*EXL* Deli Ham, 10 lb.), 4 oz.	130	20.0	0	6.0	m.q.	m.q.	1368	0
(*Holiday Glaze*, 3 lb.), 4 oz.	130	21.0	2.0	4.0	m.q.	m.q.	m.q.	0
(*Hormel* Bone-In), 4 oz.	210	17.0	1.0	15.0	m.q.	m.q.	m.q.	0
(*Hormel Cure 81*), 4 oz.	160	22.0	0	8.0	m.q.	m.q.	1322	0
(*Hormel Curemaster*), 4 oz.	140	22.0	1.0	5.0	m.q.	m.q.	1361	0
(*JM* 95% Fat Free), 2 oz.	60	10.0	1.0	2.0	m.q.	m.q.	680	0
(*Light & Lean* Boneless), 2 oz.	60	10.0	0	2.0	m.q.	m.q.	574	0
(*Oscar Mayer* Jubilee), 1 oz.	29	5.0	.1	.9	.4	14	287	0
chopped:								
1 oz.	68	4.6	.1	5.3	1.8	14	387	0
1 slice, 4¼″ × 4¼″ × ¹⁄₁₆″,								
approx. .75 oz.	50	3.4	.1	4.0	1.3	10	287	0
(*Hormel*, 8 lb.), 3 oz.	240	12.0	1.0	21.0	m.q.	m.q.	1062	0
(*Hormel*, 12 oz.), 2 oz.	120	10.0	0	9.0	m.q.	m.q.	703	0
chunk (*Hormel*), 6¾ oz.	310	32.0	0	20.0	m.q.	m.q.	2241	0
hickory smoked (*Rath Black Hawk*),								
2 oz.	60	10.0	1.0	2.0	m.q.	m.q.	720	0
roll (*Hormel*), 4 oz.	170	21.0	0	10.0	m.q.	m.q.	1338	0
spiced (*Hormel*), 3 oz.	240	13.0	1.0	21.0	m.q.	m.q.	1093	0

HAM, CHOPPED OR MINCED,
see "Ham, canned" and "Ham
luncheon meat"

HAM, CURED[1], boneless:

Food and Measure	cal.	prot. (gms)	carbo. (gms)	tot. fat (gms)	sat. fat (gms)	chol. (mgs)	sod. (mgs)	fiber (gms)
whole, separable lean and fat:								
unheated, 1 oz.	70	5.2	<.1	5.3	1.9	16	364	0
unheated, chopped or diced, 1 cup								
not packed	345	25.9	.1	25.9	9.3	78	1797	0
roasted, 4 oz.	276	24.5	0	19.0	6.8	70	1346	0
roasted, chopped or diced, 1 cup								
not packed	341	30.2	0	23.5	8.4	86	1661	0
whole, separable lean only:								
unheated, 1 oz.	42	6.3	<.1	1.6	.5	15	430	0
unheated, chopped or diced, 1 cup								
not packed	206	31.2	.1	8.0	2.7	73	2122	0
roasted, 4 oz.	178	28.4	0	6.2	2.1	62	1505	0
roasted, chopped or diced, 1 cup								
not packed	219	35.1	0	7.7	2.6	78	1858	0
whole (*JM*), 3 oz.	140	17.0	0	8.0	n.a.	n.a.	40	0

1. *Cooked meats are prepared without added ingredients.*

Food and Measure	cal.	prot. (gms)	carbo. (gms)	tot. fat (gms)	sat. fat (gms)	chol. (mgs)	sod. (mgs)	fiber (gms)
HAM, CURED *(cont.)*								
regular (approx. 11% fat):								
unheated, 1-oz. slice, 6¼" × 4" × ¹⁄₁₆"	52	5.0	.9	3.0	1.0	16	373	0
unheated, chopped or diced, 1 cup not packed	255	24.6	4.4	14.8	4.8	8	1844	0
roasted, 4 oz.	202	25.7	0	10.2	3.5	67	1701	0
roasted, chopped or diced, 1 cup not packed	249	31.7	0	12.6	4.4	83	2100	0
regular and extra lean:								
unheated, 1-oz. slice, 6¼" × 4" × ¹⁄₁₆"	46	5.2	.7	2.4	.8	15	362	0
unheated, chopped or diced, 1 cup not packed	227	25.6	3.2	11.8	3.8	74	1789	0
roasted, 4 oz.	187	24.9	.6	8.7	3.0	65	1571	0
roasted, chopped or diced, 1 cup not packed	231	30.8	.7	10.7	3.7	80	1938	0
extra lean (approx. 5% fat):								
unheated, 1-oz. slice, 6¼" × 4" × ¹⁄₁₆"	37	5.5	.3	1.4	.5	13	405	0
unheated, chopped or diced, 1 cup not packed	183	27.1	1.4	6.9	2.3	66	2000	0
roasted, 4 oz.	164	23.7	1.7	6.3	2.1	60	1364	0
roasted, chopped or diced, 1 cup not packed	203	29.3	2.1	7.7	2.5	74	1684	0
center slice, separable lean and fat, unheated, 1 oz.	57	5.7	<.1	3.7	1.3	15	393	0
country style, lean only, raw, 1 oz.	55	7.9	.1	2.4	.8	m.q.	m.q.	0
mini (*JM*), 3 oz.	90	17.0	0	3.0	m.q.	m.q.	40	0
w/natural juices (*JM* EZ Cut), 2 oz.	70	11.0	1.0	3.0	m.q.	m.q.	660	0
steak:								
unheated, 1 oz.	35	5.5	0	1.2	.4	13	360	0
unheated, 2-oz. steak	69	11.1	0	2.4	.8	26	720	0
(*Oscar Mayer* Jubilee), 2-oz. steak	57	9.7	.2	1.9	.7	31	754	0
"HAM," VEGETARIAN, frozen:								
roll or slices (*Worthington Wham*), 3 slices, approx. 2.4 oz.	120	11.0	3.0	7.0	1.0	0	940	m.q.
HAM BOLOGNA, see "Bologna"								
HAM BREAKFAST TACO, refrigerated:								
(*Owens Border Breakfasts*), 2.17 oz.	90	7.0	13.0	6.0	m.q.	50	430	m.q.
HAM DINNER, frozen:								
(*Morton*), 10 oz.	290	15.0	49.0	4.0	m.q.	45	1400	m.q.
steak:								
(*Armour Classics*), 10.75 oz.	270	15.0	36.0	7.0	m.q.	50	1320	m.q.
(*Le Menu*), 10 oz.	300	19.0	31.0	11.0	m.q.	m.q.	1500	m.q.
glazed (*Stouffer's Dinner Supreme*), 10.5 oz.	380	25.0	35.0	15.0	m.q.	m.q.	1960	m.q.

Food and Measure	cal.	prot. (gms)	carbo. (gms)	tot. fat (gms)	sat. fat (gms)	chol. (mgs)	sod. (mgs)	fiber (gms)
HAM ENTREE, frozen:								
(*Banquet* Platters), 10 oz.	400	20.0	43.0	17.0	m.q.	50	1180	m.q.
and asparagus, au gratin (*The Budget Gourmet* Slim Selects), 9 oz. ...	280	14.0	33.0	10.0	m.q.	40	1130	m.q.
and asparagus bake (*Stouffer's*), 9.5 oz.	510	18.0	31.0	35.0	m.q.	m.q.	900	m.q.
scalloped potatoes and (*Swanson* Homestyle Recipe), 9 oz.	300	19.0	26.0	13.0	m.q.	m.q.	1080	m.q.
HAM LUNCHEON MEAT (see also "Ham, cured" and "Ham, canned"):								
(*Boar's Head* Lower Salt), 1 oz.	28	5.0	<1.0	<1.0	m.q.	15	250	0
(*Healthy Deli* Deluxe), 1 oz.	31	4.7	1.1	.9	m.q.	12	245	0
(*Healthy Deli* Lessalt), 1 oz.	32	4.7	1.4	.9	m.q.	13	190	0
(*Healthy Deli* Light AM), 1 oz.	27	3.9	1.4	.6	m.q.	11	200	0
(*Healthy Deli* Taverne), 1 oz.	31	5.4	.3	.8	m.q.	15	210	0
(*JM* Slice 'n Eat 93% Fat Free), 2 oz.	70	10.0	1.0	3.0	m.q.	24	630	0
(*JM* Slice 'n Eat 95% Fat Free Presliced), 2 slices	60	9.0	1.0	2.0	m.q.	30	620	0
(*Jones Dairy Farm*), 1 slice	50	8.8	tr.	1.1	m.q.	21	381	0
(*Jones Dairy Farm* Family Ham), 1 oz.	35	5.8	tr.	1.2	m.q.	14	298	0
(*Kahn's* Low Salt), 1 slice	30	5.0	1.0	1.0	m.q.	m.q.	290	0
(*Oscar Mayer* Breakfast Ham), 1.5-oz. slice	47	7.2	1.2	1.5	.6	21	582	0
(*Oscar Mayer* Jubilee), 1 oz.	43	5.3	.1	2.4	.8	15	365	0
(*Oscar Mayer* Jubilee, 8-oz. Slice), 1 oz.	29	4.7	.1	1.1	.4	14	335	0
(*Occar Mayer* Lower Salt), .7-oz. slice	23	3.6	.6	.7	.3	10	174	0
(*Swift Premium* Hostess), 1 oz.	30	5.0	0	1.0	m.q.	m.q.	330	0
(*Swift Premium* Sugar Plum), 1 oz.	30	5.0	1.0	1.0	m.q.	m.q.	280	0
baked:								
(*Oscar Mayer*), .75-oz. slice	21	3.9	.4	.5	.1	11	238	0
Virginia (*Healthy Deli*), 1 oz.	34	4.8	1.6	.9	m.q.	12	245	0
Virginia (*Healthy Deli* Lessalt), 1 oz.	32	4.7	1.4	.9	m.q.	13	19	0
barbecue (*Light & Lean*), 2 slices ..	50	8.0	0	2.0	m.q.	m.q.	m.q.	0
Black Forest (*Healthy Deli*), 1 oz. ...	32	5.9	.4	.6	m.q.	16	220	0
boiled:								
(*Boar's Head* Deluxe), 1 oz.	28	5.0	1.0	<1.0	m.q.	15	275	0
(*Oscar Mayer*), .75-oz. slice	23	3.9	.3	.7	.1	12	275	0
(*Oscar Mayer* Thin Sliced), .4-oz. slice	13	2.2	.2	.4	.1	7	157	0
Cajun (*Hillshire Farm* Deli Select), 1 oz.	31	6.0	<1.0	.9	m.q.	m.q.	350	(0)

Food and Measure	cal.	prot. (gms)	carbo. (gms)	tot. fat (gms)	sat. fat (gms)	chol. (mgs)	sod. (mgs)	fiber (gms)
HAM LUNCHEON MEAT (cont.)								
chopped:								
1 oz.	65	4.9	0	4.9	1.6	15	389	0
1-oz. slice, 4″ × 4″ × ³⁄₃₂″	65	4.9	0	4.9	1.6	15	389	0
1 slice, 4¼″ × 4¼″ × ¹⁄₁₆″,								
.7 oz.	48	3.6	0	3.6	1.2	11	288	0
(Eckrich), 1-oz. slice	45	5.0	<1.0	2.0	m.q.	m.q.	350	0
(Eckrich Lean Supreme), 1-oz.								
slice	35	10.0	<1.0	2.0	m.q.	m.q.	350	0
(Hormel Perma-Fresh), 2 slices	88	11.0	0	5.0	m.q.	m.q.	685	0
(JM), 1-oz. slice	80	4.0	1.0	7.0	m.q.	m.q.	370	0
(Kahn's), 1 slice	50	5.0	1.0	3.0	m.q.	m.q.	360	0
(Light & Lean), 2 slices	70	8.0	.0	4.0	m.q.	m.q.	m.q.	0
(OHSE), 1 oz.	65	4.0	1.0	5.0	m.q.	m.q.	260	0
(Oscar Mayer), 1-oz. slice	41	4.4	.7	2.3	.7	14	303	0
cooked:								
(JM), 1 oz.	30	4.0	1.0	1.0	m.q.	m.q.	360	0
(OHSE), 1 oz.	30	5.0	1.0	1.0	m.q.	m.q.	260	0
fresh (Healthy Deli), 1 oz.	33	5.9	.2	.8	m.q.	13	120	0
sliced:								
regular (approx. 11% fat), 1-oz.								
slice, 6¼″ × 4″ × ¹⁄₁₆″	52	5.0	.9	3.0	1.0	16	373	0
extra lean (approx. 5% fat),								
1-oz. slice, 6¼″ × 4″ × ¹⁄₁₆″	37	5.5	.3	1.4	.5	13	405	0
(Kahn's), 1 slice	30	5.0	1.0	1.0	m.q.	m.q.	360	0
(Light & Lean), 2 slices	50	9.0	0	2.0	m.q.	m.q.	m.q.	0
glazed (Light & Lean), 2 slices	50	9.0	0	2.0	m.q.	m.q.	m.q.	0
honey:								
(Healthy Deli Honey Valley), 1 oz.	31	4.8	1.2	.8	m.q.	10	26	0
(Hillshire Farm Deli Select), 1 oz.	31	6.0	<1.0	.9	m.q.	m.q.	270	0
(Oscar Mayer), .75-oz. slice	23	3.8	.5	.6	.3	12	268	0
(Oscar Mayer Thin Sliced), .4-oz.								
slice	13	2.2	.3	.4	.2	7	153	0
jalapeño (Healthy Deli), 1 oz.	25	3.7	.8	.6	m.q.	11	260	(0)
loaf (Eckrich), 1-oz. slice	50	5.0	1.0	4.0	m.q.	m.q.	290	0
minced:								
1 oz.	75	4.6	.5	5.9	2.0	20	353	0
1 slice, 4¼″ × 4¼″ × ¹⁄₁₆″,								
approx. .75 oz.	55	3.4	.4	4.3	1.5	15	261	0
peppered:								
black (Light & Lean), 2 slices	50	9.0	0	2.0	m.q.	m.q.	m.q.	(0)
black, cracked (Oscar Mayer),								
.75-oz. slice	22	3.8	.2	.8	.3	11	284	(0)
chopped (Oscar Mayer), 1 oz.	55	4.4	.9	3.7	1.3	16	312	(0)
red (Light & Lean), 2 slices	50	9.0	0	2.0	m.q.	m.q.	m.q.	(0)
pit (OHSE), 1 oz.	40	4.0	1.0	2.0	m.q.	m.q.	300	0
smoked:								
(Eckrich Slender Sliced), 1 oz.	40	5.0	1.0	2.0	m.q.	m.q.	360	0
(Hillshire Farm Deli Select), 1 oz.	31	6.0	<1.0	.9	m.q.	m.q.	300	0

Food and Measure	cal.	prot. (gms)	carbo. (gms)	tot. fat (gms)	sat. fat (gms)	chol. (mgs)	sod. (mgs)	fiber (gms)
(*OHSE* 95% Fat Free), 1 oz.	30	5.0	1.0	1.0	m.q.	m.q.	310	0
cooked (*Light & Lean*), 2 slices ..	50	9.0	0	2.0	m.q.	m.q.	m.q.	0
cooked (*Oscar Mayer*), .75-oz.								
slice	22	3.8	.1	.7	.3	12	266	0
golden (*JM*), 2 oz.	80	8.0	1.0	5.0	m.q.	m.q.	630	0
golden, and water (*JM*), 2 oz. ...	70	8.0	4.0	2.0	m.q.	23	810	0
Virginia, see "baked," above								
HAM PATTY:								
(*Swift Premium* Brown 'N Serve),								
1 patty	130	3.0	1.0	13.0	m.q.	m.q.	260	0
unheated[1], 1 oz.	89	3.6	.5	8.0	2.9	20	308	0
unheated[1], 2.3-oz. patty	206	8.3	1.1	18.4	6.6	46	709	0
grilled:								
14.6 oz., yield from 1 lb.								
unheated	1411	54.9	7.0	127.4	45.8	297	4390	0
4 oz.	388	15.1	1.9	35.0	12.6	82	1205	0
1 patty, 2.1 oz., yield from 2.3-oz.								
unheated patty	203	7.9	1.0	18.4	6.6	43	632	0
canned (*Hormel*), 1 patty	180	7.0	0	16.0	m.q.	m.q.	456	0
HAM SALAD SPREAD:								
1 oz.	61	2.5	3.0	4.4	1.4	10	259	n.a.
1 tbsp.	32	1.3	1.6	2.3	.8	6	137	n.a.
HAM SPREAD, DEVILED,								
canned:								
(*Hormel*), 1 tbsp.	35	2.0	0	3.0	m.q.	m.q.	108	0
(*Underwood*), 2⅛ oz.	220	8.0	<1.0	19.0	6.0	50	430	n.a.
(*Underwood* Light), 2⅛ oz.	120	11.0	1.0	8.0	1.0	35	250	n.a.
smoked (*Underwood*), 2⅛ oz.	190	9.0	<1.0	18.0	6.0	65	260	n.a.
HAM STEAK, see "Ham, cured"								
and "Ham dinner"								
HAM AND ASPARAGUS AU								
GRATIN, frozen:								
(*The Budget Gourmet* Slim Selects),								
9 oz.	280	14.0	33.0	10.0	m.q.	40	1130	m.q.
HAM AND CHEESE								
BREAKFAST SANDWICH,								
refrigerated:								
(*Owens Border Breakfasts*), 2 oz. ...	150	7.0	14.0	6.0	m.q.	m.q.	600	m.q.
on bagel (*Swanson Great Starts*),								
3 oz.	240	12.0	28.0	8.0	m.q.	m.q.	600	m.q.
HAM AND CHEESE								
CASSEROLE, frozen:								
(*Pillsbury Microwave Classic*),								
1 pkg.	470	18.0	34.0	29.0	m.q.	m.q.	1300	n.a.
HAM AND CHEESE LOAF:								
1-oz. slice, 4″ × 4″ × ³/₃₂″	73	4.7	.4	5.7	2.1	16	381	0
(*Eckrich*), 1-oz. slice	50	4.0	1.0	4.0	m.q.	m.q.	300	0

1. *Product is fully cooked as purchased.*

Food and Measure	cal.	prot. (gms)	carbo. (gms)	tot. fat (gms)	sat. fat (gms)	chol. (mgs)	sod. (mgs)	fiber (gms)
HAM AND CHEESE LOAF *(cont.)*								
(*Hormel* Perma-Fresh), 2 slices	110	11.0	0	7.0	m.q.	m.q.	668	0
(*Kahn's*), 1 slice	70	4.0	1.0	6.0	m.q.	m.q.	310	0
(*Light & Lean*), 2 slices	90	8.0	0	6.0	m.q.	m.q.	m.q.	0
(*OHSE*), 1 oz.	65	4.0	2.0	5.0	m.q.	m.q.	190	0
(*Oscar Mayer*), 1-oz. slice	66	4.2	1.0	5.0	2.4	19	358	0
canned (*Hormel*, 8 lb.), 3 oz.	260	13.0	1.0	22.0	m.q.	m.q.	1135	0
HAM AND CHEESE PATTY:								
canned (*Hormel*), 1 patty	190	7.0	0	18.0	m.q.	m.q.	468	0
HAM AND CHEESE POCKET								
SANDWICH, frozen:								
(*Hot Pockets*), 5 oz.	360	19.0	36.0	16.0	m.q.	90	1320	m.q.
HAM AND CHEESE SPREAD:								
1 oz.	69	4.6	.6	5.3	2.4	17	339	0
1 tbsp.	37	2.4	.3	2.8	1.3	9	179	0
HAMBURGER, see "Beef, ground"								
and "Beef entree, frozen"								
"HAMBURGER," VEGETARIAN,								
see "Burger, vegetarian"								
HAMBURGER ENTREE MIX[1]**:**								
beef:								
noodle (*Hamburger Helper*),								
⅕ pkg. dry	140	5.0	26.0	2.0	m.q.	n.a.	1000	m.q.
noodle (*Hamburger Helper*), 1 cup	320	20.0	26.0	15.0	m.q.	m.q.	1050	m.q.
Romanoff (*Hamburger Helper*),								
⅕ pkg. dry	180	7.0	31.0	3.0	m.q.	n.a.	1030	m.q.
Romanoff (*Hamburger Helper*),								
1 cup	350	22.0	31.0	16.0	m.q.	m.q.	1070	m.q.
cheeseburger macaroni (*Hamburger*								
Helper), ⅕ pkg. dry	190	6.0	26.0	6.0	m.q.	n.a.	980	m.q.
cheeseburger macaroni (*Hamburger*								
Helper), 1 cup	370	21.0	28.0	19.0	m.q.	m.q.	1030	m.q.
chili:								
w/beans (*Hamburger Helper*),								
¼ pkg. dry	130	5.0	25.0	1.0	n.a.	n.a.	1680	m.q.
w/beans (*Hamburger Helper*),								
1¼ cup	350	24.0	25.0	17.0	m.q.	m.q.	1740	m.q.
tomato (*Hamburger Helper*),								
⅕ pkg. dry	150	5.0	31.0	1.0	n.a.	n.a.	1360	m.q.
tomato (*Hamburger Helper*), 1 cup	330	20.0	31.0	14.0	m.q.	m.q.	1410	m.q.
hamburger:								
hash (*Hamburger Helper*),								
⅕ pkg. dry	140	3.0	27.0	2.0	m.q.	n.a.	970	m.q.
hash (*Hamburger Helper*), 1 cup ..	320	18.0	27.0	15.0	m.q.	m.q.	1020	m.q.
stew (*Hamburger Helper*),								
⅕ pkg. dry	120	3.0	25.0	1.0	n.a.	n.a.	960	m.q.
stew (*Hamburger Helper*), 1 cup ..	300	18.0	25.0	14.0	m.q.	m.q.	1010	m.q.

1. *Prepared according to package directions, except as noted.*

Food and Measure	cal.	prot. (gms)	carbo. (gms)	tot. fat (gms)	sat. fat (gms)	chol. (mgs)	sod. (mgs)	fiber (gms)
Italian:								
cheesy (*Hamburger Helper*),								
⅕ pkg. dry	160	5.0	27.0	3.0	m.q.	n.a.	970	m.q.
cheesy (*Hamburger Helper*),								
1 cup[1]	360	22.0	30.0	17.0	m.q.	m.q.	1040	m.q.
zesty (*Hamburger Helper*),								
⅕ pkg. dry	170	6.0	35.0	1.0	n.a.	n.a.	940	m.q.
zesty (*Hamburger Helper*), 1 cup	340	21.0	35.0	13.0	m.q.	m.q.	980	m.q.
lasagne (*Hamburger Helper*),								
⅕ pkg. dry	160	5.0	33.0	1.0	n.a.	n.a.	1000	m.q.
lasagne (*Hamburger Helper*), 1 cup ..	340	21.0	33.0	14.0	m.q.	m.q.	1050	m.q.
meatloaf (*Hamburger Helper*),								
⅕ pkg. dry	70	2.0	13.0	1.0	n.a.	n.a.	620	m.q.
meatloaf (*Hamburger Helper*), 1 cup	360	27.0	14.0	22.0	m.q.	m.q.	710	m.q.
pizza:								
(*Hamburger Helper Pizzabake*),								
⅙ pkg. dry	150	4.0	29.0	2.0	m.q.	n.a.	800	m.q.
(*Hamburger Helper Pizzabake*),								
4.5 oz.	320	19.0	29.0	14.0	m.q.	m.q.	840	m.q.
dish (*Hamburger Helper*),								
⅕ pkg. dry	180	6.0	37.0	1.0	n.a.	n.a.	960	m.q.
dish (*Hamburger Helper*), 1 cup ..	360	21.0	37.0	14.0	m.q.	m.q.	1010	m.q.
potato:								
au gratin (*Hamburger Helper*),								
⅕ pkg. dry	150	4.0	28.0	2.0	m.q.	n.a.	860	m.q.
au gratin (*Hamburger Helper*),								
1 cup	320	19.0	28.0	15.0	m.q.	m.q.	910	m.q.
Stroganoff (*Hamburger Helper*),								
⅕ pkg. dry	140	3.0	28.0	2.0	m.q.	n.a.	900	m.q.
Stroganoff (*Hamburger Helper*),								
1 cup	320	18.0	28.0	15.0	m.q.	m.q.	950	m.q.
rice Oriental (*Hamburger Helper*),								
⅕ pkg. dry	180	4.0	38.0	1.0	n.a.	n.a.	1070	m.q.
rice Oriental (*Hamburger Helper*),								
1 cup	340	19.0	38.0	14.0	m.q.	m.q.	1120	m.q.
sloppy Joe (*Hamburger Helper Sloppy*								
Joe Bake), ⅙ pkg. dry	180	5.0	33.0	3.0	m.q.	n.a.	1060	m.q.
sloppy Joe (*Hamburger Helper Sloppy*								
Joe Bake), 5 oz.	340	18.0	33.0	15.0	m.q.	m.q.	1100	m.q.
spaghetti (*Hamburger Helper*),								
⅕ pkg. dry	170	5.0	32.0	2.0	m.q.	n.a.	1060	m.q.
spaghetti (*Hamburger Helper*), 1 cup	340	20.0	32.0	15.0	m.q.	m.q.	1110	m.q.
Stroganoff, creamy (*Hamburger*								
Helper), ⅕ pkg. dry	190	5.0	30.0	5.0	m.q.	n.a.	800	m.q.
Stroganoff, creamy (*Hamburger*								
Helper), 1 cup[2]	390	22.0	30.0	20.0	m.q.	m.q.	870	m.q.

1. *Prepared with 2% lowfat milk.*
2. *Prepared with whole milk.*

Food and Measure	cal.	prot. (gms)	carbo. (gms)	tot. fat (gms)	sat. fat (gms)	chol. (mgs)	sod. (mgs)	fiber (gms)
HAMBURGER ENTREE MIX *(cont.)*								
taco *(Hamburger Helper Tacobake)*,								
⅙ pkg. dry	170	4.0	31.0	4.0	m.q.	n.a.	920	m.q.
taco *(Hamburger Helper Tacobake)*,								
5.75 oz.	320	17.0	31.0	15.0	m.q.	m.q.	940	m.q.
tamale pie *(Hamburger Helper)*,								
⅕ pkg. dry	200	4.0	39.0	3.0	m.q.	n.a.	890	m.q.
tamale pie *(Hamburger Helper)*,								
1 cup	380	19.0	39.0	16.0	m.q.	m.q.	940	m.q.
HAMBURGER RELISH, see								
"Relish"								
HAMBURGER ROLL, see "Roll"								
HARDEE'S:								
breakfast, 1 serving:								
Big Country Breakfast:								
bacon, 7.7 oz.	660	24.0	51.0	40.0	10.0	305	1540	m.q.
country ham, 9 oz.	670	29.0	52.0	38.0	9.0	345	2870	m.q.
ham, 8.9 oz.	620	28.0	51.0	33.0	7.0	325	1780	m.q.
sausage, 9.7 oz.	850	33.0	51.0	57.0	16.0	340	1980	m.q.
biscuit:								
bacon, 3.3 oz.	360	10.0	34.0	21.0	4.0	10	950	m.q.
bacon and egg, 4.4 oz.	410	15.0	35.0	24.0	5.0	155	990	m.q.
bacon, egg, and cheese, 4.8 oz.	460	17.0	35.0	28.0	8.0	165	1220	m.q.
Biscuit 'N' Gravy, 7.8 oz.	440	9.0	45.0	24.0	6.0	15	1250	m.q.
Canadian Rise 'N' Shine,								
5.7 oz.	470	22.0	35.0	27.0	8.0	180	1550	m.q.
chicken, 5.1 oz.	430	17.0	42.0	22.0	4.0	45	1330	m.q.
Cinnamon 'N' Raisin, 2.8 oz.	320	4.0	37.0	17.0	5.0	0	510	m.q.
country ham, 3.8 oz.	350	11.0	35.0	18.0	3.0	25	1550	m.q.
country ham and egg, 4.9 oz. ..	400	16.0	35.0	22.0	4.0	175	1600	m.q.
ham, 3.7 oz.	320	10.0	34.0	16.0	2.0	15	1000	m.q.
ham and egg, 4.9 oz.	370	15.0	35.0	19.0	4.0	160	1050	m.q.
ham, egg, and cheese, 5.3 oz.	420	18.0	35.0	23.0	6.0	170	1270	m.q.
Rise 'N' Shine, 2.9 oz.	320	5.0	34.0	18.0	3.0	0	740	m.q.
sausage, 4.2 oz.	440	13.0	34.0	28.0	7.0	25	1100	m.q.
sausage and egg, 5.3 oz.	490	18.0	35.0	31.0	8.0	170	1150	m.q.
steak, 5.2 oz.	500	15.0	46.0	29.0	7.0	30	1320	m.q.
steak and egg, 6.3 oz.	550	20.0	47.0	32.0	8.0	175	1370	m.q.
Hash Rounds, 2.8 oz.	230	3.0	24.0	14.0	3.0	0	560	m.q.
margarine/butter blend, .2 oz. ...	35	0	0	4.0	<1.0	5	40	0
pancake syrup, 1.5 oz.	120	<1.0	31.0	<1.0	1.0	0	25	0
pancakes, 3 pieces:								
4.8 oz.	280	8.0	56.0	2.0	1.0	15	890	m.q.
w/2 bacon strips, 5.3 oz.	350	13.0	56.0	9.0	3.0	25	1110	m.q.
w/1 sausage patty, 6.2 oz.	430	16.0	56.0	16.0	6.0	40	1290	m.q.
sandwiches, 1 serving:								
Big Deluxe burger, 7.6 oz.	500	27.0	32.0	30.0	12.0	70	760	m.q.
Big Roast Beef, 4.7 oz.	300	18.0	32.0	11.0	5.0	45	880	m.q.
Big Twin, 6.1 oz.	450	23.0	34.0	25.0	11.0	55	580	m.q.

Food and Measure	cal.	prot. (gms)	carbo. (gms)	tot. fat (gms)	sat. fat (gms)	chol. (mgs)	sod. (mgs)	fiber (gms)
cheeseburger:								
4.3 oz.	320	16.0	33.0	14.0	7.0	30	710	m.q.
bacon, 7.7 oz.	610	34.0	31.0	39.0	16.0	80	1030	m.q.
quarter pound, 6.4 oz.	500	29.0	34.0	29.0	14.0	70	1060	m.q.
chicken breast, grilled, 6.8 oz. ...	310	24.0	34.0	9.0	1.0	60	890	m.q.
Chicken Fillet, 6.1 oz.	370	19.0	44.0	13.0	2.0	55	1060	m.q.
Fisherman's Fillet, 7.3 oz.	500	23.0	49.0	24.0	6.0	70	1030	m.q.
hamburger, 3.9 oz.	270	13.0	33.0	10.0	4.0	20	490	m.q.
hot dog, all beef, 4.2 oz.	300	11.0	25.0	17.0	8.0	25	710	m.q.
Hot Ham 'N' Cheese, 5.3 oz.	330	23.0	32.0	12.0	5.0	65	1420	m.q.
Mushroom 'N' Swiss burger,								
6.6 oz.	490	30.0	33.0	27.0	13.0	70	940	m.q.
roast beef, regular, 4 oz.	260	15.0	31.0	9.0	4.0	35	730	m.q.
Turkey Club, 7.3 oz.	390	29.0	32.0	16.0	4.0	70	1280	m.q.
salads, side dishes and special items:								
Chicken Stix, 9 pieces, 5.3 oz. ...	310	28.0	20.0	14.0	3.0	55	1020	m.q.
Chicken Stix, 6 pieces, 3.5 oz. ...	210	19.0	13.0	9.0	2.0	35	680	m.q.
Crispy Curls, 3 oz.	300	4.0	36.0	16.0	3.0	0	840	m.q.
french fries:								
big, 5.5 oz.	500	6.0	66.0	23.0	5.0	0	180	m.q.
large, 4 oz.	360	4.0	48.0	17.0	3.0	0	135	m.q.
regular, 2.5 oz.	230	3.0	30.0	11.0	2.0	0	85	m.q.
salad:								
chef, 10.4 oz.	240	22.0	5.0	15.0	9.0	115	930	m.q.
chicken 'n' pasta, 14.6 oz.	230	27.0	23.0	3.0	1.0	55	380	m.q.
garden, 8.5 oz.	210	14.0	3.0	14.0	8.0	105	270	m.q.
side, 4 oz.	20	2.0	1.0	<1.0	<1.0	0	15	m.q.
dressings, sauces, and condiments:								
barbecue dipping sauce, 1 oz. ...	30	<1.0	8.0	<1.0	<1.0	0	300	0
barbecue sauce, .5-oz. pkt.	14	<1.0	4.0	<1.0	<1.0	0	140	0
Big Twin sauce, .5 oz.	50	<1.0	4.0	4.0	<1.0	5	35	n.a.
blue cheese dressing, 2 oz.	210	1.0	10.0	18.0	3.0	20	790	0
catsup, .5 oz.	14	<1.0	3.0	<1.0	<1.0	0	135	(0)
catsup, .4-oz. pkt.	12	<1.0	3.0	<1.0	<1.0	0	115	(0)
French dressing, reduced calorie,								
2 oz.	130	1.0	21.0	5.0	1.0	0	480	0
honey sauce, .5 oz.	45	<1.0	11.0	<1.0	<1.0	0	0	0
horseradish, .25-oz. pkt.	25	<1.0	1.0	2.0	<1.0	5	35	n.a.
house dressing, 2 oz.	290	1.0	6.0	29.0	4.0	25	510	n.a.
Italian dressing, reduced calorie[1],								
2 oz.	90	<1.0	5.0	8.0	1.0	0	310	(0)
mayonnaise, .5 oz.	50	<1.0	1.0	5.0	1.0	5	75	0
mustard, .1 oz.	tr.	<1.0	<1.0	<1.0	<1.0	0	10	(0)
mustard, .3-oz. pkt.	6	<1.0	<1.0	<1.0	<1.0	0	120	(0)
sweet mustard dipping sauce,								
1 oz.	50	<1.0	10.0	<1.0	<1.0	0	160	(0)
sweet 'n' sour dipping sauce,								
1 oz.	40	<1.0	10.0	<1.0	<1.0	0	95	0

1. *Depending on supplier, dressing may contain 100 calories.*

Food and Measure	cal.	prot. (gms)	carbo. (gms)	tot. fat (gms)	sat. fat (gms)	chol. (mgs)	sod. (mgs)	fiber (gms)
HARDEE'S, DRESSINGS _(cont.)_								
tartar sauce, .7 oz.	90	<1.0	2.0	9.0	1.0	10	160	n.a.
Thousand Island dressing, 2 oz. . . .	250	1.0	9.0	23.0	3.0	35	540	n.a.
desserts and shakes:								
apple turnover, 3.2 oz.	270	3.0	38.0	12.0	4.0	0	250	m.q.
Big Cookie, 1.7 oz.	250	3.0	31.0	13.0	4.0	5	240	m.q.
Cool Twist cone:								
chocolate, 4.2 oz.	200	4.0	31.0	6.0	4.0	20	65	m.q.
vanilla, 4.2 oz.	190	5.0	28.0	6.0	4.0	15	100	m.q.
vanilla/chocolate, 4.2 oz.	190	4.0	29.0	6.0	4.0	20	80	m.q.
Cool Twist sundae:								
caramel, 6 oz.	330	6.0	54.0	10.0	5.0	20	290	(0)
hot fudge, 5.9 oz.	320	7.0	45.0	12.0	6.0	25	270	(0)
strawberry, 5.9 oz.	260	5.0	43.0	8.0	5.0	15	115	(0)
shake:								
chocolate, 12 oz.	460	11.0	85.0	8.0	5.0	45	340	(0)
strawberry, 12 oz.	440	11.0	82.0	8.0	5.0	40	300	(0)
vanilla, 12 oz.	400	13.0	66.0	9.0	6.0	50	320	0
HAWAIIAN YAM, see "Yam,								
mountain"								
HAZELNUT, see "Filbert"								
HAZELNUT OIL:								
1 oz.	251	0	0	28.4	2.1	0	0	0
½ cup	964	0	0	109.0	8.1	0	0	0
1 tbsp.	120	0	0	13.6	1.0	0	0	0
HEAD CHEESE:								
(_Oscar Mayer_), 1-oz. slice	55	4.5	.1	4.0	1.4	25	347	0
pork, 1-oz. slice, 4″ × 4″ × ³⁄₃₂″ . . .	60	4.5	.1	4.5	1.4	23	356	0
HEART[1]:								
beef:								
raw, 1 oz.	33	4.8	.7	1.1	.3	40	18	0
simmered, 9.1 oz., yield from 1 lb.								
raw	450	74.0	1.1	14.4	4.3	496	162	0
simmered, 4 oz.	198	32.6	.5	6.4	1.9	219	71	0
chicken, broiler-fryer:								
raw, 1 heart, .2 oz.	9	1.0	<.1	.6	.2	8	5	0
simmered, 4 oz.	210	29.9	.1	9.0	2.6	275	54	0
simmered, 1 heart, .1 oz.	6	.9	tr.	.3	.1	8	2	0
lamb:								
raw, 1 oz.	35	4.7	.1	1.6	.6	38	25	0
simmered, 6.7 oz., yield from								
1 lb. raw	354	47.7	3.7	15.1	6.0	476	120	0
simmered, 4 oz.	210	28.3	2.2	9.0	3.6	282	71	0
pork:								
raw, 1 oz.	33	4.9	.4	1.2	.3	37	16	0
braised:								
4.6 oz., yield from 8 oz. raw . .	191	30.4	.5	6.5	1.7	285	46	0
4 oz.	168	26.8	.5	5.7	1.5	251	40	0

1. _Cooked meats are prepared without added ingredients._

Food and Measure	cal.	prot. (gms)	carbo. (gms)	tot. fat (gms)	sat. fat (gms)	chol. (mgs)	sod. (mgs)	fiber (gms)
chopped or diced, 1 cup not packed	214	34.2	.6	7.3	1.9	320	51	0
turkey:								
raw, 1 oz.	41	5.2	.2	2.0	.6	33	25	0
simmered:								
4 oz.	201	30.3	2.3	6.9	2.0	256	62	0
.6 oz., yield from 11.2-lb.								
turkey	28	4.3	.3	1.0	.3	36	9	0
chopped or diced, 1 cup	257	38.8	3.0	8.8	2.5	327	79	0
veal:								
raw, 1 oz.	31	4.9	<.1	1.1	.3	30	22	0
simmered, 7 oz., yield from 1 lb.								
raw	368	57.7	.3	13.4	3.6	349	116	0
simmered, 4 oz.	211	33.0	.1	7.7	2.1	200	66	0
HEART NUT, see "Cashew"								
HERB AND GARLIC SAUCE:								
w/lemon juice (*Lawry's*), ¼ cup	36	3.6	3.8	.4	n.a.	n.a.	3688	<.1 c
HERB GRAVY MIX[1]**:**								
(*McCormick/Schilling*), ¼ cup	20	.5	3.0	.5	n.a.	n.a.	312	n.a.
HERB SEASONING AND COATING MIX:								
Italian (*McCormick/Schilling* Bag'n Season), 1 pkg.	94	2.0	21.0	.2	n.a.	n.a.	1367	m.q.
Italian (*Shake'n Bake*), ¼ pouch	80	2.0	14.0	1.0	n.a.	0	620	m.q.
HERB SIDE DISH MIX:								
(*Hain* 3-Grain Side Dish), ½ cup ...	80	3.0	15.0	1.0	n.a.	0	470	m.q.
HERBAL TEA, see "Tea, herbal"								
HERBS, see specific listings								
HERBS, MIXED:								
seasoning (*Lawry's* Pinch of Herbs), 1 tsp.	9	.3	.9	.5	n.a.	0	259	.2 c
HERRING, ATLANTIC, meat only:								
raw:								
1 lb.	718	81.5	0	41.0	9.3	272	407	0
1 oz.	45	5.1	0	2.6	.6	17	26	0
1 fillet, approx. 6.5 oz., yield from 1½-lb. whole fish	291	33.1	0	16.60	3.8	110	165	0
baked, broiled, or microwaved[2], 4 oz.	230	26.1	0	13.1	3.0	87	130	0
kippered, 4 oz.	246	27.9	0	14.0	3.2	93	1041	0
kippered, 1 piece, 4⅜″ × 1¾″ × ¼″	87	9.8	0	5.0	1.1	33	367	0
pickled, 4 oz.	297	16.1	10.9	20.4	2.7	15	987	0
pickled, 1 piece, 1¾″ × ⅞″ × ½″	39	2.1	1.5	2.7	.4	2	131	0
HERRING, CANNED, see "Sardine, canned"								

1. *Prepared according to package directions.*
2. *Without added ingredients.*

Food and Measure	cal.	prot. (gms)	carbo. (gms)	tot. fat (gms)	sat. fat (gms)	chol. (mgs)	sod. (mgs)	fiber (gms)
HERRING, KIPPERED, see								
"Herring, Atlantic" and								
"Sardine, canned"								
HERRING, LAKE, see "Cisco"								
HERRING, PACIFIC, meat only,								
raw:								
1 lb.	885	74.4	0	63.0	14.8	348	335	0
1 oz.	55	4.6	0	3.9	.9	22	21	0
1 fillet, approx. 6.5 oz., yield from								
1½-lb. whole fish	359	30.2	0	25.5	6.0	141	136	0
HERRING, PICKLED, see								
"Herring, Atlantic"								
HICKORY NUT, dried:								
in shell, 1 lb.	954	18.5	26.5	93.4	10.2	0	1	4.7 c
shelled, 1 oz.	187	3.6	5.2	18.3	2.0	0	tr.	.9 c
HIRATAKE MUSHROOM, see								
"Mushroom, oyster"								
HOG PLUM:								
seeded, 1 oz.	20	.2	3.9	.6	n.a.	0	n.a.	.3 c
HOLLANDAISE SAUCE:								
(*Great Impressions*), 2 tbsp.	192	.5	.3	21.0	m.q.	48	107	m.q.
(*Tone's*), 1 tsp.	15	.3	1.3	1.0	n.a.	n.a.	60	n.a.
mix:								
w/butterfat, 1.2-oz. pkt.	187	3.7	10.8	15.5	9.1	40	1230	<.1 c
w/butterfat, ½ cup[1]	119	2.4	6.9	9.9	5.8	26	783	<.1 c
w/vegetable oil, .9-oz. pkt.	93	3.4	15.5	2.3	.5	tr.	645	.1 c
w/vegetable oil, ½ cup[2]	352	4.1	9.0	34.1	20.9	95	567	<.1 c
(*McCormick/Schilling*), ¼ pkg. ..	51	1.0	3.5	3.8	m.q.	n.a.	170	m.q.
HOMESTYLE GRAVY MIX, see								
"Gravy mix"								
HOMINY, canned:								
golden:								
(*Allens*), ½ cup	80	2.0	16.0	<1.0	n.a.	0	370	m.q.
(*Van Camp's*), 1 cup	128	2.7	27.9	.6	n.a.	0	701	.8 c
w/red and green peppers (*Van*								
Camp's), 1 cup	129	2.6	28.5	.5	n.a.	0	685	.7 c
Mexican (*Allens*), ½ cup	80	2.0	16.0	<1.0	n.a.	0	330	m.q.
white:								
or yellow, 4 oz.	82	1.7	16.2	1.0	.1	0	238	.5 c
or yellow, ½ cup	57	1.2	11.4	.7	.1	0	168	.4 c
(*Allens*), ½ cup	70	2.0	16.0	<1.0	n.a.	0	430	m.q.
(*Van Camp's*), 1 cup	138	3.0	30.0	.7	n.a.	0	708	.8 c
HOMINY GRITS, see "Corn grits"								
HON SHIMEJI, see "Mushroom,								
Japanese honey"								
HONEY:								
½-oz. pkt.	43	tr.	11.5	0	0	0	1	0

1. *Prepared according to package directions, with water.*
2. *Prepared according to package directions, with whole milk and butter.*

Food and Measure	cal.	prot. (gms)	carbo. (gms)	tot. fat (gms)	sat. fat (gms)	chol. (mgs)	sod. (mgs)	fiber (gms)
(*Golden Blossom Honey*), 1 tbsp. ...	60	0	16.0	0	0	0	n.a.	0
(*Sioux Honey*), 1 tbsp.	60	0	16.0	0	0	0	n.a.	0
HONEY BUN, see "Bun, sweet"								
HONEY BUTTER:								
(*Honey Butter*), 1 tbsp. or ½ oz. ...	50	<1.0	11.0	1.0	n.a.	n.a.	5	0
HONEY LOAF:								
(*Eckrich*), 1-oz. slice	35	4.0	2.0	1.0	m.q.	m.q.	280	0
(*Eckrich Smorgas Pac*), 1-oz. slice ..	35	4.0	2.0	1.0	m.q.	m.q.	280	0
(*Hormel* Perma-Fresh), 2 slices	90	1.0	0	5.0	m.q.	m.q.	584	0
(*Kahn's*), 1 slice	40	4.0	1.0	2.0	m.q.	m.q.	320	0
(*Oscar Mayer*), 1-oz. slice	34	5.2	1.0	1.0	.4	16	378	0
pork and beef, 1-oz. slice, 4″ × 4″ × ³⁄₃₂″	36	4.5	1.5	1.3	.4	10	374	0
HONEY ROLL SAUSAGE, beef:								
1 oz.	52	5.3	.6	3.0	1.2	14	375	0
1 slice, 4″ diam. × ⅛″, approx. .8 oz.	42	4.3	.5	2.4	.9	12	304	0
HONEYDEW:								
untrimmed, 1 lb.	74	1.0	19.2	.2	(0)	0	21	1.3 c
pulp, 1 oz.	10	.1	2.6	<.1	(0)	0	3	.2 c
¹⁄₁₀ melon, 7″ × 2″ slice, approx. 8 oz.	46	.6	11.8	.1	(0)	0	13	.8 c
cubed, ½ cup	30	.4	7.8	.1	(0)	0	9	.5 c
HORSE, meat only:								
raw, 1 oz.	38	6.1	0	1.3	.4	15	15	0
roasted[1]:								
12 oz., yield from 1 lb. raw boneless	594	95.7	0	20.6	6.5	231	189	0
4 oz.	198	31.9	0	6.9	2.2	77	62	0
diced, 1 cup, approx. 4.9 oz.	245	39.4	0	8.5	2.7	95	77	0
HORSE BEAN SEEDS, dried:								
whole, 1 oz.	94	7.2	16.2	.4	n.a.	0	n.a.	tr.c
HORSERADISH, prepared:								
(*Crowley*), 1 oz.	10	<1.0	2.0	<1.0	(0)	0	25	m.q.
(*Kraft*), 1 tbsp.	10	0	1.0	0	0	0	140	m.q.
cream style (*Kraft*), 1 tbsp.	12	0	1.0	0	0	0	85	m.q.
hot (*Gold's*), 1 tsp.	4	<1.0	<1.0	<1.0	(0)	0	60	m.q.
red (*Gold's*), 1 tsp.	4	<1.0	<1.0	0	0	0	75	m.q.
white (*Gold's*), 1 tsp.	4	<1.0	<1.0	<1.0	(0)	0	55	m.q.
HORSERADISH, JAPANESE, see "Wasabi"								
HORSERADISH SAUCE:								
(*Great Impressions*), 1 tbsp.	74	0	1.4	7.6	m.q.	1	199	m.q.
(*Heinz*), 1 tbsp.	74	.2	2.0	7.4	m.q.	n.a.	113	m.q.
(*Sauceworks*), 1 tbsp.	50	0	2.0	5.0	1.0	5	105	m.q.
strong (*Life* All Natural), .25 fl. oz. or ½ tbsp.	7	<1.0	<1.0	<1.0	(0)	0	<2	m.q.

1. *Without added ingredients.*

Food and Measure	cal.	prot. (gms)	carbo. (gms)	tot. fat (gms)	sat. fat (gms)	chol. (mgs)	sod. (mgs)	fiber (gms)
HORSERADISH TREE:								
leafy tips:								
raw:								
untrimmed, 1 lb.	181	26.4	23.3	3.9	n.a.	0	26	4.2 c
trimmed, 1 oz.	18	2.7	2.3	.4	n.a.	0	3	.4 c
chopped, ½ cup	6	.9	.8	.1	n.a.	0	1	.2 c
boiled, drained, 4 oz.	68	6.0	12.6	1.1	n.a.	0	10	2.0 c
boiled, drained, chopped, ½ cup	13	1.1	2.3	.2	n.a.	0	2	.4 c
pods:								
raw:								
untrimmed, 1 lb.	88	5.0	20.1	.5	n.a.	0	99	3.1 c
trimmed, 1 oz.	10	.6	2.4	.1	n.a.	0	12	.4 c
1 pod, 15⅓″ × ½″, approx.								
.7 oz.	4	.2	.9	<.1	n.a.	0	5	.1 c
sliced, ½ cup	19	1.1	4.3	.1	n.a.	0	21	.7 c
boiled, drained, 4 oz.	41	2.4	9.3	.2	n.a.	0	49	2.1 c
boiled, drained, sliced, ½ cup . . .	21	1.2	4.8	.1	n.a.	0	25	1.1 c
HOT DOG, see "Frankfurter"								
HOT DOG BATTER MIX, see								
"Corn dog batter mix"								
HOT DOG SAUCE, see "Chili								
sauce"								
HUBBARD SQUASH:								
raw:								
untrimmed, 1 lb.	116	5.8	25.3	1.5	.3	0	20	4.1 c
trimmed, 1 oz.	11	.6	2.5	.1	<.1	0	2	.4 c
cubed, ½ cup	23	1.2	5.1	.3	.1	0	4	.8 c
baked, 4 oz.	57	2.8	12.3	.7	.1	0	9	2.0 c
baked, cubed, ½ cup	51	2.5	11.0	.6	.1	0	8	1.8 c
boiled, drained, mashed, 4 oz.	34	1.7	7.3	.4	.1	0	6	1.2 c
boiled, drained, mashed, ½ cup . . .	35	1.8	7.6	.4	.1	0	6	1.2 c
HUMMUS:								
1 oz.	48	1.4	5.7	2.4	.4	0	69	.4 c
½ cup	210	6.0	24.8	10.4	1.6	0	300	1.7 c
dip mix (*Fantastic Foods*), 2 oz. or								
¼ cup	111	4.0	9.5	6.5	m.q.	0	263	m.q.
mix (*Casbah*), 1 oz. dry	110	5.0	10.0	5.0	m.q.	0	n.a.	m.q.
HUSH PUPPY:								
frozen (*SeaPak* Regular), 4 oz.	330	6.0	56.0	9.0	m.q.	n.a.	690	m.q.
mix:								
deluxe (*Golden Dipt*), 1¼ oz.	120	3.0	26.0	0	0	0	520	m.q.
jalapeño (*Golden Dipt*), 1¼ oz. . . .	120	3.0	27.0	0	0	0	570	m.q.
w/onion (*Golden Dipt*), 1¼ oz. . . .	120	3.0	27.0	0	0	0	520	m.q.
HYACINTH BEAN:								
raw:								
untrimmed, 1 lb.	196	8.9	38.8	.8	.4	0	8	5.5 c
trimmed, 1 oz.	13	.6	2.6	.1	<.1	0	<1	.4 c
trimmed, ½ cup	19	.8	3.7	.1	<.1	0	1	.5 c

Food and Measure	cal.	prot. (gms)	carbo. (gms)	tot. fat (gms)	sat. fat (gms)	chol. (mgs)	sod. (mgs)	fiber (gms)
boiled, drained, 4 oz.	57	3.3	10.4	.3	.1	0	2	2.0 c
boiled, drained, ½ cup	22	1.3	4.1	.1	.1	0	1	.8 c
HYACINTH BEAN, MATURE, dried:								
raw, 1 oz.	98	6.8	17.2	.5	n.a.	0	6	2.0 c
raw, ½ cup	362	25.1	63.8	1.8	n.a.	0	22	7.5 c
boiled, 4 oz.	133	9.2	23.5	.7	n.a.	0	8	2.8 c
boiled, ½ cup	114	7.9	20.1	.6	n.a.	0	7	2.4 c

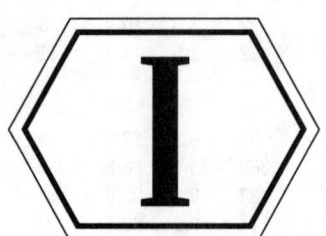

Food and Measure	cal.	prot. (gms)	carbo. (gms)	tot. fat (gms)	sat. fat (gms)	chol. (mgs)	sod. (mgs)	fiber (gms)
ICE (see also "Sherbet" and "Sorbet"):								
cherry, Italian (*Good Humor*), 6 fl. oz.	138	0	34.2	.1	(0)	0	0	(0)
daiquiri (*Baskin-Robbins*), 1 regular scoop	140	0	35.0	0	0	0	150	(0)
ICE BAR (see also "Fruit bar" and "Gelatin bar"), 1 piece:								
all flavors:								
(*Gold Bond* Twin Pop)	60	0	14.0	0	0	0	0	(0)
(*Good Humor* Ice Stripes), 1.5 fl. oz.	35	0	8.6	0	0	0	0	(0)
(*Popsicle* All Natural)	60	0	14.0	0	0	0	0	(0)
except cherry and wild berry *Popsicle* Water Ice)	50	0	12.0	0	0	0	10	(0)
cherry (*Good Humor Calippo*), 4.5 fl. oz.	138	.1	34.9	.1	(0)	0	5	(0)
cherry (*Popsicle* Water Ice)	70	0	17.0	0	0	0	15	(0)
lemon (*Good Humor Calippo*), 4.5 fl. oz.	112	0	27.6	.1	(0)	0	0	(0)
orange (*Good Humor Calippo*), 4.5 fl. oz.	111	0	27.2	.2	(0)	0	0	(0)
wildberry (*Popsicle* Water Ice)	40	0	10.0	0	0	0	10	(0)
ICE CREAM, ½ cup, except as noted:								
almond fudge (*Baskin-Robbins Jamoca*), 1 regular scoop	270	5.0	30.0	14.0	m.q.	32	115	m.q.
butter almond (*Breyers*)	170	4.0	15.0	10.0	4.0	25	125	m.q.
butter crunch (*Sealtest*)	150	2.0	18.0	7.0	4.0	25	90	(0)
butter pecan:								
(*Breyers*)	180	3.0	15.0	12.0	5.0	25	125	m.q.

Food and Measure	cal.	prot. (gms)	carbo. (gms)	tot. fat (gms)	sat. fat (gms)	chol. (mgs)	sod. (mgs)	fiber (gms)
(*Frusen Glädjé*)	280	5.0	16.0	21.0	m.q.	85	160	m.q.
(*Häagen-Dazs*)	390	5.0	29.0	24.0	9.0	110	100	m.q.
(*Lady Borden*)	180	3.0	16.0	12.0	m.q.	m.q.	65	m.q.
(*Sealtest*)	160	3.0	16.0	9.0	4.0	15	125	m.q.
caramel nut sundae (*Häagen-Dazs*)	310	5.0	26.0	21.0	m.q.	m.q.	100	m.q.
cherry vanilla (*Breyers*)	150	3.0	17.0	7.0	4.0	20	45	(0)
chocolate:								
(*Baskin-Robbins*), 1 regular scoop	270	5.0	32.0	14.0	m.q.	37	160	(0)
(*Baskin-Robbins World Class*),								
1 regular scoop	280	5.0	35.0	14.0	m.q.	36	145	(0)
(*Breyers*)	160	3.0	20.0	8.0	5.0	20	30	(0)
(*Darigold/Darigold* Alpine)	140	2.0	17.0	7.0	m.q.	m.q.	70	(0)
(*Darigold* Classic)	180	3.0	16.0	13.0	m.q.	m.q.	30	(0)
(*Frusen Glädjé*)	240	5.0	17.0	17.0	9.0	75	65	(0)
(*Häagen-Dazs*)	270	5.0	24.0	17.0	8.0	120	50	(0)
(*Sealtest*)	140	2.0	18.0	6.0	4.0	20	50	(0)
chocolate mint (*Häagen-Dazs*) ...	300	5.0	26.0	20.0	m.q.	m.q.	50	(0)
deep (*Häagen-Dazs*)	290	5.0	26.0	14.0	m.q.	m.q.	70	(0)
Dutch (*Borden Olde Fashioned*								
Recipe)	130	2.0	16.0	6.0	m.q.	m.q.	65	(0)
fudge, deep (*Häagen-Dazs*)	290	5.0	26.0	14.0	m.q.	m.q.	70	(0)
mint (*Breyers*)	170	3.0	18.0	10.0	6.0	25	45	(0)
swirl (*Borden*)	130	2.0	18.0	6.0	m.q.	m.q.	65	(0)
triple stripes (*Sealtest*)	140	2.0	17.0	7.0	m.q.	m.q.	50	(0)
chocolate, Swiss, almond (*Frusen*								
Glädjé)	270	6.0	18.0	19.0	9.0	55	60	m.q.
chocolate chip:								
(*Baskin-Robbins*), 1 regular scoop	260	4.0	27.0	15.0	m.q.	40	110	(0)
(*Dreyer's*)	150	3.0	16.0	9.0	m.q.	30	40	(0)
(*Sealtest*)	150	2.0	17.0	8.0	m.q.	15	50	(0)
chocolate:								
(*Frusen Glädjé*)	270	5.0	21.0	18.0	9.0	55	60	(0)
(*Häagen-Dazs*)	290	5.0	28.0	20.0	10.0	105	40	(0)
chocolate-marshmallow sundae								
(*Sealtest*)	150	2.0	21.0	6.0	4.0	20	40	(0)
chocolate-peanut butter, deep								
(*Häagen-Dazs*)	330	7.0	25.0	19.0	m.q.	m.q.	90	(0)
chocolate-raspberry truffle (*Baskin-*								
Robbins International Creams),								
1 regular scoop	310	4.0	35.0	17.0	m.q.	45	115	. (0)
coffee:								
(*Breyers*)	150	3.0	16.0	8.0	5.0	30	50	0
(*Häagen-Dazs*)	270	5.0	23.0	17.0	8.0	120	55	0
(*Sealtest*)	140	2.0	16.0	7.0	4.0	15	50	0
cookies n' cream (*Breyers*)	170	3.0	19.0	9.0	5.0	20	60	(0)
cookies 'n' cream (*Dreyer's*)	160	3.0	18.0	9.0	n.a.	28	80	(0)
fudge, marble (*Dreyer's*)	150	3.0	18.0	8.0	m.q.	28	50	(0)
fudge royale (*Sealtest*)	140	3.0	19.0	7.0	4.0	15	55	(0)

Food and Measure	cal.	prot. (gms)	carbo. (gms)	tot. fat (gms)	sat. fat (gms)	chol. (mgs)	sod. (mgs)	fiber (gms)
ICE CREAM *(cont.)*								
heavenly hash (*Sealtest*)	150	2.0	19.0	7.0	4.0	15	50	(0)
macadamia brittle (*Häagen-Dazs*) ...	280	4.0	25.0	18.0	m.q.	m.q.	60	m.q.
maple walnut (*Sealtest*)	160	3.0	17.0	9.0	3.0	20	40	m.q.
peach, natural (*Breyers*)	130	2.0	18.0	6.0	3.0	15	35	(0)
peanut fudge sundae (*Sealtest*)	140	3.0	17.0	7.0	4.0	20	50	m.q.
pralines 'n cream (*Baskin-Robbins*),								
1 regular scoop	280	4.0	35.0	14.0	m.q.	36	180	(0)
rocky road (*Baskin-Robbins*),								
1 regular scoop	300	5.0	39.0	14.0	m.q.	32	135	(0)
rocky road (*Dreyer's*)	170	3.0	18.0	10.0	m.q.	30	30	(0)
rum raisin (*Häagen-Dazs*)	250	4.0	21.0	17.0	8.0	110	45	(0)
strawberry:								
(*Baskin-Robbins* Very Berry),								
1 regular scoop	220	3.0	30.0	10.0	m.q.	30	95	(0)
(*Borden*)	130	2.0	18.0	6.0	m.q.	m.q.	55	(0)
(*Breyers*)	130	2.0	16.0	6.0	4.0	20	40	(0)
(*Frusen Glädjé*)	230	4.0	20.0	15.0	10.0	65	60	(0)
(*Häagen-Dazs*)	250	4.0	23.0	15.0	8.0	95	40	(0)
(*Sealtest*)	130	2.0	18.0	5.0	3.0	15	40	(0)
cream (*Borden Olde Fashioned*								
Recipe)	130	2.0	19.0	5.0	m.q.	m.q.	55	(0)
vanilla:								
regular, 10% fat, hardened, 1 oz.	57	1.0	6.8	3.1	1.9	13	25	0
regular, 10% fat, hardened	134	2.4	15.9	7.2	4.5	30	58	0
rich, 16% fat, hardened, 1 oz. ...	67	.8	6.1	4.5	2.8	17	21	0
rich, 16% fat, hardened	175	2.1	16.0	11.8	7.4	44	54	0
(*Baskin-Robbins*), 1 regular scoop	240	4.0	24.0	14.0	m.q.	52	115	0
(*Borden Olde Fashioned Recipe*) ..	130	2.0	15.0	7.0	m.q.	m.q.	55	0
(*Breyers*)	150	3.0	15.0	8.0	5.0	25	50	0
(*Darigold/Darigold* Alpine)	130	2.0	15.0	7.0	m.q.	m.q.	50	0
(*Darigold* Classic)	180	2.0	16.0	12.0	m.q.	m.q.	40	0
(*Dreyer's*)	160	2.0	14.0	10.0	m.q.	40	30	0
(*Eagle* Brand Homestyle)	150	3.0	16.0	9.0	m.q.	m.q.	55	0
(*Frusen Glädjé*)	230	5.0	16.0	17.0	9.0	65	70	0
(*Good Humor* Cup), 3 fl. oz.	98	1.5	11.6	5.1	m.q.	m.q.	35	0
(*Häagen-Dazs*)	260	5.0	23.0	17.0	8.0	120	55	0
(*Sealtest*)	140	2.0	16.0	7.0	4.0	20	50	0
French:								
(*Baskin-Robbins*), 1 regular								
scoop	280	4.0	25.0	18.0	m.q.	90	90	0
(*Sealtest*)	140	2.0	16.0	7.0	m.q.	35	50	0
soft-serve, 1 oz.	62	1.2	6.3	3.7	2.2	25	25	0
soft-serve	189	3.5	19.1	11.3	6.8	77	77	0
honey (*Häagen-Dazs*)	250	5.0	22.0	16.0	8.0	135	55	0
nuggets, dark chocolate coated								
(*Carnation Bon Bons*),								
5 pieces	170	2.0	15.0	11.0	m.q.	14	50	(0)

Food and Measure	cal.	prot. (gms)	carbo. (gms)	tot. fat (gms)	sat. fat (gms)	chol. (mgs)	sod. (mgs)	fiber (gms)
nuggets, milk chocolate coated								
(*Carnation Bon Bons*),								
5 pieces	165	2.0	14.0	11.0	m.q.	16	50	(0)
vanilla fudge (*Häagen-Dazs*)	270	5.0	26.0	17.0	m.q.	m.q.	100	(0)
vanilla fudge twirl (*Breyers*)	160	3.0	19.0	8.0	4.0	20	55	(0)
vanilla Swiss almond (*Frusen Glädjé*)	270	6.0	18.0	19.0	9.0	65	65	m.q.
vanilla Swiss almond (*Häagen-Dazs*)	290	5.0	24.0	19.0	m.q.	m.q.	55	m.q.
vanilla toffee chunk (*Frusen Glädjé*)	270	5.0	22.0	17.0	m.q.	85	160	0
vanilla-chocolate (*Breyers*)	160	3.0	17.0	8.0	5.0	25	40	(0)
vanilla-chocolate-strawberry:								
(*Breyers*)	150	3.0	17.0	8.0	4.0	20	40	(0)
(*Sealtest*)	140	2.0	18.0	6.0	3.0	20	50	(0)
(*Sealtest Cubic Scoops*)	130	2.0	17.0	6.0	3.0	20	50	(0)
vanilla-orange (*Sealtest Cubic*								
Scoops)	130	2.0	22.0	4.0	2.0	15	40	(0)
vanilla-peanut butter swirl (*Häagen-*								
Dazs)	280	5.0	19.0	21.0	8.0	110	120	(0)
vanilla-raspberry (*Sealtest Cubic*								
Scoops)	130	2.0	22.0	4.0	2.0	15	40	(0)
ICE CREAM, SUBSTITUTE AND								
IMITATION, ½ cup, except as								
noted:								
all flavors (*Lite Lite Tofutti*)	90	2.0	20.0	<1.0	n.a.	0	80	n.a.
cappuccino (*Tofutti* Love Drops)	230	3.0	26.0	12.0	3.0	0	120	n.a.
cherry, black (*Sealtest Free*)	100	2.0	25.0	0	0	0	45	(0)
chocolate:								
(*Sealtest Free*)	100	3.0	23.0	0	0	0	50	(0)
(*Simple Pleasures*), 4 oz.	140	9.0	25.0	<1.0	.3	15	n.a.	0
(*Tofutti* Love Drops)	230	3.0	26.0	13.0	5.0	0	100	(0)
(*Weight Watchers*)	80	3.0	19.0	0	0	5	75	(0)
soft-serve (*Lite Lite Tofutti*)	90	2.0	20.0	<1.0	n.a.	0	80	(0)
supreme (*Tofutti*)	210	3.0	20.0	13.0	3.0	0	130	(0)
swirl (*Weight Watchers*)	90	3.0	22.0	0	0	5	75	(0)
chocolate chip (*Low, Lite'n*								
Luscious)	100	3.0	19.0	2.0	m.q.	4	80	(0)
coffee (*Simple Pleasures*), 4 oz.	120	8.0	22.0	<1.0	.3	15	n.a.	0
Jamoca Swiss almond (*Low, Lite'n*								
Luscious)	90	3.0	19.0	2.0	m.q.	4	100	(0)
Neapolitan (*Weight Watchers*)	80	3.0	19.0	0	0	5	75	(0)
peach (*Sealtest Free*)	100	2.0	23.0	0	0	0	45	(0)
peach (*Simple Pleasures*), 4 oz.	135	9.0	24.0	<1.0	.3	5	n.a.	0
pineapple coconut (*Low, Lite'n*								
Luscious)	90	3.0	19.0	1.0	n.a.	3	70	(0)
rum raisin (*Simple Pleasures*), 4 oz.	130	7.0	25.0	<1.0	.3	10	n.a.	0
strawberry:								
(*Low, Lite'n Luscious*)	80	3.0	17.0	1.0	n.a.	3	70	(0)
(*Sealtest Free*)	100	2.0	23.0	0	0	0	40	(0)
(*Simple Pleasures*), 4 oz.	120	8.0	22.0	<1.0	.3	11	55	0

Food and Measure	cal.	prot. (gms)	carbo. (gms)	tot. fat (gms)	sat. fat (gms)	chol. (mgs)	sod. (mgs)	fiber (gms)
ICE CREAM, SUBSTITUTE AND IMITATION *(cont.)*								
vanilla:								
(*Sealtest Free*)	100	3.0	24.0	0	0	0	45	0
(*Tofutti*)	200	2.0	21.0	11.0	1.50	0	90	n.a.
(*Tofutti* Love Drops)	220	3.0	26.0	12.0	3.0	0	100	n.a.
(*Weight Watchers*)	80	3.0	20.0	0	0	5	75	0
chocolate dipped (*Tofutti O's*),								
1 piece	40	1.0	4.0	2.0	m.q.	0	20	n.a.
soft-serve (*Lite Lite Tofutti*)	90	2.0	20.0	<1.0	n.a.	0	80	n.a.
vanilla almond bark (*Tofutti*)	230	3.0	23.0	14.0	4.0	0	950	n.a.
vanilla-chocolate-strawberry (*Sealtest*								
Free)	100	3.0	23.0	0	0	0	40	(0)
vanilla-fudge royale (*Sealtest Free*) ..	100	3.0	24.0	0	0	0	50	(0)
vanilla-strawberry royale (*Sealtest*								
Free)	100	3.0	25.0	0	0	0	35	(0)
wildberry (*Tofutti*)	210	2.0	22.0	12.0	3.0	0	100	(0)
ICE CREAM BAR, 1 piece:								
(*Good Humor* Fat Frog), 3 fl. oz. ...	154	1.8	16.0	9.2	m.q.	m.q.	36	n.a.
(*Good Humor* Halo Bar), 2.5 fl. oz.	230	3.7	22.8	13.7	m.q.	m.q.	64	n.a.
(*Heath*), 3 fl. oz.	170	3.0	16.0	13.0	m.q.	m.q.	155	n.a.
(*Klondike*), 5 fl. oz.	280	4.0	23.0	19.0	m.q.	m.q.	65	n.a.
(*Klondike* Krispy), 5 fl. oz.	290	4.0	26.0	19.0	m.q.	m.q.	70	n.a.
(*Klondike* Lite), 2.5 fl. oz.	140	3.0	10.0	10.0	m.q.	10	45	n.a.
assorted (*Good Humor Whammy*),								
1.6 fl. oz.	95	.8	6.6	7.2	m.q.	m.q.	17	n.a.
almond, toasted (*Good Humor*),								
3 fl. oz.	212	1.8	24.3	11.8	m.q.	m.q.	34	m.q.
caramel almond (*Häagen-Dazs*								
Crunch Bar)	240	3.0	17.0	18.0	7.0	40	65	m.q.
chip candy crunch (*Good Humor*),								
3 fl. oz.	255	2.2	21.2	17.9	m.q.	m.q.	40	n.a.
chocolate:								
(*Klondike*), 5 fl. oz.	270	4.0	23.0	19.0	m.q.	m.q.	60	n.a.
w/dark chocolate coating (*Häagen-*								
Dazs)	390	5.0	32.0	27.0	m.q.	m.q.	60	0
fudge:								
cake (*Good Humor*), 6.3 fl. oz.	214	1.7	18.1	15.0	m.q.	m.q.	50	n.a.
sundae (*Baker's Fudgetastic*) ..	220	3.0	23.0	15.0	m.q.	20	45	n.a.
sundae, crunchy (*Baker's*								
Fudgetastic)	230	3.0	24.0	14.0	m.q.	20	40	n.a.
milk, w/almonds, milk chocolate								
coated (*Nestlé* Premium),								
3.7 fl. oz.	350	6.0	28.0	23.0	m.q.	5	45	n.a.
w/milk chocolate coating (*Nestlé*								
Quik), 3 fl. oz.	210	3.0	19.0	14.0	m.q.	m.q.	40	n.a.
chocolate eclair (*Good Humor*),								
3 fl. oz.	188	2.1	22.6	9.9	m.q.	m.q.	54	n.a.
peanut butter (*Häagen-Daz* Crunch								
Bar)	270	6.0	16.0	21.0	7.0	35	55	m.q.

Food and Measure	cal.	prot. (gms)	carbo. (gms)	tot. fat (gms)	sat. fat (gms)	chol. (mgs)	sod. (mgs)	fiber (gms)
strawberry shortcake (*Good Humor*), 3 fl. oz.	176	1.7	23.8	8.2	m.q.	m.q.	88	n.a.
vanilla:								
(*Häagen-Dazs* Crunch Bar)	220	3.0	16.0	16.0	6.0	40	55	m.q.
w/caramel peanut center, milk chocolate coated (*Oh, Henry!*), 3 fl. oz.	320	1.0	34.0	20.0	m.q.	m.q.	75	m.q.
chocolate flavor coated (*Good Humor*), 3 fl. oz.	198	1.9	16.8	13.7	m.q.	m.q.	44	n.a.
w/dark chocolate coating (*Häagen-Dazs*)	390	5.0	32.0	27.0	m.q.	m.q.	60	n.a.
w/milk chocolate coating (*Häagen-Dazs*)	360	4.0	26.0	27.0	m.q.	m.q.	55	n.a.
w/milk chocolate-almond coating (*Häagen-Dazs*)	370	5.0	27.0	27.0	m.q.	m.q.	55	m.q.
w/milk chocolate-brittle coating (*Häagen-Dazs*)	370	5.0	32.0	25.0	m.q.	m.q.	160	(0)
w/milk chocolate coating and crisps (*Nestlé Crunch*), 3 fl. oz.	180	2.0	15.0	13.0	m.q.	m.q.	m.q.	m.q.
w/white chocolate coating (*Nestlé Alpine* Premium), 3.7 fl. oz.	350	6.0	25.0	25.0	m.q.	5	50	n.a.
ICE CREAM BAR, SUBSTITUTE AND IMITATION, frozen, 1 bar:								
(*Good Humor* Cool Shark), 3 fl. oz.	68	0	17.0	.1	n.a.	m.q.	7	n.a.
(*Good Humor* Jumbo Jet Star), 4.5 fl. oz.	85	0	19.5	.7	n.a.	m.q.	0	n.a.
(*Good Humor* Milky Pop), 1.5 fl. oz.	45	1.0	8.0	0	0	n.a.	25	n.a.
amaretto-chocolate swirl (*Crystal Light Cool'n Creamy*)	60	2.0	10.0	2.0	m.q.	0	60	(0)
chocolate:								
(*Weight Watchers* Treat Bars), 2.75 oz.	100	4.0	18.0	1.0	0	0	75	(0)
dip (*Weight Watchers*), 1.7 oz.	110	2.0	10.0	7.0	3.0	5	35	(0)
fudge (*Good Humor*), 2.5 fl. oz.	127	3.7	26.5	.6	n.a.	m.q.	91	n.a.
fudge, double (*Crystal Light Cool'n Creamy*)	50	2.0	7.0	2.0	m.q.	0	60	(0)
fudge, double (*Weight Watchers*), 1.75 oz.	60	3.0	12.0	1.0	0	5	50	(0)
fudge swirl (*Sealtest Free*), 2.4 oz.	90	3.0	19.0	0	0	0	30	(0)
mousse (*Weight Watchers* Sugar Free), 1.75 oz.	35	2.0	9.0	<1.0	0	5	30	(0)
chocolate/vanilla (*Crystal Light Cool'n Creamy*)	50	2.0	7.0	2.0	m.q.	0	55	(0)
English toffee crunch (*Weight Watchers*), 1.7 oz.	120	2.0	11.0	8.0	4.0	5	45	(0)
orange-vanilla (*Crystal Light Cool'n Creamy*)	30	1.0	5.0	1.0	n.a.	0	25	(0)

Food and Measure	cal.	prot. (gms)	carbo. (gms)	tot. fat (gms)	sat. fat (gms)	chol. (mgs)	sod. (mgs)	fiber (gms)
ICE CREAM BAR, SUBSTITUTE AND IMITATION *(cont.)*								
orange-vanilla (*Weight Watchers* Sugar Free Treat Bars), 1.75 oz.	30	2.0	8.0	<1.0	0	5	40	(0)
sandwich snacks (*Weight Watchers*), 1.5 oz.	90	2.0	17.0	2.0	0	0	120	n.a.
strawberry finger (*Good Humor*), 2.5 fl. oz.	49	0	12.2	.1	n.a.	m.q.	0	n.a.
vanilla sandwich (*Weight Watchers*) ..	150	3.0	28.0	3.0	2.0	5	170	(0)
vanilla-fudge swirl (*Sealtest Free*), 2.4 oz.	80	3.0	18.0	0	0	0	30	(0)
vanilla-strawberry swirl (*Sealtest Free*), 2.4 oz.	90	2.0	17.0	2.0	0	0	120	n.a.
ICE CREAM CONE AND CUP:								
plain:								
(*Little Debbie* Ice Cream Cup), 1 cup	15	.4	3.0	.1	(0)	<1	15	m.q.
sugar (*Baskin-Robbins*), 1 cone ..	60	1.0	11.0	1.0	n.a.	0	45	m.q.
waffle (*Baskin-Robbins*), 1 cone ..	140	3.0	28.0	2.0	m.q.	0	5	m.q.
filled:								
(*Good Humor* King Cone), 5.5 fl. oz.	290	4.5	40.9	12.0	m.q.	m.q.	119	m.q.
boysenberry (*Good Humor* King Cone), 5 fl. oz.	340	3.9	51.6	13.1	m.q.	m.q.	151	m.q.
vanilla-chocolate cup (*Good Humor* Combo), 6 fl. oz.	201	3.8	25.6	9.2	m.q.	m.q.	80	m.q.
ICE CREAM MIX[1]:								
Dutch chocolate (*Salada*), 1 oz. dry	110	1.0	26.0	0	0	0	20	(0)
Dutch chocolate (*Salada*), 1 cup	310	4.0	31.0	19.0	m.q.	m.q.	75	(0)
peach, vanilla, or wild strawberry (*Salada*), 1 oz. dry	110	0	27.0	0	0	0	10	(0)
peach, vanilla, or wild strawberry (*Salada*), 1 cup	310	4.0	32.0	18.0	m.q.	m.q.	60	(0)
ICE CREAM SANDWICH, 1 piece:								
chocolate chip cookie, chocolate (*Good Humor*), 2.7 fl. oz.	204	2.2	30.1	8.3	m.q.	m.q.	166	m.q.
chocolate chip cookie, chocolate (*Good Humor*), 4 fl. oz.	246	2.9	35.1	10.5	m.q.	m.q.	181	m.q.
vanilla:								
(*Good Humor*), 3 fl. oz.	191	3.7	31.1	5.7	m.q.	m.q.	155	m.q.
(*Good Humor*), 2.5 fl. oz.	165	3.2	26.9	4.9	m.q.	m.q.	134	m.q.
(*Klondike*), 5 fl. oz.	230	5.0	33.0	9.0	m.q.	m.q.	220	m.q.
ICE CREAM AND SORBET, see "Sorbet"								
ICE MILK, ½ cup, except as noted:								
caramel nut (*Light n' Lively*)	120	3.0	18.0	4.0	2.0	10	85	(0)
chocolate:								
(*Borden*)	100	3.0	18.0	2.0	m.q.	m.q.	80	0

1. *Prepared according to package directions, except as noted.*

Food and Measure	cal.	prot. (gms)	carbo. (gms)	tot. fat (gms)	sat. fat (gms)	chol. (mgs)	sod. (mgs)	fiber (gms)
(*Breyers* Light)	120	3.0	18.0	4.0	2.0	15	55	(0)
(*Darigold* Lite)	110	3.0	19.0	3.0	m.q.	m.q.	65	(0)
(*Weight Watchers Grand*								
Collection)	110	4.0	18.0	3.0	2.0	10	75	(0)
fudge twirl (*Breyers* Light)	130	4.0	21.0	4.0	2.0	10	60	(0)
chocolate chip (*Light n' Lively*)	120	3.0	18.0	4.0	3.0	10	35	0
chocolate chip (*Weight Watchers*								
Grand Collection)	120	3.0	19.0	4.0	2.0	10	75	(0)
chocolate swirl (*Weight Watchers*								
Grand Collection)	120	3.0	19.0	3.0	2.0	5	75	(0)
coffee (*Light n' Lively*)	100	3.0	16.0	3.0	1.0	10	40	0
cookies n' cream (*Light n' Lively*) ...	110	3.0	18.0	3.0	2.0	10	65	0
heavenly hash (*Breyers* Light)	150	3.0	21.0	5.0	3.0	10	55	(0)
heavenly hash (*Light n' Lively*)	120	3.0	20.0	4.0	2.0	10	35	(0)
Neapolitan (*Weight Watchers Grand*								
Collection)	110	3.0	18.0	3.0	1.0	10	75	(0)
pecan pralines 'n creme (*Weight*								
Watchers Grand Collection)	120	3.0	20.0	4.0	3.0	10	80	(0)
praline almond (*Breyers* Light)	130	3.0	19.0	5.0	2.0	10	70	(0)
strawberry (*Borden*)	90	2.0	17.0	2.0	m.q.	m.q.	65	0
strawberry (*Breyers* Light)	110	3.0	18.0	3.0	2.0	15	50	(0)
toffee fudge parfait (*Breyers* Light) ..	140	3.0	22.0	5.0	3.0	10	90	(0)
vanilla:								
hardened, 1 oz.	40	1.1	6.3	1.2	.8	4	23	0
hardened	92	2.6	14.5	2.8	1.8	9	52	0
soft-serve, 1 oz.	36	1.3	6.2	.7	.5	2	26	0
soft-serve	112	4.0	19.2	2.3	1.4	7	81	0
(*Borden*)	90	2.0	17.0	2.0	m.q.	m.q.	65	0
(*Breyers* Light)	120	3.0	18.0	4.0	2.0	10	60	0
(*Darigold*)	110	2.0	18.0	3.0	m.q.	m.q.	66	0
(*Light n' Lively*)	100	3.0	16.0	3.0	2.0	10	40	0
(*Weight Watchers Grand*								
Collection)	100	3.0	16.0	3.0	1.0	10	75	0
vanilla-chocolate-almond (*Light n'*								
Lively)	120	3.0	17.0	4.0	1.0	10	45	(0)
vanilla-chocolate-strawberry (*Breyers*								
Light)	120	3.0	18.0	4.0	2.0	15	55	(0)
vanilla-chocolate-strawberry (*Light n'*								
Lively)	100	2.0	17.0	3.0	2.0	10	35	(0)
vanilla-fudge twirl (*Light n' Lively*) ..	110	3.0	18.0	3.0	2.0	10	45	0
vanilla-raspberry parfait (*Breyers*								
Light)	130	3.0	23.0	3.0	2.0	15	50	(0)
vanilla-raspberry swirl (*Light n'*								
Lively)	110	3.0	19.0	3.0	1.0	10	35	0
ICE MILK CONE:								
w/nuts (*Gold Bond* Olde Nut								
Sundae), 3 fl. oz.	230	5.0	36.0	8.0	n.a.	n.a.	n.a.	m.q.

ICING, CAKE, see "Frosting"
INDIAN DATE, see "Tamarind"

Food and Measure	cal.	prot. (gms)	carbo. (gms)	tot. fat (gms)	sat. fat (gms)	chol. (mgs)	sod. (mgs)	fiber (gms)
IOWA BRAND LOAF:								
(*Hormel* Perma-Fresh), 2 slices	90	10.0	0	6.0	m.q.	m.q.	607	0
IRISH MOSS, see "Seaweed"								
ITALIAN CHESTNUT, see								
"Chestnut, European"								
ITALIAN FENNEL, see "Fennel,								
fresh"								
ITALIAN SAUSAGE:								
hot (*Hillshire Farm* Links), 2 oz.	180	7.0	1.0	17.0	m.q.	m.q.	m.q.	0
mild (*Hillshire Farm* Links), 2 oz. ..	190	7.0	1.0	17.0	m.q.	m.q.	m.q.	0
pork:								
raw:								
1 oz.	98	4.0	.2	8.9	3.2	22	207	0
1 link, 3.2 oz., 5 links per lb. ..	315	13.0	.6	28.5	10.3	69	665	0
1 link, 4 oz., 4 links per lb.	391	16.0	.7	35.4	12.7	86	826	0
cooked:								
1 oz.	92	5.7	.4	7.3	2.6	22	261	0
1 link, approx. 2.4 oz., yield								
from 3.2 oz. raw	216	13.4	1.0	17.2	6.1	52	618	0
1 link, approx. 3 oz., yield from								
4 oz. raw	268	16.6	1.2	21.3	7.5	65	765	0
smoked (*Hillshire Farm* Flavorseal),								
2 oz.	200	7.0	1.0	18.0	m.q.	m.q.	500	0
ITALIAN SEASONING:								
(*McCormick/Schilling* Spice Blends),								
¼ tsp.	1	<.1	.1	n.a.	n.a.	0	<1	n.a.
(*Tone's*), 1 tsp.	3	.1	.7	.1	<.1	0	<1	.2 d
ITALIAN STONE PINE, see "Pine								
nut, pignolia"								

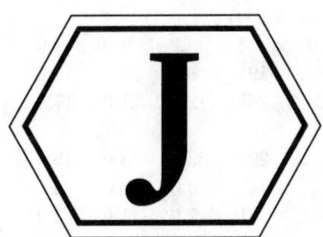

Food and Measure	cal.	prot. (gms)	carbo. (gms)	tot. fat (gms)	sat. fat (gms)	chol. (mgs)	sod. (mgs)	fiber (gms)
JACK, see "Mackerel, Pacific or jack"								
JACK BEAN SEEDS, see "Horse bean seeds"								
JACK-IN-THE-BOX:								
breakfast, 1 serving:								
Breakfast Jack, 4.4 oz.	307	18.0	30.0	13.0	5.2	203	871	m.q.
crescent:								
Canadian, 4.7 oz.	452	19.0	25.0	31.0	9.7	226	851	m.q.
sausage, 5.5 oz.	584	22.0	28.0	43.0	15.5	187	1012	m.q.
supreme, 5.1 oz.	547	20.0	27.0	40.0	13.2	178	1053	m.q.
hash browns, 2.2 oz.	116	2.0	11.0	7.0	3.6	3	211	m.q.
jelly, grape, .5 oz.	38	0	9.0	0	0	0	3	0
pancake platter, 8.1 oz.	612	15.0	87.0	22.0	8.6	99	888	m.q.
scrambled egg platter, 8.8 oz. ...	662	24.0	52.0	40.0	17.1	354	1188	m.q.
sandwiches, 1 serving:								
bacon cheeseburger, 8.1 oz.	705	35.0	48.0	39.0	15.0	85	1127	m.q.
beef fajita pita, 6.2 oz.	333	24.0	27.0	14.0	5.9	45	635	m.q.
cheeseburger:								
4 oz.	315	15.o	33.0	14.0	5.7	41	746	m.q.
double, 5.3 oz.	467	21.0	33.0	27.0	12.3	72	842	m.q.
ultimate, 10 oz.	942	47.0	33.0	69.0	26.4	127	1176	m.q.
chicken fajita pita, 6.7 oz.	292	24.0	29.0	8.0	2.9	34	703	m.q.
chicken fillet, grilled, 7.2 oz.	408	31.0	33.0	17.0	4.1	64	1130	m.q.
chicken supreme, 8.1 oz.	575	27.0	34.0	36.0	14.3	62	1525	m.q.
fish supreme, 8 oz.	554	20.0	47.0	32.0	13.5	66	1047	m.q.
hamburger, 3.4 oz.	267	13.0	28.0	11.0	4.1	26	556	m.q.
Jumbo Jack, 7.8 oz.	584	26.0	42.0	34.0	11.0	73	733	m.q.
Jumbo Jack, w/cheese, 8.5 oz. ...	677	32.0	46.0	40.0	14.0	102	1090	m.q.
Swiss and bacon burger, 6.6 oz.	678	31.0	34.0	47.0	20.0	92	1458	m.q.
Mexican food:								
guacamole, 1 oz.	55	.9	1.8	5.0	m.q.	0	130	m.q.

Food and Measure	cal.	prot. (gms)	carbo. (gms)	tot. fat (gms)	sat. fat (gms)	chol. (mgs)	sod. (mgs)	fiber (gms)
JACK-IN-THE-BOX, **MEXICAN FOOD** *(cont.)*								
salsa, 1 oz.	8	.2	2.0	<1.0	<1.0	0	129	m.q.
taco, 2.9 oz.	191	8.0	16.0	11.0	5.2	21	406	m.q.
taco, super, 4.8 oz.	288	12.0	21.0	17.0	8.0	37	765	m.q.
salads, 1 serving:								
chef, 14 oz.	295	32.0	3.0	18.0	9.4	107	812	m.q.
Mexican chicken, 14.6 oz.	442	28.0	30.0	23.0	8.6	89	1500	m.q.
side, 4 oz.	51	7.0	<1.0	3.0	2.0	<1	84	m.q.
taco, 14.2 oz.	503	34.0	28.0	31.0	13.4	92	1600	m.q.
finger foods:								
chicken strips, 4 pieces, 4.4 oz. ...	349	29.0	28.0	14.0	6.8	68	748	m.q.
chicken strips, 6 pieces, 6.6 oz. ...	523	43.0	42.0	20.0	10.0	103	1122	m.q.
egg rolls, 3 pieces, 6 oz.	405	15.0	42.0	19.0	7.2	30	903	m.q.
egg rolls, 5 pieces, 10 oz.	675	26.0	70.0	32.0	12.0	50	1505	m.q.
shrimp, 10 pieces, 3 oz.	270	10.0	22.0	16.0	7.2	84	669	m.q.
shrimp, 15 pieces, 4.4 oz.	404	15.0	34.0	24.0	10.8	126	1003	m.q.
taquitos, 5 pieces, 5 oz.	363	16.0	40.0	16.0	5.6	37	467	m.q.
taquitos, 7 pieces, 7 oz.	508	22.0	56.0	22.0	7.9	52	654	m.q.
side dishes, 1 serving:								
french fries:								
small, 2.4 oz.	221	2.0	27.0	12.0	5.0	0	164	m.q.
regular, 3.9 oz.	353	3.0	43.0	19.0	7.9	13	262	m.q.
jumbo, 4.8 oz.	442	4.0	54.0	24.0	10.0	16	328	m.q.
onion rings, 3.8 oz.	382	5.0	39.0	23.0	11.1	27	407	m.q.
dressings and sauces:								
BBQ sauce, 1 oz.	44	.5	10.6	<1.0	<1.0	0	300	0
bleu cheese dressing, 2.5 oz.	262	<1.0	14.0	22.0	4.0	18	918	0
buttermilk dressing, 2.5 oz.	362	<1.0	8.0	36.0	5.8	21	694	0
French dressing, reduced calorie								
2.5 oz.	176	<1.0	26.0	8.0	1.2	0	600	0
mayo-mustard sauce, .7 oz.	124	.5	2.0	13.0	n.a.	10	247	0
mayo-onion sauce, .7 oz.	143	.3	1.0	15.0	n.a.	20	140	0
seafood cocktail sauce, 1 oz.	32	<1.0	6.8	<1.0	<1.0	0	206	n.a.
sweet and sour sauce, 1 oz.	40	<1.0	11.0	<1.0	<1.0	<1	160	0
Thousand Island dressing, 2.5 oz.	312	<1.0	12.0	30.0	5.0	23	700	(0)
desserts and shakes:								
apple turnover, 4.2 oz.	410	4.0	45.0	24.0	10.8	15	350	m.q.
cheesecake, 3.5 oz.	309	8.0	29.0	17.5	9.0	63	208	n.a.
shake:								
chocolate, 11.4 oz.	330	11.0	55.0	7.0	4.3	25	270	(0)
strawberry, 11.6 oz.	320	10.0	55.0	7.0	4.3	25	240	(0)
vanilla, 11.2 oz.	320	10.0	57.0	6.0	3.6	25	230	0
JACKFRUIT:								
untrimmed, 1 lb.	119	1.9	30.5	.4	n.a.	0	3	1.3 c
trimmed, 1 oz.	27	.4	6.8	.1	(0)	0	1	.3 c
JALAPEÑO BEAN DIP:								
(*Wise*), 2 tbsp.	25	1.0	5.0	0	0	0	100	n.a.
medium (*Hain*), 4 tbsp.	70	4.0	10.0	1.0	n.a.	5	250	n.a.

Food and Measure	cal.	prot. (gms)	carbo. (gms)	tot. fat (gms)	sat. fat (gms)	chol. (mgs)	sod. (mgs)	fiber (gms)
JALAPEÑO LOAF:								
(*Kahn's*), 1 slice	70	3.0	2.0	6.0	m.q.	m.q.	340	n.a.
JALAPEÑO PEPPER, see								
"Pepper, jalapeño"								
JALAPEÑO PEPPER DIP:								
(*Kraft*), 2 tbsp.	50	1.0	3.0	4.0	2.0	0	160	n.a.
cheddar (*Breakstone's* Gourmet),								
2 tbsp.	70	2.0	2.0	6.0	3.0	15	90	n.a.
cheese (*Kraft* Premium), 2 tbsp. ...	50	1.0	3.0	4.0	3.0	15	160	n.a.
nacho (*Price's*), 1 oz.	80	2.6	2.0	7.1	m.q.	n.a.	m.q.	n.a.
JAM AND PRESERVES (see also								
"Fruit spreads" and								
"Marmalade"):								
all flavors:								
(*Bama*), 2 tsp.	30	0	8.0	0	0	0	5	m.q.
(*Estee*), 1 tsp.	2	0	0	0	0	0	10	m.q.
(*Featherweight*), 1 tsp.	4	0	1.0	0	0	0	0	m.q.
(*Kraft*), 1 tsp.	17	0	4.0	0	0	0	0	m.q.
(*Polaner*), 2 tsp.	35	0	9.0	0	0	0	n.a.	m.q.
(*S&W/Nutradiet*), 1 tsp.	4	0	1.0	0	0	0	0	m.q.
(*Smucker's*), 1 tsp.	18	0	4.0	0	0	0	0	m.q.
(*Smucker's Slenderella*), 1 tsp. ...	8	0	2.0	0	0	0	0	m.q.
apricot (*Finast*), 2 tsp.	35	0	9.0	0	0	0	1	m.q.
blackberry (*Finast*), 2 tsp.	16	0	4.0	0	0	0	5	m.q.
blueberry (*Finast*), 2 tsp.	16	0	4.0	0	0	0	5	m.q.
cherry (*Finast*), 2 tsp.	25	0	9.0	0	0	0	5	m.q.
grape, regular or concord (*Finast*),								
2 tsp.	35	0	9.0	0	0	0	5	(0)
grape (*Welch's*), 2 tsp.	35	0	9.0	0	0	0	5	0
peach (*Finast*), 2 tsp.	35	0	9.0	0	0	0	1	m.q.
pineapple (*Finast*), 2 tsp.	35	0	9.0	0	0	0	1	m.q.
raspberry, red (*Finast*), 2 tsp.	35	0	9.0	0	0	0	3	m.q.
raspberry-apple (*Welch's*), 2 tsp. ...	35	0	9.0	0	0	0	5	0
strawberry:								
(*Finast*), 2 tsp.	35	0	9.0	0	0	0	3	m.q.
(*Kraft* Reduced Calorie), 1 tsp. ..	6	0	2.0	0	0	0	5	m.q.
(*Smucker's* Imitation), 1 tsp.	2	0	1.0	0	0	0	2	n.a.
(*Welch's*), 2 tsp.	35	0	9.0	0	0	0	5	0
JAMBERRY, see "Tomatillo"								
JAMBOLAN, see "Java Plum"								
JAPANESE HONEY								
MUSHROOM, see								
"Mushroom, Japanese honey"								
JAPANESE WHITE RADISH, see								
"Radish, Oriental"								
JAVA PLUM:								
w/seeds, 1 lb.	222	2.7	57.2	.9	n.a.	0	50	1.0 c
seeded, 1 oz.	17	.2	4.4	.1	(0)	0	4	.1 c
seeded, ½ cup	41	.5	10.5	.2	(0)	0	9	.2 c

Food and Measure	cal.	prot. (gms)	carbo. (gms)	tot. fat (gms)	sat. fat (gms)	chol. (mgs)	sod. (mgs)	fiber (gms)
JAVA PLUM *(cont.)*								
3 medium, approx. .4 oz.	5	.1	1.4	<.1	(0)	0	1	<.1 c
JELLY:								
all flavors:								
(*Estee*), 1 tsp.	2	0	0	0	0	0	10	0
(*Kraft*), 1 tsp.	17	0	4.0	0	0	0	0	0
(*Polaner*), 2 tsp.	35	0	9.0	0	0	0	n.a.	0
(*Smucker's*), 1 tsp.	18	0	4.0	0	0	0	0	0
(*Smucker's Slenderella*), 1 tsp. ...	8	0	2.0	0	0	0	0	0
except grape (*Featherweight*),								
1 tsp.	4	0	1.0	0	0	0	0	0
apple:								
(*Bama*), 2 tsp.	30	0	8.0	0	0	0	5	0
(*Finast*), 2 tsp.	35	0	9.0	0	0	0	2	0
(*Lucky Leaf/Musselman's*), 1 oz.	80	0	20.0	0	0	0	5	0
apple-blackberry (*Musselman's*),								
1 oz.	80	0	19.0	0	0	0	0	0
apple-cherry (*Musselman's*), 1 oz. ..	80	0	19.0	0	0	0	5	0
apple-grape (*Musselman's*), 1 oz. ...	80	0	20.0	0	0	0	5	0
apple-grape (*Welch's*), 2 tsp.	35	0	9.0	0	0	0	5	0
apple-raspberry (*Musselman's*),								
1 oz.	80	0	19.0	0	0	0	0	0
apple-strawberry (*Musselman's*),								
1 oz.	80	0	20.0	0	0	0	5	0
blackberry (*Bama*), 2 tsp.	30	0	8.0	0	0	0	5	0
currant (*Finast*), 2 tsp.	35	0	9.0	0	0	0	2	0
grape:								
(*Bama*), 2 tsp.	30	0	8.0	0	0	0	5	0
(*Featherweight*), 1 tsp.	4	0	1.0	0	0	0	5	0
(*Finast*), 2 tsp.	35	0	9.0	0	0	0	5	0
(*Kraft* Reduced Calorie), 1 tsp. ..	6	0	2.0	0	0	0	5	0
(*Musselman's*), 1 oz.	80	0	20.0	0	0	0	0	0
(*Smucker's* Imitation), 1 tsp.	2	0	1.0	0	0	0	2	0
(*Welch's*), 2 tsp.	35	0	9.0	0	0	0	5	0
green pepper (*Great Impressions*),								
1 tbsp.	50	0	12.6	0	0	0	<1	n.a.
jalapeño (*Great Impressions*), 1 tbsp.	58	0	14.6	0	0	0	51	n.a.
mint (*Finast*), 2 tsp.	35	0	9.0	0	0	0	2	0
red pepper (*Great Impressions*),								
1 tbsp.	50	0	12.6	0	0	0	9	n.a.
strawberry (*Finast*), 2 tsp.	35	0	9.0	0	0	0	2	0
JELLY AND PEANUT BUTTER:								
(*Bama*), 2 tbsp.	150	3.0	20.0	7.0	m.q.	0	75	m.q.
JERUSALEM ARTICHOKE:								
untrimmed, 1 lb.	238	6.3	54.6	<.1	tr.	0	n.a.	2.5 c
trimmed, 1 oz.	22	.6	4.9	tr.	tr.	0	n.a.	.2 c
sliced, ½ cup	57	1.5	13.1	<.1	tr.	0	n.a.	.6 c

Food and Measure	cal.	prot. (gms)	carbo. (gms)	tot. fat (gms)	sat. fat (gms)	chol. (mgs)	sod. (mgs)	fiber (gms)
JEW'S EAR:								
untrimmed, 1 lb.	111	2.1	30.0	.2	(0)	0	41	9.5 c
trimmed, 1 oz.	7	.1	1.9	<.1	(0)	0	3	.6 c
1 piece, 2¼″ × ¹⁄₁₆″ × 1¾″, approx.								
.2 oz.	2	<.1	.4	tr.	(0)	0	1	.1 c
sliced, ½ cup	13	.2	3.3	<.1	(0)	0	5	1.1 c
JEW'S EAR, DRIED:								
trimmed, 1 oz.	84	1.4	23.0	.1	(0)	0	20	8.8 c
trimmed, ½ cup	36	.6	9.7	.1	(0)	0	8	3.7 c
JICAMA, see "Yam bean tuber"								
JOWL, pork:								
raw, 1 oz.	186	1.8	0	19.7	7.2	25	7	0
JUJUBE:								
raw, w/seeds, 1 lb.	331	5.1	85.3	.8	n.a.	0	11	5.9 c
raw, seeded, 1 oz.	22	.3	5.7	.1	(0)	0	1	.4 c
dried, 1 oz.	81	1.0	20.1	.3	(0)	0	3	.9 c
JUTE, potherb:								
raw:								
untrimmed, 1 lb.	96	13.1	16.3	.7	.1	0	23	3.4 c
trimmed, 1 oz.	10	1.3	1.6	.1	<.1	0	2	.3 c
trimmed, ½ cup	5	.7	.8	<.1	tr.	0	1	.2 c
boiled, drained, 4 oz.	42	4.2	8.3	.2	<.1	0	12	2.2 c
boiled, drained, ½ cup	16	1.6	3.1	.1	<.1	0	5	.8 c

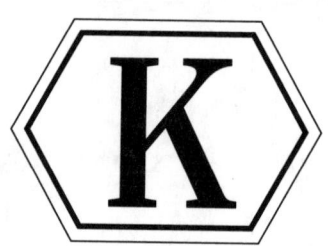

Food and Measure	cal.	prot. (gms)	carbo. (gms)	tot. fat (gms)	sat. fat (gms)	chol. (mgs)	sod. (mgs)	fiber (gms)
KALE:								
raw:								
untrimmed, 1 lb.	137	9.1	27.7	1.9	.3	0	119	4.2 c
trimmed, 1 oz.	14	.9	2.8	.2	<.1	0	12	.4 c
chopped, ½ cup	17	1.1	3.4	.2	<.1	0	15	.5 c
boiled, drained, 4 oz.	36	2.2	6.4	.5	.1	0	26	.9 c
boiled, drained, chopped, ½ cup ...	21	1.2	3.7	.3	<.1	0	15	.5 c
KALE, CANNED:								
chopped (*Allens*), ½ cup	25	2.0	3.0	<1.0	n.a.	0	15	m.q.
KALE, FROZEN:								
10-oz. pkg.	79	7.6	13.9	1.3	.2	0	43	2.5 c
boiled, drained, 4 oz.	34	3.2	5.9	.6	.1	0	17	1.1 c
boiled, drained, chopped, ½ cup ...	20	1.9	3.4	.3	<.1	0	10	.6 c
chopped:								
(*Frosty Acres*), 3.3 oz.	25	3.0	5.0	0	0	0	15	1.0 c
(*Seabrook*), 3.3 oz.	25	3.0	5.0	0	0	0	14	1.0 c
(*Southern*), 3.5 oz.	30	2.6	4.8	.5	(0)	0	30	m.q.
KALE, SCOTCH:								
raw:								
untrimmed, 1 lb.	115	7.8	23.0	1.7	.2	0	194	3.4 c
trimmed, 1 oz.	12	.8	2.4	.2	<.1	0	20	.3 c
chopped, ½ cup	14	1.0	2.8	.2	<.1	0	24	.4 c
boiled, drained, 4 oz.	32	2.2	6.4	.5	.1	0	51	1.0 c
boiled, drained, chopped, ½ cup ...	18	1.2	3.7	.3	<.1	0	29	.6 c
KAMBOKO, see "Fish paste cake, Japanese"								
KANPYO:								
1 lb.	1169	38.9	295.0	2.5	.2	0	68	41.4 c
1 oz.	73	2.4	18.4	.2	<.1	0	4	2.6 c
3 strips, 40¾″ long × ½″ diam. ...	49	1.6	12.4	.1	tr.	0	3	1.7 c
½ cup	70	2.3	17.6	.2	<.1	0	4	2.5 c

Food and Measure	cal.	prot. (gms)	carbo. (gms)	tot. fat (gms)	sat. fat (gms)	chol. (mgs)	sod. (mgs)	fiber (gms)
KASHA, see "Buckwheat groats"								
KELP, see "Seaweed"								
KENTUCKY FRIED CHICKEN:								
chicken, *Original Recipe:*								
breast, center, 4.1 oz.	283	27.5	8.8	15.3	3.8	93	672	m.q.
breast, side, 3.2 oz.	267	18.8	10.8	16.5	4.2	77	735	m.q.
drumstick, 2 oz.	146	13.1	4.2	8.5	2.2	67	275	m.q.
thigh, 3.7 oz.	294	17.9	11.1	19.7	5.3	123	619	m.q.
wing, 1.9 oz.	178	12.2	6.0	11.7	3.0	64	372	m.q.
chicken, *Extra Tasty Crispy:*								
breast, center, 4.8 oz.	342	33.0	11.7	19.7	4.8	114	790	m.q.
breast, side, 3.9 oz.	343	21.7	14.0	22.3	5.5	81	748	m.q.
drumstick, 2.4 oz.	204	13.6	6.1	13.9	3.4	71	324	m.q.
thigh, 4.2 oz.	406	20.0	14.4	29.8	7.7	129	688	m.q.
wing, 2.3 oz.	254	12.4	9.3	18.6	4.4	67	422	m.q.
chicken, Hot Wings, 6 pieces	376	22.4	m.q.	24.1	5.3	148	677	m.q.
chicken, *Kentucky Nuggets,*								
.6 oz.-piece	46	2.8	2.2	2.9	.7	12	140	m.q.
chicken, *Lite'N Crispy:*								
breast, center, 3 oz.	220	m.q.	m.q.	11.9	2.9	57	416	m.q.
breast, side, 2.6 oz.	204	m.q.	m.q.	12.4	3.2	53	417	m.q.
drumstick, 1.7 oz.	121	m.q.	m.q.	7.0	1.7	51	196	m.q.
thigh, 2.8 oz.	246	m.q.	m.q.	16.7	4.3	80	386	m.q.
Kentucky Nuggets sauces:								
barbeque, 1 oz.	35	.3	7.1	.6	.1	<1	450	n.a.
honey, .5 oz.	49	0	12.1	<.1	<.1	<1	<15	0
mustard, 1 oz.	36	.9	6.0	.9	.1	<1	346	n.a.
sweet and sour, 1 oz.	58	.1	13.0	.6	.1	<1	148	n.a.
side dishes:								
buttermilk biscuits, 2.3 oz.	232	4.2	27.1	11.9	2.8	1	539	m.q.
Chicken Littles sandwich, 1.7 oz.	169	5.7	13.8	10.1	2.0	18	331	m.q.
coleslaw, 3.2 oz.	119	1.5	13.3	6.6	1.0	5	197	m.q.
Colonel's chicken sandwich,								
5.9 oz.	482	20.8	38.6	27.3	5.7	47	1060	m.q.
corn-on-the-cob, 5 oz.	176	5.1	31.9	3.1	.5	<1	<21	m.q.
french fries, regular, 2.7 oz.	244	3.2	31.1	11.9	2.6	2	139	m.q.
mashed potatoes and gravy,								
3.5 oz.	71	2.4	11.9	1.6	.5	<1	342	m.q.
KETCHUP, see "Catsup"								
KIDNEY BEAN:								
all varieties:								
raw, 1 oz.	94	6.7	17.0	.2	.1	0	7	2.9 d
raw, ½ cup	306	21.7	55.2	.8	.1	0	22	9.6 d
boiled, 4 oz.	144	9.3	25.9	.6	.1	0	2	4.1 d
boiled, ½ cup	112	7.6	20.1	.4	.1	0	2	3.2 d
red:								
raw:								
1 oz.	96	6.4	17.4	.1	<.1	0	3	2.9 d
½ cup	310	20.7	56.4	1.0	.1	0	11	9.6 d

Food and Measure	cal.	prot. (gms)	carbo. (gms)	tot. fat (gms)	sat. fat (gms)	chol. (mgs)	sod. (mgs)	fiber (gms)
KIDNEY BEAN, RED, RAW *(cont.)*								
(Arrowhead Mills), 2 oz.	190	13.0	35.0	1.0	n.a.	0	3	11.7 d
boiled:								
4 oz.	144	9.8	25.9	.6	.1	0	2	4.1 d
½ cup	112	7.6	20.1	.4	.1	0	2	3.2 d
(A&P), 1 cup	230	17.0	41.0	1.0	n.a.	0	5	m.q.
California:								
raw, 1 oz.	94	6.9	17.0	.1	<.1	0	3	1.8 c
raw, ½ cup	304	22.4	55.0	.2	<.1	0	10	5.7 c
boiled, 4 oz.	141	10.4	25.4	.1	<.1	0	5	2.7 c
boiled, ½ cup	109	8.0	19.7	.1	<.1	0	4	2.1 c
royal:								
raw, 1 oz.	93	7.2	16.5	.1	<.1	0	4	1.7 c
raw, ½ cup	303	23.3	53.7	.4	.1	0	12	5.7 c
boiled, 4 oz.	139	10.8	24.8	.2	<.1	0	6	2.6 c
boiled, ½ cup	108	8.4	19.2	.2	<.1	0	4	2.0 c
KIDNEY BEAN, CANNED,								
½ cup, except as noted:								
all varieties, w/liquid, 4 oz.	92	5.9	16.9	.4	.1	0	393	1.1 c
all varieties, w/liquid.............	104	6.7	19.0	.4	.1	0	445	1.2 c
(A&P)	110	7.0	20.0	<1.0	(0)	0	440	m.q.
(Hunt's), 4 oz.	120	7.0	21.0	0	0	0	400	m.q.
(Pathmark)	110	7.0	20.0	0	0	0	350	m.q.
(S&W/Nutradiet)	90	7.0	16.0	1.0	(0)	0	1	m.q.
red *(Progresso)*	100	9.0	21.0	<1.0	(0)	0	210	7.0 d
red, dark:								
(Allens)	105	5.0	20.0	<1.0	(0)	0	290	m.q.
(Pathmark)	110	8.0	18.0	0	0	0	370	m.q.
(S&W Lite 50% Less Salt)	120	7.0	22.0	1.0	(0)	0	355	m.q.
(S&W Premium)	120	6.0	22.0	1.0	(0)	0	596	m.q.
(Van Camp's), 1 cup	182	11.7	35.0	.5	(0)	0	830	m.q.
red, dark or light:								
w/liquid, 4 oz.	96	6.0	17.7	.4	.1	0	387	1.1 c
w/liquid	108	6.7	20.0	.4	.1	0	437	1.2 c
(Finast)	110	6.0	20.0	2.0	n.a.	0	350	m.q.
(Joan of Arc/Green Giant)	90	7.0	20.0	0	0	0	250	5.9 d
(Stokely)	110	7.0	20.0	1.0	(0)	0	360	m.q.
red, light *(Allens)*	105	5.0	2.0	<1.0	(0)	0	290	m.q.
red, light *(Van Camp's)*, 1 cup	184	11.5	36.0	.5	(0)	0	650	m.q.
red, New Orleans style *(Van Camp's)*, 1 cup	178	12.1	34.0	.6	(0)	n.a.	940	m.q.
white *(Pathmark Cannellini)*	100	6.0	18.0	0	0	0	390	m.q.
white *(Progresso Cannellini)*	80	8.0	19.0	<1.0	(0)	0	220	6.5 d
baked, red *(B&M)*, 8 oz.	250	15.0	42.0	7.0	m.q.	5	640	11.0 d
baked, red *(Friends)*, 8 oz.	340	17.0	57.0	4.0	2.0	4	1060	11.0 d

Food and Measure	cal.	prot. (gms)	carbo. (gms)	tot. fat (gms)	sat. fat (gms)	chol. (mgs)	sod. (mgs)	fiber (gms)
KIDNEY BEAN, SPROUTED,								
mature seeds:								
raw:								
1 lb.	132	19.1	18.6	2.3	.3	0	m.q.	m.q.
1 oz.	8	1.2	1.2	.1	<.1	0	m.q.	m.q.
½ cup	27	3.9	3.8	.5	.1	0	m.q.	m.q.
boiled, drained, 4 oz.	37	5.5	5.4	.7	.1	0	m.q.	m.q.
KIDNEYS[1]:								
beef:								
raw, 1 oz.	30	4.7	.6	.9	.3	81	51	0
simmered, 6.9 oz., yield from								
1 lb. raw	283	50.2	1.9	6.8	2.2	762	264	0
simmered, 4 oz.	163	28.9	1.1	3.9	1.2	439	152	0
lamb:								
raw, 1 oz.	28	4.5	.2	.8	.3	96	44	0
braised, 9 oz., yield from 1 lb.								
raw	351	60.4	2.5	9.2	3.1	1443	384	0
braised, 4 oz.	155	26.8	1.1	4.1	1.4	641	171	0
pork:								
raw, 1 oz.	28	4.7	0	.9	.3	90	34	0
braised, 4 oz.	171	28.8	0	5.3	1.7	544	91	0
braised, chopped or diced, not								
packed, 1 cup	211	35.6	0	6.6	2.1	673	111	0
veal:								
raw, 1 oz.	28	4.5	.2	.9	.3	103	50	0
braised, 6.5 oz., yield from 1 lb.								
raw	300	48.3	0	10.4	3.2	1452	499	0
braised, 4 oz.	185	29.8	0	6.4	2.0	897	125	0
KIELBASA (see also "Polish								
sausage"):								
(*Eckrich Lean Supreme* Polska),								
1 oz.	72	4.0	1.0	6.0	m.q.	m.q.	224	0
(*Hillshire Farm* Bun Size), 2 oz.	180	8.0	2.0	16.0	m.q.	m.q.	570	0
(*Hillshire Farm* Polska Flavorseal),								
2 oz.	190	8.0	2.0	17.0	m.q.	m.q.	540	0
(*Hillshire Farm* Polska Flavorseal								
Lite), 2 oz.	160	8.0	2.0	13.0	m.q.	m.q.	m.q.	0
(*Hillshire Farm* Polska Links), 2 oz.	190	7.0	2.0	17.0	m.q.	m.q.	530	0
(*Hormel* Kolbase), 3 oz.	220	12.0	1.0	19.0	m.q.	m.q.	904	0
beef (*Hillshire Farm* Polska								
Flavorseal), 2 oz.	190	7.0	1.0	17.0	m.q.	m.q.	550	0
mild (*Hillshire Farm* Polska								
Flavorseal), 2 oz.	190	7.0	2.0	17.0	m.q.	m.q.	530	0
pork and beef[2], 1 oz.	88	3.7	.6	7.7	2.8	19	305	0
pork and beef[2], 1 slice, 6″ × 3¾″ ×								
¹⁄₁₆″, approx. .9 oz.	81	3.5	.6	7.1	2.6	17	280	0

1. *Cooked meats prepared without added ingredients.*
2. *Nonfat dry milk added.*

Food and Measure	cal.	prot. (gms)	carbo. (gms)	tot. fat (gms)	sat. fat (gms)	chol. (mgs)	sod. (mgs)	fiber (gms)
KIELBASA *(cont.)*								
skinless (*Eckrich* Polska), 1 link	180	7.0	2.0	16.0	m.q.	m.q.	420	0
skinless (*Hormel*), ½ link	180	12.0	1.0	14.0	m.q.	m.q.	826	0
KIWIFRUIT:								
w/skin, 1 lb.	237	3.9	58.1	1.7	n.a.	0	18	13.3 d
trimmed, 1 oz.	17	.3	4.2	.1	(0)	0	1	1.0 d
1 large, approx. 3.7 oz.	55	.9	13.5	.4	(0)	0	4	3.1 d
1 medium, approx. 3.1 oz.	46	.8	11.3	.3	(0)	0	4	2.6 d
KNACKWURST, see "Knockwurst"								
KNOCKWURST:								
(*Hillshire Farm* Links), 2 oz.	180	7.0	1.0	16.0	m.q.	m.q.	460	0
beef (*Hebrew National*), 3-oz. link ..	263	10.2	<1.0	25.0	m.q.	26	877	0
pork and beef, 1 oz.	87	3.4	.5	7.8	2.9	16	286	0
pork and beef, 1 link, 4" long × 1⅛", approx. 2.4 oz.	209	8.1	1.2	18.9	6.9	39	687	0
KOHLRABI:								
raw:								
untrimmed, 1 lb.	57	3.6	12.9	.2	<.1	0	42	2.3 d
trimmed, 1 oz.	8	.5	1.8	<.1	tr.	0	6	.3 d
sliced, ½ cup	19	1.2	4.3	.1	tr.	0	14	.8 d
boiled, drained, 4 oz.	33	2.0	7.6	.1	<.1	0	24	1.2 c
boiled, drained, sliced, ½ cup	24	1.5	5.5	.1	<.1	0	17	.9 c
KOLBASSY, see "Kielbasa"								
KOMBU, see "Seaweed, kelp"								
KUMQUAT:								
w/seeds, 1 lb.	266	3.8	69.3	.4	n.a.	0	25	15.6 c
seeded, 1 oz.	18	.3	4.7	<.1	(0)	0	2	1.0 c
1 medium, approx. .7 oz.	12	.2	3.1	<.1	(0)	0	1	.7 c

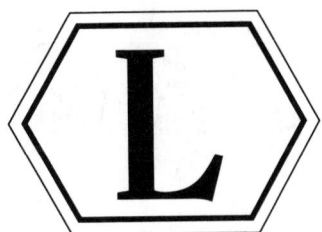

Food and Measure	cal.	prot. (gms)	carbo. (gms)	tot. fat (gms)	sat. fat (gms)	chol. (mgs)	sod. (mgs)	fiber (gms)
LAMB[1], domestic, choice grade:								
composite cuts, separable lean and fat:								
raw, 1 oz.	76	4.8	0	6.1	2.7	20	16	0
cooked, 8.5 oz., yield from 1 lb.								
raw w/bone	709	59.2	0	50.6	21.3	235	173	0
cooked, 4 oz.	333	27.8	0	23.7	10.0	110	82	0
composite cuts, separable lean only:								
raw, 1 oz.	38	5.8	0	1.5	.5	19	19	0
cooked, 6.6 oz., yield from 1 lb.								
raw w/bone and fat	385	52.7	0	17.8	6.4	172	141	0
cooked, 4 oz.	234	32.0	0	10.8	3.9	104	86	0
composite cuts, separable fat only:								
raw, 1 oz.	189	1.9	0	20.1	9.2	26	9	0
cooked, 1 oz.	166	3.4	0	16.8	7.7	32	16	0
cubed for stew or kabob (leg and shoulder):								
raw, 1 oz.	38	5.7	0	1.5	.5	18	18	0
braised or stewed, 9.6 oz., yield from 1 lb. raw	608	91.7	0	23.9	8.6	295	191	0
braised or stewed, 4 oz.	253	38.2	0	10.0	3.6	122	79	0
broiled, 11.5 oz., yield from 1 lb.								
raw	607	91.7	0	23.9	8.6	295	250	0
broiled, 4 oz.	211	31.8	0	8.3	3.0	102	86	0
foreshank, separable lean and fat:								
raw, 1 oz.	57	5.4	0	3.8	1.7	20	20	0
braised or stewed:								
5.2 oz., yield from 1 lb. raw								
w/bone	358	41.9	0	19.9	8.3	156	106	0
4 oz.	276	32.2	0	15.3	6.4	120	82	0

1. *Cooked meats are prepared without added ingredients.*

Food and Measure	cal.	prot. (gms)	carbo. (gms)	tot. fat (gms)	sat. fat (gms)	chol. (mgs)	sod. (mgs)	fiber (gms)
LAMB, FORESHANK, LEAN AND FAT *(cont.)*								
1 slice, 3″ diam. × ¼″, approx.								
1 oz.	69	8.0	0	3.8	1.6	30	20	0
diced, 1 cup, approx. 4.9 oz. . .	340	39.7	0	18.8	7.9	148	101	0
foreshank, separable lean only:								
raw, 1 oz.	34	6.0	0	.9	.3	19	22	0
braised or stewed:								
4.5 oz., yield from 1 lb. raw								
w/bone and fat	238	39.6	0	7.7	2.7	133	95	0
4 oz.	212	35.2	0	6.8	2.4	118	84	0
1 slice, 3″ diam. × ¼″, approx.								
1 oz.	53	8.8	0	1.7	.6	29	21	0
diced, 1 cup, approx. 4.9 oz. . .	262	43.4	0	8.4	3.0	146	104	0
ground:								
raw, 1 oz.	80	4.7	0	6.7	2.9	21	17	0
raw, 1 cup, approx. 8 oz.	637	37.4	0	52.9	23.0	165	133	0
broiled:								
11 oz., yield from 1 lb. raw	885	77.5	0	61.5	25.4	303	253	0
5.4 oz., approx. yield from								
1 cup raw	435	38.1	0	30.3	12.5	149	125	0
4 oz.	321	28.1	0	22.3	9.2	110	92	0
1 cup, approx. 4.1 oz.	328	28.7	0	23.1	9.4	113	94	0
leg, whole, separable lean and fat:								
raw, 1 oz.	65	5.1	0	4.8	2.1	20	16	0
roasted:								
9.3 oz., yield from 1 lb. raw								
w/bone	684	67.8	0	43.7	18.3	247	176	0
4 oz.	293	29.0	0	18.7	7.8	105	75	0
1 slice, 3″ diam. × ¼″, approx.								
1 oz.	73	7.2	0	4.7	2.0	26	19	0
diced, 1 cup, approx. 4.9 oz. . .	361	35.8	0	23.0	9.6	130	92	0
leg, whole, separable lean only:								
raw, 1 oz.	36	5.8	0	1.3	.5	18	18	0
roasted:								
7.7 oz., yield from 1 lb. raw								
w/bone and fat	416	61.7	0	16.9	6.0	194	148	0
4 oz.	217	32.1	0	8.8	3.1	101	77	0
1 slice, 3″ diam. × ¼″, approx.								
1 oz.	54	8.0	0	2.2	.8	25	19	0
diced, 1 cup, approx. 4.9 oz. . .	267	39.6	0	10.8	3.9	125	95	0
leg, shank half, separable lean and fat:								
raw, 1 oz.	57	5.3	0	3.8	1.6	19	16	0
roasted:								
9.5 oz., yield from 1 lb. raw								
w/bone	604	70.9	0	33.4	13.7	242	175	0
4 oz.	255	29.9	0	14.1	5.8	102	74	0
1 slice, 3″ diam. × ¼″, approx.								
1 oz.	64	7.5	0	3.5	1.4	26	18	0

Food and Measure	cal.	prot. (gms)	carbo. (gms)	tot. fat (gms)	sat. fat (gms)	chol. (mgs)	sod. (mgs)	fiber (gms)
diced, 1 cup, approx. 4.9 oz. ..	315	37.0	0	17.4	7.1	126	91	0
leg, shank half, separable lean only:								
raw, 1 oz.	36	5.8	0	1.2	.4	18	17	0
roasted:								
8.4 oz., yield from 1 lb. raw								
w/bone and fat	430	67.2	0	15.9	5.7	208	158	0
4 oz.	204	31.9	0	7.6	2.7	99	75	0
1 slice, 3″ diam. × ¼″, approx.								
1 oz.	51	8.0	0	1.9	.7	25	19	0
diced, 1 cup, approx. 4.9 oz. ..	252	39.4	0	9.3	3.3	122	92	0
leg, sirloin half, separable lean and								
fat:								
raw, 1 oz.	77	4.8	0	6.3	2.8	20	16	0
roasted:								
9.25 oz., yield from 1 lb. raw								
w/bone	764	64.5	0	54.2	22.9	254	178	0
4 oz.	331	27.9	0	23.4	9.9	110	77	0
1 slice, 3″ diam. × ¼″, approx.								
1 oz.	83	7.0	0	5.9	2.5	27	19	0
diced, 1 cup, approx. 4.9 oz. ..	409	34.5	0	28.9	12.2	136	95	0
leg, sirloin half, separable lean only:								
raw, 1 oz.	38	5.8	0	1.4	.5	19	18	0
roasted:								
7.1 oz., yield from 1 lb. raw								
w/bone and fat	409	56.9	0	18.4	6.6	184	142	0
4 oz.	231	32.1	0	10.4	3.7	104	81	0
1 slice, 3″ diam. × ¼″, approx.								
1 oz.	58	8.0	0	2.6	.9	26	20	0
diced, 1 cup, approx. 4.9 oz. ..	286	39.7	0	12.8	4.6	129	99	0
loin, separable lean and fat:								
raw, 1 oz.	88	4.6	0	7.6	3.3	21	16	0
broiled, 1 chop, 2.25 oz., yield								
from 4.2-oz. raw chop w/bone	201	16.1	0	14.7	6.3	64	49	0
broiled, 4 oz.	358	28.5	0	26.2	11.1	113	87	0
roasted, 9.5 oz., yield from 1 lb.								
raw w/bone	831	60.6	0	63.4	27.5	255	172	0
roasted, 4 oz.	350	25.6	0	26.8	11.6	108	73	0
loin, separable lean only:								
raw, 1 oz.	41	5.9	0	1.7	.6	19	19	0
broiled, 1 chop, 1.6 oz., yield from								
4.2-oz. raw chop w/bone and fat	100	13.9	0	4.5	1.6	44	39	0
broiled, 4 oz.	245	34.0	0	11.0	3.9	108	95	0
roasted, 6.8 oz., yield from 1 lb.								
raw w/bone and fat	389	51.3	0	18.8	7.2	168	128	0
roasted, 4 oz.	229	30.2	0	11.1	4.2	99	75	0
rib, separable lean and fat:								
raw, 1 oz.	106	4.1	0	9.8	4.3	22	16	0
broiled, 8.1 oz., yield from 1 lb.								
raw w/bone	826	50.6	0	67.6	29.0	227	173	0

Food and Measure	cal.	prot. (gms)	carbo. (gms)	tot. fat (gms)	sat. fat (gms)	chol. (mgs)	sod. (mgs)	fiber (gms)
LAMB, RIB, LEAN AND FAT *(cont.)*								
broiled, 4 oz.	409	25.1	0	33.6	14.4	112	86	0
roasted, 9 oz., yield from 1 lb. raw								
w/bone	915	53.8	0	76.0	32.5	247	186	0
roasted, 4 oz.	407	24.0	0	33.8	14.5	110	83	0
rib, separable lean only:								
raw, 1 oz.	48	5.7	0	2.6	.9	19	21	0
broiled, 5.2 oz., yield from 1 lb.								
raw w/bone and fat	345	40.7	0	19.0	6.8	134	125	0
broiled, 4 oz.	266	31.5	0	14.7	5.3	103	96	0
roasted, 5.6 oz., yield from 1 lb.								
raw w/bone and fat	369	41.6	0	21.2	7.6	139	129	0
roasted, 4 oz.	263	29.7	0	15.1	5.4	100	92	0
shoulder, whole, separable lean and fat:								
raw, 1 oz.	75	4.7	0	6.1	2.6	20	17	0
braised or stewed:								
7.7 oz., yield from 1 lb. raw								
w/bone	749	62.4	0	53.5	22.5	252	162	0
4 oz.	390	32.5	0	27.8	11.7	132	85	0
1 slice, 3″ diam. × ¼″, approx.								
1 oz.	98	8.1	0	7.0	2.9	33	21	0
diced, 1 cup, approx. 4.9 oz. ..	482	40.2	0	34.4	14.5	162	105	0
broiled:								
8.75 oz., yield from 1 lb. raw								
w/bone	690	60.6	0	47.8	20.0	240	194	0
4 oz.	315	27.7	0	21.8	9.1	110	88	0
1 slice, 3″ diam. × ¼″, approx.								
1 oz.	79	6.9	0	5.5	2.3	27	22	0
diced, 1 cup, approx. 4.9 oz. ..	389	34.2	0	27.0	11.3	136	109	0
roasted:								
9.5 oz., yield from 1 lb. raw								
w/bone	743	60.5	0	53.7	22.7	247	177	0
4 oz.	313	25.5	0	22.6	9.6	104	75	0
1 slice, 3″ diam. × ¼″, approx.								
1 oz.	78	6.4	0	5.7	2.4	26	19	0
diced, 1 cup, approx. 4.9 oz. ..	386	31.5	0	28.0	11.8	129	92	0
shoulder, whole, separable lean only:								
raw, 1 oz.	41	5.6	0	1.9	.7	19	20	0
braised or stewed:								
6.1 oz., yield from 1 lb. raw								
w/bone and fat	494	57.2	0	27.7	10.8	203	137	0
4 oz.	321	37.2	0	10.0	7.0	133	90	0
1 slice, 3″ diam. × ¼″, approx.								
1 oz.	80	9.3	0	4.5	1.7	33	22	0
diced, 1 cup, approx. 4.9 oz. ..	396	45.9	0	22.2	8.6	164	111	0
broiled:								
7.1 oz., yield from 1 lb. raw								
w/bone and fat	426	54.9	0	21.3	7.9	188	167	0

Food and Measure	cal.	prot. (gms)	carbo. (gms)	tot. fat (gms)	sat. fat (gms)	chol. (mgs)	sod. (mgs)	fiber (gms)
4 oz.	238	30.8	0	11.9	4.4	105	94	0
1 slice, 3″ diam. × ¼″, approx.								
1 oz.	60	7.7	0	3.0	1.1	26	24	0
diced, 1 cup, approx. 4.9 oz. ..	294	38.0	0	14.7	5.4	130	116	0
roasted:								
7.6 oz., yield from 1 lb. raw								
w/bone and fat	442	54.2	0	23.4	11.7	189	147	0
4 oz.	231	28.3	0	12.2	4.6	99	77	0
1 slice, 3″ diam. × ¼″, approx.								
1 oz.	58	7.1	0	3.1	1.2	25	19	0
diced, 1 cup, approx. 4.9 oz. ..	286	34.9	0	15.1	5.7	122	95	0
shoulder, arm, separable lean and								
fat:								
raw, 1 oz.	74	4.8	0	5.9	2.6	20	17	0
braised or stewed, 1 chop, 2.5 oz.,								
yield from 5.6-oz. raw chop								
w/bone	244	21.4	0	16.9	7.0	84	51	0
braised or stewed, 4 oz.	392	34.5	0	27.2	11.2	136	82	0
broiled, 1 chop, 3.3 oz., yield from								
5.6-oz. raw chop w/bone	262	22.8	0	18.2	7.8	90	72	0
broiled, 4 oz.	319	27.7	0	22.2	9.5	109	87	0
roasted, 10 oz., yield from 1 lb.								
raw w/bone	798	64.5	0	57.9	25.0	262	186	0
roasted, 4 oz.	316	25.5	0	23.0	9.9	104	74	0
shoulder, arm, separable lean only:								
raw, 1 oz.	38	5.7	0	1.5	.5	18	20	0
braised or stewed, 1 chop, 1.9 oz.,								
yield from 5.6-oz. raw w/bone								
and fat	152	19.4	0	7.7	2.8	66	41	0
braised or stewed, 4 oz.	316	40.3	0	16.0	5.7	137	86	0
broiled, 1 chop, 2.6 oz., yield from								
5.6-oz. raw w/bone and fat	147	20.4	0	6.7	2.5	68	60	0
broiled, 4 oz.	227	31.4	0	10.2	3.9	104	93	0
roasted, 7.9 oz., yield from 1 lb.								
raw w/bone and fat	431	57.0	0	20.8	8.0	192	150	0
roasted, 4 oz.	218	28.9	0	10.5	4.1	98	76	0
shoulder, blade, separable lean and								
fat:								
raw, 1 oz.	74	4.7	0	5.9	2.5	20	18	0
braised or stewed:								
7.4 oz., yield from 1 lb. raw								
w/bone	721	59.6	0	51.7	21.5	243	156	0
4 oz.	391	32.3	0	28.0	11.7	132	85	0
1 slice, 3″ diam. × ¼″, approx.								
1 oz.	98	8.1	0	7.0	2.9	33	21	0
diced, 1 cup, approx. 4.9 oz. ..	483	39.9	0	34.6	14.4	162	105	0
broiled:								
8.9 oz., yield from 1 lb. raw								
w/bone	700	58.1	0	50.2	20.6	240	208	0

Food and Measure	cal.	prot. (gms)	carbo. (gms)	tot. fat (gms)	sat. fat (gms)	chol. (mgs)	sod. (mgs)	fiber (gms)
LAMB, SHOULDER, BLADE, LEAN AND FAT, BROILED *(cont.)*								
4 oz.	315	26.1	0	22.6	9.3	108	93	0
1 slice, 3″ diam. × ¼″, approx.								
1 oz.	79	6.5	0	5.7	2.3	27	23	0
diced, 1 cup, approx. 4.9 oz. ..	389	32.3	0	27.9	11.5	133	115	0
roasted:								
9.1 oz., yield from 1 lb. raw								
w/bone	726	57.5	0	53.3	22.4	239	171	0
4 oz.	319	25.2	0	23.4	9.8	104	75	0
1 slice, 3″ diam. × ¼″, approx.								
1 oz.	80	6.3	0	5.8	2.4	26	19	0
diced, 1 cup, approx. 4.9 oz. ..	393	31.2	0	28.9	12.1	129	92	0
shoulder, blade, separable lean only:								
raw, 1 oz.	43	5.5	0	2.2	.8	19	20	0
braised or stewed:								
5.9 oz., yield from 1 lb. raw								
w/bone and fat	485	54.5	0	28.0	10.7	197	133	0
4 oz.	327	36.7	0	18.9	7.2	133	90	0
1 slice, 3″ diam. × ¼″, approx.								
1 oz.	82	9.2	0	4.7	1.8	33	22	0
diced, 1 cup, approx. 4.9 oz. ..	403	45.3	0	23.3	8.9	164	111	0
broiled:								
7.3 oz., yield from 1 lb. raw								
w/bone and fat	436	52.7	0	23.4	8.4	189	182	0
4 oz.	239	28.9	0	12.8	4.6	103	100	0
1 slice, 3″ diam. × ¼″, approx.								
1 oz.	60	7.2	0	3.2	1.1	26	25	0
diced, 1 cup, approx. 4.9 oz. ..	295	35.7	0	15.8	5.7	127	123	0
roasted:								
7.4 oz., yield from 1 lb. raw								
w/bone and fat	440	51.8	0	24.3	9.1	184	143	0
4 oz.	237	27.9	0	13.1	4.9	99	77	0
1 slice, 3″ diam. × ¼″, approx.								
1 oz.	59	7.0	0	3.3	1.2	25	19	0
diced, 1 cup, approx. 4.9 oz. ..	293	34.5	0	16.2	6.1	122	95	0
LAMB, NEW ZEALAND[1], frozen:								
composite cuts, separable lean and fat:								
raw, 1 oz.	79	4.5	0	6.5	3.3	22	11	0
cooked, 7.8 oz., yield from 1 lb.								
raw w/bone	678	54.3	0	49.5	24.6	242	103	0
cooked, 4 oz.	346	27.7	0	25.2	12.5	124	52	0
composite cuts, separable lean only:								
raw, 1 oz.	36	5.9	0	1.3	.5	21	13	0
cooked, 5.8 oz., yield from 1 lb.								
raw w/bone and fat	339	48.6	0	14.6	6.3	179	83	0
cooked, 4 oz.	234	33.6	0	10.0	4.4	124	57	0

1. *Cooked meats are prepared without added ingredients.*

Food and Measure	cal.	prot. (gms)	carbo. (gms)	tot. fat (gms)	sat. fat (gms)	chol. (mgs)	sod. (mgs)	fiber (gms)
composite cuts, separable fat only:								
raw, 1 oz.	182	2.0	0	19.2	10.0	25	6	0
cooked, 1 oz.	166	2.8	0	17.1	8.9	31	9	0
foreshank, separable lean and fat:								
raw, 1 oz.	63	5.1	0	4.6	2.3	20	13	0
braised or stewed:								
5.9 oz., yield from 1 lb. raw								
w/bone..................	433	45.3	0	26.6	13.1	171	78	0
4 oz.	293	30.6	0	18.0	8.9	116	53	0
1 slice, 3″ diam. × ¼″, approx.								
1 oz.	73	7.6	0	4.5	2.2	29	13	0
diced, 1 cup, approx. 4.9 oz. ..	361	37.8	0	22.2	10.9	143	66	0
foreshank, separable lean only:								
raw, 1 oz.	34	5.9	0	.9	.4	19	14	0
braised or stewed:								
4.85 oz., yield from 1 lb. raw								
w/bone and fat	256	42.3	0	8.3	3.6	138	68	0
4 oz.	211	34.9	0	6.8	3.0	115	56	0
1 slice, 3″ diam. × ¼″, approx.								
1 oz.	53	8.7	0	1.7	.7	29	14	0
diced, 1 cup, approx. 4.9 oz. ..	260	43.1	0	8.5	3.7	141	69	0
leg, whole, separable lean and fat:								
raw, 1 oz.	61	5.2	0	4.3	2.2	22	11	0
roasted:								
9.1 oz., yield from 1 lb. raw								
w/bone	635	64.0	0	40.1	19.6	261	112	0
4 oz.	279	28.1	0	17.6	8.6	115	49	0
1 slice, 3″ diam. × ¼″, approx.								
1 oz.	70	7.0	0	4.4	2.2	29	12	0
diced, 1 cup, approx. 4.9 oz. ..	344	34.7	0	21.8	10.7	141	60	0
leg, whole, separable lean only:								
raw, 1 oz.	35	5.9	0	1.1	.5	21	12	0
roasted:								
7.7 oz., yield from 1 lb. raw								
w/bone and fat	396	60.3	0	15.3	6.7	218	98	0
4 oz.	205	31.4	0	7.9	3.5	113	51	0
1 slice, 3″ diam. × ¼″, approx.								
1 oz.	51	7.8	0	2.0	.9	28	13	0
diced, 1 cup, approx. 4.9 oz. ..	253	38.8	0	9.8	4.3	140	63	0
loin, separable lean and fat:								
raw, 1 oz.	86	4.6	0	7.4	3.8	23	11	0
broiled, 1 chop, 1.5 oz., yield from								
3-oz. raw chop w/bone	135	10.0	0	10.2	5.2	48	21	0
broiled, 4 oz.	357	26.6	0	27.1	13.6	127	56	0
loin, separable lean only:								
raw, 1 oz.	37	6.0	0	1.3	.5	23	13	0
broiled, 1 chop, 1.1 oz., yield from								
3-oz. raw chop w/bone and fat	60	8.8	0	2.5	1.1	34	16	0
broiled, 4 oz.	226	33.2	0	9.3	4.1	129	62	0

Food and Measure	cal.	prot. (gms)	carbo. (gms)	tot. fat (gms)	sat. fat (gms)	chol. (mgs)	sod. (mgs)	fiber (gms)
LAMB, NEW ZEALAND *(cont.)*								
rib, separable lean and fat:								
raw, 1 oz.	98	4.2	0	8.9	4.5	23	11	0
roasted, 8.5 oz., yield from 1 lb.								
raw w/bone	820	45.7	0	69.3	38.4	241	104	0
roasted, 4 oz.	386	21.5	0	32.6	16.4	113	49	0
rib, separable lean only:								
raw, 1 oz.	40	5.8	0	1.7	.7	22	15	0
roasted, 5.4 oz., yield from 1 lb.								
raw w/bone and fat	298	37.1	0	15.5	6.7	143	73	0
roasted, 4 oz.	222	27.7	0	11.5	5.0	107	54	0
shoulder, whole, separable lean and fat:								
raw, 1 oz.	77	4.7	0	6.3	3.2	21	12	0
braised or stewed:								
7.3 oz., yield from 1 lb. raw								
w/bone	724	59.2	0	52.3	25.2	253	106	0
4 oz.	398	32.5	0	28.8	13.9	139	59	0
1 slice, 3″ diam. × ¼″, approx.								
1 oz.	100	8.1	0	7.2	3.5	35	15	0
diced, 1 cup, approx. 4.9 oz. ..	491	40.2	0	35.5	17.1	172	73	0
shoulder, whole, separable lean only:								
raw, 1 oz.	38	5.8	0	1.5	.7	20	13	0
braised or stewed:								
6.5 oz., yield from 1 lb. raw								
w/bone and fat	522	62.3	0	28.3	12.5	232	103	0
4 oz.	323	38.6	0	17.6	7.7	144	64	0
1 slice, 3″ diam. × ¼″, approx.								
1 oz.	81	9.7	0	4.4	1.9	36	16	0
diced, 1 cup	399	47.7	0	21.7	9.5	178	78	0
LAMB, VARIETY MEATS, see specific listings								
LAMB'S-QUARTER:								
raw, trimmed, 1 lb.	195	19.1	33.1	3.6	.3	0	m.q.	9.5 c
raw, trimmed, 1 oz.	12	1.2	2.1	.2	<.1	0	m.q.	.6 c
boiled, drained, 4 oz.	36	3.6	5.7	.8	.1	0	m.q.	2.0 c
boiled, drained, chopped, ½ cup ...	29	2.9	4.5	.6	<.1	0	m.q.	1.6 c
LARD, pork:								
1 cup	1849	0	0	205.0	80.4	195	tr.	0
1 tbsp.	115	0	0	12.8	5.0	12	tr.	0
LASAGNA, pasta, see "Pasta"								
LASAGNA, CANNED:								
(*Chef Boyardee* Microwave), 7.5 oz.	230	7.0	31.0	9.0	m.q.	18	1080	m.q.
(*Nalley's*), 7.5 oz.	180	10.0	24.0	5.0	m.q.	m.q.	720	m.q.
in garden vegetable sauce (*Chef Boyardee* Microwave), 7.5 oz.	170	5.0	14.0	1.0	<1.0	3	940	m.q.
LASAGNA DINNER, FROZEN:								
(*Banquet Extra Helping*), 16.5 oz. ..	645	24.0	88.0	23.0	m.q.	38	1582	m.q.

Food and Measure	cal.	prot. (gms)	carbo. (gms)	tot. fat (gms)	sat. fat (gms)	chol. (mgs)	sod. (mgs)	fiber (gms)
LASAGNA DINNER MIX:								
(*Chef Boyardee*), 5.97 oz.	280	15.0	42.0	8.0	m.q.	m.q.	900	m.q.
LASAGNA ENTREE, FROZEN:								
(*Celentano*), 6.25 oz.	230	13.0	22.0	14.0	m.q.	m.q.	600	m.q.
(*Celentano*), 8 oz.	370	19.0	32.0	19.0	m.q.	m.q.	700	m.q.
(*Celentano*), 10 oz.	460	24.0	40.0	24.0	m.q.	m.q.	870	m.q.
(*Green Giant* Entrees), 12 oz.	490	33.0	44.0	20.0	m.q.	m.q.	1660	m.q.
(*Stouffer's*), 10.5-oz. pkg.	360	28.0	33.0	13.0	m.q.	m.q.	1020	m.q.
(*Stouffer's* 21 oz.), 10.5 oz.	360	28.0	33.0	13.0	m.q.	m.q.	1020	m.q.
(*Tyson Gourmet Selection*), 11.5 oz.	380	20.0	47.0	14.0	m.q.	m.q.	840	m.q.
cheese:								
(*Dining Lite*), 9 oz.	260	14.0	36.0	6.0	m.q.	30	800	m.q.
Italian (*Weight Watchers*), 11 oz. ..	350	29.0	33.0	12.0	4.0	30	690	m.q.
three cheese (*The Budget*								
Gourmet), 10 oz.	400	22.0	38.0	17.0	m.q.	65	760	m.q.
fiesta (*Stouffer's*), 10.25 oz.	430	24.0	35.0	22.0	m.q.	m.q.	960	m.q.
garden (*Weight Watchers*), 11 oz. ...	290	19.0	35.0	7.0	2.0	20	670	m.q.
meat (*Buitoni* Single Serving),								
9 oz.	580	23.0	57.0	19.0	12.0	110	820	m.q.
w/meat and sauce (*Lean Cuisine*),								
10.25 oz.	270	25.0	24.0	8.0	3.0	60	970	m.q.
w/meat sauce:								
(*Banquet Family Entrees*), 7 oz. ...	270	15.0	30.0	10.0	m.q.	m.q.	m.q.	m.q.
(*The Budget Gourmet* Slim								
Selects), 10 oz.	290	18.0	32.0	10.0	m.q.	25	890	m.q.
(*Dining Lite*), 9 oz.	240	13.0	36.0	5.0	m.q.	25	800	m.q.
(*Freezer Queen Deluxe Family*								
Suppers), 7 oz.	200	8.0	28.0	6.0	m.q.	m.q.	730	m.q.
(*Healthy Choice*), 9 oz.	260	18.0	37.0	5.0	2.0	20	420	m.q.
(*Le Menu* LightStyle), 10 oz.	290	19.0	36.0	8.0	m.q.	30	510	m.q.
(*Swanson* Homestyle Recipe),								
10.5 oz.	400	26.0	39.0	15.0	m.q.	m.q.	1070	m.q.
(*Weight Watchers*), 11 oz.	320	26.0	32.0	10.0	4.0	45	630	m.q.
primavera (*Celentano*), 11 oz.	330	18.0	34.0	14.0	m.q.	n.a.	470	m.q.
in sauce (*Buitoni* Family Style),								
7.3 oz.	370	13.0	30.0	13.0	7.0	55	940	m.q.
sausage, Italian (*The Budget*								
Gourmet), 10 oz.	420	20.0	38.0	20.0	m.q.	80	950	m.q.
seafood (*Mrs. Paul's* Light), 9.5 oz.	290	14.0	39.0	8.0	3.0	57	750	m.q.
w/tofu and sauce (*Legume* Classic),								
8 oz.	210	15.0	20.0	8.0	1.3	0	410	8.2 d
tuna, w/spinach noodles and								
vegetables (*Lean Cuisine*),								
9.75 oz.	270	17.0	29.0	10.0	2.0	35	890	m.q.
vegetable:								
(*Stouffer's*), 10.5 oz.	420	23.0	29.0	24.0	m.q.	n.a.	970	m.q.
garden (*Le Menu* LightStyle),								
10.5 oz.	260	11.0	35.0	8.0	3.0	25	500	m.q.
w/tofu and sauce (*Legume*), 12 oz.	240	14.0	26.0	8.0	1.7	0	520	5.8 d

Food and Measure	cal.	prot. (gms)	carbo. (gms)	tot. fat (gms)	sat. fat (gms)	chol. (mgs)	sod. (mgs)	fiber (gms)
LASAGNA ENTREE, FROZEN *(cont.)*								
zucchini (*Lean Cuisine*), 11 oz.	260	20.0	28.0	7.0	2.0	25	950	m.q.
LASAGNA ENTREE, PACKAGED:								
Italian style (*Hormel Top Shelf*),								
1 serving	360	24.0	28.0	17.0	m.q.	40	1350	m.q.
vegetable (*Hormel Top Shelf*),								
10.6 oz.	275	18.0	34.0	8.0	m.q.	35	1024	m.q.
LAVER, see "Seaweed"								
LEAF FAT, pork:								
raw, 1 oz.	243	.5	0	26.7	12.8	31	2	0
LEBANON BOLOGNA, see "Bologna, beef"								
LEEK:								
raw:								
untrimmed, 1 lb.	122	3.0	28.2	.6	.1	0	40	2.4 d
trimmed, 1 oz.	17	.4	4.0	.1	<.1	0	6	.3 d
1 medium, approx. 9.9 oz.	76	1.9	17.6	.4	.1	0	25	1.5 d
chopped, ½ cup	32	.8	7.4	.2	<.1	0	10	.6 d
boiled, drained:								
4 oz.	35	.9	8.6	.2	<.1	0	11	.9 c
1 medium, approx. 4.4 oz.	38	1.0	9.5	.3	<.1	0	13	1.0 c
chopped, ½ cup	16	.4	4.0	.1	<.1	0	6	.4 c
LEEK, FREEZE-DRIED:								
1 oz.	91	4.3	21.2	.6	.1	0	10	2.5 c
¼ cup	3	.1	.6	<.1	tr.	0	tr.	.1 c
1 tbsp.	1	<.1	.2	tr.	tr.	0	tr.	<.1 c
LEGUMES, see specific listings								
LEMON:								
w/peel:								
whole, 1 lb.	89	5.3	47.6	1.3	.2	0	13	m.q.
1 medium, 2⅛" diam., 3.9 oz. ...	22	1.3	11.6	.3	<.1	0	3	m.q.
1-oz. wedge, ¼ medium lemon ..	5	.3	2.9	.1	<.1	0	1	m.q.
w/out peel, 1 large, 2⅜" diam.,								
5.6 oz.	25	.9	7.8	.3	<.1	0	2	.3 c
w/out peel, 1 medium, 2⅛" diam.,								
3.9 oz.	17	.6	5.4	.2	<.1	0	1	.2 c
LEMON BUTTER DILL COOKING SAUCE:								
(*Golden Dipt*), 1 fl. oz.	110	0	5.0	10.0	1.0	0	180	n.a.
LEMON AND DILL SEASONING MIX:								
(*McCormick/Schilling* Bag'n Season),								
1 pkg.	161	3.0	15.0	11.0	m.q.	0	2035	m.q.
LEMON DRINK (see also "Lemonade"):								
chilled (*Crowley*), 8 fl. oz.	130	0	32.0	0	0	0	15	(0)

Food and Measure	cal.	prot. (gms)	carbo. (gms)	tot. fat (gms)	sat. fat (gms)	chol. (mgs)	sod. (mgs)	fiber (gms)
mix[1] (*Pathmark* No Frills), 8 fl. oz.	90	0	20.0	0	0	0	55	(0)
LEMON EXTRACT:								
(*Virginia Dare*), 1 tsp.	22	0	0	0	0	0	0	0
LEMON HERB MARINADE:								
(*Golden Dipt*), 1 fl. oz.	130	0	2.0	14.0	2.0	0	210	n.a.
LEMON AND HERB SEASONING:								
(*McCormick/Schilling* Spice Blends),								
¼ tsp.	1	.1	.2	.1	(0)	0	154	n.a.
LEMON JUICE:								
fresh:								
1 fl. oz.	8	.1	2.6	0	0	0	<1	(0)
½ cup	30	.5	10.5	0	0	0	1	(0)
1 tbsp.	4	.1	1.3	0	0	0	tr.	(0)
canned or bottled:								
½ cup[2].....................	26	.5	7.9	.4	<.1	0	25	(0)
1 tbsp.[2]	3	.1	1.0	<.1	tr.	0	3	(0)
(*Lucky Leaf*), 6 fl. oz.	30	1.0	6.0	0	0	0	35	(0)
(*Minute Maid* 100% Pure),								
1 tbsp.	4	.1	1.0	.1	0	0	2	(0)
reconstituted, natural strength:								
(*A&P*), 1 fl. oz.	6	<1.0	2.0	<1.0	(0)	0	0	(0)
(*ReaLemon*), 1 fl. oz.	6	0	2.0	0	0	0	10	(0)
refrigerated (*ReaLemon* 100%),								
1 fl. oz.	6	0	2.0	0	0	0	5	(0)
frozen:								
single strength, ½ cup	27	.6	7.9	.4	.1	0	1	(0)
single strength, 1 tbsp.	3	.1	1.0	.1	tr.	0	tr.	(0)
(*Sunkist*), 1 fl. oz.	7	.1	2.0	.1	(0)	0	<1	(0)
LEMON PEEL:								
raw, 1 tbsp.	—[3]	.1	1.0	<.1	tr.	0	tr.	m.q.
raw, 1 tsp.	—[3]	<.1	.3	<.1	tr.	0	tr.	m.q.
(*Tone's*), 1 tsp.	0	tr.	.3	0	0	0	0	0
LEMON PEPPER, seasoning,								
1 tsp.:								
(*Lawry's*)	6	.2	1.2	.1	(0)	0	340	.1 c
(*McCormick/Schilling Parsley Patch*)	13	.4	1.0	.6	(0)	0	2	m.q.
(*Tone's*)	6	.1	.9	.2	<.1	0	1086	.1 d
coarse or fine ground (*Tone's Mr. Pepper*)	12	.3	2.8	.1	<.1	0	1	.3 c
LEMON AND PEPPER:								
(*McCormick/Schilling* Spice Blends),								
1 tsp.	7	.2	.8	0	0	0	618	m.q.
LEMON-LIME DRINK, bottled:								
(*Veryfine*), 8 fl. oz.	120	.1	30.0	0	0	0	<10	(0)

1. *Prepared according to package directions.*
2. *Sodium benzoate and sodium bisulfite added as preservatives.*
3. *Value cannot be calculated; no digestibility value for peel.*

Food and Measure	cal.	prot. (gms)	carbo. (gms)	tot. fat (gms)	sat. fat (gms)	chol. (mgs)	sod. (mgs)	fiber (gms)
LEMON-LIME FLAVOR DRINK MIX[1]:								
(*Crystal Light* Sugar Free), 8 fl. oz.	4	0	0	0	0	0	0	0
(*Kool-Aid*), 8 fl. oz.	100	0	25.0	0	0	0	0	0
LEMONADE:								
canned, bottled, or boxed:								
(*Hi-C*), 8.45 fl. oz.	109	.1	27.2	.1	(0)	0	73	(0)
(*Minute Maid* Light'N Juicy),								
6 fl. oz.	8	.2	1.5	.1	(0)	0	17	(0)
(*Shasta*), 12 fl. oz.	146	0	39.0	0	0	0	106	(0)
(*Sunkist*), 8 fl. oz.	141	0	36.0	0	0	0	0	(0)
(*Tropicana* Single Serve), 8 fl. oz.	120	(0)	30.0	0	0	0	<3	(0)
(*Veryfine*), 8 fl. oz.	120	.2	30.0	0	0	0	<25	(0)
(*Wylers*), 6 fl. oz.	64	0	16.5	0	0	0	33	(0)
pink (*Wyler's* Fruit Slush), 4 fl. oz.	157	0	39.3	0	0	0	10	(0)
chilled, regular, pink, or country								
style (*Minute Maid*), 6 fl. oz. ..	81	.2	21.3	0	0	0	23	(0)
frozen[2]:								
undiluted, 6 fl. oz.	397	.6	103.1	.4	.1	0	8	.2 d
1 fl. oz.	13	tr.	3.2	tr.	tr.	0	1	tr.c
8 fl. oz.	100	.1	26.0	.1	<.1	0	8	.1 c
(*Sunkist*), 8 fl. oz.	92	.1	24.2	0	0	0	1	(0)
regular or pink (*A&P*), 8 fl. oz. ..	110	<1.0	28.0	<1.0	(0)	0	0	(0)
regular, pink, or country style								
(*Minute Maid*), 6 fl. oz.	77	.2	20.1	0	0	0	23	(0)
mix, dry:								
1 oz.	107	0	28.0	tr.	tr.	0	7	0
2 tbsp. or 1 scoop	102	0	26.9	tr.	tr.	0	6	0
low-calorie[3], 1 oz.	94	1.0	23.7	.1	tr.	0	3	0
LEMONADE FLAVOR DRINK MIX[1], 8 fl. oz.								
(*Crystal Light* Sugar Free)	4	0	0	0	0	0	0	0
(*Finast*)	80	0	20.0	0	0	0	15	0
(*Kool-Aid* Presweetened)	80	0	20.0	0	0	0	0	0
(*Kool-Aid* Sugar Free)	4	0	0	0	0	0	0	0
(*Wyler's* Crystals, 4 servings/pkg.)	92	0	19.6	1.5	n.a.	0	44	0
(*Wyler's* Crystals, 32 servings/pkg.)	78	0	19.4	0	0	0	39	0
punch (*Country Time*)	80	0	20.0	0	0	0	15	0
regular or pink:								
(*Country Time*)	80	0	20.0	0	0	0	20	0
(*Country Time* Sugar Free)	4	0	0	0	0	0	0	0
(*Kool-Aid*)	100	0	25.0	0	0	0	0	0
LENTIL:								
raw:								
1 oz.	96	8.0	16.2	.3	<.1	0	3	3.2 d
½ cup	324	26.9	54.8	.9	.1	0	9	10.9 d

1. *Prepared according to package directions.*
2. *Diluted according to package directions, except as noted.*
3. *Aspartame sweetened; without added sodium.*

Food and Measure	cal.	prot. (gms)	carbo. (gms)	tot. fat (gms)	sat. fat (gms)	chol. (mgs)	sod. (mgs)	fiber (gms)
green (*Arrowhead Mills*), 2 oz. ...	190	13.0	35.0	1.0	m.q.	0	9	8.8 d
red (*Arrowhead Mills*), 2 oz.	195	14.0	34.0	1.0	m.q.	0	10	8.8 d
boiled:								
4 oz.	132	10.2	22.8	.4	.1	0	2	4.5 d
½ cup	115	8.9	19.9	.4	.1	0	2	4.0 d
(*A&P*), 1 cup	210	16.0	39.0	1.0	m.q.	0	0	m.q.
LENTIL, SPROUTED:								
raw:								
1 lb.	479	40.7	100.4	2.5	.3	0	48	13.8 c
1 oz.	30	2.5	6.3	.2	<.1	0	3	.9 c
½ cup	40	3.4	8.4	.2	<.1	0	4	1.2 c
stir-fried, w/out fat, 4 oz.	115	10.0	24.1	.5	.1	0	m.q.	1.2 c
LENTIL DINNER, canned:								
w/garden vegetables (*Health Valley*								
Fast Menu), 7½ oz.	160	13.0	18.0	4.0	m.q.	0	204	15.5 d
LENTIL PILAF MIX:								
(*Casbah*), 1 oz. dry or ½ cup								
cooked	100	5.0	20.0	0	0	0	m.q.	m.q.
LENTIL RICE LOAF, frozen:								
(*Harvest Bake*), 4 oz. or 2 slices,								
½″ each	190	8.0	18.0	9.0	1.0	0	620	m.q.
LETTUCE:								
bibb, Boston, or butterhead:								
untrimmed, 1 lb.	45	4.3	7.8	.7	.1	0	18	3.4 d
trimmed, 1 oz.	4	.4	.7	.1	tr.	0	1	.3 d
1 head, 5″ diam., approx. 7.75 oz.	21	2.1	3.8	.4	<.1	0	8	1.6 d
2 inner leaves, approx. .5 oz.	2	.2	.4	<.1	tr.	0	1	.5 d
cos or romaine:								
untrimmed, 1 lb.	68	6.9	10.1	.9	.1	0	32	7.2 d
trimmed, 1 oz.	5	.5	.7	.1	tr.	0	2	.5 d
1 inner leaf, approx. .4 oz.	2	.2	.2	<.1	tr.	0	1	.2 d
shredded, ½ cup	4	.5	.7	.1	tr.	0	2	.5 d
iceberg:								
untrimmed, 1 lb.	55	4.3	9.0	.8	.1	0	39	4.3 d
trimmed, 1 oz.	4	.3	.6	.1	tr.	0	3	.3 d
1 head, approx. 6″ diam.,								
1.25 lb.	70	5.4	11.3	1.0	.1	0	48	5.4 d
1 leaf, approx. .7 oz.	3	.2	.4	<.1	tr.	0	2	.2 d
looseleaf:								
untrimmed, 1 lb.	52	3.8	10.2	.9	.1	0	26	2.0 c
trimmed, 1 oz. or ½ cup								
shredded	5	.4	1.0	.1	<.1	0	3	.2 c
1 leaf, approx. .4 oz.	2	.1	.4	<.1	tr.	0	1	.1 c
LIMA BEAN:								
raw:								
untrimmed, 1 lb.	226	13.7	40.2	1.7	.4	0	16	7.4 d
trimmed, 1 oz.	32	1.9	5.7	.2	.1	0	2	1.0 d
trimmed, ½ cup	88	5.3	15.7	.7	.2	0	6	2.9 d
boiled, drained, 4 oz.	139	7.7	26.8	.4	.1	0	19	4.8 d

Food and Measure	cal.	prot. (gms)	carbo. (gms)	tot. fat (gms)	sat. fat (gms)	chol. (mgs)	sod. (mgs)	fiber (gms)
LIMA BEAN *(cont.)*								
boiled, drained, ½ cup	104	5.8	20.1	.3	.1	0	14	3.6 d
LIMA BEAN, CANNED, ½ cup,								
except as noted:								
w/liquid:								
4 oz.	85	5.2	15.8	.3	.1	0	282	4.8 d
½ cup	93	5.6	17.2	.4	.1	0	309	5.2 d
low-sodium, 4 oz.	85	5.2	15.8	.3	.1	0	5	4.8 d
low-sodium	93	5.6	17.2	.4	.1	0	5	5.2 d
(A&P)	110	7.0	20.0	<1.0	(0)	0	380	m.q.
(Featherweight)	80	5.0	16.0	0	0	0	25	m.q.
(Green Giant/Joan of Arc)	80	6.0	16.0	0	0	0	420	3.7 d
(S&W)	100	6.0	19.0	1.0	(0)	0	440	m.q.
(Stokely)	80	5.0	16.0	0	0	0	390	m.q.
(Stokely No Salt or Sugar Added) ...	80	5.0	16.0	0	0	0	5	m.q.
butterbeans *(Van Camp's)*, 1 cup ...	162	11.0	30.0	.5	(0)	0	710	m.q.
butterbeans, large *(Allens)*	110	5.0	18.0	<1.0	(0)	0	370	m.q.
Fordhook *(Stokely)*	80	5.0	14.0	0	0	0	300	m.q.
green:								
(A&P)	80	5.0	15.0	<1.0	(0)	0	320	m.q.
w/liquid *(Del Monte)*	70	4.0	14.0	0	0	0	355	m.q.
small *(S&W* Fancy)	80	6.0	16.0	0	0	0	390	m.q.
tiny, small, or medium *(Allens)* ..	90	5.0	15.0	<1.0	(0)	0	350	m.q.
and white *(Allens)*	90	5.0	15.0	<1.0	(0)	0	370	m.q.
green, small, w/pork *(Luck's)*,								
7.5 oz.	220	10.0	33.0	7.0	m.q.	m.q.	640	8.0 d
w/ham *(Dennison's)*, 7.5 oz.	250	14.0	33.0	7.0	m.q.	m.q.	935	9.0 d
w/pork *(Luck's)*, 7.5 oz.	230	12.0	34.0	7.0	m.q.	m.q.	720	9.0 d
LIMA BEAN, FROZEN:								
(Green Giant)), ½ cup	100	6.0	19.0	0	0	0	30	5.0 d
(Green Giant Harvest Fresh), ½ cup	80	6.0	18.0	0	0	0	170	4.0 d
(Health Valley), ½ cup	94	6.0	18.0	0	0	0	26	3.4 d
baby:								
10-oz. pkg.	376	21.6	71.4	1.3	.3	0	147	6.2 c
boiled, drained, 4 oz.	119	7.5	22.1	.3	.1	0	33	m.q.
boiled, drained, ½ cup	94	6.0	17.5	.3	.1	0	26	m.q.
(Birds Eye), 3.3 oz.	130	7.0	24.0	0	0	0	115	m.q.
(Frosty Acres), 3.3 oz.	130	7.0	24.0	0	0	0	125	2.0 c
(Seabrook), 3.3 oz.	130	7.0	24.0	0	0	0	125	2.0 c
(Southern), 3.5 oz.	135	7.3	25.2	.5	n.a.	0	125	m.q.
butter *(Seabrook)*, 3.3 oz.	140	7.0	26.0	1.0	n.a.	0	213	2.0 c
green *(A&P)*, 3.3 oz.	130	7.0	24.0	<1.0	n.a.	0	130	m.q.
Fordhook:								
10-oz. pkg.	301	18.2	56.3	1.0	.2	0	166	5.6 c
boiled, drained, 4 oz.	113	6.9	21.3	.4	.1	0	60	2.1 c
boiled, drained, ½ cup	85	5.2	16.0	.3	.1	0	45	1.6 c
(A&P), 3.3 oz.	100	6.0	19.0	<1.0	(0)	0	70	m.q.
(Birds Eye), 3.3 oz.	100	6.0	19.0	0	0	0	100	m.q.
(Frosty Acres), 3.3 oz.	100	6.0	19.0	0	0	0	71	2.0 c
(Seabrook), 3.3 oz.	100	6.0	19.0	0	0	0	71	2.0 c

Food and Measure	cal.	prot. (gms)	carbo. (gms)	tot. fat (gms)	sat. fat (gms)	chol. (mgs)	sod. (mgs)	fiber (gms)
(Southern), 3.5 oz.	105	6.4	19.1	.3	(0)	0	100	m.q.
speckled (Seabrook), 3.3 oz.	120	7.0	23.0	0	0	0	19	2.0 c
speckled (Southern), 3.5 oz.	135	7.8	25.0	.4	(0)	0	30	m.q.
tiny (Seabrook), 3.3 oz.	110	6.0	21.0	1.0	(0)	0	144	2.0 c
in butter sauce (Green Giant),								
½ cup	100	6.0	17.0	2.0	<1.0	5	310	2.0 d
in butter sauce, baby (Stokely								
Singles), 4 oz.	140	7.0	25.0	2.0	m.q.	5	450	m.q.
LIMA BEAN, MATURE, dry:								
baby:								
raw, 1 oz.	95	5.8	17.8	.3	.1	0	4	2.8 d
raw, ½ cup	338	20.8	63.5	.9	.2	0	13	10.1 d
boiled:								
4 oz.	143	9.1	26.4	.4	.1	0	3	4.9 d
½ cup	115	7.3	21.2	.3	.1	0	2	3.9 d
(A&P), 1 cup	230	16.0	40.0	1.0	n.a.	0	15	m.q.
large:								
raw, 1 oz.	96	6.1	18.0	.2	<.1	0	5	5.4 d
raw, ½ cup	301	19.1	56.4	.6	.1	0	16	16.9 d
boiled:								
4 oz.	130	8.8	23.7	.4	.1	0	2	8.2 d
½ cup	108	7.3	19.6	.4	.1	0	2	6.8 d
(A&P), 1 cup	230	15.0	35.0	1.0	m.q.	0	0	m.q.
LIMA BEAN, MATURE,								
CANNED (see also "Lima								
bean, canned"):								
w/liquid, 4 oz.	90	5.6	16.9	.2	<.1	0	381	1.4 c
w/liquid, ½ cup	95	5.9	17.9	.2	<.1	0	403	1.5 c
LIME:								
untrimmed, 1 lb.	115	2.7	40.2	.8	.1	0	8	1.9 c
peeled and seeded, 1 oz.	9	.2	3.0	.1	tr.	0	1	.1 c
1 medium, 2″ diam., approx. 2.8 oz.	20	.5	7.1	.1	<.1	0	1	.3 c
LIME JUICE:								
fresh:								
1 fl. oz.	8	.1	2.8	<.1	tr.	0	<1	(0)
½ cup	33	.5	20.4	.2	<.1	0	1	(0)
1 tbsp.	4	.1	1.4	<.1	tr.	0	tr.	(0)
canned or bottled:								
½ cup[1]	26	.3	8.2	.3	<.1	0	20	(0)
1 tbsp.[1]	3	<.1	1.0	<.1	tr.	0	2	(0)
(Rose's), 1 fl. oz.	48	0	12.0	0	0	0	6	(0)
reconstituted, natural strength								
(ReaLime), 1 fl. oz.	6	0	2.0	0	0	0	10	(0)
LIMEADE, frozen[2]:								
undiluted, 6 fl. oz.	408	.4	107.9	.2	<.1	0	n.a.	(0)
1 fl. oz.[3]	13	tr.	3.4	tr.	tr.	0	1	(0)
8 fl. oz.[3]	102	.1	27.1	.1	tr.	0	6	(0)

1. *Sodium benzoate and sodium bisulfite added as preservatives.*
2. *Diluted according to package directions, except as noted.*
3. *Sodium value for contribution from water only.*

Food and Measure	cal.	prot. (gms)	carbo. (gms)	tot. fat (gms)	sat. fat (gms)	chol. (mgs)	sod. (mgs)	fiber (gms)
LIMEADE *(cont.)*								
(Minute Maid), 6 fl. oz.	71	0	19.2	0	0	0	20	(0)
LING, meat only, raw:								
1 lb.	394	86.1	0	2.9	m.q.	m.q.	612	0
1 oz.	25	5.4	0	.2	m.q.	m.q.	38	0
1 fillet, approx. 6.8 oz., yield from								
2½-lb. whole fish	168	36.7	0	1.2	m.q.	m.q.	261	0
LINGCOD, meat only, raw:								
1 lb.	385	80.1	0	4.8	.9	236	266	0
1 oz.	24	5.0	0	.3	<.1	15	17	0
½ fillet, approx. 6.8 oz., yield from								
5-lb. whole fish	164	34.1	0	2.0	.4	100	113	0
LINGUINE, see "Pasta"								
LINGUINE ENTREE, FROZEN:								
w/clam sauce *(Lean Cuisine)*,								
9⅝ oz.	270	16.0	35.0	7.0	1.0	30	890	m.q.
w/scallops and clams *(The Budget*								
Gourmet Slim Selects), 9.5 oz.	280	16.0	28.0	11.0	m.q.	60	630	m.q.
w/shrimp *(The Budget Gourmet)*,								
10 oz.	330	15.0	33.0	15.0	m.q.	75	1250	m.q.
w/shrimp *(Healthy Choice)*, 9.5 oz.	230	12.0	40.0	2.0	1.0	55	390	m.q.
LINGUINE ENTREE,								
PACKAGED:								
w/clam sauce *(Hormel Top Shelf)*,								
1 serving	330	12.0	30.0	18.0	m.q.	85	1420	m.q.
LINSEED OIL, edible:								
1 oz.	251	0	0	28.4	2.7	0	0	0
½ cup	964	0	0	109.0	10.3	0	0	0
1 tbsp.	120	0	0	13.6	1.3	0	0	0
LIQUOR[1], 1 fl. oz.:								
80 proof	65	0	tr.	0	0	0	tr.	0
86 proof	70	0	tr.	0	0	0	tr.	0
90 proof	74	0	tr.	0	0	0	tr.	0
94 proof	77	0	tr.	0	0	0	tr.	0
100 proof	83	0	tr.	0	0	0	tr.	0
LITCHI:								
raw:								
untrimmed, 1 lb.	179	2.3	45.0	1.2	n.a.	0	2	.6 c
shelled and seeded, 1 oz.	19	.2	4.7	.1	(0)	0	<1	.1 c
shelled and seeded, ½ cup	63	.8	15.7	.4	tr.	0	1	.2 c
1 medium, approx. .6 oz.	6	.1	1.6	<.1	(0)	0	tr.	<.1 c
dried, 1 oz.	79	1.1	20.0	.3	(0)	0	1	.4 c
LITTLE CAESARS:								
Little Caesars Meals, 1 serving:								
cheese pizza and individual tossed								
salad	600	30.0	73.0	21.0	m.q.	35	1605	3.0 d

1. *Includes all pure distilled liquors (bourbon, brandy, gin, rum, rye, Scotch, tequila, vodka, whiskey).*

Food and Measure	cal.	prot. (gms)	carbo. (gms)	tot. fat (gms)	sat. fat (gms)	chol. (mgs)	sod. (mgs)	fiber (gms)
pizza, w/green peppers, onions, mushrooms, and individual tossed salad	640	34.0	76.0	22.0	m.q.	40	1715	3.6 d
pizza, single slice:								
cheese, 2.2 oz.	170	9.0	20.0	6.0	m.q.	10	285	.2 d
pepperoni, green peppers, onions, mushrooms, 2.7 oz.	190	10.0	20.0	7.0	m.q.	15	340	.8 d
sandwiches, 1 serving:								
ham and cheese	520	28.0	55.0	21.0	m.q.	45	1045	0.5 d
Italian sub	590	29.0	55.0	28.0	m.q.	60	1230	1.7 d
tuna melt	700	34.0	58.0	37.0	m.q.	65	825	0.6 d
vegetarian	620	30.0	58.0	30.0	m.q.	55	1000	1.3 d
salads, w/low-calorie dressing:								
antipasto salad, 12 oz.	170	10.0	12.0	9.0	m.q.	40	1145	m.q.
Greek salad, 11 oz.	140	8.0	8.0	8.0	m.q.	25	1075	m.q.
tossed salad, 11 oz.	80	4.0	11.0	2.0	m.q.	0	745	m.q.
LIVER[1]:								
beef:								
raw, 1 oz.	40	5.7	1.7	1.1	.4	100	21	0
braised, 11.9 oz., yield from 1 lb.								
raw	542	81.9	11.5	16.4	6.4	1307	235	0
braised, 4 oz.	183	27.6	3.9	5.5	2.2	441	79	0
pan-fried in vegetable oil, 10.4 oz., yield from 1 lb. raw	639	78.8	23.2	23.6	7.9	1422	313	0
pan-fried in vegetable oil, 4 oz. ...	246	30.3	8.9	9.1	3.0	547	120	0
calf, see "veal," below								
chicken, broiler-fryer:								
raw, 1 liver, 1.1 oz.	40	5.8	1.1	1.2	.4	140	25	0
simmered:								
4 oz.	178	27.6	1.0	6.2	2.1	716	58	0
1 liver, approx. .7 oz.	31	4.9	.2	1.1	.4	126	10	0
chopped or diced, 1 cup	219	34.1	1.2	7.6	2.6	883	71	0
duck, domesticated, raw, 1 oz.	39	5.3	1.0	1.3	.4	146	m.q.	0
goose, domesticated, raw, 1 medium, 3.3 oz.	125	15.4	5.9	4.0	1.5	m.q.	132	0
goose, domesticated, raw, 1 oz. ...	38	4.6	1.8	1.2	.5	m.q.	40	0
lamb:								
raw, 1 oz.	40	5.8	.5	1.4	.6	105	20	0
braised, 13.4 oz., yield from 1 lb.								
raw	738	102.6	8.5	29.6	11.4	1681	188	0
braised, 4 oz.	249	34.7	2.9	10.0	3.9	568	64	0
pan-fried in vegetable oil, 11.4 oz., yield from 1 lb. raw	766	82.2	12.2	40.8	15.8	1586	398	0
pan-fried in vegetable oil, 4 oz. ..	270	29.0	4.3	14.3	5.6	559	141	0
pork:								
raw, 1 oz.	38	6.1	.7	1.0	.3	85	25	0

1. *Cooked meats are prepared without added ingredients, except as noted.*

Food and Measure	cal.	prot. (gms)	carbo. (gms)	tot. fat (gms)	sat. fat (gms)	chol. (mgs)	sod. (mgs)	fiber (gms)
LIVER, PORK *(cont.)*								
braised, 12.5 oz., yield from								
1 lb. raw	585	92.1	13.3	15.6	5.0	1257	173	0
braised, 4 oz.	187	29.5	4.3	5.0	1.6	403	56	0
turkey:								
raw, 1 oz.	39	5.7	1.2	1.1	.4	132	27	0
raw, approx. 3.6 oz., from								
15.5-lb. turkey	140	20.4	4.2	4.1	1.3	475	98	0
simmered:								
4 oz.	192	27.2	3.9	6.7	2.1	710	73	0
approx. 2.6 oz., from								
11.2-lb. turkey	127	18.0	2.6	4.5	1.4	470	48	0
chopped or diced, 1 cup	237	33.6	4.8	8.3	2.6	876	89	0
veal:								
raw, 1 oz.	38	5.1	1.3	1.2	.5	88	18	0
braised, 8.8 oz., yield from								
1 lb. raw	412	54.0	6.8	17.2	6.4	1401	132	0
braised, 4 oz.	187	24.5	3.1	7.8	2.9	636	60	0
pan-fried in vegetable oil, 9.6 oz.,								
yield from 1 lb. raw	667	81.0	10.7	31.0	11.5	898	359	0
pan-fried in vegetable oil, 4 oz. . .	278	33.8	4.5	12.9	4.8	374	150	0
LIVER CHEESE:								
(JM), 1-oz. slice	70	4.0	1.0	6.0	m.q.	m.q.	m.q.	0
(Oscar Mayer), 1.34-oz. slice	116	5.8	.5	10.0	3.5	80	418	0
pork, 1 oz.	86	4.3	.6	7.3	2.5	49	347	0
pork, 1 slice, approx. 1.3 oz.,								
6 slices per 8-oz. pkg.	115	5.8	.8	9.7	3.4	66	465	0
LIVER LOAF:								
(Hormel Perma-Fresh), 2 slices	160	9.0	1.0	13.0	m.q.	m.q.	704	0
(Kahn's), 1 slice	170	6.0	3.0	15.0	m.q.	m.q.	370	0
LIVER PATE, see "Paté"								
LIVER SAUSAGE, see								
"Braunschweiger" and								
"Liverwurst"								
LIVERWURST:								
(Hickory Farms), 1 oz.	97	4.0	1.0	9.0	m.q.	74	249	0
(Jones Dairy Farm Chub), 1 oz.	80	4.5	tr.	6.3	m.q.	43	254	0
(Jones Dairy Farm Slices), 1 slice . . .	75	3.5	tr.	6.6	m.q.	43	186	0
pork, 1 oz.	92	4.0	.6	8.1	3.0	45	m.q.	0
pork, 1 slice, 2½″ diam. × ¼″,								
approx. .6 oz.	59	2.5	.4	5.1	1.9	28	m.q.	0
LIVERWURST SPREAD, canned:								
(Hormel), ½ oz.	35	2.0	0	3.0	m.q.	m.q.	m.q.	0
(Underwood), 2⅛ oz.	180	8.0	4.0	15.0	m.q.	90	470	n.a.
LOBSTER, northern, meat only:								
raw:								
1 lb.	410	85.3	2.3	4.1	m.q.	432	m.q.	0
1 oz.	26	5.3	.1	.3	m.q.	27	m.q.	0

Food and Measure	cal.	prot. (gms)	carbo. (gms)	tot. fat (gms)	sat. fat (gms)	chol. (mgs)	sod. (mgs)	fiber (gms)
5.3 oz., yield from 1½-lb. whole lobster	136	28.2	.8	1.4	m.q.	143	m.q.	0
boiled, poached, or steamed[1]:								
4 oz.	111	23.2	1.5	.7	.1	82	431	0
1 cup, approx. 5.1 oz.	142	29.7	1.9	.9	.2	104	551	0
LOBSTER, SPINY, see "Spiny lobster"								
LOBSTER ENTREE, frozen:								
Newburg (*Stouffer's*), 6½ oz.	380	14.0	9.0	32.0	m.q.	m.q.	870	m.q.
LOBSTER SAUCE, canned:								
rock (*Progresso*), ½ cup	120	4.0	11.0	8.0	1.0	10	430	2.0 d
LOGANBERRY:								
untrimmed, 1 lb.	267	4.3	64.2	2.6	m.q.	0	4	m.q.
trimmed, 1 lb.	281	4.5	67.6	2.7	m.q.	0	5	m.q.
trimmed, 1 cup	89	1.4	21.5	.9	m.q.	0	1	4.3 c
LOGANBERRY, FROZEN:								
4 oz.	62	1.7	14.8	.4	m.q.	0	1	m.q.
½ cup	40	1.1	9.6	.2	m.q.	0	1	m.q.
LONDON BROIL, see "Beef entree, frozen"								
LONGAN:								
raw:								
untrimmed, 1 lb.	144	3.2	36.4	.2	n.a.	0	1	1.0 c
shelled and seeded, 1 oz.	17	.4	4.3	<.1	(0)	0	tr.	.1 c
1 medium, approx. .2 oz.	2	<.1	.5	tr.	(0)	0	tr.	<.1 c
dried, 1 oz.	81	1.4	21.0	.1	(0)	0	14	.6 c
LOQUAT:								
untrimmed, 1 lb.	132	1.2	34.1	.6	.1	0	3	1.4 c
peeled and seeded, 1 oz.	13	.1	3.4	.1	<.1	0	<1	.1 c
1 medium, approx. .6 oz.	5	<.1	1.2	<.1	tr.	0	tr.	.1 c
LOTTE, see "Monkfish"								
LOTUS ROOT:								
raw:								
untrimmed, 1 lb.	201	9.3	61.8	.4	.1	0	145	2.9 c
trimmed, 1 oz.	16	.7	4.9	<.1	tr.	0	11	.2 c
1 root, 9½" × 1⅞", approx. 5.1 oz.	64	3.0	19.8	.1	<.1	0	47	.9 c
10 slices, ¼" thick × 2½" diam.	45	2.1	14.0	.1	<.1	0	33	.6 c
boiled, drained, 4 oz.	75	1.8	18.2	.1	<.1	0	51	1.0 c
boiled, drained, 10 slices, 3.1 oz. ..	59	1.4	14.3	.1	<.1	0	40	.8 c
LOTUS SEED[2]:								
raw, in shell, 1 lb.	214	9.9	41.5	1.3	.2	0	3	1.6 c
raw, 1 oz.	25	1.2	4.9	.2	<.1	0	tr.	.2 c
dried, 1 oz., 47 small or 36 large ...	94	4.4	18.3	.6	.1	0	1	.7 c
fried, 1 cup	106	4.9	20.6	.6	.1	0	1	.8 c

1. *Without added ingredients.*
2. *Shelled, except as noted.*

Food and Measure	cal.	prot. (gms)	carbo. (gms)	tot. fat (gms)	sat. fat (gms)	chol. (mgs)	sod. (mgs)	fiber (gms)
LOX, see "Salmon, chinook, smoked" and " 'Salmon,' smoked, imitation"								
LUFFA, see "Sponge gourd"								
LUNCHEON MEAT (see also specific listings):								
(*Oscar Mayer*), 1-oz. slice	94	3.7	.7	8.5	3.3	21	323	0
pork and beef:								
1-oz. slice, 4″ × 4″ × ³⁄₃₂″	100	3.6	.7	9.1	3.3	15	367	0
sausage, 1 oz.	74	4.4	.5	5.9	2.2	18	335	0
sausage, 1 slice, 4¼″ × 4¼″ × 4¼″ × ¹⁄₁₆″, approx. .8 oz. ...	60	3.5	.4	4.8	1.8	15	272	0
canned:								
(*Spam*, 12 oz.), 2 oz.	170	8.0	0	15.0	m.q.	m.q.	862	0
(*Spam*, 7 oz.), 1¾ oz.	150	7.0	0	14.0	m.q.	m.q.	756	0
w/cheese chunks (*Spam*), 2 oz. ..	170	8.0	0	16.0	m.q.	m.q.	811	0
deviled (*Spam*), 1 tbsp.	35	2.0	0	3.0	m.q.	m.q.	125	0
smoke flavored (*Spam*), 2 oz.	170	8.0	0	15.0	m.q.	m.q.	774	0
spiced (*Hormel*), 3 oz.	280	11.0	2.0	26.0	m.q.	m.q.	1110	0
loaf (*OHSE*), 1 oz.	75	3.0	1.0	6.0	m.q.	m.q.	320	0
loaf, spiced (*JM*), 1-oz. slice	70	4.0	1.0	6.0	m.q.	m.q.	370	0
spiced:								
(*Hormel* Perma-Fresh), 2 slices ..	118	9.0	1.0	9.0	m.q.	m.q.	702	0
(*Kahn's* Luncheon Loaf), 1 slice	80	3.0	1.0	7.0	m.q.	m.q.	240	0
(*Light & Lean*), 2 slices	120	8.0	1.0	9.0	m.q.	m.q.	m.q.	0
LUNCHEON "MEAT," VEGETARIAN, canned:								
(*Worthington Numete*), ½″ slice, 2.4 oz.	160	8.0	6.0	11.0	2.0	0	570	m.q.
(*Worthington Protose*), ½″ slice, 2.7 oz.	180	17.0	9.0	8.0	1.0	0	470	m.q.
LUNGS[1]:								
beef:								
raw, 1 oz.	26	4.6	0	.7	.2	69	56	0
braised, 10.7 oz., yield from 1 lb. raw	365	61.8	0	11.2	2.9	840	306	0
braised, 4 oz.	136	23.1	0	4.2	1.4	314	115	0
lamb:								
raw, 1 oz.	27	4.7	0	.7	m.q.	m.q.	45	0
braised, 13.4 oz., yield from 1 lb. raw	430	75.8	0	11.8	m.q.	m.q.	320	0
braised, 4 oz.	128	22.5	0	3.5	m.q.	m.q.	95	0
pork:								
raw, 1 oz.	24	4.0	0	.8	.3	91	43	0
braised, 10.6 oz., yield from 1 lb. raw untrimmed	297	49.8	0	9.3	3.3	1161	242	0

1. *Cooked meats are prepared without added ingredients.*

Food and Measure	cal.	prot. (gms)	carbo. (gms)	tot. fat (gms)	sat. fat (gms)	chol. (mgs)	sod. (mgs)	fiber (gms)
braised, 4 oz.	112	18.8	0	3.5	1.2	439	92	0
veal:								
raw, 1 oz.	26	4.6	0	.7	m.q.	m.q.	31	0
braised, 10.6 oz., yield from 1 lb.								
raw	311	56.2	0	7.9	m.q.	m.q.	167	0
braised, 4 oz.	118	21.3	0	3.0	m.q.	m.q.	64	0
LUPIN:								
raw, 1 oz.	105	10.3	11.4	2.8	.3	0	4	3.9 c
raw, ½ cup	334	32.6	36.3	8.8	1.0	0	13	12.4 c
boiled, 4 oz.	135	17.7	11.2	3.3	.4	0	5	.8 c
boiled, ½ cup	98	12.9	8.2	2.4	.3	0	3	.6 c
LUXURY LOAF:								
pork, 1-oz. slice, 4″ × 4″ × ³⁄₃₂″ ...	40	5.2	1.4	1.4	.5	10	347	0

LYCHEE, see "Litchi"

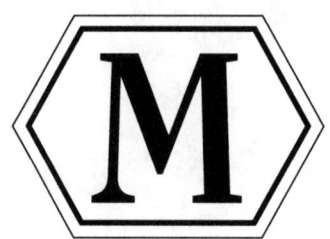

Food and Measure	cal.	prot. (gms)	carbo. (gms)	tot. fat (gms)	sat. fat (gms)	chol. (mgs)	sod. (mgs)	fiber (gms)
MACADAMIA NUT[1]:								
dried:								
in shell, 1 lb.	987	11.7	19.3	103.7	15.5	0	6	7.4 c
1 oz.	199	2.4	3.9	20.9	3.1	0	1	1.5 c
1 cup	940	11.1	18.4	98.8	14.8	0	6	7.1 c
oil-roasted:								
1 oz., 10–12 whole kernels or								
20–24 halves	204	2.1	3.7	21.7	3.3	0	2	.5 c
1 cup, 30 whole kernels or								
73 halves	962	9.7	17.3	102.5	15.4	0	9	2.3 c
chopped, 1 cup	790	8.0	14.2	84.2	12.6	0	8	1.9 c
salted:								
1 oz.	204	2.1	3.7	21.7	3.3	0	74	.5 c
1 cup	962	9.7	17.3	102.5	15.4	0	348	2.3 c
chopped, 1 cup	790	8.0	14.2	84.2	12.6	0	286	1.9 c
(*Mauna Loa*), 1 oz.	210	2.0	4.0	21.0	m.q.	0	75	m.q.
MACARONI[2] (see also "Pasta"):								
1 lb.	1682	58.0	338.8	7.2	1.0	0	33	10.9 d
2 oz.	211	7.3	42.6	.9	.1	0	4	1.4 d
elbow, 1 cup	389	13.4	78.4	1.7	.2	0	8	2.5 d
shells, small, 1 cup	345	11.9	69.5	1.5	.2	0	7	2.2 d
spirals, 1 cup	312	10.7	62.7	1.3	.2	0	6	2.0 d
(*Creamette*), 2 oz.	210	7.0	42.0	1.0	0	0	0	.1 d
(*Delmonico/P&R*), 2 oz.	210	7.0	42.0	1.0	(0)	0	0	m.q.
(*Gioia*), 2 oz.	210	7.0	41.0	1.0	(0)	0	n.a.	m.q.
(*Prince*), 2 oz.	210	7.0	43.0	1.0	0	0	5	m.q.
(*Ronzoni*), 2 oz.	210	7.0	41.0	1.0	(0)	0	<5	m.q.
(*San Giorgio* Italian/American Style),								
2 oz.	210	7.0	42.0	1.0	(0)	0	0	m.q.

1. *Shelled, except as noted.*
2. *Uncooked, except as noted.*

Food and Measure	cal.	prot. (gms)	carbo. (gms)	tot. fat (gms)	sat. fat (gms)	chol. (mgs)	sod. (mgs)	fiber (gms)
cooked:								
4 oz.	160	5.4	32.1	.8	.1	0	1	1.8 d
elbow, 1 cup	197	6.7	39.7	.9	.1	0	1	2.2 d
shells, small, 1 cup	162	5.5	32.6	.8	.1	0	1	1.8 d
spirals, 1 cup	189	6.4	38.0	.9	.1	0	1	2.1 d
protein-fortified:								
1 lb.	1699	90.1	306.5	10.1	1.5	0	37	19.5 d
2 oz.	214	11.3	38.5	1.3	.2	0	5	2.4 d
shells, 1 cup	348	18.5	62.8	2.1	.3	0	8	4.0 d
cooked, 4 oz.	186	9.2	35.9	.2	<.1	0	6	.3 c
cooked, shells, 1 cup	188	9.3	36.4	.3	<.1	0	6	.3 c
vegetable, rainbow, or tricolor:								
1 lb.	1666	59.6	339.6	4.7	.7	0	196	19.5 d
2 oz.	209	7.5	42.7	.6	.1	0	25	2.4 d
spirals, 1 cup	308	11.0	62.9	.9	.1	0	36	3.6 d
cooked, 4 oz.	145	5.1	30.2	.1	<.1	0	7	m.q.
cooked, spirals, 1 cup	171	6.1	35.7	.1	<.1	0	9	m.q.
whole wheat:								
1 lb.	1578	66.4	340.3	6.4	1.2	0	36	53.5 d
2 oz.	198	8.3	42.8	.8	.1	0	5	6.7 d
elbow, 1 cup	365	15.4	78.8	1.5	.3	0	8	12.4 d
cooked, 4 oz.	141	6.0	30.1	.6	.1	0	3	1.1 c
cooked, elbow, 1 cup	174	7.5	37.2	.8	.1	0	4	1.4 c
MACARONI AND BEEF, see "Macaroni dinner" and "Macaroni entree"								
MACARONI AND CHEESE, see "Macaroni dinner," "Macaroni dishes, mix," and "Macaroni entree"								
MACARONI AND CHEESE LOAF:								
(*Eckrich*), 1-oz. slice	75	3.0	3.0	6.0	m.q.	m.q.	320	m.q.
(*OHSE*), 1 oz.	60	4.0	4.0	3.0	m.q.	m.q.	310	m.q.
MACARONI DINNER, frozen:								
and beef (*Swanson*), 12 oz.	370	12.0	48.0	15.0	m.q.	m.q.	930	m.q.
and cheese:								
(*Banquet*), 10 oz.	420	14.0	46.0	20.0	m.q.	30	450	m.q.
(*Swanson*), 12¼ oz.	370	13.0	43.0	15.0	m.q.	m.q.	1070	m.q.
w/mini franks (*Kid Cuisine*), 9 oz.	380	9.0	55.0	14.0	m.q.	40	1000	m.q.
MACARONI DISHES, mix[1] (see also "Salad mix"):								
and cheese:								
(*Kraft* Dinner), ¾ cup	290	9.0	34.0	13.0	3.0	5	530	m.q.
(*Kraft* Deluxe Dinner), ¾ cup ...	260	11.0	36.0	8.0	4.0	20	590	m.q.
(*Kraft* Dinomac/Teddy Bears/*Wild Wheels* Dinner), ¾ cup	310	9.0	36.0	14.0	3.0	10	560	m.q.

1. *Prepared according to package directions, except as noted.*

Food and Measure	cal.	prot. (gms)	carbo. (gms)	tot. fat (gms)	sat. fat (gms)	chol. (mgs)	sod. (mgs)	fiber (gms)
MACARONI DISHES, AND CHEESE *(cont.)*								
(*Kraft* Family Size Dinner),								
¾ cup	290	9.0	34.0	13.0	3.0	5	490	m.q.
cheddar:								
(*Fantastic Foods* Traditional),								
½ cup	112	5.0	19.0	2.0	m.q.	m.q.	205	m.q.
(*Golden Grain*), 1.81 oz. dry ..	190	7.4	35.6	2.1	.8	4	466	1.4 d
(*Golden Grain*), 1 serving	310	8.0	36.0	15.0	m.q.	m.q.	620	m.q.
Parmesan and herbs (*Fantastic*								
Foods), ½ cup[1]	109	5.0	19.0	2.0	m.q.	m.q.	264	m.q.
shells:								
(*Velveeta*), ½ cup	210	10.0	25.0	8.0	4.0	20	570	m.q.
w/bacon (*Velveeta* Bits of								
Bacon), ½ cup	240	11.0	27.0	10.0	5.0	25	690	m.q.
Mexican (*Velveeta* Touch of								
Mexico), ½ cup	210	10.0	27.0	8.0	4.0	20	630	m.q.
spirals (*Kraft* Dinner), ¾ cup	340	9.0	36.0	18.0	4.0	10	600	m.q.
shells 'n curry (*Tofu Classics*),								
½ cup[2]	103	8.0	15.0	3.0	m.q.	n.a.	275	m.q.
shells 'n curry (*Tofu Classics*),								
½ cup[3]	143	8.0	15.0	7.0	m.q.	m.q.	330	m.q.
MACARONI ENTREE, CANNED:								
and beef:								
(*Chef Boyardee* Beefaroni								
Microwave), 7.5 oz.	220	7.0	31.0	7.0	1.0	18	1145	2.0 d
(*Nalley's*), 7.5 oz	180	9.0	29.0	3.0	m.q.	m.q.	900	m.q.
elbows, in beef sauce (*Chef*								
Boyardee Microwave), 7.5 oz.	210	8.0	29.0	7.0	m.q.	15	1000	m.q.
in tomato sauce (*Heinz*), 7.5 oz. ..	200	8.0	23.0	8.0	m.q.	m.q.	850	m.q.
in tomato sauce (*Pathmark* No								
Frills), 7.5 oz.	200	9.0	22.0	8.0	m.q.	m.q.	880	m.q.
and cheese:								
(*Franco-American*), 7⅜ oz.	170	6.0	24.0	6.0	m.q.	m.q.	870	m.q.
(*Heinz*), 7.5 oz.	190	5.0	26.0	8.0	m.q.	m.q.	1105	m.q.
(*Hormel Micro-Cup*), 7.5-oz.								
container	189	7.0	26.0	6.0	m.q.	17	874	m.q.
shells and cheddar (*Lipton Hearty*								
Ones), 11 oz.	367	15.4	60.0	7.4	m.q.	14	1406	m.q.
MACARONI ENTREE, FROZEN:								
and beef, w/tomatoes (*Stouffer's*),								
½ of 11.5-oz. pkg.	170	11.0	15.0	7.0	m.q.	m.q.	810	m.q.
and cheese:								
(*Banquet* Casserole), 8 oz.	350	11.0	36.0	17.0	m.q.	m.q.	930	m.q.
(*Banquet* Family Entrees), 8 oz. ..	290	12.0	32.0	13.0	m.q.	m.q.	m.q.	m.q.
(*The Budget Gourmet* Side Dish),								
5.3 oz.	210	9.0	23.0	8.0	m.q.	25	370	m.q.

1. *Prepared with whole milk.*
2. *Prepared with tofu.*
3. *Prepared with tofu and 2 tbsp. salted butter.*

Food and Measure	cal.	prot. (gms)	carbo. (gms)	tot. fat (gms)	sat. fat (gms)	chol. (mgs)	sod. (mgs)	fiber (gms)
(Freezer Queen Family Side Dish),								
4 oz.	110	3.0	19.0	2.0	m.q.	m.q.	420	m.q.
(Green Giant One Serving),								
5.7 oz.	230	9.0	28.0	9.0	4.0	25	590	m.q.
(Myers), 3.5 oz.	168	7.0	16.0	9.0	m.q.	m.q.	516	m.q.
(Stouffer's), ½ of 12-oz. pkg.	250	12.0	22.0	13.0	m.q.	m.q.	730	m.q.
(Stouffer's), ¼ of 20-oz. pkg.	210	10.0	18.0	11.0	m.q.	m.q.	610	m.q.
(Swanson Homestyle Recipe),								
10 oz.	390	17.0	37.0	19.0	m.q.	m.q.	1150	m.q.
pie *(Swanson Pot Pie),* 7 oz.	200	7.0	24.0	8.0	m.q.	m.q.	740	m.q.
MACARONI MIX, see "Macaroni dishes, mix"								
MACE, ground:								
1 oz.	135	1.9	14.3	9.2	2.7	0	23	1.4 c
1 tbsp.	25	.4	2.7	1.7	.5	0	4	.3 c
1 tsp.	8	.1	.9	.6	.2	0	1	.1 c
(Spice Islands), 1 tsp.	10	.1	.8	.7	m.q.	0	1	.1 c
(Tone's), 1 tsp.	8	.1	.9	.6	.2	0	1	.1 d
MACKEREL, ATLANTIC, meat only:								
raw:								
1 lb.	929	84.4	0	63.0	14.8	318	408	0
1 oz.	58	5.3	0	3.9	.9	20	26	0
1 fillet, approx. 3.95 oz., yield from 1½-lb. whole fish	229	20.8	0	15.6	3.6	78	101	0
baked, broiled, or microwaved[1],								
4 oz.	297	27.0	0	20.2	4.7	85	94	0
MACKEREL, CANNED, Jack, drained:								
12.7 oz., yield from No. 300 can ...	563	83.7	0	22.7	6.7	285	1368	0
4 oz.	177	26.3	0	7.1	2.1	90	430	0
1 cup	296	44.1	0	12.0	3.5	150	720	0
MACKEREL, KING, meat only, raw:								
1 lb.	475	92.0	0	9.1	1.6	242	717	0
1 oz.	30	5.7	0	.6	.1	15	45	0
½ fillet, approx. 7 oz., yield from 5-lb. whole fish	207	40.2	0	4.0	.7	106	313	0
MACKEREL, PACIFIC AND JACK, mixed species, meat only, raw:								
1 lb.	712	91.0	0	35.8	10.2	213	391	0
1 oz.	45	5.7	0	2.2	.6	13	24	0
1 fillet, approx. 7.9 oz., yield from 3-lb. whole fish	353	45.2	0	17.8	5.1	106	194	0

1. *Without added ingredients.*

Food and Measure	cal.	prot. (gms)	carbo. (gms)	tot. fat (gms)	sat. fat (gms)	chol. (mgs)	sod. (mgs)	fiber (gms)
MACKEREL, SPANISH, meat								
only:								
raw:								
1 lb.	631	87.5	0	28.6	8.3	345	266	0
1 oz.	39	5.5	0	1.8	.5	22	17	0
1 fillet, approx. 6.6 oz., yield from								
3-lb. whole fish	260	36.1	0	11.8	3.4	142	110	0
baked, broiled, or microwaved[1]:								
4 oz.	179	26.8	0	7.2	2.0	83	75	0
1 fillet, approx. 5.1 oz., yield from								
6.6-oz. raw fillet	230	34.4	0	9.2	2.6	107	96	0
MAHI MAHI, see "Dolphin fish"								
MAHOGANY APPLE, see								
"Cashew"								
MAI TAI MIX:								
bottled (*Holland House*), 1 fl. oz. ...	32	0	8.0	0	0	0	60	(0)
instant (*Holland House*), .56 oz.	64	0	16.0	0	0	0	4	(0)
MALACCA APPLE:								
seeded, 1 oz.	9	.2	2.3	<.1	tr.	0	n.a.	.2 c
MALT LIQUOR, see "Beer, ale,								
and malt liquor"								
MALTED MILK:								
chocolate flavor:								
powder, 1 oz.	112	1.8	24.1	1.3	.6	1	66	.1 c
powder, ¾ oz. or 2–3 heaping								
tsp.	83	1.4	17.8	.9	.5	1	49	.1 c
beverage, 1 cup whole milk and								
¾ oz. powder	233	9.4	29.2	9.1	5.5	34	168	.1 c
natural flavor:								
powder, 1 oz.	117	3.7	20.5	2.4	1.2	6	130	.2 c
powder, ¾ oz. or 2–3 heaping								
tsp.	86	2.7	15.2	1.8	.9	4	96	.1 c
beverage, 1 cup whole milk and								
¾ oz. powder	236	10.8	26.6	9.9	6.0	37	215	.1 c
MALTED MILK FLAVOR MIX:								
chocolate flavor:								
powder:								
1 oz.	106	1.4	24.9	1.1	.6	1	71	<.1 c
3 heaping tsp. or .7 oz.	79	1.1	18.4	.8	.5	1	53	tr.c
(*Carnation*), 3 heaping tsp. ...	80	1.0	18.0	.8	.5	0	55	n.a.
(*Kraft* Instant), 3 tsp.	90	1.0	18.0	1.0	n.a.	n.a.	45	n.a.
beverage:								
1 cup whole milk and 3 heaping								
tsp. powder	229	9.1	29.8	8.9	5.5	34	172	tr.c
1 cup lowfat 2% milk and								
3 heaping tsp. powder	200	9.2	30.1	5.5	3.4	19	175	tr.c

1. *Without added ingredients.*

Food and Measure	cal.	prot. (gms)	carbo. (gms)	tot. fat (gms)	sat. fat (gms)	chol. (mgs)	sod. (mgs)	fiber (gms)
1 cup lowfat 1% milk and 3 heaping tsp. powder	181	9.1	30.1	3.4	2.1	11	176	tr.c
1 cup skim milk and 3 heaping tsp. powder	165	9.5	30.3	1.2	.7	5	179	tr.c
chocolate flavor, w/added nutrients:								
powder, 1 oz.	101	1.4	23.9	1.0	.6	n.a.	168	tr.c
powder, 4–5 heaping tsp. or .7 oz.	75	1.0	17.7	.7	.4	n.a.	125	tr.c
beverage[1]:								
1 cup whole milk and 4–5 heaping tsp. powder	225	9.1	29.1	8.9	5.5	33	244	tr.c
1 cup lowfat 2% milk and 4–5 heaping tsp. powder	196	9.1	29.4	5.4	3.3	18	247	tr.c
1 cup lowfat 1% milk and 4–5 heaping tsp. powder	177	9.0	29.4	3.3	2.0	10	248	tr.c
1 cup skim milk and 4–5 heaping tsp. powder	161	9.3	29.6	1.1	.7	4	251	tr.c
natural flavor:								
powder:								
1 oz.	117	3.2	21.5	2.2	1.2	6	140	tr.c
3 heaping tsp. or .7 oz.	87	2.3	15.9	1.7	.9	4	103	tr.c
(Carnation Original), 3 heaping tsp.	90	3.0	15.0	1.8	1.0	0	100	n.a.
(Kraft Instant), 3 tsp.	90	3.0	16.0	2.0	m.q.	n.a.	100	n.a.
beverage:								
1 cup whole milk and 3 heaping tsp. powder	237	10.4	27.3	9.8	6.0	37	223	tr.c
1 cup lowfat 2% milk and 3 heaping tsp. powder	208	10.4	27.6	6.4	3.8	22	225	tr.c
1 cup lowfat 1% milk and 3 heaping tsp. powder	189	10.3	27.6	4.3	2.5	14	226	tr.c
1 cup skim milk and 3 heaping tsp. powder	173	10.7	27.8	2.1	1.2	8	229	tr.c
natural flavor, w/added nutrients:								
powder, 1 oz.	109	2.5	23.0	.8	.4	n.a.	115	<.1 c
powder, 4–5 heaping tsp. or .7 oz. dry	80	1.8	17.1	.6	.3	n.a.	85	tr.c
beverage[1]:								
1 cup whole milk and 4–5 heaping tsp. powder	230	9.9	28.4	8.7	5.4	33	205	tr.c
1 cup lowfat 2% milk and 4–5 heaping tsp. powder	201	9.9	28.8	5.3	3.2	18	207	tr.c
1 cup lowfat 1% milk and 4–5 heaping tsp. powder	182	9.8	28.8	3.2	1.9	10	208	tr.c
1 cup skim milk and 4–5 heaping tsp. powder	166	10.2	29.0	1.0	.6	4	211	tr.c

1. Cholesterol value for contribution from milk only.

Food and Measure	cal.	prot. (gms)	carbo. (gms)	tot. fat (gms)	sat. fat (gms)	chol. (mgs)	sod. (mgs)	fiber (gms)
MAMMY APPLE:								
untrimmed, 1 lb.	139	1.4	34.0	1.4	n.a.	0	41	2.7 c
peeled and seeded, 1 oz.	14	.1	3.5	.1	n.a.	0	4	.3 c
1 medium, approx. 3.1 lb.	431	4.2	105.8	4.2	n.a.	0	127	8.5 c
MANDARIN ORANGE, see "Tangerine"								
MANGO:								
untrimmed, 1 lb.	204	1.6	53.2	.9	.2	0	6	3.4 d
peeled and seeded, 1 oz.	18	.1	4.8	.1	<.1	0	1	.3 d
1 medium, approx. 10.6 oz.	135	1.1	35.2	.6	.1	0	4	2.2 d
sliced, ½ cup	54	.4	14.0	.2	.1	0	2	.9 d
MANGO NECTAR:								
(Libby's), 6 fl. oz.	110	0	26.0	0	0	0	0	m.q.
MANHATTAN[1]:								
1 fl. oz.	64	tr.	.9	0	0	0	1	0
MANHATTAN MIX:								
bottled (Holland House), 1 fl. oz. ...	28	0	7.0	0	0	0	5	0
MANICOTTI DINNER, frozen:								
three cheese (Le Menu), 11.75 oz.	390	19.0	44.0	15.0	m.q.	m.q.	870	m.q.
MANICOTTI ENTREE, frozen:								
(Buitoni Single Serving), 9-oz. pkg.	470	18.0	45.0	14.0	8.0	130	830	m.q.
(Celentano), 8 oz.	300	16.0	36.0	11.0	m.q.	m.q.	690	m.q.
cheese:								
(Weight Watchers), 9.25 oz.	280	17.0	33.0	8.0	4.0	75	490	m.q.
w/meat sauce (The Budget Gourmet), 10 oz.	450	20.0	33.0	26.0	m.q.	50	920	m.q.
w/sauce (Celentano), 10 oz.	380	20.0	45.0	14.0	m.q.	m.q.	860	m.q.
w/sauce (Celentano), 7 oz.	360	21.0	35.0	16.0	m.q.	m.q.	580	m.q.
w/spinach, tofu, and sauce (Legume Florentine), 11 oz.	260	18.0	30.0	7.0	1.0	0	650	8.7 d
w/tofu and sauce (Legume Classic), 8 oz.	220	17.0	24.0	11.0	1.9	0	370	7.0 d
MANIOC, see "Cassava"								
MAPLE SUGAR, see "Sugar, maple"								
MAPLE SYRUP (see also "Pancake syrup"):								
½ cup	397	0	102.4	0	0	0	16	0
1 tbsp.	50	0	12.8	0	0	0	2	0
MARGARINE, 1 tbsp., except as noted:								
(A&P Corn Oil Quarters)	100	<1.0	<1.0	11.0	2.0	0	105	0
(A&P Premium)	100	<1.0	<1.0	11.0	2.0	0	110	0
(Ann Page Quarters)	100	<1.0	<1.0	11.0	2.0	0	110	0
(Country Morning Stick), 1 tsp.	35	0	0	4.0	m.q.	5	35	0
(Country Morning Tub), 1 tsp.	30	0	0	3.0	m.q.	5	25	0
(Country Morning Unsalted Stick), 1 tsp.	35	0	0	4.0	m.q.	4	0	0

1. Recipe: 73.7% whiskey and 26.3% vermouth.

Food and Measure	cal.	prot. (gms)	carbo. (gms)	tot. fat (gms)	sat. fat (gms)	chol. (mgs)	sod. (mgs)	fiber (gms)
(*Country Morning* Unsalted Tub),								
1 tsp.	30	0	0	3.0	m.q.	5	0	0
(*Country Morning* Light Stick),								
1 tsp.	20	0	0	2.0	m.q.	3	30	0
(*Country Morning* Light Tub), 1 tsp.	20	0	0	2.0	m.q.	3	25	0
(Diet *Mazola*)	50	0	0	6.0	1.0	0	130	0
(*Hain* Safflower)	100	0	0	11.0	2.0	0	170	0
(*Hain* Safflower Unsalted)	100	0	0	11.0	2.0	0	<5	0
(*Hollywood* Safflower)	100	0	0	11.0	5.0	0	130	0
(*Hollywood* Safflower Unsalted)	100	0	0	11.0	2.0	0	2	0
(*I Can't Believe It's Not Butter* Sweet								
Unsalted)	90	0	0	10.0	2.0	0	0	0
(*Land O'Lakes* Stick or Tub), 1 tsp.	35	0	0	4.0	m.q.	0	35	0
(*Mazola*)	100	0	0	11.0	2.0	0	100	0
(*Mazola* Unsalted)	100	0	0	11.0	2.0	0	0	0
(*Nucoa*)	100	0	0	11.0	2.0	0	160	0
(*Nucoa Heart Beat*)	25	0	0	3.0	<1.0	0	110	0
(*Nucoa Heart Beat* Unsalted)	24	0	0	3.0	<1.0	0	0	0
(*Parkay*)	100	0	0	11.0	2.0	0	105	0
(*Weight Watchers* Stick)	60	0	0	7.0	1.0	0	130	0
(*Weight Watchers* Tub)	50	0	0	6.0	1.0	0	130	0
(*Weight Watchers* Unsalted)	50	0	0	6.0	1.0	0	0	0
blend, see specific brands								
soft:								
(*A&P* Soft Bowl)	100	<1.0	<1.0	11.0	2.0	0	105	0
(*Chiffon* Cup)	90	0	0	10.0	1.0	0	95	0
(*Chiffon* Stick)	100	0	0	11.0	2.0	0	105	0
(*Chiffon* Unsalted)	90	0	0	10.0	2.0	0	0	0
(Diet *Parkay*)	50	0	0	6.0	1.0	0	110	0
(*Hain* Safflower)	100	0	0	11.0	2.0	0	170	0
(*Nucoa*)	90	0	0	10.0	2.0	0	150	0
(*Parkay*)	100	0	0	11.0	2.0	0	105	0
spread:								
(*Hollywood* Soft)	90	0	1.0	10.0	1.0	0	135	0
(*Kraft* "Touch of Butter" Bowl) ..	50	0	0	6.0	1.0	0	110	0
(*Kraft* "Touch of Butter" Stick) ..	90	0	0	10.0	2.0	0	110	0
(*Land O'Lakes* Tub), 1 tsp.	25	0	0	3.0	m.q.	0	25	0
(*Mazola* Corn Oil Light)	50	0	0	6.0	1.0	0	100	0
(*Parkay* 50% Vegetable Oil)	60	0	0	7.0	1.0	0	110	0
(*Weight Watchers* Light)	50	0	0	6.0	1.0	0	130	0
w/sweet cream:								
(*Land O'Lakes* Stick), 1 tsp. ..	30	0	0	4.0	m.q.	0	35	0
(*Land O'Lakes* Tub), 1 tsp.	25	0	0	3.0	m.q.	0	25	0
(*Land O'Lakes* Unsalted),								
1 tsp.	30	0	0	4.0	m.q.	0	0	0
vegetable (*P&Q* 60% Quarters) ..	80	<1.0	<1.0	8.0	1.0	0	105	0
squeeze (*Parkay*)	90	0	0	10.0	2.0	0	110	0
whipped:								
(*Chiffon*)	70	0	0	8.0	1.0	0	80	0

Food and Measure	cal.	prot. (gms)	carbo. (gms)	tot. fat (gms)	sat. fat (gms)	chol. (mgs)	sod. (mgs)	fiber (gms)
MARGARINE, WHIPPED *(cont.)*								
(*Miracle* Brand Cup)	60	0	0	7.0	1.0	0	70	0
(*Miracle* Brand Stick)	70	0	0	7.0	1.0	0	65	0
(*Parkay* Cup)	70	0	0	7.0	1.0	0	70	0
(*Parkay* Stick)	70	0	0	7.0	1.0	0	65	0
MARGARITA MIX:								
bottled (*Holland House*), 1 fl. oz. ...	27	0	6.0	0	0	0	92	(0)
instant (*Holland House*), .5 oz.	57	0	14.0	0	0	0	4	(0)
strawberry, bottled (*Holland House*), 1 fl. oz.	31	0	7.0	0	0	0	3	n.a.
strawberry, instant (*Holland House*), .56 oz.	66	0	16.0	0	0	0	<1	(0)
MARINADE, see specific listings								
MARINARA SAUCE, see "Pasta sauce" and "Tomato sauce"								
MARJORAM, dried:								
1 oz.	77	3.6	17.2	2.0	n.a.	0	22	5.1 c
1 tbsp.	5	.2	1.0	.1	(0)	0	1	.3 c
1 tsp.	2	.1	.4	<.1	(0)	0	tr.	.1 c
(*Spice Islands*), 1 tsp.	4	.2	.7	.1	(0)	0	1	.2 c
(*Tone's*), 1 tsp.	2	.1	.3	<.1	(0)	0	<1	.1 d
MARMALADE, orange:								
(*Finast*), 2 tsp.	35	0	9.0	0	0	0	2	m.q.
(*Smucker's*), 1 tsp.	18	0	4.0	0	0	0	0	m.q.
MARMALADE PLUM, see "Sapote"								
MARROW SQUASH:								
raw, trimmed, 1 oz.	4	.2	1.0	<.1	tr.	0	n.a.	.1 c
MARSHMALLOW, see "Candy"								
MARSHMALLOW TOPPING:								
(*Marshmallow Fluff*), 1 heaping tsp., .6 oz.	59	0	15.0	0	0	0	12	0
creme (*Finast*), 1 oz.	95	0	23.0	0	0	0	45	0
creme (*Kraft*), 1 oz.	90	0	23.0	0	0	0	20	0
MARTINI[1]:								
1 fl. oz.	63	tr.	.1	0	0	0	1	0
MASA, see "Corn Flour"								
MATAI, see "Waterchestnut"								
MATZO, see "Cracker"								
MATZO MEAL, see "Cracker crumbs and meal"								
MAYONNAISE (see also "Mayonnaise, imitation" and "Salad dressing"), 1 tbsp., except as noted:								
(*Bama*)	100	0	0	11.0	m.q.	m.q.	65	0
(*Bennett's* Real)	110	0	1.0	12.0	m.q.	m.q.	65	0

1. *Recipe: 79.4% gin and 20.6% vermouth.*

Food and Measure	cal.	prot. (gms)	carbo. (gms)	tot. fat (gms)	sat. fat (gms)	chol. (mgs)	sod. (mgs)	fiber (gms)
(*Cains*)	100	0	0	11.0	2.0	10	80	0
(*Finast*)	100	0	0	11.0	2.0	10	80	0
(*Hain/Hollywood* Canola)	100	0	<1.0	11.0	1.0	5	100	0
(*Hain* Real No Salt Added)	110	0	0	12.0	2.0	5	0	0
(*Hain* Safflower)	110	0	0	12.0	1.0	5	70	0
(*Hellmann's/Best Foods*)	100	0	0	11.0	2.0	5	80	0
(*Hollywood*)	110	0	0	12.0	1.0	5	80	0
(*Hollywood* Safflower)	100	0	0	12.0	1.0	5	75	0
(*Kraft* Real)	100	0	0	12.0	2.0	5	70	0
(*Pathmark*)	100	0	0	11.0	2.0	5	70	0
(*Pathmark* Low Sodium)	100	0	0	11.0	2.0	5	70	0
(*Pathmark* No Frills)	100	0	0	11.0	2.0	10	75	0
(*Rokeach*)	100	0	0	11.0	2.0	10	70	0
cold processed (*Hain*)	110	0	0	12.0	2.0	5	70	0
reduced calorie:								
(*Estee*)	45	0	1.0	4.0	1.0	10	120	0
(*Featherweight*)	30	0	3.0	2.0	m.q.	10	40	0
(*Finast* Lite)	40	0	1.0	4.0	1.0	5	100	0
(*Hain* Light Low Sodium)	60	0	2.0	6.0	1.0	10	95	0
(*Hellmann's/Best Foods* Light) ...	50	0	1.0	5.0	1.0	5	115	0
(*Kraft* Light)	50	0	1.0	5.0	1.0	0	110	0
(*Pathmark*)	40	0	1.0	4.0	1.0	5	100	0
(*Weight Watchers*)	50	0	1.0	5.0	1.0	5	100	0
(*Weight Watchers* Low Sodium) ...	50	0	1.0	5.0	1.0	5	45	0
safflower and soybean:								
1 oz.	203	.3	.8	22.5	2.4	m.q.	161	0
1 cup	1577	2.4	6.0	174.6	18.9	m.q.	1250	0
1 tbsp.	99	.2	.4	11.0	1.2	m.q.	78	0
soybean:								
1 oz.	203	.3	.8	22.5	3.3	17	161	0
1 cup	1577	2.4	6.0	174.6	26.1	130	1250	0
1 tbsp.	99	.2	.4	11.0	1.6	8	78	0
(*Featherweight Soyamaise*)	100	0	0	11.0	m.q.	5	3	0
MAYONNAISE, IMITATION (see also "Salad dressing"):								
(*Hain* Canola Reduced Calorie), 1 tbsp.	60	0	2.0	5.0	0	0	160	0
(*Hain* Eggless No Salt Added), 1 tbsp.	110	0	0	12.0	2.0	0	<5	0
(*Hellmann's* Cholesterol Free), 1 tbsp.	50	0	1.0	5.0	1.0	0	80	0
(*Nucoa Heart Beat*), 1 tbsp.	40	0	1.0	4.0	<1.0	0	110	0
(*Weight Watchers* Cholesterol Free), 1 tbsp.	50	0	1.0	5.0	1.0	0	90	0
milk cream:								
1 oz.	27	.6	3.1	1.4	.8	12	143	0
1 cup	232	5.1	26.6	12.2	6.7	103	1210	0
1 tbsp.	15	.3	1.7	.8	.4	6	76	0

Food and Measure	cal.	prot. (gms)	carbo. (gms)	tot. fat (gms)	sat. fat (gms)	chol. (mgs)	sod. (mgs)	fiber (gms)
MAYONNAISE, IMITATION *(cont.)*								
soybean:								
1 oz.	66	.1	4.5	5.4	.9	7	141	0
1 cup	556	.6	38.4	46.1	8.0	58	1193	0
1 tbsp.	35	tr.	2.4	2.9	.5	4	75	0
no cholesterol:								
1 oz.	137	<.1	4.5	13.5	2.1	0	100	0
1 cup	1084	.2	35.6	107.3	16.9	0	794	0
1 tbsp.	68	tr.	2.2	6.7	1.1	0	49	0
sunflower (*Life* All Natural), 1 tbsp.	71	<1.0	1.0	8.0	m.q.	0	3	0
tofu (*Nasoya Nayonaise*), 1 tbsp.	40	1.0	1.0	4.0	m.q.	0	50	(0)
McDONALD'S:								
breakfast, 1 serving:								
apple bran muffin, 3 oz.	190	5.0	46.0	0	0	0	230	m.q.
biscuit:								
w/bacon, egg, and cheese, 5.5 oz.	440	17.5	33.3	26.4	8.2	253	1230	m.q.
w/biscuit spread, 2.6 oz.	260	4.6	31.9	12.7	3.4	1	730	m.q.
w/sausage, 4.3 oz.	440	13.0	31.9	29.0	9.3	49	1080	m.q.
w/sausage and egg, 6.3 oz.	520	19.9	32.6	34.5	11.2	275	1250	m.q.
danish:								
apple, 4.1 oz.	390	5.8	51.2	17.9	3.5	25	370	m.q.
cinnamon raisin, 3.9 oz.	440	6.4	57.5	21.0	4.2	34	430	m.q.
iced cheese, 3.9 oz.	390	7.4	42.3	21.8	5.9	47	420	m.q.
raspberry, 4.1 oz.	410	6.1	61.5	15.9	3.1	26	310	m.q.
Egg McMuffin, 4.9 oz.	290	18.2	28.1	11.2	3.8	226	740	m.q.
eggs, scrambled, 3.5 oz.	140	12.4	1.2	9.8	3.3	399	290	0
English muffin, w/butter, 2.1 oz.	170	5.4	26.7	4.6	2.4	9	270	m.q.
English muffin, w/out butter	140	m.q.	m.q.	m.q.	m.q.	0	235	m.q.
hash brown potatoes, 1.9 oz.	130	1.4	14.9	7.3	3.2	9	330	m.q.
hotcakes, w/butter and syrup, 6.2 oz.	410	8.2	74.4	9.2	3.7	21	640	m.q.
sausage, pork, 1.7 oz.	180	8.4	0	16.3	5.9	48	350	0
Sausage McMuffin, 4.1 oz.	370	16.5	27.3	21.9	7.8	64	830	m.q.
Sausage McMuffin, w/egg, 5.9 oz.	440	22.6	27.9	26.8	9.5	263	980	m.q.
sandwiches and chicken, 1 serving:								
Big Mac, 7.6 oz.	560	25.2	42.5	32.4	10.1	103	950	m.q.
cheeseburger, 4.1 oz.	310	15.0	31.2	13.8	5.2	53	750	m.q.
Chicken McNuggets, 4 oz.	290	19.0	16.5	16.3	4.1	65	520	m.q.
Filet-O-Fish, 5 oz.	440	13.8	37.9	26.1	5.2	50	1030	m.q.
hamburger, 3.6 oz.	260	12.3	30.6	9.5	3.6	37	500	m.q.
McChicken, 6.7 oz.	490	19.2	39.8	28.6	5.4	43	780	m.q.
McD.L.T., 8.3 oz.	580	26.3	36.0	36.8	11.5	109	990	m.q.
McLean Deluxe, 7.3 oz.	320	22.0	35.0	10.0	4.0	60	670	m.q.
McLean Deluxe, w/cheese, 7.7 oz.	370	24.0	35.0	14.0	5.0	75	890	m.q.
McLean Deluxe, patty only, 3 oz.	130	17.0	0	7.0	3.0	60	110	0
Quarter Pounder, 5.9 oz.	410	23.1	34.0	20.7	8.1	86	660	m.q.
Quarter Pounder, w/cheese, 6.8 oz.	520	28.5	35.1	29.2	11.2	118	1150	m.q.

Food and Measure	cal.	prot. (gms)	carbo. (gms)	tot. fat (gms)	sat. fat (gms)	chol. (mgs)	sod. (mgs)	fiber (gms)
Chicken McNuggets sauces:								
barbeque, 1 oz.	50	.3	12.1	.5	.1	0	340	0
honey, 1.5 oz.	45	0	11.5	0	0	0	0	0
hot mustard, 1 oz.	70	.5	8.2	3.6	.5	5	250	0
sweet and sour, 1 oz.	60	.2	13.8	.2	tr.	0	190	0
french fries:								
small, 2.4 oz.	220	3.1	25.6	12.0	2.7	0	110	m.q.
small, w/out salt, 2.4 oz.	220	3.1	25.6	12.0	2.7	0	25	m.q.
medium, 3.4 oz.	320	4.4	36.3	17.1	3.9	0	150	m.q.
medium, w/out salt, 3.4 oz.	320	4.4	36.3	17.1	3.9	0	35	m.q.
large, 4.3 oz.	400	5.6	45.9	21.6	5.0	0	200	m.q.
large, w/out salt, 4.3 oz.	400	5.6	45.9	21.6	5.0	0	45	m.q.
salads, 1 serving:								
chef, 10 oz.	230	20.5	7.5	13.3	5.9	128	490	m.q.
chunky chicken, 8.8 oz.	140	23.1	5.3	3.4	0.9	78	230	m.q.
garden, 7.5 oz.	110	7.1	6.2	6.6	2.9	83	160	m.q.
side salad, 4.1 oz.	60	3.7	3.3	3.3	1.5	41	85	m.q.
dressings and condiments:								
bacon bits, .1 oz.	16	1.3	.1	1.2	0	0	95	n.a.
bleu cheese dressing, ⅕ pkg. ...	70	.5	1.2	6.9	1.3	6	150	n.a.
croutons, .4 oz.	50	1.4	6.8	2.2	.5	0	140	m.q.
French dressing, red, reduced								
calorie, ¼ pkg.	40	.1	5.2	1.9	.3	0	110	n.a.
peppercorn dressing, ⅕ pkg.	80	.2	.1	8.7	1.4	7	85	n.a.
Thousand Island dressing,								
⅕ pkg.	78	.2	2.4	7.5	1.2	8	100	n.a.
vinaigrette dressing, lite, ¼ pkg.	15	.2	2.0	.5	.1	0	75	n.a.
desserts and shakes, 1 serving:								
apple pie, 2.9 oz.	260	2.2	30.0	14.8	4.8	6	240	m.q.
cookies, chocolaty chip, 2.3 oz. ...	330	4.2	41.9	15.6	5.0	4	280	m.q.
cookies, *McDonaldland*, 2.3 oz.	290	4.2	47.1	9.2	1.9	0	300	m.q.
milk shake, lowfat:								
chocolate, 10.3 oz.	320	11.6	66.0	1.7	.8	10	240	(0)
strawberry, 10.3 oz.	320	10.7	67.0	1.3	.6	10	170	(0)
vanilla, 10.3 oz.	290	10.8	60.0	1.3	.6	10	170	0
yogurt, lowfat, frozen:								
cone, vanilla, 3 oz.	100	4.0	22.0	.8	.4	3	80	m.q.
sundae:								
hot caramel, 6.1 oz.	270	6.6	59.3	2.8	1.5	13	180	(0)
hot fudge, 6 oz.	240	7.3	50.5	3.2	2.4	6	170	(0)
strawberry, 6 oz.	210	5.7	49.2	1.1	.6	5	95	(0)
MEAT, see specific listings								
MEAT, POTTED, canned:								
(*Hormel* Food Product), 1 tbsp.	30	2.0	0	2.0	m.q.	m.q.	145	0
(*Libby's*), 1.83 oz.	110	7.0	0	9.0	m.q.	m.q.	320	0
MEAT EXTENDER, nonmeat								
(soybean):								
1 oz.	88	10.7	10.7	.8	.1	0	3	.5 c
1 cup	275	33.5	33.7	2.6	.4	0	8	1.5 c

Food and Measure	cal.	prot. (gms)	carbo. (gms)	tot. fat (gms)	sat. fat (gms)	chol. (mgs)	sod. (mgs)	fiber (gms)
MEAT LOAF DINNER, frozen:								
(*Armour Classics*), 11.25 oz.	360	20.0	32.0	17.0	m.q.	65	1170	m.q.
(*Banquet*), 11 oz.	440	26.0	27.0	27.0	m.q.	85	770	m.q.
(*Freezer Queen*), 10 oz.	350	19.0	26.0	19.0	m.q.	m.q.	910	m.q.
(*Morton*), 10 oz.	310	11.0	26.0	17.0	m.q.	50	1520	m.q.
(*Swanson*), 10.75 oz.	360	15.0	41.0	15.0	m.q.	m.q.	960	m.q.
homestyle (*Stouffer's Dinner Supreme*), 12⅛ oz.	410	25.0	29.0	22.0	m.q.	m.q.	1170	m.q.
MEAT LOAF ENTREE, FROZEN:								
(*Banquet Cookin' Bags*), 4 oz.	200	10.0	8.0	14.0	m.q.	m.q.	m.q.	m.q.
tomato sauce and (*Freezer Queen Family Suppers*), 7 oz.	230	12.0	15.0	13.0	m.q.	m.q.	850	m.q.
MEAT LOAF ENTREE MIX:								
homestyle (*Lipton Microeasy*), ¼ pkg. dry	90	4.0	15.0	1.0	n.a.	n.a.	630	m.q.
homestyle (*Lipton Microeasy*), ¼ pkg.[1]	390	31.0	15.0	22.0	m.q.	m.q.	700	m.q.
"MEAT" LOAF ENTREE MIX, VEGETARIAN:								
(*Natural Touch* Loaf Mix), 4 oz.	180	21.0	7.0	7.0	m.q.	0	25	m.q.
MEAT LOAF SEASONING MIX:								
(*French's*), ⅛ pkg.	20	1.0	5.0	0	0	0	620	n.a.
(*Lawry's* Seasoning Blends), 1 pkg.	355	15.5	64.5	1.2	n.a.	n.a.	6547	1.8 c
MEAT MARINADE MIX:								
(*French's*), ⅛ pkg.	10	0	2.0	0	0	0	540	n.a.
MEAT TENDERIZER:								
seasoned (*Tone's*), 1 tsp.	7	<.1	1.2	.2	<.1	0	1650	<.1 d
unseasoned (*Tone's*), 1 tsp.	7	0	1.2	.2	<.1	0	1760	tr.d
"MEATBALL," VEGETARIAN, canned:								
(*Worthington Non-Meat Balls*), 3 pieces or 1.9 oz.	100	7.0	4.0	6.0	m.q.	0	220	m.q.
MEATBALL DINNER, frozen:								
Swedish (*Armour Classics*), 11.25 oz.	330	19.0	23.0	18.0	m.q.	80	720	m.q.
MEATBALL ENTREE, frozen:								
Italian style, w/noodles and peppers (*The Budget Gourmet*), 10 oz.	310	20.0	29.0	12.0	m.q.	55	1120	m.q.
stew (*Lean Cuisine*), 10 oz.	250	21.0	20.0	10.0	3.0	85	940	m.q.
Swedish:								
(*Swanson* Homestyle Recipe), 8.5 oz.	360	19.0	26.0	20.0	m.q.	m.q.	790	m.q.
in gravy, w/parsley noodles (*Stouffer's*), 11 oz.	480	24.0	37.0	26.0	m.q.	m.q.	1510	m.q.
w/noodles (*The Budget Gourmet*), 10 oz.	600	23.0	40.0	39.0	m.q.	140	1085	m.q.

1. *Prepared according to package directions, with ground beef.*

Food and Measure	cal.	prot. (gms)	carbo. (gms)	tot. fat (gms)	sat. fat (gms)	chol. (mgs)	sod. (mgs)	fiber (gms)
sauce and (*Dining Lite*), 9 oz. ...	280	14.0	34.0	10.0	m.q.	55	660	m.q.
in sauce, w/pasta and vegetables								
(*Le Menu* LightStyle), 8.5 oz.	260	18.0	30.0	8.0	3.0	40	700	m.q.
MEATBALL SEASONING MIX:								
(*French's*), ¼ pkg.	35	1.0	7.0	0	0	0	830	n.a.
MEATBALL STEW, canned:								
(*Chef Boyardee*), 8 oz.	350	9.0	24.0	24.0	m.q.	m.q.	1315	m.q.
(*Dinty Moore*), 8 oz.	240	13.0	15.0	15.0	m.q.	m.q.	m.q.	m.q.
MELON, see specific listings								
MELON BALLS, frozen:								
cantaloupe and honeydew:								
1 lb.	144	3.8	36.0	1.1	n.a.	0	139	m.q.
1 oz.	9	.2	2.3	.1	(0)	0	9	m.q.
½ cup	28	.7	6.9	.2	tr.	0	27	m.q.
MENUDO, canned:								
(*Old El Paso*), ½ can	476	15.0	14.0	52.0	21.0	176	770	2.0 d
MESQUITE SAUCE:								
w/lime juice (*Lawry's*), ¼ cup	24	3.0	3.0	.4	(0)	0	4142	.1 c
MESQUITE SEASONING:								
(*Tone's*), 1 tsp.	13	.1	3.2	<.1	(0)	0	467	n.a.
MEXICAN BEAN, canned:								
(*Old El Paso* Mexe-Beans), ½ cup ..	163	10.0	31.0	1.0	0	0	627	13.0 d
MEXICAN BEAN DIP:								
(*Hain*), 4 tbsp.	60	4.0	9.0	1.0	n.a.	5	260	n.a.
MEXICAN DINNER, frozen (see								
also specific listings):								
(*Swanson Hungry Man*), 20.25 oz.	820	25.0	88.0	41.0	m.q.	m.q.	2080	m.q.
fiesta (*Patio*), 12.25 oz.	470	16.0	55.0	20.0	m.q.	30	2040	m.q.
style:								
(*Banquet*), 12 oz.	490	18.0	62.0	18.0	m.q.	m.q.	2000	m.q.
(*Morton*), 10 oz.	300	9.0	44.0	10.0	m.q.	20	1390	m.q.
(*Patio*), 13.25 oz.	540	15.0	64.0	25.0	m.q.	45	1940	m.q.
combination (*Banquet*), 12 oz. ...	520	20.0	72.0	17.0	m.q.	m.q.	1980	m.q.
combination (*Swanson*), 14.25 oz.	490	19.0	62.0	18.0	m.q.	m.q.	1760	m.q.
MEXICAN ENTREE, frozen (see								
also specific listings):								
(*Van de Kamp's*), ½ pkg.	220	7.0	25.0	10.0	m.q.	m.q.	640	m.q.
MEXICAN POTATO, see "Yam								
bean tuber"								
MEXICAN SEASONING:								
(*Tone's*), 1 tsp.	6	.3	1.3	.1	<.1	tr.	4185	.4 d
MILK, cow, fluid:								
buttermilk, cultured:								
1 oz.	11	.9	1.4	.2	.1	1	30	0
1 quart	396	32.4	46.9	8.6	5.4	34	1028	0
1 cup	99	8.1	11.7	2.2	1.3	9	257	0
(*A&P*), 1 cup	90	8.0	12.0	1.0	m.q.	m.q.	260	0
(*Crowley*), 1 cup	110	9.0	12.0	4.0	m.q.	15	390	0
(*Crowley* Unsalted), 1 cup	110	9.0	12.0	4.0	m.q.	15	130	0

Food and Measure	cal.	prot. (gms)	carbo. (gms)	tot. fat (gms)	sat. fat (gms)	chol. (mgs)	sod. (mgs)	fiber (gms)
MILK, BUTTERMILK, CULTURED *(cont.)*								
lowfat:								
2% *(Knudsen)*, 1 cup	120	8.0	12.0	5.0	m.q.	m.q.	140	0
1.5% *(Borden* Golden Churn),								
1 cup	120	8.0	11.0	4.0	m.q.	m.q.	250	0
1.5% *(Friendship* Unsalted),								
1 cup	120	9.0	12.0	4.0	m.q.	14	125	0
whole:								
3.7% fat, producer:								
1 oz.	18	.9	1.3	1.0	.6	4	14	0
1 quart	626	32.0	45.4	35.7	22.2	140	476	0
1 cup	157	8.0	11.4	8.9	5.6	35	119	0
3.3% fat:								
1 oz.	17	.9	1.3	.9	.6	4	14	0
1 quart	600	32.1	45.5	32.6	20.3	133	478	0
1 cup	150	8.0	11.4	8.2	5.1	33	120	0
low-sodium:								
1 oz.	17	.9	1.3	1.0	.6	4	<1	0
1 quart	594	30.3	43.5	33.8	21.0	133	24	0
1 cup	149	7.6	10.9	8.4	5.3	33	6	0
(A&P), 1 cup	150	8.0	11.0	8.0	m.q.	m.q.	120	0
(Borden), 1 cup	150	8.0	11.0	8.0	m.q.	m.q.	130	0
(Borden Hi-Calcium), 1 cup	150	8.0	11.0	8.0	m.q.	m.q.	130	0
(Crowley), 1 cup	150	8.0	11.0	8.0	m.q.	30	125	0
(Darigold), 1 cup	150	8.0	11.0	8.0	4.9	33	125	0
(Knudsen), 1 cup	160	9.0	12.0	8.0	m.q.	m.q.	180	0
lowfat, 2% fat:								
1 oz.	14	.9	1.4	.5	.3	2	14	0
1 quart	485	32.5	46.9	18.7	11.7	73	487	0
1 cup	121	8.1	11.7	4.7	2.9	18	122	0
nonfat milk solids added:								
1 oz.	14	1.0	1.4	.5	.3	2	15	0
1 quart	500	34.1	48.7	18.8	11.7	74	514	0
1 cup	125	8.5	12.2	4.7	2.9	18	128	0
protein fortified:								
1 oz.	16	1.1	1.6	.6	.3	2	17	0
1 quart	546	38.9	54.0	19.5	12.1	76	579	0
1 cup	137	9.7	13.5	4.9	3.0	19	145	0
(A&P), 1 cup	120	8.0	12.0	5.0	m.q.	m.q.	120	0
(Borden Hi-Protein), 1 cup	140	10.0	13.0	5.0	m.q.	m.q.	150	0
(Crowley), 1 cup	120	8.0	11.0	5.0	m.q.	15	125	0
(Crowley Tone Acidophilus), 1 cup	120	8.0	11.0	5.0	m.q.	15	125	0
(Darigold), 1 cup	120	8.0	11.0	5.0	2.9	18	130	0
(Darigold Nutrish Acidophilus),								
1 cup	120	8.0	11.0	5.0	2.9	18	130	0
(Finast) 1 cup	130	9.0	12.0	5.0	m.q.	m.q.	130	0
(Knudsen/Knudsen Sweet								
Acidophilus), 1 cup	140	10.0	13.0	5.0	m.q.	m.q.	150	0
(Viva), 1 cup	120	8.0	11.0	5.0	m.q.	m.q.	125	0

Food and Measure	cal.	prot. (gms)	carbo. (gms)	tot. fat (gms)	sat. fat (gms)	chol. (mgs)	sod. (mgs)	fiber (gms)
lowfat, 1% fat:								
1 oz.	12	.9	1.4	.3	.2	1	14	0
1 quart	409	32.1	46.7	10.4	6.4	39	493	0
1 cup	102	8.0	11.7	2.6	1.6	10	123	0
nonfat milk solids added:								
1 oz.	12	1.0	1.4	.3	.2	1	15	0
1 quart	418	34.1	48.7	9.5	5.9	39	514	0
1 cup	104	8.5	12.2	2.4	1.5	10	128	0
protein fortified:								
1 oz.	14	1.1	1.6	.3	.2	1	16	0
1 quart	477	38.7	54.3	11.5	7.2	39	574	0
1 cup	119	9.7	13.6	2.9	1.8	10	143	0
(*Crowley*), 1 cup	120	10.0	14.0	2.0	m.q.	10	150	0
(*A&P*), 1 cup	100	8.0	12.0	3.0	m.q.	m.q.	120	0
(*Borden*), 1 cup	100	8.0	11.0	2.0	m.q.	m.q.	130	0
(*Crowley*), 1 cup	100	8.0	11.0	2.0	m.q.	10	130	0
(*Darigold*), 1 cup	100	8.0	13.0	2.0	1.6	10	130	0
(*Knudsen* Nice n' Light), 1 cup ..	130	10.0	15.0	3.0	m.q.	m.q.	153	0
calcium added (*Darigold*), 1 cup ..	100	8.0	11.0	2.0	1.6	10	130	0
w/lactose enzyme (*Crowley*								
Lactaid), 1 cup	100	8.0	11.0	2.0	m.q.	10	125	0
skim:								
1 oz.	10	1.0	1.4	<.1	<.1	<1	15	0
1 quart	342	33.4	47.5	1.8	1.1	18	505	0
1 cup	86	8.4	11.9	.4	.3	4	126	0
nonfat milk solids added:								
1 oz.	10	1.0	1.4	.1	<.1	<1	15	0
1 quart	361	35.0	49.2	2.5	1.6	20	519	0
1 cup	90	8.8	12.3	.6	.4	5	130	0
protein fortified:								
1 oz.	12	1.1	1.6	.1	<.1	<1	17	0
1 quart	400	39.0	54.7	2.5	1.6	20	578	0
1 cup	100	9.7	13.7	.6	.4	5	144	0
(*A&P*), 1 cup	90	8.0	12.0	<1.0	m.q.	m.q.	125	0
(*Borden*), 1 cup	90	8.0	12.0	1.0	m.q.	m.q.	130	0
(*Borden Skim-Line*), 1 cup	100	10.0	13.0	1.0	m.q.	m.q.	150	0
(*Crowley*), 1 cup	90	9.0	12.0	<1.0	m.q.	<1	130	0
(*Darigold*), 1 cup	80	8.0	11.0	1.0	.3	4	130	0
(*Darigold* Trim), 1 cup	80	8.0	11.0	1.0	.3	4	130	0
(*Knudsen*), 1 cup	80	9.0	12.0	m.q.	m.q.	m.q.	130	0
(*Weight Watchers*), 1 cup	90	9.0	13.0	<1.0	m.q.	m.q.	140	0
MILK, CANNED:								
condensed, sweetened:								
1 oz.	91	2.2	15.4	2.5	1.6	10	36	0
1 cup	982	24.2	166.5	26.6	16.8	104	389	0
1 tbsp.	61	1.5	10.4	1.7	1.0	6	24	0
(*Borden*), ⅓ cup	320	7.0	54.0	8.0	m.q.	m.q.	115	0
(*Carnation*), ⅓ cup	320	7.0	56.0	8.0	m.q.	m.q.	110	0
(*Diehl* Jerzee), ⅓ cup	320	7.0	52.0	9.0	m.q.	m.q.	120	0

Food and Measure	cal.	prot. (gms)	carbo. (gms)	tot. fat (gms)	sat. fat (gms)	chol. (mgs)	sod. (mgs)	fiber (gms)
MILK, CANNED, CONDENSED, SWEETENED *(cont.)*								
(*Eagle*), ⅓ cup	320	7.0	52.0	9.0	m.q.	m.q.	120	0
evaporated:								
(*Carnation*), ½ cup	170	8.0	12.0	10.0	m.q.	m.q.	135	0
(*Diehl*), ½ cup	170	8.0	12.0	10.0	m.q.	m.q.	135	0
(*Finast*), ½ cup	170	8.0	12.0	10.0	m.q.	m.q.	135	0
(*IGA*), ½ cup	170	8.0	12.0	10.0	m.q.	m.q.	140	0
(*Pathmark*), ½ cup	170	8.0	12.0	10.9	m.q.	m.q.	140	0
(*Pet*), ½ cup	170	8.0	12.0	10.0	m.q.	36	140	0
filled (*Pet*), ½ cup	150	8.0	12.0	8.0	1.0	5	140	0
imitation, filled (*Diehl*), ½ cup ...	150	8.0	12.0	8.0	2.0	5	135	0
whole:								
1 oz.	38	1.9	2.8	2.1	1.3	8	30	0
1 cup	338	17.2	25.3	19.1	11.6	73	267	0
1 tbsp.	21	1.1	1.6	1.2	.7	5	17	0
lowfat (*Carnation*), ½ cup	110	9.0	12.0	3.0	m.q.	m.q.	130	0
skim:								
1 oz.	22	2.1	3.2	<.1	<.1	1	33	0
1 cup	200	19.3	29.1	.5	.3	10	294	0
1 tbsp.	12	1.2	1.8	<.1	<.1	<1	18	0
(*Carnation*), ½ cup	100	9.0	14.0	.3	m.q.	m.q.	147	0
(*Diehl*), ½ cup	100	9.0	14.0	<1.0	m.q.	m.q.	150	0
(*Finast*), ½ cup	100	9.0	14.0	<1.0	m.q.	m.q.	150	0
(*Pathmark*), ½ cup	100	9.0	14.0	0	0	m.q.	15	0
(*Pet* Light), ½ cup	100	9.0	14.0	<1.0	m.q.	10	150	0
MILK, CHOCOLATE, see "Chocolate milk"								
MILK, CONDENSED, see "Milk, canned"								
MILK, DRY:								
buttermilk, sweet cream:								
1 oz.	110	9.7	13.9	1.6	1.0	20	147	0
1 cup	464	41.2	58.8	6.9	4.3	83	621	0
1 tbsp.	25	2.2	3.2	.4	.2	5	34	0
whole, 1 oz.	141	7.5	10.9	7.6	4.7	27	105	0
whole, 1 cup	635	33.7	49.2	34.2	21.4	124	475	0
nonfat:								
regular, 1 oz.	103	10.3	14.7	.2	.1	6	152	0
regular, 1 cup	435	43.4	62.4	.9	.6	24	642	0
instant:								
1 oz.	101	10.0	14.8	.2	.1	5	156	0
1 cup	326	31.9	47.5	.7	.4	17	499	0
3.2-oz. envelope or 1⅓ cup ...	244	23.9	35.5	.5	.3	12	373	0
(*Carnation*), 5 level tbsp.	80	8.0	12.0	.2	.1	5	125	0
(*Sanalac* Dairy Fresh), .8 oz. ..	80	8.0	12.0	.1	<.1	5	85	0
(*Weight Watchers* Dairy Creamer), 1 pkt.	10	1.0	1.0	0	0	n.a.	15	0
calcium reduced, 1 oz.	100	10.1	14.7	.1	<.1	1	646	0

Food and Measure	cal.	prot. (gms)	carbo. (gms)	tot. fat (gms)	sat. fat (gms)	chol. (mgs)	sod. (mgs)	fiber (gms)
MILK, EVAPORATED, see "Milk, canned"								
MILK, GOAT, fluid, whole:								
1 oz.	20	1.0	1.3	1.2	.8	3	14	0
1 cup	168	8.7	10.9	10.1	6.5	28	122	0
MILK, HUMAN, fluid, whole:								
1 oz.	20	.3	2.0	1.2	.6	4	5	0
1 cup	171	2.5	17.0	10.8	4.9	34	42	0
1 tbsp.	11	.2	1.1	.7	.3	2	3	0
MILK, IMITATION:								
fluid[1]:								
1 oz.	17	.5	1.7	1.0	.2	tr.	22	0
1 quart	600	17.1	60.1	33.3	7.5	2	764	0
1 cup	150	4.3	15.0	8.3	1.9	tr.	191	0
fluid[2]:								
1 oz.	17	.5	1.7	1.0	.9	tr.	22	0
1 quart	600	17.1	60.1	33.3	29.6	2	764	0
1 cup	150	4.3	15.0	8.3	7.4	tr.	191	0
soy, see "Soy milk"								
MILK, INDIAN BUFFALO, fluid, whole:								
1 oz.	27	1.1	1.5	2.0	1.3	5	15	0
1 cup	236	9.2	12.6	16.8	11.2	46	127	0
MILK, MALTED, see "Malted milk"								
MILK, SHEEP, fluid, whole:								
1 oz.	31	1.7	1.5	2.0	1.3	m.q.	12	0
1 cup	264	14.7	13.1	17.2	11.3	m.q.	108	0
MILK, SOY, see "Soy milk"								
MILK BEVERAGE, CANNED OR MIX, see specific flavors								
MILK BEVERAGE, FROZEN, see "Milkshake"								
MILKFISH, meat only, raw:								
1 lb.	673	93.1	0	30.5	m.q.	235	m.q.	0
1 oz.	42	5.8	0	1.9	m.q.	15	m.q.	0
MILKSHAKE:								
frozen:								
chocolate (*MicroMagic*), 11.5 fl. oz.	340	5.0	55.0	8.0	m.q.	40	120	(0)
chocolate (*MicroMagic*), 7 fl. oz.	200	2.0	32.0	4.0	m.q.	25	70	(0)
strawberry (*MicroMagic*), 11.5 fl. oz.	340	5.0	54.0	9.0	m.q.	40	120	(0)
vanilla (*MicroMagic*), 11.5 fl. oz.	380	8.0	60.0	13.0	m.q.	45	150	0
mix, chocolate fudge (*Weight Watchers*), 1 pkt.	70	6.0	11.0	1.0	n.a.	n.a.	170	(0)

1. *Containing blend of hydrogenated vegetable oils.*
2. *Containing lauric acid oil (lauric oils include modified coconut oil, hydrogenated coconut oil, and/or palm kernel oil).*

Food and Measure	cal.	prot. (gms)	carbo. (gms)	tot. fat (gms)	sat. fat (gms)	chol. (mgs)	sod. (mgs)	fiber (gms)
MILKSHAKE *(cont.)*								
mix, orange sherbet (*Weight*								
Watchers), 1 pkt.	70	6.0	11.0	0	0	0	210	(0)
MILLET:								
raw:								
1 oz.	107	3.1	20.7	1.2	.2	0	1	.3 c
1 cup	756	22.0	145.7	8.4	1.4	0	10	2.1 c
hulled (*Arrowhead Mills*), 1 oz. ..	90	3.0	21.0	1.0	m.q.	0	1	1.8 d
cooked, 4 oz.	135	4.0	26.8	1.1	.2	0	2	.4 c
cooked, 1 cup	287	8.4	56.8	2.4	.4	0	5	.9 c
MILLET FLOUR:								
whole-grain (*Arrowhead Mills*),								
2 oz.	185	6.0	41.0	2.0	m.q.	0	1	3.7 d
MINCEMEAT, see "Pie filling,								
canned"								
MISO:								
1 oz.	58	3.3	7.9	1.7	.2	0	1034	1.5 d
½ cup	284	16.3	38.6	8.4	1.2	0	5032	7.6 d
w/barley malt (mugi-koji), 1 oz.	56	2.7	8.0	1.2	m.q.	0	1191	m.q.
w/rice malt (kome-koji), sweet,								
1 oz.	62	2.7	10.4	.9	m.q.	0	680	m.q.
w/rice malt (kome-koji), dark yellow,								
1 oz.	53	3.7	5.4	1.6	m.q.	0	1446	m.q.
w/soybean malt (mame-koji), 1 oz.	62	4.9	3.2	3.9	m.q.	0	1219	m.q.
MIXED FRUIT, see "Fruit, mixed"								
MIXED NUTS, see "Nuts, mixed"								
MIXED VEGETABLES, see								
"Vegetables, mixed"								
MOCHI, see "Rice, glutinous"								
MOLASSES, 1 tbsp.:								
dark (*Br'er Rabbit*)	60	0	14.0	0	0	0	15	(0)
gold (*Grandma's*)	70	0	17.0	0	0	0	28	(0)
green (*Grandma's*)	70	0	16.0	0	0	0	57	(0)
light (*Br'er Rabbit*)	60	0	14.0	0	0	0	10	(0)
MONKFISH, meat only, raw:								
1 lb.	343	65.7	0	6.9	m.q.	115	84	0
1 oz.	22	4.1	0	.4	m.q.	7	5	0
MONOSODIUM GLUTAMATE:								
(*Tone's*), 1 tsp.	0	0	0	0	0	0	638	0
MOOSE, meat only:								
raw, 1 oz.	29	6.3	0	.2	.1	17	19	0
roasted[1]:								
12 oz., yield from 1 lb. raw								
boneless	455	99.6	0	3.3	1.0	266	234	0
4 oz.	152	33.2	0	1.1	.3	88	78	0
diced, 1 cup, approx. 4.9 oz.	188	41.0	0	1.4	.4	109	97	0

1. *Without added ingredients.*

Food and Measure	cal.	prot. (gms)	carbo. (gms)	tot. fat (gms)	sat. fat (gms)	chol. (mgs)	sod. (mgs)	fiber (gms)
MORTADELLA, beef and pork:								
1 oz.	88	4.6	.9	7.2	2.7	16	353	0
1 slice, approx. .5 oz.	47	2.5	.5	3.8	1.4	8	187	0
MOSTACCIOLI ENTREE, frozen:								
and meat sauce (*Banquet Family*								
Entrees), 7 oz.	170	7.0	28.0	3.0	m.q.	m.q.	m.q.	m.q.
MOTH BEAN:								
raw, 1 oz.	97	6.5	17.4	.5	.1	0	9	1.1 c
raw, ½ cup	337	22.5	60.3	1.6	.4	0	29	3.9 c
boiled, 4 oz.	133	8.9	23.8	.6	.1	0	11	1.5 c
boiled, ½ cup	103	6.9	18.4	.5	.1	0	8	1.2 c
MOTHER'S LOAF LUNCHEON								
MEAT:								
pork, 1 oz.	80	3.4	2.1	6.3	2.3	13	320	(0)
pork, 1 slice, 4¼″ × 4¼″ × ¹⁄₁₆″,								
approx. .7 oz.	59	2.5	1.6	4.7	1.7	9	237	(0)
MOUNTAIN YAM, HAWAIIAN,								
see "Yam, mountain"								
MOUSSE, FROZEN:								
chocolate:								
(*Weight Watchers*), ½ pkg. or								
2.5 oz.	170	6.0	24.0	6.0	<1.0	5	190	n.a.
praline pecan (*Weight Watchers*),								
½ pkg. or 2.71 oz.	190	5.0	27.0	7.0	1.0	5	180	n.a.
MOUSSE CAKE, see "Cake"								
MOUSSE MIX, ½ cup[1]:								
cheesecake (*Weight Watchers*)[2]	60	4.0	12.0	2.0	m.q.	m.q.	75	n.a.
chocolate:								
(*Jell-O Rich & Luscious*)[3]	150	5.0	21.0	6.0	m.q.	10	75	n.a.
(*Weight Watchers*)[2]	60	3.0	9.0	3.0	m.q.	m.q.	45	n.a.
fudge (*Jell-O Rich & Luscious*)[3] ..	140	5.0	20.0	6.0	m.q.	10	75	n.a.
white, almond (*Weight Watchers*)[2]	60	3.0	6.0	3.0	m.q.	m.q.	50	n.a.
raspberry (*Weight Watchers*)[2]	60	3.0	12.0	3.0	m.q.	m.q.	75	n.a.
MUFFIN (see also "Toaster muffins								
and pastries"), 1 piece, except								
as noted:								
apple:								
(*Awrey's*), 2.5 oz.	220	3.0	30.0	10.0	2.0	35	350	1.0 d
(*Awrey's*), 1.5 oz.	130	2.0	17.0	6.0	1.0	20	210	0
streusel (*Awrey's Grande*), 4.2 oz.	340	6.0	50.0	13.0	2.0	35	540	1.0 d
banana nut (*Awrey's Grande*),								
4.2 oz.	260	3.0	27.0	16.0	2.0	40	160	.6 d
banana walnut, mini (*Hostess*								
Breakfast Bake Shop), 5 pieces	160	2.0	17.0	9.0	m.q.	0	90	m.q.
blueberry:								
(*Awrey's*), 2.5 oz.	210	3.0	31.0	8.0	1.0	20	280	1.0 d
(*Awrey's*), 1.5 oz.	130	2.0	18.0	5.0	1.0	10	180	1.0 d

1. *Prepared according to package directions.*
2. *Prepared with skim milk.*
3. *Prepared with whole milk.*

Food and Measure	cal.	prot. (gms)	carbo. (gms)	tot. fat (gms)	sat. fat (gms)	chol. (mgs)	sod. (mgs)	fiber (gms)
MUFFIN, BLUEBERRY *(cont.)*								
(Awrey's Grande), 4.2 oz.	360	5.0	52.0	14.0	2.0	35	480	2.0 d
mini *(Hostess Breakfast Bake Shop)*, 5 pieces	240	3.0	29.0	13.0	2.0	40	180	.7 d
cinnamon apple, mini *(Hostess Breakfast Bake Shop)*, 5 pieces	260	3.0	27.0	16.0	2.0	45	180	.6 d
corn *(Awrey's)*, 2.5 oz.	220	4.0	33.0	8.0	1.0	25	430	1.0 d
corn *(Awrey's)*, 1.5 oz.	130	2.0	20.0	5.0	1.0	15	270	0
cranberry *(Awrey's)*, 1.5 oz.	120	2.0	20.0	4.0	0	10	210	0
English:								
(Hi Fiber)	110	5.0	21.0	1.0	n.a.	0	280	5.0 d
(Pepperidge Farm)	140	5.0	27.0	1.0	0	0	220	m.q.
(Roman Meal Original)	146	6.4	28.5	1.8	m.q.	0	350	2.7 d
(Thomas')	130	4.3	25.4	1.3	n.a.	0	206	m.q.
(Wonder)	130	4.0	26.0	1.0	n.a.	0	280	1.2 d
cinnamon apple *(Pepperidge Farm)*	140	4.0	27.0	1.0	0	0	210	m.q.
cinnamon chip *(Pepperidge Farm)*	160	4.0	28.0	3.0	0	0	180	m.q.
cinnamon raisin *(Hi Fiber)*	110	4.0	21.0	1.0	n.a.	0	275	5.0 d
cinnamon raisin *(Pepperidge Farm)*	150	4.0	29.0	2.0	0	0	200	m.q.
cinnamon and raisin oatmeal *(Oatmeal Goodness)*	140	5.0	26.0	2.0	m.q.	0	160	1.5 d
honey and oatmeal *(Oatmeal Goodness)*	140	5.0	26.0	2.0	m.q.	0	160	1.5 d
multigrain *(Hi Fiber)*	120	4.0	23.0	1.0	n.a.	0	240	4.0 d
oat bran *(Thomas')*	116	4.2	26.0	1.2	n.a.	0	192	2.9 d
raisin *(Thomas')*	153	4.5	30.4	1.5	m.q.	0	200	.2 c
rye *(Thomas')*	120	5.0	27.0	1.0	n.a.	0	210	3.0 d
sourdough *(Pepperidge Farm)*	135	4.0	27.0	1.0	0	0	260	m.q.
wheat, honey *(Thomas')*	129	5.0	24.0	1.1	n.a.	0	200	.4 c
oat bran:								
(Awrey's), 2.75 oz.	180	5.0	27.0	7.0	1.0	0	330	2.0 d
(Hostess Breakfast Bake Shop) ...	160	2.0	21.0	7.0	1.0	0	150	1.5 d
almond and date *(Health Valley Oat Bran Fancy Fruit Muffins)*	180	4.0	31.0	4.0	m.q.	0	81	8.2 d
banana nut *(Hostess Breakfast Bake Shop)*	140	2.0	20.0	5.0	1.0	0	160	1.0 d
blueberry *(Health Valley Oat Bran Fancy Fruit Muffins)*	180	4.0	32.0	4.0	m.q.	0	99	7.5 d
raisin *(Health Valley Oat Bran Fancy Fruit Muffins)*	180	4.0	31.0	5.0	m.q.	0	90	7.8 d
pineapple raisin oat bran *(Awrey's)*, 2.75 oz.	180	5.0	26.0	6.0	1.0	0	320	2.0 d
raisin *(Wonder* Raisin Rounds)	140	4.0	27.0	2.0	m.q.	0	280	1.2 d
raisin bran:								
(Awrey's), 2.5 oz.	190	3.0	30.0	7.0	1.0	20	280	2.0 d
(Awrey's), 1.5 oz.	110	2.0	18.0	4.0	1.0	15	170	1.0 d
(Awrey's Grande), 4.2 oz.	320	5.0	50.0	12.0	2.0	35	470	3.0 d
rice bran, raisin *(Health Valley Rice Bran Fancy Fruit Muffins)*	215	5.0	35.0	7.0	m.q.	0	124	5.5 d

Food and Measure	cal.	prot. (gms)	carbo. (gms)	tot. fat (gms)	sat. fat (gms)	chol. (mgs)	sod. (mgs)	fiber (gms)
sourdough (*Wonder*)	130	4.0	27.0	1.0	n.a.	0	250	1.2 d
MUFFIN, FROZEN, 1 piece:								
apple spice (*Sara Lee*),								
2.5 oz.	220	4.0	36.0	8.0	m.q.	0	280	m.q.
apple spice (*Weight Watchers*								
Microwave), 2.5 oz.	160	3.0	29.0	5.0	1.0	n.a.	260	m.q.
banana nut (*Weight Watchers*								
Microwave), 2.5 oz.	170	3.0	32.0	5.0	1.0	10	250	m.q.
blueberry:								
(*Pepperidge Farm* Old Fashioned)	170	2.0	27.0	7.0	1.0	25	250	1.0 d
(*Sara Lee*), 2.5 oz.	200	3.0	34.0	8.0	m.q.	0	290	m.q.
(*Sara Lee Free & Light*)	120	3.0	28.0	0	0	0	140	m.q.
(*Weight Watchers* Microwave),								
2.5 oz.	170	3.0	32.0	5.0	1.0	10	220	m.q.
cheese streusel (*Sara Lee*), 2.1 oz.	220	4.0	27.0	11.0	m.q.	n.a.	170	m.q.
chocolate chunk (*Sara Lee*), 2.1 oz.	220	3.0	33.0	8.0	m.q.	n.a.	210	m.q.
cinnamon swirl (*Pepperidge Farm* Old								
Fashioned)	190	2.0	30.0	6.0	1.0	35	170	1.0 d
corn (*Pepperidge Farm* Old								
Fashioned)	180	3.0	27.0	7.0	1.0	30	260	2.0 d
corn, golden (*Sara Lee*), 2.5 oz.	250	4.0	31.0	13.0	m.q.	0	310	m.q.
oat bran (*Sara Lee*), 2.5 oz.	210	4.0	35.0	8.0	m.q.	0	320	m.q.
oat bran, w/apple (*Pepperidge Farm*								
Old Fashioned Cholesterol								
Free)	190	3.0	29.0	7.0	1.0	0	200	2.0 d
oat bran, apple (*Sara Lee*), 2.5 oz.	210	4.0	35.0	8.0	m.q.	0	320	m.q.
raisin bran (*Pepperidge Farm* Old								
Fashioned Cholesterol Free)	170	4.0	30.0	6.0	1.0	0	280	3.0 d
raisin bran (*Sara Lee*), 2.5 oz.	220	4.0	37.0	7.0	m.q.	0	400	m.q.
MUFFIN, REFRIGERATED:								
English (*Roman Meal*), ½ piece	71	2.3	14.3	.5	.1	0	88	1.3 d
English, honey nut and oat bran								
(*Roman Meal*), ½ piece	81	2.5	14.7	1.3	.2	0	114	1.1 d
MUFFIN MIX[1]:								
apple cinnamon:								
(*Betty Crocker*), 1/12 pkg.[2]	120	2.0	18.0	4.0	1.0	25	140	m.q.
(*Betty Crocker*), 1/12 pkg.[3]	110	2.0	18.0	3.0	1.0	0	140	m.q.
(*Martha White*), 1/6 pkg.	140	2.0	25.0	3.0	m.q.	3	250	m.q.
apple streusel, Dutch (*Betty Crocker*								
Bake Shop), 1/12 pkg.[4]	200	3.0	32.0	7.0	m.q.	m.q.	240	m.q.
applesauce (*Robin Hood/Gold Medal*								
Pouch Mix), 1/6 pkg.[4]	160	3.0	26.0	5.0	m.q.	m.q.	240	m.q.
banana:								
(*Robin Hood/Gold Medal* Pouch								
Mix), 1/6 pkg.[4]	150	3.0	24.0	5.0	m.q.	m.q.	240	m.q.

1. *Prepared according to package directions, except as noted.*
2. *Prepared with egg and 2% lowfat milk.*
3. *Prepared with egg white and skim milk.*
4. *Prepared with egg and whole milk.*

Food and Measure	cal.	prot. (gms)	carbo. (gms)	tot. fat (gms)	sat. fat (gms)	chol. (mgs)	sod. (mgs)	fiber (gms)
MUFFIN, MIX, BANANA *(cont.)*								
nut (*Betty Crocker*), $\frac{1}{12}$ pkg. [1]	120	2.0	17.0	5.0	1.0	25	140	m.q.
nut (*Betty Crocker*), $\frac{1}{12}$ pkg. [2]	110	2.0	17.0	4.0	1.0	0	140	m.q.
blackberry (*Martha White*), $\frac{1}{6}$ pkg.	140	2.0	25.0	3.0	m.q.	3	250	m.q.
blueberry:								
(*Duncan Hines* Bakery Style),								
1 piece	190	2.0	32.0	6.0	m.q.	n.a.	250	m.q.
(*Martha White*), $\frac{1}{6}$ pkg.	140	2.0	25.0	3.0	m.q.	3	260	m.q.
(*Robin Hood/Gold Medal* Pouch								
Mix), $\frac{1}{6}$ pkg. [3]	170	3.0	26.0	6.0	m.q.	m.q.	240	m.q.
streusel (*Betty Crocker* Bake								
Shop), $\frac{1}{12}$ pkg. [3]	210	3.0	31.0	8.0	m.q.	m.q.	230	m.q.
wild:								
(*Betty Crocker*), $\frac{1}{12}$ pkg. [1]	120	2.0	18.0	4.0	1.0	25	150	m.q.
(*Betty Crocker*), $\frac{1}{12}$ pkg. [2]	110	2.0	18.0	3.0	<1.0	0	150	m.q.
(*Duncan Hines*), 1 piece	110	2.0	17.0	3.0	m.q.	n.a.	155	m.q.
bran (*Martha White*), $\frac{1}{6}$ pkg.	150	3.0	24.0	5.0	m.q.	14	330	m.q.
bran and honey (*Duncan Hines*),								
1 piece	120	2.0	18.0	4.0	m.q.	n.a.	170	m.q.
bran and honey (*Duncan Hines*								
Bakery Style), 1 piece	200	2.0	32.0	7.0	m.q.	n.a.	220	m.q.
caramel (*Robin Hood/Gold Medal*								
Pouch Mix), $\frac{1}{6}$ pkg. [3]	150	3.0	23.0	5.0	m.q.	m.q.	250	m.q.
carrot nut (*Betty Crocker*), $\frac{1}{12}$ pkg. [1]	150	3.0	22.0	5.0	1.0	25	160	m.q.
carrot nut (*Betty Crocker*), $\frac{1}{12}$ pkg. [2]	150	3.0	22.0	5.0	1.0	0	160	m.q.
chocolate chip (*Betty Crocker*),								
$\frac{1}{12}$ pkg. [1]	150	2.0	22.0	6.0	2.0	20	180	m.q.
chocolate chip (*Betty Crocker*),								
$\frac{1}{12}$ pkg. [2]	140	2.0	22.0	5.0	2.0	0	180	m.q.
cinnamon streusel (*Betty Crocker*),								
$\frac{1}{10}$ pkg. [1]	200	3.0	27.0	9.0	2.0	30	240	m.q.
cinnamon swirl (*Duncan Hines*								
Bakery Style), 1 piece	200	2.0	32.0	7.0	m.q.	n.a.	245	m.q.
corn:								
(*Dromedary*), 3½ tbsp. dry	110	1.0	20.0	3.0	m.q.	n.a.	250	m.q.
(*Dromedary*), 1 piece	120	3.0	20.0	4.0	m.q.	n.a.	270	m.q.
(*Flako*), 1 serving	116	1.8	19.8	3.3	.6	n.a.	351	.7 d
(*Robin Hood/Gold Medal*), $\frac{1}{6}$ pkg. [3]	130	3.0	24.0	2.0	m.q.	m.q.	250	m.q.
blue (*Arrowhead Mills*), 1 piece ..	110	4.0	15.0	4.0	m.q.	n.a.	n.a.	2.6 d
cranberry-orange nut (*Duncan Hines*								
Bakery Style), 1 piece	200	2.0	30.0	8.0	m.q.	n.a.	215	m.q.
honey bran (*Robin Hood/Gold Medal*								
Pouch Mix), $\frac{1}{6}$ pkg. [3]	170	5.0	25.0	6.0	m.q.	m.q.	240	m.q.
oat (*Robin Hood/Gold Medal* Pouch								
Mix), $\frac{1}{6}$ pkg. [1]	150	4.0	23.0	5.0	1.0	45	220	m.q.

1. *Prepared with egg and 2% lowfat milk.*
2. *Prepared with egg white and skim milk.*
3. *Prepared with egg and whole milk.*

Food and Measure	cal.	prot. (gms)	carbo. (gms)	tot. fat (gms)	sat. fat (gms)	chol. (mgs)	sod. (mgs)	fiber (gms)
oat bran:								
(*Betty Crocker*), ⅛ pkg [1]	190	4.0	25.0	8.0	2.0	35	240	m.q.
(*Betty Crocker*), ⅛ pkg. [2]	180	4.0	25.0	7.0	2.0	0	240	m.q.
apple cinnamon (*Hain*), 1 piece ..	140	4.0	28.0	3.0	m.q.	0	200	5.0 d
apple spice (*Arrowhead Mills*),								
1 piece	120	6.0	15.0	4.0	m.q.	n.a.	m.q.	5.4 d
banana nut (*Hain*), 1 piece	140	4.0	26.0	4.0	m.q.	0	190	4.0 d
raspberry spice (*Hain*), 1 piece ..	140	5.0	27.0	3.0	m.q.	0	190	4.0 d
wheat free (*Arrowhead Mills*),								
1 piece	100	5.0	11.0	5.0	m.q.	n.a.	m.q.	4.5 d
oatmeal raisin (*Betty Crocker*),								
1/12 pkg. [1]	140	3.0	22.0	4.0	1.0	25	125	m.q.
oatmeal raisin (*Betty Crocker*),								
1/12 pkg. [2]	130	3.0	22.0	3.0	1.0	0	125	m.q.
orangeberry (*Martha White*),								
⅙ pkg.	140	2.0	25.0	3.0	m.q.	2	220	m.q.
pecan crunch (*Duncan Hines* Bakery								
Style), 1 piece	220	3.0	27.0	11.0	m.q.	n.a.	250	m.q.
raspberry (*Martha White*), ⅙ pkg. ...	140	2.0	25.0	3.0	m.q.	3	184	m.q.
strawberry:								
(*Martha White*), ⅙ pkg.	140	2.0	25.0	3.0	m.q.	3	270	m.q.
crown (*Betty Crocker*), 1/10 pkg. [1]	150	2.0	24.0	5.0	2.0	25	170	m.q.
crown (*Betty Crocker*), 1/10 pkg. [2]	140	2.0	24.0	4.0	1.0	0	170	m.q.
wheat bran (*Arrowhead Mills*),								
2 pieces	270	10.0	43.0	7.0	m.q.	n.a.	m.q.	10.5 d
MULBERRY:								
1 lb.	197	6.5	44.5	1.8	n.a.	0	46	4.4 c
1 oz.	12	.4	2.8	.1	(0)	0	3	.3 c
10 berries, approx. .5 oz.	7	.2	1.5	.1	(0)	0	2	.1 c
½ cup	31	1.0	6.9	.3	(0)	0	7	.7 c
MULLANGI, see "Radish, Oriental"								
MULLET, striped, meat only:								
raw:								
1 lb.	530	87.8	0	17.2	5.1	224	294	0
1 oz.	33	5.5	0	1.1	.3	14	18	0
1 fillet, approx. 4.2 oz., yield from								
1½-lb. whole fish	139	23.0	0	4.5	1.3	59	77	0
baked, broiled, or microwaved[3],								
4 oz.	170	28.1	0	5.5	1.6	71	81	0
MUNG BEAN:								
raw:								
1 oz.	98	6.8	17.8	.3	.1	0	4	2.7 d
½ cup	361	24.8	65.1	1.2	.4	0	15	10.0 d
boiled, 4 oz.	119	8.0	21.7	.4	.1	0	2	2.8 d
boiled, ½ cup	107	7.1	19.3	.4	.1	0	2	2.5 d

1. *Prepared with egg and 2% lowfat milk.*
2. *Prepared with egg white and skim milk.*
3. *Without added ingredients.*

Food and Measure	cal.	prot. (gms)	carbo. (gms)	tot. fat (gms)	sat. fat (gms)	chol. (mgs)	sod. (mgs)	fiber (gms)
MUNG BEAN, SPROUTED,								
mature seeds:								
raw:								
1 lb.	136	13.8	26.9	.8	.2	0	26	5.0 d
1 oz.	9	.9	1.7	.1	<.1	0	2	.3 d
½ cup	16	1.6	3.1	.1	<.1	0	3	.6 d
boiled, drained, 4 oz.	24	2.3	4.8	.1	<.1	0	11	.6 c
boiled, drained, ½ cup	13	1.3	2.6	.1	<.1	0	6	.3 c
stir-fried, 4 oz.	57	4.9	12.0	.2	<.1	0	m.q.	.8 c
stir-fried, ½ cup	31	2.7	6.6	.1	<.1	0	m.q.	.4 c
MUNG BEAN, SPROUTED,								
CANNED:								
drained, 4 oz.	14	1.6	2.4	.1	<.1	0	m.q.	.3 c
drained, ½ cup	8	.9	1.3	<.1	<.1	0	m.q.	.2 c
(*La Choy*), 2 oz.	8	.8	1.0	.1	n.a.	0	20	.7 d
MUNG BEAN LONG RICE,								
dehydrated:								
1 oz.	99	<.1	24.4	tr.	tr.	0	3	tr.c
½ cup	246	.1	60.3	<.1	tr.	0	7	tr.c
MUNGO BEAN:								
raw, 1 oz.	100	7.1	17.3	.5	<.1	0	7	1.3 c
raw, ½ cup	365	26.1	63.5	1.9	.1	0	27	4.6 c
boiled, 4 oz.	119	8.6	20.8	.6	<.1	0	8	1.5 c
boiled, ½ cup	95	6.8	16.5	.5	<.1	0	7	1.2 c
MUSHROOM:								
raw:								
untrimmed, 1 lb.	111	9.2	20.5	1.9	.2	0	16	5.7 d
trimmed, 1 oz.	7	.6	1.3	.1	<.1	0	1	.4 d
1 medium, approx. .7 oz.	5	.4	.8	.1	<.1	0	1	.3 d
pieces, ½ cup	9	.7	1.6	.2	<.1	0	1	.5 d
boiled, drained:								
4 oz.	31	2.5	5.8	.5	.1	0	2	2.5 d
1 medium, approx. .4 oz.	3	.3	.6	.1	tr.	0	tr.	.3 d
pieces, ½ cup	21	1.7	4.0	.4	<.1	0	2	1.7 d
MUSHROOM, CANNED:								
drained:								
4 oz.	27	2.1	5.6	.3	<.1	0	m.q.	m.q.
1 medium, approx. .4 oz.	3	.2	.6	<.1	tr.	0	m.q.	m.q.
pieces, ½ cup	19	1.5	3.9	.2	<.1	0	m.q.	m.q.
(*B in B*), ¼ cup	12	1.0	2.0	0	0	0	240	1.0 d
whole, pieces, and stems (*Green*								
Giant), ¼ cup	12	1.0	2.0	0	0	0	220	1.0 d
pieces and stems (*Allens*), ½ cup ..	20	2.0	3.0	<1.0	(0)	0	450	m.q.
pieces and stems (*Empress*), 2 oz. ...	14	1.0	2.0	n.a.	n.a.	0	260	m.q.
in butter sauce (*Green Giant*),								
½ cup	30	2.0	4.0	1.0	n.a.	n.a.	330	.6 d
w/garlic (*B in B*), ¼ cup	12	1.0	2.0	0	0	0	200	1.0 d

Food and Measure	cal.	prot. (gms)	carbo. (gms)	tot. fat (gms)	sat. fat (gms)	chol. (mgs)	sod. (mgs)	fiber (gms)
MUSHROOM, FROZEN:								
whole (*Birds Eye* Deluxe), 2.6 oz. ..	20	2.0	4.0	0	0	0	0	2.0 d
battered (*Stilwell Quick Krisp*),								
2 oz.	140	2.0	15.0	8.0	m.q.	5	280	m.q.
MUSHROOM, JAPANESE								
HONEY, trimmed:								
(*Frieda* of California), 1 lb.	136	9.5	20.0	1.4	n.a.	0	m.q.	m.q.
(*Frieda* of California), 1 oz.	9	.6	1.2	<.1	(0)	0	m.q.	m.q.
MUSHROOM, ORIENTAL								
STRAW, canned:								
(*Green Giant*), 2 oz.	12	1.0	2.0	0	0	0	290	1.0 d
MUSHROOM, OYSTER:								
(*Frieda* of California), 1 lb.	113	9.5	20.9	1.8	n.a.	0	18	3.6 d
(*Frieda* of California), 1 oz.	7	.6	1.3	.1	(0)	0	1	.2 d
MUSHROOM, SHIITAKE:								
cooked, 4 oz.	62	1.8	16.2	.2	.1	0	5	2.2 c
cooked, 4 medium or ½ cup pieces	40	1.1	10.4	.2	<.1	0	3	1.4 c
MUSHROOM, SHIITAKE,								
DRIED:								
1 lb.	1343	43.5	341.9	4.5	1.1	0	60	52.2 c
1 oz.	84	2.7	21.4	.3	.1	0	4	3.3 c
4 medium, approx. .5 oz.	44	1.4	11.3	.2	<.1	0	2	1.7 c
MUSHROOM GRAVY:								
canned:								
¼ cup	30	.8	3.3	1.6	.2	0	340	n.a.
(*Franco-American*), 2 oz.	25	0	3.0	1.0	n.a.	n.a.	290	n.a.
(*Heinz* HomeStyle), 2 oz. or ¼ cup	25	1.0	3.0	1.0	n.a.	n.a.	340	n.a.
mix:								
1 oz. dry	93	2.8	18.3	1.1	.7	1	1865	n.a.
¼ cup[1]	18	.5	3.4	.2	.1	<1	351	n.a.
(*French's*), w/water, ¼ cup[1]	20	1.0	3.0	1.0	n.a.	n.a.	250	n.a.
(*McCormick/Schilling*), ¼ cup ...	19	.5	3.0	.5	n.a.	n.a.	270	n.a.
MUSHROOM AND HERB DIP:								
(*Breakstone's* Gourmet), 2 tbsp.	50	1.0	2.0	4.0	3.0	10	150	n.a.
MUSHROOM SAUCE MIX:								
1-oz. pkt. dry	99	4.1	15.5	2.7	.4	0	1766	.3 c
w/whole milk, ½ cup	114	5.6	11.9	5.2	2.7	17	767	.1 c
MUSKMELON, see "Cantaloupe"								
MUSKRAT, meat only:								
raw, 1 oz.	46	5.9	0	2.3	m.q.	m.q.	23	0
roasted[2]:								
14 oz., yield from 1 lb. raw								
boneless	734	94.2	0	36.8	m.q.	m.q.	298	0
4 oz.	209	26.8	0	10.4	m.q.	m.q.	85	0
diced, 1 cup, approx. 4.9 oz.	258	33.0	0	12.9	m.q.	m.q.	105	0
MUSSEL, blue, meat only:								
raw:								
1 lb.	391	54.0	16.8	10.2	1.9	127	1296	0

1. *Prepared according to package directions, with water.*
2. *Without added ingredients.*

Food and Measure	cal.	prot. (gms)	carbo. (gms)	tot. fat (gms)	sat. fat (gms)	chol. (mgs)	sod. (mgs)	fiber (gms)
MUSSEL *(cont.)*								
1 oz.	24	3.4	1.0	.7	.1	8	81	0
1 cup	129	17.9	5.5	3.4	.6	42	429	0
boiled or steamed[1], 4 oz.	195	27.0	8.4	5.1	1.0	64	418	0
MUSTARD, prepared:								
(*Featherweight*), 1 tsp.	5	0	0	0	0	0	0	0
(*Hain* Stone Ground), 1 tbsp.	14	1.0	1.0	1.0	n.a.	0	185	n.a.
(*Hain* Stone Ground No Salt Added),								
1 tbsp.	14	1.0	1.0	1.0	n.a.	0	10	n.a.
(*Kraft* Pure), 1 tbsp.	11	0	1.0	1.0	0	0	160	0
brown, spicy (*Gulden's*), ¼ oz.	8	0	0	0	0	0	45	0
Dijon (*French's*), 1 tsp.	8	0	0	1.0	n.a.	0	140	0
Dijon (*Grey Poupon*), 1 tbsp.	18	0	0	1.0	n.a.	0	450	0
English (*Life* All Natural), 1 tbsp.	22	2.0	<1.0	2.0	n.a.	0	<2	n.a.
w/horseradish (*French's*), 1 tbsp.	16	1.0	1.0	1.0	n.a.	0	265	n.a.
horseradish (*Kraft*), 1 tbsp.	14	1.0	1.0	1.0	0	0	135	0
hot (*Gulden's* Diablo), ¼ oz.	8	0	0	0	0	0	55	0
jalapeño (*Great Impressions*), 2 tsp.	7	.4	.7	.3	n.a.	0	173	n.a.
Medford (*French's*), 1 tbsp.	16	1.0	1.0	1.0	n.a.	0	240	n.a.
mild (*Heinz*), 1 tsp.	5	.3	.5	.2	n.a.	0	70	0
mild, creamy (*Gulden's*), ¼ oz.	6	0	0	0	0	0	60	0
w/onion (*French's*), 1 tsp.	8	0	2.0	0	0	0	70	n.a.
spicy (*French's* Bold'n Spicy), 1 tsp.	6	0	0	0	0	0	50	n.a.
yellow (*French's*), 1 tbsp.	10	1.0	1.0	1.0	n.a.	0	180	n.a.
yellow (*Heinz*), 1 tsp.	3	.2	.2	.2	n.a.	0	55	n.a.
MUSTARD GREENS:								
raw, untrimmed, 1 lb.	109	11.4	20.7	.8	<.1	0	107	2.5 d
raw, trimmed, 1 oz. or ½ cup								
chopped	7	.8	1.4	.1	tr.	0	7	.2 d
boiled, drained, 4 oz.	17	2.6	2.4	.3	<.1	0	18	.8 c
boiled, drained, chopped, ½ cup	11	1.6	1.5	.2	tr.	0	11	.5 c
MUSTARD GREENS, CANNED:								
chopped (*Allens*), ½ cup	20	1.0	2.0	<1.0	n.a.	0	35	m.q.
MUSTARD GREENS, FROZEN:								
10-oz. pkg.	58	7.1	9.7	.8	<.1	0	83	2.3 c
boiled, drained, 4 oz.	22	2.6	3.5	.3	<.1	0	28	.8 c
boiled, drained, chopped, ½ cup	14	1.7	2.3	.2	<.1	0	19	.6 c
(*Frosty Acres*), 3.3 oz.	20	2.0	3.0	0	0	0	20	1.0 c
chopped (*Seabrook*), 3.3 oz.	20	2.0	3.0	0	0	0	20	1.0 c
chopped (*Southern*), 3.5 oz.	25	2.5	3.6	.3	(0)	0	40	m.q.
MUSTARD OIL:								
1 oz.	251	0	0	28.4	3.3	0	0	0
½ cup	964	0	0	109.0	12.6	0	0	0
1 tbsp.	124	0	0	14.0	1.6	0	0	0
MUSTARD POWDER:								
(*Spice Islands*), 1 tsp.	9	.5	.3	.6	n.a.	0	<1	<.1 c
MUSTARD SEED, yellow:								
1 oz.	133	7.1	9.9	8.2	.4	0	1	1.9 c

1. *Without added ingredients.*

Food and Measure	cal.	prot. (gms)	carbo. (gms)	tot. fat (gms)	sat. fat (gms)	chol. (mgs)	sod. (mgs)	fiber (gms)
1 tbsp.	53	2.8	3.9	3.2	.2	0	<1	.7 c
1 tsp.	15	.8	1.2	1.0	.1	0	tr.	.2 c
MUSTARD SPINACH:								
raw:								
untrimmed, 1 lb.	93	9.3	16.5	1.3	n.a.	0	m.q.	4.2 c
trimmed, 1 oz.	6	.6	1.1	.1	n.a.	0	m.q.	.3 c
chopped, ½ cup	17	1.7	2.9	.2	n.a.	0	m.q.	.8 c
boiled, drained, 4 oz.	18	1.9	3.2	.2	n.a.	0	m.q.	.9 c
boiled, drained, chopped, ½ cup ...	14	1.5	2.5	.2	n.a.	0	m.q.	.7 c
MUSTARD TALLOW:								
1 oz.	256	0	0	28.4	13.4	29	0	0
½ cup	925	0	0	102.5	48.5	105	0	0
1 tbsp.	115	0	0	12.8	6.1	13	0	0

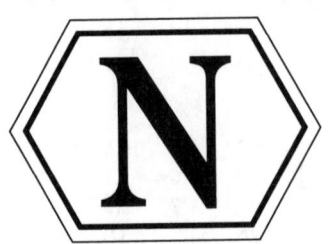

Food and Measure	cal.	prot. (gms)	carbo. (gms)	tot. fat (gms)	sat. fat (gms)	chol. (mgs)	sod. (mgs)	fiber (gms)
NACHO CHIPS, see "Corn chips, puffs, and similar snacks"								
NACHO DIP, see "Cheese dip"								
NACHO MIX:								
(*Tio Sancho* Microwave Snacks):								
cheese sauce, 3.5 oz.	247	14.5	2.3	20.0	m.q.	m.q.	995	.4 c
chips, 4 oz.	567	8.5	74.4	26.1	m.q.	n.a.	590	4.0 c
NACHO SAUCE, see "Cheese sauce"								
NACHO SEASONING:								
(*Lawry's* Seasoning Blends), 1 pkg.	141	6.7	15.0	6.8	m.q.	n.a.	2168	1.6 c
NATAL PLUM, see "Carissa"								
NATTO:								
1 oz.	60	5.0	4.1	3.1	.5	0	2	.5 c
½ cup	187	15.6	12.6	9.7	1.4	0	6	1.4 c
NAVY BEAN:								
raw, 1 oz.	95	6.3	17.2	.4	.1	0	4	2.7 d
raw, ½ cup	348	23.2	63.1	1.3	.3	0	15	10.1 d
boiled, 4 oz.	161	9.9	29.8	.6	.2	0	1	4.1 d
boiled, ½ cup	129	7.9	24.0	.5	.1	0	1	3.3 d
cooked (*A&P* Michigan #1), 1 cup	220	15.0	40.0	1.0	m.q.	0	15	m.q.
NAVY BEAN, CANNED:								
(*Allens*), ½ cup	160	8.0	24.0	<1.0	.1	0	440	m.q.
w/liquid, 4 oz.	128	8.5	23.2	.5	.1	0	508	2.1 c
w/liquid, ½ cup	148	9.9	26.8	.6	.1	0	587	2.4 c
NAVY BEAN, SPROUTED, mature seeds:								
raw:								
1 lb.	306	27.9	59.2	3.2	.4	0	m.q.	11.3 c
1 oz.	19	1.7	3.7	.2	<.1	0	m.q.	.7 c
½ cup	35	3.2	6.8	.4	<.1	0	m.q.	1.3 c
boiled, drained, 4 oz.	88	8.0	17.0	.9	.1	0	m.q.	3.3 c

Food and Measure	cal.	prot. (gms)	carbo. (gms)	tot. fat (gms)	sat. fat (gms)	chol. (mgs)	sod. (mgs)	fiber (gms)
NECTARINE:								
whole, 1 lb.	204	3.9	48.6	1.9	n.a.	0	1	6.6 d
pitted, 1 oz.	14	.3	3.3	.1	n.a.	0	tr.	.5 d
1 medium, 2½″ diam., approx.								
5.3 oz.	67	1.3	16.0	.6	n.a.	0	tr.	2.2 d
sliced, ½ cup	34	.7	8.1	.3	n.a.	0	tr.	1.1 d
NEW ENGLAND BRAND								
SAUSAGE:								
(*Eckrich*), 1 oz. or 1 slice	35	5.0	1.0	1.0	m.q.	m.q.	370	(0)
(*Light & Lean*), 2 slices	90	10.0	0	6.0	m.q.	m.q.	m.q.	0
(*Oscar Mayer*), .8-oz. slice	29	3.9	.4	1.3	.6	14	291	(0)
pork and beef, 1 oz.	46	4.9	1.4	2.2	.7	14	346	(0)
pork and beef, 1 slice, 4″ × ⅛″,								
approx. .8 oz.	37	4.0	1.1	1.7	.6	11	281	(0)
NEW ZEALAND SPINACH:								
raw, untrimmed, 1 lb.	47	4.9	8.2	.7	.1	0	425	2.3 c
raw, trimmed, 1 oz. or ½ cup								
chopped	4	.4	.7	.1	tr.	0	37	.2 c
boiled, drained, 4 oz.	14	1.5	2.5	.2	<.1	0	121	.7 c
boiled, drained, chopped, ½ cup ...	11	1.2	2.0	.2	<.1	0	97	.6 c
NEWBERG SAUCE:								
w/sherry, canned (*Snow's*), ⅓ cup ..	120	3.0	10.0	8.0	m.q.	n.a.	520	n.a.
NOODLE, egg[1]:								
plain:								
1 lb.	1730	63.6	322.6	19.1	4.0	432	96	12.2 d
2 oz.	217	8.0	40.5	2.4	.5	54	12	1.5 d
(*Creamette*), 2 oz.	221	8.0	40.0	2.5	.8	70	3	.8 d
(*Gioia*), 2 oz.	220	8.0	40.0	3.0	m.q.	m.q.	m.q.	m.q.
(*Golden Grain*), 2 oz.	210	8.2	39.3	2.2	.8	65	10	1.8 d
(*Goodman's* Country Style), 2 oz.	220	8.0	40.0	3.0	m.q.	m.q.	15	m.q.
(*Mrs. Grass*), 2 oz.	220	8.0	40.0	3.0	m.q.	m.q.	200	m.q.
(*Mueller's*), 2 oz.	220	8.0	40.0	3.0	m.q.	55	10	m.q.
(*P&R*), 2 oz.	220	8.0	42.0	3.0	m.q.	m.q.	15	m.q.
(*Prince*), 2 oz.	210	8.0	40.0	2.0	m.q.	65	35	m.q.
(*San Giorgio*), 2 oz.	220	8.0	42.0	3.0	m.q.	m.q.	15	m.q.
cooked, 4 oz.	151	5.4	28.2	1.7	.4	37	8	2.5 d
cooked, 1 cup	212	7.6	39.7	2.4	.5	53	11	3.5 d
spinach:								
1 lb.	1732	66.3	319.0	20.7	4.7	431	326	10.0 d
2 oz.	218	8.3	40.1	2.6	.6	54	41	1.2 d
cooked, 4 oz.	150	5.7	27.5	1.8	.4	37	14	m.q.
cooked, 1 cup	211	8.1	38.8	2.5	.6	52	20	m.q.
NOODLE, CHINESE:								
cellophane or long rice, dehydrated,								
1 lb.	1594	.7	390.6	.3	.1	0	44	.3 c
cellophane or long rice, dehydrated,								
2 oz.	199	.1	48.8	<.1	tr.	0	6	<.1 c

1. *Uncooked, except as noted.*

Food and Measure	cal.	prot. (gms)	carbo. (gms)	tot. fat (gms)	sat. fat (gms)	chol. (mgs)	sod. (mgs)	fiber (gms)
NOODLE, CHINESE *(cont.)*								
chow mein, 1 oz.	149	2.4	16.3	8.7	1.2	0	124	1.1 d
chow mein, 1 cup	237	3.8	25.9	13.8	2.0	0	197	1.8 d
NOODLE, JAPANESE:								
soba (buckwheat):								
dry, 1 lb.	1526	65.2	338.5	3.2	.6	0	3593	m.q.
dry, 2 oz.	192	8.2	42.5	.4	.1	0	449	m.q.
cooked, 1 cup, approx. 4 oz.	113	5.8	24.4	.1	<.1	0	40	m.q.
somen (wheat):								
dry, 1 lb.	1617	51.5	336.1	3.7	.5	0	8346	19.5 d
dry, 2 oz.	203	6.5	42.2	.5	.1	0	1043	2.4 d
cooked, 4 oz.	149	4.5	31.2	.2	<.1	0	183	.3 c
cooked, 1 cup	230	7.0	48.5	.3	<.1	0	284	.4 c
udon (wheat):								
dry, 2 oz.	159	3.9	32.3	.7	m.q.	0	340	m.q.
cooked, 4 oz.	115	2.8	23.0	.6	m.q.	0	51	m.q.
NOODLE DINNER, and chicken,								
frozen:								
(Banquet), 10 oz.	350	10.0	42.0	15.0	m.q.	45	460	m.q.
(Banquet Family Favorites), 10 oz. . .	340	11.0	42.0	15.0	m.q.	45	455	m.q.
(Swanson), 10½ oz.	280	7.0	45.0	8.0	m.q.	m.q.	740	m.q.
NOODLE DISHES, MIX[1]:								
Alfredo (see also "carbonara								
Alfredo," below):								
(Lipton Noodles and Sauce),								
¼ pkg. dry	150	6.0	22.0	4.0	m.q.	m.q.	510	m.q.
(Lipton Noodles and Sauce),								
½ cup[2]	220	7.0	24.0	10.0	m.q.	m.q.	580	m.q.
(Lipton Noodles and Sauce),								
½ cup[3]	180	7.0	24.0	7.0	m.q.	m.q.	550	m.q.
(Minute Microwave Family Size),								
½ cup[4]	170	7.0	23.0	6.0	m.q.	45	670	m.q.
(Minute Microwave Single Size),								
½ cup[4]	160	7.0	23.0	5.0	m.q.	40	660	m.q.
(Mueller's Chef's Series), ½ cup . .	190	5.0	23.0	9.0	m.q.	m.q.	580	m.q.
beef:								
(Lipton Noodles and Sauce),								
¼ pkg. dry	120	5.0	23.0	2.0	m.q.	m.q.	640	m.q.
(Lipton Noodles and Sauce),								
½ cup[5]	180	5.0	23.0	7.0	m.q.	m.q.	700	m.q.
(Lipton Noodles and Sauce),								
½ cup[6]	150	5.0	23.0	5.0	m.q.	m.q.	680	m.q.
butter:								
(Lipton Noodles and Sauce),								
¼ pkg. dry	150	6.0	23.0	4.0	m.q.	m.q.	450	m.q.

1. *Prepared according to package directions, except as noted.*
2. *Prepared with ½ cup whole milk and 2 tbsp. butter.*
3. *Prepared with ½ cup skim milk and 1 tbsp. margarine.*
4. *Prepared with salted butter.*
5. *Prepared with 2 tbsp. butter.*
6. *Prepared with 1 tbsp. margarine.*

Food and Measure	cal.	prot. (gms)	carbo. (gms)	tot. fat (gms)	sat. fat (gms)	chol. (mgs)	sod. (mgs)	fiber (gms)
(*Lipton* Noodles and Sauce),								
½ cup[1]	200	6.0	23.0	10.0	m.q.	m.q.	510	m.q.
(*Lipton* Noodles and Sauce),								
½ cup[2]	180	6.0	23.0	7.0	m.q.	m.q.	480	m.q.
butter and herb:								
(*Lipton* Noodles and Sauce),								
¼ pkg. dry	140	5.0	23.0	3.0	m.q.	m.q.	460	m.q.
(*Lipton* Noodles and Sauce),								
½ cup[1]	190	5.0	23.0	9.0	m.q.	m.q.	520	m.q.
(*Lipton* Noodles and Sauce),								
½ cup[2]	170	5.0	23.0	6.0	m.q.	m.q.	490	m.q.
carbonara Alfredo:								
(*Lipton* Noodles and Sauce),								
¼ pkg. dry	140	5.0	20.0	4.0	m.q.	m.q.	460	m.q.
(*Lipton* Noodles and Sauce),								
½ cup[3]	210	6.0	22.0	11.0	m.q.	m.q.	530	m.q.
(*Lipton* Noodles and Sauce),								
½ cup[4]	180	6.0	22.0	7.0	m.q.	m.q.	510	m.q.
cheese (see also "Parmesan,"								
below):								
(*Kraft* Dinner), ¾ cup	340	10.0	37.0	17.0	4.0	50	670	m.q.
(*Lipton* Noodles and Sauce),								
¼ pkg. dry	140	5.0	25.0	2.0	m.q.	m.q.	470	m.q.
(*Lipton* Noodles and Sauce),								
½ cup[1]	190	5.0	25.0	8.0	m.q.	m.q.	530	m.q.
(*Lipton* Noodles and Sauce),								
½ cup[2]	170	5.0	25.0	5.0	m.q.	m.q.	500	m.q.
chicken or chicken flavor:								
(*Kraft* Dinner), ¾ cup	240	8.0	32.0	9.0	2.0	45	1050	m.q.
(*Lipton* Noodles and Sauce),								
¼ pkg. dry	130	5.0	23.0	2.0	m.q.	m.q.	390	m.q.
(*Lipton* Noodles and Sauce),								
½ cup[1]	180	5.0	23.0	8.0	m.q.	m.q.	450	m.q.
(*Lipton* Noodles and Sauce),								
½ cup[2]	160	5.0	23.0	5.0	m.q.	m.q.	430	m.q.
(*Minute* Microwave Family Size),								
½ cup[5]	160	6.0	23.0	5.0	m.q.	35	570	m.q.
(*Minute* Microwave Single Size),								
½ cup[5]	160	6.0	25.0	4.0	m.q.	35	610	m.q.
(*Mueller's Chef's Series*), ½ cup	160	3.0	21.0	8.0	m.q.	m.q.	550	m.q.
broccoli:								
(*Lipton* Noodles and Sauce),								
¼ pkg. dry	130	5.0	22.0	2.0	m.q.	m.q.	430	m.q.

1. *Prepared with 2 tbsp. butter.*
2. *Prepared with 1 tbsp. margarine.*
3. *Prepared with ½ cup whole milk and 2 tbsp. butter.*
4. *Prepared with ½ cup skin milk and 1 tbsp. margarine.*
5. *Prepared according to package directions.*

Food and Measure	cal.	prot. (gms)	carbo. (gms)	tot. fat (gms)	sat. fat (gms)	chol. (mgs)	sod. (mgs)	fiber (gms)
NOODLE DISHES, MIX, CHICKEN BROCCOLI *(cont.)*								
(*Lipton* Noodles and Sauce),								
½ cup[1]	200	6.0	24.0	9.0	m.q.	m.q.	500	m.q.
(*Lipton* Noodles and Sauce),								
½ cup[2]	160	6.0	24.0	5.0	m.q.	m.q.	480	m.q.
mushroom (*Golden Grain/Noodle*								
Roni), 1.2 oz. dry	134	4.7	23.6	2.4	.6	19	531	1.2 d
mushroom (*Golden Grain/Noodle*								
Roni), ½ cup	160	6.0	25.0	4.0	m.q.	m.q.	550	m.q.
fettuccini (*Golden Grain/Noodle*								
Roni), 1.5 oz. dry	181	6.1	27.8	5.1	1.5	27	411	1.4 d
fettuccini (*Golden Grain/Noodle*								
Roni), ½ cup	300	7.0	29.0	18.0	m.q.	m.q.	560	m.q.
garlic, creamy (*Golden Grain/Noodle*								
Roni), 1.5 oz. dry	172	6.1	27.4	4.2	1.5	29	472	1.3 d
garlic, creamy (*Golden Grain/Noodle*								
Roni), ½ cup	300	7.0	29.0	17.0	m.q.	m.q.	630	m.q.
garlic and butter (*Mueller's Chef's*								
Series), ½ cup	170	3.0	21.0	7.0	m.q.	m.q.	480	m.q.
herb and butter (*Golden Grain/*								
Noodle Roni), 1 oz. dry	114	4.0	18.4	2.7	.8	19	228	1.0 d
herb and butter (*Golden Grain/*								
Noodle Roni), ½ cup	160	5.0	19.0	7.0	m.q.	m.q.	290	m.q.
Parmesan:								
(*Golden Grain/Noodle Roni*),								
1.2 oz. dry	135	5.6	21.5	2.9	.9	19	340	1.1 d
(*Golden Grain/Noodle Roni*),								
½ cup	240	7.0	23.0	13.0	m.q.	m.q.	470	m.q.
(*Lipton* Noodles and Sauce),								
¼ pkg. dry	140	6.0	21.0	4.0	m.q.	m.q.	410	m.q.
(*Lipton* Noodles and Sauce),								
½ cup[1]	210	7.0	23.0	11.0	m.q.	m.q.	480	m.q.
(*Lipton* Noodles and Sauce),								
½ cup[2]	180	7.0	23.0	7.0	m.q.	m.q.	460	m.q.
(*Minute* Microwave Family Size),								
½ cup[3]	170	6.0	23.0	6.0	m.q.	45	470	m.q.
(*Minute* Microwave Single Size),								
½ cup[3]	160	6.0	23.0	5.0	m.q.	40	460	m.q.
Romanoff (*Golden Grain/Noodle*								
Roni), 1.5 oz. dry	168	6.7	26.1	4.1	1.6	23	647	1.2 d
Romanoff (*Golden Grain/Noodle*								
Roni), ½ cup	240	8.0	28.0	11.0	m.q.	m.q.	730	m.q.
sour cream and chives:								
(*Lipton* Noodles and Sauce),								
¼ pkg. dry	150	5.0	24.0	3.0	m.q.	m.q.	440	m.q.

1. *Prepared with ½ cup whole milk and 2 tbsp. butter.*
2. *Prepared with ½ cup skim milk and 1 tbsp. margarine.*
3. *Prepared with salted butter.*

Food and Measure	cal.	prot. (gms)	carbo. (gms)	tot. fat (gms)	sat. fat (gms)	chol. (mgs)	sod. (mgs)	fiber (gms)
(*Lipton* Noodles and Sauce),								
½ cup[1]	200	5.0	24.0	9.0	m.q.	m.q.	500	m.q.
(*Lipton* Noodles and Sauce),								
½ cup[2]	170	5.0	24.0	6.0	m.q.	m.q.	480	m.q.
(*Mueller's Chef's Series*), ½ cup ..	190	4.0	22.0	8.0	m.q.	m.q.	470	m.q.
Stroganoff:								
(*Golden Grain/Noodle Roni*), 2 oz.								
dry	225	8.7	33.0	6.4	2.2	42	1058	1.8 d
(*Golden Grain/Noodle Roni*),								
½ cup	350	11.0	37.0	17.0	m.q.	m.q.	1190	m.q.
(*Lipton* Noodles and Sauce),								
¼ pkg. dry	130	6.0	22.0	3.0	m.q.	m.q.	330	m.q.
(*Lipton* Noodles and Sauce),								
½ cup[3]	200	7.0	23.0	9.0	m.q.	m.q.	410	m.q.
(*Lipton* Noodles and Sauce),								
½ cup[4]	170	7.0	23.0	5.0	m.q.	m.q.	380	m.q.
(*Mueller's Chef's Series*), ½ cup ..	190	5.0	22.0	9.0	m.q.	m.q.	620	m.q.
NOODLE ENTREE, CANNED:								
and beef, in sauce (*Heinz*), 7.5 oz. ...	170	8.0	17.0	8.0	m.q.	m.q.	825	m.q.
and chicken:								
(*Heinz*), 7.5 oz.	160	6.0	19.0	7.0	m.q.	m.q.	930	m.q.
(*Hormel/Dinty Moore Micro-Cup*),								
7.5 oz.	180	7.0	18.0	8.0	m.q.	20	1000	m.q.
(*Nalley's*), 7⅜ oz.	150	9.0	17.0	5.0	m.q.	m.q.	1000	m.q.
w/vegetables (*Nalley's*), 7⅜ oz. ...	160	10.0	18.0	5.0	m.q.	m.q.	1450	m.q.
w/franks (*Van Camp's Noodle*								
Weenee), 1 cup	245	9.3	32.9	8.5	m.q.	m.q.	1245	.5 c
and tuna (*Heinz*), 7.5 oz.	170	11.0	20.0	5.0	m.q.	m.q.	950	m.q.
NOODLE ENTREE, FREEZE-								
DRIED[5]:								
and chicken (*Mountain House*),								
1 cup	270	10.0	34.0	10.0	m.q.	m.q.	201	m.q.
NOODLE ENTREE, FROZEN:								
and beef, w/gravy (*Banquet Family*								
Entrees), 8 oz.	200	13.0	22.0	7.0	m.q.	m.q.	m.q.	m.q.
and julienne beef, w/sauce (*Banquet*								
Family Entrees), 7 oz.	170	12.0	22.0	3.0	m.q.	m.q.	m.q.	m.q.
Romanoff (*Stouffer's*), ⅓ of 12-oz.								
pkg.	170	7.0	15.0	9.0	m.q.	m.q.	840	m.q.
NOODLE MIX, see "Noodle dishes,								
mix"								
NORI, see "Seaweed, laver"								
NUT, PINE, see "Pine nut, piñon"								
NUT TOPPING:								
(*Planters*), 1 oz.	180	5.0	6.0	16.0	2.0	0	0	m.q.

1. *Prepared with 2 tbsp. butter.*
2. *Prepared with 1 tbsp. margarine.*
3. *Prepared with ½ cup whole milk and 2 tbsp. butter.*
4. *Prepared with ½ cup skim milk and 1 tbsp. margarine.*
5. *Prepared according to package directions.*

Food and Measure	cal.	prot. (gms)	carbo. (gms)	tot. fat (gms)	sat. fat (gms)	chol. (mgs)	sod. (mgs)	fiber (gms)
NUTMEG, ground:								
1 oz.	149	1.7	14.0	10.3	7.4	0	5	1.1 c
1 tbsp.	37	.4	3.5	2.5	1.8	0	1	.3 c
1 tsp.	12	.1	1.1	.8	.6	0	tr.	.1 c
(*Spice Islands*), 1 tsp.	11	.1	.9	.7	m.q.	0	<1	.1 c
NUTMEG BUTTER OIL:								
1 oz.	251	0	0	28.4	25.5	0	0	0
½ cup	964	0	0	109.0	98.1	0	0	0
1 tbsp.	120	0	0	13.6	12.2	0	0	0
NUTS, see specific listings								
NUTS, MIXED, 1 oz., except as noted:								
w/peanuts (*Guy's*)	170	8.0	3.0	14.0	m.q.	0	140	m.q.
dry-roasted (*Planters*)	160	5.0	7.0	14.0	2.0	0	250	m.q.
dry-roasted (*Planters* Unsalted)	170	6.0	7.0	15.0	2.0	0	0	m.q.
dry-roasted, w/peanuts:								
1 oz.	169	4.9	7.2	14.6	2.0	0	3	.3 c
1 cup	814	23.7	34.7	70.5	9.5	0	16	1.2 c
salted:								
1 oz.	169	4.9	7.2	14.6	2.0	0	190	.3 c
1 cup	814	23.7	34.7	70.5	9.5	0	917	1.2 c
(*Finast* No Frills)	180	5.0	7.0	14.0	m.q.	0	150	m.q.
(*Pathmark* No Frills)	180	6.0	7.0	14.0	2.0	0	220	m.q.
oil-roasted (*Flavor House*)	180	5.0	6.0	18.0	m.q.	0	125	m.q.
oil-roasted, w/peanuts:								
1 oz.	175	4.8	6.1	16.0	2.5	0	3	2.6 d
1 cup	876	23.8	30.4	80.0	12.4	0	16	12.8 d
salted:								
1 oz.	175	4.8	6.1	16.0	2.5	0	185	2.6 d
1 cup	876	23.8	30.4	80.0	12.4	0	926	12.8 d
(*Pathmark* No Frills)	180	6.0	5.0	15.0	0	0	150	m.q.
oil-roasted, w/out peanuts:								
1 oz.	175	4.4	6.3	16.0	2.6	0	3	.6 c
1 cup	886	22.4	32.1	80.9	13.1	0	16	3.2 c
salted:								
1 oz.	175	4.4	6.3	16.0	2.6	0	198	.6 c
1 cup	886	22.4	32.1	80.9	13.1	0	1008	3.2 c
(*Pathmark* No Frills Fancy)	180	4.0	7.0	15.0	m.q.	0	150	m.q.

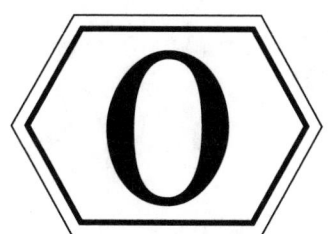

Food and Measure	cal.	prot. (gms)	carbo. (gms)	tot. fat (gms)	sat. fat (gms)	chol. (mgs)	sod. (mgs)	fiber (gms)
OAT (see also "Cereal"):								
whole-grain, 1 oz.	110	4.8	18.8	2.0	.3	0	1	m.q.
whole-grain, 1 cup	607	26.3	103.4	10.8	1.9	0	3	m.q.
flaked, see "Oat flakes"								
rolled or oatmeal:								
dry, 1 oz.	109	4.5	19.0	1.8	.3	0	1	2.9 d
dry, 1 cup	311	13.0	54.2	5.1	.9	0	3	8.3 d
cooked:								
unsalted, 4 oz.	70	2.9	12.2	1.1	.2	0	1	.2 c
unsalted, 1 cup	145	6.0	25.2	2.4	.4	0	1	.4 c
salted, 4 oz.	70	2.9	12.2	1.1	.2	0	181	.2 c
salted, 1 cup	145	6.0	25.2	2.4	.4	0	374	.4 c
steel cut (*Arrowhead Mills*), 2 oz. ...	220	10.0	37.0	4.0	m.q.	0	1	2.8 d
OAT BRAN (see also "Cereal"):								
raw, 1 oz.	70	4.9	18.8	2.0	.4	0	1	4.5 d
raw, 1 cup	231	16.3	62.2	6.6	1.2	0	4	14.9 d
cooked, 4 oz.	45	3.6	13.0	1.0	.2	0	1	.4 c
cooked, 1 cup	87	7.0	25.1	1.9	.4	0	2	.8 c
OAT BRAN PILAF DINNER, canned:								
w/garden vegetables (*Health Valley Fast Menu*), 7½ oz.	210	8.0	31.0	7.0	m.q.	0	445	5.8 d
OAT BRAN SNACK BAR, see "Snack bar"								
OAT FLAKES:								
(*Arrowhead Mills*), 2 oz.	220	10.0	39.0	4.0	m.q.	0	1	8.1 d
OAT FLOUR:								
whole-grain (*Arrowhead Mills*), 2 oz.	200	7.0	43.0	1.0	m.q.	0	1	8.3 d
blend (*Gold Medal*), 4 oz. or 1 cup ..	390	14.0	81.0	3.0	m.q.	0	0	4.0 d
OAT GROATS:								
(*Arrowhead Mills*), 2 oz.	220	8.0	38.0	4.0	m.q.	0	1	5.6 d

Food and Measure	cal.	prot. (gms)	carbo. (gms)	tot. fat (gms)	sat. fat (gms)	chol. (mgs)	sod. (mgs)	fiber (gms)
OATMEAL, see "Cereal" and "Oat"								
OCEAN PERCH, Atlantic, meat								
only:								
raw:								
1 lb.	427	84.5	0	7.4	1.1	191	339	0
1 oz.	27	5.3	0	.5	.1	12	21	0
1 fillet, approx. 2.25 oz., yield								
from 1-lb. whole fish	60	11.9	0	1.0	.2	27	48	0
baked, broiled, or microwaved[1],								
4 oz.	137	27.1	0	2.4	.4	61	109	0
OCEAN PERCH, FROZEN:								
(*Booth*), 4 oz.	100	20.0	0	1.0	m.q.	m.q.	250	0
(*Gorton's* Fishmarket Fresh), 5 oz. ...	140	25.0	2.0	3.0	m.q.	m.q.	100	0
(*Van de Kamp's* Natural), 4 oz.	130	20.0	0	5.0	2.0	40	65	0
OCEAN PERCH ENTREE,								
frozen:								
breaded (*Van de Kamp's* Light),								
1 piece	280	17.0	21.0	14.0	3.0	35	450	m.q.
OCTOBER BEAN, canned:								
w/pork (*Luck's*), 7.25 oz.	230	12.0	32.0	6.0	m.q.	m.q.	550	10.0 d
OCTOPUS, meat only:								
raw, 1 lb.	372	67.6	10.0	4.7	1.0	219	m.q.	0
raw, 1 oz.	23	4.2	.6	.3	.1	14	m.q.	0
OHELOBERRY:								
1 lb.	126	1.7	31.0	1.0	n.a.	0	6	6.0 c
1 oz.	8	.1	1.9	.1	(0)	0	<1	.4 c
10 berries, .4 oz.	3	<.1	.8	<.1	(0)	0	tr.	.2 c
½ cup	20	.3	4.8	.2	(0)	0	1	.9 c
OIL, see specific listings								
OKARA, see "Tofu"								
OKRA:								
raw:								
untrimmed, 1 lb.	148	7.8	29.8	.4	.1	0	32	3.7 c
trimmed, 1 oz.	11	.6	2.2	<.1	tr.	0	2	.3 c
8 pods, 3″ × ⅝″, approx. 3.9 oz.	36	1.9	7.3	.1	<.1	0	8	.9 c
sliced, ½ cup	19	1.0	3.8	.1	<.1	0	4	.5 c
boiled, drained:								
4 oz.	36	2.1	8.2	.2	.1	0	6	1.0 c
8 pods, 3″ × ⅝″	27	1.6	6.1	.1	<.1	0	5	.8 c
sliced, ½ cup	25	1.5	5.8	.1	<.1	0	4	.7 c
OKRA, FROZEN:								
10-oz. pkg.	85	4.8	18.8	.7	.2	0	7	2.4 c
boiled, drained, 4 oz.	42	2.4	9.3	.3	.1	0	3	1.2 c
boiled, drained, sliced, ½ cup	34	1.9	7.5	.3	.1	0	3	.9 c
whole:								
(*Seabrook*), 3.3 oz.	30	2.0	7.0	0	0	0	2	1.0 c
(*Southern*), 3.5 oz.	35	1.9	7.4	.2	(0)	0	20	m.q.

1. *Without added ingredients.*

Food and Measure	cal.	prot. (gms)	carbo. (gms)	tot. fat (gms)	sat. fat (gms)	chol. (mgs)	sod. (mgs)	fiber (gms)
baby (*Frosty Acres*), 3.3 oz.	30	2.0	7.0	0	0	0	2	1.0 c
cut (*Seabrook*), 3.3 oz.	25	1.0	6.0	0	0	0	3	1.0 c
cut (*Southern*), 3.5 oz.	31	1.6	6.5	.2	(0)	0	20	m.q.
OLD-FASHIONED DRINK MIX:								
bottled (*Holland House*), 1 fl. oz. ...	33	0	8.0	0	0	0	6	0
OLD-FASHIONED LOAF (see also "Dutch brand loaf"):								
(*Oscar Mayer*), 1-oz. slice	62	4.0	2.4	4.0	1.6	16	337	(0)
OLIVE, pickled (see also "Olive, green" and "Olive, ripe"), canned or bottled:								
all varieties, all sizes (*S&W*), 1 oz.	46	0	0	5.1	m.q.	0	215	m.q.
salad (*Progresso*), ½ cup	120	1.0	1.0	15.0	2.0	0	2400	4.0 d
OLIVE, GREEN, pickled, canned or bottled:								
w/pits:								
10 small, select, or standard, approx. 1.2 oz.	33	.4	.4	3.6	m.q.	0	686	.7 d
10 large, approx. 1.6 oz.	45	.5	.5	4.9	m.q.	0	926	1.0 d
10 giant, approx. 2.75 oz.	76	.9	.9	8.3	m.q.	0	1572	1.7 d
pitted, 1 oz.	33	.4	.4	3.6	m.q.	0	680	.7 d
OLIVE, RIPE, pickled, canned or bottled:								
Manzanilla or Mission varieties, pitted:								
all sizes, 1 oz.	33	.2	1.8	3.0	.4	0	247	.9 d
all sizes (*Lindsay*), 1 oz.	32	.2	1.8	3.0	.5	0	247	.9 d
10 small, approx. 1.1 oz.	37	.3	2.0	3.4	.5	0	279	1.0 d
10 large, approx. 1.6 oz.	51	.5	2.8	4.7	.6	0	384	1.3 d
(*Lindsay*), 10 small	37	.3	2.0	3.5	.6	0	283	1.0 d
(*Lindsay*), 10 medium	44	.3	2.4	4.1	.7	0	336	1.2 d
(*Lindsay*), 10 large	50	.4	2.8	4.8	.8	0	388	1.4 d
(*Lindsay*), 10 extra large	63	.5	3.5	5.9	1.1	0	484	1.8 d
mixed varieties:								
pitted (*Vlasic*), 1 oz.	37	.3	.7	3.9	m.q.	0	230	.4 c
sliced or chopped (*Lindsay*), 1 oz.	29	.2	1.7	2.7	.5	0	249	.8 d
sliced (*Lindsay*), ½ cup	70	.6	4.1	6.5	1.1	0	598	2.0 d
salt-cured, oil-coated, Greek style:								
10 medium, approx. .8 oz. w/pits	65	.4	1.7	6.9	m.q.	0	631	m.q.
10 extra large, approx. 1.2 oz. w/pits	89	.6	2.3	9.5	m.q.	0	868	m.q.
pitted, 1 oz.	96	.6	2.5	10.2	m.q.	0	932	m.q.
Sevillano and Ascolano varieties, pitted:								
all sizes, 1 oz.	23	.3	1.6	1.9	.3	0	255	.9 d
all sizes (*Lindsay*), 1 oz.	23	.3	1.6	1.9	.3	0	255	.7 d
10 jumbo, approx. 2.9 oz.	67	.8	4.7	5.7	.8	0	745	2.5 d
10 super colossal, approx. 5.4 oz.	123	1.5	8.5	10.4	1.4	0	1365	4.6 d
(*Lindsay*), 10 jumbo	66	.8	4.7	5.7	1.0	0	745	2.1 d

Food and Measure	cal.	prot. (gms)	carbo. (gms)	tot. fat (gms)	sat. fat (gms)	chol. (mgs)	sod. (mgs)	fiber (gms)
OLIVE, RIPE *(cont.)*								
(Lindsay), 10 colossal	90	1.1	6.3	7.7	1.3	0	1010	2.8 d
(Lindsay), 10 super colossal	122	1.5	8.5	10.4	1.8	0	1365	3.8 d
OLIVE APPETIZER:								
(Progresso), ½ cup	180	1.0	6.0	21.0	3.0	0	1600	2.5 d
(Progresso Condite), ½ cup	130	<1.0	5.0	14.0	2.0	0	870	2.0 d
OLIVE LOAF:								
(Boar's Head), 1 oz.	60	3.0	1.0	4.5	m.q.	10	360	(0)
(Eckrich), 1-oz. slice	80	3.0	2.0	6.0	m.q.	m.q.	320	(0)
(Hormel Perma-Fresh), 2 slices	110	7.0	5.0	7.0	m.q.	m.q.	810	(0)
(Oscar Mayer), 1-oz. slice	63	2.9	3.2	4.3	1.5	8	392	(0)
pork, 1-oz. slice, 4″ × 4″ × ³⁄₃₂″ ...	67	3.4	2.6	4.7	1.7	11	421	(0)
OLIVE OIL:								
1 oz.	251	0	0	28.4	3.8	0	tr.	0
½ cup	955	0	0	108.0	14.6	0	tr.	0
1 tbsp.	119	0	0	13.5	1.8	0	tr.	0
(Amore Pure or Extra Virgin), 1 tbsp.	130	0	0	14.0	2.0	0	0	0
(Bertolli), 1 tbsp.	120	0	0	14.0	m.q.	0	(0)	0
(Filippo Berio), 1 tbsp.	120	0	0	14.0	2.0	0	(0)	0
(Hain), 1 tbsp.	120	0	0	14.0	2.0	0	0	0
all varieties *(Progresso)*, 1 tbsp.	119	0	0	14.0	2.0	0	0	0
spray *(Pam)*, ⅓ of 10″ skillet	2	0	0	1.0	n.a.	0	0	0
OMELET, see "Egg" and "Egg breakfast"								
ONION, mature:								
raw:								
untrimmed, 1 lb.	154	4.7	35.2	.7	.1	0	12	6.5 d
trimmed, 1 oz.	11	.3	2.4	<.1	<.1	0	1	.5 d
chopped, ½ cup	30	.9	6.9	0.1	<.1	0	2	1.3 d
chopped, 1 tbsp.	4	.1	.9	<.1	tr.	0	tr.	.2 d
boiled, drained:								
4 oz.	50	1.5	11.5	.2	<.1	0	3	.8 c
chopped, ½ cup	47	1.4	10.7	.2	<.1	0	3	.7 c
chopped, 1 tbsp.	7	.2	1.5	<.1	tr.	0	tr.	.1 c
ONION, CANNED:								
w/liquid:								
4 oz.	22	1.0	4.5	.1	<.1	0	421	1.2 d
1 medium, approx. 1″ diam.	12	.5	2.5	.1	<.1	0	234	.7 d
chopped, ½ cup	21	1.0	4.5	.1	<.1	0	416	1.2 d
whole, small *(Pathmark)*, ½ cup ...	35	2.0	7.0	0	0	0	280	m.q.
whole, small *(S&W)*, ½ cup	35	1.0	9.0	0	0	0	345	m.q.
sweet *(Heinz)*, 1 oz.	40	0	9.0	0	0	0	165	m.q.
ONION, COCKTAIL:								
lightly spiced *(Vlasic)*, 1 oz.	4	0	1.0	0	0	0	365	m.q.
ONION, DRIED OR DEHYDRATED:								
flakes:								
1 oz.	92	2.5	23.6	.1	<.1	0	6	1.3 c

Food and Measure	cal.	prot. (gms)	carbo. (gms)	tot. fat (gms)	sat. fat (gms)	chol. (mgs)	sod. (mgs)	fiber (gms)
¼ cup	45	1.3	11.7	.1	<.1	0	3	.6 c
1 tbsp.	16	.5	4.2	<.1	tr.	0	1	.2 c
minced, w/green onion (*Lawry's*),								
1 tsp.	7	.4	1.6	.2	(0)	0	1	.6 c
ONION, FROZEN:								
whole:								
10-oz. pkg.	101	2.5	24.0	.2	<.1	0	27	2.0 c
boiled, drained, 4 oz.	32	.8	7.6	.1	<.1	0	9	.6 c
small (*Birds Eye*), 4 oz.	40	1.0	10.0	0	0	0	10	2.0 d
small (*Seabrook*), 3.3 oz.	35	1.0	8.0	0	0	0	9	1.0 c
chopped:								
10-oz. pkg.	83	2.2	19.4	.3	<.1	0	35	2.3 d
boiled, drained, 4 oz.	32	.9	7.5	.1	<.1	0	14	.5 c
boiled, drained, ½ cup	30	.8	6.9	.1	<.1	0	13	.5 c
boiled, drained, 1 tbsp.	4	.1	1.0	<.1	tr.	0	2	.1 c
(*Ore-Ida*), 2 oz.	20	0	4.0	<1.0	(0)	0	10	m.q.
(*Seabrook*), 1 oz.	8	0	2.0	0	0	0	2	0
w/cream sauce, small (*Birds Eye*								
Combinations), 5 oz.	140	2.0	12.0	10.0	m.q.	0	400	1.0 d
rings, see "Onion ring"								
ONION, GREEN (scallion):								
untrimmed, 1 lb.	140	8.0	32.0	.8	.1	0	71	10.5 d
trimmed, w/top:								
1 oz.	19	.5	2.1	<.1	tr.	0	5	.7 d
chopped, ½ cup	16	.9	3.7	.1	<.1	0	8	1.2 d
chopped, 1 tbsp.	2	.1	.4	<.1	tr.	0	1	.1 d
ONION, WELSH:								
untrimmed, 1 lb.	100	5.6	19.2	1.2	.2	0	n.a.	3.0 c
trimmed, 1 oz.	10	.5	1.8	.1	<.1	0	n.a.	.3 c
ONION DIP:								
bean (*Hain*), 4 tbsp.	70	4.0	10.0	1.0	m.q.	5	270	m.q.
creamy (*Kraft* Premium), 2 tbsp. ...	45	1.0	2.0	4.0	2.0	10	160	n.a.
French:								
(*Bison*), 1 oz.	60	1.0	2.0	5.0	m.q.	20	180	n.a.
(*Breakstone's/Sealtest*), 2 tbsp. ...	50	1.0	2.0	5.0	3.0	15	140	n.a.
(*Kraft*), 2 tbsp.	60	1.0	3.0	4.0	2.0	0	240	n.a.
(*Kraft* Premium), 2 tbsp.	45	1.0	2.0	4.0	2.0	10	150	n.a.
(*Nasoya Vegi-Dip*), 1 oz.	50	2.0	4.0	3.0	m.q.	0	100	n.a.
green (*Kraft*), 2 tbsp.	60	1.0	3.0	4.0	2.0	0	170	n.a.
toasted (*Breakstone's* Gourmet),								
2 tbsp.	50	1.0	2.0	5.0	3.0	10	170	n.a.
ONION FLAKES, see "Onion,								
dried or dehydrated"								
ONION-FLAVORED SNACK:								
(*Funyuns*), 1 oz.	140	2.0	18.0	6.0	m.q.	0	275	m.q.
rings (*Wise*), 1 oz.	130	<1.0	21.0	5.0	m.q.	0	360	m.q.

Food and Measure	cal.	prot. (gms)	carbo. (gms)	tot. fat (gms)	sat. fat (gms)	chol. (mgs)	sod. (mgs)	fiber (gms)
ONION GRAVY MIX[1]:								
.8-oz. pkg. dry[2]	77	2.2	16.2	.7	.5	tr.	1005	n.a.
¼ cup[2]	19	.5	4.1	.2	.1	tr.	253	n.a.
(French's), ¼ cup	25	1.0	4.0	1.0	n.a.	n.a.	270	n.a.
(McCormick/Schilling), ¼ cup	22	.6	3.6	.6	n.a.	n.a.	337	n.a.
ONION POWDER:								
(Spice Islands), 1 tsp.	8	.2	1.7	<.1	tr.	0	1	.1 c
(Tone's), 1 tsp.	5	.2	1.8	<.1	tr.	0	1000	.1 d
ONION RING, frozen:								
(Ore-Ida Onion Ringers), 2 oz.	140	2.0	18.0	7.0	3.0	0	190	m.q.
battered (Stilwell), 3 oz.	250	2.0	22.0	16.0	m.q.	<1.0	300	m.q.
battered, precooked (Farm Rich								
Batter Dipt), 4 oz.	260	3.0	32.0	13.0	m.q.	n.a.	580	m.q.
breaded[3]:								
9-oz. pkg.	658	8.0	77.8	36.0	11.6	0	627	m.q.
oven-heated, 4 oz.	462	6.1	43.3	30.3	9.7	0	425	.5 c
oven-heated, 2 rings, .7 oz.	81	1.1	7.6	5.3	1.7	0	75	.1 c
crispy (Farm Rich Onion O's),								
5 rings	190	3.0	26.0	9.0	m.q.	0	480	m.q.
crispy (Mrs. Paul's), 2½ oz.	190	2.0	19.0	12.0	m.q.	n.a.	230	m.q.
ONION RING BATTER MIX:								
(Golden Dipt), 1 oz.	100	2.0	22.0	0	0	0	570	m.q.
ONION SALT:								
(Tone's), 1 tsp.	1	.1	.4	tr.	tr.	0	1599	<.1 d
OPOSSUM, roasted[4], meat only:								
14 oz., yield from 1 lb. raw boneless	882	120.6	0	40.7	m.q.	m.q.	m.q.	0
4 oz.	251	34.2	0	11.6	m.q.	m.q.	m.q.	0
diced, 1 cup, approx. 4.9 oz.	309	42.3	0	14.3	m.q.	m.q.	m.q.	0
ORANGE:								
all commercial varieties:								
untrimmed, 1 lb.	156	3.1	38.9	.4	.1	0	0	7.9 d
peeled and seeded, 1 oz.	13	.3	3.3	<.1	tr.	0	0	.7 d
1 medium, 2⅝″ diam., approx.								
6.3 oz.	62	1.2	15.4	.2	<.1	0	0	3.1 d
sections w/out membrane, ½ cup	43	.8	10.6	.1	<.1	0	0	2.2 d
California navel:								
untrimmed, 1 lb.	142	3.2	35.9	.3	<.1	0	2	1.4 c
peeled and seeded, 1 oz.	13	.3	3.3	<.1	tr.	0	<1	.1 c
1 medium, 2⅞″ diam., approx.								
7.3 oz.	65	1.4	16.3	.1	<.1	0	1	.6 c
sections w/out membrane, ½ cup	38	.9	9.6	.1	tr.	0	1	.4 c
California Valencia:								
untrimmed, 1 lb.	167	3.5	40.5	1.0	.1	0	0	1.7 c
peeled and seeded, 1 oz.	14	.3	3.4	.1	tr.	0	0	.1 c

1. *Prepared according to package directions, with water, except as noted.*
2. *Contains beef fat and coconut oil.*
3. *Par-fried in vegetable oil.*
4. *Without added ingredients.*

Food and Measure	cal.	prot. (gms)	carbo. (gms)	tot. fat (gms)	sat. fat (gms)	chol. (mgs)	sod. (mgs)	fiber (gms)
1 medium, 2⅝″ diam., approx.								
5.7 oz.	59	1.3	14.4	.4	<.1	0	0	.6 c
sections w/out membrane, ½ cup	44	.9	10.7	.3	<.1	0	0	.5 c
Florida:								
untrimmed, 1 lb.	153	2.4	38.7	.7	.1	0	2	1.2 c
peeled and seeded, 1 oz.	13	.2	3.3	.1	tr.	0	tr.	.1 c
1 medium, 2¹¹⁄₁₆″ diam., approx.								
7.2 oz.	69	1.1	17.4	.3	<.1	0	1	.5 c
sections w/out membrane, ½ cup	42	.7	10.7	.2	<.1	0	1	.3 c
ORANGE, CANNED, see								
"Tangerine, canned"								
ORANGE, MANDARIN, see								
"Tangerine"								
ORANGE BREAKFAST DRINK,								
see "Orange drink" and								
"Orange flavor drink"								
ORANGE DRINK (see also								
"Orange flavor drink"):								
canned, bottled, or boxed:								
1 fl. oz.	16	0	4.0	tr.	tr.	0	5	(0)
8 fl. oz.	128	0	32.0	tr.	tr.	0	40	(0)
(Bama), 8.45 fl. oz.	120	0	29.0	0	0	0	60	(0)
(Crowley), 8 fl. oz.	130	0	32.0	0	0	0	15	(0)
(Hawaiian Punch), 6 fl. oz.	100	0	24.0	0	0	0	20	(0)
(Hi-C), 8.45 fl. oz.	134	.2	32.9	<.1	(0)	0	24	(0)
(Hi-C), 6 fl. oz.	95	.1	23.3	<.1	(0)	0	17	(0)
(Pathmark No Frills Sodium Free),								
6 fl. oz.	80	0	22.0	0	0	0	0	(0)
(Tropicana Single Serve), 10 fl. oz.	132	(0)	33.0	0	0	0	<3	(0)
(Veryfine), 8 fl. oz.	130	<1.0	33.0	0	0	0	<70	(0)
(Wylers Fruit Slush), 4 fl. oz.	157	0	39.3	0	0	0	10	(0)
frozen, breakfast:								
w/orange juice and pulp, undiluted,								
12 fl. oz.	669	1.6	169.9	.1	tr.	0	113	.9 d
w/orange pulp, 1 fl. oz.¹	14	tr.	3.5	tr.	tr.	0	3	<.1 d
mix², 8 fl. oz., except as noted:								
(Kool-Aid)	100	0	25.0	0	0	0	0	(0)
(Kool-Aid Presweetened)	80	0	20.0	0	0	0	0	(0)
(Kool-Aid Sugar Free)	4	0	0	0	0	0	0	0
breakfast (Finast)	80	0	20.0	0	0	0	15	(0)
breakfast (Pathmark No Frills),								
4 fl. oz.	60	0	15.0	0	0	0	0	(0)
ORANGE EXTRACT:								
(Virginia Dare), 1 tsp.	22	0	0	0	0	0	0	0

1. *Diluted according to package directions.*
2. *Prepared according to package directions.*

Food and Measure	cal.	prot. (gms)	carbo. (gms)	tot. fat (gms)	sat. fat (gms)	chol. (mgs)	sod. (mgs)	fiber (gms)
ORANGE FLAVOR DRINK,								
breakfast (see also "Orange drink"):								
frozen:								
w/orange pulp, undiluted,								
12 fl. oz.	729	.3	182.0	2.2	.3	0	103	.4 d
w/orange pulp, 1 fl. oz.[1]	15	tr.	3.8	tr.	tr.	0	3	m.q.
frozen[1] or chilled (*Bright & Early*),								
6 fl. oz.	90	.1	20.8	.2	n.a.	0	18	m.q.
mix:								
powder, 1 oz.	109	<.1	28.0	<.1	<.1	0	5	(0)
powder, 3 rounded tsp. or .8 oz.	93	tr.	23.7	tr.	<.1	0	4	(0)
beverage[2], 6 fl. oz.:								
(*Finast* Instant Breakfast Drink)	90	0	22.0	0	0	0	20	(0)
crystals (*Tang*)	90	0	22.0	0	0	0	0	(0)
crystals (*Tang* Sugar Free)	6	0	1.0	0	0	0	0	(0)
ORANGE FLAVOR GELATIN, see "Gelatin drink mix"								
ORANGE FRUIT JUICE BLEND:								
(*Mott's*), 10-fl.-oz. bottle	144	1.0	35.0	0	0	0	6	(0)
(*Mott's*), 9.5-fl.-oz. can	139	1.0	34.0	0	0	0	6	(0)
ORANGE JUICE, 6 fl. oz., except as noted:								
fresh:								
1 fl. oz.	14	.2	3.2	.1	tr.	0	<1	<.1 c
6 fl. oz.	83	1.3	19.3	.4	<.1	0	2	.2 c
juice from 2⅝"-diam. orange	39	.6	8.9	.2	<.1	0	1	.1 c
canned, bottled, or boxed:								
1 fl. oz.	13	.2	3.1	<.1	tr.	0	1	<.1 c
6 fl. oz.	78	1.1	18.4	.3	<.1	0	5	.2 c
(*Del Monte* Unsweetened)	80	1.0	19.0	0	0	0	<10	m.q.
(*Minute Maid*), 8.45 fl. oz.	129	1.9	30.8	.2	(0)	0	20	m.q.
(*Ocean Spray*)	90	1.0	18.0	1.0	(0)	0	5	m.q.
(*S&W*)	83	2.0	18.0	0	0	0	2	m.q.
(*Sippin' Pak*), 8.45 fl. oz.	110	1.0	26.0	0	0	0	25	m.q.
(*Stokely* Unsweetened)	89	1.0	21.0	1.0	(0)	0	5	m.q.
(*Tree Top*)	90	1.0	22.0	0	0	0	5	m.q.
(*TreeSweet*)	78	1.0	18.0	0	0	0	15	m.q.
(*Tropicana* 100% Pure), 8 fl. oz.	109	m.q.	24.9	0	0	0	3	m.q.
(*Veryfine* 100%), 8 fl. oz.	121	1.5	24.0	0	0	0	<10	m.q.
blend:								
(*Minute Maid* Juices to Go), 11.5 fl. oz.	178	2.1	44.5	.7	(0)	0	37	m.q.
(*Minute Maid* Juices to Go), 9.6 fl. oz.	149	1.7	37.1	.6	(0)	0	31	m.q.

1. *Diluted according to package directions.*
2. *Prepared according to package directions.*

Food and Measure	cal.	prot. (gms)	carbo. (gms)	tot. fat (gms)	sat. fat (gms)	chol. (mgs)	sod. (mgs)	fiber (gms)
(Minute Maid On The Go),								
10 fl. oz.	155	1.8	38.7	.6	(0)	0	32	m.q.
(Veryfine 100%), 8 fl. oz.	120	<1.0	30.0	0	0	0	<35	m.q.
canned or chilled *(Sunkist)*	84	1.3	20.0	.1	(0)	0	2	m.q.
chilled:								
1 fl. oz.	14	.3	3.1	.1	tr.	0	tr.	m.q.
6 fl. oz.	83	1.5	18.8	.5	.1	0	2	m.q.
(Citrus Hill Plus Calcium)	90	<1.0	20.0	<1.0	(0)	0	10	m.q.
(Citrus Hill Select)	90	<1.0	20.0	<1.0	(0)	0	10	m.q.
(Crowley), 8 fl. oz.	110	2.0	26.0	0	0	0	5	m.q.
(Kraft Pure 100% Unsweetened)	80	1.0	19.0	0	0	0	0	m.q.
(Sunkist)	84	1.3	20.1	.1	(0)	0	2	m.q.
(Sunkist Fresh Squeezed)	77	1.2	17.7	.3	(0)	0	2	m.q.
chilled or frozen[1]:								
(Minute Maid)	91	1.4	21.9	.1	(0)	0	19	m.q.
calcium fortified *(Minute Maid)* ..	93	1.4	21.9	.1	(0)	0	19	m.q.
reduced acid *(Minute Maid)*	89	1.4	21.9	.1	(0)	0	19	m.q.
frozen[2]:								
undiluted	339	5.1	81.3	.4	.1	0	7	1.7 d
1 fl. oz.	14	.2	3.4	<.1	tr.	0	tr.	<.1 d
6 fl. oz.	84	1.3	20.1	.1	<.1	0	2	.4 d
(A&P)	80	1.0	19.0	<1.0	(0)	0	0	m.q.
(Sunkist, 8/16 servings per pkg.)	112	1.7	26.8	.1	(0)	0	3	m.q.
(TreeSweet)	84	1.0	20.0	0	0	0	15	m.q.
ORANGE JUICE COCKTAIL:								
(Welch's Orchard), 10 fl. oz.	150	0	37.0	0	0	0	0	0
ORANGE JUICE DRINK:								
(Citrus Hill Lite Premium),								
6 fl. oz.	60	<1.0	14.0	<1.0	(0)	0	10	(0)
(Kool-Aid Koolers), 8.45 fl. oz.	110	0	30.0	0	0	0	10	(0)
(Minute Maid Light'n Juicy), 6 fl. oz.	16	.3	3.8	<.1	(0)	0	17	(0)
(Tang Fruit Box), 8.45 fl. oz.	130	0	31.0	0	0	0	10	(0)
tropical *(Tang* Fruit Box), 8.45 fl. oz.	150	0	37.0	0	0	0	10	(0)
tropical *(Tropicana* Juice Sparkler),								
8 fl. oz.	110	m.q.	26.0	0	0	0	50	(0)
ORANGE PEEL, fresh:								
1 oz.	—[3]	.4	7.1	.1	tr.	0	1	m.q.
1 tbsp.	—[3]	.1	1.5	<.1	tr.	0	tr.	m.q.
1 tsp.	—[3]	<.1	.5	tr.	tr.	0	tr.	m.q.
ORANGE SAUCE:								
Mandarin *(La Choy)*, 1 tbsp.	24	<.1	6.1	tr.	0	0	38	.1 d
ORANGE-APRICOT JUICE COCKTAIL:								
(Musselman's Breakfast), 6 fl. oz. ..	90	0	21.0	0	0	0	20	(0)

1. *Diluted according to package directions.*
2. *Diluted according to package directions, except as noted.*
3. *Value cannot be calculated; no digestibility value for peel.*

Food and Measure	cal.	prot. (gms)	carbo. (gms)	tot. fat (gms)	sat. fat (gms)	chol. (mgs)	sod. (mgs)	fiber (gms)
ORANGE-APRICOT JUICE DRINK:								
1 fl. oz.	16	.1	4.0	tr.	tr.	0	n.a.	.1 c
1 cup	128	.8	31.8	.3	<.1	0	n.a.	.5 c
(*Tropicana Twister*), 8 fl. oz.	115	m.q.	30.0	0	0	0	2	m.q.
ORANGE-BANANA JUICE:								
(*Smucker's* Naturally 100%), 8 fl. oz.	120	0	30.0	0	0	0	10	m.q.
ORANGE-CRANBERRY JUICE DRINK:								
(*Tropicana* Single Serve), 10 fl. oz.	175	m.q.	43.0	0	0	0	<3	m.q.
(*Tropicana Twister*), 8 fl. oz.	115	m.q.	30.0	0	0	0	1	m.q.
ORANGE-GRAPEFRUIT JUICE:								
canned, 1 fl. oz.	13	.2	3.2	<.1	tr.	0	1	m.q.
canned, 6 fl. oz.	80	1.1	19.1	.2	<.1	0	6	m.q.
chilled (*Kraft* Pure 100%), 6 fl. oz.	80	1.0	19.0	0	0	0	0	m.q.
ORANGE-GRAPEFRUIT JUICE COCKTAIL:								
(*Musselman's* Breakfast), 6 fl. oz. ..	90	1.0	22.0	0	0	0	20	(0)
ORANGE-PASSION FRUIT JUICE DRINK:								
(*Tropicana Twister*), 8 fl. oz.	90	m.q.	22.0	0	0	0	1	m.q.
ORANGE-PEACH FRUIT JUICE DRINK:								
(*Tropicana Twister*), 8 fl. oz.	115	m.q.	30.0	0	0	0	2	m.q.
ORANGE-PINEAPPLE JUICE:								
(*Kraft* Pure 100%), 6 fl. oz.	80	1.0	19.0	0	0	0	0	m.q.
(*Tropicana* 100% Pure), 8 fl. oz. ...	111	m.q.	27.0	0	0	0	2	m.q.
ORANGE-PINEAPPLE JUICE COCKTAIL:								
(*Musselman's* Breakfast), 6 fl. oz. ..	90	1.0	23.0	0	0	0	15	(0)
ORANGE-RASPBERRY FRUIT JUICE DRINK:								
(*Tropicana Twister*), 8 fl. oz.	110	m.q.	28.0	0	0	0	1	m.q.
ORANGE-STRAWBERRY-BANANA JUICE:								
(*Tropicana* 100% Pure), 8 fl. oz. ...	141	m.q.	27.3	0	0	0	3	m.q.
ORANGE-STRAWBERRY-BANANA JUICE DRINK:								
(*Tropicana Twister*), 8 fl. oz.	95	m.q.	28.0	0	0	0	<1	m.q.
OREGANO, dried:								
(*Spice Islands*), 1 tsp.	6	.2	1.0	.1	n.a.	0	<1	.2 c
ground (*Tone's*), 1 tsp.	5	.2	1.0	.2	<.1	0	<1	.2 d
ORIENTAL FOODS, see specific listings								
ORIENTAL SPICE:								
5-spice (*Tone's*), 1 tsp.	9	.3	1.9	.3	<.1	0	2	.5 d
OYSTER, CANNED:								
Eastern, w/liquid, 4 oz.	78	8.0	4.4	2.8	.7	62	127	0

Food and Measure	cal.	prot. (gms)	carbo. (gms)	tot. fat (gms)	sat. fat (gms)	chol. (mgs)	sod. (mgs)	fiber (gms)
Eastern, w/liquid, 1 cup, approx.								
8.7 oz.	170	17.5	9.7	6.1	1.6	136	277	0
(*Bumble Bee*), 1 cup	218	25.4	15.4	5.3	m.q.	m.q.	185	0
whole (*S&W Fancy*), 2 oz.	95	12.0	4.0	3.0	m.q.	m.q.	m.q.	0
OYSTER, EASTERN, meat only:								
raw:								
1 lb.	311	32.0	17.7	11.2	2.9	248	507	0
1 oz.	20	2.0	1.1	.7	.2	16	32	0
1 cup	170	17.5	9.7	6.1	1.6	136	277	0
6 medium, approx. 3 oz. or 70								
per quart	58	5.9	3.3	2.1	.5	46	94	0
boiled, poached, or steamed[1]:								
4 oz.	155	16.0	8.9	5.6	1.4	124	254	0
6 medium, approx. 1.5 oz., yield								
from 3 oz. raw	58	5.9	3.3	2.1	.5	46	94	0
breaded[2], fried:								
4 oz.	223	9.9	13.2	14.3	3.6	92	473	.2 c
6 medium, approx. 3.1 oz., yield								
from 3 oz. raw, unbreaded	173	7.7	10.2	11.0	2.8	72	367	.1 c
OYSTER, PACIFIC, meat only,								
raw:								
1 lb.	370	42.9	22.5	10.4	2.3	m.q.	481	0
1 oz.	23	2.7	1.4	.7	.1	m.q.	30	0
1 medium, approx. 1.75 oz. or 20								
per quart	41	4.7	2.5	1.2	.3	m.q.	53	0
OYSTER MUSHROOM, see								
"Mushroom, oyster"								
OYSTER PLANT, see "Salsify"								
OYSTER STEW, see "Soup"								

1. *Without added ingredients.*
2. *Recipe: 84.2% oysters, 9.3% bread crumbs, 4.6% egg, 1.4% milk, and .5% salt.*

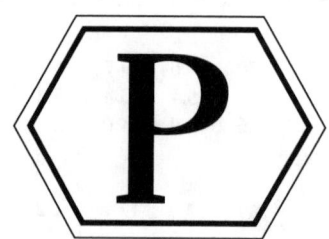

Food and Measure	cal.	prot. (gms)	carbo. (gms)	tot. fat (gms)	sat. fat (gms)	chol. (mgs)	sod. (mgs)	fiber (gms)
P&B LOAF:								
(*JM*), 1-oz. slice	70	3.0	2.0	5.0	m.q.	m.q.	330	0
(*Kahn's*), 1 slice	40	5.0	1.0	2.0	m.q.	m.q.	270	0
PAK-CHOI, see "Cabbage, Chinese, bok-choy"								
PALM KERNEL OIL:								
1 oz.	251	0	0	28.4	23.1	0	0	0
½ cup	964	0	0	109.0	88.7	0	0	0
1 tbsp.	120	0	0	13.6	11.1	0	0	0
PALM OIL:								
1 oz.	251	0	0	28.4	14.0	0	0	0
½ cup	964	0	0	109.0	53.7	0	0	0
1 tbsp.	120	0	0	13.6	6.7	0	0	0
PANCAKE, frozen:								
(*Aunt Jemima* Original Microwave), 3.5 oz.	211	6.2	40.3	3.6	m.q.	n.a.	801	1.8 d
(*Downyflake*), 3 pieces	280	5.0	45.0	9.0	m.q.	n.a.	920	m.q.
(*Pillsbury* Original Microwave), 3 pieces	240	6.0	47.0	4.0	m.q.	n.a.	550	m.q.
blueberry:								
(*Aunt Jemima*), 3.5 oz.	220	6.2	42.3	3.7	.7	21	826	1.7 d
(*Downyflake*), 3 pieces	290	5.0	48.0	9.0	m.q.	n.a.	920	m.q.
(*Pillsbury* Microwave), 3 pieces ..	250	5.0	49.0	4.0	m.q.	n.a.	540	m.q.
buttermilk:								
(*Aunt Jemima* Lite Microwave), 3.5 oz.	140	7.0	28.0	3.0	m.q.	n.a.	660	m.q.
(*Aunt Jemima* Microwave), 3.5 oz.	210	6.4	41.3	3.0	.7	20	860	1.8 d
(*Downyflake*), 3 pieces	280	5.0	45.0	9.0	m.q.	n.a.	920	m.q.
(*Pillsbury* Microwave), 3 pieces ..	260	6.0	51.0	4.0	m.q.	n.a.	590	m.q.
(*Weight Watchers* Microwave), ½ pkg. or 2.5 oz.	140	5.0	22.0	3.0	1.0	10	270	m.q.

Food and Measure	cal.	prot. (gms)	carbo. (gms)	tot. fat (gms)	sat. fat (gms)	chol. (mgs)	sod. (mgs)	fiber (gms)
wheat, harvest (*Pillsbury* Microwave), 3 pieces	240	6.0	48.0	4.0	m.q.	n.a.	420	m.q.
PANCAKE BATTER, frozen, 3.6 oz.:								
(*Aunt Jemima* Original)	183	5.7	36.5	2.4	.6	19	763	1.8 d
blueberry (*Aunt Jemima*)	204	5.0	38.7	4.0	.7	27	688	1.8 d
buttermilk (*Aunt Jemima*)	180	5.5	36.0	2.3	.7	27	778	1.8 d
PANCAKE BREAKFAST, frozen:								
w/bacon (*Swanson Great Starts*), 4.5 oz.	400	11.0	47.0	20.0	m.q.	m.q.	1000	m.q.
w/blueberry topping (*Weight Watchers* Microwave), 4.75 oz.	200	5.0	37.0	3.0	1.0	10	300	m.q.
w/links (*Weight Watchers* Microwave), 4 oz.	220	12.0	21.0	10.0	4.0	15	510	m.q.
lite, w/lite links (*Aunt Jemima* Homestyle), 6 oz.	310	14.0	43.0	10.0	m.q.	m.q.	970	m.q.
lite, w/lite syrup (*Aunt Jemima* Homestyle), 6 oz.	260	10.0	53.0	3.0	m.q.	n.a.	860	m.q.
and sausages:								
(*Aunt Jemima* Homestyle), 6 oz.	420	12.0	57.0	16.0	m.q.	m.q.	1140	m.q.
(*Downyflake*), 5.5 oz.	430	11.0	47.0	23.0	m.q.	m.q.	1170	m.q.
(*Swanson Great Starts*), 6 oz.	460	15.0	52.0	22.0	m.q.	m.q.	920	m.q.
silver dollar, and sausage (*Swanson Great Starts*), 3.75 oz.	310	10.0	37.0	14.0	m.q.	m.q.	680	m.q.
w/strawberry topping (*Weight Watchers* Microwave), 4.75 oz.	200	5.0	37.0	3.0	1.0	10	360	m.q.
whole wheat, w/lite links (*Swanson Great Starts*), 5.5 oz.	350	15.0	39.0	16.0	m.q.	m.q.	600	m.q.
PANCAKE AND WAFFLE MIX[1], 3 pieces, 4″ each, except as noted:								
(*Arrowhead Mills* Griddle Lite), ½ cup	260	8.0	50.0	3.0	m.q.	0	m.q.	m.q.
(*Aunt Jemima* Original)	116	3.4	25.4	.8	.1	0	609	1.4 d
(*Aunt Jemima* Original Complete) ...	253	7.0	50.2	3.6	.8	16	1024	2.1 d
(*Bisquick Shake 'n Pour*)	260	6.0	48.0	5.0	m.q.	0	850	m.q.
(*Estee*), 3 pieces, 3″ each	100	3.0	21.0	0	0	0	130	m.q.
(*Featherweight*)	140	6.0	24.0	2.0	m.q.	5	90	m.q.
(*Hungry Jack Extra Lights*)	210	6.0	30.0	7.0	m.q.	n.a.	490	m.q.
(*Hungry Jack Extra Lights* Complete)	190	4.0	37.0	2.0	m.q.	n.a.	700	m.q.
(*Hungry Jack* Panshakes)	250	7.0	43.0	6.0	m.q.	n.a.	880	m.q.
(*Martha White FlapStax*), 1 piece ..	100	3.0	18.0	2.0	m.q.	2	320	m.q.
(*Martha White* Light Crust), 2 oz. dry	120	4.0	20.0	3.0	m.q.	25	290	m.q.
(*Robin Hood/Gold Medal* Pouch Mix), ⅛ pouch[2]	100	3.0	17.0	2.0	m.q.	n.a.	280	m.q.

1. *Prepared according to package directions, except as noted.*
2. *Prepared with egg.*

Food and Measure	cal.	prot. (gms)	carbo. (gms)	tot. fat (gms)	sat. fat (gms)	chol. (mgs)	sod. (mgs)	fiber (gms)
PANCAKE AND WAFFLE MIX *(cont.)*								
apple cinnamon *(Bisquick Shake 'n*								
Pour)	270	6.0	49.0	5.0	m.q.	0	870	m.q.
blueberry *(Bisquick Shake 'n Pour)*	280	6.0	53.0	5.0	m.q.	0	860	m.q.
blueberry *(Hungry Jack)*	320	6.0	41.0	15.0	m.q.	n.a.	820	m.q.
buckwheat *(Arrowhead Mills),*								
½ cup	270	11.0	53.0	2.0	m.q.	n.a.	m.q.	m.q.
buckwheat *(Aunt Jemima)*	143	5.5	31.7	1.6	.2	n.a.	773	5.0 d
buttermilk:								
(Aunt Jemima)	122	4.2	26.1	.7	.1	1	698	1.3 d
(Aunt Jemima Complete)	231	7.2	46.4	2.8	.7	9	950	2.0 d
(Aunt Jemima Lite Complete)	130	7.0	25.0	2.0	m.q.	n.a.	570	m.q.
(Betty Crocker)	280	8.0	39.0	10.0	m.q.	n.a.	810	m.q.
(Betty Crocker Complete), ½ cup								
dry	210	5.0	41.0	3.0	m.q.	n.a.	500	m.q.
(Bisquick Shake 'n Pour)	260	7.0	47.0	5.0	m.q.	0	860	m.q.
(Hungry Jack)	240	7.0	29.0	11.0	m.q.	n.a.	570	m.q.
(Hungry Jack Complete)	180	4.0	39.0	1.0	m.q.	n.a.	710	m.q.
(Hungry Jack Complete Packets)	180	4.0	35.0	3.0	m.q.	n.a.	680	m.q.
corn, blue *(Arrowhead Mills),* ½ cup	330	10.0	36.0	5.0	m.q.	0	m.q.	1.2 d
multigrain *(Arrowhead Mills),* ½ cup	350	12.0	70.0	2.0	m.q.	n.a.	m.q.	.8 d
oat bran *(Arrowhead Mills),* ½ cup	200	9.0	64.0	2.0	m.q.	n.a.	m.q.	1.8 d
oat bran *(Bisquick Shake 'n Pour)*	240	7.0	45.0	4.0	m.q.	0	580	1.0 d
whole wheat *(Aunt Jemima)*	161	7.0	34.5	1.0	.2	0	892	3.6 d
PANCAKE SYRUP (see also								
"Maple syrup"):								
table blends:								
cane and maple, ½ cup	397	0	102.4	0	0	0	6	0
cane and maple, 1 tbsp.	50	0	12.8	0	0	0	tr.	0
chiefly corn, light and dark, ½ cup	476	0	123.0	0	0	0	n.a.	0
chiefly corn, light and dark,								
1 tbsp.	59	0	15.4	0	0	0	n.a.	0
(Aunt Jemima ButterLite), 1 fl. oz.	50	0	13.0	0	0	0	65	(0)
(Aunt Jemima Lite), 1 fl. oz.	54	.1	13.1	.1	(0)	0	92	.3 d
(Aunt Jemima Original), 1 fl. oz.	109	0	27.1	0	0	0	32	(0)
(Estee), 1 tbsp.	4	0	1.0	0	0	0	25	(0)
(Featherweight), 1 tbsp.	16	0	4.0	0	0	0	25	(0)
(Log Cabin Country Kitchen),								
1 fl. oz.	100	0	26.0	0	0	0	20	(0)
(Log Cabin Lite), 1 fl. oz.	50	0	13.0	0	0	0	90	(0)
(Log Cabin Pancake and Waffle),								
1 fl. oz.	100	0	26.0	0	0	0	35	(0)
(Vermont Maid), 1 tbsp.	50	0	13.0	0	0	0	5	(0)
maple flavored[1] *(S&W),* 1 tsp.	4	0	1.0	0	0	0	25	(0)
PANCREAS[2]:								
beef:								
raw, 1 oz.	67	4.5	0	5.3	m.q.	m.q.	86	0

1. *Saccharin sweetened.*
2. *Cooked meats are prepared without added ingredients.*

Food and Measure	cal.	prot. (gms)	carbo. (gms)	tot. fat (gms)	sat. fat (gms)	chol. (mgs)	sod. (mgs)	fiber (gms)
braised, 7.8 oz., yield from 1 lb.								
raw	601	60.2	0	38.2	m.q.	m.q.	133	0
braised, 4 oz.	307	30.7	0	19.5	m.q.	m.q.	68	0
lamb:								
raw, 1 oz.	43	4.2	0	2.8	1.3	74	21	0
braised, 13.4 oz., yield from 1 lb.								
raw	541	52.8	0	35.0	15.8	925	120	0
braised, 4 oz.	265	25.9	0	17.1	7.8	454	59	0
pork:								
raw, 1 oz.	56	5.3	0	3.8	m.q.	55	12	0
braised, 8.6 oz., yield from 1 lb.								
raw	537	69.8	0	26.5	m.q.	772	102	0
braised, 4 oz.	248	32.3	0	12.2	m.q.	357	48	0
veal:								
raw, 1 oz.	52	4.3	0	3.7	m.q.	m.q.	m.q.	0
braised, 8.5 oz., yield from 1 lb.								
raw	615	70.0	0	35.1	m.q.	m.q.	m.q.	0
braised, 4 oz.	290	33.0	0	16.6	m.q.	m.q.	m.q.	0
PAPAYA:								
untrimmed, 1 lb. or 1 medium,								
3½″ × 5⅛″	117	1.9	29.8	.4	.1	0	8	2.8 d
peeled and seeded, 1 oz.	11	.2	2.8	<.1	<.1	0	1	.3 d
cubed, ½ cup	27	.4	6.9	.1	<.1	0	2	.6 d
(Calavo Growers), ½ medium	80	0	19.0	0	0	0	15	2.7 d
(Del Monte), ⅓ medium	60	0	15.0	0	0	0	<5	m.q.
PAPAYA NECTAR, canned or								
bottled:								
1 fl. oz.	18	.1	4.5	.1	<.1	0	2	m.q.
6 fl. oz.	107	.3	27.2	.3	.1	0	11	m.q.
(Libby's), 6 fl. oz.	110	0	28.0	0	0	0	10	m.q.
PAPAYA PUNCH:								
(Veryfine), 8 fl. oz.	120	<1.0	30.0	0	0	0	<10	m.q.
PAPRIKA:								
1 oz.	82	4.2	15.8	3.7	.6	0	10	5.9 c
1 tbsp.	20	1.0	3.9	.9	.1	0	2	1.4 c
1 tsp.	6	.3	1.2	.3	<.1	0	1	.4 c
(Spice Islands), 1 tsp.	7	.3	1.1	.2	(0)	0	<1	.4 c
PARANUT, see "Brazil nut"								
PARROT FISH, meat only:								
raw, 1 lb.	390	87.5	0	1.8	m.q.	m.q.	m.q.	0
raw, 1 oz.	24	5.5	0	.1	m.q.	m.q.	m.q.	0
PARSLEY, raw:								
untrimmed, 1 lb.	140	9.5	29.8	1.3	n.a.	0	169	19.0 d
trimmed, 1 oz.	9	.6	2.0	.1	(0)	0	11	1.2 d
10 sprigs, approx. .4 oz.	3	.2	.7	<.1	(0)	0	4	.4 d
chopped, ½ cup	10	.7	2.1	.1	(0)	0	12	1.3 d
PARSLEY, DRIED:								
1 oz.	78	6.4	14.6	1.3	n.a.	0	128	2.9 c
1 tbsp.	4	.3	.7	.6	(0)	0	6	.1 c

Food and Measure	cal.	prot. (gms)	carbo. (gms)	tot. fat (gms)	sat. fat (gms)	chol. (mgs)	sod. (mgs)	fiber (gms)
PARSLEY, DRIED *(cont.)*								
1 tsp.	1	.1	.2	.1	(0)	0	1	tr.c
flakes (*Spice Islands*), 1 tsp.	4	.2	.6	.1	(0)	0	6	.1 c
freeze-dried:								
1 oz.	77	8.9	12.0	1.5	n.a.	0	111	2.9 c
¼ cup	4	.4	.6	.1	(0)	0	5	.1 c
1 tbsp.	1	.1	.2	<.1	(0)	0	2	<.1 c
PARSLEY ROOT:								
1 lb.	50	12.7	10.4	2.7	n.a.	0	454	5.9 d
1 oz.	3	.8	.7	.2	(0)	0	28	.4 d
PARSLEY SEASONING:								
all purpose (*McCormick/Schilling*								
Parsley Patch), 1 tsp.	6	.3	1.0	0	0	0	3	m.q.
PARSNIP:								
raw:								
untrimmed, 1 lb.	289	4.6	69.4	1.2	.2	0	39	7.7 c
trimmed, 1 oz.	21	.3	5.1	.1	<.1	0	3	.6 c
sliced, ½ cup	50	.8	12.1	.2	<.1	0	7	1.3 c
boiled, drained:								
4 oz.	92	1.5	22.1	.3	.1	0	11	3.1 d
1 medium, 9″ × 2¼″ diam.	130	2.1	31.3	.5	.1	0	17	4.3 d
sliced, ½ cup	63	1.0	15.2	.2	<.1	0	8	2.1 d
PARTY MIX, see "Snack mix"								
PASSION FRUIT, purple:								
untrimmed, 1 lb.	230	5.2	55.1	1.7	n.a.	0	n.a.	25.8 c
trimmed, 1 oz.	27	.6	6.6	.2	(0)	0	n.a.	3.1 c
1 medium, approx. 1.2 oz.	18	.4	4.2	.1	(0)	0	n.a.	2.0 c
PASSION FRUIT JUICE, fresh:								
purple, 1 fl. oz.	16	.1	4.2	<.1	(0)	0	n.a.	<.1 c
purple, 6 fl. oz.	95	.7	25.2	.1	(0)	0	n.a.	.3 c
yellow, 1 fl. oz.	19	.2	4.5	.1	(0)	0	2	.1 c
yellow, 6 fl. oz.	112	1.2	26.8	.3	(0)	0	11	.3 c
PASSION FRUIT JUICE COCKTAIL:								
(*Welch's Orchard Tropicals* Cocktails-In-A-Box), 8.45 fl. oz.	140	0	34.0	0	0	0	20	0
bottled or frozen[1] (*Welch's Orchard Tropicals*), 6 fl. oz.	100	0	25.0	0	0	0	20	0
PASSION FRUIT-ORANGE REFRESHER:								
tropical (*Veryfine*), 8 fl. oz.	110	<1.0	26.0	0	0	0	<25	n.a.
PASTA[2] (see also "Macaroni" and "Noodles"):								
1 lb.	1682	58.0	338.8	7.2	1.0	0	33	10.9 d
2 oz.	211	7.3	42.6	.9	.1	0	4	1.4 d
(*Antoine's* Penne Rigati), 2 oz.	210	7.0	41.0	1.0	n.a.	0	0	m.q.
(*Creamette*), 2 oz.	210	7.0	42.0	1.0	0	0	0	.1 d

1. *Diluted according to package directions.*
2. *Uncooked, except as noted. (Includes angel hair, fettuccine, fusilli, linguine, penne, spaghetti, ziti, etc.).*

Food and Measure	cal.	prot. (gms)	carbo. (gms)	tot. fat (gms)	sat. fat (gms)	chol. (mgs)	sod. (mgs)	fiber (gms)
(*Golden Grain*), 2 oz.	203	8.0	41.2	.7	.1	0	26	m.q.
(*Ronzoni*), 2 oz.	210	7.0	41.0	1.0	n.a.	0	<5	m.q.
cooked, 4 oz.	160	5.4	32.1	.8	.1	0	1	2.5 d
cooked, 1 cup	197	6.7	39.7	.9	.1	0	1	3.1 d
protein-fortified:								
1 lb.	1699	90.1	306.5	10.1	1.5	0	37	19.5 d
2 oz.	214	11.3	38.5	1.3	.2	0	5	2.4 d
cooked, 4 oz.	186	9.2	35.9	.2	<.1	0	1	.3 c
cooked, 1 cup	229	11.3	44.3	.3	<.1	0	7	.4 c
amaranth (*Health Valley* Spaghetti),								
2 oz.	170	7.0	40.0	1.0	n.a.	0	10	8.8 d
basil (*Al Dente* Fettucine), 2 oz.	220	8.0	40.0	2.0	m.q.	m.q.	20	m.q.
corn:								
1 lb.	1620	33.8	359.5	9.4	1.3	0	13	m.q.
2 oz.	204	4.3	45.2	1.2	.2	0	2	m.q.
cooked, 4 oz.	143	3.0	31.6	.8	.1	0	tr.	m.q.
cooked, 1 cup	176	3.7	39.1	1.0	.1	0	1	m.q.
wheat-free (*De Boles*), 2 oz.	210	4.0	44.0	2.0	m.q.	n.a.	30	m.q.
curry (*Al Dente* Fettucine), 2 oz. ...	220	8.0	40.0	2.0	m.q.	m.q.	20	m.q.
dill (*Al Dente* Fettucine), 2 oz.	220	8.0	40.0	2.0	m.q.	m.q.	20	m.q.
w/egg (*Creamette*), 2 oz.	221	8.0	40.0	2.5	.8	7	3	.8 d
garlic and parsley (*De Boles*), 2 oz.	210	8.0	43.0	1.0	n.a.	0	3	m.q.
Jerusalem artichoke (*De Boles*),								
2 oz.	210	8.0	43.0	1.0	n.a.	0	3	m.q.
mushroom, wild (*Al Dente*), 2 oz. ..	220	8.0	40.0	2.0	m.q.	m.q.	20	m.q.
oat bran (*Health Valley* Spaghetti),								
2 oz.	120	4.0	23.0	1.0	n.a.	0	2	3.8 d
pepper (*Al Dente* Three Pepper								
Pasta), 2 oz.	220	8.0	40.0	2.0	m.q.	m.q.	20	m.q.
spicy (*Antoine's* Spirals), 2 oz.	210	7.0	41.0	1.0	n.a.	0	40	m.q.
spinach:								
1 lb.	1688	60.6	339.3	7.1	1.0	0	163	48.1 d
1 cup	212	7.6	42.6	.9	.1	0	20	6.0 d
(*Al Dente* Fettucine), 2 oz.	220	8.0	40.0	2.0	m.q.	m.q.	20	m.q.
(*De Boles*), 2 oz.	210	8.0	43.0	1.0	n.a.	0	3	m.q.
cooked, 4 oz.	147	5.2	29.7	.7	.1	0	16	1.3 c
cooked, 1 cup	183	6.4	36.6	.9	.1	0	20	1.7 c
w/egg (*Creamette*), 2 oz.	220	8.0	40.0	3.0	m.q.	70	65	.8 d
tarragon (*Al Dente* Fettucine), 2 oz.	220	8.0	40.0	2.0	m.q.	m.q.	20	m.q.
tomato and basil (*De Boles*), 2 oz. ..	200	8.0	41.0	1.0	n.a.	0	8	m.q.
vegetable, rainbow, or tricolor (see								
also "Macaroni"):								
(*Antoine's* Fusilli), 2 oz.	210	7.0	41.0	1.0	n.a.	0	20	m.q.
(*Creamette*), 2 oz.	210	8.0	42.0	1.0	0	0	5	1.3 d
(*De Boles* Primavera), 2 oz.	200	8.0	41.0	1.0	n.a.	0	8	m.q.
whole wheat:								
1 lb.	1578	66.4	340.3	6.4	1.2	0	36	53.5 d
1 cup	198	8.3	42.8	.8	.1	0	5	6.7 d
(*Al Dente* Fettucine), 2 oz.	210	8.0	42.0	1.0	n.a.	0	10	m.q.

Food and Measure	cal.	prot. (gms)	carbo. (gms)	tot. fat (gms)	sat. fat (gms)	chol. (mgs)	sod. (mgs)	fiber (gms)
PASTA, WHOLE WHEAT *(cont.)*								
(*De Boles* Natural Gourmet), 2 oz.	200	7.0	40.0	<1.0	n.a.	0	0	6.0 d
(*Health Valley* Lasagna/Spaghetti),								
2 oz.	170	9.0	40.0	1.0	n.a.	0	10	7.2 d
w/bran (*Misura*), 2 oz.	197	6.0	40.0	1.0	n.a.	0	16	m.q.
cooked, 4 oz.	141	6.0	30.1	.6	.1	0	3	1.1 c
cooked, 1 cup	174	7.5	37.2	.6	.1	0	4	1.4 c
whole-wheat spinach (*Health Valley*								
Lasagna), 2 oz.	170	9.0	40.0	1.0	n.a.	0	15	7.2 d
whole-wheat spinach (*Health Valley*								
Spaghetti), 2 oz.	170	9.0	40.0	1.0	n.a.	0	10	7.2 d
PASTA, FRESH,								
REFRIGERATED[1] (see also								
specific listings):								
w/egg:								
1 lb.	1305	51.3	248.3	10.4	1.5	331	118	m.q.
2 oz.	163	6.4	31.0	1.3	.2	41	15	m.q.
cooked, 4 oz.	149	5.8	28.3	1.2	.2	37	7	m.q.
spinach, w/egg:								
1 lb.	1309	51.1	252.8	9.5	2.2	331	122	m.q.
2 oz.	164	6.4	31.6	1.2	.3	41	15	m.q.
cooked, 4 oz.	147	5.7	28.4	1.1	.2	37	7	m.q.
PASTA, HOMEMADE:								
w/egg[2], cooked, 4 oz.	147	6.0	26.7	2.0	.5	46	94	0
w/out egg[3], cooked, 4 oz.	141	5.0	28.5	1.1	.2	0	84	0
PASTA DINNER, frozen (see also								
specific pasta listings):								
shells, stuffed, 3-cheese (*Le Menu*								
LightStyle), 10 oz.	280	17.0	34.0	8.0	m.q.	25	690	m.q.
PASTA DISHES, CANNED (see								
also specific pasta listings),								
7.5 oz., except as noted:								
in chicken sauce (*Chef Boyardee* Pac								
Man)	170	6.0	22.0	7.0	m.q.	n.a.	905	m.q.
garden medley (*Lipton Hearty Ones*),								
11 oz.	323	15.1	63.4	3.8	m.q.	6	914	m.q.
Italiano (*Lipton Hearty Ones*), 11 oz.	328	13.9	63.4	1.9	m.q.	n.a.	1241	m.q.
w/meatballs:								
(*Chef Boyardee* Dinosaurs								
Microwave)	240	8.0	32.0	9.0	3.0	17	900	4.0 d
(*Chef Boyardee* Tic Tac Toes								
Microwave)	250	7.0	32.0	10.0	3.0	16	1035	3.0 d
(*Franco-American* TeddyO's),								
7⅜ oz.	210	9.0	25.0	8.0	m.q.	m.q.	950	m.q.
mini (*Chef Boyardee* ABC's/123's								
Microwave)	260	7.0	32.0	11.0	4.0	17	1005	2.0 d

1. *Uncooked, except as noted.*
2. *Recipe: 75% enriched semolina, 22% whole eggs, 1.1% water, 1% vegetable oil, and .9% salt.*
3. *Recipe: 67% enriched semolina, 31% water, 1.2% vegetable oil, and .7% salt.*

Food and Measure	cal.	prot. (gms)	carbo. (gms)	tot. fat (gms)	sat. fat (gms)	chol. (mgs)	sod. (mgs)	fiber (gms)
in tomato sauce (*Franco-American* CircusO's/SportyO's), 7⅜ oz.	210	9.0	25.0	8.0	m.q.	m.q.	950	m.q.
rings, in sauce (*Buitoni*)	150	5.0	24.0	4.0	1.0	5	650	m.q.
rings or twists and meatballs, in sauce (*Buitoni*)	210	8.0	28.0	7.0	5.0	20	850	m.q.
shells, in meat sauce (*Chef Boyardee* Microwave)	210	8.0	32.0	6.0	m.q.	15	1090	m.q.
shells, in mushroom sauce (*Chef Boyardee* Microwave)	170	6.0	35.0	1.0	<1.0	2	1080	m.q.
in spaghetti sauce w/cheese flavor:								
(*Chef Boyardee* ABC's/123's Microwave)	180	5.0	37.0	1.0	<1.0	3	940	m.q.
(*Chef Boyardee* Dinosaurs Microwave)	180	6.0	36.0	1.0	<1.0	3	880	3.0 d
(*Chef Boyardee* Tic Tac Toes Microwave)	170	5.0	36.0	1.0	<1.0	2	930	3.0 d
in tomato and cheese sauce:								
(*Franco-American* CircusO's/ SportyO's), 7⅜ oz.	170	5.0	38.0	2.0	m.q.	n.a.	860	m.q.
(*Franco-American* TeddyO's), 7⅜ oz.	170	5.0	33.0	2.0	m.q.	n.a.	900	m.q.
twists, in sauce (*Buitoni*)	150	5.0	24.0	4.0	1.0	0	610	m.q.
PASTA DISHES, FROZEN (see also "Pasta entree" and specific pasta listings), ½ cup, except as noted:								
Alfredo, w/broccoli (*The Budget Gourmet* Side Dish), 5.5 oz. ...	200	14.0	17.0	8.0	m.q.	25	390	m.q.
creamy cheddar (*Green Giant Pasta Accents*)	100	4.0	12.0	5.0	2.0	5	310	m.q.
Dijon (*Green Giant* Garden Gourmet), 1 pkg.	260	7.0	21.0	17.0	9.0	55	630	4.0 d
Florentine (*Green Giant* Garden Gourmet), 1 pkg.	230	14.0	27.0	9.0	5.0	25	840	4.0 d
garden herb (*Green Giant Pasta Accents*)	80	3.0	11.0	3.0	<1.0	5	220	m.q.
garlic seasoning (*Green Giant Pasta Accents*)	110	3.0	13.0	5.0	2.0	5	280	m.q.
marinara (*Green Giant* One Serving), 5.5 oz.	180	5.0	29.0	5.0	<1.0	0	440	m.q.
Parmesan, w/sweet peas (*Green Giant* One Serving), 5.5 oz. ...	170	9.0	23.0	5.0	2.0	10	510	m.q.
primavera (*Green Giant Pasta Accents*)	110	5.0	13.0	5.0	2.0	5	180	m.q.
and vegetables, in creamy Stroganoff sauce (*Birds Eye Custom Cuisine*), 4.6 oz.[1]	120	5.0	15.0	5.0	m.q.	30	700	m.q.

1. *Prepared without added ingredients.*

Food and Measure	cal.	prot. (gms)	carbo. (gms)	tot. fat (gms)	sat. fat (gms)	chol. (mgs)	sod. (mgs)	fiber (gms)
PASTA DISHES, FROZEN *(cont.)*								
and vegetables, w/white cheese sauce *(Birds Eye Custom Cuisine)*, 4.6 oz.[1]	150	7.0	19.0	6.0	m.q.	15	440	1.0 d
PASTA DISHES, MIX[2] (see also "Salad mix" and specific pasta listings), ½ cup, except as noted:								
(Kraft Light Rancher's Choice Pasta Salad)	170	5.0	23.0	7.0	1.0	0	350	m.q.
(Kraft Rancher's Choice Pasta Salad)	250	5.0	21.0	16.0	3.0	10	350	m.q.
Alfredo *(McCormick/Schilling Pasta Prima)*, 1 pkg. dry	169	7.0	12.0	0	0	0	4199	m.q.
Alfredo *(McCormick/Schilling Pasta Prima)*	253	7.0	27.0	13.0	m.q.	n.a.	1178	m.q.
bacon vinaigrette *(Country Recipe Pasta Salad)*[1]	110	4.0	24.0	1.0	n.a.	n.a.	210	m.q.
bacon vinaigrette *(Country Recipe Pasta Salad)*	140	4.0	24.0	4.0	m.q.	n.a.	210	m.q.
broccoli:								
cheddar w/fusilli:								
(Lipton Pasta & Sauce), ¼ pkg. dry	140	6.0	24.0	2.0	m.q.	n.a.	450	m.q.
(Lipton Pasta & Sauce)[3]	200	7.0	25.0	9.0	m.q.	m.q.	520	m.q.
(Lipton Pasta & Sauce)[4]	170	7.0	25.0	5.0	m.q.	n.a.	500	m.q.
creamy *(Lipton* Pasta Salad), ¼ pkg. dry	120	5.0	22.0	1.0	n.a.	n.a.	120	m.q.
creamy *(Lipton* Pasta Salad)[5]	200	5.0	23.0	10.0	m.q.	m.q.	190	m.q.
and vegetable *(Kraft* Pasta Salad)	210	4.0	15.0	16.0	2.0	10	290	m.q.
buttermilk, country *(Mueller's* Salad Bar)	250	5.0	22.0	16.0	m.q.	n.a.	410	m.q.
carbonara Alfredo *(Lipton* Pasta & Sauce)	140	4.6	20.2	4.2	m.q.	n.a.	459	m.q.
cheese:								
cheddar:								
(Minute Microwave Family Size)[6]	160	6.0	20.0	7.0	m.q.	15	530	m.q.
(Minute Microwave Single Size)[6]	160	6.0	20.0	6.0	m.q.	15	620	m.q.
tangy *(Hain* Pasta & Sauce), ¼ pkg.	180	6.0	24.0	6.0	m.q.	3	350	m.q.
and broccoli *(Kraft* Pasta & Cheese)	180	6.0	19.0	8.0	3.0	30	620	m.q.
Parmesan *(Kraft* Pasta & Cheese)	180	6.0	19.0	8.0	2.0	30	630	m.q.
Parmesan, creamy *(Hain* Pasta & Sauce), ¼ pkg.	150	8.0	22.0	3.0	m.q.	10	400	m.q.

1. *Prepared without added ingredients.*
2. *Prepared according to package directions, except as noted.*
3. *Prepared with ½ cup whole milk and 2 tbsp. butter.*
4. *Prepared with ½ cup skim milk and 1 tbsp. margarine.*
5. *Prepared with 3 tbsp. milk and 3 tbsp. mayonnaise or salad dressing.*
6. *Prepared with salted butter.*

Food and Measure	cal.	prot. (gms)	carbo. (gms)	tot. fat (gms)	sat. fat (gms)	chol. (mgs)	sod. (mgs)	fiber (gms)
supreme (*Lipton* Pasta & Sauce)	139	5.8	24.0	2.3	m.q.	n.a.	406	.2 c
three cheese, w/vegetables (*Kraft* Pasta & Cheese)	180	6.0	19.0	8.0	3.0	25	630	m.q.
chicken broccoli (*Lipton* Pasta & Sauce)	129	5.4	22.4	2.0	m.q.	n.a.	425	m.q.
chicken w/herbs (*Kraft* Pasta & Cheese)	170	5.0	21.0	7.0	2.0	25	550	m.q.
cucumber, creamy (*Mueller's* Salad Bar)	250	4.0	22.0	16.0	m.q.	n.a.	460	m.q.
Dijon, creamy (*Country Recipe* Pasta Salad)[1]	110	4.0	24.0	1.0	n.a.	n.a.	240	m.q.
Dijon, creamy (*Country Recipe* Pasta Salad)	190	4.0	24.0	10.0	m.q.	n.a.	310	m.q.
garlic, creamy:								
(*Lipton* Pasta & Sauce), ¼ pkg. dry	140	5.0	25.0	3.0	m.q.	n.a.	550	m.q.
(*Lipton* Pasta & Sauce)[2]	210	6.0	27.0	10.0	m.q.	m.q.	620	m.q.
(*Lipton* Pasta & Sauce)[3]	180	6.0	27.0	6.0	m.q.	n.a.	600	m.q.
(*McCormick/Schilling Pasta Prima*), 1 pkg. dry	107	5.0	9.8	5.3	m.q.	n.a.	3183	m.q.
herb:								
Italian (*Fantastic* Pasta Salad),[4] ...	167	4.0	19.0	9.0	m.q.	n.a.	176	m.q.
Italian (*Hain* Pasta & Sauce), ⅕ pkg.	110	4.0	17.0	2.0	m.q.	n.a.	160	m.q.
and garlic (*McCormick/Schilling Pasta Prima*), 1 pkg. dry	65	3.0	8.0	0	0	0	3391	m.q.
and garlic (*McCormick/Schilling Pasta Prima*)	326	9.0	45.0	12.0	m.q.	n.a.	869	m.q.
herb tomato:								
(*Lipton* Pasta & Sauce), ¼ pkg. dry	130	5.0	26.0	<1.0	n.a.	n.a.	360	m.q.
(*Lipton* Pasta & Sauce)[5]	180	5.0	26.0	7.0	m.q.	m.q.	420	m.q.
(*Lipton* Pasta & Sauce)[6]	160	5.0	26.0	4.0	m.q.	n.a.	390	m.q.
homestyle (*Kraft* Pasta Salad)	240	4.0	21.0	16.0	2.0	10	300	m.q.
homestyle (*Mueller's* Salad Bar)	250	4.0	22.0	16.0	m.q.	n.a.	390	m.q.
Italian:								
creamy:								
(*Country Recipe* Pasta Salad)[1]	100	4.0	22.0	1.0	n.a.	n.a.	290	m.q.
(*Country Recipe* Pasta Salad)	160	4.0	22.0	7.0	m.q.	n.a.	340	m.q.
(*Kraft Light* Pasta Salad)	130	5.0	20.0	3.0	1.0	0	420	m.q.
(*Mueller's* Salad Bar)	290	3.0	20.0	22.0	m.q.	n.a.	550	m.q.
robust:								
(*Lipton* Pasta Salad), ¼ pkg. dry	130	5.0	25.0	1.0	n.a.	n.a.	300	m.q.

1. *Prepared without added ingredients.*
2. *Prepared with ½ cup whole milk and 2 tbsp. butter.*
3. *Prepared with ½ cup skim milk and 1 tbsp. margarine.*
4. *Prepared with oil, vinegar, and tomato.*
5. *Prepared with 2 tbsp. butter.*
6. *Prepared with 1 tbsp. margarine.*

Food and Measure	cal.	prot. (gms)	carbo. (gms)	tot. fat (gms)	sat. fat (gms)	chol. (mgs)	sod. (mgs)	fiber (gms)
PASTA DISHES, FROZEN, ITALIAN, ROBUST *(cont.)*								
(*Lipton* Pasta Salad)[1]	190	5.0	25.0	8.0	m.q.	n.a.	300	m.q.
(*Lipton* Pasta Salad)[2]	160	5.0	25.0	4.0	m.q.	n.a.	300	m.q.
zesty (*Mueller's* Salad Bar)	140	3.0	21.0	5.0	m.q.	n.a.	400	m.q.
marinara:								
(*McCormick/Schilling Pasta*								
Prima), 1 pkg. dry	74	1.0	16.0	0	0	0	690	m.q.
(*McCormick/Schilling Pasta Prima*)	329	9.0	55.0	8.0	m.q.	n.a.	432	m.q.
mushroom, creamy:								
(*Lipton* Pasta & Sauce), ¼ pkg.								
dry	140	5.0	25.0	3.0	m.q.	m.q.	420	m.q.
(*Lipton* Pasta & Sauce)[3]	210	6.0	26.0	9.0	m.q.	m.q.	500	m.q.
(*Lipton* Pasta & Sauce)[4]	190	6.0	26.0	5.0	m.q.	n.a.	470	m.q.
mushroom and chicken flavors								
(*Lipton* Pasta & Sauce)	124	5.8	23.4	.8	n.a.	n.a.	435	.2 c
Oriental, w/fusilli (*Lipton* Pasta and								
Sauce)	130	5.4	25.5	.7	n.a.	n.a.	506	.3 c
Oriental, spicy (*Fantastic* Pasta								
Salad)[5]	175	3.0	19.0	10.0	m.q.	n.a.	168	m.q.
pasta salad (*McCormick/Schilling*								
Pasta Prima), 1 pkg. dry	78	2.0	16.0	0	0	0	3997	m.q.
pasta salad (*McCormick/Schilling*								
Pasta Prima)	390	7.0	41.0	23.0	m.q.	n.a.	822	m.q.
pesto (*McCormick/Schilling Pasta*								
Prima), 1 pkg. dry	37	2.0	5.0	0	0	0	2055	m.q.
pesto (*McCormick/Schilling Pasta*								
Prima)	193	6.0	29.0	6.0	m.q.	n.a.	356	m.q.
primavera (*Hain* Pasta & Sauce),								
¼ pkg.	140	7.0	20.0	4.0	m.q.	10	430	m.q.
primavera, garden (*Kraft* Pasta								
Salad)	170	5.0	21.0	7.0	2.0	0	450	m.q.
ranch (*Country Recipe* Pasta Salad)[6]	90	4.0	19.0	1.0	n.a.	n.a.	260	m.q.
ranch (*Country Recipe* Pasta Salad)	140	4.0	19.0	5.0	m.q.	n.a.	300	m.q.
seafood, creamy (*McCormick/*								
Schilling Pasta Prima), 1 pkg.								
dry	135	2.3	27.4	1.8	m.q.	n.a.	3016	m.q.
sour cream and chives (*Kraft* Pasta								
& Cheese)	180	5.0	22.0	8.0	2.0	25	360	m.q.
Swiss, creamy (*Hain* Pasta &								
Sauce), ⅕ pkg.	170	6.0	26.0	4.0	m.q.	n.a.	360	m.q.
PASTA ENTREE, frozen (see also "Pasta dishes" and specific pasta listings):								
angel hair (*Weight Watchers*), 10 oz.	210	12.0	23.0	5.0	1.0	20	420	m.q.
baked, and cheese (*Celentano*),								
6 oz.	290	12.0	29.0	13.0	m.q.	m.q.	350	m.q.

1. *Prepared with 2 tbsp. oil.*
2. *Prepared with 1 tbsp. oil.*
3. *Prepared with ½ cup whole milk and 2 tbsp. butter.*
4. *Prepared with ½ cup skim milk and 1 tbsp. margarine.*
5. *Prepared with oil, vinegar, and green onions.*
6. *Prepared without added ingredients.*

Food and Measure	cal.	prot. (gms)	carbo. (gms)	tot. fat (gms)	sat. fat (gms)	chol. (mgs)	sod. (mgs)	fiber (gms)
carbonara (*Stouffer's*), 9.75-oz. pkg.	620	19.0	34.0	45.0	m.q.	m.q.	780	m.q.
casino (*Stouffer's*), 9.25-oz. pkg. ...	300	9.0	44.0	10.0	m.q.	m.q.	800	m.q.
Dijon (*Green Giant* Microwave Garden Gourmet), 1 pkg.	300	7.0	24.0	20.0	m.q.	n.a.	560	3.0 d
Mexicali (*Stouffer's*), 10-oz. pkg. ...	490	16.0	36.0	31.0	m.q.	n.a.	1020	m.q.
Oriental (*Stouffer's*), 9⅞-oz. pkg. ..	300	8.0	35.0	14.0	m.q.	n.a.	760	m.q.
primavera (*Stouffer's*), 10⅝-oz. pkg.	540	14.0	26.0	42.0	m.q.	n.a.	1160	m.q.
primavera (*Weight Watchers*), 8.5 oz.	260	15.0	22.0	11.0	<1.0	5	800	m.q.
rigati (*Weight Watchers*), 10.63 oz.	300	20.0	35.0	9.0	2.0	25	490	m.q.
shells:								
and beef (*The Budget Gourmet*), 10 oz.	340	20.0	34.0	14.0	m.q.	35	985	m.q.
cheese, w/tomato sauce (*Stouffer's*), 9.25 oz.	330	17.0	32.0	15.0	m.q.	m.q.	850	m.q.
stuffed:								
(*Buitoni* Single Serving), 9 oz.	460	18.0	46.0	13.0	7.0	80	840	m.q.
(*Celentano*), 8 oz.	330	18.0	41.0	11.0	m.q.	m.q.	680	m.q.
w/sauce (*Celentano*), 10 oz. ...	410	23.0	51.0	14.0	m.q.	m.q.	850	m.q.
w/sauce (*Celentano*), 6.25 oz.	340	17.0	31.0	16.0	m.q.	m.q.	420	m.q.
w/vegetables, tofu, and sauce (*Legume* Provencale), 11 oz.	240	15.0	26.0	12.0	1.9	0	660	6.2 d
trio (*Tyson Gourmet Selection*), 11 oz.	450	21.0	53.0	17.0	m.q.	n.a.	890	m.q.
PASTA SALAD, see "Pasta dishes, mix" and specific pasta listings								
PASTA SAUCE, canned or in jars (see also "Tomato sauce" and specific sauce listings):								
(*Enrico's* All Natural), 4 oz.	60	2.0	9.0	1.0	n.a.	0	345	m.q.
(*Enrico's* All Natural No Salt Added), 4 oz.	60	2.0	9.0	1.0	n.a.	0	30	m.q.
(*Estee*), 4 oz.	60	2.0	9.0	1.0	<1.0	0	30	m.q.
(*Featherweight*), 4 oz.	60	2.0	11.0	1.0	n.a.	0	310	m.q.
(*Hunt's* Traditional), 4 oz.	70	2.0	12.0	2.0	m.q.	0	530	m.q.
(*Pastorelli Italian Chef*), 4 oz.	81	3.0	11.0	3.0	m.q.	n.a.	430	1.1 c
(*Prego*), 4 oz.	130	2.0	20.0	5.0	m.q.	n.a.	630	m.q.
(*Prego* No Salt Added), 4 oz.	110	2.0	11.0	6.0	m.q.	n.a.	25	m.q.
(*Progresso* Spaghetti Sauce), ½ cup	110	3.0	13.0	5.0	1.0	2	660	m.q.
(*Ragu*), 4 oz.	80	2.0	9.0	4.0	m.q.	0	740	m.q.
(*Ragu* Chunky Garden Style), 4 oz.	70	2.0	10.0	3.0	m.q.	0	440	m.q.
(*Ragu* Fresh Italian), 4 oz.	90	2.0	13.0	3.0	m.q.	0	490	m.q.
(*Ragu* Homestyle), 4 oz.	50	2.0	6.0	2.0	m.q.	0	390	m.q.
(*Ragu* Thick & Hearty), 4 oz.	100	2.0	15.0	3.0	m.q.	0	460	m.q.
w/beef, ground (*Chef Boyardee* Jars), 4 oz.	90	2.0	14.0	3.0	m.q.	m.q.	605	m.q.
cheese, three (*Prego*), 4 oz.	100	3.0	17.0	2.0	m.q.	m.q.	410	n.a.
garden combination (*Prego*), 4 oz. ..	80	2.0	14.0	2.0	m.q.	n.a.	420	m.q.
marinara:								
15½ oz.	300	7.0	44.7	14.7	2.1	0	2760	2.9 c

Food and Measure	cal.	prot. (gms)	carbo. (gms)	tot. fat (gms)	sat. fat (gms)	chol. (mgs)	sod. (mgs)	fiber (gms)
PASTA SAUCE, MARINARA *(cont.)*								
4 oz.	77	1.8	11.5	3.8	.5	0	713	.7 c
½ cup	86	2.0	12.7	4.2	.6	0	786	.8 c
(Buitoni), ½ cup	70	1.0	11.0	3.0	<1.0	0	570	m.q.
(Pathmark All Natural), ½ cup ...	80	2.0	12.0	2.0	m.q.	0	710	m.q.
(Pathmark No Frills), ½ cup	80	1.0	12.0	3.0	m.q.	0	620	m.q.
(Prego), 4 oz.	100	1.0	10.0	6.0	m.q.	0	620	m.q.
(Progresso), ½ cup	90	4.0	9.0	5.0	1.0	1	520	m.q.
(Progresso Authentic Pasta								
Sauces), ½ cup	110	4.0	10.0	6.0	1.5	4	250	2.4 d
(Rokeach), 3 oz.	60	1.0	9.0	2.0	m.q.	0	257	m.q.
meat or meat flavor:								
(Chef Boyardee), 3.75 oz.	80	2.0	11.0	3.0	m.q.	n.a.	650	m.q.
(Chef Boyardee Original), 3.75 oz.	120	3.0	13.0	6.0	m.q.	n.a.	650	m.q.
(Hunt's), 4 oz.	70	2.0	12.0	2.0	m.q.	n.a.	570	m.q.
(P&Q), ½ cup	70	1.0	11.0	2.0	m.q.	n.a.	510	m.q.
(Pathmark All Natural), ½ cup ...	80	2.0	11.0	3.0	m.q.	n.a.	790	m.q.
(Pathmark No Frills), ½ cup	90	2.0	11.0	5.0	m.q.	n.a.	620	m.q.
(Prego), 4 oz.	140	2.0	20.0	6.0	m.q.	n.a.	660	m.q.
(Progresso), ½ cup	110	4.0	13.0	5.0	1.0	5	660	m.q.
(Weight Watchers), ⅓ cup	50	2.0	9.0	1.0	m.q.	n.a.	440	m.q.
meatless:								
(Chef Boyardee Jars), 4 oz.	60	1.0	11.0	1.0	n.a.	n.a.	790	m.q.
(P&Q), ½ cup	70	1.0	14.0	1.0	n.a.	n.a.	540	m.q.
(Pathmark All Natural), ½ cup ...	70	2.0	11.0	2.0	m.q.	n.a.	710	m.q.
(Pathmark No Frills), ½ cup	80	1.0	11.0	3.0	m.q.	n.a.	583	m.q.
mushroom or mushroom flavor:								
(Chef Boyardee), 3.75 oz.	60	1.0	11.0	1.0	n.a.	n.a.	790	m.q.
(Chef Boyardee Jars), 4 oz.	70	1.0	11.0	2.0	m.q.	n.a.	655	m.q.
(Chef Boyardee Original), 3.75 oz.	80	1.0	13.0	3.0	m.q.	n.a.	680	m.q.
(Enrico's), 4 oz.	60	2.0	9.0	1.0	n.a.	0	m.q.	m.q.
(Featherweight), 4 oz.	60	2.0	11.0	1.0	n.a.	0	310	m.q.
(Hunt's), 4 oz.	70	2.0	12.0	2.0	m.q.	0	560	m.q.
(P&Q), ½ cup	70	1.0	14.0	1.0	n.a.	n.a.	580	m.q.
(Pathmark All Natural), ½ cup ...	70	2.0	11.0	2.0	m.q.	n.a.	730	m.q.
(Prego), 4 oz.	130	2.0	20.0	5.0	m.q.	n.a.	630	m.q.
(Progresso), ½ cup	110	3.0	13.0	5.0	1.0	5	630	m.q.
(Weight Watchers), ⅓ cup	40	1.0	9.0	0	0	0	430	m.q.
w/extra spice *(Prego* Extra								
Chunky), 4 oz.	100	2.0	17.0	3.0	m.q.	n.a.	450	m.q.
w/fresh sliced mushrooms								
(Enrico's Pasta Sauce), 4 oz. ..	60	2.0	9.0	1.0	n.a.	0	336	m.q.
mushroom and green pepper:								
(Enrico's All Natural), 4 oz.	60	2.0	9.0	1.0	n.a.	0	345	m.q.
(Enrico's All Natural No Salt								
Added), 4 oz.	60	2.0	9.0	1.0	n.a.	0	30	m.q.
(Prego Extra Chunky), 4 oz.	100	2.0	14.0	4.0	m.q.	n.a.	410	m.q.
mushroom and onion *(Prego* Extra								
Chunky), 4 oz.	100	2.0	13.0	4.0	m.q.	n.a.	490	m.q.

Food and Measure	cal.	prot. (gms)	carbo. (gms)	tot. fat (gms)	sat. fat (gms)	chol. (mgs)	sod. (mgs)	fiber (gms)
mushroom and tomato (*Prego* Extra Chunky), 4 oz.	110	1.0	14.0	5.0	m.q.	n.a.	500	m.q.
onion and garlic (*Prego*), 4 oz.	110	1.0	16.0	4.0	m.q.	n.a.	510	m.q.
primavera, creamy (*Progresso* Authentic Pasta Sauces), ½ cup	190	5.0	8.0	17.0	10.0	54	410	1.0 d
sausage and green pepper (*Prego* Extra Chunky), 4 oz.	160	3.0	19.0	8.0	m.q.	m.q.	500	m.q.
Sicilian (*Progresso* Authentic Pasta Sauces), ½ cup	30	<1.0	2.0	2.5	<1.0	0	660	<1.0 d
tomato or tomato-based:								
15½ oz.	479	8.0	69.9	20.9	3.0	0	2179	4.1 c
4 oz.	124	2.1	18.1	5.4	.8	0	562	1.1 c
½ cup	136	2.3	19.8	5.9	.9	0	618	1.2 c
and basil (*Prego*), 4 oz.	100	2.0	18.0	2.0	m.q.	n.a.	370	m.q.
and onion (*Prego* Extra Chunky), 4 oz.	110	2.0	14.0	5.0	m.q.	n.a.	490	m.q.
PASTA SAUCE MIX:								
1.5-oz. pkg.	118	2.5	27.4	.4	.3	0	3562	m.q.
(*Lawry's* Rich & Thick), 1 pkg.	147	3.5	28.1	2.2	m.q.	n.a.	2172	.5 c
(*McCormick/Schilling*), ¼ pkg.	32	1.0	6.0	.3	n.a.	n.a.	615	m.q.
cheese and garlic (*French's Pasta Toss*), 2 tsp.	25	1.0	2.0	2.0	m.q.	n.a.	320	m.q.
Italian (*French's Pasta Toss*), 2 tsp. ...	25	1.0	2.0	2.0	m.q.	n.a.	340	m.q.
Italian style (*French's*), ⅝ cup[1]	100	2.0	15.0	4.0	m.q.	n.a.	790	m.q.
w/mushrooms:								
1.4-oz. pkg.	118	3.9	19.1	3.5	2.2	11	3674	m.q.
(*French's*), ⅝ cup[1]	100	2.0	13.0	4.0	m.q.	n.a.	1050	m.q.
imported (*Lawry's*), 1 pkg.	143	5.2	26.0	1.5	m.q.	n.a.	2015	2.1 c
Romanoff (*French's Pasta Toss*), 2 tsp.	30	1.0	1.0	2.0	m.q.	n.a.	310	m.q.
PASTA SNACK CHIP:								
(*Bachman Pastapazazz*), 1 oz.	150	2.0	15.0	9.0	m.q.	n.a.	340	m.q.
PASTRAMI:								
(*Boar's Head* Round), 1 oz.	40	6.0	<1.0	1.5	m.q.	16	270	0
(*Healthy Deli* Round), 1 oz.	34	5.3	.8	1.1	m.q.	14	195	0
(*Hillshire Farm* Deli Select), 1 oz. ...	31	6.0	<1.0	.4	m.q.	m.q.	290	0
(*Oscar Mayer*), .6-oz. slice	16	3.4	.1	.3	.2	7	217	0
beef, 1-oz. slice	99	4.9	.9	8.3	3.0	26	348	0
turkey, see "Turkey pastrami"								
PASTRY, see specific listings								
PASTRY POCKET, refrigerated:								
(*Pillsbury*), 1 piece	240	4.0	25.0	13.0	3.0	0	520	m.q.
PÂTÉ, canned:								
1 oz.	90	4.0	.4	7.9	m.q.	m.q.	198	0
1 tbsp.	41	1.9	.2	3.6	m.q.	m.q.	91	0
chicken liver, 1 oz.	57	3.8	1.9	3.7	m.q.	m.q.	m.q.	0
chicken liver, 1 tbsp.	26	1.8	.9	1.7	m.q.	m.q.	m.q.	0
goose liver, smoked, 1 oz.	131	3.2	1.3	12.4	m.q.	43	m.q.	0

1. *Prepared according to package directions.*

Food and Measure	cal.	prot. (gms)	carbo. (gms)	tot. fat (gms)	sat. fat (gms)	chol. (mgs)	sod. (mgs)	fiber (gms)
PÂTÉ *(cont.)*								
goose liver, smoked, 1 tbsp.	60	1.5	.6	5.7	m.q.	20	m.q.	0
liver *(Sells)*, 2⅛ oz.	190	8.0	4.0	16.0	m.q.	90	470	0
PATTY SHELL, see "Puff Pastry, frozen"								
PEA BEAN, see "Baked beans"								
PEA POD, CHINESE, see "Peas, edible-podded"								
PEACH:								
untrimmed, 1 lb.	148	2.4	38.2	.3	<.1	0	2	5.5 d
peeled and pitted, 1 oz.	12	.2	3.1	<.1	tr.	0	tr.	.5 d
1 medium, 2½" diam., approx.								
4 per lb.	37	.6	9.7	.1	tr.	0	tr.	1.4 d
peeled, sliced, ½ cup	37	.6	9.4	.1	tr.	0	1	1.4 d
PEACH, CANNED, ½ cup, except as noted:								
(Mott's Peach Fruit Pak), 3.75 oz. ..	75	0	18.0	0	0	0	7	m.q.
freestone, halves or slices:								
(Del Monte)	90	0	23.0	0	0	0	<10	m.q.
(Del Monte Lite)	60	0	13.0	0	0	0	<10	m.q.
(S&W/Nutradiet)	30	0	7.0	0	0	0	10	m.q.
yellow cling (clingstone):								
diced *(Del Monte* Fruit Cup), 5 oz.	110	0	28.0	0	0	0	<10	m.q.
halves *(S&W/Nutradiet)*	30	0	8.0	0	0	0	5	m.q.
halves or slices:								
(Del Monte)	80	0	22.0	0	0	0	<10	m.q.
(Del Monte Lite)	50	0	13.0	0	0	0	<10	m.q.
no sugar added *(Finast* Lite) ..	50	0	14.0	0	0	0	10	m.q.
sliced, unsweetened *(S&W/Nutradiet)*	30	0	8.0	0	0	0	5	m.q.
spiced, w/pits *(Del Monte)*, 3½ oz.	80	0	20.0	0	0	0	<10	m.q.
in water, yellow cling:								
4 oz.	27	.5	6.9	.1	tr.	0	3	.4 c
halves or slices	29	.5	7.5	.1	tr.	0	4	.4 c
1 half and 1⅔ tbsp. liquid	18	.3	4.7	<.1	tr.	0	3	.2 c
in juice:								
freestone or yellow cling:								
4 oz.	50	.7	13.1	<.1	tr.	0	5	.5 d
halves or slices	55	.8	14.3	<.1	tr.	0	6	.6 d
1 half and 1⅔ tbsp. liquid	34	.5	8.9	<.1	tr.	0	3	.3 d
yellow cling:								
in pear juice *(A&P)*	50	<1.0	12.0	<1.0	tr.	0	10	m.q.
halves, in pear juice *(A&P)*	50	<1.0	12.0	<1.0	tr.	0	10	m.q.
halves or slices *(Featherweight)*	50	0	14.0	0	0	0	<10	m.q.
halves or slices *(Libby Lite)*	50	0	13.0	0	0	0	10	m.q.
sliced:								
(IGA)	50	1.0	14.0	0	0	0	10	m.q.
(Pathmark)	50	0	14.0	0	0	0	10	m.q.

Food and Measure	cal.	prot. (gms)	carbo. (gms)	tot. fat (gms)	sat. fat (gms)	chol. (mgs)	sod. (mgs)	fiber (gms)
sweetened (*S&W*)	90	0	20.0	0	0	0	10	m.q.
in extra light syrup, yellow cling:								
4 oz.	48	.5	12.6	.1	<.1	0	6	.2 c
halves or slices	52	.5	13.7	.1	<.1	0	6	.2 c
1 half and 1⅔ tbsp. liquid	32	.3	8.6	.1	tr.	0	4	.2 c
in light syrup, yellow cling:								
4 oz.	61	.5	16.5	<.1	tr.	0	6	.3 c
halves or slices	68	.6	18.3	<.1	tr.	0	7	.4 c
1 half and 1¾ tbsp. liquid	44	.4	11.8	<.1	tr.	0	4	.2 c
sliced (*Pathmark* No Frills), 1 cup	140	1.0	36.0	0	0	0	15	m.q.
in heavy syrup:								
freestone, halves or slices (*S&W*)	100	0	26.0	0	0	0	10	m.q.
freestone or yellow cling:								
4 oz.	84	.5	22.6	.1	<.1	0	7	.3 c
halves or slices	95	.6	25.5	.1	<.1	0	8	.4 c
1 half and 1¾ tbsp. liquid	60	.4	16.2	.1	tr.	0	5	.2 c
yellow cling:								
halves or slices (*A&P*)	100	<1.0	25.0	<1.0	n.a.	0	10	m.q.
halves or slices (*S&W*)	100	0	25.0	0	0	0	10	m.q.
sliced:								
(*Finast*)	100	0	25.0	0	0	0	6	m.q.
(*Pathmark*)	100	0	25.0	0	0	0	<10	m.q.
(*Pathmark*), 1 cup	190	1.0	50.0	0	0	0	20	m.q.
whole, spiced (*S&W*)	90	0	23.0	0	0	0	10	m.q.
in extra heavy syrup, freestone:								
4 oz.	109	.5	29.6	<.1	tr.	0	9	.3 c
halves or slices	126	.6	34.1	<.1	tr.	0	11	.4 c
1 half and 1¾ tbsp. liquid	77	.4	21.1	<.1	tr.	0	6	.2 c
spiced, in heavy syrup:								
4 oz.	85	.5	22.8	.1	<.1	0	5	.3 c
whole	90	.5	24.3	.1	<.1	0	5	.3 c
1 peach and 2 tbsp. liquid	66	.4	17.7	.1	<.1	0	3	.2 c
PEACH, DEHYDRATED,								
sulfured[1]:								
uncooked, 4 oz.	369	5.5	94.3	1.2	.1	0	11	4.5 c
uncooked, ½ cup	188	2.8	48.2	.6	.1	0	6	2.3 c
cooked, 4 oz.	151	2.3	38.7	.5	.1	0	5	1.8 c
cooked, ½ cup	161	2.4	41.3	.5	.1	0	5	2.0 c
PEACH, DRIED:								
(*Sun•Maid/Sunsweet*), 2 oz.	140	2.0	38.0	0	0	0	<10	m.q.
uncooked (*Del Monte*), 2 oz.	140	2.0	35.0	0	0	0	<10	m.q.
sulfured:								
uncooked:								
4 oz.	271	4.1	69.5	.9	.1	0	8	9.3 d
halves, ½ cup	192	2.9	49.1	.6	.1	0	6	6.6 d
10 halves, approx. 4.6 oz.	311	4.7	79.7	1.0	.1	0	9	10.7 d
cooked:								
unsweetened, 4 oz.	87	1.3	22.3	.3	<.1	0	2	1.1 c

1. *Sodium bisulfite used to preserve color.*

Food and Measure	cal.	prot. (gms)	carbo. (gms)	tot. fat (gms)	sat. fat (gms)	chol. (mgs)	sod. (mgs)	fiber (gms)
PEACH, DRIED, COOKED *(cont.)*								
unsweetened, halves, ½ cup ..	91	1.5	25.4	.3	<.1	0	3	1.2 c
sweetened, 4 oz.	117	1.2	30.2	.2	<.1	0	2	1.0 c
sweetened, halves, ½ cup	139	1.4	35.9	.3	<.1	0	3	1.2 c
PEACH, FREEZE-DRIED:								
(*Mountain House*), ¼ cup[1]	50	1.0	12.0	0	0	0	<1	m.q.
PEACH, FROZEN, sliced, sweetened:								
10-oz. pkg.	267	1.8	68.1	.4	<.1	0	18	1.1 c
4 oz.	107	.7	27.2	.1	<.1	0	7	.5 c
½ cup	118	.8	30.0	.2	<.1	0	8	.5 c
PEACH BUTTER:								
(*Smucker's*), 1 tsp.	15	0	4.0	0	0	0	0	m.q.
PEACH COBBLER, see "Cobbler, frozen"								
PEACH DRINK:								
(*Hi-C*), 6 fl. oz.	101	.1	24.8	<.1	(0)	0	18	(0)
PEACH JUICE:								
(*Smucker's* Naturally 100%), 8 fl. oz.	120	1.0	30.0	0	0	0	10	m.q.
orchard blend (*Dole Pure & Light*), 6 fl. oz.	90	0	24.0	0	0	0	10	m.q.
PEACH NECTAR, canned or bottled:								
1 fl. oz.	17	.1	4.3	<.1	tr.	0	2	<.1 d
6 fl. oz.	101	.5	26.0	<.1	<.1	0	13	.3 d
(*Libby's*), 6 fl. oz.	100	0	24.0	0	0	0	5	m.q.
PEACH TURNOVER, see "Turnover"								
PEANUT[2] (see also "Candy"):								
(*Beer Nuts*), 1 oz.	180	7.0	7.0	14.0	m.q.	0	60	m.q.
(*Pathmark* Sweet and Crunchy), 1 oz.	140	4.0	15.0	8.0	m.q.	0	30	m.q.
(*Weight Watchers*), 1 pouch	100	8.0	4.0	7.0	m.q.	0	50	m.q.
all varieties:								
raw, in shell, 1 lb.	1877	85.4	53.4	163.0	22.6	0	60	19.5 d
raw, 1 oz.	159	7.2	4.5	13.8	1.9	0	5	1.7 d
raw, ½ cup	414	18.8	11.8	35.9	5.0	0	14	8.6 d
boiled, salted, 1 oz.	90	3.8	6.0	6.2	.9	0	213	.6 c
boiled, salted, ½ cup	102	4.3	6.8	7.0	1.0	0	240	.6 c
dry-roasted:								
1 oz.	164	6.6	6.0	13.9	1.9	0	2	2.3 d
½ cup	428	17.3	15.7	36.3	5.0	0	4	5.8 d
salted, 1 oz.	164	6.6	6.0	13.9	1.9	0	228	2.3 d
salted, ½ cup	428	17.3	15.7	36.3	5.0	0	594	5.8 d
oil-roasted:								
1 oz.	163	7.4	5.3	13.8	1.9	0	2	2.5 d
½ cup	419	19.0	13.6	35.5	4.9	0	4	6.3 d

1. *Prepared according to package directions.*
2. *Shelled, except as noted.*

Food and Measure	cal.	prot. (gms)	carbo. (gms)	tot. fat (gms)	sat. fat (gms)	chol. (mgs)	sod. (mgs)	fiber (gms)
salted, 1 oz.	163	7.4	5.3	13.8	1.9	0	121	2.5 d
salted, ½ cup	419	19.0	13.6	35.5	4.9	0	312	6.3 d
cocktail, oil-roasted (*Planters*), 1 oz.	170	7.0	5.0	15.0	3.0	0	160	m.q.
cocktail, oil-roasted, unsalted								
(*Planters*), 1 oz.	170	7.0	5.0	15.0	3.0	0	0	m.q.
dry-roasted:								
(*Finast*), 1 oz.	160	7.0	5.0	14.0	m.q.	0	15	m.q.
(*Flavor House*), 1 oz.	180	8.0	5.0	14.0	m.q.	0	0	m.q.
(*Pathmark*), 1 oz.	170	7.0	5.0	14.0	m.q.	0	0	m.q.
(*Pathmark No Frills*), 1 oz.	180	8.0	5.0	14.0	2.0	0	0	m.q.
(*Planters*), 1 oz.	170	7.0	5.0	15.0	2.0	0	0	m.q.
salted:								
(*Finast*), 1 oz.	160	8.0	6.0	14.0	m.q.	0	120	m.q.
(*Flavor House*), 1 oz.	180	8.0	5.0	14.0	m.q.	0	200	m.q.
(*Frito-Lay's*), 1⅛ oz.	190	7.0	7.0	16.0	m.q.	0	300	m.q.
(*Guy's*), 1 oz.	170	8.0	3.0	14.0	m.q.	0	310	m.q.
(*Pathmark*), 1 oz.	170	7.0	5.0	14.0	m.q.	0	150	m.q.
(*Planters*), 1 oz.	160	7.0	6.0	14.0	2.0	0	250	m.q.
honey-roasted:								
(*Eagle Honey Roast*), 1 oz.	170	7.0	7.0	13.0	m.q.	0	140	m.q.
(*Flavor House*), 1 oz.	160	6.0	9.0	11.0	m.q.	0	120	m.q.
(*Little Debbie*), 1.13 oz.	190	8.0	9.0	13.0	m.q.	<1	15	m.q.
(*Pathmark*), 1 oz.	170	6.0	8.0	13.0	m.q.	0	75	m.q.
(*Planters*), 1 oz.	170	6.0	8.0	13.0	2.0	0	180	m.q.
dry-roasted (*Planters*), 1 oz.	160	7.0	7.0	13.0	2.0	0	90	m.q.
oil-roasted, salted:								
(*Flavor House*), 1 oz.	170	7.0	5.0	15.0	m.q.	0	125	m.q.
(*Pathmark*), 1 oz.	180	8.0	5.0	14.0	m.q.	0	150	m.q.
(*Planters*), 1 oz.	170	7.0	5.0	15.0	3.0	0	160	m.q.
redskin, oil-roasted (*Planters*), 1 oz.	170	7.0	5.0	15.0	5.0	0	150	m.q.
salted (*Little Debbie*), 1.25 oz.	230	10.0	5.0	18.0	m.q.	<1	90	m.q.
Spanish:								
raw, 1 oz.	160	7.3	4.4	13.9	2.1	0	6	1.4 c
raw, ½ cup	417	19.1	11.6	36.2	5.6	0	16	3.5 c
dry-roasted (*Planters*), 1 oz.	160	7.0	6.0	14.0	3.0	0	200	m.q.
oil-roasted:								
1 oz.	162	7.8	4.9	13.7	2.1	0	2	1.4 c
½ cup	426	20.6	12.8	36.0	5.6	0	4	3.7 c
salted, 1 oz.	162	7.8	4.9	13.7	2.1	0	121	1.4 c
salted, ½ cup	426	20.6	12.8	36.0	5.6	0	319	3.7 c
salted (*Flavor House*), 1 oz. ...	170	7.0	5.0	15.0	m.q.	0	125	m.q.
salted (*Guy's*), 1 oz.	170	8.0	3.0	14.0	m.q.	0	170	m.q.
Valencia:								
raw, 1 oz.	160	7.0	5.9	13.3	2.1	0	0	.6 c
raw, ½ cup	417	18.3	15.3	34.7	5.4	0	<1	1.6 c
oil-roasted:								
1 oz.	165	7.6	4.6	14.4	2.2	0	2	.6 c
½ cup	424	19.5	11.7	36.9	5.7	0	4	1.6 c
salted, 1 oz.	165	7.6	4.6	14.4	2.2	0	216	.6 c

Food and Measure	cal.	prot. (gms)	carbo. (gms)	tot. fat (gms)	sat. fat (gms)	chol. (mgs)	sod. (mgs)	fiber (gms)
PEANUT, VALENCIA, OIL ROASTED *(cont.)*								
salted, ½ cup	424	19.5	11.7	36.9	5.7	0	556	1.6 c
Virginia:								
raw, 1 oz.	158	7.1	4.6	13.7	1.8	0	3	1.4 c
raw, ½ cup	411	18.4	12.1	35.6	4.6	0	8	3.6 c
oil-roasted:								
1 oz.	161	8.3	4.5	13.6	1.8	0	2	1.5 c
½ cup	413	18.5	14.2	34.8	4.5	0	4	3.8 c
salted, 1 oz.	161	8.3	4.5	13.6	1.8	0	121	1.5 c
salted, ½ cup	413	18.5	14.2	34.8	4.5	0	310	3.8 c
PEANUT BUTTER, 2 tbsp.,								
except as noted:								
(Estee), 1 tbsp.	100	4.0	3.0	8.0	1.0	0	2	m.q.
(Hollywood Unsalted), 1 tbsp.	35	2.0	1.0	3.0	0	0	0	1.0 d
(Pathmark Natural)	200	9.0	5.0	17.0	m.q.	0	130	m.q.
(S&W/Nutradiet), 1 tbsp.	93	3.0	2.0	8.0	m.q.	0	<10	m.q.
chunk style:								
1 oz.	167	6.8	6.1	14.2	2.7	0	5	1.9 d
½ cup	760	31.0	27.9	64.4	12.4	0	22	8.5 d
2 tbsp.	188	7.7	6.9	16.0	3.1	0	5	2.1 d
(Bama)	200	7.0	6.0	17.0	m.q.	0	115	m.q.
(Featherweight), 1 tbsp.	90	4.0	2.0	7.0	m.q.	0	5	m.q.
(Finast Crunchy)	195	9.0	6.0	17.0	m.q.	0	175	m.q.
(JIF)	190	9.0	6.0	16.0	3.0	0	155	m.q.
(Pathmark Super Chunky)	200	7.0	6.0	17.0	m.q.	0	140	m.q.
(Peter Pan Extra Crunchy)	190	9.1	5.1	16.3	2.3	0	122	m.q.
(Skippy Super Chunk)	190	9.0	4.0	17.0	3.0	0	130	.6 d
(Smucker's Chunky Natural)	200	8.0	6.0	16.0	1.0	0	125	m.q.
salted (see also specific brands):								
1 oz.	167	6.8	6.1	14.2	2.7	0	138	1.9 d
½ cup	760	31.0	27.9	64.4	12.4	0	628	8.5 d
2 tbsp.	188	7.7	6.9	16.0	3.1	0	156	2.1 d
chunk or creamy:								
(Arrowhead Mills)	190	9.0	6.0	16.0	m.q.	0	<1	4.5 d
(Health Valley No Salt Added)	180	8.0	6.0	14.0	m.q.	0	2	2.6 d
(Hollywood), 1 tbsp.	35	2.1	1.0	3.0	0	0	25	1.0 d
smooth style:								
1 oz.	167	7.0	5.9	14.2	2.7	0	5	1.7 d
½ cup	759	31.7	26.7	64.5	12.4	0	22	7.7 d
2 tbsp.	188	7.9	6.6	16.0	3.1	0	5	1.9 d
(Algood)	190	m.q.	6.0	16.0	m.q.	0	150	m.q.
(Bama)	200	7.0	6.0	17.0	m.q.	0	140	m.q.
(Featherweight), 1 tbsp.	90	4.0	2.0	7.0	m.q.	0	<3	m.q.
(Finast)	195	9.0	6.0	17.0	m.q.	0	175	m.q.
(JIF)	190	9.0	6.0	16.0	3.0	0	155	m.q.
(Pathmark Creamy)	200	7.0	6.0	17.0	m.q.	0	170	m.q.
(Pathmark No Frills Creamy)	200	7.0	6.0	17.0	m.q.	0	170	m.q.
(Peter Pan Creamy)	190	8.6	5.7	16.4	2.2	0	150	m.q.
(Peter Pan Creamy Salt Free)	195	8.7	5.3	17.1	2.4	0	1	m.q.

Food and Measure	cal.	prot. (gms)	carbo. (gms)	tot. fat (gms)	sat. fat (gms)	chol. (mgs)	sod. (mgs)	fiber (gms)
(*Skippy* Creamy)	190	9.0	4.0	17.0	3.0	0	150	.6 d
(*Smucker's* Natural)	200	8.0	6.0	16.0	1.0	0	125	m.q.
(*Smucker's* No Salt Added								
Natural)	200	8.0	6.0	17.0	1.0	0	<10	m.q.
(*Woodstock* Old Fashioned								
Unsalted)	200	9.0	6.0	16.0	m.q.	0	3	m.q.
salted (see also specific brands):								
1 oz.	167	7.0	5.9	14.2	2.7	0	136	1.7 d
½ cup	759	31.7	26.7	64.5	12.4	0	617	7.7 d
2 tbsp.	188	7.9	6.6	16.0	3.1	0	153	1.9 d
jelly and, see "Jelly and peanut butter"								
PEANUT BUTTER FLAVOR								
BAKING CHIPS:								
(*Reese's*), 1.5 oz. or ¼ cup	230	7.0	19.0	13.0	m.q.	5	90	m.q.
PEANUT BUTTER TOPPING:								
caramel (*Smucker's*), 2 tbsp.	150	3.0	29.0	2.0	m.q.	0	105	m.q.
PEANUT FLOUR:								
defatted:								
1 oz.	93	14.8	9.8	.2	<.1	0	5	1.1 c
1 cup	196	31.3	20.8	.3	<.1	0	9	2.4 c
1 tbsp.	13	2.1	1.4	<.1	tr.	0	1	.2 c
salted:								
1 oz.	93	14.8	9.8	.2	<.1	0	51	1.1 c
1 cup	196	31.3	20.8	.3	<.1	0	108	2.4
1 tbsp.	13	2.1	1.4	<.1	tr.	0	7	.2 c
low-fat, 1 oz.	120	9.5	8.8	6.1	.9	0	0	m.q.
low-fat, 1 cup	257	20.3	18.8	13.1	1.8	0	0	m.q.
PEANUT OIL:								
1 oz.	251	0	0	28.4	4.8	0	0	0
½ cup	955	0	0	108.0	18.3	0	0	0
1 tbsp.	119	0	0	13.5	2.3	0	0	0
(*Hain*), 1 tbsp.	120	0	0	14.0	2.0	0	0	0
(*Planters*), 1 tbsp.	120	0	0	14.0	2.0	0	0	0
PEAR:								
untrimmed, 1 lb.	247	1.6	63.1	1.7	.1	0	2	10.9 d
trimmed, w/skin, 1 oz.	17	.1	4.3	.1	tr.	0	tr.	.7 d
w/skin, sliced, ½ cup	49	.3	12.5	.3	<.1	0	1	2.1 d
Bartlett, 2½" diam. × 3½", approx.								
2½ per lb.	98	.7	25.1	.7	<.1	0	1	4.3 d
PEAR, CANNED, ½ cup, except								
as noted:								
Bartlett:								
halves, unsweetened (*IGA*)	60	0	15.0	0	0	0	10	m.q.
halves or slices:								
(*Del Monte*)	80	0	22.0	0	0	0	<10	m.q.
(*Del Monte Lite*)	50	0	14.0	0	0	0	<10	m.q.
(*Finast* Lite No Sugar Added)	60	0	15.0	0	0	0	10	m.q.
peeled, unsweetened (*S&W/								
Nutradiet*)	35	0	10.0	0	0	0	10	m.q.

Food and Measure	cal.	prot. (gms)	carbo. (gms)	tot. fat (gms)	sat. fat (gms)	chol. (mgs)	sod. (mgs)	fiber (gms)
PEAR, CANNED, BARTLETT *(cont.)*								
peeled, halves or quarters *(S&W/*								
Nutradiet)	35	0	10.0	0	0	0	10	m.q.
in water:								
4 oz.	33	.2	8.9	<.1	tr.	0	2	.7 c
halves	36	.2	9.5	<.1	tr.	0	3	.7 c
1 half and 1⅔ tbsp. liquid	22	.2	6.0	<.1	tr.	0	2	.5 c
in juice:								
4 oz.	57	.4	14.7	.1	tr.	0	5	1.0 d
halves	62	.4	16.0	.1	tr.	0	5	1.1 d
1 half and 1⅔ tbsp. liquid	38	.3	10.0	.1	tr.	0	3	.7 d
halves *(Featherweight)*	60	0	15.0	0	0	0	<10	m.q.
halves or slices *(A&P)*	60	<1.0	15.0	<1.0	(0)	0	10	m.q.
halves or slices *(Libby Lite)*	60	0	19.0	0	0	0	10	m.q.
slices, sweetened *(S&W* Natural								
Style)	80	0	20.0	0	0	0	10	m.q.
Bartlett, halves *(Pathmark)*	60	0	15.0	0	0	0	10	m.q.
in extra light syrup:								
4 oz.	53	.3	13.8	.1	tr.	0	2	.7 c
halves	58	.4	15.1	.1	tr.	0	3	.7 c
1 half and 1⅔ tbsp. liquid	36	.2	9.4	.1	tr.	0	2	.5 c
in light syrup:								
4 oz.	65	.2	17.2	<.1	<.1	0	6	.7 c
halves	72	.2	19.0	<.1	<.1	0	7	.7 c
1 half and 1¾ tbsp. liquid	45	.2	12.0	<.1	tr.	0	4	.5 c
halves or slices *(A&P)*	70	<1.0	20.0	<1.0	(0)	0	10	m.q.
Bartlett *(Pathmark* No Frills),								
1 cup	140	0	38.0	0	0	0	10	m.q.
in heavy syrup:								
4 oz.	84	.2	21.7	.1	tr.	0	6	.7 c
halves	94	.3	24.4	.2	tr.	0	7	.7 c
1 half and 1¾ tbsp. liquid	58	.2	15.1	.1	tr.	0	4	.5 c
halves *(S&W)*	100	0	25.0	0	0	0	<10	m.q.
halves or slices *(A&P)*	95	<1.0	25.0	<1.0	(0)	0	10	m.q.
Bartlett:								
halves *(Pathmark)*	90	0	23.0	0	0	0	10	m.q.
halves or slices *(Finast)*	100	0	25.0	0	0	0	10	m.q.
slices *(Pathmark)*, 1 cup	180	0	46.0	0	0	0	20	m.q.
in extra heavy syrup:								
4 oz.	110	.2	28.6	.1	tr.	0	6	.7 c
halves	127	.3	33.0	.2	tr.	0	7	.8 c
1 half and 1¾ tbsp. liquid	77	.2	20.0	.1	tr.	0	4	.5 c
PEAR, DRIED, sulfured:								
uncooked, 4 oz.	297	2.1	79.0	.7	<.1	0	7	6.5 c
uncooked, halves, ½ cup	236	1.7	62.7	.6	<.1	0	5	5.1 c
cooked:								
unsweetened, 4 oz.	144	1.0	38.3	.4	<.1	0	3	3.1 c
unsweetened, halves, ½ cup	163	1.2	43.3	.4	<.1	0	4	3.5 c
sweetened, 4 oz.	159	1.0	42.1	.3	<.1	0	3	3.0 c

Food and Measure	cal.	prot. (gms)	carbo. (gms)	tot. fat (gms)	sat. fat (gms)	chol. (mgs)	sod. (mgs)	fiber (gms)
sweetened, halves, ½ cup	196	1.2	52.0	.4	<.1	0	4	3.7 c
PEAR NECTAR, canned:								
1 fl. oz.	19	<.1	4.9	tr.	tr.	0	1	.2 d
6 fl. oz.	112	.2	29.6	<.1	<.1	0	7	1.2 d
PEAS, see specific listings								
PEAS, BLACK-EYED, see "Cowpea"								
PEAS, CREAM, canned:								
(*Allens* Fresh), ½ cup	90	7.0	14.0	<1.0	n.a.	0	440	m.q.
PEAS, CROWDER, CANNED:								
(*Allens* Fresh), ½ cup	80	5.0	15.0	<1.0	n.a.	0	370	m.q.
PEAS, CROWDER, FROZEN:								
(*Seabrook*), 3 oz.	130	8.0	23.0	1.0	n.a.	0	n.a.	1.0 c
PEAS, EDIBLE-PODDED:								
raw:								
untrimmed, 1 lb.	180	11.9	32.2	.9	.2	0	18	11.1 d
trimmed, 1 oz.	12	.8	2.1	.1	<.1	0	1	.7 d
trimmed, ½ cup	30	2.0	5.4	.1	<.1	0	3	1.9 d
boiled, drained, 4 oz.	48	3.7	8.0	.3	<.1	0	5	3.2 d
boiled, drained, ½ cup	34	2.6	5.6	.2	<.1	0	3	2.2 d
PEAS, EDIBLE-PODDED, FROZEN:								
10-oz. pkg.	118	8.0	20.5	.9	.2	0	11	6.8 c
boiled, drained, 4 oz.	59	4.0	10.2	.4	.1	0	6	3.4 c
boiled, drained, ½ cup	42	2.8	7.2	.3	.1	0	4	2.4 c
Chinese (*Chun King*), 1.5 oz.	20	1.0	3.0	0	0	0	<10	m.q.
Chinese (*Seabrook*), 2 oz.	20	2.0	4.0	0	0	0	n.a.	m.q.
snow (*Birds Eye* Deluxe), 3 oz.	35	2.0	6.0	0	0	0	0	3.0 d
sugar snap:								
(*Birds Eye* Deluxe), 2.6 oz.	45	2.0	9.0	0	0	0	5	4.0 d
(*Green Giant*), ½ cup	30	2.0	8.0	0	0	0	0	2.0 d
(*Green Giant Harvest Fresh*), ½ cup	30	2.0	8.0	0	0	0	100	2.0 d
w/baby carrots and water chestnuts (*Birds Eye* Farm Fresh), 3.2 oz.	50	2.0	11.0	0	0	0	20	4.0 d
PEAS, FIELD, canned:								
(*Allens* Fresh), ½ cup	100	7.0	18.0	<1.0	n.a.	0	370	m.q.
w/snaps (*Allens* Fresh), ½ cup	100	5.0	20.0	<1.0	n.a.	0	370	m.q.
tiny, w/snaps (*Allens* Fresh), ½ cup	70	6.0	13.0	<1.0	n.a.	0	340	m.q.
PEAS, GREEN OR SWEET:								
raw:								
in pod, 1 lb.	140	9.3	24.9	.7	.1	0	8	5.9 d
shelled, 1 oz.	23	1.5	4.1	.1	<.1	0	1	1.0 d
shelled, ½ cup	58	3.9	10.4	.3	.1	0	3	2.4 d
boiled, drained, 4 oz.	95	6.1	17.7	.2	<.1	0	3	4.2 d
boiled, drained, ½ cup	67	4.3	12.5	.2	<.1	0	2	3.0 d

Food and Measure	cal.	prot. (gms)	carbo. (gms)	tot. fat (gms)	sat. fat (gms)	chol. (mgs)	sod. (mgs)	fiber (gms)
PEAS, GREEN OR SWEET, CANNED, ½ cup, except as noted:								
w/liquid:								
4 oz.	56	3.4	10.2	.3	.1	0	311	2.3 d
½ cup	61	3.7	11.1	.4	.1	0	340	2.5 d
low-sodium, 4 oz.	56	3.4	10.2	.3	.1	0	2	2.3 d
low-sodium	61	3.7	11.1	.4	.1	0	2	2.5 d
(Del Monte)	60	3.0	10.0	0	0	0	355	m.q.
(Del Monte No Salt Added)	60	3.0	11.0	0	0	0	<10	m.q.
drained:								
4 oz.	78	5.0	14.3	.4	.1	0	248	3.9 d
½ cup	59	3.8	10.7	.3	.1	0	186	2.9 d
low-sodium, 4 oz.	78	5.0	14.3	.4	.1	0	2	3.9 d
low-sodium	59	3.8	10.7	.3	.1	0	2	2.9 d
(Green Giant 50% Less Salt)	50	4.0	11.0	0	0	0	160	3.0 d
(Stokely No Salt or Sugar Added) ...	50	4.0	9.0	0	0	0	5	m.q.
dry early June (Allens)	80	5.0	15.0	<1.0	(0)	0	320	m.q.
early:								
(A&P)	70	4.0	15.0	<1.0	(0)	0	350	m.q.
(Stokely)	60	4.0	12.0	0	0	0	320	m.q.
June (Green Giant)	50	3.0	12.0	0	0	0	330	3.0 d
June (S&W Petit Pois)	70	4.0	12.0	0	0	0	330	m.q.
mixed sizes (A&P)	60	4.0	12.0	<1.0	(0)	0	350	m.q.
mixed (IGA No Salt or Sugar Added)	50	4.0	10.0	0	0	0	<10	m.q.
seasoned[1], w/liquid, 4 oz. or ½ cup	57	3.5	10.5	.3	.1	0	288	1.9 c
seasoned, w/liquid (Del Monte)	60	3.0	11.0	0	0	0	355	m.q.
small, w/liquid (Del Monte)	50	3.0	9.0	0	0	0	355	m.q.
sweet:								
(Featherweight)	70	5.0	12.0	0	0	0	<10	m.q.
(Finast)	70	4.0	13.0	1.0	(0)	0	300	m.q.
(Finast No Salt Added)	60	4.0	12.0	0	0	0	10	m.q.
(Green Giant)	50	4.0	11.0	0	0	0	320	4.0 d
(Pathmark Little Gem)	70	4.0	12.0	1.0	(0)	0	350	m.q.
(Pathmark No Frills), 1 cup	120	8.0	25.0	1.0	(0)	0	640	m.q.
(S&W Perfection)	70	4.0	12.0	0	0	0	330	m.q.
(S&W/Nutradiet)	40	3.0	8.0	0	0	0	5	m.q.
(Stokely)	60	4.0	10.0	0	0	0	320	m.q.
garden, fancy (Pathmark)	70	4.0	12.0	1.0	(0)	0	350	m.q.
large, tender (Pathmark)	70	4.0	12.0	1.0	(0)	0	350	m.q.
mini (Green Giant)	50	4.0	12.0	0	0	0	340	4.0 d
mini, in brine (Green Giant)	60	4.0	12.0	<1.0	n.a.	0	240	4.0 d
mixed sizes (Pathmark No Salt Added)	50	4.0	10.0	0	0	0	10	m.q.
small (Pathmark)	70	4.0	12.0	1.0	(0)	0	350	m.q.
tiny, early June (IGA)	70	4.0	12.0	0	0	0	340	m.q.

1. *Mixture includes peas, onions, red peppers, garlic, and salt.*

Food and Measure	cal.	prot. (gms)	carbo. (gms)	tot. fat (gms)	sat. fat (gms)	chol. (mgs)	sod. (mgs)	fiber (gms)
PEAS, GREEN OR SWEET, FREEZE-DRIED:								
(*Mountain House*), ½ cup[1]	70	4.0	12.0	1.0	(0)	0	21	m.q.
PEAS, GREEN OR SWEET, FROZEN:								
10-oz. pkg.	219	14.8	38.9	1.1	.2	0	319	10.8 d
boiled, drained, 4 oz.	88	5.8	16.2	.3	.1	0	99	4.3 d
boiled, drained, ½ cup	63	4.1	11.4	.2	<.1	0	70	3.0 d
(*Birds Eye*), 3.3 oz.	80	5.0	13.0	0	0	0	130	4.0 d
(*Birds Eye* Portion Pack), 3 oz.	70	5.0	12.0	0	0	0	120	4.0 d
(*Frosty Acres*), 3.3 oz.	80	5.0	13.0	0	0	0	91	2.0 c
(*Health Valley*), ½ cup	65	4.0	11.0	0	0	0	70	3.0 d
(*Seabrook*), 3.3 oz.	80	5.0	13.0	0	0	0	91	2.0 c
(*Southern*), 3.5 oz.	79	5.5	14.0	.5	(0)	0	130	m.q.
(*Stokely Singles*), 3 oz.	65	4.0	12.0	1.0	(0)	0	95	m.q.
early June (*Green Giant Harvest Fresh*), ½ cup	60	4.0	12.0	1.0	(0)	0	140	3.0 d
petite (*Southern*), 3.5 oz.	64	4.7	11.0	.4	(0)	0	50	m.q.
sweet:								
(*Finast*), 3.3 oz.	80	5.0	13.0	0	0	0	125	m.q.
(*Green Giant*), ½ cup	50	4.0	11.0	0	0	0	95	4.0 d
(*Green Giant Harvest Fresh*), ½ cup	50	4.0	12.0	0	0	0	135	3.0 d
tender tiny (*Birds Eye* Deluxe), 3.3 oz.	60	4.0	11.0	0	0	0	120	4.0 d
tiny (*Frosty Acres*), 3.3 oz.	60	4.0	11.0	0	0	0	127	2.0 c
tiny (*Seabrook*), 3.3 oz.	60	4.0	11.0	0	0	0	127	2.0 c
in butter sauce:								
(*Finast*), ½ cup	80	8.0	15.0	4.0	m.q.	n.a.	400	m.q.
early (*Green Giant* One Serving), 4.5 oz.	90	6.0	16.0	2.0	<1.0	5	500	5.0 d
early (*LeSueur*), ½ cup	80	5.0	14.0	2.0	<1.0	5	440	3.0 d
sweet (*Green Giant*), ½ cup	80	5.0	14.0	2.0	<1.0	5	410	4.0 d
sweet (*Stokely Singles*), 4 oz.	90	5.0	16.0	1.0	n.a.	5	335	m.q.
w/cream sauce (*Birds Eye* Combinations), 5 oz.	180	5.0	16.0	11.0	m.q.	0	480	3.0 d
PEAS, GREEN, COMBINATIONS, frozen:								
and carrots, see "Peas and carrots"								
and cauliflower, in cream sauce (*The Budget Gourmet* Side dish), 5.75 oz.	170	6.0	16.0	7.0	m.q.	20	280	m.q.
LeSueur style (*Green Giant Valley Combination*), ½ cup	70	4.0	12.0	2.0	m.q.	0	400	2.1 d
mini, w/pea pods and water chestnuts, in butter sauce (*LeSueur*), ½ cup	80	4.0	10.0	2.0	m.q.	n.a.	410	3.0 d

1. *Prepared according to package directions.*

Food and Measure	cal.	prot. (gms)	carbo. (gms)	tot. fat (gms)	sat. fat (gms)	chol. (mgs)	sod. (mgs)	fiber (gms)
PEAS, GREEN, COMBINATIONS *(cont.)*								
and onions, see "Peas and onions"								
w/onions and carrots, in butter sauce								
(*LeSueur*), ½ cup	80	4.0	11.0	3.0	m.q.	n.a.	470	3.0 d
and potatoes, w/cream sauce (*Birds*								
Eye Combinations), 5 oz.	190	4.0	17.0	12.0	m.q.	0	490	2.0 d
and water chestnuts Oriental (*The*								
Budget Gourmet Side Dish),								
5 oz.	120	5.0	15.0	3.0	m.q.	5	240	m.q.
PEAS, PIGEON, see "Pigeon pea"								
PEAS, PURPLE HULL,								
CANNED:								
(*Allens* Fresh), ½ cup	100	6.0	16.0	<1.0	(0)	0	370	m.q.
PEAS, PURPLE HULL,								
FROZEN:								
(*Frosty Acres*), 3.3 oz.	130	9.0	23.0	0	0	0	6	m.q.
PEAS, SNOW, see "Peas, edible-								
podded"								
PEAS, SPLIT, see "Split pea"								
PEAS, SPROUTED, mature seeds:								
raw:								
1 lb.	581	39.9	128.2	3.1	.6	0	89	12.6 c
1 oz.	36	2.5	8.0	.2	<.1	0	6	.8 c
½ cup	77	5.3	17.0	.4	.1	0	12	1.7 c
boiled, drained, 4 oz.	134	8.0	24.8	.6	.1	0	3	3.7 d
PEAS, SUGAR SNAP, see "Peas,								
edible-podded"								
PEAS, WHITE ACRE, canned:								
fresh (*Allens*), ½ cup	90	7.0	14.0	<1.0	(0)	0	440	m.q.
PEAS AND CARROTS,								
CANNED, ½ cup, except								
as noted:								
(*Finast*)	55	3.0	9.0	0	0	0	315	m.q.
(*Kohl's*)	50	3.0	20.0	<1.0	(0)	0	330	m.q.
(*Pathmark*)	60	3.0	18.0	1.0	(0)	0	330	m.q.
(*S&W*)	50	3.0	9.0	0	0	0	310	m.q.
(*S&W/Nutradiet*)	35	2.0	7.0	0	0	0	5	m.q.
(*Stokely*)	50	3.0	9.0	0	0	0	320	m.q.
w/liquid:								
4 oz.	43	2.5	9.6	.3	.1	0	295	1.3 c
½ cup	48	2.8	10.9	.4	.1	0	332	1.5 c
(*Del Monte*)	50	2.0	10.0	0	0	0	355	m.q.
low-sodium, 4 oz.	43	2.5	9.6	.3	.1	0	5	1.3 c
low-sodium	48	2.8	10.9	.4	.1	0	5	1.5 c
diced carrots (*Stokely* No Salt or								
Sugar Added)	45	3.0	8.0	0	0	0	20	m.q.
sliced carrots (*Stokely* No Salt or								
Sugar Added)	45	3.0	8.0	0	0	0	25	m.q.
early June (*A&P* No Salt Added) . . .	60	4.0	12.0	<1.0	(0)	0	10	m.q.

Food and Measure	cal.	prot. (gms)	carbo. (gms)	tot. fat (gms)	sat. fat (gms)	chol. (mgs)	sod. (mgs)	fiber (gms)
mixed sizes (*A&P*)	60	4.0	12.0	<1.0	(0)	0	10	m.q.
PEAS AND CARROTS, FROZEN:								
10-oz. pkg.	150	9.7	31.7	1.3	.2	0	225	4.3 c
boiled, drained, 4 oz.	54	3.5	11.5	.5	.1	0	77	1.6 c
boiled, drained, ½ cup	38	2.5	8.1	.3	.1	0	55	1.1 c
(*A&P*), 3.3 oz.	60	3.0	11.0	<1.0	(0)	0	75	m.q.
(*Frosty Acres*), 3.3 oz.	60	3.0	11.0	0	0	0	75	1.0 c
(*Seabrook*), 3.3 oz.	60	3.0	11.0	0	0	0	75	1.0 c
(*Southern*), 3.5 oz.	64	3.2	11.7	0	0	0	80	m.q.
sweet (*A&P*), ½ cup	80	5.0	13.0	<1.0	(0)	0	90	m.q.
PEAS AND ONIONS, CANNED,								
w/liquid:								
4 oz.	58	3.7	9.7	.4	.1	0	501	1.4 c
½ cup	30	2.0	5.1	.2	<.1	0	265	.7 c
w/pearl onions (*Green Giant*)	50	4.0	11.0	0	0	0	510	4.0 d
w/tiny pearl onions (*S&W*)	60	3.0	10.0	1.0	(0)	0	490	m.q.
PEAS AND ONIONS, FROZEN:								
10-oz. pkg.	199	11.3	38.4	.9	.2	0	n.a.	m.q.
(*Seabrook*), 3.3 oz.	70	4.0	13.0	0	0	0	n.a.	m.q.
boiled, drained, 4 oz.	51	2.9	9.8	.2	<.1	0	n.a.	m.q.
boiled, drained, ½ cup	40	2.3	7.8	.2	<.1	0	n.a.	m.q.
and pearl onions:								
(*Birds Eye* Combinations), 3.3 oz.	70	5.0	13.0	0	0	0	440	3.0 d
(*Frosty Acres*), 3.3 oz.	70	4.0	13.0	0	0	0	80	m.q.
w/cheese sauce (*Birds Eye* Cheese								
Sauce Combinations), 5 oz. ...	140	6.0	17.0	5.0	m.q.	5	470	3.0 d
PECAN[1]:								
halves, pieces, or chips (*Planters*),								
1 oz.	190	2.0	5.0	20.0	2.0	0	0	m.q.
dried:								
in shell, 1 lb.	1604	18.6	43.8	162.6	13.0	0	3	15.6 d
1 oz., approx. 31 large, 20 jumbo								
or 16 mammoth halves	190	2.2	5.2	19.2	1.5	0	tr.	1.8 d
halves, 1 cup	721	8.4	19.7	73.1	5.9	0	1	7.0 d
chopped, 1 cup	794	9.2	21.7	80.5	6.4	0	1	7.7 d
ground, 1 cup	634	7.4	17.3	64.3	5.1	0	1	6.2 d
dry-roasted, 1 oz.	187	2.3	6.3	18.4	1.5	0	tr.	.5 c
dry-roasted, salted, 1 oz.	187	2.3	6.3	18.4	1.5	0	221	.5 c
oil-roasted:								
1 oz., approx. 15 halves	195	2.0	4.6	20.2	1.6	0	tr.	.5 c
1 cup	754	7.7	17.7	78.3	6.3	0	1	1.8 c
salted, 1 oz.	195	2.0	4.6	20.2	1.6	0	214	.5 c
salted, 1 cup	754	7.7	17.7	78.3	6.3	0	832	1.8 c
PECAN FLOUR:								
1 oz.	93	9.1	14.4	.4	<.1	0	tr.	.4 c
PECAN TOPPING:								
in syrup (*Smucker's*), 2 tbsp.	130	2.0	28.0	1.0	n.a.	0	0	m.q.

1. *Shelled, except as noted.*

Food and Measure	cal.	prot. (gms)	carbo. (gms)	tot. fat (gms)	sat. fat (gms)	chol. (mgs)	sod. (mgs)	fiber (gms)
PEPEAO, see "Jew's-ear"								
PEPPER, ground:								
coarse grind (*Tone's Mr. Pepper*),								
1 tsp.	8	.3	2.0	<.1	<.1	0	1	.5 d
fine grind (*Tone's Mr. Pepper*), 1 tsp.	8	.3	1.9	.1	<.1	0	1	.4 d
black:								
1 oz.	72	3.1	18.4	.9	.4	0	12	3.7 c
1 tbsp.	16	.7	4.2	.2	.1	0	3	.8 c
1 tsp.	5	.2	1.4	.1	<.1	0	1	.3 c
(*Spice Islands*), 1 tsp.	9	.2	1.5	.2	(0)	0	<1	.2 c
chili (*Spice Islands*), 1 tsp.	9	.3	1.2	.3	(0)	0	<1	.3 c
red or cayenne:								
1 oz.	90	3.4	16.1	4.9	.9	0	9	7.1 c
1 tbsp.	17	.6	3.0	.9	.2	0	2	1.3 c
1 tsp.	6	.2	1.0	.3	.1	0	1	.5 c
(*Spice Islands*), 1 tsp.	9	.3	1.1	.3	(0)	0	<1	.5 c
white:								
1 oz.	84	2.9	19.5	.6	n.a.	0	1	1.2 c
1 tbsp.	21	.7	4.9	.2	(0)	0	tr.	.3 c
1 tsp.	7	.3	1.7	.1	(0)	0	tr.	.1 c
(*Spice Islands*), 1 tsp.	9	.3	1.5	.2	(0)	0	<1	.1 c
seasoned:								
(*Lawry's*), 1 tsp.	9	.3	1.8	.1	(0)	0	5	.2 c
(*McCormick/Schilling* All Pepper),								
¼ tsp.	1	<.1	.3	0	0	0	106	m.q.
lemon, see "Lemon pepper seasoning"								
PEPPER, BELL, see "Pepper, sweet"								
PEPPER, CHERRY:								
hot:								
(*Progresso*), ½ cup	190	0	3.0	20.0	3.0	0	130	1.0 d
(*Vlasic*), 1 oz.	10	0	2.0	0	0	0	425	m.q.
pickled (*Progresso*), ½ cup	130	0	3.0	12.0	2.0	0	110	1.0 d
mild (*Vlasic*), 1 oz.	8	0	2.0	0	0	0	410	m.q.
PEPPER, CHILI, HOT:								
green and red, raw:								
untrimmed, 1 lb.	134	6.6	31.3	.7	.1	0	23	6.0 c
trimmed, 1 oz.	11	.6	2.7	.1	tr.	0	2	.5 c
1 medium, approx. 1.6 oz.	18	.9	4.3	.1	tr.	0	3	.8 c
chopped, ½ cup	30	1.5	7.1	.2	<.1	0	5	1.4 c
PEPPER, CHILI, HOT, CANNED:								
green and red, seeded, w/liquid:								
4 oz.	28	1.0	6.9	.1	<.1	0	m.q.	1.4 c
1 medium, approx. 2.6 oz.	18	.7	4.5	.1	tr.	0	m.q.	.9 c
chopped, ½ cup	17	.6	4.2	.1	tr.	0	m.q.	.8 c

Food and Measure	cal.	prot. (gms)	carbo. (gms)	tot. fat (gms)	sat. fat (gms)	chol. (mgs)	sod. (mgs)	fiber (gms)
green:								
whole or diced, w/liquid (*Del*								
Monte), ½ cup	20	0	5.0	0	0	0	690	m.q.
whole (*Old El Paso*), 1 chili	8	<1.0	1.0	<1.0	n.a.	0	105	m.q.
whole, diced, sliced, or strips								
(*Ortega*), 1 oz.	10	0	3.0	0	0	0	20	m.q.
chopped (*Old El Paso*), 2 tbsp. ...	8	<1.0	2.0	<1.0	n.a.	0	70	m.q.
PEPPER, GREEN, see "Pepper,								
sweet"								
PEPPER, HOT (see also specific								
listings):								
whole or diced (*Ortega*), 1 oz.	8	0	2.0	0	0	0	m.q.	m.q.
tiny, Mexican (*Vlasic*), 1 oz.	6	0	2.0	0	0	0	430	m.q.
PEPPER, JALAPENO, canned or								
in jars:								
w/liquid, 4 oz.	27	.9	5.6	.7	.1	0	1659	2.6 c
w/liquid, chopped, ½ cup	17	.5	3.3	.4	<.1	0	995	1.6 c
whole:								
(*Old El Paso*), 2 peppers	14	0	1.0	1.0	(0)	0	480	m.q.
or diced (*Ortega*), 1 oz.	10	0	3.0	0	0	0	20	m.q.
or sliced, w/liquid (*Del Monte*),								
½ cup	30	1.0	6.0	1.0	(0)	0	1690	m.q.
hot Mexican (*Vlasic*), 1 oz.	8	0	2.0	0	0	0	380	m.q.
marinated (*La Victoria*), 1 tbsp.	4	<1.0	1.0	<1.0	(0)	0	251	m.q.
nacho (*La Victoria*), 1 tbsp.	2	<1.0	1.0	<1.0	(0)	0	335	m.q.
PEPPER, PEPPERONCINI:								
mild Greek salad (*Vlasic*), 1 oz.	4	0	1.0	0	0	0	450	m.q.
Tuscan (*Progresso*), ½ cup	20	0	7.0	0	0	0	5	1.0 d
PEPPER, PICCALILLI:								
(*Progresso*), ½ cup	190	<1.0	4.0	20.0	3.0	0	220	1.0 d
PEPPER, STUFFED, ENTREE,								
frozen:								
green, w/beef, in tomato sauce								
(*Stouffer's*), 7¾ oz.	200	11.0	19.0	9.0	m.q.	m.q.	940	m.q.
sweet red (*Celentano*), 13 oz.	350	28.0	28.0	20.0	m.q.	m.q.	810	m.q.
PEPPER, SWEET, green and red:								
raw:								
untrimmed, 1 lb.	99	3.3	23.9	.7	.1	0	7	6.0 d
trimmed, 1 oz.	8	.3	1.8	.1	<.1	0	<1	.5 d
1 medium, 3¾" × 3" diam.,								
approx. 3.2 oz.	20	.7	4.8	.1	<.1	0	1	1.2 d
chopped, ½ cup	13	.4	3.2	.1	<.1	0	1	.8 d
boiled, drained:								
4 oz.	32	1.0	7.6	.2	<.1	0	2	.5 c
1 medium, approx. 2.6 oz.	20	.7	4.9	.1	<.1	0	1	.3 c
chopped, ½ cup	19	.6	4.6	.1	<.1	0	1	.3 c
PEPPER, SWEET, CANNED (see								
also "Pimiento"):								
w/liquid, 4 oz.	20	.9	4.4	.3	.1	0	1552	.9 c

Food and Measure	cal.	prot. (gms)	carbo. (gms)	tot. fat (gms)	sat. fat (gms)	chol. (mgs)	sod. (mgs)	fiber (gms)
PEPPER, SWEET, CANNED *(cont.)*								
w/liquid, halves, ½ cup	13	.6	2.7	.2	<.1	0	958	.6 c
(*Heinz* Sweet Pepper Mementos),								
1 oz.	6	0	1.0	0	0	0	320	m.q.
fried (*Progresso*), ½ jar	37	<1.0	4.0	3.0	<1.0	0	17	1.0 d
roasted (*Progresso*), ½ cup	20	<1.0	5.0	<1.0	<1.0	0	2	1.7 d
PEPPER, SWEET, FREEZE-DRIED:								
1 oz.	89	5.1	19.5	.9	.1	0	55	4.6 c
¼ cup	5	.3	1.1	.1	tr.	0	3	.3 c
1 tbsp.	1	.1	.3	<.1	tr.	0	1	<.1 c
PEPPER, SWEET, FROZEN:								
10-oz. pkg.	58	3.1	12.6	.6	.1	0	15	2.8 c
boiled, drained, chopped, 4 oz.	20	1.1	4.4	.2	<.1	0	5	1.0 c
green (*Seabrook*), 1 oz.	6	0	1.0	0	0	0	1	m.q.
red (*Seabrook*), 1 oz.	8	0	1.0	0	0	0	n.a.	m.q.
PEPPER RINGS:								
hot, banana (*Vlasic*), 1 oz.	4	0	1.0	0	0	0	465	m.q.
PEPPER SAUCE, HOT:								
(*Gebhardt* Louisiana Style), ½ tsp. ...	0	0	(0)	0	0	0	45	(0)
(*Tabasco*), ¼ tsp.	<1	tr.	<1.0	tr.	(0)	0	9	(0)
PEPPER STEAK, see "Beef dinner, frozen" and "Beef entree, frozen"								
PEPPERED LOAF:								
(*Eckrich*), 1-oz. slice	35	5.0	2.0	1.0	m.q.	m.q.	340	(0)
(*Kahn's*), 1 slice	40	5.0	1.0	2.0	m.q.	m.q.	340	(0)
(*Oscar Mayer*), 1-oz. slice	39	5.1	1.2	1.5	.8	14	367	(0)
pork and beef, 1-oz. slice, 4" × 4" × ³⁄₃₂"	42	4.9	1.3	1.8	.7	13	432	(0)
PEPPERONI:								
(*Hickory Farms*), 1 oz.	140	6.0	1.0	13.0	m.q.	23	578	0
(*Hormel*), 1 oz.	140	6.0	0	13.0	m.q.	m.q.	462	0
(*Hormel* Chunk), 1 oz.	140	6.0	0	12.0	m.q.	m.q.	423	0
(*Hormel* Leoni Brand), 1 oz.	130	6.0	0	12.0	m.q.	m.q.	508	0
(*Hormel* Perma-Fresh), 2 slices	80	3.0	0	7.0	m.q.	m.q.	281	0
(*Hormel* Rosa), 1 oz.	140	6.0	0	13.0	m.q.	m.q.	626	0
(*Hormel* Rosa Grande), 1 oz.	140	6.0	0	13.0	m.q.	m.q.	512	0
(*JM*), 8 slices, approx. ½ oz.	70	3.0	1.0	6.0	m.q.	m.q.	290	0
pork and beef:								
1 oz.	141	6.0	.8	12.5	4.6	m.q.	578	0
1 sausage, 10¼" long × 1⅜", approx. 9 oz.	1248	52.6	7.1	110.4	40.5	m.q.	5120	0
1 slice, 1⅜" diam. × ⅛", approx. .2 oz.	27	1.2	.2	2.4	.9	m.q.	112	0
PEPPERONI BITS:								
(*Hormel*), 1 tbsp.	35	2.0	0	3.0	m.q.	m.q.	m.q.	0

Food and Measure	cal.	prot. (gms)	carbo. (gms)	tot. fat (gms)	sat. fat (gms)	chol. (mgs)	sod. (mgs)	fiber (gms)
PERCH, mixed species, meat only:								
raw:								
1 lb.	413	87.9	0	4.2	.8	407	280	0
1 oz.	26	5.5	0	.3	<.1	26	18	0
1 fillet, approx. 2.1 oz., yield from								
¾-lb. whole fish	54	11.4	0	.5	.1	53	36	0
baked, broiled, or microwaved[1],								
4 oz.	133	28.2	0	1.3	.3	130	90	0
PERCH, FROZEN:								
(*Booth*), 4 oz.	100	20.0	0	1.0	m.q.	m.q.	90	0
(*SeaPak*), 4 oz.	100	19.0	0	2.0	m.q.	m.q.	80	0
PERCH, OCEAN, see "Ocean perch"								
PERCH ENTREE, frozen:								
battered (*Van de Kamp's*), 2 pieces	310	12.0	18.0	21.0	4.0	30	500	m.q.
PERSIMMON:								
Japanese:								
fresh:								
untrimmed, 1 lb.	268	2.2	70.8	.7	n.a.	0	6	5.6 c
trimmed, 1 oz.	20	.2	5.3	.1	(0)	0	<1	.4 c
1 medium, 2½″ × 3½″, approx.								
7.1 oz.	118	1.0	31.2	.3	(0)	0	3	2.5 c
dried, 1 oz.	78	.4	20.8	.2	(0)	0	1	1.0 c
dried, 1 medium, approx. 1.3 oz.	93	.5	25.0	.2	(0)	0	1	1.2 c
native, fresh:								
untrimmed, 1 lb.	472	3.0	124.6	1.5	n.a.	0	4	5.6 c
trimmed, 1 oz.	36	.2	9.5	.1	(0)	0	<1	.4 c
1 medium, approx. 1.1 oz.	32	.2	8.4	.1	(0)	0	tr.	.4 c
PESTO SAUCE:								
mix (*French's Pasta Toss*), 2 tsp. dry	20	1.0	1.0	1.0	n.a.	n.a.	280	m.q.
refrigerated (*Contadina Fresh*),								
2⅓ oz.	350	6.0	6.0	34.0	m.q.	10	420	m.q.
PHEASANT, fresh, raw:								
meat, w/skin:								
½ pheasant, 14.1 oz., yield from								
1 lb. w/bone	723	90.8	0	37.2	10.8	m.q.	161	0
1 lb.	821	103.0	0	42.1	12.2	m.q.	181	0
1 oz.	51	6.4	0	2.6	.8	m.q.	11	0
meat only:								
½ pheasant, 12.4 oz., yield from								
1 lb. w/bone and skin	470	83.0	0	12.8	4.4	m.q.	131	0
1 lb.	603	106.9	0	16.5	5.6	m.q.	168	0
1 oz.	38	6.7	0	1.0	.4	m.q.	10	0
breast, ½ breast, approx. 6.4 oz.	243	44.4	0	5.9	2.0	m.q.	60	0
breast, 1 oz.	38	6.9	0	.9	.3	m.q.	9	0
leg, 1 leg, approx. 3.8 oz.	143	23.8	0	4.6	1.6	m.q.	48	0
leg, 1 oz.	38	6.3	0	1.2	.4	m.q.	13	0

1. *Without added ingredients.*

Food and Measure	cal.	prot. (gms)	carbo. (gms)	tot. fat (gms)	sat. fat (gms)	chol. (mgs)	sod. (mgs)	fiber (gms)
PICANTE SAUCE (see also "Salsa"):								
(*Estee*), 2 tbsp.	8	<1.0	2.0	0	0	0	60	m.q.
(*Gebhardt*), 1 tbsp.	4	0	1.0	0	0	0	120	m.q.
(*Pace*), 2 tsp.	3	.1	.6	.1	(0)	0	111	m.q.
(*Wise*), 2 tbsp.	12	0	3.0	0	0	0	130	m.q.
all varieties (*Old El Paso*), 2 tbsp.	8	<1.0	2.0	<1.0	n.a.	0	310	m.q.
all varieties (*Old El Paso* Chunky), 2 tbsp.	7	0	2.0	0	0	0	270	m.q.
mild (*Azteca*), 1 tbsp.	4	0	1.0	0	0	0	85	m.q.
mild (*Rosarita* Chunky), 3.5 oz.	45	2.0	9.0	<1.0	n.a.	0	1015	m.q.
PICCALILLI, see "Relish"								
PICKLE:								
bread and butter:								
(*Vlasic* Deli), 1 oz.	25	0	6.0	0	0	0	120	m.q.
slices:								
(*Claussen* Bread 'n Butter), 1 oz.	20	.2	4.7	.1	(0)	0	172	m.q.
(*Claussen* Bread 'n Butter), .4-oz. piece	7	.1	1.7	tr.	(0)	0	61	m.q.
(*Heinz* Cucumber Slices), 1 oz.	25	0	6.0	0	0	0	170	m.q.
(*Mrs. Fanning's*), 2 slices, approx. ⅔ oz.	16	0	3.0	0	0	0	140	m.q.
chunks (*Vlasic* Old-Fashion), 1 oz.	25	0	6.0	0	0	0	120	m.q.
sweet (*Vlasic* Sweet Butter Chips), 1 oz.	30	0	7.0	0	0	0	160	m.q.
sweet (*Vlasic* Sweet Butter Stix), 1 oz.	18	0	5.0	0	0	0	110	m.q.
dill:								
1 lb.	81	2.8	18.7	.9	.2	0	5813	5.4 d
1 oz.	5	.2	1.2	.1	<.1	0	363	.3 d
1 medium, 3¾" long, approx. 2.3 oz.	12	.4	2.7	.1	<.1	0	833	.8 d
1 slice, approx. .2 oz.	1	<.1	.3	<.1	tr.	0	77	.1 d
(*Vlasic* Original), 1 oz.	4	0	1.0	0	0	0	375	m.q.
whole:								
(*Featherweight*), 1 piece	4	0	1.0	0	0	0	5	m.q.
(*Heinz* Genuine), 1 oz.	2	0	0	0	0	0	420	m.q.
processed (*Heinz*), 1 oz.	2	0	0	0	0	0	435	m.q.
halves (*Heinz* Deli Style), 1 oz.	4	0	1.0	0	0	0	280	m.q.
halves (*Vlasic* Deli), 1 oz.	4	0	1.0	0	0	0	290	m.q.
spears (*Claussen*), 1 oz.	4	.1	.5	.1	(0)	0	330	m.q.
spears (*Claussen*), 1.1-oz. piece	4	.2	.6	.1	(0)	0	373	m.q.
hamburger chips, half salt (*Vlasic*), 1 oz.	2	0	1.0	0	0	0	175	m.q.
hamburger slices (*Heinz*), 1 oz.	2	0	0	0	0	0	405	m.q.
kosher:								
whole or spears (*Heinz*), 1 oz.	4	0	1.0	0	0	0	295	m.q.
spears (*Vlasic*), 1 oz.	4	0	1.0	0	0	0	175	m.q.

Food and Measure	cal.	prot. (gms)	carbo. (gms)	tot. fat (gms)	sat. fat (gms)	chol. (mgs)	sod. (mgs)	fiber (gms)
baby (*Heinz*), 1 oz.	4	0	1.0	0	0	0	285	m.q.
baby, crunchy, or gherkins								
(*Vlasic*), 1 oz.	4	0	1.0	0	0	0	210	m.q.
chips (*Heinz*), 1 oz.	4	0	1.0	0	0	0	275	m.q.
chunks, snack (*Vlasic*), 1 oz. ..	4	0	1.0	0	0	0	220	m.q.
half salt, crunchy (*Vlasic*), 1 oz.	4	0	1.0	0	0	0	125	m.q.
half salt, spears (*Vlasic*), 1 oz.	4	0	1.0	0	0	0	120	m.q.
low sodium:								
1 lb.	81	2.8	18.7	.9	.2	0	82	5.4 d
1 oz.	5	.2	1.2	.1	<.1	0	5	.3 d
1 medium, 3¾″ long, approx.								
2.3 oz.	12	.4	2.7	.1	<.1	0	12	.8 d
1 slice, approx. .2 oz.	1	<.1	.3	<.1	tr.	0	1	.1 d
no garlic:								
(*Claussen*), 1 oz.	6	.2	1.0	.1	(0)	0	313	m.q.
(*Claussen*), 2.9-oz. piece	17	.6	2.8	.3	(0)	0	895	m.q.
spears (*Vlasic*), 1 oz.	4	0	1.0	0	0	0	210	m.q.
Polish snack chunks (*Vlasic*), 1 oz.	4	0	1.0	0	0	0	300	m.q.
Polish style, whole (*Heinz*), 1 oz.	4	0	1.0	0	0	0	285	m.q.
Polish style, spears (*Heinz*), 1 oz.	4	0	1.0	0	0	0	285	m.q.
zesty, spears (*Vlasic*), 1 oz.	4	0	1.0	0	0	0	230	m.q.
zesty crunchy (*Vlasic*), 1 oz.	4	0	1.0	0	0	0	250	m.q.
zesty snack chunks (*Vlasic*), 1 oz.	4	0	1.0	0	0	0	290	m.q.
kosher (see also "dill," above):								
whole:								
(*Claussen*), 1 oz.	3	.2	.5	.1	(0)	0	332	m.q.
(*Claussen*), 2.5-oz. piece	9	.4	1.3	.2	(0)	0	832	m.q.
(*Heinz* Old Fashioned), 1 oz. ...	4	0	1.0	0	0	0	280	m.q.
halves:								
(*Claussen*), 1 oz.	4	.1	.5	.1	(0)	0	330	m.q.
(*Claussen*), 2.3-oz. piece	9	.3	1.3	.2	(0)	0	769	m.q.
(*Heinz* Old Fashioned Deli								
Halves), 1 oz.	4	0	1.0	0	0	0	275	m.q.
slices (*Claussen*), 1 oz.	3	.1	.5	.1	(0)	0	319	m.q.
slices (*Claussen*), .3-oz. piece ...	1	tr.	.2	tr.	(0)	0	107	m.q.
chips (*Heinz* Old Fashioned),								
1 oz.	4	0	1.0	0	0	0	270	m.q.
mixed, garden, hot and spicy								
(*Vlasic*), 1 oz.	4	0	1.0	0	0	0	380	m.q.
salad cubes, sweet (*Heinz*), 1 oz. ...	30	0	7.0	0	0	0	270	m.q.
sour:								
1 lb.	48	1.5	10.2	.9	.2	0	5477	2.8 c
1 oz.	3	.1	.6	.1	<.1	0	342	.2 c
1 medium, 3¾″ long, approx.								
1.2 oz.	4	.1	.8	.1	<.1	0	423	.2 c
1 slice, approx. .25 oz.	1	<.1	.2	<.1	tr.	0	85	<.1 c
low sodium:								
1 lb.	48	1.5	10.2	.9	.2	0	82	2.8 c
1 oz.	3	.1	.6	.1	<.1	0	5	.2 c

Food and Measure	cal.	prot. (gms)	carbo. (gms)	tot. fat (gms)	sat. fat (gms)	chol. (mgs)	sod. (mgs)	fiber (gms)
PICKLE, SOUR, LOW SODIUM *(cont.)*								
1 medium, 3¾″ long, approx.								
1.2 oz.	4	.1	.8	.1	<.1	0	6	.2 c
1 slice, approx. .25 oz.	1	<.1	.2	<.1	tr.	0	1	<.1 c
sweet:								
1 lb.	529	1.7	144.3	1.2	.3	0	4257	5.0 d
1 oz.	33	.1	9.0	.1	<.1	0	266	.3 d
1 large, 3″ long, approx. 1.2 oz.	41	.1	11.1	.1	<.1	0	328	.4 d
1 slice, approx. .2 oz.	7	<.1	1.9	<.1	tr.	0	56	.1 d
(Heinz), 1 oz.	35	0	8.0	0	0	0	210	m.q.
(Heinz Cucumber Stix), 1 oz.	25	0	6.0	0	0	0	145	m.q.
gherkins *(Heinz)*, 1 oz.	35	0	8.0	0	0	0	210	m.q.
gherkins, midget *(Heinz)*, 1 oz.	35	0	8.0	0	0	0	205	m.q.
half salt *(Vlasic* Sweet Butter								
Chips), 1 oz.	30	0	7.0	0	0	0	80	m.q.
low sodium:								
1 lb.	529	1.7	144.3	1.2	.3	0	82	5.0 d
1 oz.	33	.1	9.0	.1	<.1	0	5	.3 d
1 large, 3″ long, approx. 1.2 oz.	41	.1	11.1	.1	<.1	0	6	.4 d
1 slice, approx. .2 oz.	7	<.1	1.9	<.1	tr.	0	1	.1 d
mixed *(Heinz)*, 1 oz.	40	0	9.0	0	0	0	200	m.q.
sliced:								
(Featherweight), 3–4 slices	24	0	6.0	0	0	0	5	m.q.
(Heinz), 1 oz.	35	0	8.0	0	0	0	205	m.q.
(Heinz Cucumber Slices), 1 oz.	20	0	5.0	0	0	0	195	m.q.
PICKLE LOAF:								
(Eckrich), 1-oz. slice	80	3.0	2.0	6.0	m.q.	m.q.	270	(0)
(Eckrich Smorgas Pac), 1-oz. slice	80	3.0	2.0	6.0	m.q.	m.q.	270	(0)
(Hormel Perma-Fresh), 2 slices	102	8.0	3.0	7.0	m.q.	m.q.	752	(0)
(Kahn's), 1 slice	80	3.0	2.0	7.0	m.q.	m.q.	280	(0)
(Kahn's Family Pack), 1 slice	70	3.0	2.0	6.0	m.q.	m.q.	220	(0)
(Light & Lean), 2 slices	100	8.0	3.0	6.0	m.q.	m.q.	m.q.	(0)
(OHSE), 1 oz.	60	3.0	2.0	4.0	m.q.	m.q.	330	(0)
beef *(Kahn's* Family Pack), 1 slice	60	2.0	1.0	5.0	m.q.	m.q.	210	(0)
PICKLE AND PIMIENTO LOAF:								
(Oscar Mayer), 1-oz. slice	66	3.1	4.1	4.1	1.5	13	370	m.q.
pork, 1-oz. slice, 4″ × 4″ × ³⁄₃₂″	74	3.3	1.7	6.0	2.2	10	394	m.q.
PICKLE RELISH, see "Relish"								
PICKLING SPICE:								
(Tone's), 1 tsp.	10	.3	1.2	.6	.1	0	1	.3 d
PICNIC LOAF:								
(Oscar Mayer), 1-oz. slice	61	4.3	1.2	4.3	1.6	16	337	0
pork and beef, 1-oz. slice, 4″ ×								
4″ × ³⁄₃₂″	66	4.2	1.4	4.7	1.7	11	330	0
PIE, FROZEN (see also "Cobbler"								
and "Pie, snack"):								
apple:								
(Banquet Family Size), ⅙ pie,								
3⅓ oz.	250	2.0	37.0	11.0	m.q.	n.a.	290	m.q.

Food and Measure	cal.	prot. (gms)	carbo. (gms)	tot. fat (gms)	sat. fat (gms)	chol. (mgs)	sod. (mgs)	fiber (gms)
(*Mrs. Smith's "Pie In Minutes"*),								
⅛ of 8" pie	210	2.0	29.0	9.0	2.0	0	250	m.q.
(*Pet-Ritz*), ⅙ pie	330	2.0	53.0	12.0	m.q.	n.a.	385	m.q.
(*Sara Lee* Homestyle), ⅒ of 9" pie	280	2.0	42.0	12.0	m.q.	0	220	m.q.
(*Sara Lee* Homestyle High), ⅒ of								
10" pie	400	3.0	46.0	23.0	m.q.	0	450	m.q.
(*Weight Watchers*), ½ pkg.,								
3.5 oz.	200	2.0	39.0	5.0	1.0	5	280	m.q.
Dutch (*Sara Lee* Homestyle),								
⅒ of 9" pie	300	2.0	45.0	12.0	m.q.	0	310	m.q.
streusel (*Sara Lee Free & Light*),								
⅛ pie	170	1.0	36.0	2.0	m.q.	0	140	m.q.
banana cream:								
(*Banquet*), ⅙ pie, 2⅓ oz.	180	2.0	21.0	10.0	m.q.	n.a.	150	m.q.
(*Pet-Ritz*), ⅙ pie, 2⅓ oz.	170	2.0	22.0	9.0	m.q.	n.a.	155	m.q.
blackberry (*Banquet* Family Size),								
⅙ pie, 3⅓ oz.	270	3.0	40.0	11.0	m.q.	n.a.	350	m.q.
blueberry:								
(*Banquet* Family Size), ⅙ pie,								
3⅓ oz.	270	3.0	40.0	11.0	m.q.	n.a.	350	m.q.
(*Mrs. Smith's "Pie In Minutes"*),								
⅛ of 8" pie	220	2.0	32.0	9.0	2.0	0	240	m.q.
(*Pet-Ritz*), ⅙ pie	370	3.0	50.0	12.0	m.q.	n.a.	330	m.q.
(*Sara Lee* Homestyle), ⅒ of 9" pie	300	2.0	45.0	12.0	m.q.	0	210	m.q.
Boston cream, see "Cake, frozen"								
cherry:								
(*Banquet* Family Size), ⅙ pie,								
3⅓ oz.	250	3.0	36.0	11.0	m.q.	n.a.	260	m.q.
(*Mrs. Smith's "Pie In Minutes"*),								
⅛ of 8" pie	220	2.0	32.0	9.0	2.0	0	200	m.q.
(*Pet-Ritz*), ⅙ pie	300	3.0	48.0	12.0	m.q.	n.a.	330	m.q.
(*Sara Lee* Homestyle), ⅒ of 9" pie	270	2.0	37.0	13.0	m.q.	0	270	m.q.
streusel (*Sara Lee Free & Light*),								
⅒ pie	160	2.0	34.0	2.0	m.q.	0	140	m.q.
chocolate cream:								
(*Banquet*), ⅙ pie, 2⅓ oz.	190	2.0	24.0	10.0	m.q.	n.a.	110	m.q.
(*Pet-Ritz*), ⅙ pie, 2⅓ oz.	190	1.0	27.0	8.0	m.q.	n.a.	145	m.q.
chocolate mocha (*Weight Watchers*),								
½ pkg. or 2.75 oz.	160	5.0	23.0	5.0	3.0	5	150	m.q.
coconut cream:								
(*Banquet*), ⅙ pie, 2⅓ oz.	190	2.0	22.0	11.0	m.q.	n.a.	120	m.q.
(*Pet-Ritz*), ⅙ pie, 2⅓ oz.	190	2.0	27.0	8.0	m.q.	n.a.	145	m.q.
egg custard (*Pet-Ritz*), ⅙ pie	200	5.0	28.0	8.0	m.q.	m.q.	m.q.	m.q.
lemon:								
cream (*Banquet*), ⅙ pie, 2⅓ oz.	170	2.0	23.0	9.0	m.q.	n.a.	120	m.q.
cream (*Pet-Ritz*), ⅙ pie, 2⅓ oz. ..	190	2.0	26.0	9.0	m.q.	n.a.	150	m.q.
meringue (*Mrs. Smith's*), ⅛ of								
8" pie	210	2.0	38.0	5.0	m.q.	n.a.	130	m.q.

Food and Measure	cal.	prot. (gms)	carbo. (gms)	tot. fat (gms)	sat. fat (gms)	chol. (mgs)	sod. (mgs)	fiber (gms)
PIE, FROZEN *(cont.)*								
mince (*Pet-Ritz*), ⅙ pie	280	2.0	48.0	9.0	m.q.	n.a.	m.q.	m.q.
mince (*Sara Lee* Homestyle), ⅒ of								
9″ pie	300	3.0	43.0	13.0	m.q.	0	340	m.q.
mincemeat (*Banquet* Family Size),								
⅙ pie, 3⅓ oz.	260	3.0	38.0	11.0	m.q.	n.a.	370	m.q.
Neapolitan cream (*Pet-Ritz*), ⅙ pie,								
2⅓ oz.	180	1.0	17.0	10.0		n.a.	185	m.q.
peach:								
(*Banquet* Family Size), ⅙ pie,								
3⅓ oz.	245	3.0	35.0	11.0	m.q.	n.a.	280	m.q.
(*Mrs. Smith's "Pie In Minutes"*),								
⅛ of 8″ pie	210	2.0	29.0	9.0	2.0	0	190	m.q.
(*Pet Ritz*), ⅙ pie	320	2.0	51.0	12.0	m.q.	n.a.	320	m.q.
(*Sara Lee* Homestyle), ⅒ of 9″ pie	280	2.0	41.0	12.0	m.q.	0	170	m.q.
pecan (*Mrs. Smith's "Pie In*								
Minutes"), ⅛ of 8″ pie	330	3.0	51.0	13.0	2.0	35	200	m.q.
pecan (*Sara Lee* Homestyle), ⅒ of								
9″ pie	400	4.0	56.0	18.0	m.q.	55	290	m.q.
pumpkin:								
(*Banquet* Family Size), ⅙ pie,								
3⅓ oz.	200	3.0	29.0	8.0	m.q.	n.a.	350	m.q.
(*Mrs. Smith's "Pie In Minutes"*),								
⅛ of 8″ pie	190	3.0	30.0	6.0	2.0	35	230	m.q.
(*Sara Lee* Homestyle), ⅒ of 9″ pie	240	4.0	34.0	10.0	m.q.	40	250	m.q.
custard (*Pet-Ritz*), ⅙ pie	250	4.0	39.0	9.0	m.q.	n.a.	m.q.	m.q.
raspberry (*Sara Lee* Homestyle),								
⅒ of 9″ pie	280	2.0	39.0	13.0	m.q.	0	150	m.q.
strawberry cream:								
(*Banquet*), ⅙ pie, 2⅓ oz.	170	2.0	22.0	9.0	m.q.	n.a.	120	m.q.
(*Pet-Ritz*), ⅙ pie, 2⅓ oz.	170	2.0	20.0	9.0	m.q.	n.a.	145	m.q.
sweet potato (*Pet-Ritz*), ⅙ pie	150	2.0	21.0	7.0	m.q.	n.a.	110	m.q.
PIE, SNACK, 1 piece:								
apple:								
(*Drake's*), approx. 2 oz.	210	2.0	29.0	10.0	2.0	0	135	m.q.
(*Hostess*)	430	3.0	60.0	20.0	9.0	15	390	2.0 d
(*Tastykake*), 4 oz.	296	3.0	46.0	12.3	2.6	0	339	2.5 d
Dutch (*Little Debbie*), 2.17 oz. ...	230	2.0	42.0	8.0	m.q.	<1	150	m.q.
Dutch (*Little Debbie*), 2.5 oz.	270	2.0	48.0	8.0	m.q.	<1	170	m.q.
French (*Hostess*)	430	3.0	60.0	20.0	9.0	15	390	2.0 d
French (*Tastykake*), 4.2 oz	353	3.0	63.0	10.7	2.5	0	225	1.9 d
banana cream (*Tastykake*), 4.2 oz. ..	382	5.2	53.9	16.1	5.7	26	428	1.7 d
blackberry (*Hostess*)	420	4.0	59.0	18.0	9.0	15	360	2.4 d
blueberry:								
(*Hostess*)	420	4.0	59.0	18.0	9.0	15	360	2.4 d
(*Tastykake*), 4 oz.	308	2.8	55.0	9.4	2.1	0	410	2.1 d
apple (*Drake's*), approx. 2 oz. ...	210	2.0	30.0	10.0	2.0	0	135	m.q.
cherry:								
(*Hostess*)	460	4.0	65.0	20.0	9.0	15	380	2.4 d

Food and Measure	cal.	prot. (gms)	carbo. (gms)	tot. fat (gms)	sat. fat (gms)	chol. (mgs)	sod. (mgs)	fiber (gms)
(*Tastykake*), 4 oz.	298	3.0	48.8	9.7	2.2	0	306	2.0 d
apple (*Drake's*), approx. 2 oz. ...	220	2.0	30.0	10.0	2.0	0	135	m.q.
chocolate pudding (*Hostess*)	490	5.0	76.0	19.0	m.q.	21	439	m.q.
chocolate pudding (*Tastykake*), 4.2 oz.	443	6.0	68.3	16.2	m.q.	n.a.	m.q.	m.q.
coconut creme (*Tastykake*), 4 oz. ...	377	4.9	46.0	20.2	5.2	65	416	2.3 d
lemon:								
(*Drake's*), approx. 2 oz.	210	2.0	27.0	11.0	2.0	0	115	m.q.
(*Hostess*)	440	4.0	60.0	20.0	10.0	30	370	1.4 d
(*Tastykake*), 4 oz.	319	3.6	48.1	13.2	2.9	39	375	1.7 d
lemon-lime (*Tastykake*), 4 oz.	310	3.3	54.1	8.8	m.q.	55	329	.2 d
marshmallow:								
banana (*Little Debbie*), 3 oz.	360	3.0	60.0	12.0	m.q.	<1	180	m.q.
banana or chocolate (*Little Debbie*), 1.4 oz.	170	1.0	28.0	6.0	m.q.	<1	85	m.q.
chocolate (*Little Debbie*), 3 oz. ...	370	3.0	59.0	13.0	m.q.	<1	170	m.q.
oatmeal creme (*Little Debbie*), 1.33 oz.	160	2.0	25.0	6.0	m.q.	<1	125	m.q.
oatmeal creme (*Little Debbie*), 2.75 oz.	350	4.0	51.0	14.0	m.q.	<1	260	m.q.
peach (*Hostess*)	420	4.0	60.0	19.0	9.0	15	360	2.0 d
peach (*Tastykake*), 4 oz.	310	3.3	54.1	8.8	m.q.	55	329	.2 d
pecan (*Little Debbie*), 1.83 oz.	170	2.0	37.0	2.0	m.q.	<1	200	m.q.
pecan (*Little Debbie*), 3 oz.	280	3.0	60.0	3.0	m.q.	<1	340	m.q.
pineapple cheese (*Tastykake*), 4.2 oz.	343	4.5	53.9	13.2	3.3	19	405	2.2 d
pumpkin (*Tastykake*), 4 oz.	324	4.5	46.5	14.2	4.1	28	520	1.9 d
raisin creme (*Little Debbie*), 1.17 oz.	140	1.0	21.0	6.0	m.q.	<1	90	m.q.
raisin creme (*Little Debbie*), 2.5 oz.	290	2.0	47.0	10.0	m.q.	<1	190	m.q.
strawberry (*Hostess*)	410	4.0	56.0	19.0	9.0	15	360	2.2 d
strawberry (*Tastykake*), 4 oz.	342	3.1	57.4	11.4	2.7	0	303	.6 d
(*Tastykake* Tasty Klair), 4 oz.	402	5.8	51.2	20.1	3.8	56	315	1.8 d
PIE, SNACK, FROZEN:								
Boston cream, see "Cake, snack, frozen"								
Mississippi mud (*Pepperidge Farm American Collection*), 1 ramekin	310	3.0	23.0	23.0	12.0	60	45	m.q.
PIE CRUST SHELL, frozen or refrigerated (see also "Puff pastry, frozen")								
(*Mrs. Smith's, 8"*), ⅛ shell	80	1.0	8.0	5.0	1.0	0	105	m.q.
(*Mrs. Smith's 9"*), ⅛ shell	90	1.0	10.0	5.0	1.0	0	125	m.q.
(*Mrs. Smith's 9⅝"*), ⅛ shell	120	2.0	12.0	7.0	2.0	0	160	m.q.
(*Pet-Ritz*), ⅙ shell, .83 oz.	110	1.0	11.0	7.0	m.q.	7	110	m.q.
(*Pet-Ritz, 9⅝"*), ⅙ shell, 1.25 oz. ..	170	2.0	15.0	11.0	m.q.	7	180	m.q.
(*Pillsbury All Ready*), ⅛ of 2 crust pie	240	2.0	24.0	15.0	m.q.	15	210	m.q.
all vegetable shortening (*Pet-Ritz*), ⅙ shell	110	2.0	10.0	8.0	2.0	0	60	m.q.

Food and Measure	cal.	prot. (gms)	carbo. (gms)	tot. fat (gms)	sat. fat (gms)	chol. (mgs)	sod. (mgs)	fiber (gms)
PIE CRUST SHELL *(cont.)*								
deep dish:								
(*Pet-Ritz*), ⅙ shell, 1 oz.	130	1.0	12.0	8.0	m.q.	7	120	m.q.
all vegetable shortening (*Pet-Ritz*),								
⅙ shell	140	2.0	12.0	9.0	2.0	0	75	m.q.
whole grain (*Pet-Ritz*),								
⅙ shell, 1 oz.	130	1.0	14.0	8.0	m.q.	n.a.	125	m.q.
graham cracker (*Pet-Ritz*), ⅙ shell,								
.83 oz.	110	1.0	8.0	6.0	m.q.	7	80	m.q.
PIE CRUST SHELL MIX:								
(*Betty Crocker*), 1/16 pkg.	120	1.0	10.0	8.0	2.0	0	140	m.q.
(*Flako*), 1 serving[1]	247	3.7	24.4	15.0	4.5	9	393	1.2 d
PIE CRUST STICK:								
(*Betty Crocker*), ⅛ stick	120	1.0	10.0	8.0	2.0	0	140	m.q.
PIE FILLING, canned:								
apple:								
(*Comstock*), 3.5 oz.	120	0	30.0	0	0	0	15	.4 d
(*Comstock* Lite), 3.5 oz.	80	0	20.0	0	0	0	10	.4 d
(*Lucky Leaf/Musselman's*), 4 oz.	120	0	30.0	0	0	0	60	m.q.
(*Lucky Leaf/Musselman's* Plus),								
4 oz.	121	.3	30.2	0	0	0	24	m.q.
(*Pathmark* No Frills), 4 oz.	130	0	33.0	0	0	0	60	m.q.
(*White House*), 3.5 oz.	121	0	29.0	1.0	(0)	0	44	m.q.
deluxe (*Lucky Leaf/Musselman's*),								
4 oz.	120	0	35.0	0	0	0	40	m.q.
turnover, diced (*Lucky Leaf/*								
Musselman's), 4 oz.	120	0	30.0	0	0	0	60	m.q.
apricot (*Comstock*), 3.5 oz.	110	0	29.0	0	0	0	100	.4 d
apricot (*Lucky Leaf/Musselman's*),								
4 oz.	150	0	39.0	0	0	0	90	m.q.
banana (*Comstock*), 3.5 oz.	110	1.0	22.0	2.0	(0)	0	300	.5 d
blackberry (*Lucky Leaf/*								
Musselman's), 4 oz.	120	1.0	31.0	0	0	0	140	m.q.
blackberry (*Lucky Leaf/Musselman's*								
Plus), 4 oz.	121	.9	30.1	0	0	0	20	m.q.
blueberry:								
(*Comstock*), 3.5 oz.	110	0	28.0	0	0	0	15	.5 d
(*Comstock* Lite), 3.5 oz.	75	0	17.0	0	0	0	15	.6 d
(*Lucky Leaf/Musselman's* Plus),								
4 oz.	145	.3	35.2	0	0	0	17	m.q.
(*White House*), 3.5 oz.	118	0	28.0	1.0	(0)	0	48	m.q.
cultivated (*Lucky Leaf/*								
Musselman's), 4 oz.	120	1.0	31.0	0	0	0	150	m.q.
boysenberry (*Lucky Leaf/*								
Musselman's), 4 oz.	120	1.0	31.0	0	0	0	140	m.q.
cherry:								
(*Comstock*), 3.5 oz.	110	0	28.0	0	0	0	15	.3 d
(*Comstock* Lite), 3.5 oz.	75	0	19.0	0	0	0	15	.3 d
(*Lucky Leaf/Musselman's*), 4 oz.	120	1.0	29.0	0	0	0	50	m.q.

1. *Prepared according to package directions.*

Food and Measure	cal.	prot. (gms)	carbo. (gms)	tot. fat (gms)	sat. fat (gms)	chol. (mgs)	sod. (mgs)	fiber (gms)
(*Lucky Leaf/Musselman's* Plus),								
4 oz.	108	.8	26.0	.2	(0)	0	10	m.q.
(*Pathmark* No Frills), 4 oz.	130	0	33.0	0	0	0	60	m.q.
(*White House*), 3.5 oz.	141	0	33.0	1.0	(0)	0	54	m.q.
chocolate (*Comstock*), 3.5 oz.	130	1.0	26.0	3.0	m.q.	0	240	.2 d
coconut (*Comstock*), 3.5 oz.	120	1.0	22.0	3.0	m.q.	0	290	.2 d
gooseberry (*Lucky Leaf/*								
Musselman's), 4 oz.	180	0	45.0	0	0	0	30	m.q.
lemon:								
(*Comstock*), 3.5 oz.	140	0	34.0	1.0	(0)	0	110	.1 d
(*Lucky Leaf/Musselman's*), 4 oz.	200	0	48.0	2.0	m.q.	n.a.	235	m.q.
French (*Lucky Leaf/Musselman's*),								
4 oz.	180	0	42.0	1.0	(0)	n.a.	140	m.q.
mincemeat:								
(*Comstock*), 3.5 oz.	150	0	39.0	1.0	(0)	0	180	.7 d
(*Lucky Leaf/Musselman's*), 4 oz.	190	0	48.0	1.0	(0)	n.a.	145	m.q.
w/brandy (*S&W* Old Fashioned),								
4 oz.	234	1.1	55.6	2.3	m.q.	n.a.	234	m.q.
condensed (*Borden None Such*),								
¼ pkg.	220	1.0	50.0	2.0	m.q.	n.a.	310	m.q.
ready-to-use (*Borden None Such*),								
⅓ cup	200	1.0	48.0	1.0	(0)	n.a.	280	m.q.
ready-to-use, w/brandy and rum								
(*Borden None Such*), ⅓ cup . . .	220	1.0	48.0	2.0	m.q.	n.a.	260	m.q.
peach:								
(*Comstock*), 3.5 oz.	110	0	26.0	0	0	0	20	.2 d
(*Lucky Leaf/Musselman's*), 4 oz.	150	0	37.0	0	0	0	65	m.q.
(*Lucky Leaf/Musselman's* Plus),								
4 oz.	113	.7	27.4	0	0	0	16	m.q.
(*White House*), 3.5 oz.	117	0	28.0	1.0	(0)	0	30	m.q.
pineapple (*Comstock*), 3.5 oz.	100	0	28.0	0	0	0	65	.4 d
pineapple (*Lucky Leaf/Musselman's*),								
4 oz.	110	0	30.0	0	0	0	65	m.q.
pumpkin:								
(*Comstock*), 3.5 oz.	100	0	24.0	0	0	0	180	m.q.
(*Lucky Leaf/Musselman's*), 4 oz.	170	1.0	33.0	4.0	m.q.	n.a.	200	m.q.
(*Stokely*), ½ cup	170	1.0	44.0	0	0	0	420	m.q.
pie mix:								
4 oz.	118	1.2	29.9	.1	.1	0	236	1.3 c
½ cup	141	1.5	35.6	.2	.1	0	280	1.6 c
(*Libby's*), 1 cup	260	2.0	64.0	.3	0	0	440	m.q.
raisin (*Comstock*), 3.5 oz.	120	0	32.0	0	0	0	80	m.q.
raisin (*Lucky Leaf/Musselman's*),								
4 oz.	130	1.0	34.0	1.0	(0)	n.a.	120	m.q.
raspberry, black (*Lucky Leaf/*								
Musselman's), 4 oz.	190	0	43.0	0	0	0	50	m.q.
raspberry, red (*Lucky Leaf/*								
Musselman's), 4 oz.	190	0	46.0	0	0	0	80	m.q.

Food and Measure	cal.	prot. (gms)	carbo. (gms)	tot. fat (gms)	sat. fat (gms)	chol. (mgs)	sod. (mgs)	fiber (gms)
PIE FILLING *(cont.)*								
strawberry:								
(*Comstock*), 3.5 oz.	100	0	25.0	0	0	0	20	.6 d
(*Lucky Leaf/Musselman's*), 4 oz.	120	0	30.0	0	0	0	75	m.q.
(*Lucky Leaf/Musselman's* Plus),								
4 oz.	138	.9	33.5	0	0	0	17	m.q.
strawberry-rhubarb (*Lucky Leaf/*								
Musselman's), 4 oz.	120	0	31.0	0	0	0	95	m.q.
vanilla creme (*Lucky Leaf/*								
Musselman's), 4 oz.	150	0	32.0	3.0	m.q.	n.a.	145	m.q.
PIE FILLING MIX, see "Pudding mix"								
PIE MIX[1], ⅛ pie, except as noted:								
banana cream (*Jell-O* No Bake)	240	3.0	27.0	14.0	m.q.	30	300	m.q.
chocolate:								
mint (*Royal No-Bake*)	260	5.0	25.0	15.0	m.q.	n.a.	280	m.q.
mousse (*Jell-O* No Bake)	260	4.0	25.0	17.0	m.q.	30	430	m.q.
mousse (*Royal No-Bake*)	230	4.0	27.0	12.0	m.q.	n.a.	260	m.q.
coconut cream (*Jell-O* No Bake)	260	3.0	27.0	16.0	m.q.	30	300	m.q.
lemon meringue (*Royal No-Bake*) . . .	310	3.0	50.0	11.0	m.q.	n.a.	250	m.q.
pumpkin (*Jell-O* No Bake)	250	4.0	31.0	13.0	m.q.	30	450	m.q.
pumpkin (*Libby's*), ⅙ pie	390	7.0	53.0	17.0	5.0	70	380	m.q.
PIGEON, see "Squab"								
PIGEON PEA[2]:								
raw:								
in pods, 1 lb.	296	15.7	52.0	3.6	.8	0	11	5.8 c
1 oz.	39	2.0	6.8	.5	.1	0	1	.8 c
10 peas, approx. .1 oz.	5	.3	1.0	.1	<.1	0	tr.	.1 c
½ cup	105	5.5	18.4	1.3	.3	0	4	2.1 c
boiled, drained:								
4 oz.	126	6.8	22.1	1.5	.1	0	5	3.3 c
½ cup	86	4.6	15.0	1.1	.1	0	3	2.2 c
PIGEON PEA, MATURE, dried:								
raw, 1 oz.	97	6.2	17.8	.4	.1	0	5	3.8 d
raw, ½ cup	350	22.1	64.0	1.5	.3	0	17	13.8 d
boiled, 4 oz.	137	7.8	26.4	.4	.1	0	6	5.3 d
boiled, ½ cup	102	5.7	19.5	.3	.1	0	5	3.9 d
PIGNOLIA, see "Pine nut"								
PIG'S EAR[3], frozen:								
raw, 1 oz.	66	6.4	0	4.3	m.q.	23	54	0
simmered, 4 oz.	188	18.1	0	12.2	m.q.	102	189	0
simmered, 3.9 oz., yield from 4-oz.								
raw whole ear	183	17.6	0	11.9	m.q.	99	183	0
PIG'S FEET[3]:								
raw, 1 oz.	75	6.3	0	5.3	1.8	30	18	0

1. *Prepared according to package directions.*
2. *Shelled, except as noted.*
3. *Cooked meats are prepared without added ingredients.*

Food and Measure	cal.	prot. (gms)	carbo. (gms)	tot. fat (gms)	sat. fat (gms)	chol. (mgs)	sod. (mgs)	fiber (gms)
simmered, 4 oz.	220	21.8	0	14.1	4.9	113	m.q.	0
simmered, 2.5 oz., yield from 8-oz.								
raw whole foot	138	13.6	0	8.8	3.0	71	m.q.	0
pickled:								
(*Penrose*), 1 piece, approx. 6 oz.	220	19.0	2.0	15.0	m.q.	m.q.	2890	0
cured, 1 lb.	923	61.3	.1	73.2	25.3	419	m.q.	0
cured, 1 oz.	58	3.8	<.1	4.6	1.6	26	m.q.	0
PIG'S KNUCKLES, pickled:								
(*Penrose*), 1 piece, approx. 6 oz. ...	290	23.0	1.0	21.0	m.q.	m.q.	2380	0
PIG'S TAIL[1]:								
raw, 1 oz.	107	5.0	0	9.5	3.3	28	n.a.	0
simmered, 4 oz.	449	19.3	0	40.6	14.1	146	n.a.	0
simmered, 9.7 oz., yield from 1 lb.								
raw untrimmed	1088	46.8	0	98.5	34.2	355	n.a.	0
PIKE, NORTHERN, meat only:								
raw:								
1 lb.	401	87.3	0	3.1	.5	177	177	0
1 oz.	25	5.5	0	.2	<.1	11	11	0
½ fillet, approx. 7 oz., yield from								
5-lb. whole fish	175	38.1	0	1.4	.2	77	77	0
baked, broiled, or microwaved[2],								
4 oz.	128	28.0	0	1.0	.2	57	56	0
PIKE, WALLEYE, meat only, raw:								
1 lb.	420	86.8	0	5.5	1.1	390	230	0
1 oz.	26	5.4	0	.3	<.1	24	14	0
1 fillet, approx. 5.6 oz., yield from								
2-lb. whole fish	147	30.4	0	1.9	.4	137	81	0
PILI NUT, CANARY TREE, dried:								
in shell, 1 lb.	619	9.3	3.4	68.5	26.8	0	3	2.4 c
shelled, 1 oz., approx. 15 kernels ..	204	3.1	1.1	22.6	8.9	0	1	.8 c
shelled, 1 cup	863	13.0	4.8	95.5	37.4	0	4	3.4 c
PIMIENTO, canned or in jars:								
2 oz.	13	.6	2.9	.2	<.1	0	8	.6 c
1 tbsp.	3	.1	.6	<.1	tr.	0	2	.1 c
all varieties, drained (*Dromedary*),								
1 oz.	10	0	2.0	0	0	0	5	m.q.
PIMIENTO SPREAD:								
(*Price's*), 1 oz.	80	3.0	2.0	6.0	m.q.	n.a.	m.q.	n.a.
PIÑA COLADA:								
1 fl. oz.[3]	58	.1	8.9	.6	.3	0	2	m.q.
canned, 1 fl. oz.	77	.2	9.0	2.5	2.1	0	23	m.q.
PIÑA COLADA MIX:								
bottled (*Holland House*), 1 fl. oz. ...	33	0	8.0	0	0	0	4	n.a.
instant (*Holland House*), .56 oz.	82	0	12.0	3.0	n.a.	0	<1	n.a.

1. *Cooked meats and prepared without added ingredients.*
2. *Without added ingredients.*
3. *Recipe: 44.2% canned pineapple juice, 29.7% rum, 15.7% sugar, 10.4% coconut cream.*

Food and Measure	cal.	prot. (gms)	carbo. (gms)	tot. fat (gms)	sat. fat (gms)	chol. (mgs)	sod. (mgs)	fiber (gms)
PINE NUT[1], dried:								
pignolia:								
in shell, 1 lb.	1798	83.8	49.7	177.0	27.2	0	14	2.8 c
1 oz.	146	6.8	4.0	14.4	2.2	0	1	.2 c
1 tbsp.	51	2.4	1.4	5.1	.8	0	tr.	.1 c
piñon:								
in shell, 1 lb.	1468	29.9	49.9	157.6	24.2	0	186	12.2 c
1 oz.	161	3.3	5.5	17.3	2.7	0	20	1.3 c
10 kernels	6	.1	.2	.6	.1	0	1	.1 c
PINEAPPLE:								
untrimmed, 1 lb.	117	.9	29.2	1.0	.1	0	2	2.8 d
trimmed, 1 oz.	14	.1	3.5	.1	tr.	0	<1	.3 d
sliced, 1 slice, 3½" diam. × ¾",								
approx. 3 oz.	42	.3	10.4	.4	<.1	0	1	1.0 d
sliced (*Del Monte*), 2 slices,								
3½" × ¾"	90	1.0	24.0	0	0	0	<5	m.q.
diced, ½ cup	39	.3	9.6	.3	<.1	0	<1	.9 d
PINEAPPLE, CANNED:								
(*Mott's* Pineapple Fruit Pak),								
3.75 oz.	86	0	21.0	0	0	0	2	m.q.
in water:								
4 oz.	36	.5	9.4	.1	tr.	0	1	.5 c
1 slice, 3" × 5⁄16" and 1¼ tbsp.								
liquid	19	.3	4.8	.1	tr.	0	1	.3 c
tidbits, ½ cup	40	.5	10.2	.1	tr.	0	2	.6 c
in juice:								
4 oz.	68	.5	17.8	.1	tr.	0	1	.9 d
all cuts (*Dole*), ½ cup	70	.5	17.5	.5	(0)	0	1	m.q.
slices:								
1 slice, 3" × 5⁄16" and 1¼ tbsp.								
liquid	35	.2	9.1	.1	tr.	0	1	.4 d
(*A&P*), 2 slices	70	<1.0	18.0	<1.0	(0)	0	10	m.q.
(*Featherweight*), ½ cup	70	0	18.0	0	0	0	<10	m.q.
(*S&W* 100% Hawaiian), ½ cup	70	0	17.0	0	0	0	10	m.q.
chunks, tidbits or crushed (*Del*								
Monte), ½ cup	70	0	18.0	0	0	0	<10	m.q.
spears (*Del Monte*), 2 spears,								
3.1 oz.	50	0	14.0	0	0	0	10	m.q.
chunks or crushed (*A&P*), ½ cup	70	<1.0	18.0	<1.0	(0)	0	10	m.q.
chunks or tidbits, ½ cup	75	.5	19.6	.1	tr.	0	2	.9 d
crushed (*Empress*), ½ cup	70	0	18.0	0	0	0	<10	m.q.
in syrup, all cuts (*Del Monte*), ½ cup	90	0	23.0	0	0	0	<10	m.q.
in syrup, all cuts (*Dole*), ½ cup	95	.4	24.8	.2	(0)	0	2	m.q.
in light syrup:								
4 oz.	59	.4	15.3	.1	<.1	0	1	.5 c
1 slice, 3" × 5⁄16" and 1¼ tbsp.								
liquid	30	.20	7.8	.1	tr.	0	1	.3 c

1. *Shelled, except as noted.*

Food and Measure	cal.	prot. (gms)	carbo. (gms)	tot. fat (gms)	sat. fat (gms)	chol. (mgs)	sod. (mgs)	fiber (gms)
½ cup	66	.5	16.9	.1	<.1	0	2	.6 c
in heavy syrup:								
4 oz.	88	.4	22.9	.1	<.1	0	1	.5 c
slices:								
1 slice, 3″ × ⁵⁄₁₆″ and 1¼ tbsp.								
liquid	45	.2	11.7	.1	tr.	0	1	.3 c
(A&P), 2 slices	90	<1.0	23.0	<1.0	(0)	0	10	m.q.
(S&W 100% Hawaiian), 2 slices	90	0	23.0	0	0	0	0	m.q.
chunks or crushed (A&P), ½ cup	90	<1.0	23.0	<1.0	(0)	0	10	m.q.
chunks or slices (Pathmark								
Hawaiian), ½ cup	90	0	23.0	0	0	0	10	m.q.
chunks, tidbits or crushed, ½ cup	100	.5	25.8	.1	<.1	0	2	.6 c
in extra heavy syrup:								
4 oz.	94	.4	24.4	.1	<.1	0	1	.5 c
1 slice, 3″ × ⁵⁄₁₆″ and 1¼ tbsp.								
liquid	48	.2	12.5	.1	tr.	0	1	.3 c
chunks or crushed, ½ cup	109	.4	28.0	.1	<.1	0	2	.6 c
unsweetened, spears, slices, chunks,								
or crushed, (Pathmark								
Hawaiian), ½ cup	70	0	18.0	0	0	0	10	m.q.
unsweetened, slices, (S&W/								
Nutradiet), ½ cup	60	0	15.0	0	0	0	10	m.q.
PINEAPPLE, FROZEN,								
sweetened:								
chunks, 4 oz.	96	.5	25.2	.1	tr.	0	2	.3 c
chunks, ½ cup	104	.5	27.1	.1	tr.	0	2	.4 c
PINEAPPLE DANISH, see								
"Danish pastry"								
PINEAPPLE JUICE, 6 fl. oz.,								
except as noted:								
canned, bottled, or boxed:								
1 fl. oz.	17	.1	4.3	<.1	tr.	0	tr.	<.1 c
6 fl. oz.	104	.6	25.8	.2	<.1	0	2	.2 c
(Del Monte Unsweetened)	100	0	25.0	0	0	0	<10	m.q.
(Dole)	103	.8	25.4	.2	(0)	0	2	m.q.
(IGA Unsweetened)	100	0	25.0	0	0	0	10	m.q.
(Minute Maid), 8.45 fl. oz.	139	1.1	34.1	.8	(0)	0	27	m.q.
(Minute Maid On The Go),								
10 fl. oz.	165	.3	40.4	.1	(0)	0	32	m.q.
(Mott's), 9.5-fl.-oz. can	169	0	42.0	0	0	0	0	m.q.
(Pathmark Hawaiian)	100	0	25.0	0	0	0	10	m.q.
(Pathmark No Frills								
Unsweetened)	100	0	25.0	0	0	0	0	m.q.
(S&W Unsweetened)	100	0	25.0	0	0	0	0	m.q.
(Veryfine 100%), 8 fl. oz.	125	.7	31.0	0	0	0	<10	m.q.
chilled or frozen[1]:								
(Dole)	100	0	25.0	n.a.	n.a.	0	7	m.q.

1. *Diluted according to package directions.*

Food and Measure	cal.	prot. (gms)	carbo. (gms)	tot. fat (gms)	sat. fat (gms)	chol. (mgs)	sod. (mgs)	fiber (gms)
PINEAPPLE JUICE, CHILLED OR FROZEN *(cont.)*								
(*Minute Maid*)	99	.8	24.2	.1	(0)	0	19	m.q.
frozen[1]:								
undiluted	387	2.8	95.7	.2	<.1	0	6	.7 c
1 fl. oz.	16	.1	4.0	<.1	tr.	0	tr.	<.1 c
6 fl. oz.	97	.8	23.9	.1	<.1	0	2	.2 c
PINEAPPLE NECTAR:								
(*Libby's*), 6 fl. oz.	110	0	27.0	0	0	0	30	m.q.
PINEAPPLE TOPPING:								
(*Kraft*), 1 tbsp.	50	0	13.0	0	0	0	0	m.q.
(*Smucker's*), 2 tbsp.	130	0	32.0	0	0	0	0	m.q.
PINEAPPLE-BANANA JUICE COCKTAIL:								
bottled or frozen[2] (*Welch's Orchard Tropicals*), 6 fl. oz.	100	0	24.0	0	0	0	20	0
boxed (*Welch's Orchard Tropicals Cocktails-In-A-Box*), 8.45 fl. oz.	140	0	34.0	0	0	0	20	0
PINEAPPLE-GRAPEFRUIT JUICE:								
(*Dole*), 6 fl. oz.	90	1.0	23.0	n.a.	n.a.	0	8	m.q.
(*Tropicana* 100% Pure), 8 fl. oz. ...	120	m.q.	29.3	0	0	0	3	m.q.
w/pink grapefruit (*Dole*), 6 fl. oz. ...	101	.4	25.4	.1	(0)	0	tr.	m.q.
PINEAPPLE-GRAPEFRUIT JUICE COCKTAIL:								
(*Ocean Spray*), 6 fl. oz.	110	0	26.0	0	0	0	5	m.q.
PINEAPPLE-GRAPEFRUIT JUICE DRINK:								
1 fl. oz.	15	.1	3.6	tr.	tr.	0	4	tr.c
6 fl. oz.	90	.6	21.6	.2	<.1	0	24	tr.c
(*Del Monte*), 6 fl. oz.	90	0	24.0	0	0	0	50	m.q.
(*Pathmark*), 6 fl. oz.	80	0	21.0	0	0	0	0	m.q.
(*Tropicana* Single Serve), 10 fl. oz.	159	(0)	39.0	0	0	0	<3	m.q.
(*Tropicana Twister*), 8 fl. oz.	125	(0)	32.0	0	0	0	2	m.q.
pink grapefruit (*Del Monte*), 6 fl. oz.	90	0	24.0	0	0	0	50	m.q.
PINEAPPLE-ORANGE DRINK:								
(*Veryfine*), 8 fl. oz.	130	0	32.0	0	0	0	<10	m.q.
PINEAPPLE-ORANGE JUICE:								
(*Dole*), 6 fl. oz.	100	1.0	23.0	n.a.	n.a.	0	8	m.q.
chilled or frozen[2] (*Minute Maid*), 6 fl. oz.	98	.8	23.9	.1	(0)	0	19	m.q.
PINEAPPLE-ORANGE JUICE DRINK, canned:								
1 fl. oz.	16	.4	3.7	0	0	0	1	0
6 fl. oz.	96	2.4	22.2	0	0	0	6	0
(*Del Monte*), 6 fl. oz.	90	0	24.0	0	0	0	20	0

1. *Diluted according to package directions, except as noted.*
2. *Diluted according to package directions.*

Food and Measure	cal.	prot. (gms)	carbo. (gms)	tot. fat (gms)	sat. fat (gms)	chol. (mgs)	sod. (mgs)	fiber (gms)
PINEAPPLE-ORANGE-BANANA								
JUICE:								
(*Dole*), 6 fl. oz.	90	.8	23.0	.1	(0)	0	5	m.q.
PINK BEAN:								
raw, 1 oz.	97	5.9	18.2	.3	.1	0	2	2.5 d
raw, ½ cup	361	22.0	67.4	1.2	.3	0	8	9.3 d
boiled, 4 oz.	169	10.3	31.6	.6	.1	0	2	5.0 d
boiled, ½ cup	125	7.6	23.5	.4	.1	0	2	3.7 d
PINOCCHIO, see "Pine nut,								
pignolia"								
PIÑON, see "Pine nut"								
PINTO BEAN:								
raw:								
1 oz.	96	5.9	18.0	.3	.1	0	3	3.4 d
½ cup	326	20.1	60.9	1.1	.2	0	10	11.5 d
(*Arrowhead Mills*), 2 oz.	200	13.0	36.0	1.0	n.a.	0	3	11.2 d
boiled:								
4 oz.	155	9.3	29.1	.6	.1	0	2	4.5 d
½ cup	117	7.0	21.8	.4	.1	0	1	3.4 d
(*A&P*), 1 cup	230	17.0	42.0	1.0	n.a.	0	5	n.a.
PINTO BEAN, CANNED:								
w/liquid, 4 oz.	88	5.2	16.5	.4	.1	0	472	1.4 c
w/liquid, ½ cup	93	5.5	17.5	.4	.1	0	499	1.5 c
(*Allens*), ½ cup	105	5.0	18.0	<1.0	n.a.	0	480	m.q.
(*Gebhardt*), 4 oz.	197	12.8	35.7	.5	n.a.	0	608	m.q.
(*Green Giant/Joan of Arc*), ½ cup ...	90	6.0	20.0	1.0	n.a.	0	280	5.2 d
(*Old El Paso*), ½ cup	100	6.0	19.0	0	0	0	320	8.0 d
(*Progresso*), ½ cup	110	8.0	21.0	<1.0	n.a.	0	410	6.5 d
baked style:								
w/pork (*Luck's*, 29 oz.), 7.25 oz.	220	11.0	30.0	6.0	m.q.	m.q.	520	11.0 d
w/pork (*Luck's*, 15 oz.), 7.5 oz. ..	220	12.0	30.0	6.0	m.q.	m.q.	787	7.0 d
and great northern, w/pork								
(*Luck's*), 7.25 oz.	200	12.0	29.0	5.0	m.q.	m.q.	822	m.q.
Picante style (*Green Giant/Joan of*								
Arc), ½ cup	100	7.0	21.0	1.0	n.a.	0	580	6.6 d
PINTO BEAN, FROZEN:								
10-oz. pkg.	484	27.8	92.3	1.4	.2	0	n.a.	m.q.
boiled, drained, 4 oz.	184	10.6	35.0	.5	.1	0	n.a.	m.q.
(*Seabrook*), 3.2 oz.	160	9.0	29.0	0	0	0	n.a.	m.q.
PINTO BEAN, SPROUTED,								
mature seeds:								
raw, 1 lb.	280	23.8	52.6	4.1	.5	0	694	12.3 c
raw, 1 oz.	18	1.5	3.3	.3	<.1	0	43	.8 c
boiled, drained, 4 oz.	25	2.1	4.6	.4	<.1	0	58	1.1 c
PINYON, see "Pine nut"								
PISTACHIO NUT[1]:								
dried:								
in shell, 1 lb.	1309	46.7	56.3	109.7	13.9	0	13	24.5 d

1. *Shelled, except as noted.*

Food and Measure	cal.	prot. (gms)	carbo. (gms)	tot. fat (gms)	sat. fat (gms)	chol. (mgs)	sod. (mgs)	fiber (gms)
PISTACHIO NUT, DRIED *(cont.)*								
1 oz., approx. 47 kernels	164	5.8	7.1	13.7	1.7	0	2	3.1 d
1 cup	739	26.3	31.8	61.9	7.8	0	7	13.8 d
dry-roasted:								
in shell, 1 lb.	1429	35.2	64.9	124.5	15.8	0	14	4.3 c
in shell, salted, 1 lb.	1429	35.2	64.9	124.5	15.8	0	1840	4.3 c
1 oz.	172	4.2	7.8	15.0	1.9	0	2	.5 c
1 cup	776	19.1	35.2	67.6	8.6	0	8	2.3 c
salted, 1 oz.	172	4.2	7.8	15.0	1.9	0	221	.5 c
salted, 1 cup	776	19.1	35.2	67.6	8.6	0	998	2.3 c
(Planters), 1 oz.	170	5.0	6.0	15.0	2.0	0	250	m.q.
roasted *(Dole)*, 1 oz.	163	6.0	7.0	14.0	m.q.	0	2	m.q.
PITA, see "Bread"								
PITANGUA:								
untrimmed, 1 lb.	132	3.2	29.9	1.6	n.a.	0	11	2.4 c
trimmed, 1 oz.	9	.2	2.1	.1	(0)	0	1	.2 c
trimmed, ½ cup	29	.7	6.5	.3	(0)	0	3	.5 c
1 medium, approx. .3 oz.	2	.1	.5	<.1	(0)	0	tr.	<.1 c
PIZZA, frozen:								
Canadian bacon:								
(Jeno's Crisp'n Tasty), ½ pie	250	11.0	27.0	11.0	m.q.	m.q.	880	m.q.
(Tombstone), ¼ pie	340	22.0	34.0	13.0	5.0	40	910	m.q.
(Totino's Party), ½ pie	290	12.0	38.0	10.0	2.0	10	860	2.0 d
(Celentano 9-Slice Pizza), 2.7 oz. ..	150	6.0	22.0	4.0	m.q.	m.q.	390	m.q.
(Celentano Thick Crust), 4.3 oz. ...	290	13.0	35.0	11.0	m.q.	m.q.	700	m.q.
(Celeste Suprema), ¼ pie	381	16.8	29.2	24.1	7.0	15	1090	3.0 d
(Celeste Suprema Pizza For One),								
1 pie	678	26.5	54.0	39.3	12.0	20	1610	4.5 d
cheese:								
(Celeste), ¼ pie	317	14.2	27.8	16.6	7.0	20	770	2.2 d
(Celeste Pizza For One), 1 pie	497	21.2	48.0	24.5	11.0	40	1070	3.6 d
(Jeno's Crisp'n Tasty), ½ pie	270	10.0	28.0	14.0	m.q.	m.q.	770	m.q.
(Jeno's 4-Pack), 1 pie	160	6.0	17.0	8.0	m.q.	m.q.	460	m.q.
(John's 3-Pack), 1 pie	300	14.0	33.0	12.0	m.q.	m.q.	1040	m.q.
(Pillsbury Microwave), ½ pie	240	10.0	28.0	10.0	m.q.	m.q.	540	m.q.
(Stouffer's), ½ of 8½-oz. pkg. ...	320	14.0	32.0	15.0	m.q.	m.q.	640	m.q.
(Stouffer's Extra Cheese), ½ of								
9¼-oz. pkg.	370	17.0	33.0	19.0	m.q.	m.q.	720	m.q.
(Tombstone), ¼ pie	330	20.0	34.0	13.0	6.0	30	700	m.q.
(Totino's Microwave), 1 pie	250	11.0	30.0	10.0	4.0	15	550	2.0 d
(Totino's Party), ½ pie	280	15.0	35.0	10.0	3.0	15	570	3.0 d
(Totino's Party Family Size), ⅓ pie	310	16.0	38.0	11.0	4.0	20	620	3.0 d
(Weight Watchers), 5.86-oz. pkg.	300	22.0	37.0	7.0	3.0	35	630	m.q.
dinner, see "Pizza dinner, frozen"								
snack tray *(Jeno's* Snacks), 4 pies								
or ⅓ pkg.	130	5.0	12.0	7.0	m.q.	m.q.	440	m.q.
three cheese:								
(Tombstone Double Top), ¼ pie	490	30.0	36.0	25.0	13.0	65	1110	m.q.

Food and Measure	cal.	prot. (gms)	carbo. (gms)	tot. fat (gms)	sat. fat (gms)	chol. (mgs)	sod. (mgs)	fiber (gms)
(*Tombstone* Microwave),								
7.7-oz. pkg.	520	29.0	41.0	27.0	13.0	60	1130	m.q.
two cheese (*Tombstone* Thin								
Crust), ¼ pie	330	20.0	25.0	16.0	7.0	35	670	m.q.
cheese combination:								
double cheese, ¼ pie:								
and hamburger (*Tombstone*								
Double Top)	530	37.0	35.0	27.0	12.0	75	1480	m.q.
and sausage (*Tombstone* Double								
Top)	510	38.0	35.0	25.0	11.0	80	1360	m.q.
and sausage (*Tombstone* Double								
Top Deluxe)	520	38.0	36.0	25.0	11.0	80	1360	m.q.
and hamburger (*Tombstone*),								
¼ pie	360	21.0	34.0	16.0	6.0	40	910	m.q.
and hamburger (*Tombstone* Italian								
Thin Crust), ¼ pie	320	19.0	23.0	17.0	7.0	40	810	m.q.
and pepperoni:								
(*Tombstone*), ¼ pie	380	20.0	34.0	18.0	7.0	30	950	m.q.
(*Tombstone* Microwave),								
7.5-oz. pkg.	530	30.0	39.0	29.0	12.0	50	1300	m.q.
(*Tombstone* Thin Crust), ¼ pie	330	18.0	23.0	19.0	8.0	30	820	m.q.
and sausage (*Tombstone*), ¼ pie ..	350	22.0	34.0	14.0	6.0	40	850	m.q.
and sausage, Italian (*Tombstone*								
Thin Crust), ¼ pie	330	19.0	23.0	18.0	7.0	40	710	m.q.
sausage and mushroom								
(*Tombstone*), ¼ pie	360	23.0	35.0	15.0	6.0	40	860	m.q.
combination:								
(*Jeno's* 4-Pack), 1 pie	180	7.0	17.0	9.0	m.q.	m.q.	470	m.q.
(*Mr. P's*), ½ pie	260	10.0	26.0	13.0	m.q.	m.q.	640	m.q.
(*Pappalo's* Pan Pizza), ⅙ pie	340	17.0	34.0	15.0	m.q.	m.q.	700	m.q.
(*Pappalo's* Thin Crust), ⅙ pie	260	13.0	29.0	10.0	m.q.	m.q.	590	m.q.
(*Pillsbury* Microwave), ½ pie	310	14.0	29.0	15.0	m.q.	m.q.	780	m.q.
(*Totino's* Microwave), 1 pie	290	9.0	34.0	13.0	3.0	15	780	3.0 d
(*Totino's* Party), ½ pie	340	13.0	39.0	15.0	4.0	15	860	3.0 d
(*Totino's Party* Family Size), ⅓ pie	290	9.0	34.0	13.0	3.0	15	780	3.0 d
(*Weight Watchers* Deluxe),								
7.15-oz. pkg.	330	26.0	35.0	10.0	3.0	25	650	m.q.
deluxe:								
(*Celeste*), ¼ pie	378	15.5	29.3	22.1	7.0	20	910	3.1 d
(*Celeste* Pizza For One), 1 pie	582	22.7	51.2	31.8	10.0	20	1370	4.4 d
(*Stouffer's*), ½ of 10-oz. pkg.	370	16.0	33.0	19.0	m.q.	m.q.	590	m.q.
golden topping:								
(*Fox Deluxe*), ½ pie	240	9.0	25.0	11.0	m.q.	m.q.	600	m.q.
(*John's*), ½ pie	240	9.0	25.0	11.0	m.q.	m.q.	600	m.q.
(*Mr. P's*), ½ pie	240	9.0	25.0	11.0	m.q.	m.q.	600	m.q.
hamburger:								
(*Fox Deluxe*), ½ pie	260	11.0	26.0	12.0	m.q.	m.q.	700	m.q.
(*Jeno's* Crisp'n Tasty), ½ pie	290	12.0	28.0	15.0	m.q.	m.q.	810	m.q.

Food and Measure	cal.	prot. (gms)	carbo. (gms)	tot. fat (gms)	sat. fat (gms)	chol. (mgs)	sod. (mgs)	fiber (gms)
PIZZA, HAMBURGER *(cont.)*								
(Jeno's 4-Pack), 1 pie	180	8.0	17.0	9.0	m.q.	m.q.	500	m.q.
(Mr. P's), ½ pie	260	11.0	26.0	12.0	m.q.	m.q.	700	m.q.
(Pappalo's Pan Pizza), ⅙ pie	310	17.0	34.0	12.0	m.q.	m.q.	580	m.q.
(Pappalo's Thin Crust), ⅙ pie	240	14.0	28.0	8.0	m.q.	m.q.	470	m.q.
(Totino's Party), ½ pie	320	13.0	37.0	13.0	3.0	15	840	3.0 d
Mexican style *(Totino's* Party Pizza), ½ pie	380	13.0	35.0	21.0	m.q.	m.q.	970	m.q.
Mexican style *(Totino's* Temptin' Toppings), ¼ pie	220	8.0	21.0	12.0	m.q.	m.q.	530	m.q.
pepperoni:								
(Celeste), ¼ pie	368	15.0	29.2	21.3	7.0	15	1000	m.q.
(Celeste Pizza For One), 1 pie	546	20.2	49.7	29.6	9.0	20	1360	3.9 d
(Fox Deluxe), ½ pie	250	8.0	26.0	13.0	m.q.	m.q.	640	m.q.
(Jeno's Crisp'n Tasty), ½ pie	280	10.0	27.0	15.0	m.q.	m.q.	760	m.q.
(Jeno's 4-Pack), 1 pie	170	6.0	17.0	9.0	m.q.	m.q.	460	m.q.
(Mr. P's), ½ pie	250	8.0	26.0	13.0	m.q.	m.q.	640	m.q.
(Pappalo's Pan Pizza), ⅙ pie	330	16.0	34.0	14.0	m.q.	m.q.	710	m.q.
(Pappalo's Thin Crust), ⅙ pie	270	13.0	28.0	11.0	m.q.	m.q.	600	m.q.
(Pillsbury Microwave), ½ pie	300	13.0	29.0	15.0	m.q.	m.q.	790	m.q.
(Stouffer's), ½ of 8¾-oz. pkg. ...	350	15.0	34.0	18.0	m.q.	m.q.	820	m.q.
(Tombstone Real Deluxe), ¼ pie ..	380	20.0	34.0	18.0	7.0	30	940	m.q.
(Totino's Microwave), 1 pie	270	10.0	29.0	13.0	3.0	15	680	1.0 d
(Totino's Party), ½ pie	330	13.0	38.0	13.0	3.0	20	890	2.0 d
(Totino's Party Family Size), ⅓ pie	360	15.0	42.0	15.0	4.0	20	980	2.0 d
(Weight Watchers), 6.09-oz. pkg.	320	26.0	31.0	10.0	3.0	35	710	m.q.
double cheese *(Tombstone* Double Top), ¼ pie	560	35.0	35.0	31.0	14.0	60	1490	m.q.
double cheese *(Tombstone* Double Top Deluxe), ¼ pie	550	33.0	36.0	30.0	13.0	55	1430	m.q.
snack tray *(Jeno's* Snacks), 4 pies or ⅓ pkg.	140	5.0	12.0	8.0	m.q.	m.q.	470	m.q.
sausage:								
(Celeste), ¼ pie	376	15.6	29.7	21.7	7.0	15	910	3.3 d
(Celeste Pizza For One), 1 pie	571	22.6	48.8	31.7	10.0	20	1370	4.2 d
(Fox Deluxe), ½ pie	260	10.0	26.0	13.0	m.q.	m.q.	630	m.q.
(Jeno's Crisp'n Tasty), ½ pie	300	11.0	28.0	16.0	m.q.	m.q.	850	m.q.
(Jeno's 4-Pack), 1 pie	180	7.0	17.0	9.0	m.q.	m.q.	460	m.q.
(John's), ½ pie	260	10.0	26.0	13.0	m.q.	m.q.	630	m.q.
(John's Deluxe), ½ pie	260	10.0	26.0	13.0	m.q.	m.q.	630	m.q.
(John's 3-Pack), 1 pie	300	15.0	34.0	11.0	m.q.	m.q.	910	m.q.
(Mr. P's), ½ pie	260	10.0	26.0	13.0	m.q.	m.q.	630	m.q.
(Pappalo's Pan Pizza), ⅙ pie	360	14.0	34.0	18.0	m.q.	m.q.	550	m.q.
(Pappalo's Thin Crust), ⅙ pie	250	12.0	28.0	9.0	m.q.	m.q.	490	m.q.
(Pillsbury Microwave), ½ pie	280	13.0	29.0	13.0	m.q.	m.q.	680	m.q.
(Stouffer's), ½ of 9⅜-oz. pkg. ...	360	16.0	32.0	18.0	m.q.	m.q.	830	m.q.
(Tombstone Deluxe), ¼ pie	350	22.0	34.0	14.0	6.0	40	840	m.q.
(Tombstone Deluxe Microwave), 8.7-oz. pkg.	520	34.0	40.0	25.0	10.0	65	1280	m.q.

Food and Measure	cal.	prot. (gms)	carbo. (gms)	tot. fat (gms)	sat. fat (gms)	chol. (mgs)	sod. (mgs)	fiber (gms)
(*Totino's* Microwave), 1 pie	280	10.0	31.0	13.0	3.0	10	680	2.0 d
(*Totino's Party*), ½ pie	340	13.0	39.0	15.0	3.0	15	840	3.0 d
(*Totino's Party* Family Size), ⅓ pie	370	14.0	43.0	16.0	4.0	20	920	4.0 d
(*Weight Watchers*), 6.26-oz. pkg.	320	24.0	35.0	10.0	2.0	35	630	m.q.
Italian (*Tombstone* Microwave), 8-oz. pkg.	550	32.0	39.0	29.0	12.0	65	1220	m.q.
smoked, w/pepperoni seasoning (*Tombstone*), ¼ pie	350	21.0	34.0	14.0	6.0	40	900	m.q.
snack tray (*Jeno's* Snacks), 4 pies or ⅓ pkg.	140	5.0	13.0	8.0	m.q.	m.q.	430	m.q.
sausage combination: (*Tombstone*), ¼ pie	370	23.0	33.0	16.0	7.0	45	98	m.q.
and mushroom (*Celeste* Pizza For One), 1 pie	592	23.9	51.3	32.3	11.0	20	1180	4.5 d
and pepperoni: (*Fox Deluxe*), ½ pie	260	10.0	26.0	13.0	m.q.	m.q.	640	m.q.
(*Jeno's* Crisp'n Tasty), ½ pie ...	300	10.0	27.0	16.0	m.q.	m.q.	840	m.q.
(*Stouffer's*), ½ of 9⅜-oz. pkg.	380	16.0	33.0	21.0	m.q.	m.q.	860	m.q.
(*Tombstone* Double Top), ¼ pie	540	36.0	35.0	29.0	13.0	70	1460	m.q.
(*Tombstone* Microwave), 8-oz. pkg.	560	34.0	39.0	29.0	12.0	65	1430	m.q.
(*Tombstone* Thin Crust Supreme), ¼ pie	340	19.0	24.0	18.0	7.0	35	770	m.q.
vegetable (*Celeste*), ¼ pie	310	13.0	28.0	16.0	m.q.	m.q.	840	m.q.
vegetable (*Celeste* Pizza For One), 1 pie	490	20.0	44.0	26.0	m.q.	m.q.	1260	m.q.

PIZZA, CROISSANT PASTRY, frozen, 1 pie:

Food and Measure	cal.	prot. (gms)	carbo. (gms)	tot. fat (gms)	sat. fat (gms)	chol. (mgs)	sod. (mgs)	fiber (gms)
cheese (*Pepperidge Farm*)	430	15.0	41.0	23.0	m.q.	m.q.	640	m.q.
deluxe (*Pepperidge Farm*)	440	16.0	43.0	23.0	m.q.	m.q.	790	m.q.
pepperoni (*Pepperidge Farm*)	420	14.0	43.0	22.0	m.q.	m.q.	690	m.q.

PIZZA, FRENCH BREAD, frozen:

Food and Measure	cal.	prot. (gms)	carbo. (gms)	tot. fat (gms)	sat. fat (gms)	chol. (mgs)	sod. (mgs)	fiber (gms)
Canadian style bacon (*Stouffer's*), ½ pkg.	360	18.0	41.0	14.0	m.q.	m.q.	960	m.q.
cheese: (*Banquet Zap*), 4.5 oz.	310	14.0	41.0	10.0	m.q.	35	800	m.q.
(*Lean Cuisine*), 5⅛-oz. pkg.	310	16.0	40.0	10.0	3.0	15	750	m.q.
(*Lean Cuisine* Extra Cheese), 5½-oz. pkg.	350	21.0	39.0	12.0	4.0	20	850	m.q.
(*Pappalo's*), 1 piece	360	16.0	40.0	15.0	m.q.	m.q.	830	m.q.
(*Pillsbury* Microwave), 1 piece ...	370	18.0	41.0	15.0	m.q.	m.q.	680	m.q.
(*Stouffer's*), ½ pkg.	340	15.0	41.0	13.0	m.q.	m.q.	840	m.q.
(*Stouffer's* Double Cheese), ½ pkg.	410	19.0	43.0	18.0	m.q.	m.q.	950	m.q.
combination (*Pappalo's*), 1 piece	430	19.0	41.0	21.0	m.q.	m.q.	1120	m.q.
deluxe: (*Banquet Zap*), 4.8 oz.	330	13.0	39.0	13.0	m.q.	25	890	m.q.
(*Lean Cuisine*), 6⅛-oz. pkg.	350	20.0	40.0	12.0	3.0	35	990	m.q.
(*Stouffer's*), ½ pkg.	430	18.0	41.0	21.0	m.q.	m.q.	1130	m.q.

Food and Measure	cal.	prot. (gms)	carbo. (gms)	tot. fat (gms)	sat. fat (gms)	chol. (mgs)	sod. (mgs)	fiber (gms)
PIZZA, FRENCH BREAD *(cont.)*								
(Weight Watchers), 6.12-oz. pkg.	330	20.0	27.0	12.0	3.0	30	800	m.q.
hamburger *(Stouffer's)*, ½ pkg.	410	19.0	40.0	19.0	m.q.	m.q.	1010	m.q.
pepperoni:								
(Banquet Zap), 4.5 oz.	350	15.0	36.0	16.0	m.q.	40	1060	m.q.
(Lean Cuisine), 5¼-oz. pkg.	340	18.0	40.0	12.0	4.0	30	970	m.q.
(Pappalo's), 1 piece	410	16.0	41.0	20.0	m.q.	m.q.	1130	m.q.
(Pillsbury Microwave), 1 piece ...	430	19.0	45.0	19.0	m.q.	m.q.	940	m.q.
(Stouffer's), ½ pkg.	410	17.0	41.0	20.0	m.q.	m.q.	1120	m.q.
(Weight Watchers), 6.09-oz. pkg.	320	21.0	27.0	11.0	3.0	30	830	m.q.
pepperoni and mushroom								
(Stouffer's), ½ pkg.	430	18.0	40.0	22.0	m.q.	m.q.	1340	m.q.
sausage:								
(Lean Cuisine), 6-oz. pkg.	350	23.0	40.0	11.0	3.0	45	960	m.q.
(Pappalo's), 1 piece	410	18.0	41.0	18.0	m.q.	m.q.	1000	m.q.
(Pillsbury Microwave), 1 piece ...	410	18.0	48.0	16.0	m.q.	m.q.	860	m.q.
(Stouffer's), ½ pkg.	420	18.0	41.0	20.0	m.q.	m.q.	1110	m.q.
sausage combination:								
and mushroom *(Stouffer's)*,								
½ pkg.	410	17.0	42.0	19.0	m.q.	m.q.	1050	m.q.
and pepperoni *(Pillsbury*								
Microwave), 1 piece	450	19.0	47.0	21.0	m.q.	m.q.	950	m.q.
and pepperoni *(Stouffer's)*, ½ pkg.	450	20.0	40.0	23.0	m.q.	m.q.	1350	m.q.
vegetable deluxe *(Stouffer's)*, ½ pkg.	420	18.0	41.0	20.0	m.q.	m.q.	830	m.q.
PIZZA CRUST:								
(Pillsbury All Ready), ⅛ of crust ...	90	3.0	16.0	1.0	0	0	170	m.q.
mix *(Chef Boyardee* Q & Easy),								
⅙ pkg.	150	6.0	26.0	2.0	m.q.	n.a.	300	m.q.
mix *(Robin Hood/Gold Medal* Pouch								
Mix), ⅙ pkg.	110	3.0	22.0	1.0	m.q.	n.a.	220	m.q.
PIZZA DINNER, frozen:								
(Kid Cuisine), 6.5 oz.	240	10.0	41.0	4.0	m.q.	20	390	m.q.
PIZZA HUT:								
hand-tossed, 2 slices of medium pie:								
cheese, 7.8 oz.	518	34.0	55.0	20.0	13.6	55	1276	7.0
pepperoni, 6.9 oz.	500	28.0	50.0	23.0	12.9	50	1267	6.0
supreme, 8.4 oz.	540	32.0	50.0	26.0	13.8	55	1470	7.0
super supreme, 8.6 oz.	463	29.0	44.0	21.0	10.3	56	1336	5.0
pan pizza, 2 slices of medium pie:								
cheese, 7.2 oz.	492	30.0	57.0	18.0	9.0	34	940	5.0
pepperoni, 7.4 oz.	540	29.0	62.0	22.0	9.2	42	1127	5.0
supreme, 9 oz.	589	32.0	53.0	30.0	13.8	48	1363	7.0
super supreme, 9.1 oz.	563	33.0	53.0	26.0	12.0	55	1447	6.0
Personal Pan Pizza, 1 whole pie:								
pepperoni, 9 oz.	675	37.0	76.0	29.0	12.5	53	1335	8.0
supreme, 9.3 oz.	647	33.0	76.0	28.0	11.2	49	1313	9.0
Thin 'n Crispy, 2 slices of medium pie:								

Food and Measure	cal.	prot. (gms)	carbo. (gms)	tot. fat (gms)	sat. fat (gms)	chol. (mgs)	sod. (mgs)	fiber (gms)
cheese, 5.2 oz.	398	28.0	37.0	17.0	10.4	33	867	4.0
pepperoni, 5.1 oz.	413	26.0	36.0	20.0	10.5	46	986	4.0
supreme, 7.1 oz.	459	28.0	41.0	22.0	11.0	42	1328	5.0
super supreme, 7.2 oz.	463	29.0	44.0	21.0	10.3	56	1336	5.0
PIZZA MIX:								
plain (*Chef Boyardee*), ¼ pkg.	180	6.0	32.0	3.0	m.q.	n.a.	640	m.q.
cheese (*Chef Boyardee* Complete),								
¼ pkg.	230	9.0	36.0	6.0	m.q.	n.a.	740	m.q.
cheese (*Chef Boyardee* 2 Complete),								
⅛ pkg.	210	10.0	31.0	5.0	m.q.	m.q.	650	m.q.
pepperoni (*Chef Boyardee*								
Complete), ¼ pkg.	250	13.0	31.0	9.0	m.q.	m.q.	870	m.q.
pepperoni (*Chef Boyardee*								
2 Complete), ⅛ pkg.	210	10.0	31.0	7.0	m.q.	m.q.	595	m.q.
sausage (*Chef Boyardee*), ¼ pkg.	270	14.0	34.0	10.0	m.q.	m.q.	930	m.q.
PIZZA POCKET SANDWICH,								
frozen:								
(*Lean Pockets* Pizza Deluxe), 1 pkg.	280	14.0	34.0	9.0	m.q.	n.a.	500	m.q.
pepperoni (*Hot Pockets*), 5 oz.	380	17.0	40.0	17.0	m.q.	45	1240	m.q.
sausage (*Hot Pockets*), 5 oz.	360	15.0	40.0	16.0	m.q.	65	590	m.q.
PIZZA ROLL, frozen, 3 oz.,								
approx. 6 rolls:								
cheese (*Jeno's*)	240	8.0	23.0	12.0	m.q.	m.q.	350	m.q.
hamburger (*Jeno's*)	240	9.0	21.0	13.0	m.q.	m.q.	280	m.q.
pepperoni and cheese (*Jeno's*)	230	7.0	22.0	13.0	m.q.	m.q.	390	m.q.
pepperoni and cheese (*Jeno's*								
Microwave)	240	7.0	23.0	13.0	m.q.	m.q.	440	m.q.
sausage and cheese (*Jeno's*								
Microwave)	250	8.0	24.0	13.0	m.q.	m.q.	440	m.q.
sausage and pepperoni (*Jeno's*)	230	7.0	22.0	13.0	m.q.	m.q.	380	m.q.
PIZZA SAUCE:								
(*Contadina* Pizza Squeeze), ¼ cup	30	1.0	5.0	1.0	n.a.	n.a.	330	m.q.
canned or in jars:								
(*Contadina* Quick & Easy								
Original), ¼ cup	30	1.0	5.0	1.0	n.a.	n.a.	330	m.q.
(*Enrico's* Homemade Style All								
Natural), 4 oz.	60	2.0	9.0	1.0	n.a.	0	m.q.	m.q.
(*Enrico's* Homemade Style All								
Natural No Salt), 4 oz.	60	2.0	9.0	1.0	n.a.	0	30	m.q.
(*Pastorelli Italian Chef*), 4 oz.	90	3.0	12.0	3.0	n.a.	n.a.	430	m.q.
(*Ragu Pizza Quick*), 3 tbsp.	35	1.0	3.0	2.0	n.a.	0	330	m.q.
w/cheese (*Chef Boyardee*),								
2.63 oz.	70	1.0	7.0	4.0	m.q.	m.q.	385	m.q.
w/cheese (*Chef Boyardee* Jars),								
3.88 oz.	90	1.0	10.0	6.0	m.q.	m.q.	565	m.q.
w/Italian cheese (*Contadina*),								
¼ cup	30	1.0	5.0	1.0	m.q.	m.q.	380	m.q.
w/pepperoni (*Contadina*), ¼ cup	40	1.0	5.0	2.0	m.q.	m.q.	390	m.q.

Food and Measure	cal.	prot. (gms)	carbo. (gms)	tot. fat (gms)	sat. fat (gms)	chol. (mgs)	sod. (mgs)	fiber (gms)
PLANTAIN:								
raw:								
untrimmed, 1 lb.	360	3.8	94.0	1.1	n.a.	0	12	1.5 c
trimmed, 1 oz.	35	.4	9.0	.1	n.a.	0	1	.1 c
1 medium, approx. 9.7 oz.	218	2.3	57.1	.7	n.a.	0	7	.9 c
sliced, ½ cup	91	1.0	23.6	.3	n.a.	0	3	.4 c
cooked, 4 oz.	132	.9	35.3	.2	n.a.	0	6	m.q.
cooked, sliced, ½ cup	89	.6	24.0	.1	n.a.	0	4	m.q.
PLUM:								
w/pits, 1 lb.	235	3.4	55.5	2.6	.2	0	2	2.6 c
pitted, 1 oz.	16	.2	3.7	.2	<.1	0	tr.	.2 c
pitted, sliced, ½ cup	46	.7	10.7	.5	.4	0	1	.5 c
Japanese or hybrid, 1 medium, 2⅛″								
diam., approx. 2.5 oz.	36	.5	8.6	.4	<.1	0	tr.	.4 c
PLUM, CANNED:								
halves or whole, unpeeled (*S&W/*								
Nutradiet), ½ cup	52	0	13.0	0	0	0	0	m.q.
purple, in water:								
pitted, 4 oz.	46	.4	12.5	<.1	tr.	0	1	.3 c
½ cup	51	.5	13.7	<.1	tr.	0	1	.3 c
3 plums and 2 tbsp. liquid	39	.4	10.5	<.1	tr.	0	1	.2 c
purple, in juice:								
pitted, 4 oz.	66	.6	17.2	<.1	tr.	0	1	.4 d
½ cup	73	.7	19.1	<.1	tr.	0	2	.5 d
3 plums and 2 tbsp. liquid	55	.5	14.4	<.1	tr.	0	1	.4 d
whole (*Featherweight*), ½ cup	80	1.0	18.0	0	0	0	<10	m.q.
purple, in light syrup:								
pitted, 4 oz.	71	.4	18.5	.1	tr.	0	23	.4 c
½ cup	79	.5	20.5	.1	<.1	0	25	.4 c
3 plums and 2¾ tbsp. liquid	83	.5	21.7	.1	<.1	0	26	.5 c
(*Stokely*), ½ cup	100	0	16.0	0	0	0	20	m.q.
purple, in heavy syrup:								
pitted, 4 oz.	101	.4	26.4	.1	tr.	0	22	.4 c
½ cup	115	.5	30.0	.1	<.1	0	25	.4 c
3 plums and 2¾ tbsp. liquid	119	.5	30.9	.1	<.1	0	26	.4 c
(*Stokely*), ½ cup	130	0	30.0	0	0	0	25	m.q.
purple, in extra heavy syrup:								
pitted, 4 oz.	115	.4	29.8	.1	tr.	0	22	.4 c
½ cup	133	.5	34.3	.1	<.1	0	25	.4 c
3 plums and 2¾ tbsp. liquid	135	.5	35.0	.1	<.1	0	25	.4 c
halves or whole, unpeeled (*S&W*								
Fancy), ½ cup	135	0	35.0	0	0	0	25	m.q.
PLUM, JAVA, see "Java plum"								
PLUM SAUCE:								
tangy (*La Choy*), 1 oz.	45	.1	10.8	.1	(0)	0	17	m.q.
POCKET SANDWICH, see								
specific listings								
POHA, see "Ground cherry"								

Food and Measure	cal.	prot. (gms)	carbo. (gms)	tot. fat (gms)	sat. fat (gms)	chol. (mgs)	sod. (mgs)	fiber (gms)
POI:								
1 oz.	32	.1	7.7	<.1	tr.	0	3	.2 c
½ cup	134	.5	32.7	.2	<.1	0	14	.7 c
POKEBERRY SHOOTS:								
raw, trimmed, 4 oz.	26	2.9	4.2	.5	n.a.	0	n.a.	m.q.
raw, trimmed, ½ cup	18	2.1	3.0	.3	n.a.	0	n.a.	m.q.
boiled, drained, 4 oz.	23	2.6	3.5	.5	n.a.	0	n.a.	m.q.
boiled, drained, ½ cup	16	1.9	2.5	.3	n.a.	0	n.a.	m.q.
POLENTA MIX[1]:								
(*Fantastic Polenta*), ½ cup	106	3.0	18.0	2.0	m.q.	n.a.	246	m.q.
POLISH SAUSAGE (see also "Kielbasa"):								
1 oz.	92	4.0	.5	8.1	2.9	20	248	0
1 large link, 10″ long × 1¼″, approx. 8 oz.	739	32.0	3.7	65.2	23.4	158	1989	0
(*Hillshire Farm* Links), 2 oz.	190	7.0	2.0	17.0	m.q.	m.q.	520	0
(*Hormel*), 2 links	170	9.0	0	14.0	m.q.	m.q.	574	0
(*OHSE*), 1 oz.	80	4.0	1.0	7.0	m.q.	m.q.	290	0
(*Pilgrim's Pride*), 3 oz.	131	13.2	2.3	7.7	m.q.	72	780	0
hot (*OHSE*), 1 oz.	70	4.0	3.0	5.0	m.q.	m.q.	270	0
POLLACK, ALASKA, see "Pollack, walleye"								
POLLACK, ATLANTIC, meat only, raw:								
1 lb.	416	88.2	0	4.4	.6	320	391	0
1 oz.	26	5.5	0	.3	<.1	20	24	0
½ fillet, approx. 6.8 oz., yield from 5-lb. whole fish	177	37.5	0	1.9	.3	136	166	0
POLLACK, WALLEYE, meat only: raw:								
1 lb.	365	77.9	0	3.6	.7	323	449	0
1 oz.	23	4.9	0	.2	<.1	20	28	0
1 fillet, approx. 2.7 oz., yield from 1-lb. whole fish	62	13.2	0	.6	.1	55	76	0
baked, broiled, or microwaved[2], 4 oz.	128	26.7	0	1.3	.3	109	132	0
POMEGRANATE:								
untrimmed, 1 lb.	172	2.4	43.6	.8	n.a.	0	8	.5 c
trimmed, 1 oz.	19	.3	4.9	.1	n.a.	0	1	.1 c
1 medium, 3⅜″ × 3¾″, 9.7 oz.	104	1.5	26.4	.5	n.a.	0	5	.3 c
POMPANO, Florida, meat only: raw:								
1 lb.	745	83.8	0	42.9	15.9	227	294	0
1 oz.	46	5.2	0	2.7	1.0	14	18	0
1 fillet, approx. 4 oz., yield from 1½-lb. whole fish	184	20.7	0	10.6	3.9	56	73	0
baked, broiled, or microwaved[2], 4 oz.	239	26.4	0	13.8	5.1	73	86	0

1. *Prepared according to package directions.*
2. *Without added ingredients.*

Food and Measure	cal.	prot. (gms)	carbo. (gms)	tot. fat (gms)	sat. fat (gms)	chol. (mgs)	sod. (mgs)	fiber (gms)
PONDEROSA:								
entrees:								
chicken breast, 5.5 oz.	98	19.9	.9	2.1	m.q.	54	400	0
chicken wings, 2 pieces	213	10.7	10.7	9.0	m.q.	75	610	m.q.
fish, baked:								
bake 'r broil, 5.2 oz.	230	19.0	10.0	13.0	m.q.	50	330	m.q.
baked scrod, 7 oz.	120	27.0	0	1.0	m.q.	65	80	0
fish, broiled:								
halibut, 6 oz.	170	35.0	0	2.4	m.q.	m.q.	68	0
roughy, 5 oz.	138	20.6	n.a.	4.8	m.q.	28	88	0
salmon, 6 oz.	192	37.0	3.0	2.7	m.q.	60	72	0
swordfish, 5.9 oz.	271	43.7	0	9.4	m.q.	85	0	0
trout, 5 oz.	228	29.4	1.0	3.9	m.q.	110	51	0
fish, fried, 3.2 oz.	190	9.0	17.0	9.0	m.q.	15	170	m.q.
fish nuggets, 1 piece	31	1.7	1.9	1.7	m.q.	8	52	m.q.
hot dog, 1.6 oz.	144	5.0	1.0	13.0	m.q.	27	460	n.a.
Kansas City Strip, 5 oz.								
precooked	138	21.0	.9	5.7	m.q.	76	850	0
New York Strip, choice, 8 oz.								
precooked	314	44.5	1.4	10.5	m.q.	50	570	0
New York Strip, choice, 10 oz.								
precooked	384	33.5	1.8	14.5	m.q.	62	1420	0
porterhouse, choice, 16 oz.								
precooked	640	56.7	2.8	30.9	m.q.	82	1130	0
rib-eye, choice, 6 oz. precooked	282	28.6	.1	14.2	m.q.	60	570	0
rib-eye, nongraded, 5 oz.								
precooked	219	25.2	.9	12.8	m.q.	75	1130	0
shrimp, fried, 7 pieces	231	21.5	31.3	.5	m.q.	105	612	m.q.
shrimp, mini, 6 pieces	47	4.4	.9	1.7	m.q.	11	8	0
sirloin, choice, 7 oz. precooked ..	241	34.6	1.4	10.8	m.q.	63	570	0
sirloin tips, choice, 5 oz.								
precooked	473	29.2	1.5	8.2	m.q.	72	280	0
steak, chopped, 4 oz. precooked	225	18.5	.7	16.2	m.q.	80	150	0
steak, chopped, 5.3 oz.								
precooked	296	24.7	.9	21.5	m.q.	105	296	0
steak kabobs, meat only, 3 oz.								
precooked	153	25.8	1.7	4.8	m.q.	67	280	0
steak sandwich, 4 oz.	408	19.6	1.6	11.1	m.q.	62	850	m.q.
steak teriyaki, 5 oz. precooked ..	174	31.5	5.1	3.1	m.q.	64	1420	0
T-bone, choice, 10 oz.								
precooked	444	33.7	1.7	18.4	m.q.	80	850	0
T-bone, nongraded, 8 oz.								
precooked	178	24.7	.6	8.5	m.q.	71	850	0
side dishes, sauces, and condiments:								
BBQ sauce, 1 tbsp.	25	0	5.0	0	0	0	260	n.a.
beans, baked, 4 oz.	170	6.0	21.0	6.0	m.q.	0	330	m.q.
beans, green, 3.5 oz.	20	.9	3.1	0	0	0	391	m.q.
carrots, 3.5 oz.	31	.9	7.0	.2	n.a.	0	33	m.q.
cauliflower, breaded, 4 oz.	115	4.1	23.0	.7	n.a.	1	446	m.q.

Food and Measure	cal.	prot. (gms)	carbo. (gms)	tot. fat (gms)	sat. fat (gms)	chol. (mgs)	sod. (mgs)	fiber (gms)
cheese, herb, garlic spread,								
1 tbsp.	100	0	0	10.0	m.q.	0	120	n.a.
cheese sauce, 2 oz.	52	1.2	6.4	2.0	m.q.	4	355	n.a.
corn, 3.5 oz.	90	3.0	21.0	.4	n.a.	0	5	m.q.
gravy, brown, 2 oz.	25	.6	3.9	1.0	n.a.	0	167	n.a.
gravy, turkey, 2 oz.	25	.7	5.1	.2	n.a.	0	228	n.a.
macaroni and cheese, 1 oz.	17	.7	4.4	.5	n.a.	1	80	m.q.
margarine, liquid, 1 tbsp.	100	0	0	11.0	m.q.	0	110	0
margarine, whipped, 1 tbsp.	34	0	0	1.2	m.q.	0	65	0
okra, breaded, 4 oz.	124	2.9	22.5	1.0	n.a.	1	483	m.q.
onion rings, breaded, 4 oz.	213	3.2	30.3	8.8	m.q.	2	620	m.q.
peas, 3.5 oz.	67	5.1	11.7	.3	n.a.	0	121	m.q.
potatoes, baked, 7.2 oz.	145	4.0	32.8	.2	n.a.	0	6	m.q.
potatoes, french fried, 3 oz.	120	1.7	16.7	4.3	m.q.	3	39	m.q.
potatoes, mashed, 4 oz.	62	1.8	13.4	.2	n.a.	20	191	m.q.
potato wedges, 3.5 oz.	130	3.0	16.0	6.0	m.q.	n.a.	171	m.q.
rice pilaf, 4 oz.	160	4.0	26.0	4.0	m.q.	22	450	m.q.
rolls, dinner, 1 piece	184	5.0	33.0	3.4	m.q.	0	311	m.q.
rolls, sourdough, 1 piece	110	4.0	22.0	1.0	n.a.	0	230	m.q.
salad oil, 1 tbsp.	120	0	0	14.0	m.q.	0	0	0
shells, pasta, 2 oz.	78	2.4	16.1	.3	n.a.	0	1	m.q.
shortening, liquid, 1 oz.	249	0	0	28.3	m.q.	0	0	0
sour cream, 1 tbsp.	26	.4	.5	2.5	m.q.	5	6	0
spaghetti, 2 oz.	78	2.4	16.1	.3	n.a.	0	1	m.q.
spaghetti sauce, 4 oz.	110	2.0	17.0	4.0	m.q.	0	520	n.a.
stuffing, 4 oz.	230	6.0	27.0	11.0	m.q.	22	800	m.q.
sweet and sour sauce, 1 oz.	37	.2	7.7	.5	n.a.	0	80	n.a.
tortilla chips, 1 oz.	150	3.0	16.0	8.0	m.q.	0	80	m.q.
winter mix, 3.5 oz.	25	2.0	4.0	0	0	0	371	m.q.
zucchini, breaded, 4 oz.	102	3.1	17.8	.7	n.a.	1	584	m.q.
salad bar and condiments:								
apple, 1 medium	80	0	20.0	1.0	n.a.	0	1	m.q.
apple, canned, 4 oz.	90	0	22.0	0	0	0	15	m.q.
apple rings, spiced, 4 oz.	100	0	24.0	0	0	0	20	m.q.
applesauce, 4 oz.	80	0	20.0	0	0	0	20	m.q.
banana, 1 medium	87	1.1	22.6	.2	(0)	0	1	m.q.
banana chips, .2 oz.	25	.2	3.3	1.3	n.a.	0	tr.	m.q.
beets, diced, 4 oz.	55	.4	12.5	.4	n.a.	0	307	m.q.
breadsticks, Italian, 1 piece	100	4.0	19.0	1.0	n.a.	0	200	m.q.
breadsticks, sesame, 2 pieces	35	1.0	6.0	0	0	0	60	n.a.
broccoli, 1 oz.	9	1.0	1.7	.9	n.a.	0	4	m.q.
cabbage, green, 1 oz.	9	1.0	1.9	0	0	0	7	m.q.
cabbage, red, 1 oz.	1	.1	.3	0	0	0	1	m.q.
cantalope, 1 wedge	13	.3	3.3	0	0	0	5	m.q.
carrots, 1 oz.	12	.3	2.8	.1	(0)	0	13	m.q.
cauliflower, 1 oz.	8	.8	1.5	.1	(0)	0	4	m.q.
celery, 1 oz.	4	.3	1.1	0	0	0	36	m.q.
cheese, imitation, shredded,								
1 oz.	90	6.0	1.0	7.0	m.q.	5	420	0

Food and Measure	cal.	prot. (gms)	carbo. (gms)	tot. fat (gms)	sat. fat (gms)	chol. (mgs)	sod. (mgs)	fiber (gms)
PONDEROSA, SALAD BAR AND CONDIMENTS (cont.)								
cheese spread, 1 oz.	98	4.0	3.6	6.7	m.q.	26	188	n.a.
cherry peppers, 2 pieces	7	.2	1.4	.2	(0)	0	415	m.q.
chicken salad, 3.5 oz.	213	11.2	7.6	15.4	m.q.	42	335	n.a.
chow mein noodles, .2 oz.	25	.6	3.0	1.2	n.a.	0	42	m.q.
cocktail sauce, 1 oz.	34	.4	6.2	1.0	n.a.	0	453	n.a.
coconut, shredded, .2 oz.	25	.2	2.0	1.9	m.q.	0	14	m.q.
cottage cheese, 4 oz.	120	15.5	4.8	5.0	m.q.	17	330	0
crackers, Melba snacks, 2 pieces	18	1.0	4.0	0	0	0	60	m.q.
croutons, 1 oz.	115	3.7	18.1	3.7	m.q.	0	351	m.q.
cucumber, 1 oz.	4	.3	1.0	0	0	0	2	m.q.
eggs, diced, 2 oz.	94	7.4	1.0	6.6	m.q.	260	75	0
fruit cocktail, 4 oz.	97	.5	25.1	.2	(0)	0	7	m.q.
garbanzo beans, 1 oz.	102	5.8	17.3	0	0	0	7	m.q.
gelatin, plain, 4 oz.	71	1.3	17.0	0	0	0	73	0
granola, .2 oz.	24	.6	3.1	1.0	n.a.	0	n.a.	m.q.
grapes, 10 pieces	34	.3	8.7	.2	(0)	0	2	m.q.
ham, diced, 2 oz.	120	9.0	1.0	10.0	m.q.	76	780	0
honeydew, 1 wedge	25	.6	5.8	.2	(0)	0	9	m.q.
lemon, 1 wedge	3	.1	.8	.1	(0)	0	0	m.q.
lettuce, 1 oz.	5	0	2.0	0	0	0	5	m.q.
macaroni salad, 3.5 oz.	335	7.6	49.2	11.7	m.q.	9	431	m.q.
mushrooms, 1 oz.	8	.8	1.3	.1	(0)	0	4	m.q.
olives, black, 1 piece	4	0	.1	.4	n.a.	0	24	m.q.
olives, green, 1 piece	3	0	0	.4	n.a.	0	69	m.q.
onion, green, 1 piece	7	.2	1.6	.1	(0)	0	1	m.q.
onion, red and yellow, 1 oz.	11	.4	2.5	0	0	0	3	m.q.
oranges, 1 piece	45	1.2	11.3	.1	(0)	0	1	m.q.
pasta salad, premade, 3.5 oz.	269	6.4	34.3	11.7	m.q.	tr.	441	m.q.
peaches, canned, 4 oz.	70	0	18.0	0	0	0	10	m.q.
peanuts, granulated, .2 oz.	30	1.2	1.1	2.3	m.q.	0	0	m.q.
pears, canned, 4 oz.	98	.5	25.0	.5	n.a.	0	7	m.q.
pepper, green, 1 oz.	6	.3	1.4	.1	(0)	0	4	m.q.
pickles, dill spears, .14 oz.	<1	0	.1	0	0	0	54	m.q.
pickles, sweet chips. .14 oz.	4	.1	1.0	0	0	0	1	m.q.
pineapple, fresh, 1 wedge	11	.1	2.9	.1	(0)	0	tr.	m.q.
pineapple, tidbits, 4 oz.	95	.4	24.8	.2	n.a.	0	2	m.q.
potato salad, 3.5 oz.	126	1.4	16.1	5.9	m.q.	7	300	m.q.
radishes, 1 oz.	4	.3	.9	0	0	0	5	m.q.
spinach, 1 oz.	7	.9	1.2	.1	(0)	0	20	m.q.
sprouts, alfalfa, 1 oz.	10	1.0	1.0	0	0	0	0	m.q.
sprouts, bean, 1 oz.	10	1.1	1.9	tr.	0	0	1	m.q.
strawberries, 2 oz.	14	.3	3.1	.2	(0)	tr.	61	m.q.
sunflower seeds, .2 oz.	31	1.1	.7	m.q.	m.q.	0	n.a.	m.q.
tartar sauce, 1 oz.	85	.1	11.1	10.9	m.q.	9	477	n.a.
tomatoes, 1 oz.	6	.3	1.3	.1	(0)	0	1	m.q.
turkey, julienne, 1 oz.	29	5.1	.8	.6	m.q.	15	192	0
turkey-ham salad, 3.5 oz.	186	7.5	10.1	12.8	m.q.	12	655	n.a.

Food and Measure	cal.	prot. (gms)	carbo. (gms)	tot. fat (gms)	sat. fat (gms)	chol. (mgs)	sod. (mgs)	fiber (gms)
watermelon, 1 wedge	111	2.1	27.3	.9	n.a.	0	4	m.q.
yogurt, fruit, 4 oz.	115	4.5	23.0	1.0	m.q.	5	70	n.a.
yogurt, vanilla, 4 oz.	110	5.0	18.0	2.0	m.q.	6	75	0
zucchini, 1 oz.	5	.3	1.0	0	0	0	tr.	m.q.
desserts:								
banana pudding, 1 oz.	52	.4	6.4	2.4	m.q.	0	29	n.a.
ice milk, chocolate, 3.5 oz.	152	3.8	29.6	2.9	m.q.	22	70	(0)
ice milk, vanilla, 3.5 oz.	150	4.0	29.7	2.6	m.q.	20	58	0
mousse, chocolate, 1 oz.	78	0	6.9	4.4	m.q.	0	18	n.a.
mousse, strawberry, 1 oz.	74	0	6.3	4.6	m.q.	0	17	n.a.
strawberry glaze, 1 oz.	37	0	9.5	0	0	0	4	n.a.
toppings:								
caramel, 1 oz.	100	.4	26.2	.7	n.a.	2.4	72	n.a.
chocolate, 1 oz.	89	.5	24.3	.3	n.a.	0	37	n.a.
sprinkles, chocolate, .18 oz. ...	24	.1	n.a.	16.0	m.q.	0	4	n.a.
sprinkles, rainbow, .18 oz.	24	0	n.a.	16.0	m.q.	0	1	n.a.
strawberry, 1 oz.	71	.1	23.6	.2	n.a.	0	29	n.a.
whipped, 1 oz.	80	0	4.8	6.4	m.q.	0	16	0
wafer, vanilla, 2 cookies	35	0	6.0	1.0	n.a.	5	25	m.q.
beverages:								
coffee, 6 oz.	2	0	.5	0	0	0	26	0
milk, chocolate, 8 oz.	208	7.9	25.9	8.5	m.q.	33	149	0
milk, white, 8 oz.	159	8.5	12.0	8.6	m.q.	34	122	0
tea, 6 oz.	2	.1	.5	0	0	0	0	0
POPCORN popped, except as noted:								
(*Bachman*), ½ oz.	80	1.0	7.0	6.0	m.q.	0	160	m.q.
(*Bachman* Lite), ½ oz.	50	1.0	10.0	1.0	m.q.	0	35	2.0 d
(*Bearitos* Organic Lite), 1 oz.	132	2.8	14.7	6.9	m.q.	0	39	2.7 d
(*Bearitos* Organic No Salt), 1 oz. ...	108	3.6	21.7	.8	n.a.	0	1	.7 d
(*Bearitos* Organic Traditional), 1 oz.	140	2.4	12.0	9.2	m.q.	0	85	3.0 d
(*Bonnie Lee*), popped w/out oil and salt, 1 oz. or 1 quart popped ..	109	3.0	20.0	1.0	n.a.	0	<1	m.q.
(*Bonnie Lee*), popped w/oil and salt, 1 oz. or 1 quart popped	172	3.0	20.0	8.0	m.q.	n.a.	230	m.q.
(*Frito-Lay's*) ½ oz.	70	1.0	9.0	3.0	m.q.	0	200	m.q.
(*Jiffy Pop* Pan Popcorn), 4 cups	130	3.0	16.0	6.0	m.q.	0	270	2.0 d
(*Laura Scudder's* Tender Baby White Corn), ½ oz.	80	1.0	6.0	6.0	m.q.	0	140	m.q.
(*Orville Redenbacher* Natural), 3 cups	80	2.0	8.0	5.0	1.1	0	19	3.1 d
(*Orville Redenbacher* Natural Salt Free), 3 cups	90	2.0	8.0	6.0	1.3	0	0	3.1 d
(*Tone's*), 1 cup	30	1.0	6.0	.4	.1	0	1	1.5 d
(*Weight Watchers* Lightly Salted), .66-oz. pkg.	80	2.0	12.0	4.0	m.q.	0	65	m.q.
(*Wise* Tender Baby White Corn), ½ oz.	80	1.0	6.0	6.0	m.q.	0	140	m.q.

Food and Measure	cal.	prot. (gms)	carbo. (gms)	tot. fat (gms)	sat. fat (gms)	chol. (mgs)	sod. (mgs)	fiber (gms)
POPCORN *(cont.)*								
(*Wise* Tender Eating Baby Popcorn),								
½ oz.	70	1.0	4.0	6.0	m.q.	0	120	m.q.
butter flavor:								
(*Jiffy Pop* Pan Popcorn), 4 cups ...	130	3.0	16.0	6.0	m.q.	0	270	2.0 d
(*Orville Redenbacher*), 3 cups	80	2.0	8.0	5.0	1.0	0	150	3.1 d
(*Orville Redenbacher* Salt Free),								
3 cups	80	2.0	8.0	5.0	1.2	0	0	3.1 d
(*Wise*), ½ oz., approx. 1 cup	80	1.0	7.0	5.0	m.q.	0	140	m.q.
caramel coated, see "Candy"								
cheese and cheese flavor:								
(*Bachman*), ½ oz.	90	1.0	7.0	6.0	m.q.	n.a.	165	m.q.
(*Bearitos* Organic), 1 oz.	137	3.1	13.2	8.0	m.q.	n.a.	122	2.0 d
(*Frito-Lay's*), ½ oz.	80	1.0	7.0	5.0	m.q.	0	180	m.q.
cheddar:								
(*Orville Redenbacher*), 3 cups ..	160	3.0	12.0	12.0	m.q.	2	310	3.1 d
white:								
(*Bachman*), ½ oz.	70	1.0	7.0	4.0	m.q.	n.a.	150	m.q.
(*Cape Cod*), ½ oz.	80	2.0	6.0	5.0	m.q.	n.a.	150	m.q.
(*Clover Club*), ½ oz.	70	1.0	6.0	5.0	m.q.	n.a.	140	m.q.
(*Keebler* Deluxe), 1 oz.	140	1.0	13.0	10.0	2.0	5	270	m.q.
(*Laura Scudder's*), ½ oz. ...	70	1.0	6.0	5.0	m.q.	n.a.	140	m.q.
(*Smartfood*), ½ oz.	80	2.0	7.0	5.0	m.q.	n.a.	150	m.q.
(*Weight Watchers*),								
.66-oz. bag	100	2.0	10.0	6.0	m.q.	n.a.	85	m.q.
(*Wise*), ½ oz.	70	1.0	6.0	5.0	m.q.	n.a.	140	m.q.
honey caramel (*Keebler* Pop Deluxe),								
1 oz.	120	<1.0	22.0	3.0	1.0	0	180	m.q.
microwave, 3 cups, except as noted:								
(*Betty Crocker Pop•Secret* Natural)	100	2.0	11.0	6.0	2.0	0	170	2.0 d
(*Betty Crocker Pop•Secret* Natural								
Light)	70	2.0	12.0	3.0	<1.0	0	160	2.0 d
(*Featherweight* Natural Low Salt)	80	3.0	14.0	1.0	n.a.	0	0	m.q.
(*Jiffy Pop*), 4 cups	140	3.0	17.0	7.0	m.q.	0	270	3.0 d
(*Jolly Time* Natural)	150	2.0	15.0	10.0	m.q.	0	180	m.q.
(*Orville Redenbacher* Light								
Natural)	50	2.0	9.0	1.0	n.a.	0	85	3.1 d
(*Pillsbury* Original)	210	3.0	20.0	13.0	m.q.	0	410	m.q.
(*Planters* Natural)	140	2.0	14.0	9.0	1.0	0	560	m.q.
(*Pop Weaver's* Natural), 4 cups ...	140	3.0	20.0	8.0	m.q.	0	230	4.0 d
(*Pops-Rite* Natural)	90	2.0	13.0	5.0	m.q.	0	190	m.q.
(*Weight Watchers*), 1-oz. pkg.	100	4.0	22.0	1.0	n.a.	0	5	m.q.
butter flavor:								
(*Betty Crocker Pop•Secret*)	100	2.0	11.0	6.0	1.0	0	170	2.0 d
(*Betty Crocker Pop•Secret* Light)	70	2.0	12.0	3.0	<1.0	0	115	2.0 d
(*Featherweight* Low Salt)	100	3.0	14.0	3.0	m.q.	0	70	m.q.
(*Jiffy Pop*), 4 cups	140	3.0	17.0	7.0	m.q.	0	270	3.0 d
(*Jolly Time*)	150	3.0	18.0	7.0	m.q.	0	130	m.q.
(*Orville Redenbacher* Lite)	50	2.0	9.0	2.0	m.q.	0	70	3.1 d

Food and Measure	cal.	prot. (gms)	carbo. (gms)	tot. fat (gms)	sat. fat (gms)	chol. (mgs)	sod. (mgs)	fiber (gms)
(*Pillsbury*)	210	3.0	20.0	13.0	m.q.	n.a.	410	m.q.
(*Planters*)	140	2.0	13.0	10.0	1.0	0	560	m.q.
(*Pop Weaver's*), 4 cups	140	3.0	20.0	8.0	m.q.	0	230	4.0 d
(*Pops-Rite*)	90	2.0	13.0	5.0	m.q.	0	140	m.q.
cheddar cheese flavor								
(*Jolly Time*)	180	3.0	17.0	11.0	m.q.	0	200	m.q.
cheese flavor (*Betty Crocker*								
Pop•Secret), ⅓ pkg. unpopped	170	3.0	15.0	11.0	m.q.	0	260	2.0 d
frozen:								
(*Pillsbury* Original)	210	3.0	20.0	13.0	m.q.	n.a.	420	m.q.
(*Pillsbury* Salt-Free)	170	3.0	23.0	7.0	m.q.	n.a.	0	m.q.
butter flavor (*Pillsbury*)	210	3.0	20.0	13.0	m.q.	n.a.	480	m.q.
white, prepared w/out salt								
(*Jolly Time*), 4 cups	75	3.0	16.0	1.0	n.a.	0	tr.	3.5 d
air popped (*Pops-Rite*), 1 oz.								
kernels	100	3.0	20.0	2.0	m.q.	n.a.	0	.6 c
oil popped (*Pops-Rite*), 1 oz.								
kernels	220	3.0	20.0	15.0	m.q.	n.a.	0	.6 c
yellow, prepared w/out salt:								
(*Jolly Time*), 4 cups	88	3.0	19.0	1.0	n.a.	0	tr.	3.0 d
air popped (*Pops-Rite*), 1 oz.								
kernels	100	2.0	21.0	2.0	m.q.	n.a.	0	.6 c
oil popped (*Pops-Rite*), 1 oz.								
kernels	220	2.0	21.0	15.0	m.q.	n.a.	0	.6 c
POPCORN SEASONING:								
(*McCormick/Schilling Parsley Patch*),								
1 tsp.	10	.6	3.0	.1	(0)	0	4	n.a.
(*Tone's*), 1 tsp.	0	0	0	0	0	0	2455	0
POPPY SEED:								
1 oz.	151	5.1	6.7	12.6	1.4	0	6	1.8 c
1 tbsp.	47	1.6	2.1	3.9	.4	0	2	.6 c
1 tsp.	15	.5	.7	1.3	.1	0	1	.2 c
(*Spice Islands*), 1 tsp.	13	.6	.8	.9	n.a.	0	<1	.2 c
POPPY SEED OIL:								
1 oz.	251	0	0	28.4	3.8	0	0	0
½ cup	964	0	0	109.0	14.7	0	0	0
1 tbsp.	120	0	0	13.6	1.8	0	0	0
PORGY, see "Scup"								
PORK[1], fresh (see also "Ham" and								
"Pork, boneless"):								
back rib, raw (*JM Gourmet*),								
5.5 oz.	220	15.0	0	18.0	m.q.	m.q.	50	0
loin, whole, separable lean and fat:								
raw, 1 oz.	82	4.8	0	6.8	2.5	19	15	0
braised:								
4 oz.	417	30.8	0	31.6	11.4	116	74	0
2.5 oz., yield from 3.1-oz. raw								
chop w/bone	261	19.3	0	19.8	7.2	73	46	0

1. *Cooked meats are prepared without added ingredients, except as noted.*

Food and Measure	cal.	prot. (gms)	carbo. (gms)	tot. fat (gms)	sat. fat (gms)	chol. (mgs)	sod. (mgs)	fiber (gms)
PORK, LOIN, WHOLE, LEAN AND FAT *(cont.)*								
chopped or diced, 1 cup not packed	515	38.0	0	39.1	14.1	143	91	0
broiled:								
4 oz.	392	26.7	0	30.9	11.1	107	75	0
2.9 oz., yield from 3.7-oz. raw chop w/bone	284	19.3	0	22.3	8.1	77	54	0
chopped or diced, 1 cup not packed	484	33.0	0	38.1	13.8	132	92	0
roasted:								
4 oz.	362	26.6	0	27.5	10.0	102	71	0
2.9 oz., yield from 3.7-oz. raw chop w/bone	262	19.2	0	19.9	7.2	74	52	0
chopped or diced, 1 cup not packed	447	32.8	0	34.0	12.3	126	88	0
loin, whole, separable lean only:								
raw, 1 oz.	44	5.9	0	2.1	.7	17	18	0
braised:								
4 oz.	310	37.4	0	16.6	5.7	119	85	0
1.9 oz., yield from 3.1-oz. raw chop w/bone and fat	150	18.1	0	8.0	2.8	58	41	0
chopped or diced, 1 cup not packed	382	46.2	0	20.4	7.1	147	105	0
broiled:								
4 oz.	291	31.6	0	17.3	6.0	108	85	0
2.3 oz., yield from 3.7-oz. raw chop w/bone and fat	169	18.4	0	10.1	3.5	63	49	0
chopped or diced, 1 cup not packed	360	39.0	0	21.4	7.4	133	105	0
roasted:								
4 oz.	272	30.5	0	15.8	5.4	102	78	0
2.4 oz., yield from 3.7-oz. raw chop w/bone and fat	166	18.6	0	9.6	3.3	62	48	0
chopped or diced, 1 cup not packed	336	37.7	0	19.5	6.7	126	97	0
loin, blade, separable lean and fat:								
raw, 1 oz.	92	4.4	0	8.1	2.9	20	15	0
braised:								
4 oz.	465	27.2	0	38.7	13.9	122	78	0
2.4 oz., yield from 3.1-oz. raw chop w/bone	275	16.1	0	22.8	8.2	72	46	0
chopped or diced, 1 cup not packed	574	33.5	0	47.7	17.2	151	97	0
broiled:								
4 oz.	446	23.4	0	38.4	14.2	111	76	0
2.1 oz., yield from 3.7-oz. raw chop w/bone	303	15.9	0	26.1	9.4	75	52	0
chopped or diced, 1 cup not packed	550	28.9	0	47.4	17.0	137	94	0

Food and Measure	cal.	prot. (gms)	carbo. (gms)	tot. fat (gms)	sat. fat (gms)	chol. (mgs)	sod. (mgs)	fiber (gms)
pan-fried in hydrogenated soybean and cottonseed oil:								
4 oz.	469	21.3	0	41.9	15.1	108	69	0
3.1 oz., yield from 4.3-oz. raw chop w/bone	368	16.7	0	32.9	11.8	85	55	0
chopped or diced, 1 cup not packed	580	26.3	0	51.7	18.6	133	85	0
roasted:								
4 oz.	413	23.9	0	34.5	12.4	102	69	0
3.1 oz., yield from 4.2-oz. raw chop w/bone	321	18.5	0	26.8	9.6	79	54	0
chopped or diced, 1 cup not packed	510	29.5	0	42.6	15.3	126	85	0
loin, blade, separable lean only:								
raw, 1 oz.	52	5.5	0	3.1	1.1	18	18	0
braised:								
4 oz.	355	33.7	0	23.3	8.1	128	92	0
1.8 oz., yield from 3.1-oz. raw chop w/bone and fat	156	14.9	0	10.3	3.6	57	41	0
chopped or diced, 1 cup not packed	438	41.6	0	28.8	9.9	158	113	0
broiled:								
4 oz.	340	28.2	0	24.3	8.4	113	87	0
2.1 oz., yield from 3.7-oz. raw chop w/bone and fat	177	14.7	0	12.7	4.4	59	45	0
chopped or diced, 1 cup not packed	420	34.9	0	30.1	10.4	140	108	0
pan-fried in hydrogenated soybean and cottonseed oil:								
4 oz.	321	27.6	0	22.5	7.7	110	84	0
2.2 oz., yield from 4.3-oz. raw chop w/bone and fat	175	15.1	0	12.3	4.2	60	46	0
chopped or diced, 1 cup not packed	396	34.0	0	27.8	9.5	136	104	0
roasted:								
4 oz.	316	28.0	0	21.9	7.5	101	77	0
2.5 oz., yield from 4.2-oz. raw chop w/bone and fat	198	17.5	0	13.7	4.7	63	48	0
chopped or diced, 1 cup not packed	391	34.6	0	27.0	9.3	125	95	0
loin, center, separable lean and fat:								
raw, 1 oz.	80	5.2	0	6.2	2.2	20	16	0
braised:								
4 oz.	401	33.3	0	28.7	10.4	121	58	0
2.6 oz., yield from 3.2-oz. raw chop w/bone	266	22.1	0	19.0	6.9	81	38	0
chopped or diced, 1 cup not packed	496	41.2	0	35.5	12.8	150	71	0

Food and Measure	cal.	prot. (gms)	carbo. (gms)	tot. fat (gms)	sat. fat (gms)	chol. (mgs)	sod. (mgs)	fiber (gms)
PORK, LOIN, CENTER, LEAN AND FAT *(cont.)*								
broiled:								
4 oz.	358	31.1	0	25.1	9.1	110	79	0
3.1 oz., yield from 3.7-oz. raw chop w/bone	275	23.9	0	19.2	7.0	84	61	0
chopped or diced, 1 cup not packed	442	38.4	0	30.9	11.3	136	98	0
pan-fried in hydrogenated soybean and cottonseed oil:								
4 oz.	425	26.4	0	34.6	12.0	117	82	0
3.1 oz., yield from 4-oz. raw chop w/bone	333	20.7	0	27.2	9.8	92	64	0
chopped or diced, 1 cup not packed	525	32.6	0	42.7	15.4	144	101	0
roasted:								
4 oz.	346	28.8	0	24.7	8.9	103	73	0
3.1 oz., yield from 3.8-oz. raw chop w/bone	268	22.4	0	19.1	6.9	80	56	0
chopped or diced, 1 cup not packed	427	35.6	0	30.5	11.0	127	90	0
loin, center, separable lean only:								
raw, 1 oz.	45	6.2	0	2.0	.7	18	19	0
braised:								
4 oz.	308	39.4	0	15.5	5.4	126	62	0
2.2 oz., yield from 3.2-oz. raw chop w/bone and fat	166	21.2	0	8.4	2.9	68	33	0
chopped or diced, 1 cup not packed	381	48.7	0	19.2	6.6	155	77	0
broiled:								
4 oz.	262	36.3	0	11.9	4.1	111	88	0
2.5 oz., yield from 3.7-oz. raw chop w/bone and fat	166	23.0	0	7.5	2.6	71	56	0
chopped or diced, 1 cup not packed	323	44.8	0	14.7	5.1	137	109	0
pan-fried in hydrogenated soybean and cottonseed oil:								
4 oz.	302	32.6	0	14.0	6.2	121	96	0
2.4 oz., yield from 4-oz. raw chop w/bone and fat	178	19.3	0	10.7	3.7	71	57	0
chopped or diced, 1 cup not packed	372	40.3	0	22.3	7.6	150	119	0
roasted:								
4 oz.	272	32.3	0	14.8	5.1	103	78	0
2.5 oz., yield from 3.8-oz. raw chop w/bone and fat	180	21.4	0	9.8	3.4	68	52	0
chopped or diced, 1 cup not packed	336	39.9	0	18.3	6.3	127	97	0
loin, center rib, separable lean and fat:								
raw, 1 oz.	82	5.1	0	6.6	2.4	18	11	0

Food and Measure	cal.	prot. (gms)	carbo. (gms)	tot. fat (gms)	sat. fat (gms)	chol. (mgs)	sod. (mgs)	fiber (gms)
braised:								
4 oz.	416	32.4	0	30.8	11.1	108	54	0
2.4 oz., yield from 3.1-oz. raw chop w/bone	246	19.2	0	18.2	6.6	64	32	0
chopped or diced, 1 cup not packed	514	40.0	0	38.0	13.7	133	67	0
broiled:								
4 oz.	389	27.9	0	29.9	10.8	106	69	0
2.7 oz., yield from 3.7-oz. raw chop w/bone	264	18.9	0	20.3	7.3	72	47	0
chopped or diced, 1 cup not packed	480	34.4	0	36.9	13.3	130	85	0
pan-fried in hydrogenated soybean and cottonseed oil:								
4 oz.	442	24.5	0	37.4	13.5	95	51	0
3.1 oz., yield from 4.2-oz. raw chop w/bone	343	19.0	0	29.0	10.5	74	40	0
chopped or diced, 1 cup not packed	546	30.3	0	46.2	16.7	118	63	0
roasted:								
4 oz.	361	28.1	0	26.8	9.7	92	50	0
2.8 oz., yield from 3.8-oz. raw chop w/bone	252	19.6	0	18.6	6.7	64	35	0
chopped or diced, 1 cup not packed	445	34.6	0	33.0	11.9	113	62	0
loin, center rib, separable lean only:								
raw, 1 oz.	46	6.2	0	2.1	.7	16	13	0
braised:								
4 oz.	314	39.1	0	16.4	5.6	110	59	0
1.9 oz., yield from 3.1-oz. raw chop w/bone and fat	147	18.3	0	7.7	2.6	51	28	0
chopped or diced, 1 cup not packed	388	48.2	0	20.2	7.0	136	73	0
broiled:								
4 oz.	293	32.7	0	16.9	5.8	107	76	0
2.2 oz., yield from 3.7-oz. raw chop w/bone and fat	162	18.2	0	9.4	3.2	59	42	0
chopped or diced, 1 cup not packed	361	40.3	0	20.9	7.2	132	94	0
pan-fried in hydrogenated soybean and cottonseed oil:								
4 oz.	291	31.7	0	17.4	6.0	92	57	0
2.2 oz., yield from 4.2-oz. raw chop w/bone and fat	160	17.3	0	9.5	3.3	50	31	0
chopped or diced, 1 cup not packed	360	39.1	0	21.4	7.4	113	70	0
roasted:								
4 oz.	278	32.0	0	15.6	5.4	86	52	0

Food and Measure	cal.	prot. (gms)	carbo. (gms)	tot. fat (gms)	sat. fat (gms)	chol. (mgs)	sod. (mgs)	fiber (gms)
PORK, LOIN, CENTER RIB, LEAN ONLY *(cont.)*								
2.3 oz., yield from 3.8-oz. raw								
chop w/bone and fat	162	18.6	0	9.1	3.1	52	30	0
chopped or diced, 1 cup not								
packed	343	39.5	0	19.3	6.7	111	64	0
loin, sirloin, separable lean and fat:								
raw, 1 oz.	78	4.9	0	6.3	2.3	20	12	0
braised:								
4 oz.	399	31.7	0	29.2	10.6	120	61	0
2.5 oz., yield from 3.1-oz. raw								
chop w/bone	250	19.9	0	18.3	6.6	75	38	0
chopped or diced, 1 cup not								
packed	493	39.2	0	36.0	13.0	148	76	0
broiled:								
4 oz.	375	27.4	0	28.6	10.4	110	62	0
3 oz., yield from 3.7-oz. raw								
chop w/bone	278	20.3	0	21.2	7.7	81	46	0
chopped or diced, 1 cup not								
packed	463	33.8	0	35.4	12.8	136	77	0
roasted:								
4 oz.	330	28.4	0	23.1	8.4	103	67	0
3 oz., yield from 3.8-oz. raw								
chop w/bone	244	21.0	0	17.1	6.2	76	49	0
chopped or diced, 1 cup not								
packed	407	35.1	0	28.6	10.3	127	83	0
loin, sirloin, separable lean only:								
raw, 1 oz.	43	6.0	0	1.9	.7	18	14	0
braised:								
4 oz.	296	38.0	0	14.8	5.1	125	67	0
2 oz., yield from 3.1-oz. raw								
chop w/bone and fat	149	19.1	0	7.4	2.6	63	34	0
chopped or diced, 1 cup not								
packed	365	46.9	0	18.2	6.3	154	83	0
broiled:								
4 oz.	276	32.1	0	15.4	5.3	111	68	0
2.4 oz., yield from 3.7-oz. raw								
chop w/bone and fat	165	19.2	0	9.2	3.2	67	41	0
chopped or diced, 1 cup not								
packed	340	39.6	0	19.0	6.6	137	84	0
roasted:								
4 oz.	268	31.2	0	14.9	5.2	102	70	0
2.6 oz., yield from 3.8-oz. raw								
chop w/bone and fat	175	20.3	0	9.8	3.4	67	46	0
chopped or diced, 1 cup not								
packed	330	38.5	0	18.4	6.4	126	87	0
loin, top, separable lean and fat:								
raw, 1 oz.	86	4.9	0	7.3	2.6	18	11	0
braised:								
4 oz.	432	31.4	0	33.1	12.0	108	53	0

Food and Measure	cal.	prot. (gms)	carbo. (gms)	tot. fat (gms)	sat. fat (gms)	chol. (mgs)	sod. (mgs)	fiber (gms)
2.5 oz., yield from 3.1-oz. raw chop w/bone	267	19.4	0	20.4	7.4	67	33	0
chopped or diced, 1 cup not packed	533	38.7	0	40.8	14.8	133	66	0
broiled:								
4 oz.	408	26.9	0	32.5	11.7	105	67	0
3 oz., yield from 3.7-oz. raw chop w/bone	295	19.5	0	23.5	8.5	76	49	0
chopped or diced, 1 cup not packed	504	33.2	0	40.1	14.5	130	83	0
pan-fried in hydrogenated soybean and cottonseed oil:								
4 oz.	445	24.4	0	37.7	13.6	95	51	0
3 oz., yield from 4.1-oz. raw chop w/bone	337	18.5	0	28.6	10.3	72	39	0
chopped or diced, 1 cup not packed	549	30.1	0	46.5	16.8	118	63	0
roasted:								
4 oz.	374	27.4	0	28.5	10.3	93	50	0
2.9 oz., yield from 3.8-oz. raw chop w/bone	274	20.1	0	20.9	7.5	68	36	0
chopped or diced, 1 cup not packed	462	33.9	0	35.2	12.7	115	62	0
loin, top, separable lean only:								
raw, 1 oz.	46	6.2	0	2.1	.7	16	13	0
braised:								
4 oz.	314	39.1	0	16.4	5.6	110	59	0
1.9 oz., yield from 3.1-oz. raw chop w/bone and fat	147	18.3	0	7.7	2.6	51	28	0
chopped or diced, 1 cup not packed	388	48.2	0	20.2	7.0	136	73	0
broiled:								
4 oz.	293	32.7	0	16.9	5.8	107	76	0
2.3 oz., yield from 3.7-oz. raw chop w/bone and fat	165	18.4	0	9.6	3.3	60	43	0
chopped or diced, 1 cup not packed	361	40.3	0	20.9	7.2	132	94	0
pan-fried in hydrogenated soybean and cottonseed oil:								
4 oz.	291	31.7	0	17.4	6.0	92	57	0
2.2 oz., yield from 4.1-oz. raw chop w/bone and fat	157	17.1	0	9.3	3.2	49	31	0
chopped or diced, 1 cup not packed	360	39.1	0	21.4	7.4	113	70	0
roasted:								
4 oz.	278	32.0	0	15.6	5.4	90	52	0
2.4 oz., yield from 3.8-oz. raw chop w/bone and fat	167	19.2	0	9.4	3.2	54	31	0

Food and Measure	cal.	prot. (gms)	carbo. (gms)	tot. fat (gms)	sat. fat (gms)	chol. (mgs)	sod. (mgs)	fiber (gms)
PORK, LOIN, TOP, LEAN ONLY, ROASTED *(cont.)*								
chopped or diced, 1 cup not packed	343	39.5	0	19.3	6.7	111	64	0
shoulder, whole, separable lean and fat:								
raw, 1 oz.	78	4.6	0	6.5	2.3	21	18	0
roasted, 4 oz.	370	25.0	0	29.1	10.5	109	77	0
roasted, chopped or diced, 1 cup not packed	456	30.8	0	36.0	13.0	134	96	0
shoulder, whole separable lean only:								
raw, 1 oz.	44	5.5	0	2.2	.8	19	21	0
roasted, 4 oz.	277	28.8	0	17.0	5.9	110	86	0
roasted, chopped or diced, 1 cup not packed	341	35.5	0	21.0	7.2	135	107	0
shoulder, arm (picnic), separable lean and fat:								
raw, 1 oz.	77	4.6	0	6.3	2.3	20	19	0
braised, 4 oz.	391	30.4	0	29.0	10.5	124	100	0
braised, chopped or diced, 1 cup not packed	483	37.5	0	35.7	13.0	153	123	0
roasted, 4 oz.	375	25.3	0	29.6	10.7	107	79	0
roasted, chopped or diced, 1 cup not packed	463	31.3	0	36.5	13.3	132	97	0
shoulder, arm (picnic), separable lean only:								
raw, 1 oz.	40	5.6	0	1.8	.6	18	23	0
braised, 4 oz.	281	36.6	0	13.8	4.8	129	116	0
braised, chopped or diced, 1 cup not packed	347	45.2	0	17.1	5.9	160	143	0
roasted, 4 oz.	259	30.3	0	14.3	4.9	108	91	0
roasted, chopped or diced, 1 cup not packed	319	37.4	0	17.7	6.1	133	112	0
shoulder, Boston blade, separable lean and fat:								
raw, 1 oz.	79	4.5	0	6.6	2.4	21	17	0
braised:								
4 oz.	421	29.9	0	32.5	11.7	126	76	0
5.6 oz., yield from 6.3-oz. raw steak w/bone	594	42.4	0	45.9	16.5	178	107	0
chopped or diced, 1 cup not packed	519	37.0	0	40.1	14.4	155	94	0
broiled:								
4 oz.	397	24.8	0	32.3	11.6	117	85	0
6.5 oz., yield from 7.4-oz. raw steak w/bone	647	40.5	0	52.6	18.9	190	138	0
chopped or diced, 1 cup not packed	490	30.6	0	39.8	14.3	144	105	0
shoulder, Boston blade, separable lean only:								
raw, 1 oz.	47	5.4	0	2.6	.9	19	20	0

Food and Measure	cal.	prot. (gms)	carbo. (gms)	tot. fat (gms)	sat. fat (gms)	chol. (mgs)	sod. (mgs)	fiber (gms)
braised:								
4 oz.	333	35.3	0	19.9	6.9	132	85	0
4.6 oz., yield from 6.3-oz. raw steak w/bone and fat	382	40.5	0	22.9	7.9	151	98	0
chopped or diced, 1 cup not packed	412	43.6	0	24.6	8.5	162	105	0
broiled:								
4 oz.	311	28.5	0	20.9	7.2	119	95	0
5.2 oz., yield from 7.4-oz. raw steak w/bone and fat	413	38.0	0	27.8	9.6	159	126	0
chopped or diced, 1 cup not packed	384	35.2	0	25.8	8.9	147	118	0
roasted:								
4 oz.	290	27.6	0	19.1	6.6	111	83	0
5.6 oz., yield from 7.5-oz. raw steak w/bone and fat	404	38.5	0	26.6	9.2	155	116	0
chopped or diced, 1 cup not packed	358	34.1	0	23.6	8.1	137	102	0
spareribs, separable lean and fat:								
raw, 1 oz.	81	4.9	0	6.7	2.7	22	21	0
raw (JM Gourmet), 4.5 oz.	250	14.0	0	22.0	m.q.	m.q.	70	0
braised, 6.3 oz., yield from 1 lb. raw w/bone	703	51.4	0	53.6	20.8	214	165	0
tenderloin, separable lean only:								
raw, 1 oz.	32	6.0	0	.7	.2	18	14	0
roasted:								
4 oz.	188	32.6	0	5.5	1.9	105	76	0
12.6 oz., yield from 1 lb. raw lean only	596	103.2	0	17.2	5.9	333	238	0
chopped or diced, 1 cup not packed	232	40.3	0	6.7	2.3	130	94	0
PORK, BONELESS:								
chop (JM America's Cut), 6-oz. chop	330	38.0	0	20.0	m.q.	m.q.	90	0
loin, whole or half, center cut (JM), 3 oz.	190	16.0	0	13.0	m.q.	m.q.	50	0
shoulder butt (JM), 3 oz.	210	13.0	0	18.0	m.q.	m.q.	60	0
tenderloin (JM), 3 oz.	120	17.0	0	5.0	m.q.	m.q.	40	0
PORK, CANNED:								
1 oz.	95	3.5	.6	8.6	3.1	18	365	0
1 slice, 4¼″ × 4¼″ × ¹⁄₁₆″, approx. .75 oz.	70	2.6	.4	6.4	2.3	13	271	0
(Hormel), 3 oz.	240	11.0	2.0	21.0	m.q.	m.q.	1056	0
chopped (Hormel), 3 oz.	200	12.0	2.0	16.0	m.q.	m.q.	1073	0

Food and Measure	cal.	prot. (gms)	carbo. (gms)	tot. fat (gms)	sat. fat (gms)	chol. (mgs)	sod. (mgs)	fiber (gms)
PORK, CURED[1] (see also "Ham"), shoulder:								
arm (picnic), separable lean and fat:								
roasted, 4 oz.	318	23.2	0	24.2	8.7	66	1216	0
roasted, chopped or diced, 1 cup								
not packed	392	28.6	0	29.9	10.7	82	1501	0
arm (picnic), separable lean only:								
roasted, 4 oz.	193	28.3	0	8.0	2.7	54	1396	0
roasted, chopped or diced, 1 cup								
not packed	238	34.9	0	9.9	3.3	68	1723	0
blade roll, separable lean and fat:								
unheated, 1 oz.	76	4.7	0	6.2	2.3	15	354	0
unheated, chopped or diced, 1 cup								
not packed	377	23.1	0	30.8	11.1	74	1750	0
roasted:								
13.3 oz., yield from 1 lb.								
unheated	1079	65.0	1.4	88.3	31.5	251	3657	0
4 oz.	325	19.6	.4	26.6	9.5	76	1103	0
chopped or diced, 1 cup not								
packed	402	24.2	.5	32.9	11.7	94	1362	0
PORK, GROUND:								
(*JM*), 3 oz.	190	15.0	0	14.0	m.q.	m.q.	40	0
PORK, SALT, see "Salt pork"								
PORK VARIETY MEATS, see specific listings								
PORK BACKFAT:								
raw, 1 oz.	230	.8	0	25.1	9.1	16	3	0
PORK BELLY:								
raw, 1 oz.	147	2.7	0	15.1	5.4	20	9	0
PORK COATING MIX, see "Pork seasoning and coating mix"								
PORK DINNER, frozen:								
loin of (*Swanson*), 10¾ oz.	280	20.0	27.0	12.0	m.q.	m.q.	790	m.q.
PORK EAR, see "Pig's ear, frozen"								
PORK ENTREE, CANNED:								
chow mein (*La Choy* Bi-Pack),								
¾ cup	80	6.0	7.0	3.0	m.q.	14	970	2.0 d
PORK ENTREE, FROZEN OR REFRIGERATED:								
barbecued:								
back ribs (*John Morrell Pork Classics*), 4¾ oz.	240	12.0	8.0	17.0	m.q.	62	480	0
chops, center cut (*John Morrell Pork Classics*), 4½ oz.	230	29.0	7.0	9.0	m.q.	90	410	0
loin, thin sliced (*John Morrell Pork Classics*), 5 slices or 3 oz.	150	17.0	5.0	6.0	m.q.	52	440	0
spare ribs (*John Morrell Pork*								

1. *Fully cooked as purchased. Roasted meats are prepared without added ingredients.*

Food and Measure	cal.	prot. (gms)	carbo. (gms)	tot. fat (gms)	sat. fat (gms)	chol. (mgs)	sod. (mgs)	fiber (gms)
Classics), 4½ oz.	250	12.0	7.0	18.0	m.q.	51	470	0
tenderloin (*John Morrell Pork*								
Classics), 3 oz.	130	18.0	3.0	5.0	m.q.	53	220	0
steak, breaded (*Hormel*), 3 oz.	220	12.0	11.0	15.0	m.q.	m.q.	m.q.	m.q.
sweet and sour (*Chun King*), 13 oz.	400	11.0	78.0	5.0	m.q.	m.q.	1460	n.a.
PORK FAT[1] (see also "Lard"):								
unheated, 1 oz.	164	1.6	<.1	17.4	6.4	19	143	0
roasted, 1 oz.	167	2.2	0	17.5	6.4	24	177	0
PORK GRAVY:								
canned:								
(*Franco-American*), 2 oz.	40	0	3.0	3.0	m.q.	n.a.	330	n.a.
(*Heinz* HomeStyle), 2 oz. or ¼ cup	25	1.0	3.0	1.0	n.a.	n.a.	310	n.a.
w/chunky pork (*Hormel Great*								
Beginnings), 5 oz.	140	14.0	5.0	8.0	m.q.	m.q.	567	n.a.
mix[2]:								
1 oz. dry	101	2.6	17.9	2.6	1.0	3	1644	n.a.
¼ cup	19	.5	3.4	.5	.2	1	309	n.a.
(*French's*), ¼ cup	20	1.0	4.0	1.0	n.a.	n.a.	250	n.a.
(*McCormick/Schilling*), ¼ cup ...	20	.6	4.0	.6	n.a.	n.a.	297	n.a.
PORK LUNCHEON MEAT (see								
also "Pork, canned):								
(*Eckrich* Slender Sliced), 1 oz.	45	5.0	1.0	2.0	m.q.	m.q.	320	0
PORK RIND SNACK:								
(*Baken-ets*), 1 oz.	160	12.0	2.0	10.0	m.q.	25	850	n.a.
PORK SAUCE, see "Pork gravy"								
PORK SEASONING AND								
COATING MIX:								
(*Shake 'n Bake* Original Recipe),								
⅛ pouch	40	1.0	8.0	1.0	n.a.	0	300	m.q.
barbecue (*Shake 'n Bake* Original								
Recipe), ⅛ pouch	40	0	7.0	1.0	n.a.	0	350	m.q.
chop (*McCormick/Schilling* Bag'n								
Season), 1 pkg.	103	1.1	23.6	.4	n.a.	0	3126	m.q.
extra crispy (*Shake 'n Bake Oven*								
Fry), ¼ pouch	120	3.0	21.0	3.0	m.q.	0	690	m.q.
PORK TAIL, see "Pig's tail"								
PORK AND BEANS, see "Baked								
beans" and specific bean listings								
PORT, see "Wine"								
POT ROAST, see "Beef dinner,								
frozen" and "Beef entree,								
frozen"								
POT ROAST SEASONING MIX:								
(*Lawry's* Seasoning Blends), 1 pkg.	122	3.7	25.0	.7	n.a.	0	4008	.5 c
(*McCormick/Schilling* Bag'n Season),								
1 pkg.	55	3.9	8.5	.6	n.a.	0	3030	n.a.

1. *Separable fat from fully cooked, as-purchased ham and arm (picnic).*
2. *Prepared according to package directions, with water, except as noted.*

Food and Measure	cal.	prot. (gms)	carbo. (gms)	tot. fat (gms)	sat. fat (gms)	chol. (mgs)	sod. (mgs)	fiber (gms)
POTATO:								
raw:								
unpeeled, 1 lb.	269	7.1	61.2	.3	.1	0	21	5.4 d
peeled:								
1 oz.	22	.6	5.1	<.1	tr.	0	2	.5 d
1 medium, 2½″ diam., approx.								
5.3 oz. w/skin	88	2.3	20.1	.1	<.1	0	7	1.8 d
diced, ½ cup	59	1.6	13.5	.1	<.1	0	5	1.2 d
skin only, 2 oz.	33	1.5	7.1	.1	<.1	0	6	1.0 c
baked in skin:								
4 oz.	124	2.6	28.6	.1	<.1	0	9	.7 c
1 medium, 4¾″ × 2⅓″ diam.,								
approx. 7.1 oz.	220	4.7	51.0	.2	.1	0	16	1.3 c
pulp only, 4 oz.	105	2.2	24.4	.1	<.1	0	6	1.7 d
pulp only, ½ cup, approx. 2.2 oz.	57	1.2	13.2	.1	<.1	0	3	.9 d
skin only, 2 oz.	112	2.4	26.1	.1	<.1	0	12	2.3 d
boiled in skin:								
pulp only, 4 oz.	99	2.1	22.8	.1	<.1	0	5	1.7 d
pulp only, ½ cup, approx.								
2.75 oz.	68	1.5	15.7	.1	<.1	0	3	1.2 d
skin only, 2 oz.	44	1.6	9.8	.1	<.1	0	8	2.1 c
boiled w/out skin:								
4 oz.	98	1.9	22.7	.1	<.1	0	6	.4 c
1 potato, 2½″ diam., 4.8 oz.	116	2.3	27.0	.1	<.1	0	7	.5 c
½ cup, approx. 2.75 oz.	67	1.3	15.6	.1	<.1	0	4	.3 c
microwaved in skin:								
4 oz.	119	2.8	27.4	.1	<.1	0	9	.9 c
1 medium, 4¾″ × 2⅓″ diam.,								
7.1 oz.	212	4.9	48.7	.2	.1	0	16	1.6 c
pulp only, 4 oz.	113	2.4	26.4	.1	<.1	0	8	.5 c
pulp only, ½ cup, approx.								
2.75 oz.	78	1.6	18.2	.1	<.1	0	5	.3 c
skin only, 2 oz.	75	2.5	16.8	.1	<.1	0	9	1.8 c
hash brown[1]:								
4 oz.	237	2.7	24.2	15.8	6.2	0	27	.5 c
½ cup	163	1.9	16.6	10.9	4.2	0	19	.3 c
mashed, w/whole milk:								
4 oz.	87	2.2	19.9	.7	.4	2	344	.4 c
½ cup	81	2.0	18.4	.6	.4	2	318	.3 c
and butter, 4 oz.	120	2.1	18.9	4.8	1.2	14	335	.4 c
and butter, ½ cup	111	2.0	17.5	4.4	1.1	13	309	.3 c
and margarine, 4 oz.	120	2.1	18.9	4.8	1.2	2	335	.4 c
and margarine, ½ cup	111	2.0	17.5	4.4	1.1	2	309	.3 c
O'Brien[2]:								
4 oz.	92	2.7	17.5	1.5	.9	5	246	.5 c
½ cup	79	2.3	15.0	1.2	.8	4	211	.4 c

1. *Prepared in vegetable oil.*
2. *Recipe: 63% potatoes, 19% whole milk, 8% onions, 7% green pepper, 2% bread crumbs, 2% salt, 1% butter, and black pepper.*

Food and Measure	cal.	prot. (gms)	carbo. (gms)	tot. fat (gms)	sat. fat (gms)	chol. (mgs)	sod. (mgs)	fiber (gms)
scalloped[1]:								
w/butter, 4 oz.	98	3.3	12.2	4.2	2.6	14	380	.3 c
w/butter, ½ cup	105	3.5	13.2	4.5	2.8	14	409	.4 c
w/margarine, 4 oz.	98	3.3	12.2	4.2	2.6	7	380	.3 c
w/margarine, ½ cup	105	3.5	13.2	4.5	2.8	7	409	.4 c
POTATO, CANNED (see also "Potato dishes, canned"), ½ cup, except as noted:								
(Stokely)	50	2.0	11.0	0	0	0	360	m.q.
w/liquid, 4 oz.	45	1.5	9.8	.2	<.1	0	341	.3 c
drained:								
4 oz.	68	1.6	15.4	.2	.1	0	m.q.	.3 c
½ cup	54	1.3	12.3	.2	<.1	0	m.q.	.2 c
1 potato, 1.2 oz.	21	.5	4.8	.1	<.1	0	m.q.	.1 c
whole:								
w/liquid	60	2.0	13.0	.2	.1	0	452	.4 c
new, small (IGA)	45	2.0	9.0	0	0	0	300	n.a.
new, extra small (S&W)	45	2.0	9.0	0	0	0	310	n.a.
whole or sliced:								
w/liquid (Del Monte)	45	1.0	10.0	0	0	0	355	m.q.
white:								
(A&P)	45	2.0	11.0	<1.0	(0)	0	320	m.q.
(Pathmark No Salt Added),								
1 cup	100	3.0	20.0	0	0	0	15	m.q.
small (Finast)	55	1.0	13.0	0	0	0	375	m.q.
sliced or diced, white (Allens)	45	2.0	10.0	<1.0	(0)	0	360	m.q.
sliced or diced (Taylor's Brand),								
1 cup	90	3.0	25.0	0	0	0	292	m.q.
double diced, white (Allens)	45	2.0	10.0	<1.0	(0)	0	540	m.q.
POTATO, FREEZE-DRIED:								
hash brown (Mountain House),								
1 cup[2]	150	2.0	36.0	0	0	n.a.	m.q.	m.q.
POTATO, FROZEN (see also "Potato dishes, frozen")								
whole:								
peeled, 10 oz.	221	6.7	49.6	.5	.1	0	71	1.1 c
peeled, boiled, drained, 4 oz.	74	2.2	16.5	.1	<.1	0	23	.4 c
small (Ore-Ida), 3 oz.	70	2.0	16.0	<1.0	(0)	0	45	m.q.
white (Southern), 3.5 oz.	69	2.0	15.0	.1	(0)	0	20	m.q.
white, boiled (Seabrook), 3.2 oz.	60	2.0	13.0	0	0	0	5	m.q.
diced and hash-shred (Seabrook),								
4 oz.	80	2.0	19.0	0	0	0	41	m.q.
fried and french-fried:								
9-oz. pkg.[3]	419	6.5	63.8	16.5	7.8	0	58	1.3 c
heated in oven[3], 4 oz.	252	3.9	38.4	9.9	4.7	0	35	4.8 d
heated in oven[3], 10 strips, approx.								
1.75 oz.	111	1.7	17.0	4.4	2.1	0	15	2.1 d

1. *Recipe: 59% potatoes, 36% whole milk, 2% butter or margarine, 2% flour, and 1% salt.*
2. *Prepared according to package directions.*
3. *Par-fried in vegetable oil.*

Food and Measure	cal.	prot. (gms)	carbo. (gms)	tot. fat (gms)	sat. fat (gms)	chol. (mgs)	sod. (mgs)	fiber (gms)
POTATO, FROZEN, FRIED *(cont.)*								
(*Heinz* Deep Fries), 3 oz.	160	2.0	23.0	6.0	3.0	0	20	m.q.
(*MicroMagic*), 3 oz.	290	3.0	40.0	13.0	m.q.	n.a.	30	m.q.
(*Ore-Ida* Lites), 3 oz.	90	2.0	16.0	2.0	<1.0	0	30	m.q.
(*Ore-Ida Country Style Dinner*								
Fries), 3 oz.	110	2.0	19.0	3.0	2.0	0	30	m.q.
(*Ore-Ida Crispers!*), 3 oz.	230	2.0	25.0	15.0	8.0	0	545	m.q.
(*Ore-Ida Crispy Crowns*), 3 oz. ..	160	2.0	20.0	9.0	4.0	0	525	m.q.
(*Ore-Ida Golden Fries*), 3 oz.	120	2.0	19.0	4.0	2.0	0	35	m.q.
(*Seabrook*), 3 oz.	120	2.0	20.0	4.0	m.q.	n.a.	25	m.q.
cottage cut:								
9-oz. pkg.	391	6.2	61.1	14.8	7.0	0	82	1.3 c
heated in oven, 4 oz.	247	3.9	38.6	9.3	4.4	0	51	.8 c
heated in oven, 10 strips,								
1.8 oz.	109	1.7	17.0	4.1	1.9	0	23	.4 c
(*Ore-Ida*), 3 oz.	120	2.0	19.0	5.0	2.0	0	25	m.q.
(*Seabrook*), 2.8 oz.	110	1.0	17.0	4.0	m.q.	n.a.	14	m.q.
crinkle cut:								
or regular (*A&P*), 3.5 oz.	140	2.0	25.0	4.0	m.q.	0	25	m.q.
(*Heinz* Deep Fries), 3 oz.	150	2.0	22.0	6.0	3.0	0	30	m.q.
(*Ore-Ida* Lites), 3 oz.	90	1.0	16.0	2.0	m.q.	0	35	m.q.
(*Ore-Ida Golden Crinkles*),								
3 oz.	120	2.0	19.0	4.0	2.0	0	35	m.q.
(*Ore-Ida Pixie Crinkles*), 3 oz.	140	2.0	21.0	6.0	3.0	0	40	m.q.
(*Quick'n Crispy*), 4 oz.	370	3.0	44.0	19.0	m.q.	n.a.	50	m.q.
(*Seabrook*), 3 oz.	120	2.0	20.0	4.0	m.q.	n.a.	24	m.q.
microwave (*Ore-Ida*), 3.5 oz. ..	180	2.0	26.0	8.0	4.0	0	35	m.q.
w/onions (*Ore-Ida Crispy Crowns*),								
3 oz.	170	1.0	20.0	9.0	5.0	0	570	m.q.
shoestring:								
(*A&P*), 3.5 oz.	170	2.0	24.0	6.0	m.q.	0	50	m.q.
(*Heinz* Deep Fries), 3 oz.	200	2.0	25.0	10.0	5.0	0	20	m.q.
(*Ore-Ida*), 3 oz.	140	2.0	21.0	6.0	3.0	0	30	m.q.
(*Ore-Ida* Lites), 3 oz.	90	1.0	15.0	4.0	2.0	0	25	m.q.
(*Quick'n Crispy*), 4 oz.	390	3.0	48.0	20.0	m.q.	n.a.	50	m.q.
(*Seabrook*), 3 oz.	140	2.0	20.0	6.0	m.q.	n.a.	45	m.q.
skinny (*MicroMagic*), 3 oz.	350	4.0	49.0	15.0	m.q.	n.a.	40	m.q.
steak fries (*A&P*), 3.5 oz.	140	2.0	24.0	4.0	m.q.	0	30	m.q.
thin cuts (*Quick'n Crispy*), 4 oz.	370	3.0	44.0	19.0	m.q.	n.a.	50	m.q.
wedges (*Ore-Ida Home Style Potato*								
Wedges), 3 oz.	100	2.0	17.0	3.0	1.0	0	45	m.q.
hash brown:								
12-oz. pkg.	280	7.0	60.3	2.1	.6	n.a.	76	1.2 c
prepared in vegetable oil, 4 oz. ..	247	3.6	31.9	13.0	5.1	0	39	2.3 d
prepared in vegetable oil, ½ cup	170	2.5	21.9	9.0	3.5	0	27	1.6 d
(*A&P*), 3.5 oz.	80	2.0	17.0	0	0	0	20	m.q.
(*Ore-Ida* Southern Style), 3 oz. ..	70	1.0	16.0	<1.0	n.a.	0	35	m.q.
(*Ore-Ida Golden Patties*), 2.5 oz.	140	1.0	15.0	8.0	4.0	0	295	m.q.

Food and Measure	cal.	prot. (gms)	carbo. (gms)	tot. fat (gms)	sat. fat (gms)	chol. (mgs)	sod. (mgs)	fiber (gms)
w/butter sauce, 6-oz. pkg.	229	3.2	31.1	11.3	4.3	m.q.	130	m.q.
w/butter sauce, prepared, 4 oz. ...	202	2.8	27.4	10.0	3.8	26	115	m.q.
w/butter and onions (*Heinz* Deep Fries), 3 oz.	110	1.0	14.0	7.0	4.0	5	80	m.q.
w/cheddar (*Ore-Ida Cheddar Browns*), 3 oz.	90	2.0	13.0	2.0	1.0	10	415	m.q.
microwave (*Ore-Ida*), 2 oz.	130	1.0	12.0	8.0	4.0	0	170	m.q.
shredded (*Ore-Ida*), 3 oz.	70	1.0	15.0	<1.0	n.a.	0	40	m.q.
morsels (*A&P*), 3.5 oz.	140	2.0	23.0	4.0	m.q.	0	30	m.q.
O'Brien:								
10 oz.	215	5.2	49.5	.4	.1	n.a.	94	m.q.
prepared, 4 oz.	231	2.5	24.8	15.0	3.8	n.a.	49	m.q.
(*Ore-Ida*), 3 oz.	60	1.0	14.0	<1.0	n.a.	0	25	m.q.
puffs:								
10 oz.[1]	502	7.6	68.9	24.2	11.5	0	1687	1.4 c
prepared[1], 4 oz.	252	3.8	34.6	12.2	5.8	0	846	.7 c
prepared[1], ½ cup	138	2.1	18.9	6.7	3.2	0	462	.4 c
prepared[1], 1 puff, approx. .2 oz.	16	.2	2.1	.8	.4	0	52	<.1 c
(*Ore-Ida Tater Tots*), 3 oz.	140	1.0	19.0	7.0	3.0	0	550	m.q.
w/bacon flavored vegetable protein (*Ore-Ida Tater Tots*), 3 oz.	140	2.0	19.0	6.0	3.0	0	625	m.q.
microwave (*Ore-Ida Tater Tots*), 4 oz.	200	2.0	29.0	9.0	4.0	0	670	m.q.
w/onion (*Ore-Ida Tater Tots*), 3 oz.	140	2.0	19.0	6.0	3.0	0	715	m.q.
sticks (*MicroMagic* Tater Sticks), 4 oz.	390	2.0	43.0	22.0	m.q.	n.a.	620	m.q.
wedges (*Quick'n Crispy*), 4 oz.	280	3.0	36.0	13.0	m.q.	n.a.	40	m.q.
POTATO MIX[2] (see also "Potato dishes, mix"):								
(*Betty Crocker Potato Buds*), ⅓ cup flakes	70	2.0	16.0	0	0	0	20	m.q.
(*Betty Crocker Potato Buds*), ½ cup	130	3.0	17.0	6.0	m.q.	m.q.	360	m.q.
(*Betty Crocker Potato Buds*), ½ cup[3]	130	3.0	17.0	6.0	m.q.	m.q.	90	m.q.
au gratin:								
dry mix, 5½-oz. pkg.	490	13.1	15.5	.8	3.6	n.a.	3268	1.5 c
prepared[4], yield from 5½-oz. pkg.	764	18.0	105.5	33.9	21.3	m.q.	3609	1.4 c
prepared[4], 4 oz.	105	2.6	14.6	4.7	2.9	m.q.	498	.2 c
(*Betty Crocker*), ⅙ pkg. dry	100	3.0	19.0	1.0	n.a.	n.a.	540	m.q.
(*Betty Crocker*), ½ cup[5]	150	4.0	21.0	5.0	m.q.	m.q.	600	m.q.
(*Fantastic Foods*), ½ cup[6]	156	6.0	25.0	4.0	m.q.	m.q.	440	m.q.
(*Fantastic Foods*), ½ cup[7]	196	6.0	25.0	8.0	m.q.	m.q.	495	m.q.
(*Idahoan*), ½ cup	130	3.0	18.0	5.0	m.q.	m.q.	475	m.q.
tangy (*French's*), ½ cup	130	4.0	20.0	5.0	m.q.	n.a.	480	m.q.

1. *Par-fried in vegetable oil.*
2. *Prepared according to package directions, except as noted.*
3. *Prepared without added salt.*
4. *Water, whole milk, and margarine added.*
5. *Prepared with margarine and skim milk.*
6. *Prepared with whole milk.*
7. *Prepared with whole milk and 2 tbsp. salted butter.*

Food and Measure	cal.	prot. (gms)	carbo. (gms)	tot. fat (gms)	sat. fat (gms)	chol. (mgs)	sod. (mgs)	fiber (gms)
POTATO MIX *(cont.)*								
bacon and cheddar (*Betty Crocker* Twice Baked), ⅙ pkg. dry	110	3.0	19.0	2.0	m.q.	n.a.	500	m.q.
bacon and cheddar (*Betty Crocker* Twice Baked), ½ cup	210	6.0	21.0	11.0	m.q.	m.q.	600	m.q.
butter, herbed (*Betty Crocker* Twice Baked), ⅙ pkg. dry	100	2.0	18.0	2.0	m.q.	n.a.	440	m.q.
butter, herbed (*Betty Crocker* Twice Baked), ½ cup	220	5.0	20.0	13.0	m.q.	m.q.	540	m.q.
cheddar:								
mild, w/onion (*Betty Crocker* Twice Baked), ⅙ pkg. dry	100	2.0	18.0	2.0	m.q.	n.a.	540	m.q.
mild, w/onion (*Betty Crocker* Twice Baked), ½ cup	190	5.0	19.0	11.0	m.q.	m.q.	640	m.q.
smokey (*Betty Crocker*), ⅙ pkg. dry	100	2.0	20.0	1.0	n.a.	n.a.	620	m.q.
smokey (*Betty Crocker*), ½ cup ..	140	3.0	21.0	5.0	m.q.	m.q.	68	m.q.
spicy (*Idahoan*), ⅙ pkg. dry	90	2.0	17.0	1.0	n.a.	n.a.	450	m.q.
spicy (*Idahoan*), ½ cup	140	3.0	21.0	5.0	m.q.	m.q.	500	m.q.
cheddar and bacon:								
(*Betty Crocker*), ⅙ pkg. dry	90	2.0	19.0	1.0	n.a.	n.a.	460	m.q.
(*Betty Crocker*), ½ cup	140	3.0	21.0	5.0	m.q.	m.q.	520	m.q.
casserole (*French's*), ½ cup	130	4.0	18.0	5.0	m.q.	n.a.	390	m.q.
country style (*Fantastic Foods*), ½ cup	85	3.0	19.0	.3	n.a.	n.a.	316	m.q.
country style (*Fantastic Foods*), ½ cup[1]	118	3.0	19.0	4.0	m.q.	m.q.	362	m.q.
hash brown:								
(*Idahoan* Quick One-Pan), ½ cup	140	2.0	18.0	7.0	m.q.	n.a.	400	m.q.
(*Idahoan* Quick One-Pan), ½ cup[2]	140	2.0	18.0	7.0	m.q.	n.a.	50	m.q.
w/onions:								
(*Betty Crocker*), ⅙ pkg.	110	2.0	24.0	1.0	n.a.	n.a.	40	m.q.
(*Betty Crocker*), ½ cup[3]	160	2.0	24.0	6.0	m.q.	n.a.	100	m.q.
(*Betty Crocker*), ½ cup[4]	160	2.0	24.0	6.0	m.q.	n.a.	460	m.q.
herb and butter (*Idahoan*), ⅙ pkg. dry	90	2.0	16.0	2.0	m.q.	n.a.	425	m.q.
herb and butter (*Idahoan*), ½ cup ..	150	2.0	21.0	6.0	m.q.	m.q.	475	m.q.
julienne (*Betty Crocker*), ⅙ pkg. dry	90	2.0	17.0	1.0	n.a.	n.a.	520	m.q.
julienne (*Betty Crocker*), ½ cup[5] ...	130	3.0	18.0	5.0	m.q.	m.q.	580	m.q.
mashed:								
dehydrated flakes:								
dry, 1 oz.	100	2.4	23.0	.1	<.1	0	30	.5 c
dry, ½ cup	78	1.8	17.9	.1	<.1	0	24	.4 c
dry (*Arrowhead Mills*), 2 oz. ..	140	5.0	44.0	0	0	0	24	m.q.

1. *Prepared with 2 tbsp. salted butter.*
2. *Prepared without salt, using unsalted butter or margarine.*
3. *Prepared with margarine, without salt.*
4. *Prepared with margarine and salt.*
5. *Prepared with margarine and skim milk.*

Food and Measure	cal.	prot. (gms)	carbo. (gms)	tot. fat (gms)	sat. fat (gms)	chol. (mgs)	sod. (mgs)	fiber (gms)
prepared[1], 4 oz.	128	2.2	17.0	6.4	3.9	16	376	.5 c
prepared[1], ½ cup	118	2.0	15.8	5.9	3.6	15	349	.5 c
granules, w/out milk:								
dry, 1 oz.	105	2.3	24.2	.2	<.1	0	19	.5 c
dry, ½ cup	372	8.2	85.5	.5	.1	0	67	2.4 c
prepared[1], 4 oz.	122	2.3	16.3	5.6	3.5	16	291	.4 c
prepared[1], ½ cup	137	2.0	17.6	6.5	1.2	18	358	m.q.
granules, w/milk:								
dry, 1 oz.	101	3.1	22.0	.3	.1	1	23	.4 c
dry, ½ cup	358	10.9	77.7	1.1	.5	2	82	1.5 c
prepared[2], 4 oz.	90	2.3	14.9	2.5	.8	2	265	.3 c
prepared[2], ½ cup	83	2.1	13.8	2.3	.7	2	246	.3 c
(*Country Store* Flakes), ⅓ cup								
flakes	70	1.0	16.0	0	0	0	10	m.q.
(*French's Idaho*), ½ cup	130	2.0	16.0	6.0	m.q.	n.a.	320	m.q.
(*French's Idaho* Spuds), ½ cup	140	3.0	17.0	7.0	m.q.	n.a.	380	m.q.
(*Hungry Jack* Flakes), ½ cup	140	3.0	17.0	7.0	m.q.	n.a.	380	m.q.
(*Idahoan*), ½ cup	140	3.0	16.0	7.0	m.q.	m.q.	320	m.q.
(*Idahoan*), ½ cup[3]	140	3.0	16.0	7.0	m.q.	m.q.	55	m.q.
microwave (*Idahoan Instamash*),								
¼ pkg. or ½ cup	80	1.0	17.0	1.0	n.a.	n.a.	175	m.q.
scalloped:								
dry, 5½-oz. pkg.	558	12.1	115.3	7.2	1.9	n.a.	2462	2.2 c
dry, 1 oz.	101	2.2	21.0	1.3	.3	n.a.	447	.4 c
prepared[4], yield from 5½-oz. pkg.	764	17.4	105.0	35.4	21.6	m.q.	2803	2.2 c
prepared[4], 4 oz.	105	2.4	14.5	4.9	3.0	m.q.	387	.3 c
(*Betty Crocker*), ⅙ pkg. dry	90	2.0	19.0	1.0	n.a.	n.a.	520	m.q.
(*Betty Crocker*), ½ cup	140	3.0	20.0	5.0	m.q.	m.q.	580	m.q.
(*Idahoan*), ½ cup	140	3.0	20.0	5.0	m.q.	m.q.	425	m.q.
cheese, real (*French's*), ½ cup	140	4.0	19.0	5.0	m.q.	n.a.	380	m.q.
cheesy (*Betty Crocker*), ⅙ pkg.								
dry	90	2.0	19.0	1.0	n.a.	n.a.	500	m.q.
cheesy (*Betty Crocker*), ½ cup	140	3.0	20.0	5.0	m.q.	m.q.	560	m.q.
creamy Italian (*French's*), ½ cup	120	4.0	19.0	3.0	m.q.	n.a.	430	m.q.
crispy top w/savory onion mix								
(*French's*), ½ cup	140	3.0	20.0	5.0	m.q.	n.a.	430	n.a.
and ham (*Betty Crocker*), ⅕ pkg.	100	2.0	20.0	1.0	m.q.	m.q.	470	m.q.
and ham (*Betty Crocker*), ½ cup	160	4.0	22.0	6.0	m.q.	m.q.	540	m.q.
sour cream and chives:								
(*Betty Crocker*), ⅙ pkg. dry	100	2.0	19.0	2.0	m.q.	n.a.	460	m.q.
(*Betty Crocker*), ½ cup	140	3.0	21.0	5.0	m.q.	m.q.	520	m.q.
(*Betty Crocker* Twice Baked),								
⅙ pkg. dry	90	2.0	17.0	2.0	m.q.	n.a.	480	m.q.
(*Betty Crocker* Twice Baked),								
½ cup	200	5.0	19.0	11.0	m.q.	m.q.	570	m.q.

1. *Whole milk and butter added.*
2. *Water and vegetable table fat added.*
3. *Prepared without salt, using unsalted butter or margarine.*
4. *Water, whole milk, and butter added.*

Food and Measure	cal.	prot. (gms)	carbo. (gms)	tot. fat (gms)	sat. fat (gms)	chol. (mgs)	sod. (mgs)	fiber (gms)
POTATO MIX, SCALLOPED *(cont.)*								
(*French's*), ½ cup	150	3.0	19.0	7.0	m.q.	n.a.	550	m.q.
(*Idahoan*), ⅙ pkg. dry	90	2.0	15.0	2.0	m.q.	n.a.	340	m.q.
(*Idahoan*), ½ cup	130	2.0	18.0	5.0	m.q.	m.q.	400	m.q.
Stroganoff, creamy (*French's*),								
½ cup	130	3.0	20.0	4.0	m.q.	n.a.	520	m.q.
Western (*Idahoan*), ⅙ pkg. dry	90	2.0	17.0	1.0	n.a.	n.a.	340	m.q.
Western (*Idahoan*), ½ cup	120	2.0	18.0	4.0	m.q.	m.q.	400	m.q.
POTATO, STUFFED, see "Potato dishes, frozen"								
POTATO, SWEET, see "Sweet potato"								
POTATO, YELLOW, FINNISH, raw:								
(*Frieda* of California), 3½ oz.	100	3.3	22.0	n.a.	n.a.	0	n.a.	m.q.
POTATO CHIPS AND CRISPS, 1 oz., except as noted:								
1 oz.	148	1.8	14.7	10.1	2.6	0	133	1.4 d
10 chips, approx. .7 oz.	105	1.3	10.4	7.1	1.8	0	94	1.0 d
no salt added	148	1.8	14.7	10.1	2.6	0	2	1.4 d
no salt added, 10 chips, approx. .7 oz.	105	1.3	10.4	7.1	1.8	0	2	1.0 d
reformulated from dried potatoes ..	164	1.6	12.4	13.1	4.0	0	216	1.0 d
(*Bachman*)	160	2.0	14.0	10.0	m.q.	0	270	m.q.
(*Bachman* Kettle Cooked)	140	2.0	16.0	8.0	m.q.	0	115	m.q.
(*Bachman* Ridge/Ruffled)	160	2.0	14.0	10.0	m.q.	0	260	m.q.
(*Bachman* Unsalted)	160	2.0	14.0	10.0	m.q.	0	5	m.q.
(*Barrel O'Fun*)	150	2.0	14.0	10.0	m.q.	0	160	.4 d
(*Cape Cod/Cape Cod* Waves)	150	2.0	16.0	8.0	m.q.	0	120	m.q.
(*Cape Cod* No Salt Added)	150	2.0	16.0	8.0	m.q.	0	0	m.q.
(*Cottage Fries* No Salt Added)	160	2.0	14.0	11.0	m.q.	0	5	m.q.
(*Eagle* Extra Crunchy/Idaho Russet)	150	2.0	16.0	8.0	m.q.	0	180	m.q.
(*Eagle* Ridged/*Eagle* Thins)	150	2.0	15.0	10.0	m.q.	0	220	m.q.
(*Featherweight* Low Salt)	160	2.0	14.0	11.0	m.q.	0	4	m.q.
(*Health Valley* Country/Country Ripple/Dip/Natural)	160	2.0	15.0	10.0	m.q.	0	60	.9 d
(*Health Valley* Country/Country Ripple/Dip/Natural No Salt Added)	160	2.0	15.0	10.0	m.q.	0	1	.9 d
(*King Kold*)	150	2.0	16.0	9.0	m.q.	0	160	m.q.
(*King Kold* Rip-L)	150	2.0	16.0	9.0	m.q.	0	150	m.q.
(*Lay's*)	150	1.0	15.0	10.0	m.q.	0	200	m.q.
(*Lay's* Unsalted)	150	2.0	15.0	10.0	m.q.	0	10	m.q.
(*Munchos*)	150	1.0	16.0	9.0	m.q.	0	290	m.q.
(*O'Boisies*)	150	1.0	16.0	9.0	2.0	0	180	m.q.
(*Pringle's* Light)	150	2.0	17.0	8.0	m.q.	n.a.	120	m.q.
(*Pringle's* Regular)	170	2.0	12.0	13.0	m.q.	n.a.	170	m.q.
(*Pringle's Idaho Rippled*)	170	2.0	13.0	12.0	m.q.	n.a.	150	m.q.

Food and Measure	cal.	prot. (gms)	carbo. (gms)	tot. fat (gms)	sat. fat (gms)	chol. (mgs)	sod. (mgs)	fiber (gms)
(*Ruffles*)	150	1.0	15.0	10.0	m.q.	0	190	m.q.
(*Ruffles* Light)	130	1.0	19.0	6.0	m.q.	0	190	m.q.
(*Snacktime Krunchers!*)	150	2.0	16.0	9.0	m.q.	0	170	m.q.
(*Wise* Plain or Rippled)	150	2.0	14.0	10.0	m.q.	0	190	m.q.
(*Wise New York Deli*)	160	2.0	14.0	11.0	m.q.	0	120	m.q.
(*Wise Ridgies*)	150	2.0	14.0	10.0	m.q.	0	190	m.q.
(*Wise Ridgies* Super Crispy)	150	2.0	14.0	10.0	m.q.	0	220	m.q.
(*Zapp's* Lite/Original Kettle)	150	2.0	16.0	8.0	m.q.	0	45	m.q.
(*Zapp's* Lite/Original Kettle No Salt Added)	150	2.0	16.0	8.0	m.q.	0	<1	m.q.
au gratin (*King Kold*)	150	2.0	15.0	8.0	m.q.	n.a.	220	m.q.
barbecue flavor:								
(*Bachman*)	150	2.0	14.0	9.0	m.q.	0	280	m.q.
(*Eagle* Extra Crunchy)	150	2.0	16.0	8.0	m.q.	0	220	m.q.
(*Eagle* Extra Crunchy Louisiana)	150	2.0	16.0	8.0	m.q.	0	140	m.q.
(*Eagle* Thins)	150	2.0	15.0	10.0	m.q.	0	220	m.q.
(*King Kold* BBQ)	140	2.0	16.0	8.0	m.q.	n.a.	360	m.q.
(*Lay's* Bar-B-Q)	150	2.0	15.0	9.0	m.q.	0	310	m.q.
(*Pringle's* Light)	150	2.0	17.0	8.0	m.q.	n.a.	125	m.q.
(*Ruffles*)	150	1.0	16.0	9.0	m.q.	0	320	m.q.
(*Wise*)	150	2.0	14.0	10.0	m.q.	0	240	m.q.
(*Wise Ridgies*)	150	2.0	14.0	10.0	m.q.	0	240	m.q.
mesquite:								
(*Ruffles* Mesquite Grille)	160	2.0	14.0	10.0	m.q.	0	260	m.q.
(*Snacktime Krunchers!*)	150	2.0	16.0	9.0	m.q.	0	200	m.q.
(*Zapp's* Lite/Original Kettle)	150	2.0	16.0	8.0	m.q.	0	87	m.q.
Cajun (*Ruffles Cajun Spice*)	150	1.0	15.0	10.0	m.q.	0	240	m.q.
Cajun (*Zapp's* Lite/Original Kettle)	150	2.0	16.0	8.0	m.q.	0	94	m.q.
cheddar and sour cream (*Ruffles*)	150	2.0	16.0	9.0	m.q.	0	260	m.q.
cheese flavor (*Pringle's* Cheez-ums)	170	2.0	12.0	13.0	m.q.	n.a.	200	m.q.
dill (*King Kold*)	150	2.0	16.0	8.0	m.q.	n.a.	340	m.q.
dill and sour cream (*Cape Cod*)	150	2.0	16.0	8.0	m.q.	0	160	m.q.
dill and sour cream (*Cape Cod* No Salt)	150	2.0	16.0	8.0	m.q.	0	15	m.q.
hot (*Bachman*)	150	2.0	14.0	9.0	m.q.	0	200	m.q.
hot (*Wise*)	160	2.0	14.0	11.0	m.q.	0	290	m.q.
jalapeño flavor (*Snacktime Krunchers!*)	150	2.0	16.0	9.0	m.q.	0	270	m.q.
jalapeño flavor (*Zapp's* Original Kettle)	150	2.0	16.0	8.0	m.q.	n.a.	85	m.q.
onion, French (*Pringle's Idaho Rippled*)	170	2.0	13.0	12.0	m.q.	n.a.	175	m.q.
onion-garlic (*King Kold*)	150	2.0	15.0	9.0	m.q.	n.a.	420	m.q.
onion-garlic flavor (*Wise*)	150	2.0	14.0	10.0	m.q.	0	250	m.q.
ranch (*Pringle's* Light)	150	2.0	17.0	8.0	m.q.	n.a.	135	m.q.
ranch (*Ruffles*)	160	2.0	15.0	10.0	m.q.	0	240	m.q.
salt and vinegar (*Lay's*)	150	1.0	15.0	9.0	m.q.	0	460	m.q.
Saratoga style (*Bachman* Kettle Cooked)	140	2.0	16.0	8.0	m.q.	0	115	m.q.

Food and Measure	cal.	prot. (gms)	carbo. (gms)	tot. fat (gms)	sat. fat (gms)	chol. (mgs)	sod. (mgs)	fiber (gms)
POTATO CHIPS AND CRISPS *(cont.)*								
skins:								
baked potato (*Tato Skins*)	150	1.0	17.0	8.0	1.0	0	160	m.q.
cheese n' bacon (*Tato Skins*)	150	1.0	17.0	8.0	1.0	0	180	m.q.
sour cream n' chives (*Tato Skins*)	150	1.0	17.0	8.0	1.0	0	180	m.q.
sour cream and onion flavor:								
(*Bachman*)	150	2.0	14.0	9.0	m.q.	0	200	m.q.
(*Eagle* Ridged)	150	2.0	15.0	10.0	m.q.	0	280	m.q.
(*King Kold*)	150	2.0	15.0	10.0	m.q.	n.a.	220	m.q.
(*Lay's*)	160	2.0	15.0	10.0	m.q.	0	250	m.q.
(*O'Boisies*)	150	2.0	15.0	9.0	2.0	0	190	m.q.
(*Pringle's*)	170	2.0	13.0	12.0	m.q.	n.a.	135	m.q.
(*Ruffles*)	150	2.0	15.0	9.0	m.q.	0	240	m.q.
(*Wise Ridgies*)	160	2.0	14.0	11.0	m.q.	n.a.	240	m.q.
(*Zapp's* Lite)	150	2.0	16.0	8.0	m.q.	n.a.	79	m.q.
taco and cheddar (*Pringle's Idaho Rippled*)	170	2.0	13.0	12.0	m.q.	n.a.	160	m.q.
vinegar (*Bachman*)	150	2.0	15.0	9.0	m.q.	0	610	m.q.
POTATO DISHES, CANNED:								
au gratin (*Green Giant Pantry Express*), ½ cup	120	3.0	17.0	5.0	2.0	5	430	1.5 d
scalloped, and ham (*Hormel Micro-Cup*), 7.5 oz.	260	8.0	21.0	16.0	m.q.	25	810	m.q.
POTATO DISHES, FROZEN:								
au gratin:								
(*Birds Eye For One*), 5.5 oz.	240	8.0	24.0	13.0	m.q.	30	590	1.0 d
(*Freezer Queen Family Side Dish*), 4 oz.	100	2.0	19.0	2.0	m.q.	n.a.	440	m.q.
(*Green Giant* One Serving), 5.5 oz.	200	7.0	20.0	10.0	4.0	20	560	m.q.
(*Stouffer's*), ⅓ of 11.5-oz. pkg. ..	110	4.0	10.0	6.0	m.q.	n.a.	510	m.q.
and broccoli, in cheese flavored sauce (*Green Giant* One Serving), 5.5 oz.	130	4.0	19.0	5.0	1.0	5	720	m.q.
and broccoli, w/cheese sauce (*Freezer Queen Family Side Dish*), 5.5 oz.	140	3.0	25.0	3.0	m.q.	n.a.	79	m.q.
cheddared (*The Budget Gourmet* Side Dish), 5.5 oz.	230	7.0	22.0	13.0	m.q.	35	450	m.q.
cheddared, and broccoli (*The Budget Gourmet* Side Dish), 5 oz.	130	6.0	18.0	4.0	m.q.	25	340	m.q.
nacho (*The Budget Gourmet* Side Dish), 5 oz.	180	10.0	14.0	10.0	m.q.	30	360	m.q.
new, in sour cream sauce (*The Budget Gourmet* Side Dish), 5 oz.	120	3.0	15.0	6.0	m.q.	20	300	m.q.
scalloped (*Stouffer's*), ⅓ of 11.5-oz. pkg.	90	3.0	11.0	4.0	m.q.	m.q.	420	m.q.

Food and Measure	cal.	prot. (gms)	carbo. (gms)	tot. fat (gms)	sat. fat (gms)	chol. (mgs)	sod. (mgs)	fiber (gms)
shredded, 'n vegetables, in cheese sauce (*Stokely Singles*), 4.5 oz.	130	5.0	15.0	6.0	m.q.	15	480	m.q.
sliced, 'n bacon, in cheddar cheese sauce (*Stokely Singles*), 4.5 oz.	150	3.0	24.0	5.0	m.q.	10	460	m.q.
stuffed:								
baked:								
w/broccoli and cheese (*Weight Watchers*), 10.5 oz.	290	13.0	43.0	8.0	2.0	25	600	m.q.
w/cheese flavored topping (*Green Giant*), 5 oz.	200	4.0	33.0	6.0	m.q.	n.a.	520	m.q.
w/chicken divan (*Weight Watchers*), 11 oz.	280	18.0	42.0	4.0	2.0	40	730	m.q.
ham Lorraine (*Weight Watchers*), 11 oz.	250	20.0	31.0	4.0	2.0	15	670	m.q.
w/sour cream and chives (*Green Giant*), 5 oz.	230	5.0	31.0	10.0	m.q.	n.a.	580	m.q.
turkey, homestyle (*Weight Watchers*), 12 oz.	300	21.0	39.0	6.0	3.0	60	670	m.q.
w/real bacon (*Oh Boy!*), 6 oz.	116	4.0	18.0	3.0	m.q.	5	641	m.q.
w/cheddar cheese (*Oh Boy!*), 6 oz.	142	4.0	23.0	4.0	m.q.	6	612	m.q.
w/sour cream & chives (*Oh Boy!*), 6 oz.	129	3.0	18.0	5.0	m.q.	2	418	m.q.
three cheese (*The Budget Gourmet* Side Dish), 5.75 oz.	230	8.0	25.0	11.0	m.q.	30	410	m.q.
POTATO DISHES, MIX[1] (see also "Potato, mix"):								
broccoli au gratin (*Betty Crocker* Potato Medleys), 1/5 pkg. dry ..	110	2.0	22.0	1.0	n.a.	n.a.	550	m.q.
broccoli au gratin (*Betty Crocker* Potato Medleys), 1/2 cup[2]	140	3.0	23.0	4.0	m.q.	m.q.	590	m.q.
cheddar, w/mushrooms (*Betty Crocker* Potato Medleys), 1/5 pkg. dry	110	2.0	22.0	1.0	n.a.	n.a.	490	m.q.
cheddar, w/mushrooms (*Betty Crocker* Potato Medleys), 1/2 cup[3]	140	3.0	23.0	4.0	m.q.	m.q.	530	m.q.
and cheese:								
au gratin (*Kraft* Potatoes & Cheese), 1/2 cup	130	4.0	19.0	5.0	2.0	40	570	m.q.
broccoli au gratin (*Kraft* Potatoes & Cheese), 1/2 cup	150	5.0	20.0	5.0	2.0	40	530	m.q.
scalloped (*Kraft* Potatoes & Cheese), 1/2 cup	140	4.0	20.0	5.0	2.0	25	500	m.q.
scalloped, and ham (*Kraft* Potatoes & Cheese), 1/2 cup	150	5.0	20.0	5.0	2.0	15	510	m.q.

1. *Prepared according to package directions, except as noted.*
2. *Prepared with margarine and 2% lowfat milk.*
3. *Prepared with margarine and whole milk.*

Food and Measure	cal.	prot. (gms)	carbo. (gms)	tot. fat (gms)	sat. fat (gms)	chol. (mgs)	sod. (mgs)	fiber (gms)
POTATO DISHES, MIX, AND CHEESE *(cont.)*								
sour cream and chive (*Kraft* Potatoes & Cheese), ½ cup ...	150	5.0	20.0	5.0	2.0	10	610	m.q.
two cheese (*Kraft* Potatoes & Cheese), ½ cup	130	4.0	19.0	4.0	2.0	10	540	m.q.
scalloped:								
w/broccoli (*Betty Crocker* Potato Medleys), ⅕ pkg. dry	100	2.0	19.0	2.0	m.q.	n.a.	460	m.q.
w/broccoli (*Betty Crocker* Potato Medleys), ½ cup	140	3.0	21.0	5.0	m.q.	m.q.	500	m.q.
w/green beans and mushrooms (*Betty Crocker* Potato Medleys), ⅕ pkg. dry	110	2.0	20.0	2.0	m.q.	n.a.	460	m.q.
w/green beans and mushrooms (*Betty Crocker* Potato Medleys), ½ cup	140	3.0	21.0	5.0	m.q.	m.q.	500	m.q.
POTATO FLAKES, see "Potato mix"								
POTATO FLOUR:								
1 oz.	100	2.3	22.7	.2	.1	0	10	.5 c
1 cup	628	14.3	143.0	1.4	.4	0	61	2.9 c
POTATO JUICE, bottled:								
(*Biotta*), 6 fl. oz.	144	2.3	30.7	.1	(0)	0	222	m.q.
POTATO PANCAKE[1]**:**								
4 oz.	738	6.9	39.3	18.8	5.1	139	579	.7 c
1 cake, 2.7 oz.	495	4.6	26.4	12.6	3.4	93	388	.5 c
POTATO PANCAKE MIX[2]**:**								
dinner (*French's Idaho*), 3 cakes, 3″ each	90	3.0	16.0	2.0	m.q.	n.a.	420	m.q.
POTATO SALAD[3]**:**								
4 oz.	162	3.0	12.7	9.3	1.6	77	600	.4 c
½ cup	179	3.4	14.0	10.3	1.8	86	661	.5 c
POTATO SALAD, CANNED:								
German (*Joan of Arc/Read*), ½ cup	120	2.0	23.0	3.0	m.q.	n.a.	550	1.6 d
homestyle (*Joan of Arc/Read*), ½ cup	340	4.0	32.0	22.0	m.q.	n.a.	1070	3.0 d
POTATO SALAD SEASONING:								
(*Tone's*), 1 tsp.	5	.2	.3	.2	<.1	0	1498	.1 d
POTATO STARCH:								
(*Featherweight*), 1 cup	620	0	154.0	1.0	n.a.	0	51	n.a.
POTATO STICKS:								
1-oz. pkg.	148	1.9	15.2	10.0	2.5	0	71	.3 c
½ cup	94	1.2	9.6	6.2	1.6	0	45	.2 c
canned, shoestring (*Allens*), 1 oz. ..	140	2.0	16.0	8.0	m.q.	n.a.	190	m.q.
canned, shoestring (*Allens* No Salt), 1 oz.	140	1.0	16.0	8.0	m.q.	n.a.	10	m.q.
POULTRY, see specific listings								

1. *Recipe 72% potatoes, 12% egg, 7% onion, 7% margarine, 2% flour, and 1% salt.*
2. *Prepared according to package directions.*
3. *Recipe 62% potatoes, 12% egg, 8% mayonnaise, 7% celery, 6% sweet pickle relish, 2% onion, 1% green pepper, 1% pimiento, 1% salt, and dry mustard.*

Food and Measure	cal.	prot. (gms)	carbo. (gms)	tot. fat (gms)	sat. fat (gms)	chol. (mgs)	sod. (mgs)	fiber (gms)
POULTRY SALAD SPREAD, chicken and turkey:								
1 oz.	57	3.3	2.1	3.8	1.0	9	107	n.a.
1 tbsp.	26	1.5	1.0	1.8	.5	4	49	n.a.
POULTRY SEASONING (see also specific poultry listings):								
1 oz.	87	2.7	18.6	2.1	n.a.	0	8	3.2 c
1 tbsp.	11	.4	2.4	.3	n.a.	0	1	.4 c
1 tsp.	5	.1	1.0	.1	n.a.	0	tr.	.2 c
POUT, OCEAN, meat only, raw:								
1 lb.	360	75.5	0	4.1	1.5	236	277	0
1 oz.	22	4.7	0	.3	.1	15	17	0
½ fillet, approx. 6.2 oz., yield from 5-lb. whole fish	140	29.3	0	1.6	.6	92	107	0
PRESERVES, see "Jam and preserves"								
PRETZEL, 1 oz., except as noted:								
(*A & Eagle*)	110	3.0	22.0	2.0	m.q.	0	570	m.q.
(*Bachman* Nutzels)	110	3.0	21.0	2.0	m.q.	0	470	m.q.
(*Bachman* Petite)	110	3.0	21.0	2.0	m.q.	0	410	m.q.
(*Bachman* Petite Sodium Free)	110	3.0	21.0	2.0	m.q.	0	2	m.q.
(*Estee* Unsalted), 5 pieces	25	<1.0	5.0	<1.0	<1.0	0	<5	<1.0
(*Featherweight* Low Salt), 20 pieces	110	3.0	23.0	1.0	n.a.	0	30	m.q.
(*Mr. Salty* Mini)	110	3.0	21.0	1.0	n.a.	n.a.	450	m.q.
(*Mr. Salty Juniors*)	110	2.0	22.0	2.0	m.q.	n.a.	500	m.q.
(*Rokeach* Party Cannister)	110	2.0	23.0	1.0	n.a.	0	n.a.	m.q.
(*Rold Gold* Tiny Tim)	110	2.0	23.0	1.0	n.a.	0	610	m.q.
baldies or Dutch (*Rokeach* Unsalted)	110	2.0	20.0	0	0	0	30	m.q.
beer (*Quinlan*)	110	2.6	21.6	1.4	n.a.	0	446	.1 d
braids (*Keebler* Butter Pretzels)	110	3.0	21.0	1.0	<1.0	0	620	m.q.
cheddar flavor (*Combos*), 1.8 oz.	240	5.0	34.0	9.0	m.q.	n.a.	580	m.q.
Dutch (*Mr. Salty*), 2 pieces	110	3.0	22.0	1.0	n.a.	n.a.	440	m.q.
Dutch style (*Rokeach*)	110	3.0	24.0	0	0	0	n.a.	m.q.
hard (*Bachman*)	110	3.0	23.0	<1.0	n.a.	0	290	m.q.
hard (*Bachman* Unsalted)	110	3.0	23.0	<1.0	n.a.	0	50	m.q.
knots (*Keebler* Butter Pretzels)	110	3.0	21.0	1.0	<1.0	0	530	m.q.
logs (*Bachman*)	110	3.0	21.0	2.0	m.q.	0	470	m.q.
logs (*Quinlan*)	103	2.7	21.5	.8	n.a.	0	388	.3 d
mixed (*Mr. Salty* Mini)	110	3.0	23.0	1.0	n.a.	n.a.	480	m.q.
oat bran (*Quinlan*)	115	3.5	21.8	1.5	n.a.	0	156	.3 d
rice bran (*Quinlan* No-Salt)	101	2.6	19.5	2.3	m.q.	0	52	2.0 d
rings:								
(*Bachman*)	110	3.0	21.0	2.0	m.q.	0	410	m.q.
(*Mr. Salty*)	110	3.0	21.0	2.0	m.q.	n.a.	510	m.q.
butter flavor (*Mr. Salty*)	110	3.0	21.0	2.0	m.q.	n.a.	570	m.q.
rods:								
(*Bachman*)	110	3.0	21.0	2.0	m.q.	0	240	m.q.
(*Rold Gold*)	110	3.0	22.0	2.0	m.q.	0	550	m.q.
butter (*Seyfert's*)	110	3.0	21.0	1.0	n.a.	n.a.	530	m.q.

Food and Measure	cal.	prot. (gms)	carbo. (gms)	tot. fat (gms)	sat. fat (gms)	chol. (mgs)	sod. (mgs)	fiber (gms)
PRETZEL *(cont.)*								
sticks:								
(Mr. Salty)	110	3.0	22.0	1.0	n.a.	n.a.	620	m.q.
(Quinlan)	105	2.7	22.3	.6	n.a.	0	538	.3 d
(Rold Gold)	110	2.0	23.0	1.0	n.a.	0	760	m.q.
butter flavor *(Mr. Salty)*	110	3.0	22.0	1.0	n.a.	n.a.	620	m.q.
thins:								
(Bachman Thin'n Light)	110	3.0	21.0	2.0	m.q.	0	410	m.q.
(Mr. Salty Veri-Thin)	110	3.0	22.0	1.0	n.a.	n.a.	770	m.q.
(Quinlan)	104	2.8	22.0	.6	n.a.	0	765	.1 d
(Quinlan Ultra Thins)	106	2.7	22.5	.6	n.a.	0	618	.1 d
tiny *(Quinlan)*	109	2.6	21.2	1.5	n.a.	0	601	.2 d
tiny *(Quinlan* No-Salt)	115	2.7	22.4	1.6	n.a.	0	10	.2 d
thins or treats *(Bachman)*	110	3.0	21.0	2.0	m.q.	0	410	m.q.
twists:								
(Bachman)	110	3.0	21.0	2.0	m.q.	0	410	m.q.
(Mr. Salty), 5 pieces	110	3.0	21.0	2.0	m.q.	n.a.	590	m.q.
(Rold Gold)	110	2.0	23.0	1.0	n.a.	0	470	m.q.
PRICKLY PEAR:								
untrimmed, 1 lb.	140	2.5	32.6	1.7	n.a.	0	18	6.2 c
trimmed, 1 oz.	12	.2	2.7	.1	n.a.	0	1	.5 c
1 medium, approx. 4.8 oz.	42	.8	9.9	.5	n.a.	0	6	1.9 c
PROSCIUTTO:								
boneless *(Hormel)*, 1 oz.	90	7.0	0	7.0	m.q.	m.q.	502	0
PRUNE, CANNED, in heavy syrup:								
4 oz. pitted	119	1.0	31.5	.2	<.1	0	3	.8 c
½ cup	123	1.0	32.5	.2	<.1	0	3	.8 c
5 medium and 2 tbsp. liquid	90	.8	23.9	.2	<.1	0	2	.6 c
PRUNE, DEHYDRATED:								
uncooked, 4 oz.	384	4.2	101.0	.8	.1	0	6	3.3 c
uncooked, ½ cup	224	2.4	58.8	.5	<.1	0	4	1.9 c
cooked, 4 oz.	128	1.4	33.7	.3	<.1	0	2	1.1 c
cooked, ½ cup	158	1.7	41.6	.3	<.1	0	3	1.4 c
PRUNE, DRIED:								
(Del Monte Moist Pak), 2 oz.	120	1.0	30.0	0	0	0	<10	m.q.
(Sunsweet), 2 oz.	120	1.0	32.0	0	0	0	<10	m.q.
uncooked:								
w/pits, ½ cup	193	2.1	50.5	.4	<.1	0	3	5.8 d
w/pits *(Del Monte)*, 2 oz.	120	1.0	31.0	0	0	0	<10	m.q.
pitted:								
4 oz.	271	3.0	71.1	.6	<.1	0	5	8.2 d
10 prunes, approx. 3 oz.	201	2.2	52.7	.4	<.1	0	3	6.0 d
(Del Monte), 2 oz.	140	1.0	35.0	0	0	0	<10	m.q.
(Sunsweet), 2 oz.	140	1.0	36.0	0	0	0	<10	m.q.
cooked, stewed:								
unsweetened, w/pits, ½ cup	113	1.2	29.8	.2	<.1	0	2	7.0 d
unsweetened, pitted, 4 oz.	121	1.3	31.8	.3	<.1	0	2	7.5 d
sweetened, w/pits, ½ cup	147	1.3	39.1	.3	<.1	0	2	1.0 c
sweetened, pitted, 4 oz.	141	1.2	37.3	.2	<.1	0	2	1.0 c

Food and Measure	cal.	prot. (gms)	carbo. (gms)	tot. fat (gms)	sat. fat (gms)	chol. (mgs)	sod. (mgs)	fiber (gms)
PRUNE JUICE, canned or bottled, 6 fl. oz., except as noted:								
1 fl. oz.	23	.2	5.6	<.1	tr.	0	1	.3 d
6 fl. oz.	136	1.2	33.5	.1	<.1	0	8	1.9 d
(*Del Monte* Unsweetened)	120	1.0	33.0	0	0	0	<10	m.q.
(*Lucky Leaf*)	150	0	36.0	0	0	0	0	m.q.
(*Mott's*)	130	1.0	32.0	0	0	0	8	m.q.
(*Mott's* Country Style)	130	1.0	32.0	0	0	0	7	m.q.
(*Pathmark* All Natural)	120	1.0	30.0	0	0	0	10	m.q.
(*S&W* Unsweetened)	120	1.0	31.0	0	0	0	20	m.q.
(*Sunsweet*)	130	1.0	33.0	0	0	0	<20	m.q.
w/prune pulp (*Pathmark* Homestyle)	130	1.0	32.0	0	0	0	10	m.q.
PUDDING, ready-to-serve:								
banana (*Del Monte* Pudding Cup), 5 oz.	180	3.0	30.0	5.0	m.q.	n.a.	285	n.a.
banana (*Lucky Leaf/Musselman's*), 4 oz.	150	2.0	24.0	5.0	m.q.	n.a.	110	n.a.
butterscotch:								
(*Crowley*), 4.5 oz.	150	3.0	27.0	3.0	m.q.	10	210	n.a.
(*Del Monte* Pudding Cup), 5 oz. ..	180	3.0	31.0	5.0	m.q.	n.a.	285	n.a.
(*Featherweight*), ½ cup	100	0	21.0	1.0	n.a.	0	160	n.a.
(*Lucky Leaf/Musselman's*), 4 oz.	170	2.0	26.0	7.0	m.q.	n.a.	135	n.a.
(*White House*), 3.5 oz.	113	1.0	20.0	3.0	m.q.	n.a.	195	n.a.
butterscotch-chocolate-vanilla swirl (*Jell-O* Pudding Snacks), 4 oz.	180	3.0	28.0	5.0	m.q.	0	140	n.a.
chocolate:								
(*Crowley*), 4.5 oz.	190	4.0	29.0	3.0	m.q.	10	100	n.a.
(*Del Monte* Pudding Cup), 5 oz. ..	190	4.0	31.0	6.0	m.q.	n.a.	280	n.a.
(*Estee*), ½ cup	70	5.0	13.0	1.0	<1.0	2	75	n.a.
(*Featherweight*), ½ cup	100	1.0	21.0	1.0	n.a.	0	110	n.a.
(*Hunt's Snack Pack*), 4.25 oz. ...	160	2.0	28.0	5.0	m.q.	0	125	n.a.
(*Hunt's Snack Pack* Lite), 4 oz. ..	100	3.0	20.1	2.0	m.q.	0	120	n.a.
(*Jell-O* Light Pudding Snacks), 4 oz.	100	3.0	21.0	2.0	m.q.	5	125	n.a.
(*Jell-O* Pudding Snacks), 5.5 oz. ...	230	4.0	38.0	8.0	m.q.	0	170	n.a.
(*Jell-O* Pudding Snacks), 4 oz. ...	170	3.0	28.0	6.0	m.q.	0	130	n.a.
(*Lucky Leaf/Musselman's*), 4 oz.	180	2.0	27.0	7.0	m.q.	n.a.	100	n.a.
(*Pathmark* No Frills), 5 oz.	200	2.0	30.0	8.0	m.q.	n.a.	140	n.a.
(*Swiss Miss*), 4 oz.	180	3.0	27.0	6.0	m.q.	1	200	n.a.
(*Swiss Miss* Lite), 4 oz.	100	3.0	20.1	m.q.	n.a.	0	120	n.a.
(*White House*), 3.5 oz.	120	2.0	22.0	4.0	m.q.	n.a.	130	n.a.
fudge:								
(*Del Monte* Pudding Cup), 5 oz.	190	4.0	31.0	6.0	m.q.	n.a.	260	n.a.
(*Jell-O* Light Pudding Snacks), 4 oz.	100	3.0	22.0	1.0	n.a.	5	125	n.a.
(*Jell-O* Pudding Snacks), 4 oz.	170	3.0	28.0	6.0	m.q.	0	130	n.a.
(*Lucky Leaf/Musselman's*), 4 oz.	180	2.0	25.0	8.0	m.q.	n.a.	105	n.a.
milk (*Jell-O* Pudding Snacks), 4 oz.	170	4.0	29.0	6.0	m.q.	0	135	n.a.

Food and Measure	cal.	prot. (gms)	carbo. (gms)	tot. fat (gms)	sat. fat (gms)	chol. (mgs)	sod. (mgs)	fiber (gms)
PUDDING, READY-TO-SERVE *(cont.)*								
chocolate-caramel swirl *(Jell-O*								
Pudding Snacks), 4 oz.	170	3.0	28.0	6.0	m.q.	0	130	n.a.
chocolate, milk chocolate-fudge swirl								
(Jell-O Pudding Snacks), 4 oz.	170	3.0	28.0	6.0	m.q.	0	135	n.a.
chocolate fudge-milk chocolate swirl								
(Jell-O Pudding Snacks), 4 oz.	170	3.0	28.0	6.0	m.q.	0	135	n.a.
chocolate-vanilla:								
combo *(Jell-O* Light Pudding								
Snacks), 4 oz.	100	3.0	21.0	2.0	m.q.	5	125	n.a.
swirl *(Jell-O* Pudding Snacks),								
5.5 oz.	240	4.0	39.0	8.0	m.q.	0	180	n.a.
swirl *(Jell-O* Pudding Snacks),								
4 oz.	170	3.0	28.0	6.0	m.q.	0	135	n.a.
lemon *(White House),* 3.5 oz.	152	0	37.0	1.0	n.a.	n.a.	65	n.a.
rice:								
(Crowley), 4.5 oz.	125	4.0	22.0	2.0	m.q.	10	80	n.a.
(Lucky Leaf/Musselman's), 4 oz.	120	3.0	20.0	3.0	m.q.	n.a.	95	n.a.
(White House), 3.5 oz.	111	1.0	20.0	3.0	m.q.	n.a.	135	n.a.
tapioca:								
(Crowley), 4.5 oz.	135	4.0	27.0	1.0	n.a.	5	70	n.a.
(Del Monte Pudding Cup), 5 oz. . .	180	3.0	30.0	4.0	m.q.	n.a.	250	n.a.
(Hunt's Snack Pack), 4.25 oz. . . .	160	2.0	28.0	4.0	1.1	0	200	n.a.
(Hunt's Snack Pack Lite), 4 oz. . .	100	2.0	18.1	2.0	m.q.	0	105	n.a.
(Jell-O Pudding Snacks), 4 oz. . . .	170	3.0	27.0	4.0	m.q.	0	140	n.a.
(Lucky Leaf/Musselman's), 4 oz.	140	1.0	20.0	6.0	m.q.	n.a.	95	n.a.
(Swiss Miss), 4 oz.	150	2.0	26.0	4.0	m.q.	1	190	n.a.
(Swiss Miss Lite), 4 oz.	100	2.0	18.1	2.0	m.q.	0	105	n.a.
(White House), 3.5 oz.	131	1.0	19.0	6.0	m.q.	n.a.	105	n.a.
vanilla:								
(Crowley), 4.5 oz.	140	3.0	26.0	3.0	m.q.	10	130	n.a.
(Del Monte Pudding Cup), 5 oz. . .	180	3.0	32.0	5.0	m.q.	n.a.	285	n.a.
(Estee), ½ cup	70	4.0	13.0	<1.0	<1.0	2	75	n.a.
(Featherweight), ½ cup	100	0	20.0	2.0	m.q.	0	150	n.a.
(Hunt's Snack Pack), 4.25 oz. . . .	170	1.0	28.0	6.0	1.6	0	180	n.a.
(Hunt's Snack Pack Lite), 4 oz. . .	100	2.0	18.1	2.0	m.q.	0	110	n.a.
(Jell-O Light Pudding Snacks),								
4 oz.	100	3.0	20.0	2.0	m.q.	5	130	n.a.
(Jell-O Pudding Snacks), 5.5 oz. . . .	250	4.0	38.0	9.0	m.q.	0	190	n.a.
(Jell-O Pudding Snacks), 4 oz. . . .	180	3.0	28.0	7.0	m.q.	0	140	n.a.
(Lucky Leaf/Musselman's), 4 oz.	170	2.0	25.0	7.0	m.q.	n.a.	135	n.a.
(Pathmark No Frills), 5 oz.	200	2.0	28.0	8.0	m.q.	n.a.	150	n.a.
(Swiss Miss), 4 oz.	160	2.0	26.0	6.0	m.q.	n.a.	200	n.a.
(Swiss Miss Lite), 4 oz.	100	2.0	18.1	2.0	m.q.	0	110	n.a.
(White House), 3.5 oz.	111	1.0	20.0	3.0	m.q.	n.a.	135	n.a.
vanilla-chocolate swirl *(Jell-O*								
Pudding Snacks), 4 oz.	180	3.0	28.0	6.0	m.q.	0	140	n.a.

Food and Measure	cal.	prot. (gms)	carbo. (gms)	tot. fat (gms)	sat. fat (gms)	chol. (mgs)	sod. (mgs)	fiber (gms)
PUDDING, FROZEN:								
butterscotch flavored (*Rich's*), 3 oz.	130	2.0	18.0	6.0	m.q.	0	130	n.a.
chocolate flavored (*Rich's*), 3 oz. ...	140	2.0	18.0	7.0	m.q.	0	135	n.a.
vanilla flavored (*Rich's*), 3 oz.	130	2.0	18.0	6.0	m.q.	0	160	n.a.
PUDDING BAR, frozen, 1 bar:								
chocolate:								
(*Jell-O Pudding Pops*)	80	2.0	13.0	2.0	m.q.	0	85	n.a.
double, swirl (*Jell-O Pudding Pops*)	80	2.0	13.0	2.0	m.q.	0	90	n.a.
fudge or milk (*Jell-O Pudding Pops*)	80	2.0	13.0	2.0	m.q.	0	90	n.a.
chocolate-peanut butter swirl (*Jell-O Pudding Pops*)	80	2.0	12.0	3.0	m.q.	0	75	n.a.
chocolate-vanilla swirl (*Jell-O Pudding Pops*)	80	2.0	13.0	2.0	m.q.	0	70	n.a.
vanilla (*Jell-O Pudding Pops*)	80	2.0	13.0	2.0	m.q.	0	55	n.a.
PUDDING MIX[1], ½ cup, except as noted:								
banana (*Jell-O* Instant Sugar Free), w/2% lowfat milk	80	4.0	11.0	2.0	m.q.	10	390	n.a.
banana cream:								
(*Jell-O* Instant)	160	4.0	28.0	4.0	m.q.	15	410	n.a.
(*Jell-O* Microwave)	150	4.0	25.0	4.0	m.q.	15	220	n.a.
(*Royal*)	160	4.0	27.0	4.0	m.q.	m.q.	210	n.a.
(*Royal* Instant)	180	4.0	29.0	5.0	m.q.	m.q.	390	n.a.
butter almond, toasted (*Royal* Instant)	170	4.0	30.0	4.0	m.q.	m.q.	350	n.a.
butter pecan (*Jell-O* Instant)	170	4.0	28.0	5.0	m.q.	15	410	n.a.
butterscotch:								
(*D-Zerta*), w/skim milk	70	4.0	12.0	0	0	0	65	n.a.
(*Featherweight*)[2]................	12	0	3.0	0	0	0	6	n.a.
(*Featherweight* Instant)[2]	100	4.0	19.0	0	0	5	190	n.a.
(*Jell-O*)	170	4.0	30.0	4.0	m.q.	15	190	n.a.
(*Jell-O* Instant)	160	4.0	28.0	4.0	m.q.	15	450	n.a.
(*Jell-O* Instant Sugar Free), w/2% lowfat milk	90	4.0	12.0	2.0	m.q.	10	390	n.a.
(*Jell-O* Microwave)	170	4.0	28.0	4.0	m.q.	15	180	n.a.
(*Royal*)	160	4.0	27.0	4.0	m.q.	m.q.	210	n.a.
(*Royal* Instant)	180	4.0	29.0	5.0	m.q.	m.q.	390	n.a.
(*Royal* Instant Sugar Free), w/2% lowfat milk	100	4.0	16.0	2.0	m.q.	m.q.	470	n.a.
chocolate:								
(*D-Zerta*), w/skim milk	60	5.0	11.0	0	0	0	70	n.a.
(*Featherweight*)[2]................	12	0	3.0	0	0	0	15	n.a.
(*Featherweight* Instant)[2]	110	5.0	22.0	0	0	5	190	n.a.
(*Jell-O*)	160	5.0	28.0	4.0	m.q.	15	170	n.a.
(*Jell-O* Instant)	180	4.0	31.0	4.0	m.q.	15	480	n.a.

1. *Prepared according to package directions, with whole milk, except as noted.*
2. *Prepared according to package directions.*

Food and Measure	cal.	prot. (gms)	carbo. (gms)	tot. fat (gms)	sat. fat (gms)	chol. (mgs)	sod. (mgs)	fiber (gms)
PUDDING MIX, CHOCOLATE *(cont.)*								
(Jell-O Instant Sugar Free), w/2%								
lowfat milk	90	4.0	13.0	3.0	m.q.	10	380	n.a.
(Jell-O Microwave)	170	5.0	28.0	5.0	m.q.	15	190	n.a.
(Jell-O Cook'n Serve Sugar Free),								
w/2% lowfat milk	90	5.0	13.0	3.0	m.q.	10	160	n.a.
(Royal)	180	5.0	33.0	4.0	m.q.	m.q.	150	n.a.
(Royal Instant)	190	4.0	35.0	4.0	m.q.	m.q.	390	n.a.
(Royal Instant Sugar Free), w/2%								
lowfat milk	110	5.0	17.0	3.0	m.q.	m.q.	480	n.a.
(Weight Watchers Instant), w/skim								
milk	90	6.0	18.0	1.0	n.a.	n.a.	420	n.a.
chocolate chip *(Royal* Instant)	190	4.0	35.0	4.0	m.q.	m.q.	390	n.a.
dark'n sweet *(Royal)*	180	5.0	33.0	4.0	m.q.	m.q.	150	n.a.
dark'n sweet *(Royal* Instant)	190	4.0	35.0	4.0	m.q.	m.q.	390	n.a.
fudge:								
(Jell-O)	160	5.0	28.0	4.0	m.q.	15	170	n.a.
(Jell-O Instant)	180	5.0	31.0	5.0	m.q.	15	440	n.a.
(Jell-O Instant Sugar Free),								
w/2% lowfat milk	100	5.0	14.0	3.0	m.q.	10	330	n.a.
milk:								
(Jell-O)	160	4.0	28.0	4.0	m.q.	15	170	n.a.
(Jell-O Instant)	180	5.0	31.0	5.0	m.q.	15	470	n.a.
(Jell-O Microwave)	160	4.0	27.0	5.0	m.q.	15	190	n.a.
chocolate mint *(Royal* Instant)	190	4.0	35.0	4.0	m.q.	m.q.	390	n.a.
coconut, toasted *(Royal* Instant)	170	4.0	30.0	4.0	m.q.	m.q.	350	n.a.
coconut cream *(Jell-O* Instant)	180	4.0	27.0	6.0	m.q.	15	320	n.a.
custard:								
(Royal)	150	4.0	22.0	5.0	m.q.	m.q.	115	n.a.
egg, golden *(Jell-O Americana)*	160	5.0	23.0	5.0	m.q.	80	200	n.a.
lemon or vanilla *(Featherweight)*	40	1.0	8.0	0	0	0	40	n.a.
flan *(Jell-O)*	150	4.0	26.0	4.0	m.q.	15	65	n.a.
flan, w/caramel sauce *(Royal)*	150	4.0	22.0	5.0	m.q.	m.q.	115	n.a.
lemon:								
(French's)[1]	110	1.0	22.0	1.0	n.a.	n.a.	110	n.a.
(Jell-O Instant)	170	4.0	29.0	4.0	m.q.	15	360	n.a.
(Royal)	160	1.0	30.0	3.0	m.q.	m.q.	120	n.a.
(Royal Instant)	180	1.0	29.0	5.0	m.q.	m.q.	350	n.a.
lime, key *(Royal)*	160	1.0	30.0	3.0	m.q.	m.q.	120	n.a.
pistachio:								
(Jell-O Instant)	170	4.0	28.0	5.0	m.q.	15	410	n.a.
(Jell-O Instant Sugar Free), w/2%								
lowfat milk	90	4.0	12.0	3.0	m.q.	10	39	n.a.
nut *(Royal* Instant)	170	4.0	30.0	4.0	m.q.	m.q.	350	n.a.
raspberry, pie glaze and pudding								
(Salada Danish Dessert)	130	0	32.0	0	0	0	5	n.a.

1. *Prepared according to package directions.*

Food and Measure	cal.	prot. (gms)	carbo. (gms)	tot. fat (gms)	sat. fat (gms)	chol. (mgs)	sod. (mgs)	fiber (gms)
rennet custard:								
chocolate:								
(*Junket*), ⅜ oz. dry	40	1.0	10.0	0	0	0	5	n.a.
(*Junket*)	120	5.0	15.0	4.0	m.q.	m.q.	65	n.a.
(*Junket*), w/skim milk	90	5.0	15.0	0	0	(0)	70	n.a.
raspberry or strawberry:								
(*Junket*), ⅜ oz. dry	40	0	10.0	0	0	0	0	n.a.
(*Junket*)	120	4.0	16.0	4.0	m.q.	m.q.	60	n.a.
(*Junket*), w/skim milk	90	4.0	16.0	0	0	(0)	65	n.a.
vanilla:								
(*Junket*), ⅜ oz. dry	40	0	10.0	0	0	0	5	n.a.
(*Junket*)	120	4.0	16.0	4.0	m.q.	m.q.	65	n.a.
(*Junket*), w/skim milk	90	4.0	16.0	0	0	(0)	70	n.a.
rice (*Jell-O Americana*)	170	5.0	30.0	4.0	m.q.	15	160	n.a.
strawberry, pie glaze and pudding								
(*Salada Danish Dessert*)	130	0	32.0	0	0	0	5	n.a.
tapioca, vanilla (*Jell-O Americana*) ..	160	4.0	27.0	4.0	m.q.	15	170	n.a.
tapioca, vanilla (*Royal*)	160	4.0	27.0	4.0	m.q.	m.q.	150	n.a.
vanilla:								
(*D-Zerta*), w/skim milk	70	4.0	12.0	0	0	(0)	65	n.a.
(*Featherweight*)[1]	12	0	3.0	0	0	0	6	n.a.
(*Featherweight* Instant)[1]	100	4.0	19.0	0	0	5	190	n.a.
(*Jell-O*)	160	4.0	26.0	4.0	m.q.	15	200	n.a.
(*Jell-O* Instant)	170	4.0	29.0	4.0	m.q.	15	410	n.a.
(*Jell-O* Instant Sugar Free), w/2%								
lowfat milk	90	4.0	12.0	2.0	m.q.	10	390	n.a.
(*Jell-O* Microwave)	160	4.0	26.0	4.0	m.q.	15	180	n.a.
(*Jell-O* Cook'n Serve Sugar Free),								
w/2% lowfat milk	80	4.0	11.0	2.0	m.q.	10	200	n.a.
(*Royal*)	160	4.0	27.0	4.0	m.q.	m.q.	210	n.a.
(*Royal* Instant)	180	4.0	29.0	5.0	m.q.	m.q.	390	n.a.
(*Royal* Instant Sugar Free), w/2%								
lowfat milk	100	4.0	16.0	2.0	m.q.	m.q.	470	n.a.
French (*Jell-O*)	170	4.0	30.0	4.0	m.q.	15	190	n.a.
French (*Jell-O* Instant)	160	4.0	28.0	4.0	m.q.	15	400	n.a.
PUFF PASTRY, frozen:								
sheets (*Pepperidge Farm*), ¼ sheet	260	4.0	22.0	17.0	m.q.	n.a.	290	m.q.
shells, mini (*Pepperidge Farm*),								
1 shell	50	1.0	4.0	4.0	m.q.	n.a.	40	m.q.
shells, patty (*Pepperidge Farm*),								
1 shell	210	3.0	16.0	15.0	m.q.	n.a.	180	m.q.
PUMMELO:								
untrimmed, 1 lb.	95	1.9	24.4	.1	(0)	0	3	.5 c
trimmed, 1 oz.	11	.2	2.7	<.1	(0)	0	1	.1 c
1 medium, 5½″ diam., approx.								
2.4 lbs.	228	4.6	58.6	.2	(0)	0	7	1.1 c
sections, ½ cup	36	.7	9.1	<.1	(0)	0	1	.2 c

1. *Prepared according to package directions.*

Food and Measure	cal.	prot. (gms)	carbo. (gms)	tot. fat (gms)	sat. fat (gms)	chol. (mgs)	sod. (mgs)	fiber (gms)
PUMPKIN:								
raw:								
untrimmed, 1 lb.	83	3.2	20.6	.3	.2	0	3	3.5 c
trimmed, 1 oz.	7	.3	1.8	<.1	<.1	0	<1	.3 c
1" cubes, ½ cup	15	.6	3.8	.1	<.1	0	1	.6 c
boiled, drained, 4 oz.	23	.8	5.5	.1	<.1	0	1	.9 c
boiled, drained, mashed, ½ cup	24	.9	6.0	.1	<.1	0	2	1.0 c
PUMPKIN, CANNED:								
(Del Monte), ½ cup	35	1.0	9.0	0	0	0	<10	m.q.
(Libby's), ½ cup	42	1.4	10.1	.4	n.a.	0	6	3.8 d
(Stokely), ½ cup	40	2.0	10.0	0	0	0	15	m.q.
w/or w/out winter squash, 4 oz.	39	1.2	9.2	.3	.2	0	6	1.8 c
w/or w/out winter squash, ½ cup ..	41	1.3	9.9	.3	.2	0	6	2.0 c
PUMPKIN FLOWER:								
raw:								
untrimmed, 1 lb.	23	1.6	5.2	.1	.1	0	7	1.0 c
trimmed, 1 oz.	4	.3	.9	<.1	<.1	0	1	.2 c
trimmed, ½ cup	3	.2	.5	<.1	tr.	0	1	.1 c
boiled, drained, 4 oz.	17	1.2	3.7	.1	<.1	0	7	1.0 c
boiled, drained, ½ cup	10	.7	2.2	.1	<.1	0	4	.6 c
PUMPKIN LEAF:								
raw:								
untrimmed, 1 lb.	36	5.9	4.3	.7	.4	0	20	1.9 c
trimmed, 1 oz.	5	.9	.7	.1	.1	0	3	.3 c
trimmed, ½ cup	4	.6	.5	.1	<.1	0	2	.2 c
boiled, drained, 4 oz.	24	3.1	3.8	.2	.1	0	9	1.2 c
boiled, drained, ½ cup	7	1.0	1.2	.1	<.1	0	3	.4 c
PUMPKIN PIE, see "Pie"								
PUMPKIN PIE FILLING OR								
MIX, see "Pie filling"								
PUMPKIN PIE SPICE:								
1 oz.	97	1.6	19.6	3.6	m.q.	0	15	4.2 c
1 tbsp.	19	.3	3.9	.7	n.a.	0	3	.8 c
1 tsp.	6	.1	1.2	.2	n.a.	0	1	.3 c
PUMPKIN SEED[1]:								
roasted, whole, in shell:								
1 lb.	2021	84.1	243.8	88.0	16.6	0	82	162.8 c
1 oz., approx. 85 seeds	127	5.3	15.3	5.5	1.0	0	5	10.2 c
1 cup	285	11.9	34.4	12.4	2.3	0	12	23.0 c
salted:								
1 lb.	2021	84.1	243.8	88.0	16.6	0	2608	162.8 c
1 oz.	127	5.3	15.3	5.5	1.0	0	163	10.2 c
1 cup	285	11.9	34.4	12.4	2.3	0	368	23.0 c
roasted:								
1 oz.	148	9.4	3.8	12.0	2.2	0	5	.5 c
1 cup	1184	74.8	30.5	95.6	18.1	0	40	4.1 c
salted, 1 oz.	148	9.4	3.8	12.0	2.2	0	163	.5 c

1. *Shelled, except as noted.*

Food and Measure	cal.	prot. (gms)	carbo. (gms)	tot. fat (gms)	sat. fat (gms)	chol. (mgs)	sod. (mgs)	fiber (gms)
salted, 1 cup	1184	74.8	30.5	95.6	18.1	0	1305	4.1 c
dried:								
in shell, 1 lb.	1817	82.4	59.8	153.9	29.1	0	59	7.5 c
1 oz., approx. 142 kernels	154	7.0	5.1	13.0	2.5	0	5	.6 c
1 cup	747	33.9	24.6	63.3	12.0	0	24	3.1 c

PUMPKINSEED FISH, see
    "Sunfish"

PUNCH, see "Fruit punch" and
    specific fruit listings

PURSLANE:

raw:

Food and Measure	cal.	prot. (gms)	carbo. (gms)	tot. fat (gms)	sat. fat (gms)	chol. (mgs)	sod. (mgs)	fiber (gms)
untrimmed, 1 lb.	56	4.5	11.8	.3	(0)	0	156	2.8 c
trimmed, 1 oz.	5	.4	1.0	<.1	(0)	0	13	.2 c
trimmed, ½ cup	4	.3	.7	<.1	(0)	0	10	.2 c
1 plant, approx. .1 oz.	1	<.1	.1	tr.	(0)	0	1	<.1 c
boiled, drained, 4 oz.	20	1.7	4.0	.2	(0)	0	50	.9 c
boiled, drained, ½ cup	10	.9	2.1	.1	(0)	0	26	.5 c

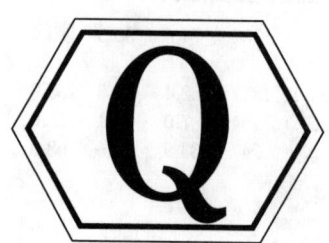

Food and Measure	cal.	prot. (gms)	carbo. (gms)	tot. fat (gms)	sat. fat (gms)	chol. (mgs)	sod. (mgs)	fiber (gms)
QUAIL, raw:								
meat w/skin:								
1 quail, 3.8 oz., yield from 4.3 oz.								
w/bone	210	21.4	0	13.1	3.7	m.q.	58	0
1 lb.	871	89.0	0	54.7	15.3	m.q.	240	0
1 oz.	54	5.6	0	3.4	1.0	m.q.	15	0
meat only:								
1 quail, 3.2 oz., yield from 4.3 oz.								
w/bone and skin	123	20.0	0	4.2	1.2	m.q.	47	0
1 lb.	608	98.7	0	20.5	6.0	m.q.	231	0
1 oz.	38	6.2	0	1.3	.4	m.q.	14	0
breast, meat only, 1 breast, approx.								
2 oz.	69	12.7	0	1.8	.5	m.q.	31	0
breast, meat only, 1 oz.	35	6.4	0	.8	.2	m.q.	16	0
QUEENSLAND NUT, see								
"Macadamia nut"								
QUINCE:								
untrimmed, 1 lb.	158	1.1	42.3	.3	<.1	0	11	4.7 c
trimmed, 1 oz.	16	.1	4.3	<.1	tr.	0	1	.5 c
1 medium, 5.3 oz.	53	.4	14.1	.1	tr.	0	4	1.6 c
QUINCY'S:								
main dishes, 1 serving:								
catfish fillets, 2 pieces, 6.9 oz. ...	309	26.0	19.0	12.0	m.q.	m.q.	101	m.q.
chicken breast, grilled, 5 oz.	145	35.0	0	.4	m.q.	72	140	0
chicken strips, 4 pieces, 4.5 oz. ..	318	39.0	4.0	15.0	m.q.	m.q.	m.q.	m.q.
hamburger, ¼ lb., 6.7 oz.	403	25.0	32.0	19.0	m.q.	m.q.	284	m.q.
hamburger, ¼ lb., w/cheese,								
7.2 oz.	451	28.0	32.0	23.0	m.q.	m.q.	432	m.q.
shrimp, 7 pieces, 3.9 oz.	248	22.0	11.0	12.0	m.q.	m.q.	205	m.q.
steak:								
chopped, 5.8 oz.	466	40.0	0	34.0	m.q.	m.q.	96	0

Food and Measure	cal.	prot. (gms)	carbo. (gms)	tot. fat (gms)	sat. fat (gms)	chol. (mgs)	sod. (mgs)	fiber (gms)
chopped, luncheon, 4 oz.	350	30.0	0	25.0	m.q.	m.q.	72	0
country style, w/mushroom								
sauce, 6 oz.	288	18.0	17.0	19.0	m.q.	m.q.	315	m.q.
filet, 5.6 oz.	331	51.0	0	12.0	m.q.	m.q.	159	0
rib-eye, 7.3 oz.	665	31.0	0	60.0	m.q.	m.q.	205	0
sirloin, 5.9 oz.	649	38.0	0	54.0	m.q.	m.q.	206	0
sirloin, large, 7.7 oz.	852	50.0	0	70.0	m.q.	m.q.	241	0
sirloin, petite, 4 oz.	446	26.0	0	37.0	m.q.	m.q.	118	0
sirloin club, 4.8 oz.	283	44.0	0	10.0	m.q.	m.q.	160	0
sirloin tips, 4 oz.	236	37.0	0	9.0	m.q.	m.q.	113	0
T-bone, 7.8 oz.	1045	43.0	0	95.0	m.q.	m.q.	222	0
side dishes, 1 serving:								
beans, green, 4.3 oz.	40	2.0	7.0	1.0	n.a.	0	500	m.q.
coleslaw, 2.1 oz.	60	<1.0	4.0	5.0	m.q.	n.a.	75	m.q.
cornbread, 1.9 oz.	178	4.0	28.0	6.0	m.q.	n.a.	263	m.q.
margarine, 1 oz.	204	<1.0	<1.0	22.0	m.q.	0	268	0
mushroom sauce, 3 oz.	27	1.0	5.0	<1.0	n.a.	n.a.	366	n.a.
peppers and onions, 4 oz.	80	1.0	8.0	5.0	m.q.	n.a.	11	m.q.
potato, baked, w/out butter,								
8.8 oz.	181	5.0	41.0	<1.0	n.a.	0	8	m.q.
steak fries, 5.5 oz.	426	7.0	56.0	21.0	m.q.	n.a.	90	m.q.
soups, 1 serving:								
broccoli, cream of, 9.2 oz.	193	3.0	13.0	14.0	m.q.	n.a.	1045	m.q.
chili w/beans, 9.2 oz.	346	20.0	32.0	16.0	m.q.	m.q.	1380	m.q.
clam chowder, 9.2 oz.	198	6.0	15.0	14.0	m.q.	m.q.	1185	m.q.
vegetable beef, 8.6 oz.	78	5.0	10.0	2.0	m.q.	m.q.	1045	m.q.
QUINOA:								
1 oz.	106	3.7	19.5	1.6	.2	0	n.a.	m.q.
1 cup	637	22.3	117.1	9.9	1.0	0	n.a.	m.q.
QUINOA SEED:								
(*Arrowhead Mills*), 2 oz.	200	9.0	35.0	3.0	n.a.	0	3	5.3 d

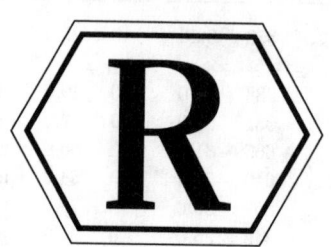

Food and Measure	cal.	prot. (gms)	carbo. (gms)	tot. fat (gms)	sat. fat (gms)	chol. (mgs)	sod. (mgs)	fiber (gms)
RABBIT[1], domesticated, composite cuts, meat only:								
raw, 1 oz.	39	5.7	0	1.6	.5	16	12	0
roasted:								
14 oz., yield from 1 lb. raw								
boneless	616	91.0	0	25.2	7.5	257	147	0
4 oz.	175	25.8	0	7.2	2.1	73	42	0
diced, 1 cup, approx. 4.9 oz.	216	31.9	0	8.8	2.6	90	52	0
stewed:								
10.5 oz., yield from 1 lb. raw								
boneless	616	91.0	0	25.2	7.5	257	111	0
4 oz.	234	34.5	0	9.5	2.8	98	42	0
diced, 1 cup, approx. 4.9 oz.	288	42.5	0	11.8	3.5	120	52	0
RABBIT, WILD, meat only:								
raw, 1 oz.	32	6.2	0	.7	.2	23	14	0
stewed[2]:								
10.5 oz., yield from 1 lb. raw								
boneless	517	98.9	0	10.5	3.1	367	135	0
4 oz.	196	37.4	0	4.0	1.2	139	51	0
diced, 1 cup, approx. 4.9 oz.	242	46.2	0	4.9	1.5	172	63	0
RACCOON, roasted[2], meat only:								
14 oz., yield from 1 lb. raw boneless	1020	116.6	0	57.9	m.q.	m.q.	m.q.	0
4 oz.	289	33.1	0	16.4	m.q.	m.q.	m.q.	0
diced, 1 cup, approx. 4.9 oz.	357	40.9	0	20.3	m.q.	m.q.	m.q.	0
RADISH:								
untrimmed, 1 lb.	68	2.5	14.6	2.2	.1	0	98	2.2 c
trimmed, 1 oz.	5	.2	1.0	.2	tr.	0	7	.2 c
10 medium, ¾"–1" diam., approx.								
1.8 oz.	7	.3	1.6	.2	<.1	0	11	.2 c
sliced, ½ cup	10	.4	2.1	.3	<.1	0	14	.3 c

1. *Cooked meats are prepared without added ingredients.*
2. *Without added ingredients.*

Food and Measure	cal.	prot. (gms)	carbo. (gms)	tot. fat (gms)	sat. fat (gms)	chol. (mgs)	sod. (mgs)	fiber (gms)
RADISH, BLACK, trimmed:								
1 lb.	77	4.5	16.3	.5	m.q.	0	82	m.q.
1 oz.	5	.3	1.0	<.1	tr.	0	5	m.q.
RADISH, ORIENTAL:								
raw:								
untrimmed, 1 lb.	65	2.2	14.7	.4	.1	0	75	2.3 c
trimmed:								
1 oz.	5	.2	1.2	<.1	tr.	0	6	.2 c
sliced, ½ cup	8	.3	1.8	<.1	<.1	0	9	.3 c
(*Frieda* of California), 1 lb.	86	4.1	19.1	.5	m.q.	0	m.q.	m.q.
(*Frieda* of California), 1 oz.	5	.3	1.2	<.1	tr.	0	m.q.	m.q.
1 medium, 7″ × 2¼″ diam.,								
approx. 15.1 oz.	62	2.0	13.9	.3	.1	0	71	2.2 c
boiled, drained, 4 oz.	19	.8	3.9	.3	.1	0	15	.6 c
boiled, drained, sliced, ½ cup	13	.5	2.5	.2	.1	0	10	.4 c
dried, 1 oz.	77	2.2	18.0	.2	.1	0	79	2.4 c
dried, ½ cup	157	4.6	36.8	.4	.1	0	161	4.9 c
RADISH, WHITE ICICLE:								
untrimmed, 1 lb.	41	3.2	7.7	.3	.1	0	47	2.1 c
trimmed, 1 oz.	4	.3	.7	<.1	tr.	0	5	.2 c
1 medium, approx. .6 oz.	2	.2	.5	<.1	tr.	0	3	.1 c
sliced, ½ cup	7	.6	1.3	.1	<.1	0	8	.4 c
RADISH, WINTER, see "Radish, black"								
RADISH JUICE, bottled:								
(*Biotta*), 6 fl. oz.	39	1.6	7.5	<.1	tr.	0	101	m.q.
RADISH LEAVES:								
trimmed, 1 oz.	15	.8	2.8	.1	tr.	0	m.q.	.4 c
RADISH SEED, sprouted:								
1 lb.	186	17.3	13.9	11.5	3.5	0	28	m.q.
1 oz.	12	1.1	.9	.7	.2	0	2	m.q.
½ cup	8	.7	.6	.5	.1	0	1	m.q.
RAISIN:								
golden (*Del Monte*), 3 oz.	260	3.0	68.0	0	0	0	<10	m.q.
golden seedless:								
1 lb.	1368	15.4	360.7	2.1	.7	0	54	6.5 c
1 oz.	86	1.0	22.5	.1	<.1	0	3	.4 c
½ cup not packed	219	2.5	57.7	.3	.1	0	9	1.0 c
½ cup packed	249	2.8	65.6	.4	.1	0	10	1.2 c
(*Dole*), ½ cup	260	3.0	63.0	0	0	0	25	m.q.
natural (*Del Monte*), 3 oz.	250	3.0	68.0	0	0	0	15	m.q.
seeded:								
1 lb.	1340	11.4	355.9	2.5	.8	0	128	3.1 c
1 oz.	84	.7	22.2	.2	.1	0	8	.2 c
½ cup not packed	214	1.8	56.9	.4	.1	0	21	.5 c
½ cup packed	244	2.1	64.7	.5	.1	0	24	.6 c
seedless:								
1 lb.	1359	14.6	358.9	2.1	.7	0	53	24.0 d
1 oz.	85	.9	22.4	.1	<.1	0	3	1.5 d

Food and Measure	cal.	prot. (gms)	carbo. (gms)	tot. fat (gms)	sat. fat (gms)	chol. (mgs)	sod. (mgs)	fiber (gms)
RAISIN, SEEDLESS *(cont.)*								
½ cup not packed	217	2.3	57.4	.3	.1	0	9	3.8 d
½ cup packed	247	2.7	65.3	.4	.1	0	10	4.4 d
(*Cinderella* Thompson), ½ cup . .	250	3.0	66.0	0	0	0	15	5.8 d
(*Dole*), ½ cup	260	3.0	63.0	0	0	0	25	m.q.
(*Finast*), ½ oz.	45	0	11.0	0	0	0	5	m.q.
(*Sun•Maid*), ½ cup	290	3.0	69.0	0	0	0	<15	m.q.
RAMONS, see "Breadnut tree seed"								
RASPBERRY:								
untrimmed, 1 lb.	215	4.0	50.4	2.4	.1	0	1	20.5 d
untrimmed, 1 pint, 11.5 oz.	154	2.8	36.1	1.7	.1	0	tr.	15.3 d
trimmed, 1 oz.	14	.3	3.3	.2	tr.	0	tr.	1.3 d
trimmed, ½ cup	31	.6	7.1	.3	<.1	0	tr.	2.9 d
RASPBERRY, CANNED:								
red, in heavy syrup, 4 oz.	103	.9	26.5	.1	tr.	0	3	m.q.
red, in heavy syrup, ½ cup	117	1.1	29.9	.2	tr.	0	4	m.q.
RASPBERRY, FROZEN:								
sweetened:								
10-oz. pkg.	291	2.0	74.3	.5	<.1	0	1	6.3 c
4 oz.	117	.8	29.7	.2	tr.	0	1	2.5 c
½ cup	128	.9	32.7	.2	tr.	0	1	2.8 c
in lite syrup, red (*Birds Eye* Quick Thaw Pouch), 5 oz.	100	1.0	25.0	1.0	tr.	0	0	4.0 d
RASPBERRY DANISH, see "Danish pastry"								
RASPBERRY DRINK MIX[1], 8 fl. oz.:								
(*Kool-Aid*)	100	0	25.0	0	0	0	25	0
(*Kool-Aid* Presweetened)	80	0	20.0	0	0	0	25	0
RASPBERRY FRUIT ROLL, see "Fruit snack"								
RASPBERRY JUICE:								
blend (*Dole Pure & Light* Country Raspberry), 6 fl. oz.	87	.3	24.0	.2	(0)	0	15	(0)
red (*Smucker's* Naturally 100%), 8 fl. oz.	120	0	30.0	0	0	0	10	(0)
RASPBERRY JUICE COCKTAIL:								
(*Welch's Orchard*), 10-fl.-oz. bottle	160	0	40.0	0	0	0	10	0
RASPBERRY MOUSSE, see "Mousse"								
RASPBERRY-CRANBERRY DRINK, 6 fl. oz.:								
(*A&P*)	110	<1.0	27.0	<1.0	(0)	0	0	(0)
(*Finast*)	110	0	27.0	0	0	0	10	(0)
(*Pathmark*)	110	0	27.0	0	0	0	10	(0)
(*Pathmark* Sodium Free)	110	0	27.0	0	0	0	0	(0)

1. *Prepared according to package directions.*

Food and Measure	cal.	prot. (gms)	carbo. (gms)	tot. fat (gms)	sat. fat (gms)	chol. (mgs)	sod. (mgs)	fiber (gms)
RASPBERRY-CRANBERRY JUICE:								
(*Apple & Eve*), 6 fl. oz.	90	0	21.0	0	0	0	10	m.q.
RAVIOLI, CANNED, 7.5 oz., except as noted:								
beef:								
(*Chef Boyardee* Microwave)	190	7.0	31.0	4.0	2.0	11	1160	2.0 d
(*Estee*)	230	8.0	25.0	11.0	4.0	10	100	m.q.
(*Nalley's*)	180	8.0	30.0	3.0	m.q.	m.q.	1040	m.q.
bite size, in tomato sauce (*Pathmark* No Frills)	180	7.0	28.0	4.0	m.q.	m.q.	890	m.q.
in meat sauce (*Franco-American* RavioliO's)	250	10.0	35.0	8.0	m.q.	m.q.	920	m.q.
in sauce (*Finast*)	250	7.0	33.0	10.0	m.q.	m.q.	1165	m.q.
in tomato sauce (*Hormel Micro-Cup*)	247	8.0	28.0	11.0	m.q.	21	951	m.q.
in tomato sauce (*Pathmark* No Frills)	180	7.0	28.0	4.0	m.q.	m.q.	890	m.q.
cheese:								
in meat sauce (*Chef Boyardee* Microwave)	200	6.0	37.0	3.0	m.q.	10	1010	m.q.
in sauce (*Buitoni*)	190	7.0	27.0	6.0	2.0	5	790	m.q.
in tomato sauce (*Pathmark* No Frills)	185	7.0	27.0	6.0	m.q.	m.q.	790	m.q.
meat, in sauce (*Buitoni*)	180	7.0	28.0	4.0	1.0	5	890	m.q.
RAVIOLI, FROZEN:								
(*Celentano*), 6.5 oz.	380	21.0	50.0	11.0	m.q.	m.q.	510	m.q.
cheese (*Buitoni*), ¼ pkg. or 4 oz. ..	360	12.0	31.0	8.0	5.0	65	220	m.q.
mini (*Celentano*), 4 oz.	250	13.0	39.0	5.0	m.q.	m.q.	210	m.q.
RAVIOLI DINNER, frozen:								
mini cheese (*Kid Cuisine*), 8.75 oz.	250	6.0	52.0	2.0	m.q.	20	730	m.q.
RAVIOLI ENTREE, frozen:								
cheese (*The Budget Gourmet* Slim Selects), 10 oz.	260	12.0	36.0	7.0	m.q.	45	960	m.q.
cheese, baked (*Weight Watchers*), 9 oz.	290	18.0	34.0	9.0	4.0	85	630	m.q.
RAX:								
sandwiches, 1 serving:								
BBC (beef, bacon, and cheddar), 8 oz.	720	30.0	40.0	49.0	m.q.	137	1873	m.q.
BBQ, 5.7 oz.	420	21.0	53.0	14.0	m.q.	24	1343	m.q.
fish, 7 oz.	460	14.0	58.0	17.0	m.q.	<1	935	m.q.
ham and Swiss, 7.9 oz.	430	23.0	42.0	23.0	m.q.	37	1,737	m.q.
Philly beef and cheese, 8.25 oz. ..	480	25.0	44.0	22.0	m.q.	49	1346	m.q.
roast beef:								
large, 8 oz.	570	22.0	41.0	35.0	m.q.	36	1169	m.q.
regular, 5.25 oz.	320	20.0	33.0	11.0	m.q.	36	969	m.q.
small (*Uncle Al*), 3.1 oz.	260	12.0	21.0	14.0	m.q.	19	562	m.q.
turkey bacon club, 9 oz.	670	29.0	41.0	43.0	m.q.	87	1878	m.q.

Food and Measure	cal.	prot. (gms)	carbo. (gms)	tot. fat (gms)	sat. fat (gms)	chol. (mgs)	sod. (mgs)	fiber (gms)
RAX *(cont.)*								
sandwich condiments and ingredients:								
American cheese slices, .5 oz.	60	3.0	<1.0	5.0	m.q.	15	180	0
bacon, .5-oz. slice	80	4.0	<1.0	7.0	m.q.	30	321	0
BBC sauce, .75 oz.	140	<1.0	<1.0	16.0	m.q.	41	163	n.a.
BBQ meat topping, 3.25 oz.	140	13.0	13.0	4.0	m.q.	24	898	n.a.
BBQ sauce, regular or smokey, 1 oz.	40	<1.0	10.0	<1.0	m.q.	<1	396	n.a.
bun, hoagie, 6″, 3 oz.	280	8.0	40.0	10.0	m.q.	<1	544	m.q.
bun, kaiser, 4″, 2.25 oz.	180	6.0	33.0	2.0	m.q.	<1	445	m.q.
bun, small, 1.7 oz.	180	4.0	21.0	3.0	m.q.	<1	282	m.q.
catsup, 1 tbsp.	6	<1.0	2.0	<1.0	(0)	0	50	m.q.
fish, 3.5 oz.	230	8.0	23.0	12.0	m.q.	<1	356	n.a.
ham, 2.5 oz.	70	13.0	1.0	2.0	m.q.	24	850	0
horseradish sauce, .75 oz.	10	<1.0	2.0	<1.0	(0)	<1	46	n.a.
lettuce, shredded, ¼ cup	2	<1.0	<1.0	<1.0	(0)	0	1	m.q.
mayonnaise, .75 oz.	150	<1.0	1.0	16.0	m.q.	<1	100	0
Philly vegetables, 2 oz.	30	1.0	4.0	1.0	m.q.	<1	36	m.q.
pickle, 2.3-oz. spear	8	<1.0	2.0	<1.0	(0)	0	928	m.q.
roast beef, 2.8 oz.	140	14.0	<1.0	9.0	m.q.	36	524	0
Swiss cheese slices, .5 oz.	30	2.0	<1.0	2.0	m.q.	13	242	0
tartar sauce, .5 oz.	50	<1.0	2.0	5.0	m.q.	<1	133	n.a.
tomatoes, .5-oz. slice	2	<1.0	<1.0	<1.0	(0)	0	<1	m.q.
turkey, 2.5 oz.	80	13.0	<1.0	3.0	m.q.	27	591	0
french fries, 1 serving:								
large, salted, 4.5 oz.	390	3.0	50.0	20.0	m.q.	16	104	m.q.
large, unsalted (on request), 4.5 oz.	390	3.0	50.0	20.0	m.q.	16	66	m.q.
regular, salted, 3 oz.	260	2.0	33.0	13.0	m.q.	10	69	m.q.
regular, unsalted (on request), 3 oz.	260	2.0	33.0	13.0	m.q.	10	44	m.q.
potatoes, 1 serving:								
plain, 8.8 oz.	270	8.0	60.0	<1.0	m.q.	0	70	m.q.
plain, w/margarine, 9.3 oz.	370	8.0	60.0	11.0	m.q.	0	170	m.q.
BBQ, w/cheese (2 oz.), 14.3 oz.	730	24.0	104.0	24.0	m.q.	18	1071	m.q.
cheese (3 oz.) and bacon, 12.8 oz.	780	22.0	110.0	28.0	m.q.	23	910	m.q.
cheese (3 oz.) and broccoli, 13.8 oz.	760	19.0	112.0	26.0	m.q.	11	489	m.q.
chili and cheese (2 oz.), 14.3 oz.	700	22.0	101.0	23.0	m.q.	25	599	m.q.
potato topping ingredients:								
bacon bits, .5 oz.	40	5.0	<1.0	2.0	m.q.	12	427	0
BBQ meat sauce, 2.5 oz.	110	10.0	10.0	3.0	m.q.	18	692	n.a.
broccoli, 1.5 oz.	16	2.0	2.0	<1.0	(0)	0	7	m.q.
cheese sauce, 3 oz.	370	9.0	50.0	15.0	m.q.	11	313	n.a.
chili, 3 oz.	80	8.0	8.0	2.0	m.q.	18	221	m.q.
liquid margarine, 1 tbsp.	100	<1.0	<1.0	11.0	m.q.	0	100	0
onion, diced, .5 oz.	10	<1.0	1.0	<1.0	(0)	0	1	m.q.

Food and Measure	cal.	prot. (gms)	carbo. (gms)	tot. fat (gms)	sat. fat (gms)	chol. (mgs)	sod. (mgs)	fiber (gms)
sour topping, 3.5 oz.	130	3.0	5.0	11.0	m.q.	<1	79	n.a.
drive-thru salad, w/out dressing,								
1 serving:								
chef salad, 12.5 oz.	230	22.0	4.0	14.0	m.q.	322	1048	m.q.
garden salad, 10.5 oz.	160	12.0	4.0	11.0	m.q.	273	362	m.q.
salad bar:								
alfalfa sprouts, 1 oz.	8	<1.0	2.0	<1.0	(0)	0	<1	m.q.
applesauce, 1 cup	100	<1.0	26.0	<1.0	(0)	0	5	m.q.
bacon bits, .5 oz.	40	5.0	>1.0	2.0	m.q.	12	427	0
banana chips, 1 oz.	100	1.0	25.0	<1.0	(0)	0	1	m.q.
beets, 1 cup	60	2.0	12.0	<1.0	(0)	0	73	m.q.
broccoli, ½ cup	16	2.0	2.0	<1.0	(0)	0	7	m.q.
cabbage, 1 cup	16	<1.0	4.0	<1.0	(0)	0	18	m.q.
cantaloupe, 2 pieces	16	<1.0	4.0	<1.0	(0)	0	6	m.q.
carrots, ¼ cup	8	<1.0	2.0	<1.0	(0)	0	<1	m.q.
cauliflower, ½ cup	16	2.0	2.0	<1.0	(0)	0	6	m.q.
celery, 1 tbsp.	<1	<1.0	<1.0	<1.0	(0)	0	10	m.q.
cheddar cheese, imitation,								
shredded, 1 oz.	90	6.0	2.0	6.0	m.q.	6	310	n.a.
cheddar cheese tidbits, 1 oz.	160	3.0	12.0	11.0	m.q.	<1	445	0
cherry peppers, 1 tbsp.	6	<1.0	<1.0	<1.0	(0)	0	180	m.q.
chow mein noodles, 1 oz.	140	4.0	17.0	6.0	m.q.	<1	242	m.q.
coconut, 1 oz.	160	<1.0	15.0	11.0	m.q.	0	<1	m.q.
coleslaw, 3.5 oz.	70	1.0	8.0	4.0	m.q.	<1	187	m.q.
cottage cheese, 1 cup	250	33.0	7.0	10.0	m.q.	47	561	m.q.
crackers (*Saltines*), 2 pieces	16	<1.0	4.0	<1.0	m.q.	<1	70	m.q.
croutons, .5 oz.	40	2.0	8.0	<1.0	m.q.	<1	155	m.q.
cucumbers, 2 slices	2	<1.0	<1.0	<1.0	(0)	0	<1	m.q.
eggs, 1.5 oz.	70	6.0	<1.0	5.0	m.q.	267	52	0
garbanzo beans, ½ cup	360	20.0	60.0	5.0	m.q.	0	26	m.q.
gelatin, lime or strawberry,								
½ cup	90	2.0	20.0	<1.0	(0)	0	90	0
grapefruit sections, 1 cup	80	2.0	18.0	<1.0	(0)	0	10	m.q.
grapes, 1 cup	100	<1.0	25.0	<1.0	(0)	0	5	m.q.
green pepper, ¼ cup	8	<1.0	1.0	<1.0	(0)	0	5	m.q.
honeydew melon, 2 pieces	25	<1.0	6.0	<1.0	(0)	0	5	m.q.
kale, 1 oz.	16	2.0	2.0	<1.0	(0)	0	21	m.q.
kidney beans, 1 cup	220	14.0	40.0	1.0	m.q.	0	8	m.q.
lettuce, 1 leaf	2	<1.0	<1.0	<1.0	(0)	0	<1	m.q.
macaroni salad, 3.5 oz.	160	2.0	21.0	7.0	m.q.	<1	216	m.q.
mushrooms, ¼ cup	4	<1.0	<1.0	<1.0	(0)	0	<1	m.q.
onions, ¼ cup	12	<1.0	3.0	<1.0	(0)	0	3	m.q.
pasta salad, 3.5 oz.	80	2.0	16.0	1.0	m.q.	<1	322	m.q.
peaches, 2 slices	16	<1.0	4.0	<1.0	(0)	0	<1	m.q.
peas, 1 oz.	25	2.0	4.0	<1.0	(0)	0	35	m.q.
pickle, 1 spear	8	<1.0	2.0	<1.0	(0)	0	928	m.q.
pineapple, fresh, 3-oz. slice	45	<1.0	12.0	<1.0	(0)	0	1	m.q.
pineapple, canned, 3.5 oz.	100	<1.0	25.0	<1.0	(0)	0	10	m.q.
potato salad, 1 cup	260	7.0	41.0	17.0	m.q.	7	127	m.q.

Food and Measure	cal.	prot. (gms)	carbo. (gms)	tot. fat (gms)	sat. fat (gms)	chol. (mgs)	sod. (mgs)	fiber (gms)
RAX, SALAD BAR *(cont.)*								
pudding, butterscotch, 3.5 oz. ...	140	2.0	20.0	6.0	m.q.	2	150	(0)
pudding, chocolate or vanilla,								
3.5 oz.	140	2.0	20.0	6.0	m.q.	2	120	(0)
radish, .5 oz.	2	<1.0	<1.0	<1.0	(0)	0	<1	m.q.
red cabbage, ¼ cup	4	<1.0	<1.0	<1.0	(0)	0	6	m.q.
sesame sticks, 1 oz.	150	3.0	13.0	10.0	m.q.	0	405	m.q.
soynuts, 1 oz.	120	10.0	5.0	7.0	m.q.	0	151	m.q.
strawberries, 2 oz.	18	<1.0	4.0	<1.0	(0)	0	<1	m.q.
sunflower seeds, w/raisins, 1 oz.	130	5.0	6.0	10.0	m.q.	0	5	m.q.
three-bean salad, ½ cup	100	3.0	23.0	<1.0	m.q.	0	450	m.q.
tomatoes, 1 oz.	6	<1.0	2.0	<1.0	(0)	0	6	m.q.
turkey bits, 2 oz.	70	10.0	<1.0	3.0	m.q.	49	686	0
watermelon, 2 pieces	18	<1.0	4.0	<1.0	(0)	0	<1	m.q.
dressings, 1 tbsp.:								
blue cheese	50	<1.0	1.0	5.0	m.q.	8	110	n.a.
blue cheese, "lite"	35	<1.0	2.0	3.0	m.q.	3	240	n.a.
French	60	<1.0	6.0	4.0	m.q.	0	140	n.a.
French, "lite"	40	<1.0	5.0	2.0	m.q.	0	122	n.a.
Italian	50	<1.0	3.0	4.0	m.q.	0	159	n.a.
Italian, "lite"	30	<1.0	1.0	3.0	m.q.	0	152	n.a.
poppy seed	60	<1.0	5.0	4.0	m.q.	6	107	n.a.
ranch	45	<1.0	<1.0	5.0	m.q.	5	103	n.a.
Thousand Island	70	<1.0	6.0	6.0	m.q.	8	110	n.a.
Thousand Island, "lite"	40	<1.0	3.0	3.0	m.q.	5	143	n.a.
oil	130	<1.0	<1.0	14.0	m.q.	0	<1	0
vinegar	2	<1.0	<1.0	<1.0	(0)	0	5	0
Mexican bar:								
banana pepper rings, 1 tbsp.	2	<1.0	<1.0	<1.0	(0)	0	20	m.q.
cheese sauce, 3.5 oz.	420	10.0	58.0	17.0	n.a.	11	365	n.a.
cheese sauce, nacho, 3.5 oz.	470	10.0	57.0	22.0	n.a.	11	190	n.a.
green onions, ¼ cup	10	<1.0	2.0	<1.0	(0)	0	1	m.q.
jalapeño peppers, 1 oz.	6	<1.0	1.0	<1.0	(0)	0	231	m.q.
olives, 3.5 oz.	110	<1.0	6.0	10.0	m.q.	0	880	m.q.
refried beans, 3 oz.	120	6.0	16.0	4.0	m.q.	2	375	m.q.
sour topping, 3.5 oz.	130	3.0	5.0	11.0	m.q.	<1	79	n.a.
Spanish rice, 3.5 oz.	90	3.0	20.0	<1.0	n.a.	0	442	m.q.
spicy meat sauce, 3.5 oz.	80	5.0	6.0	4.0	m.q.	12	751	n.a.
taco sauce, 3.5 oz.	30	1.0	6.0	<1.0	(0)	0	806	n.a.
taco shells, 1 piece	40	<1.0	6.0	2.0	m.q.	0	53	m.q.
tomatoes, 1 oz.	6	<1.0	2.0	<1.0	(0)	0	6	m.q.
tortilla, 1 piece	110	3.0	19.0	2.0	m.q.	0	284	m.q.
tortilla chips, 1 oz.	140	2.0	17.0	7.0	m.q.	0	100	m.q.
pasta bar:								
Alfredo sauce, 3.5 oz.	80	2.0	12.0	3.0	m.q.	10	70	m.q.
chicken noodle soup, 3.5 oz.	40	2.0	8.0	<1.0	m.q.	10	1040	m.q.
creme of broccoli soup, 3.5 oz. ..	50	1.0	6.0	2.0	m.q.	<1	219	m.q.
Parmesan cheese substitute,								
1 oz.	80	8.0	2.0	4.0	m.q.	<1	1000	m.q.

Food and Measure	cal.	prot. (gms)	carbo. (gms)	tot. fat (gms)	sat. fat (gms)	chol. (mgs)	sod. (mgs)	fiber (gms)
pasta shells, 3.5 oz.	170	7.0	27.0	4.0	m.q.	0	2	m.q.
pasta/vegetable blend, 3.5 oz. ...	100	4.0	12.0	4.0	m.q.	0	11	m.q.
rainbow rotini, 3.5 oz.	180	6.0	30.0	4.0	m.q.	2	9	m.q.
spaghetti, 3.5 oz.	140	3.0	23.0	4.0	m.q.	0	1	m.q.
spaghetti sauce, 3.5 oz.	80	1.0	19.0	<1.0	m.q.	<1	635	m.q.
spaghetti sauce, w/meat, 3.5 oz.	150	7.0	12.0	8.0	m.q.	<1	419	m.q.
desserts, 1 serving:								
chocolate chip cookie, 1 piece ...	130	1.0	17.0	6.0	m.q.	<1	65	m.q.
milkshake, w/out whipped topping:								
chocolate	560	13.0	97.0	13.0	m.q.	63	239	(0)
strawberry	560	13.0	97.0	13.0	m.q.	62	226	(0)
vanilla	500	13.0	81.0	14.0	m.q.	58	286	0
whipped topping, 1 dollop	50	<1.0	4.0	4.0	m.q.	2	6	0
hot cocoa mix, 6 fl. oz.	110	2.0	<1.0	11.0	m.q.	<1	120	m.q.
RED BEAN, canned:								
(*A&P*), ½ cup	120	7.0	23.0	<1.0	tr.	0	400	m.q.
(*Allens*), ½ cup	115	7.0	20.0	<1.0	tr.	0	350	m.q.
(*Green Giant/Joan of Arc*), ½ cup ...	90	6.0	19.0	1.0	tr.	0	340	5.0 d
(*Van Camp's*), 1 cup	194	11.0	38.0	.6	tr.	0	928	m.q.
small (*Hunt's*), 4 oz.	91	5.7	18.1	0	0	0	578	m.q.
small, baked-style (*B&M*), 8 oz. ...	223	9.0	36.0	5.0	2.0	5	725	11.0 d
RED CABBAGE, see "Cabbage, red"								
RED SNAPPER, see "Snapper"								
REDFISH, see "Ocean perch"								
REFRIED BEANS:								
(*Little Pancho*), ½ cup	80	6.0	15.0	0	0	n.a.	330	m.q.
canned:								
4 oz.	121	7.1	21.0	1.2	.5	n.a.	481	3.6 c
½ cup	134	7.9	23.3	1.4	.5	n.a.	534	4.0 c
(*Bearitos* Organic), 1 oz.	30	1.7	4.8	.5	m.q.	0	61	.3 d
(*Bearitos* Organic No Salt), 1 oz.	29	1.7	4.7	.5	m.q.	0	2	.2 d
(*Del Monte*), ½ cup	130	6.0	20.0	2.0	m.q.	n.a.	530	m.q.
(*Gebhardt*), 4 oz.	130	7.0	20.0	2.0	m.q.	n.a.	490	m.q.
(*Old El Paso*), ¼ cup	55	3.0	8.0	<1.0	m.q.	1	200	2.5 d
(*Rosarita*), 4 oz.	120	7.0	19.0	2.0	m.q.	n.a.	470	m.q.
w/cheese (*Old El Paso*), ¼ cup ..	36	2.0	4.0	1.0	1.0	2	280	2.0 d
w/green chilies (*Old El Paso*), ¼ cup	49	3.0	8.0	<1.0	m.q.	n.a.	252	2.5 d
jalapeño (*Gebhardt*), 4 oz.	110	7.0	18.0	2.0	m.q.	n.a.	320	m.q.
w/sausage (*Old El Paso*), ¼ cup	180	6.0	8.0	8.0	m.q.	m.q.	300	m.q.
spicy:								
(*Bearitos* Organic), 1 oz.	31	1.6	4.9	.6	m.q.	0	56	.5 d
(*Del Monte*), ½ cup	130	6.0	20.0	2.0	m.q.	n.a.	480	m.q.
(*Old El Paso*), ¼ cup	35	1.0	5.0	1.0	0	1	280	2.0 d
(*Rosarita*), 4 oz.	120	8.0	20.0	2.0	m.q.	n.a.	465	m.q.
vegetarian (*Old El Paso*), ¼ cup	70	6.0	15.0	1.0	n.a.	0	730	5.0 d
vegetarian (*Rosarita*), 4 oz.	120	7.0	19.0	2.0	m.q.	0	470	m.q.

Food and Measure	cal.	prot. (gms)	carbo. (gms)	tot. fat (gms)	sat. fat (gms)	chol. (mgs)	sod. (mgs)	fiber (gms)
REFRIED BEANS *(cont.)*								
mix, instant *(Fantastic Foods)*,								
½ cup[1]	157	10.0	28.0	2.0	m.q.	0	400	m.q.
mix, instant *(Fantastic Foods)*,								
½ cup[2]	207	10.0	28.0	8.0	m.q.	n.a.	469	m.q.
RELISH:								
dill *(Vlasic)*, 1 oz.	2	0	1.0	0	0	0	415	m.q.
hamburger *(Heinz)*, 1 oz.	40	0	9.0	0	0	0	255	m.q.
hot dog *(Heinz)*, 1 oz.	35	0	8.0	0	0	0	200	m.q.
hot dog *(Vlasic)*, 1 oz.	40	0	8.0	1.0	(0)	0	255	m.q.
India *(Heinz)*, 1 oz.	35	0	9.0	0	0	0	215	m.q.
India *(Vlasic)*, 1 oz.	30	0	8.0	0	0	0	205	m.q.
jalapeño *(Old El Paso)*, 2 tbsp.	16	1.0	4.0	0	0	0	100	1.0 d
piccalilli *(Heinz)*, 1 oz.	30	0	7.0	0	0	0	145	m.q.
piccalilli, hot *(Vlasic)*, 1 oz.	35	0	8.0	0	0	0	165	m.q.
pickle *(Claussen)*, 1 oz.	26	.3	5.6	.3	(0)	0	170	m.q.
pickle *(Claussen)*, 1 tbsp.	14	.2	2.9	.2	(0)	0	90	m.q.
sweet:								
1 cup	338	1.2	83.3	1.5	n.a.	0	1744	m.q.
1 tbsp.	21	.1	5.1	.1	(0)	0	107	m.q.
1 pkt., approx. ⅔ tbsp.	14	.1	3.4	.1	(0)	0	71	m.q.
(Heinz), 1 oz.	35	0	9.0	0	0	0	205	m.q.
(Vlasic), 1 oz.	30	0	8.0	0	0	0	220	m.q.
RENNET CUSTARD, see "Pudding mix"								
RESTAURANTS, see specific listings								
RHUBARB:								
untrimmed, 1 lb.	71	3.0	15.4	.7	n.a.	0	14	2.4 c
trimmed, 1 oz.	6	.3	1.3	.1	(0)	0	1	.2 c
diced, ½ cup	13	.6	2.8	.1	(0)	0	2	.4 c
RHUBARB, FROZEN:								
4 oz.	24	.6	5.8	.1	(0)	0	2	m.q.
½ cup	14	.4	3.5	.1	(0)	0	1	m.q.
cooked, sweetened, 4 oz.	132	.4	35.4	.1	(0)	0	1	.9 c
cooked, sweetened, ½ cup	139	.5	37.4	.1	(0)	0	2	1.0 c
RIB SAUCE:								
(Dip n'Joy Saucey Rib), 1 oz.	60	0	14.0	0	0	0	250	n.a.
RICE, ARBORIO:								
(Colavita), 1 oz. dry	100	2.0	22.0	0	0	0	5	m.q.
RICE, BASMATI, cooked[3], ½ cup, except as noted:								
(Fantastic Foods)[4]	103	2.0	23.0	0	0	0	1	m.q.
(Fantastic Foods)[5]	116	2.0	23.0	1.0	m.q.	m.q.	18	m.q.

1. *Prepared according to package directions, without added ingredients.*
2. *Prepared according to package directions, with 2 tbsp. salted butter.*
3. *Prepared according to package directions, without salt and butter, except as noted.*
4. *If adding ½ tsp. salt to basic recipe, increase sodium value by 125 mg.*
5. *Prepared with 1 tbsp. salted butter.*

Food and Measure	cal.	prot. (gms)	carbo. (gms)	tot. fat (gms)	sat. fat (gms)	chol. (mgs)	sod. (mgs)	fiber (gms)
brown:								
(*Fastastic Foods*)[1]	102	3.0	22.0	.5	n.a.	0	3	m.q.
(*Fantastic Foods*)[2]	115	3.0	22.0	2.0	m.q.	m.q.	20	m.q.
long (*Arrowhead Mills*), 2 oz. dry ..	200	4.0	44.0	1.0	n.a.	0	3	3.1 d
white, long grain (*Texmati*)	82	3.0	31.0	0	0	0	0	m.q.
RICE, BROWN:								
long grain:								
raw:								
1 oz.	105	2.3	21.9	.8	.2	0	2	1.0 d
1 cup	684	14.7	142.9	5.4	1.1	0	14	6.5 d
(*Arrowhead Mills*), 2 oz.	200	4.0	44.0	1.0	n.a.	0	3	3.1 d
cooked[3]:								
4 oz.	126	2.9	26.0	1.0	.2	0	6	1.9 d
1 cup	216	5.0	44.8	1.8	.4	0	9	3.3 d
(*Carolina*), ½ cup	110	2.0	23.0	0	0	0	0	m.q.
(*Mahatma*), ½ cup	110	2.0	23.0	0	0	0	<10	m.q.
(*River*), approx. ½ cup	110	2.0	23.0	0	0	0	n.a.	m.q.
(*S&W*), 3.5 oz.	119	3.0	26.0	0	0	0	0	m.q.
(*Uncle Ben's* Whole Grain),								
⅔ cup	130	3.0	27.0	1.0	n.a.	0	0	m.q.
quick (*S&W*), 3.5 oz.	110	2.0	25.0	0	0	0	0	m.q.
medium grain:								
raw:								
1 oz.	103	2.1	21.6	.8	.2	0	1	.3 c
1 cup	687	14.3	144.7	5.1	1.0	0	8	1.8 c
or short (*Arrowhead Mills*),								
2 oz.	200	4.0	44.0	1.0	n.a.	0	3	3.4 d
cooked, 4 oz.[3]	127	2.6	26.7	.9	.2	0	1	.3 c
cooked, 1 cup[3]	218	4.5	45.8	1.6	.3	0	2	.6 c
precooked (*Uncle Ben's*), ½ cup[3] ...	90	2.0	21.0	1.0	n.a.	0	11	1.0 d
RICE, GLUTINOUS:								
raw, 1 oz.	105	1.9	23.2	.2	<.1	0	2	.8 d
raw, 1 cup	685	12.6	151.1	1.0	.2	0	13	5.2 d
cooked[3], 4 oz.	110	2.3	23.9	.2	<.1	0	6	.1 c
cooked[3], 1 cup	234	4.9	50.8	.5	.1	0	13	.2 c
RICE, SWEET, see "Rice, glutinous"								
RICE, WHITE:								
arborio, see "Rice, arborio"								
basmati, see "Rice, basmati"								
glutinous, see "Rice, glutinous"								
long grain, regular:								
raw, 1 oz.	103	2.0	22.7	.2	<.1	0	1	.3 d
raw, 1 cup	676	13.2	147.9	1.2	.3	0	8	1.9 d
cooked[4]:								
4 oz.	146	3.1	31.6	.3	.1	0	2	.1 c

1. *If adding ½ tsp. salt to basic recipe, increase sodium value by 125 mg.*
2. *Prepared with 1 tbsp. salted butter.*
3. *Prepared according to package directions, without salt and butter.*
4. *Prepared according to package directions, without salt and butter, except as noted.*

Food and Measure	cal.	prot. (gms)	carbo. (gms)	tot. fat (gms)	sat. fat (gms)	chol. (mgs)	sod. (mgs)	fiber (gms)
RICE, WHITE, LONG GRAIN *(cont.)*								
1 cup	264	5.5	57.2	.6	.2	0	4	.2 c
(Carolina/Mahatma/River),								
½ cup	100	2.0	22.0	0	0	0	<10	m.q.
(Finast), ½ cup	115	2.0	26.0	0	0	0	0	m.q.
(Uncle Ben's Natural Whole								
Grain), ⅔ cup	130	3.0	28.0	1.0	n.a.	0	0	m.q.
(Uncle Ben's Natural Whole								
Grain), ⅔ cup[1]	150	3.0	28.0	3.0	m.q.	m.q.	420	m.q.
(Water Maid), ½ cup	100	2.0	22.0	0	0	0	<10	m.q.
long grain, parboiled:								
dry, 1 oz.	105	1.9	23.2	.2	<.1	0	1	.5 d
dry, 1 cup	686	12.6	151.2	1.0	.3	0	9	3.3 d
cooked[2],								
4 oz.	129	2.6	28.0	3.1	.1	0	3	.6 d
1 cup	199	4.0	43.3	.5	.1	0	6	.9 d
(Uncle Ben's Converted), ⅔ cup	120	2.0	28.0	<1.0	n.a.	0	0	m.q.
(Uncle Ben's Converted),								
⅔ cup[1]	140	2.0	28.0	2.0	m.q.	m.q.	410	m.q.
long grain, precooked or instant:								
dry, 1 oz.	107	2.2	23.7	.1	<.1	0	2	.5 d
dry, 1 cup	360	7.3	79.4	.3	.1	0	6	1.5 d
cooked[2],								
4 oz.	111	2.3	24.1	.2	<.1	0	3	.9 d
1 cup	161	3.4	35.1	.3	.1	0	4	1.3 d
(Carolina/Mahatma Instant								
Enriched), ½ cup	110	2.0	23.0	0	0	0	n.a.	m.q.
(Minute Rice/Minute Rice								
Premium), ⅔ cup	120	3.0	27.0	0	0	0	0	m.q.
(Minute Rice Boil-in-Bag),								
½ cup	90	2.0	20.0	0	0	0	0	m.q.
(S&W), 3.5 oz.	106	2.0	23.0	0	0	0	0	m.q.
(Success Boil-in-Bag Enriched),								
½ cup	100	2.0	21.0	0	0	0	0	m.q.
(Uncle Ben's Boil-in-Bag),								
½ cup	90	2.0	20.0	<1.0	n.a.	0	10	m.q.
(Uncle Ben's Rice In An								
Instant), ⅔ cup	120	3.0	27.0	<1.0	n.a.	0	10	m.q.
(Uncle Ben's Rice In An								
Instant), ⅔ cup[1]	130	3.0	27.0	2.0	m.q.	m.q.	310	m.q.
medium grain:								
raw, 1 oz.	102	1.9	22.5	.2	<.1	0	<1	.4 d
raw, 1 cup	702	12.9	154.7	1.1	.3	0	2	2.7 d
cooked, 4 oz.[2]	147	2.7	32.4	.2	.1	0	tr.	.1 c
cooked, 1 cup[2]	266	4.9	58.6	.4	.1	0	1	.2 c
short grain:								
raw, 1 oz.	101	1.8	22.4	.1	<.1	0	<1	.1 c

1. *Prepared with salt and butter.*
2. *Prepared according to package directions, without salt and butter, except as noted.*

Food and Measure	cal.	prot. (gms)	carbo. (gms)	tot. fat (gms)	sat. fat (gms)	chol. (mgs)	sod. (mgs)	fiber (gms)
raw, 1 cup	717	13.0	158.3	1.0	.3	0	2	.6 c
cooked, 4 oz.[1]	147	2.7	32.6	.2	.1	0	tr.	.1 c
cooked, 1 cup[1]	267	4.8	58.9	.4	.1	0	1	.2 c
RICE, WILD, see "Wild rice"								
RICE, WAXY, see "Rice, glutinous"								
RICE BEVERAGE, FLAVORED:								
chocolate (*Rice Dream*), 6 fl. oz. ...	170	1.0	39.0	2.0	m.q.	0	35	n.a.
RICE BRAN, crude:								
1 oz.	90	3.8	14.1	5.9	1.2	0	1	6.2 d
1 cup	262	11.1	41.2	17.3	3.5	0	4	18.0 d
RICE BRAN BAR, see "Snack bar"								
RICE BRAN OIL:								
1 oz.	251	0	0	28.4	5.6	0	0	0
½ cup	964	0	0	109.0	21.5	0	0	0
1 tbsp.	120	0	0	13.6	2.7	0	0	0
(*Hain*), 1 tbsp.	120	0	0	14.0	3.0	0	0	0
RICE CAKE:								
all varieties (*Lundberg* Sodium Free),								
1 piece	60	1.4	14.0	.5	(0)	0	3	m.q.
all varieties (*Lundberg* Very Low								
Sodium), 1 piece	60	1.4	14.0	.5	(0)	0	30	m.q.
plain:								
(*Hain*), 1 piece	40	<1.0	8.0	<1.0	(0)	0	10	m.q.
(*Hain* Unsalted), 1 piece	40	<1.0	8.0	<1.0	(0)	0	<5	m.q.
(*Quaker*), .32-oz. piece	35	.8	7.1	.3	.1	0	36	.3 d
(*Quaker* Unsalted), .32-oz. piece	35	.8	7.2	.3	.1	0	0	.3 d
mini (*Hain*), .5 oz.	60	1.0	12.0	<1.0	(0)	0	20	0
mini (*Hain* Unsalted), .5 oz.	60	1.0	12.0	<1.0	(0)	0	5	0
apple cinnamon, mini (*Hain*), ½ cup	60	1.0	12.0	<1.0	(0)	0	10	0
barbecue, mini (*Hain*), .5 oz.	70	1.0	10.0	3.0	n.a.	0	50	0
brown rice (*Konriko* Original								
Unsalted), 1 piece	30	0	7.0	0	0	0	<1	m.q.
cheese, mini (*Hain*), .5 oz.	60	1.0	10.0	2.0	n.a.	0	80	0
cheese, nacho, mini (*Hain*), .5 oz. ..	70	1.0	10.0	2.0	n.a.	<5	90	0
corn (*Quaker*), .32-oz. piece	35	.8	7.2	.3	.1	0	31	.3 d
five grain (*Hain*), 1 piece	40	<1.0	8.0	<1.0	(0)	0	10	m.q.
honey nut, mini (*Hain*), .5 oz.	60	1.0	11.0	<1.0	(0)	0	30	0
multigrain (*Quaker*), .32-oz. piece ..	34	.9	6.9	.4	.1	0	29	.4 d
ranch, mini (*Hain*), .5 oz.	70	1.0	9.0	3.0	n.a.	0	90	m.q.
rye (*Quaker*), .32-oz. piece	34	.8	6.9	.4	.1	0	12	.4 d
sesame:								
(*Hain*), 1 piece	40	<1.0	8.0	<1.0	(0)	0	10	m.q.
(*Hain* Unsalted), 1 piece	40	<1.0	8.0	<1.0	(0)	0	<5	m.q.
(*Quaker*), .32-oz. piece	35	.8	7.1	.3	.1	0	36	.3 d
(*Quaker*), .32-oz. piece	35	.8	7.1	.3	.1	0	1	.3 d
teriyaki, mini (*Hain*), .5 oz.	50	1.0	12.0	<1.0	(0)	0	75	0

1. *Prepared according to package directions, without salt or butter.*

Food and Measure	cal.	prot. (gms)	carbo. (gms)	tot. fat (gms)	sat. fat (gms)	chol. (mgs)	sod. (mgs)	fiber (gms)
RICE DISHES, CANNED (see also specific listings):								
fried (*La Choy*), ¾ cup	180	4.0	40.0	1.0	n.a.	0	930	1.4 d
Spanish:								
(*Featherweight*), 7½ oz.	140	4.0	30.0	0	0	0	32	m.q.
(*Heinz*), 7¼ oz.	150	3.0	26.0	5.0	m.q.	n.a.	1045	m.q.
(*Old El Paso*), ½ cup	70	1.0	15.0	1.0	0	0	400	1.0 d
(*Van Camp's*), 1 cup	160	3.1	27.0	4.0	m.q.	n.a.	1270	m.q.
RICE DISHES, FROZEN:								
and broccoli:								
au gratin (*Birds Eye For One*), 5.75 oz.	180	6.0	27.0	6.0	m.q.	5	430	1.0 d
in cheese sauce (*Green Giant* One Serving), 5.5 oz.	180	5.0	25.0	6.0	2.0	5	550	m.q.
in flavored cheese sauce (*Green Giant Rice Originals*), ½ cup ..	120	3.0	18.0	4.0	m.q.	n.a.	510	.2 c
country style (*Birds Eye* International Rice Recipes), 3.3 oz.	90	2.0	19.0	0	0	0	380	1.0 d
French style (*Birds Eye* International Rice Recipes), 3.3 oz.	110	3.0	23.0	0	0	0	610	m.q.
fried, w/chicken (*Chun King*), 8 oz.	260	14.0	41.0	4.0	m.q.	m.q.	1460	m.q.
fried, w/pork (*Chun King*), 8 oz. ...	270	10.0	44.0	6.0	m.q.	m.q.	1210	m.q.
Italian blend white rice and spinach, in cheese sauce (*Green Giant Rice Originals*), ½ cup	140	4.0	22.0	4.0	2.0	10	400	m.q.
medley (*Green Giant Rice Originals*), ½ cup	100	3.0	19.0	1.0	<1.0	5	310	m.q.
peas and mushrooms, w/sauce (*Green Giant* One Serving), 5.5 oz.	130	4.0	27.0	2.0	<1.0	5	410	m.q.
pilaf (*Green Giant Rice Originals*), ½ cup	110	2.0	21.0	1.0	<1.0	2	530	m.q.
pilaf, w/green beans (*The Budget Gourmet* Side Dish), 5.5 oz. ...	240	4.0	35.0	9.0	m.q.	10	350	m.q.
Oriental, and vegetables (*The Budget Gourmet* Side Dish), 5.75 oz. ..	210	4.0	27.0	10.0	m.q.	20	310	m.q.
Spanish style (*Birds Eye* International Rice Recipes), 3.3 oz.	110	3.0	24.0	0	0	0	540	m.q.
white and wild rice (*Green Giant Rice Originals*), ½ cup	130	3.0	24.0	2.0	<1.0	0	540	m.q.
wild, sherry (*Green Giant* Microwave Garden Gourmet), 1 pkg.	210	6.0	40.0	4.0	2.0	10	580	3.0 d
RICE DISHES, MIX[1]:								
Alfredo (*Country Inn*), ½ cup[2]	140	4.0	23.0	4.0	m.q.	n.a.	570	m.q.
almondine (*Hain* 3-Grain Side Dish), ½ cup	130	3.0	17.0	5.0	m.q.	0	260	m.q.

1. *Prepared according to package directions, except as noted.*
2. *Prepared without butter.*

Food and Measure	cal.	prot. (gms)	carbo. (gms)	tot. fat (gms)	sat. fat (gms)	chol. (mgs)	sod. (mgs)	fiber (gms)
asparagus:								
au gratin (*Country Inn*), ½ cup[1]	130	4.0	22.0	3.0	m.q.	n.a.	310	m.q.
w/hollandaise sauce (*Lipton* Rice and Sauce), ¼ pkg. dry	120	4.0	25.0	1.0	n.a.	n.a.	460	m.q.
w/hollandaise sauce (*Lipton* Rice and Sauce), ½ cup[2]	170	4.0	25.0	7.0	m.q.	m.q.	530	m.q.
w/hollandaise sauce (*Lipton* Rice and Sauce), ½ cup[3]	150	4.0	25.0	4.0	m.q.	n.a.	500	m.q.
au gratin, herbed (*Country Inn*), ½ cup[1]	140	4.0	25.0	3.0	m.q.	n.a.	450	m.q.
au gratin herb (*Success*), ½ cup[4] ...	100	2.0	20.0	0	0	0	260	m.q.
beef flavor:								
(*Finast*), 1.3 oz. dry	130	4.0	26.0	1.0	n.a.	n.a.	780	m.q.
(*Lipton* Rice and Sauce), ½ pkg. dry	120	3.0	26.0	<1.0	n.a.	n.a.	570	m.q.
(*Lipton* Rice and Sauce), ½ cup[5]	150	3.0	26.0	3.0	m.q.	m.q.	600	m.q.
(*Mahatma*), ½ cup	100	2.0	20.0	0	0	0	340	m.q.
(*Minute* Microwave Family Size), ½ cup[6]	160	4.0	28.0	3.0	m.q.	10	560	m.q.
(*Minute* Microwave Single Size), ½ cup[6]	150	4.0	28.0	2.0	m.q.	5	550	m.q.
(*Rice-A-Roni*), 1.13 oz. dry	110	3.0	24.0	1.0	n.a.	n.a.	560	m.q.
(*Rice-A-Roni*), ½ cup	140	4.0	24.0	4.0	m.q.	n.a.	610	m.q.
(*Success*), ½ cup[4]	100	2.0	19.0	0	0	0	370	m.q.
and mushroom (*Rice-A-Roni*), 1.27 oz. dry	120	4.0	26.0	<1.0	n.a.	n.a.	710	m.q.
and mushroom (*Rice-A-Roni*), ½ cup	150	4.0	26.0	3.0	m.q.	n.a.	740	m.q.
and vermicelli (*Make-it-easy*), 1.3 oz. dry	130	3.0	28.0	1.0	n.a.	0	m.q.	m.q.
broccoli almondine (*Country Inn*), ½ cup[1]	130	4.0	23.0	2.0	m.q.	n.a.	600	m.q.
broccoli au gratin:								
(*Country Inn*), ½ cup[1]	130	4.0	22.0	3.0	m.q.	n.a.	300	m.q.
(*Golden Grain/Rice-A-Roni Savory Classics*), 1.12 oz. dry	129	3.6	20.9	3.4	1.1	4	372	1.1 d
(*Golden Grain/Rice-A-Roni Savory Classics*), ½ cup	180	4.0	21.0	9.0	m.q.	m.q.	440	m.q.
broccoli stir-fry (*Suzi Wan* Dinner Recipe), 7.5 oz.[7]	200	5.0	37.0	3.0	m.q.	n.a.	750	m.q.
broccoli stir-fry (*Suzi Wan* Dinner Recipe), 7.5 oz.	370	22.0	37.0	15.0	m.q.	n.a.	800	m.q.
brown and wild:								
(*Success*), ½ cup[4]	120	3.0	23.0	0	0	0	500	m.q.

1. *Prepared without butter.*
2. *Prepared with 2 tbsp. butter.*
3. *Prepared with 1 tbsp. margarine.*
4. *Prepared without butter or margarine.*
5. *Prepared with 1 tbsp. butter.*
6. *Prepared with salted butter.*
7. *Prepared without added ingredients.*

Food and Measure	cal.	prot. (gms)	carbo. (gms)	tot. fat (gms)	sat. fat (gms)	chol. (mgs)	sod. (mgs)	fiber (gms)
RICE DISHES, MIX, BROWN AND WILD *(cont.)*								
(Uncle Ben's), ½ cup [1]	130	4.0	27.0	1.0	n.a.	0	500	m.q.
(Uncle Ben's), ½ cup [2]	150	4.0	27.0	4.0	m.q.	m.q.	520	m.q.
mushroom recipe *(Uncle Ben's)*, ½ cup	130	4.0	27.0	1.0	n.a.	n.a.	500	m.q.
Spanish style *(Arrowhead Mills Quick Brown Rice)*, 2 oz. dry ..	150	4.0	30.0	1.0	n.a.	0	145	2.8 d
vegetable herb *(Arrowhead Mills Quick Brown Rice)*, 2 oz. dry ..	150	4.0	30.0	1.0	n.a.	0	85	4.0 d
wild rice and herb *(Arrowhead Mills* Quick Brown Rice), 2 oz. dry	140	4.0	28.0	1.0	n.a.	0	128	4.0 d
Cajun *(Lipton* Rice and Sauce), ¼ pkg. dry	120	4.0	26.0	<1.0	n.a.	0	600	m.q.
Cajun *(Lipton* Rice and Sauce), ½ cup [3]	150	4.0	26.0	3.0	m.q.	m.q.	630	m.q.
cauliflower au gratin:								
(Country Inn), ½ cup [4]	130	4.0	23.0	3.0	m.q.	n.a.	570	m.q.
(Golden Grain/Rice-A-Roni Savory Classics), ½ oz. dry	141	4.4	22.7	3.6	1.1	5	372	1.1 d
(Golden Grain/Rice-A-Roni Savory Classics), ½ cup	170	4.0	23.0	7.0	m.q.	m.q.	410	m.q.
cheddar:								
and broccoli *(Minute* Microwave Family Size), ½ cup [5]	160	4.0	26.0	5.0	m.q.	10	530	m.q.
and broccoli *(Minute* Microwave Single Size), ½ cup [5]	160	4.0	26.0	4.0	m.q.	10	520	m.q.
zesty *(Golden Grain/Rice-A-Roni Savory Classics)*, 1.3 oz. dry ..	151	4.6	24.7	3.8	1.3	6	541	.9 d
zesty *(Golden Grain/Rice-A-Roni Savory Classics)*, ½ cup	180	5.0	25.0	7.0	m.q.	m.q.	580	m.q.
chicken and chicken flavor:								
(Finast), 1.6 oz. dry	160	4.0	31.0	2.0	m.q.	n.a.	950	m.q.
(Lipton Rice and Sauce), ¼ pkg. dry	130	3.0	25.0	1.0	n.a.	n.a.	440	m.q.
(Lipton Rice and Sauce), ½ cup [3]	150	3.0	25.0	4.0	m.q.	m.q.	470	m.q.
(Mahatma), ½ cup	100	2.0	20.0	0	0	0	620	m.q.
(Minute Microwave Family Size), ½ cup [5]	160	3.0	27.0	4.0	m.q.	10	670	m.q.
(Minute Microwave Single Size), ½ cup [5]	150	3.0	27.0	3.0	m.q.	5	660	m.q.
(Rice-A-Roni), 1.13 oz. dry	110	3.0	24.0	1.0	n.a.	n.a.	520	m.q.
(Rice-A-Roni), ½ cup	150	3.0	24.0	4.0	m.q.	n.a.	560	m.q.
(Success), ½ cup [6]	110	3.0	18.0	2.0	m.q.	n.a.	420	m.q.
and broccoli:								
(Rice-A-Roni), 1.23 oz. dry ...	120	3.0	25.0	1.0	n.a.	n.a.	670	m.q.

1. *Prepared without salt and butter.*
2. *Prepared with salt and butter.*
3. *Prepared with 1 tbsp. butter.*
4. *Prepared without butter.*
5. *Prepared with salted butter.*
6. *Prepared without butter or margarine.*

Food and Measure	cal.	prot. (gms)	carbo. (gms)	tot. fat (gms)	sat. fat (gms)	chol. (mgs)	sod. (mgs)	fiber (gms)
(*Rice-A-Roni*), ½ cup	150	3.0	25.0	3.0	m.q.	n.a.	710	m.q.
(*Suzi Wan*), ½ cup[1]	120	4.0	23.0	1.0	n.a.	n.a.	500	m.q.
drumstick (*Minute*), ½ cup[2]	150	3.0	25.0	4.0	m.q.	10	690	m.q.
honey lemon (*Suzi Wan* Dinner								
Recipe), 7.5 oz.[3]	200	3.0	44.0	1.0	n.a.	n.a.	600	m.q.
honey lemon (*Suzi Wan* Dinner								
Recipe), 7.5 oz.	370	23.0	45.0	11.0	m.q.	n.a.	640	m.q.
and mushroom:								
(*Rice-A-Roni*), 1.17 oz. dry ...	130	4.0	26.0	1.0	n.a.	n.a.	790	m.q.
(*Rice-A-Roni*), ½ cup	180	4.0	26.0	7.0	m.q.	n.a.	840	m.q.
creamy (*Country Inn*), ½ cup[3]	140	3.0	25.0	3.0	m.q.	n.a.	510	m.q.
royale (*Country Inn*), ½ cup[3]	120	4.0	25.0	1.0	n.a.	n.a.	560	m.q.
stock (*Country Inn*), ½ cup[3]	130	4.0	25.0	1.0	n.a.	n.a.	560	m.q.
and vegetables:								
(*Rice-A-Roni*), 1.2 oz. dry	120	3.0	25.0	<1.0	n.a.	n.a.	760	m.q.
(*Rice-A-Roni*), ½ cup	140	3.0	25.0	3.0	m.q.	n.a.	790	m.q.
(*Suzi Wan*), ½ cup[1]	120	3.0	24.0	1.0	n.a.	n.a.	550	m.q.
homestyle (*Country Inn*),								
½ cup[3]	140	4.0	25.0	3.0	m.q.	n.a.	490	m.q.
and vermicelli (*Make-it-easy*),								
1.3 oz. dry	130	3.0	28.0	1.0	n.a.	n.a.	m.q.	m.q.
Florentine:								
(*Country Inn*), ½ cup[3]	140	4.0	24.0	3.0	n.a.	n.a.	380	m.q.
chicken (*Golden Grain/Rice-A-*								
Roni Savory Classics), 1.12 oz.								
dry	108	3.7	21.7	.8	.1	1	874	1.2 d
chicken (*Golden Grain/Rice-A-*								
Roni Savory Classics), ½ cup ..	130	4.0	22.0	4.0	m.q.	m.q.	910	m.q.
fried:								
(*Minute*), ½ cup	160	3.0	25.0	5.0	m.q.	0	550	m.q.
(*Rice-A-Roni*), 1.04 oz. dry	110	3.0	21.0	1.0	n.a.	n.a.	670	m.q.
(*Rice-A-Roni*), ½ cup	110	3.0	21.0	5.0	m.q.	n.a.	700	m.q.
green bean almondine:								
(*Golden Grain/Rice-A-Roni Savory*								
Classics), 1.25 oz. dry	152	4.8	22.3	4.8	1.4	6	416	1.0 d
(*Golden Grain/Rice-A-Roni Savory*								
Classics), ½ cup	210	5.0	22.0	11.0	m.q.	m.q.	490	m.q.
casserole (*Country Inn*), ½ cup[4]	120	3.0	23.0	2.0	n.a.	n.a.	370	m.q.
herb, au gratin, see "au gratin,"								
above								
herb and butter:								
(*Lipton* Rice and Sauce), ½ cup[5]	150	3.0	24.0	5.0	m.q.	m.q.	470	m.q.
(*Rice-A-Roni*), 1.04 oz. dry	110	2.0	22.0	1.0	n.a.	n.a.	760	m.q.
(*Rice-A-Roni*), ½ cup	130	2.0	22.0	4.0	m.q.	n.a.	790	m.q.

1. *Prepared without butter or margarine.*
2. *Prepared with salted butter.*
3. *Prepared without added ingredients.*
4. *Prepared without butter.*
5. *Prepared with 1 tbsp. butter.*

Food and Measure	cal.	prot. (gms)	carbo. (gms)	tot. fat (gms)	sat. fat (gms)	chol. (mgs)	sod. (mgs)	fiber (gms)

RICE DISHES, MIX *(cont.)*

long grain and wild:

(*Lipton* Rice and Sauce Original), ¼ pkg. dry	120	4.0	26.0	<1.0	n.a.	n.a.	530	m.q.
(*Lipton* Rice and Sauce Original), ½ cup[1]	150	4.0	26.0	3.0	m.q.	m.q.	560	m.q.
(*Mahatma*), ½ cup	100	2.0	20.0	0	0	0	480	m.q.
(*Minute*), ½ cup[2]	150	3.0	25.0	4.0	m.q.	10	570	m.q.
(*Near East*), ½ cup	130	3.0	21.0	4.0	m.q.	n.a.	430	m.q.
(*Rice-A-Roni* Original), 1.1 oz. dry	110	3.0	23.0	0	0	n.a.	620	m.q.
(*Rice-A-Roni* Original), ½ cup . . .	130	3.0	23.0	3.0	m.q.	n.a.	660	m.q.
(*Uncle Ben's* Fast Cooking), ½ cup[3]	100	3.0	21.0	<1.0	n.a.	0	410	m.q.
(*Uncle Ben's* Fast Cooking), ½ cup[4]	130	3.0	21.0	4.0	m.q.	m.q.	450	m.q.
(*Uncle Ben's* Original), ½ cup[3] . . .	100	3.0	22.0	<1.0	n.a.	0	500	m.q.
(*Uncle Ben's* Original), ½ cup[4] . . .	120	3.0	22.0	2.0	m.q.	m.q.	520	m.q.
chicken w/almonds (*Rice-A-Roni*), 1.2 oz. dry	120	3.0	23.0	1.0	n.a.	n.a.	660	m.q.
chicken w/almonds (*Rice-A-Roni*), ½ cup	140	3.0	24.0	4.0	m.q.	n.a.	690	m.q.
chicken stock sauce (*Uncle Ben's*), ½ cup[3]	140	4.0	27.0	2.0	m.q.	0	650	m.q.
chicken stock sauce (*Uncle Ben's*), ½ cup[4]	160	4.0	27.0	5.0	m.q.	m.q.	680	m.q.
mushrooms and herbs (*Lipton* Rice and Sauce), ¼ pkg. dry	120	4.0	26.0	<1.0	n.a.	n.a.	330	m.q.
mushrooms and herbs (*Lipton* Rice and Sauce), ½ cup[1]	150	4.0	26.0	3.0	m.q.	m.q.	360	m.q.
Mexican (*Old El Paso*), ½ cup	140	2.0	28.0	2.0	m.q.	0	370	m.q.
mushroom:								
(*Lipton* Rice and Sauce), ¼ pkg. dry	120	3.0	26.0	<1.0	n.a.	n.a.	550	m.q.
(*Lipton* Rice and Sauce), ½ cup[1] . .	150	3.0	26.0	3.0	m.q.	m.q.	580	m.q.
creamy, and wild rice (*Country Inn*), ½ cup[5]	140	3.0	24.0	3.0	m.q.	n.a.	310	m.q.
Oriental (*Hain* 3-Grain Goodness), ½ cup	120	4.0	15.0	5.0	m.q.	n.a.	300	m.q.
Parmesan, creamy, and herbs (*Golden Grain/Rice-A-Roni Savory Classics*), 1.22 oz. dry	145	4.8	22.0	4.2	1.4	7	432	.8 d
Parmesan, creamy, and herbs (*Golden Grain/Rice-A-Roni Savory Classics*), ½ cup	170	5.0	22.0	7.0	m.q.	m.q.	470	m.q.

1. *Prepared with 1 tbsp. butter.*
2. *Prepared with salted butter.*
3. *Prepared without salt and butter.*
4. *Prepared with salt and butter.*
5. *Prepared without butter.*

Food and Measure	cal.	prot. (gms)	carbo. (gms)	tot. fat (gms)	sat. fat (gms)	chol. (mgs)	sod. (mgs)	fiber (gms)
pilaf:								
(*Casbah*), 1 oz. dry or ½ cup								
cooked	90	2.0	20.0	0	0	0	m.q.	m.q.
(*Lipton* Rice and Sauce), ¼ pkg.								
dry	120	3.0	25.0	<1.0	n.a.	n.a.	400	m.q.
(*Lipton* Rice and Sauce), ½ cup[1]	170	3.0	25.0	6.0	m.q.	m.q.	470	m.q.
(*Lipton* Rice and Sauce), ½ cup[2]	140	3.0	25.0	3.0	m.q.	n.a.	440	m.q.
(*Near East*), ½ cup	140	3.0	21.0	5.0	m.q.	n.a.	450	m.q.
(*Rice-A-Roni*), 1.2 oz. dry	120	4.0	25.0	0	0	n.a.	570	m.q.
(*Rice-A-Roni*), ½ cup	150	4.0	25.0	4.0	m.q.	n.a.	550	m.q.
(*Success*), ½ cup[3]	120	2.0	24.0	0	0	0	410	m.q.
beef flavored (*Near East*), ½ cup	140	3.0	21.0	5.0	m.q.	n.a.	470	m.q.
brown, w/miso (*Quick Pilaf*),								
½ cup	105	3.0	21.0	1.0	n.a.	n.a.	240	m.q.
brown, w/miso (*Quick Pilaf*),								
½ cup[4]	145	3.0	21.0	5.5	m.q.	m.q.	295	m.q.
chicken flavored (*Near East*),								
½ cup	140	3.0	21.0	5.0	m.q.	n.a.	420	m.q.
French style (*Minute* Microwave								
Family Size), ½ cup[5]	130	2.0	24.0	3.0	m.q.	10	420	m.q.
French style (*Minute* Microwave								
Single Size), ½ cup[5]	120	2.0	24.0	2.0	m.q.	5	410	m.q.
garden (*Golden Grain/Rice-A-Roni*								
Savory Classics), 1.12 oz. dry	113	3.6	22.9	.8	.2	1	964	1.1 d
garden (*Golden Grain/Rice-A-Roni*								
Savory Classics), ½ cup	140	4.0	23.0	4.0	m.q.	m.q.	1000	m.q.
lentil (*Near East*), ½ cup	170	6.0	21.0	7.0	m.q.	n.a.	430	m.q.
long grain and wild (*Rice-A-Roni*),								
1.06 oz. dry	100	2.0	23.0	0	0	n.a.	510	m.q.
long grain and wild (*Rice-A-Roni*),								
½ cup	130	3.0	23.0	3.0	m.q.	n.a.	550	m.q.
nutted (*Casbah*), 1 oz. dry or								
½ cup cooked	160	4.0	30.0	2.0	m.q.	0	m.q.	m.q.
Spanish:								
(*Casbah*), 1 oz. dry or ½ cup								
cooked	90	2.0	20.0	0	0	0	m.q.	m.q.
brown (*Quick Pilaf*), ½ cup ...	98	2.0	21.0	.7	n.a.	n.a.	314	m.q.
brown (*Quick Pilaf*), ½ cup[4] ..	136	2.0	21.0	5.0	m.q.	m.q.	369	m.q.
vegetable (*Country Inn*), ½ cup[6]	120	3.0	25.0	1.0	n.a.	n.a.	280	m.q.
wheat (*Near East*), ½ cup	150	3.0	21.0	6.0	m.q.	n.a.	380	m.q.
rib roast (*Minute*), ½ cup[5]	150	3.0	25.0	4.0	m.q.	10	720	m.q.
risotto:								
(*Rice-A-Roni*), 1.5 oz. dry	160	4.0	32.0	1.0	n.a.	n.a.	1070	m.q.

1. *Prepared with 2 tbsp. butter.*
2. *Prepared with 1 tbsp. margarine.*
3. *Prepared without butter or margarine.*
4. *Prepared with 2 tbsp. salted butter.*
5. *Prepared with salted butter.*
6. *Prepared without butter.*

Food and Measure	cal.	prot. (gms)	carbo. (gms)	tot. fat (gms)	sat. fat (gms)	chol. (mgs)	sod. (mgs)	fiber (gms)
RICE DISHES, MIX, RISOTTO *(cont.)*								
(*Rice-A-Roni*), ½ cup	200	4.0	32.0	6.0	m.q.	n.a.	1130	m.q.
chicken and cheese (*Country Inn*),								
½ cup[1]	120	3.0	23.0	2.0	m.q.	n.a.	410	m.q.
Spanish:								
(*Lipton* Rice and Sauce), ¼ pkg.								
dry	120	3.0	26.0	<1.0	n.a.	n.a.	540	m.q.
(*Lipton* Rice and Sauce), ½ cup[2]	140	3.0	26.0	3.0	m.q.	m.q.	570	m.q.
(*Mahatma*), ½ cup	100	2.0	20.0	0	0	0	190	m.q.
(*Near East*), ½ cup	170	3.0	24.0	7.0	m.q.	n.a.	540	m.q.
(*Rice-A-Roni*), .97 oz. dry	110	3.0	22.0	1.0	n.a.	n.a.	950	m.q.
(*Rice-A-Roni*), ½ cup	150	4.0	25.0	4.0	m.q.	n.a.	1090	m.q.
Stroganoff (*Rice-A-Roni*), 1.35 oz.								
dry	150	4.0	27.0	3.0	m.q.	n.a.	770	m.q.
Stroganoff (*Rice-A-Roni*), ½ cup ...	200	4.0	27.0	8.0	m.q.	n.a.	810	m.q.
sweet and sour:								
(*Suzi Wan*), ½ cup[1]	130	3.0	28.0	1.0	n.a.	n.a.	460	m.q.
(*Suzi Wan* Dinner Recipe),								
7.5 oz.[3]	220	4.0	48.0	1.0	n.a.	n.a.	240	m.q.
(*Suzi Wan* Dinner Recipe), 7.5 oz.	340	24.0	49.0	5.0	m.q.	m.q.	290	m.q.
teriyaki:								
(*Suzi Wan*), ½ cup[1]	120	3.0	25.0	1.0	n.a.	n.a.	690	m.q.
(*Suzi Wan* Dinner Recipe),								
7.5 oz.[3]	180	5.0	39.0	1.0	n.a.	n.a.	910	m.q.
(*Suzi Wan* Dinner recipe), 7.5 oz.	360	22.0	39.0	12.0	m.q.	m.q.	970	m.q.
three-flavor (*Suzi Wan*), ½ cup[1]	120	4.0	24.0	1.0	n.a.	n.a.	570	m.q.
vegetable medley (*Country Inn*),								
½ cup[1]	140	4.0	28.0	1.0	n.a.	n.a.	390	m.q.
w/vegetables, broccoli, and cheddar:								
(*Lipton* Rice and Sauce), ¼ pkg.								
dry	130	3.0	26.0	2.0	m.q.	n.a.	420	m.q.
(*Lipton* Rice and Sauce), ½ cup[4]	180	3.0	26.0	7.0	m.q.	m.q.	490	m.q.
(*Lipton* Rice and Sauce), ½ cup[5]	160	3.0	26.0	5.0	m.q.	n.a.	450	m.q.
vegetables, spring, and cheese								
(*Golden Grain/Rice-A-Roni Savory*								
Classics), 1.22 oz. dry	141	4.4	22.8	3.5	1.2	6	388	1.2 d
vegetables, spring, and cheese								
(*Golden Grain/Rice-A-Roni Savory*								
Classics), ½ cup	170	4.0	23.0	7.0	m.q.	m.q.	420	m.q.
white, w/pasta and seasoning:								
dry, 1 oz.	104	2.7	21.4	.7	.1	<1	529	.2 c
dry, 1 cup	601	15.3	122.8	4.0	.7	4	3041	.9 c

1. *Prepared without butter.*
2. *Prepared with 1 tbsp. butter.*
3. *Prepared without added ingredients.*
4. *Prepared with 2 tbsp. butter.*
5. *Prepared with 1 tbsp. margarine.*

Food and Measure	cal.	prot. (gms)	carbo. (gms)	tot. fat (gms)	sat. fat (gms)	chol. (mgs)	sod. (mgs)	fiber (gms)
cooked[1], 4 oz.	138	2.9	24.3	3.2	.6	1	644	.2 c
cooked[1], 1 cup	247	5.1	43.3	5.7	1.1	1	1147	.4 c
yellow:								
(*Mahatma*/*Success*), ½ cup[2]	100	2.0	21.0	0	0	0	480	m.q.
(*Rice-A-Roni*), 1.16 oz. dry	110	2.0	25.0	0	0	n.a.	730	m.q.
(*Rice-A-Roni*), ½ cup	140	2.0	25.0	4.0	m.q.	n.a.	780	m.q.
RICE ENTREE, freeze-dried:								
and chicken (*Mountain House*),								
1 cup	400	13.0	41.0	13.0	m.q.	m.q.	241	m.q.
RICE FLOUR:								
(*Featherweight*), 1 cup	500	11.0	113.0	1.0	n.a.	0	7	m.q.
brown:								
1 oz.	103	2.0	21.7	.8	.2	0	2	1.3 d
1 cup	574	11.4	120.8	4.4	.9	0	12	7.3 d
(*Arrowhead Mills*), 2 oz.	200	4.0	44.0	1.0	n.a.	0	3	3.1 d
white, 1 oz.	104	1.7	22.7	.4	.1	0	tr.	.7 d
white, 1 cup	578	9.4	126.6	2.2	.6	0	1	3.9 d
RICE MIX, see "Rice dishes, mix"								
RICE SEASONING:								
Mexican (*Lawry's* Seasoning Blends),								
1 pkg.	94	3.9	17.0	2.0	m.q.	n.a.	3246	2.1 c
RIGATONI, canned:								
(*Chef Boyardee* Microwave), 7.5 oz.	210	8.0	31.0	6.0	m.q.	17	1080	m.q.
RIGATONI ENTREE, frozen:								
bake, w/meat sauce and cheese								
(*Lean Cuisine*), 9¾ oz.	260	18.0	25.0	10.0	3.0	40	870	m.q.
RISOTTO, see "Rice mix"								
ROAST, VEGETARIAN, frozen:								
(*Worthington* Dinner Roast), 2 oz. ..	120	7.0	5.0	8.0	1.0	0	440	m.q.
ROAST BEEF, see "Beef" and								
"Beef luncheon meat"								
ROBERT SAUCE:								
(*Escoffier* Sauce Robert), 1 tbsp. ...	20	0	5.0	0	0	0	70	n.a
ROCKET SALAD, see "Arugula"								
ROCKFISH, Pacific, mixed species,								
meat only:								
raw:								
1 lb.	427	85.1	0	7.1	1.7	156	272	0
1 oz.	27	5.3	0	.4	.1	10	17	0
1 fillet, approx. 6.7 oz., yield from								
3-lb. whole fish	180	35.8	0	3.0	.7	66	114	0
baked, broiled, or microwaved[3],								
4 oz.	137	27.3	0	2.3	.5	50	87	0
ROE, mixed species:								
1 lb.	635	101.2	6.8	29.1	6.6	1696	m.q.	0

1. *Prepared with margarine.*
2. *Prepared without butter or margarine.*
3. *Without added ingredients.*

Food and Measure	cal.	prot. (gms)	carbo. (gms)	tot. fat (gms)	sat. fat (gms)	chol. (mgs)	sod. (mgs)	fiber (gms)
ROE *(cont.)*								
1 oz.	40	6.3	.4	1.8	.4	106	m.q.	0
1 tbsp.	22	3.6	.2	1.0	.2	60	m.q.	0
ROLL, 1 piece, except as noted:								
assorted (*Brownberry* Hearth)	124	4.4	23.7	2.3	m.q.	7	247	1.5 d
brown and serve:								
(*Pepperidge Farm* Hearth)	50	2.0	10.0	1.0	0	0	100	tr.d
club (*Pepperidge Farm* Deli								
Classic)	100	3.0	19.0	1.0	0	0	190	.5 d
French (*Pepperidge Farm* Deli								
Classic, 3/pkg.), ½ piece	120	4.0	24.0	1.0	0	0	250	.5 d
French, petite (*du Jour*)	230	9.0	45.0	2.0	m.q.	0	490	1.8 d
gem style (*Wonder*)	80	2.0	13.0	2.0	m.q.	n.a.	140	.6 d
Italian, crusty (*du Jour*)	80	3.0	16.0	1.0	n.a.	0	200	.6 d
w/buttermilk (*Wonder*)	80	2.0	13.0	2.0	m.q.	n.a.	140	.6 d
cinnamon, see "Roll, sweet"								
crescent, butter (*Pepperidge Farm*								
Deli Classic)	110	2.0	13.0	6.0	3.0	15	150	tr.d
croissant, see "Croissant"								
dinner:								
(*Arnold* 24 Dinner Party)	51	1.9	9.4	1.2	m.q.	1	81	.8 d
(*Pepperidge Farm* Old Fashioned)	50	2.0	7.0	2.0	1.0	5	85	tr.d
(*Pepperidge Farm* Party)	30	1.0	5.0	1.0	n.a.	0	50	tr.d
(*Roman Meal*)	69	2.9	13.0	1.2	m.q.	0	140	1.2 d
(*Wonder*)	80	2.0	14.0	1.0	n.a.	n.a.	140	.6 d
Black Forest (*Awrey's*)	50	2.0	10.0	1.0	0	0	110	0
country style (*Pepperidge Farm*								
Classic)	50	2.0	9.0	1.0	0	0	90	0
cracked wheat (*Awrey's*)	50	2.0	10.0	1.0	0	0	120	0
crusty (*Awrey's*)	70	2.0	12.0	1.0	0	0	150	0
plain (*Awrey's*)	60	2.0	11.0	1.0	0	0	115	0
poppy seed (*Awrey's*)	59	2.0	11.0	1.0	0	0	115	0
sesame seed (*Awrey's*)	60	2.0	11.0	1.0	0	0	115	0
wheat (*Home Pride*)	70	3.0	12.0	1.0	n.a.	0	140	.6 d
white (*Home Pride*)	80	2.0	14.0	2.0	m.q.	0	170	.6 d
egg (*Levy's* Old Country Deli), 1 oz.	146	5.3	28.1	2.8	m.q.	11	431	2.0 d
egg, sandwich (*Arnold* Dutch)	123	4.5	21.6	3.3	m.q.	1	203	1.9 d
finger, w/poppy seeds (*Pepperidge*								
Farm)	50	2.0	8.0	2.0	0	<5	80	tr.d
49er, sour (*Colombo* Brand), 1.2-oz.								
piece	90	4.8	16.4	.6	n.a.	n.a.	189	m.q.
49er, sweet (*Colombo* Brand),								
1.2-oz. piece	96	4.5	15.4	1.8	m.q.	n.a.	196	m.q.
frankfurter, see "hot dog," below								
French style:								
(*Francisco* International)	108	4.2	21.3	1.5	n.a.	0	285	1.2 d
(*Pepperidge Farm* Deli Classic,								
9/pkg)	100	4.0	20.0	1.0	0	0	230	.5 d

Food and Measure	cal.	prot. (gms)	carbo. (gms)	tot. fat (gms)	sat. fat (gms)	chol. (mgs)	sod. (mgs)	fiber (gms)
(*Pepperidge Farm* Deli Classic, 4/pkg), ½ piece	120	4.0	22.0	2.0	m.q.	n.a.	250	.5 d
sourdough (*Pepperidge Farm*)	100	4.0	19.0	1.0	n.a.	0	240	.5 d
hamburger:								
(*Arnold*)	115	4.3	22.0	2.2	m.q.	0	223	1.8 d
(*Pepperidge Farm*)	130	5.0	22.0	2.0	1.0	0	240	.5 d
(*Roman Meal* Original)	113	4.7	21.1	1.9	m.q.	0	228	2.0 d
(*Wonder*)	120	4.0	21.0	2.0	m.q.	n.a.	230	.9 d
(*Wonder* Light)	80	5.0	13.0	1.0	n.a.	n.a.	210	4.0 d
hoagie (*Wonder*)	400	13.0	73.0	7.0	m.q.	n.a.	800	3.0 d
hoagie, soft (*Pepperidge Farm* Deli Classic)	210	8.0	34.0	5.0	1.0	0	320	1.0 d
honey bun, see "Bun, sweet"								
hot dog:								
(*Arnold*)	100	3.2	19.6	1.8	m.q.	0	162	1.2 d
(*Arnold* New England Style)	108	3.7	20.9	2.0	m.q.	0	178	1.4 d
(*Country Grain*)	100	4.0	18.0	1.0	n.a.	n.a.	230	.9 d
(*Pepperidge Farm*)	140	5.0	24.0	3.0	1.0	0	270	.5 d
(*Roman Meal* Original)	104	4.3	19.5	1.9	m.q.	0	210	1.8 d
(*Wonder*)	80	2.0	14.0	1.0	n.a.	n.a.	150	.6 d
(*Wonder* Light)	80	5.0	13.0	1.0	n.a.	n.a.	210	4.0 d
Dijon (*Pepperidge Farm*)	160	5.0	23.0	5.0	1.0	0	230	2.0 d
oat bran (*Awrey's*)	110	4.0	20.0	2.0	0	0	210	1.0 d
kaiser (*Arnold* Francisco)	184	7.0	35.4	2.9	m.q.	5	338	2.0 d
kaiser (*Brownberry* Hearth)	152	5.4	29.3	2.8	m.q.	9	318	1.9 d
Luigi (*Colombo Brand*-Twin Pack), 2-oz. piece	146	7.6	25.4	1.6	m.q.	n.a.	334	m.q.
onion (*Levy's* Old Country Deli), 1 oz.	153	6.1	30.8	1.9	m.q.	11	380	1.8 d
pan (*Wonder*)	80	2.0	14.0	1.0	n.a.	n.a.	140	.6 d
Parker House (*Pepperidge Farm*)	60	2.0	9.0	1.0	0	5	80	tr.d
party (*Pepperidge Farm*)	30	1.0	5.0	1.0	0	0	50	tr.d
potato (*Pepperidge Farm* Hearty Classic)	90	2.0	14.0	3.0	m.q.	0	125	tr.d
sandwich:								
oat bran (*Awrey's*)	120	4.0	22.0	2.0	0	0	250	1.0 d
onion, w/poppy seeds (*Pepperidge Farm*)	150	5.0	26.0	3.0	1.0	0	260	.5 d
potato (*Pepperidge Farm*)	160	4.0	28.0	4.0	1.0	0	260	1.0 d
salad (*Pepperidge Farm* Deli Classic)	110	4.0	16.0	4.0	m.q.	10	150	m.q.
w/sesame seeds (*Pepperidge Farm*)	140	5.0	23.0	3.0	1.0	0	230	.5 d
soft (*Pepperidge Farm* Family)	100	4.0	18.0	2.0	1.0	0	190	.5 d
steak, sour (*Colombo* Brand), 2.6-oz. piece	200	10.1	35.1	2.2	m.q.	n.a.	413	m.q.
steak, sweet (*Colombo* Brand), 2.6-oz. piece	206	10.0	34.2	3.3	m.q.	0	439	m.q.

Food and Measure	cal.	prot. (gms)	carbo. (gms)	tot. fat (gms)	sat. fat (gms)	chol. (mgs)	sod. (mgs)	fiber (gms)
ROLL *(cont.)*								
twist, golden (*Pepperidge Farm* Heat 'n Serve)	110	2.0	14.0	5.0	2.0	5	150	tr.d
ROLL, FROZEN:								
apple, sweet (*Weight Watchers* Microwave), ½ pkg. or 2.25 oz.	160	3.0	27.0	4.0	<1.0	5	100	m.q.
cheese (*Weight Watchers* Microwave), ½ pkg. or 2.25 oz.	180	5.0	32.0	4.0	<1.0	5	210	m.q.
cinnamon:								
(*Pepperidge Farm*, 2/pkg.), 1 piece	280	4.0	34.0	14.0	m.q.	n.a.	190	m.q.
all butter (*Sara Lee*), 2-oz. piece	230	3.0	31.0	11.0	m.q.	n.a.	220	m.q.
all butter, icing packet (*Sara Lee*), .5-oz. pkt.	50	0	12.0	0	0	0	0	m.q.
Parkerhouse (*Bridgford*), 1-oz. piece	85	2.5	15.8	1.3	n.a.	0	172	m.q.
strawberry (*Weight Watchers* Microwave), ½ pkg. or 2.25 oz.	170	3.0	29.0	5.0	1.0	20	90	m.q.
ROLL, REFRIGERATED:								
butterflake (*Pillsbury*), 1 piece	140	3.0	20.0	5.0	1.0	0	530	m.q.
cinnamon:								
iced (*Hungry Jack*), 2 pieces	290	3.0	37.0	14.0	m.q.	n.a.	570	m.q.
iced (*Pillsbury*), 1 piece	110	1.0	17.0	5.0	1.0	0	260	m.q.
crescent (*Pillsbury*), 1 piece	100	2.0	11.0	6.0	2.0	5	230	m.q.
ROLL, SWEET see also "Bun, sweet"), 1 piece:								
cinnamon:								
(*Hostess Breakfast Bake Shop*) ...	140	3.0	24.0	4.0	2.0	20	170	.9 d
homestyle (*Awrey's*)	240	4.0	40.0	7.0	1.0	5	200	1.0 d
swirl (*Awrey's Grande*)	340	4.0	46.0	16.0	3.0	10	370	1.0 d
orange swirl (*Hostess Breakfast Bake Shop*)	230	3.0	26.0	12.0	6.0	10	150	1.1 d
pecan spinner (*Hostess Breakfast Bake Shop*)	220	3.0	30.0	10.0	2.0	5	135	1.4 d
pecan-caramel swirl (*Hostess Breakfast Bake Shop*)	240	3.0	23.0	15.0	7.0	10	160	1.8 d
ROLL MIX[1], hot:								
(*Dromedary*), ⅛ pkg. dry	209	6.0	41.0	2.0	m.q.	n.a.	363	m.q.
(*Dromedary*), 2 pieces	239	6.0	41.0	5.0	m.q.	n.a.	410	m.q.
(*Pillsbury*), 2 pieces	270	4.0	25.0	17.0	m.q.	n.a.	420	m.q.
ROMAN BEAN, canned:								
(*Progresso*), ½ cup	110	7.0	18.0	<1.0	n.a.	0	420	12.0 d
ROQUETTE, see "Arugula"								
ROSÉ, see "Wine"								
ROSE APPLE:								
untrimmed, 1 lb.	76	1.8	17.3	.9	n.a.	0	1	3.3 c
trimmed, 1 oz.	7	.2	1.6	.1	(0)	0	tr.	.3 c
ROSELLE:								
untrimmed, 1 lb.	136	2.7	31.3	1.8	n.a.	0	16	3.2 c

1. *Prepared according to package directions, except as noted.*

Food and Measure	cal.	prot. (gms)	carbo. (gms)	tot. fat (gms)	sat. fat (gms)	chol. (mgs)	sod. (mgs)	fiber (gms)
trimmed, 1 oz. or ½ cup	14	.3	3.2	.2	(0)	0	2	.3 c
ROSEMARY, dried:								
1 oz.	94	1.4	18.2	4.3	n.a.	0	14	5.0 c
1 tbsp.	11	.2	2.1	.5	(0)	0	2	.6 c
1 tsp.	4	.1	.8	.2	(0)	0	1	.2 c
(*Spice Islands*), 1 tsp.	5	.1	.8	.2	(0)	0	1	.2 c
ROTINI, see "Pasta"								
ROTINI ENTREE, frozen:								
cheddar (*Green Giant* Microwave								
Garden Gourmet), 1 pkg.	230	9.0	32.0	10.0	6.0	20	570	4.5 d
seafood (*Mrs. Paul's* Light), 9 oz. ...	240	12.0	34.0	6.0	2.0	25	570	m.q.
ROUGHY, orange, meat only, raw:								
1 lb.	571	66.7	0	31.8	.6	91	286	0
1 oz.	36	4.2	0	2.0	<.1	6	18	0
ROY ROGERS:								
breakfast, 1 piece or serving:								
apple swirls	328	5.0	62.0	7.0	m.q.	n.a.	279	m.q.
cheese swirls	383	8.0	54.0	15.0	m.q.	n.a.	369	m.q.
cinnamon roll	376	5.0	55.0	15.0	m.q.	n.a.	339	m.q.
crescent roll	287	5.0	27.0	18.0	m.q.	<5	547	m.q.
crescent sandwich:								
regular	408	13.0	28.0	27.0	m.q.	207	820	m.q.
w/bacon	446	15.0	28.0	30.0	m.q.	212	982	m.q.
w/ham	456	20.0	29.0	29.0	m.q.	227	1243	m.q.
w/sausage	564	19.0	28.0	42.0	m.q.	248	1145	m.q.
egg and biscuit platter:								
regular	557	18.0	44.0	34.0	m.q.	417	1020	m.q.
w/bacon	607	21.0	44.0	39.0	m.q.	424	1236	m.q.
w/ham	605	25.0	44.0	36.0	m.q.	437	1442	m.q.
w/sausage	713	25.0	44.0	49.0	m.q.	458	1345	m.q.
pancake platter, w/syrup and								
butter:								
regular	386	5.0	63.0	13.0	m.q.	51	547	m.q.
and bacon	436	8.0	63.0	17.0	m.q.	58	763	m.q.
and ham	434	11.0	64.0	15.0	m.q.	71	969	m.q.
and sausage	542	11.0	63.0	28.0	m.q.	92	872	m.q.
chicken, fried, 1 serving:								
breast	412	33.0	17.0	24.0	m.q.	118	609	m.q.
breast and wing	604	44.0	25.0	37.0	m.q.	165	894	m.q.
leg (drumstick)	140	12.0	6.0	8.0	m.q.	40	190	m.q.
leg and thigh	436	30.0	17.0	28.0	m.q.	125	596	m.q.
nuggets, 6 pieces	288	10.0	21.0	18.0	m.q.	63	548	m.q.
thigh	296	18.0	12.0	20.0	m.q.	85	406	m.q.
wing	192	11.0	9.0	13.0	m.q.	47	285	m.q.
sandwiches, 1 serving:								
bacon cheeseburger	552	32.0	31.0	33.0	m.q.	83	1025	m.q.
bar burger	573	36.0	38.0	31.0	m.q.	96	1252	m.q.
cheeseburger	525	29.0	37.0	29.0	m.q.	76	830	m.q.
cheeseburger, small	275	15.0	24.0	13.0	m.q.	36	558	m.q.

Food and Measure	cal.	prot. (gms)	carbo. (gms)	tot. fat (gms)	sat. fat (gms)	chol. (mgs)	sod. (mgs)	fiber (gms)
ROY ROGERS, SANDWICHES *(cont.)*								
*Express*burger	561	27.0	42.0	32.0	m.q.	70	899	m.q.
Express bacon cheeseburger	641	33.0	36.0	41.0	m.q.	89	1317	m.q.
Express cheeseburger	613	30.0	42.0	37.0	m.q.	82	1122	m.q.
fish sandwich	514	18.0	58.0	24.0	m.q.	62	857	m.q.
hamburger	472	26.0	37.0	25.0	m.q.	64	607	m.q.
hamburger, small	222	12.0	23.0	9.0	m.q.	26	336	m.q.
roast beef sandwich:								
regular	350	26.0	37.0	11.0	m.q.	68	732	m.q.
w/cheese	403	29.0	37.0	15.0	m.q.	70	954	m.q.
large	373	35.0	31.0	12.0	m.q.	82	840	m.q.
large, w/cheese	427	38.0	31.0	17.0	m.q.	94	1062	m.q.
side dishes, 1 serving:								
biscuit	231	4.0	26.0	12.0	m.q.	<5	575	m.q.
coleslaw	110	1.0	11.0	7.0	m.q.	<5	261	m.q.
french fries:								
4 oz.	320	4.0	39.0	16.0	m.q.	13	164	m.q.
small, 3 oz.	238	3.0	29.0	12.0	m.q.	10	122	m.q.
large, 5.5 oz.	440	6.0	54.0	22.0	m.q.	19	225	m.q.
salad bar:								
alfalfa sprouts, 2 tbsp.	1	tr.	tr.	tr.	(0)	0	<1	m.q.
bacon bits, 1 tsp.	33	3.0	2.0	1.0	n.a.	0	189	n.a.
bean sprouts, 2 tbsp.	4	tr.	1.0	tr.	(0)	0	<1	m.q.
beets, sliced, ¼ cup	18	1.0	4.0	tr.	(0)	0	162	m.q.
broccoli, ¼ cup	6	1.0	1.0	tr.	(0)	0	6	m.q.
cabbage, ¼ cup	5	tr.	1.0	tr.	(0)	0	2	m.q.
cantaloupe cubes, ¼ cup	14	tr.	3.0	tr.	(0)	0	4	m.q.
carrots, shredded, ¼ cup	12	tr.	3.0	tr.	(0)	0	2	m.q.
cauliflower, raw, ¼ cup	6	1.0	1.0	tr.	(0)	0	4	m.q.
cheddar cheese, ¼ cup	100	7.0	tr.	8.0	m.q.	15	275	0
Chinese noodles, ¼ cup	55	2.0	7.0	3.0	m.q.	1	113	m.q.
cottage cheese, 2 tbsp.	29	4.0	<1.0	1.0	m.q.	4	114	0
croutons, 2 tbsp.	14	1.0	3.0	tr.	(0)	0	50	m.q.
cucumbers, 5–6 slices	4	tr.	1.0	0	0	0	2	m.q.
eggs, chopped, 2 tbsp.	55	4.0	1.0	4.0	m.q.	m.q.	41	0
fruit cocktail, ¼ cup	46	tr.	12.0	tr.	(0)	0	1	m.q.
garbanzo beans, ¼ cup	55	3.0	9.0	1.0	m.q.	0	240	m.q.
gelatin parfait, ¼ cup	50	1.0	10.0	2.0	m.q.	0	23	(0)
granola, ¼ cup	65	2.0	9.0	3.0	m.q.	0	8	m.q.
grapes, 5 grapes	20	tr.	5.0	tr.	(0)	0	<1	m.q.
green peas, ¼ cup	28	2.0	5.0	tr.	(0)	0	41	m.q.
green pepper, 2 tbsp.	3	tr.	1.0	tr.	(0)	0	tr.	m.q.
honeydew cubes, ¼ cup	15	tr.	4.0	tr.	(0)	0	4	m.q.
iceburg lettuce, 1 cup	7	1.0	1.0	tr.	(0)	0	5	m.q.
macaroni salad, ¼ cup	93	2.0	10.0	5.0	m.q.	n.a.	301	m.q.
onions, chopped, 2 tbsp.	7	tr.	2.0	tr.	(0)	0	tr.	m.q.
Greek pasta salad, ¼ cup	159	3.0	19.0	9.0	m.q.	n.a.	328	m.q.
peach slices, ¼ cup	48	tr.	13.0	tr.	(0)	0	5	m.q.
pineapple chunks, fresh, ¼ cup ..	19	tr.	5.0	tr.	(0)	0	<1	m.q.

Food and Measure	cal.	prot. (gms)	carbo. (gms)	tot. fat (gms)	sat. fat (gms)	chol. (mgs)	sod. (mgs)	fiber (gms)
pineapple chunks, canned, ¼ cup	48	tr.	12.0	tr.	(0)	0	5	m.q.
potato salad, ¼ cup	54	1.0	5.0	3.0	m.q.	n.a.	348	m.q.
radishes, slices, 2 tbsp.	2	tr.	1.0	tr.	(0)	0	4	m.q.
romaine lettuce, 1 cup	9	1.0	1.0	tr.	(0)	0	5	m.q.
strawberries, fresh, ¼ cup	11	tr.	3.0	tr.	(0)	0	<1	m.q.
tomatoes, 3 slices	20	1.0	5.0	tr.	(0)	0	1	m.q.
watermelon, diced, ¼ cup	13	tr.	3.0	tr.	(0)	0	1	m.q.
salad dressings, 2 tbsp:								
bacon and tomato	136	tr.	6.0	12.0	m.q.	n.a.	150	n.a.
blue cheese	150	2.0	2.0	16.0	m.q.	n.a.	153	n.a.
Italian, lo-cal	70	tr.	2.0	6.0	m.q.	n.a.	100	n.a.
ranch	155	tr.	4.0	14.0	m.q.	n.a.	100	n.a.
Thousand Island	160	tr.	4.0	16.0	m.q.	n.a.	150	n.a.
desserts and shakes, 1 serving:								
shake:								
chocolate	358	8.0	61.0	10.0	m.q.	37	290	(0)
strawberry	315	8.0	49.0	10.0	m.q.	37	261	(0)
vanilla	306	8.0	45.0	11.0	m.q.	40	282	0
sundae:								
caramel	293	7.0	52.0	9.0	m.q.	23	193	(0)
hot fudge	337	7.0	53.0	13.0	m.q.	23	186	(0)
strawberry	216	6.0	33.0	7.0	m.q.	23	99	(0)
Vitari, 1 oz.	30	m.q.	7.0	m.q.	n.a.	9	m.q.	(0)
RUCOLO OR RUGULA, see "Arugula"								
RUM, see "Liquor"								
RUTABAGA:								
raw:								
untrimmed, 1 lb.	140	4.6	31.4	.8	.1	0	77	4.2 c
trimmed, 1 oz.	10	.3	2.3	.1	tr.	0	6	.3 c
cubed, ½ cup	25	.8	5.7	.1	<.1	0	14	.8 c
boiled, drained:								
4 oz.	39	1.2	8.8	.2	<.1	0	20	1.2 c
cubed, ½ cup	29	.9	6.6	.2	<.1	0	15	.9 c
mashed, ½ cup	41	1.3	9.3	.2	<.1	0	22	1.3 c
RUTABAGA, CANNED:								
diced (*Allens*), ½ cup	20	1.0	4.0	<1.0	(0)	0	260	m.q.
RYE, whole-grain:								
1 oz.	95	4.2	19.8	.7	.1	0	2	.4 c
1 cup	567	25.0	117.9	4.2	.5	0	10	2.5 c
(*Arrowhead Mills*), 2 oz.	190	7.0	42.0	1.0	m.q.	0	1	7.6 d
RYE CAKE:								
(*Quaker* Grain Cakes), .32-oz. piece	35	1.4	6.5	.3	0	0	52	.8 d
RYE FLAKES:								
(*Arrowhead Mills*), 2 oz.	190	7.0	42.0	1.0	m.q.	0	1	7.6 d
RYE FLOUR:								
dark, 1 oz.	92	4.0	19.5	.8	.1	0	<1	m.q.
dark, 1 cup	415	18.0	88.0	3.4	.4	0	2	m.q.
light, 1 oz.	104	2.4	22.7	.4	<.1	0	<1	4.1 d

Food and Measure	cal.	prot. (gms)	carbo. (gms)	tot. fat (gms)	sat. fat (gms)	chol. (mgs)	sod. (mgs)	fiber (gms)
RYE FLOUR *(cont.)*								
light, 1 cup	374	8.6	81.8	1.4	.1	0	2	14.9 d
medium:								
1 oz.	100	2.7	22.0	.5	.1	0	1	4.1 d
1 cup	361	9.9	79.0	1.8	.2	0	3	14.9 d
(Pillsbury's Best), 1 cup	400	12.0	83.0	2.0	m.q.	0	0	m.q.
stone ground *(Robin Hood)*, 4 oz. or								
1 cup	360	13.0	86.0	2.0	m.q.	0	10	13.0 d
whole grain *(Arrowhead Mills)*, 2 oz.	190	9.0	39.0	1.0	m.q.	0	1	7.6 d
RYE LIQUOR, see "Liquor"								
RYE AND WHEAT FLOUR:								
(Pillsbury's Best Bohemian Style),								
1 cup	400	11.0	86.0	1.0	m.q.	0	0	m.q.

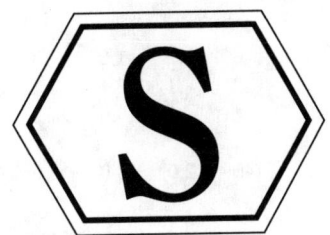

Food and Measure	cal.	prot. (gms)	carbo. (gms)	tot. fat (gms)	sat. fat (gms)	chol. (mgs)	sod. (mgs)	fiber (gms)
SABLEFISH, meat only:								
raw:								
1 lb.	886	60.8	0	69.4	14.5	222	254	0
1 oz.	55	3.8	0	4.3	.9	14	16	0
½ fillet, approx. 6.8 oz., yield								
from 5-lb. whole fish	377	25.9	0	29.5	6.2	95	108	0
smoked, 4 oz.	291	20.0	0	22.8	4.8	73	836	0
smoked, 1 oz.	73	5.0	0	5.7	1.2	18	209	0
SACCHARIN, see "Sugar, substitute"								
SAFFLOWER OIL:								
(*Hain*), 1 tbsp.	120	0	0	14.0	1.0	0	0	0
linoleic:								
1 oz.	251	0	0	28.4	2.6	0	0	0
½ cup	964	0	0	109.0	0	0	0	0
1 tbsp.	120	0	0	13.6	1.2	0	0	0
oleic:								
1 oz.	251	0	0	28.4	1.7	0	0	0
½ cup	964	0	0	109.0	6.7	0	0	0
1 tbsp.	120	0	0	13.6	.8	0	0	0
(*Hain* Hi-Oleic), 1 tbsp.	120	0	0	14.0	1.0	0	0	0
unrefined (*Hain*), 1 tbsp.	120	0	0	m.q.	1.2	0	0	0
SAFFLOWER SEED KERNEL:								
dried, unsalted, 1 oz.	147	4.6	9.7	10.9	1.0	0	(0)	.7 c
SAFFLOWER SEED MEAL:								
partially defatted, 1 oz.	97	10.1	13.8	.7	.1	0	n.a.	2.2 c
SAFFRON:								
1 oz.	88	3.2	18.5	1.7	n.a.	0	42	1.0 c
1 tbsp.	7	.2	1.4	.1	(0)	0	3	.1 c
1 tsp.	2	.1	.5	<.1	(0)	0	1	tr.c
SAGE, ground:								
1 oz.	89	3.0	17.2	3.6	2.0	0	3	5.1 c

Food and Measure	cal.	prot. (gms)	carbo. (gms)	tot. fat (gms)	sat. fat (gms)	chol. (mgs)	sod. (mgs)	fiber (gms)
SAGE *(cont.)*								
1 tbsp.	6	.2	1.2	.3	.1	0	tr.	.4 c
1 tsp.	2	.1	.4	.1	<.1	0	tr.	.1 c
(*Spice Islands*), 1 tsp.	4	.1	.6	.1	<.1	0	<1	.1 c
SALAD DIP:								
egg-free (*Nasoya Vegi-Dip*), 1 oz.	45	2.0	3.0	3.0	m.q.	0	110	n.a.
SALAD DRESSING, 1 tbsp.,								
except as noted:								
bacon, creamy, (*Kraft* Reduced								
Calorie)	30	0	2.0	2.0	0	0	150	n.a.
bacon and tomato:								
(*Estee*)	8	<1.0	1.0	<1.0	<1.0	5	35	n.a.
(*Kraft*)	70	0	1.0	7.0	1.0	0	130	n.a.
(*Kraft* Reduced Calorie)	30	0	2.0	2.0	0	0	150	n.a.
blue cheese:								
1 oz.	143	1.4	2.1	14.8	2.8	m.q.	m.q.	<.1 c
1 cup	1235	11.8	18.1	128.1	24.1	m.q.	m.q.	.2 c
1 tbsp.	77	.7	1.1	8.0	1.5	m.q.	m.q.	tr.c
(*Estee*)	8	<1.0	1.0	<1.0	<1.0	0	50	n.a.
(*Featherweight Neu Bleu*)	4	0	1.0	0	0	0	110	n.a.
(*Roka* Brand)	60	1.0	1.0	6.0	1.0	10	170	n.a.
(*Roka* Brand Reduced Calorie)	16	1.0	1.0	1.0	1.0	5	280	n.a.
(*S&W/Nutradiet*)	25	0	2.0	2.0	n.a.	0	200	n.a.
chunky:								
(*Kraft*)	60	1.0	2.0	6.0	1.0	<5	230	n.a.
(*Kraft* Reduced Calorie)	30	0	2.0	2.0	1.0	<5	240	n.a.
(*Wish-Bone*)	75	.4	.7	7.9	1.2	1	149	n.a.
(*Wish-Bone* Lite)	40	.3	1.5	3.7	.8	1	197	n.a.
buttermilk:								
(*Hain* Old Fashioned)	70	0	0	7.0	m.q.	0	100	n.a.
(*Hollywood* Old Fashion)	75	0	1.0	8.0	1.0	0	40	0
(*Seven Seas Buttermilk Recipe*)	80	0	1.0	8.0	1.0	5	130	n.a.
creamy (*Kraft*)	80	0	1.0	8.0	1.0	<5	120	0
creamy (*Kraft* Reduced Calorie)	30	0	1.0	3.0	0	<5	125	n.a.
Caesar:								
(*Hollywood*)	70	1.0	2.0	7.0	1.0	0	65	0
(*Lawry's* Classic), 1 oz.	130	.8	1.0	13.5	1.8	n.a.	337	.1 c
(*Weight Watchers*)	4	0	1.0	0	0	0	200	n.a.
(*Weight Watchers* Single Serve),								
1 pkt.	6	0	1.0	0	0	0	270	n.a.
(*Wish-Bone*)	77	.4	.9	8.0	1.2	1	248	n.a.
creamy (*Hain*)	60	0	1.0	6.0	m.q.	<5	220	n.a.
creamy (*Hain* Low Salt)	60	0	1.0	6.0	m.q.	<5	15	n.a.
golden (*Kraft*)	70	0	1.0	7.0	1.0	0	180	n.a.
Chinese vinegar w/sesame and								
ginger (*Lawry's* Classic), 1 oz.	145	.2	2.4	15.0	2.1	0	325	0
citrus, tangy (*Hain* Canola)	50	0	1.0	5.0	m.q.	0	75	n.a.
coleslaw (*Kraft*)	70	0	4.0	6.0	1.0	10	200	n.a.
coleslaw (*Miracle Whip*)	70	0	3.0	6.0	1.0	5	105	n.a.

Food and Measure	cal.	prot. (gms)	carbo. (gms)	tot. fat (gms)	sat. fat (gms)	chol. (mgs)	sod. (mgs)	fiber (gms)
creamy (see also specific listings):								
(*Rancher's Choice*)	90	0	1.0	10.0	1.0	5	140	n.a.
(*Rancher's Choice* Reduced								
Calorie)	30	0	1.0	3.0	0	5	150	n.a.
egg-free (*Life* All Natural)	39	<1.0	2.0	4.0	m.q.	0	4	n.a.
cucumber:								
creamy:								
(*Featherweight*)	4	0	1.0	0	0	0	80	n.a.
(*Kraft*)	70	0	1.0	8.0	1.0	0	190	n.a.
(*Kraft* Reduced Calorie)	25	0	1.0	2.0	0	0	220	n.a.
(*Weight Watchers*)	18	m.q.	4.0	0	0	n.a.	85	n.a.
dill (*Hain*)	80	0	0	8.0	m.q.	5	210	n.a.
Dijon:								
creamy (*Estee*)	8	<1.0	<1.0	<1.0	<1.0	5	100	n.a.
creamy (*Featherweight*)	20	0	1.0	2.0	m.q.	0	80	n.a.
mustard (*Great Impressions*)	57	.4	.3	6.1	m.q.	18	103	n.a.
vinaigrette:								
(*Hain*)	50	0	0	5.0	m.q.	<5	180	n.a.
(*Hollywood*)	60	0	2.0	6.0	1.0	0	40	0
(*Wish-Bone* Classic)	60	.2	1.0	6.1	.9	<1	171	n.a.
(*Wish-Bone* Lite Classic)	30	.1	1.1	2.8	m.q.	0	176	n.a.
dill, creamy (*Nasoya Vegi-Dressing*)	40	1.0	1.0	3.0	m.q.	0	50	n.a.
French:								
1 tbsp.	67	.1	2.7	6.4	1.5	n.a.	214	.1 c
1 oz.	122	.2	5.0	11.6	2.7	n.a.	388	.2 c
1 cup	1074	1.4	43.6	102.4	23.7	n.a.	3425	1.9 c
(*Catalina*)	60	0	4.0	5.0	1.0	0	180	n.a.
(*Catalina* Reduced Calorie)	18	0	3.0	1.0	0	0	120	n.a.
(*Estee*)	4	0	1.0	0	0	0	10	n.a.
(*Featherweight*)	14	0	3.0	0	0	0	15	n.a.
(*Kraft*)	60	0	2.0	6.0	1.0	0	125	n.a.
(*Kraft Free*)	20	0	4.0	0	0	0	120	n.a.
(*Kraft Free Catalina*)	16	0	3.0	0	0	0	120	n.a.
(*Kraft Miracle*)	70	0	3.0	6.0	1.0	0	240	n.a.
(*Kraft* Reduced Calorie)	20	0	3.0	1.0	0	0	120	n.a.
(*Pathmark* Reduced Calorie)	20	0	3.0	1.0	0	0	160	n.a.
(*S&W/Nutradiet*)	18	0	3.0	0	0	0	120	n.a.
(*Seven Seas French! Light*)	35	0	2.0	3.0	0	0	210	n.a.
(*Wish-Bone* Deluxe)	60	.1	2.3	5.4	.8	0	83	n.a.
(*Wish-Bone* Deluxe Food Service)	61	.1	2.4	5.6	m.q.	0	86	0
(*Wish-Bone* Lite)	31	0	2.1	2.5	m.q.	0	70	0
(*Wish-Bone* Lite Sweet'n Spicy) ..	18	0	3.2	.5	n.a.	0	110	n.a.
(*Wish-Bone* Sweet'n Spicy)	63	.1	2.9	5.7	.8	0	156	n.a.
creamy:								
(*Hain*)	60	0	1.0	6.0	m.q.	0	80	n.a.
(*Hollywood*)	70	0	2.0	7.0	1.0	0	45	0
(*Pathmark*)	60	0	2.0	5.0	1.0	0	90	n.a.
(*Seven Seas*)	60	0	2.0	6.0	1.0	0	240	n.a.
garlic (*Wish-Bone*)	55	.1	1.8	5.3	m.q.	0	158	.1 c

Food and Measure	cal.	prot. (gms)	carbo. (gms)	tot. fat (gms)	sat. fat (gms)	chol. (mgs)	sod. (mgs)	fiber (gms)
SALAD DRESSING, FRENCH *(cont.)*								
low-calorie (see also specific								
brands):								
1 tbsp.	22	tr.	3.5	.9	.1	1	128	tr.c
1 oz.	38	.1	6.2	1.6	.2	2	223	.1 c
1 cup	349	.6	56.4	15.1	2.2	15	2046	.7 c
red (*Wish-Bone* Lite)	17	.2	3.2	.4	n.a.	0	155	n.a.
style (*Weight Watchers*)	10	0	2.0	0	0	0	170	n.a.
style (*Wish-Bone* Lite)	30	.1	1.9	2.5	.1	0	67	n.a.
w/green pepper (*Great*								
Impressions)	64	.2	4.1	5.2	m.q.	0	188	n.a.
garlic:								
creamy:								
(*Estee*)	2	0	0	0	0	0	10	n.a.
(*Kraft*)	50	0	1.0	5.0	1.0	0	170	n.a.
(*Wish-Bone*)	74	.1	.5	8.0	m.q.	0	158	.6 c
French (*Wish-Bone*)	55	.1	1.8	5.3	m.q.	0	158	.1 c
herb (*Nasoya Vegi-Dressing*)	40	1.0	1.0	3.0	m.q.	0	50	n.a.
and sour cream (*Hain*)	70	0	0	7.0	m.q.	0	100	n.a.
herb:								
(*Featherweight*)	6	0	1.0	0	0	0	5	n.a.
garden (*Featherweight*)	25	0	2.0	2.0	m.q.	0	65	n.a.
savory (*Hain* No Salt Added)	90	0	0	10.0	m.q.	0	25	n.a.
herb and spice (*Seven Seas Viva*)	60	0	1.0	6.0	1.0	0	170	n.a.
herb and spice (*Seven Seas Viva*								
Herbs & Spices! Light)	30	0	1.0	3.0	0	0	200	n.a.
homestyle (*Dorothy Lynch*)	55	.1	5.0	3.8	.5	0	85	n.a.
homestyle (*Dorothy Lynch* Reduced								
Calorie)	30	0	7.0	<1.0	m.q.	0	80	n.a.
honey and sesame (*Hain*)	60	0	2.0	5.0	m.q.	0	210	n.a.
Italian:								
1 tbsp.	69	.1	1.5	7.1	1.0	n.a.	116	tr.c
1 oz.	132	.2	2.9	13.7	2.0	n.a.	223	.1 c
1 cup	1098	1.5	24.0	113.5	16.3	n.a.	1849	.5 c
(*Featherweight*)	4	0	1.0	0	0	0	120	n.a.
(*Hain* Canola)	50	0	1.0	5.0	m.q.	0	150	n.a.
(*Hain* Traditional)	80	0	0	8.0	m.q.	0	330	n.a.
(*Hain* Traditional No Salt Added)	60	0	1.0	6.0	m.q.	0	20	n.a.
(*Hollywood*)	90	0	1.0	9.0	1.0	0	300	0
(*Kraft Free*)	6	0	1.0	0	0	0	210	n.a.
(*Kraft Presto*)	70	0	1.0	7.0	1.0	0	150	n.a.
(*Nasoya Vegi-Dressing*)	40	1.0	1.0	3.0	m.q.	0	50	n.a.
(*Ott's*)	80	<.1	.2	9.1	m.q.	<1	87	tr.d
(*Seven Seas Free Viva*)	4	0	1.0	0	0	0	220	n.a.
(*Seven Seas Viva*)	50	0	1.0	5.0	1.0	0	240	n.a.
(*Seven Seas Viva Italian! Light*)	30	0	1.0	3.0	0	0	230	n.a.
(*Wish-Bone*)	46	0	1.5	4.5	.6	0	280	n.a.
(*Wish-Bone* Lite)	7	.2	.9	.3	n.a.	0	212	n.a.
(*Wish-Bone* Robusto)	47	.1	1.8	4.5	.6	0	288	n.a.

Food and Measure	cal.	prot. (gms)	carbo. (gms)	tot. fat (gms)	sat. fat (gms)	chol. (mgs)	sod. (mgs)	fiber (gms)
blended (*Wish-Bone*)	37	0	1.2	3.6	.5	0	199	n.a.
w/bleu cheese (*Lawry's* Classic),								
1 oz.	186	.1	1.9	2.0	m.q.	n.a.	385	.1 c
cheese (*Featherweight*)	20	0	1.0	2.0	m.q.	0	70	n.a.
cheese (*Hollywood*)	80	0	2.0	8.0	1.0	0	60	0
w/cheese (*Wish-Bone*)	89	.2	1.0	9.2	1.3	<1	170	n.a.
cheese vinaigrette (*Hain*)	55	0	0	6.0	m.q.	<5	130	n.a.
creamy:								
(*Hain*)	80	0	0	8.0	m.q.	0	100	n.a.
(*Hain* No Salt Added)	80	0	1.0	8.0	m.q.	0	25	n.a.
(*Hollywood*)	90	0	2.0	9.0	1.0	0	140	0
(*Kraft* Reduced Calorie)	25	0	1.0	2.0	0	0	120	n.a.
(*Pathmark*)	70	0	1.0	7.0	1.0	0	260	n.a.
(*S&W/Nutradiet*)	10	0	1.0	1.0	n.a.	n.a.	180	n.a.
(*Seven Seas*)	70	0	1.0	7.0	1.0	0	240	n.a.
(*Seven Seas Viva Creamy*								
Italian! Light)	45	0	1.0	4.0	1.0	0	230	n.a.
(*Weight Watchers*)	50	0	2.0	5.0	1.0	5	80	n.a.
(*Wish-Bone*)	56	.1	1.5	5.5	.9	<1	149	n.a.
(*Wish-Bone* Lite)	26	.1	2.0	2.0	.4	<1	148	n.a.
w/real sour cream (*Kraft*)	50	0	1.0	5.0	1.0	0	120	n.a.
creamy or regular (*Estee*)	4	0	1.0	0	0	0	13	n.a.
herbal (*Wish-Bone* Classics)	70	0	1.2	7.3	m.q.	0	228	n.a.
house (*Kraft*)	60	0	1.0	6.0	1.0	0	115	n.a.
house (*Kraft* Reduced Calorie) ...	30	0	1.0	2.0	0	0	115	n.a.
low-calorie (see also specific								
brands):								
1 tbsp.	16	tr.	.7	1.5	.2	1	118	tr.c
1 oz.	30	<.1	1.4	2.8	.4	2	223	.1 c
1 cup	253	.2	11.6	23.6	3.2	14	1889	.7 c
no oil (*Kraft* Reduced Calorie) ...	4	0	1.0	0	0	0	220	n.a.
no oil (*S&W/Nutradiet*)	2	0	0	0	0	0	290	n.a.
w/Parmesan cheese (*Lawry's*								
Classic), 1 oz.	156	0	4.5	15.1	2.1	n.a.	178	.1 c
style (*Weight Watchers*)	6	0	1.0	0	0	0	310	n.a.
style (*Weight Watchers* Single								
Serve), 1 pkt.	9	0	2.0	0	0	0	430	n.a.
zesty:								
(*Kraft*)	50	0	1.0	5.0	1.0	0	260	n.a.
(*Kraft* Reduced Calorie)	20	0	1.0	2.0	0	0	230	n.a.
(*Pathmark*)	70	0	1.0	8.0	1.0	0	370	n.a.
(*Pathmark* Reduced Calorie) ...	6	0	1.0	0	0	0	190	n.a.
mayonnaise, see "Mayonnaise"								
mayonnaise type (see also specific								
brands):								
1 tbsp.	57	.1	3.5	4.9	.7	4	104	0
1 oz.	110	.3	6.8	9.5	1.4	7	202	0
1 cup	916	2.1	56.2	78.4	11.6	60	1670	0
(*A&P*)	70	<1.0	2.0	7.0	1.0	8	105	0

Food and Measure	cal.	prot. (gms)	carbo. (gms)	tot. fat (gms)	sat. fat (gms)	chol. (mgs)	sod. (mgs)	fiber (gms)
SALAD DRESSING, MAYONNAISE TYPE *(cont.)*								
(*Bama*)	50	0	3.0	4.0	m.q.	n.a.	105	0
(*Finast*)	70	0	2.0	7.0	m.q.	n.a.	90	0
(*Kraft Free*)	12	0	3.0	0	0	0	190	0
(*Miracle Whip*)	70	0	2.0	7.0	1.0	5	85	0
(*Miracle Whip* Free)	20	0	5.0	0	0	0	210	0
(*Miracle Whip* Light)	45	0	2.0	4.0	1.0	0	125	0
(*P&Q*)	50	<1.0	3.0	5.0	1.0	8	110	0
(*Pathmark* No Frills)	50	0	3.0	5.0	1.0	5	120	0
(*Spin Blend*)	60	0	3.0	5.0	1.0	10	110	0
cholesterol free (*Spin Blend*)	40	0	2.0	4.0	1.0	0	110	0
whipped (*Weight Watchers*)	45	0	3.0	4.0	1.0	0	100	0
mustard, spicy French (*Hain* Canola)	50	1.0	1.0	5.0	m.q.	5	190	n.a.
oil and vinegar (*Kraft*)	70	0	1.0	8.0	1.0	0	210	0
olive oil:								
Italian (*Wish-Bone* Classic)	34	0	1.7	3.0	.4	0	190	0
vinaigrette (*Wish-Bone*)	28	0	1.8	2.3	m.q.	0	111	0
vinaigrette (*Wish-Bone* Lite)	16	.1	1.9	.9	.1	0	111	0
onion and chive (*Wish-Bone* Lite)	37	.2	1.6	3.3	m.q.	0	164	n.a.
onion and chives, creamy (*Kraft*)	70	0	1.0	7.0	1.0	0	150	n.a.
orange marmalade fruit salad (*Great Impressions*)	87	.2	5.4	7.1	m.q.	11	48	n.a.
Oriental style (*Featherweight*)	20	0	1.0	2.0	m.q.	0	75	n.a.
(*Ott's Famous*)	40	.1	4.1	2.7	m.q.	<1	195	<.1 d
(*Ott's* Reduced Calorie *Famous*)	26	.2	3.6	1.3	m.q.	0	60	<.1 d
peppercorn, creamy (*Weight Watchers*)	8	0	2.0	0	0	n.a.	85	n.a.
poppyseed (*Great Impressions*), 2 tbsp.	131	.1	8.0	11.0	m.q.	0	130	n.a.
poppyseed (*Hain* Rancher's)	60	0	0	7.0	m.q.	<5	105	n.a.
Ranch:								
(*Kraft Free*)	16	0	3.0	0	0	0	150	n.a.
(*Seven Seas* Buttermilk Recipe Ranch! Light)	50	0	1.0	5.0	1.0	0	135	n.a.
(*Seven Seas* Free)	16	0	4.0	0	0	0	120	n.a.
(*Seven Seas* Viva)	80	0	1.0	8.0	1.0	5	135	n.a.
(*Seven Seas* Viva Ranch! Light)	50	0	2.0	5.0	1.0	5	125	n.a.
(*Wish-Bone*)	78	.1	1.1	8.3	1.2	4	156	n.a.
(*Wish-Bone* Lite)	42	.2	2.5	3.5	.7	5	148	n.a.
creamy (*Weight Watchers*)	25	0	6.0	0	0	0	100	n.a.
creamy (*Weight Watchers* Single Serve), 1 pkt.	35	0	8.0	0	0	0	140	n.a.
red wine (see also "vinegar and oil," below):								
vinaigrette (*Wish-Bone*)	51	0	4.2	3.8	.5	0	216	(0)
vinegar:								
(*Estee*)	2	0	0	0	0	0	10	0
(*Featherweight*)	6	0	1.0	0	0	0	100	0
(*Seven Seas* Free)	6	0	1.0	0	0	0	190	n.a.

Food and Measure	cal.	prot. (gms)	carbo. (gms)	tot. fat (gms)	sat. fat (gms)	chol. (mgs)	sod. (mgs)	fiber (gms)
w/Cabernet (*Lawry's* Classics),								
1 oz.	138	0	4.9	13.7	1.0	n.a.	178	0
Russian:								
1 tbsp.	76	.2	1.6	7.8	1.1	n.a.	133	tr.c
1 oz.	140	.5	2.9	14.4	2.1	n.a.	246	.1 c
1 cup	1210	3.9	25.5	124.5	17.9	n.a.	2127	.7 c
(*Featherweight*)	6	0	1.0	0	0	0	125	m.q.
(*Kraft*)	60	0	4.0	5.0	1.0	0	130	m.q.
(*Kraft* Reduced Calorie)	30	0	4.0	1.0	0	0	130	m.q.
(*S&W/Nutradiet*)	25	0	4.0	1.0	m.q.	0	120	m.q.
(*Weight Watchers*)	50	0	2.0	5.0	1.0	5	80	m.q.
(*Wish-Bone*)	46	.1	6.0	2.5	.4	0	147	m.q.
(*Wish-Bone* Food Service)	47	.1	6.0	2.5	m.q.	0	147	m.q.
(*Wish-Bone* Lite)	22	.1	3.9	.6	.1	0	126	m.q.
creamy (*Kraft*)	60	0	2.0	5.0	1.0	5	150	m.q.
low-calorie (see also specific								
brands):								
1 tbsp.	23	.1	4.5	.7	.1	1	141	.1 c
1 oz.	40	.1	7.8	1.1	.2	2	246	.1 c
1 cup	368	1.3	71.8	10.4	1.5	15	2257	.9 c
w/pure honey (*Kraft*)	60	0	4.0	5.0	1.0	0	130	m.q.
San Francisco, w/Romano cheese								
(*Lawry's* Classic), 1 oz.	136	.6	2.0	14.0	1.9	n.a.	547	.1 c
sesame garlic (*Nasoya Vegi-Dressing*)	40	1.0	1.0	3.0	m.q.	0	50	m.q.
sesame seed:								
1 tbsp.	68	.5	1.3	6.9	.9	0	153	.1 c
1 oz.	126	.9	2.4	12.8	1.8	0	284	.1 c
1 cup	1086	7.6	21.0	110.8	15.1	0	2450	.9 c
sour (*Friendship Sour Treat*), 1 oz. ...	36	1.0	2.0	3.0	m.q.	0	15	n.a.
Swiss cheese vinaigrette (*Hain*)	60	0	0	7.0	m.q.	<5	160	n.a.
Thousand Island:								
1 tbsp.	59	.1	2.4	5.6	.9	n.a.	109	.3 c
1 oz.	107	.3	4.3	10.1	1.7	n.a.	198	.6 c
1 cup	943	2.3	38.0	89.3	15.1	n.a.	1750	5.0 c
(*Estee*)	8	0	2.0	0	0	0	30	m.q.
(*Featherweight*)	18	0	3.0	0	0	0	70	m.q.
(*Hain*)	50	0	0	5.0	m.q.	0	85	m.q.
(*Hollywood*)	60	0	3.0	6.0	1.0	5	15	0
(*Kraft*)	60	0	2.0	5.0	1.0	5	150	m.q.
(*Kraft Free*)	20	0	5.0	0	0	0	135	m.q.
(*Kraft* Reduced Calorie)	20	0	3.0	1.0	0	0	135	m.q.
(*S&W/Nutradiet*)	25	0	2.0	2.0	m.q.	n.a.	105	m.q.
(*Seven Seas Thousand Island!*								
Light)	30	0	3.0	2.0	0	5	160	m.q.
(*Weight Watchers*)	50	0	2.0	5.0	1.0	5	80	m.q.
(*Wish-Bone*)	63	.1	3.1	5.6	.8	7	158	m.q.
(*Wish-Bone* Food Service)	40	.2	2.6	3.2	m.q.	9	107	0
(*Wish-Bone* Lite)	36	.2	1.9	3.0	.4	9	99	m.q.
and bacon (*Kraft*)	60	0	2.0	6.0	1.0	0	100	m.q.

Food and Measure	cal.	prot. (gms)	carbo. (gms)	tot. fat (gms)	sat. fat (gms)	chol. (mgs)	sod. (mgs)	fiber (gms)
SALAD DRESSING, THOUSAND ISLAND *(cont.)*								
creamy *(Seven Seas)*	50	0	2.0	5.0	1.0	5	150	m.q.
low-calorie (see also specific brands):								
1 tbsp.	24	.1	2.5	1.6	.2	2	153	.2 c
1 oz.	45	.2	4.6	3.0	.5	4	284	.3 c
1 cup	389	1.9	39.6	26.1	3.9	38	2450	2.9 c
tomato, zesty *(Featherweight)*	2	0	0	0	0	0	5	0
tomato vinaigrette *(Weight Watchers)*	8	0	2.0	0	0	0	150	n.a.
tomato vinaigrette, garden *(Hain Canola)*	60	0	1.0	6.0	m.q.	0	150	n.a.
vinaigrette, see specific listings								
vinegar and oil:								
balsamic vinegar *(Great Impressions)*	67	<1.0	2.3	6.5	m.q.	0	367	n.a.
red wine vinegar:								
(Great Impressions)	64	<1.0	2.5	6.1	m.q.	0	277	n.a.
(Kraft)	60	0	4.0	4.0	1.0	0	200	n.a.
(Pathmark)	70	0	2.0	7.0	1.0	0	235	n.a.
(Seven Seas Viva)	70	0	1.0	7.0	1.0	0	290	n.a.
(Seven Seas Viva Red Wine! Vinegar & Oil Light)	45	0	1.0	4.0	1.0	0	190	n.a.
white wine vinegar *(Great Impressions)*	63	<1.0	.8	6.6	m.q.	0	242	n.a.
vintage, w/sherry wine *(Lawry's Classic)*, 1 oz.	110	4.3	2.5	10.5	2.1	0	415	.1 c
white wine, w/Chardonnay *(Lawry's Classic)*, 1 oz.	153	0	2.7	15.7	2.0	0	178	.1 c
SALAD DRESSING MIX:								
dry:								
bacon *(Lawry's)*, 1 pkg.	65	5.2	9.1	.8	n.a.	n.a.	1820	.5 c
blue cheese *(Tone's)*, 1 tsp.	13	.3	2.4	.2	n.a.	n.a.	146	n.a.
buttermilk *(Tone's)*, 1 tsp.	10	.2	2.1	.2	<.1	<1	389	<.1 d
Caesar *(Lawry's)*, 1 pkg.	75	3.4	8.7	3.1	m.q.	n.a.	1962	.3 c
Italian:								
(Lawry's), 1 pkg.	45	1.6	9.3	.2	n.a.	n.a.	2255	.3 c
(Tone's), 1 tsp.	12	.2	2.9	<.1	tr.	0	323	.1 d
w/cheese *(Lawry's)*, 1 pkg.	74	2.2	11.6	2.1	m.q.	n.a.	1624	.2 c
creamy *(Tone's)*, 1 tsp.	13	.1	3.1	.1	n.a.	n.a.	251	n.a.
Thousand Island *(Tone's)*, 1 tsp. ...	19	.2	3.0	n.a.	n.a.	n.a.	46	n.a.
prepared[1], 1 tbsp.:								
bleu cheese *(Hain No Oil)*	14	1.0	1.0	1.0	n.a.	<5	180	n.a.
bleu cheese and herbs *(Good Seasons)*	70	0	1.0	8.0	m.q.	0	150	n.a.
buttermilk *(Good Seasons* Farm Style)	60	1.0	1.0	6.0	m.q.	5	135	n.a.
buttermilk *(Hain No Oil)*	11	1.0	1.0	<1.0	n.a.	0	150	n.a.

1. *Prepared according to package directions.*

Food and Measure	cal.	prot. (gms)	carbo. (gms)	tot. fat (gms)	sat. fat (gms)	chol. (mgs)	sod. (mgs)	fiber (gms)
Caesar (*Hain* No Oil)	6	0	1.0	<1.0	n.a.	0	200	n.a.
cheese garlic (*Good Seasons*)	70	0	1.0	8.0	m.q.	0	170	n.a.
cheese Italian (*Good Seasons*)	70	0	1.0	8.0	m.q.	0	130	n.a.
French (*Hain* No Oil)	12	0	3.0	0	0	0	340	n.a.
garlic and cheese (*Hain* No Oil) ..	6	<1.0	1.0	<1.0	n.a.	0	180	n.a.
garlic and herbs (*Good Seasons*) ..	70	0	1.0	8.0	m.q.	0	190	n.a.
herb (*Good Seasons* Classic)	70	0	1.0	8.0	m.q.	0	150	n.a.
herb (*Hain* No Oil)	2	0	1.0	0	0	0	140	n.a.
Italian:								
(*Good Seasons*)	70	0	1.0	8.0	m.q.	0	170	n.a.
(*Good Seasons* Lite)	25	0	1.0	3.0	m.q.	0	180	n.a.
(*Good Seasons* No Oil)	6	0	2.0	0	0	0	30	n.a.
(*Hain* No Oil)	2	0	1.0	0	0	0	170	n.a.
cheese (*Good Seasons* Lite) ...	25	0	1.0	3.0	m.q.	0	135	n.a.
mild (*Good Seasons*)	70	0	1.0	8.0	m.q.	0	190	n.a.
zesty (*Good Seasons*)	70	0	1.0	8.0	m.q.	0	120	n.a.
zesty (*Good Seasons* Lite)	25	0	1.0	3.0	m.q.	0	135	n.a.
lemon and herbs (*Good Seasons*)	70	0	1.0	8.0	m.q.	0	140	n.a.
ranch (*Good Seasons*)	60	0	1.0	6.0	m.q.	5	110	n.a.
ranch (*Good Seasons* Lite)	30	1.0	2.0	2.0	m.q.	5	115	n.a.
Thousand Island (*Hain* No Oil) ...	12	0	3.0	0	0	<1	150	n.a.
SALAD MIX[1]:								
Caesar (*Suddenly Salad*), ⅙ pkg.								
dry	110	4.0	20.0	1.0	n.a.	n.a.	450	n.a.
Caesar (*Suddenly Salad*), ½ cup ...	170	4.0	20.0	8.0	m.q.	n.a.	450	m.q.
macaroni, creamy (*Suddenly Salad*),								
⅙ pkg. dry	100	4.0	20.0	1.0	n.a.	n.a.	210	n.a.
macaroni, creamy (*Suddenly Salad*),								
½ cup	200	4.0	21.0	10.0	m.q.	n.a.	280	m.q.
pasta:								
classic (*Suddenly Salad*), ⅙ pkg.								
dry	120	4.0	23.0	1.0	n.a.	n.a.	530	n.a.
classic (*Suddenly Salad*), ½ cup ..	160	4.0	23.0	6.0	m.q.	n.a.	530	m.q.
Italian (*Suddenly Salad*), ⅙ pkg.								
dry	110	5.0	20.0	1.0	n.a.	n.a.	380	n.a.
Italian (*Suddenly Salad*), ½ cup ..	150	5.0	20.0	6.0	m.q.	n.a.	380	m.q.
primavera (*Suddenly Salad*),								
⅙ pkg. dry	90	3.0	19.0	1.0	n.a.	n.a.	270	n.a.
primavera (*Suddenly Salad*),								
½ cup	190	4.0	20.0	10.0	m.q.	n.a.	340	m.q.
ranch and bacon (*Suddenly Salad*),								
⅙ pkg. dry	110	5.0	21.0	1.0	n.a.	n.a.	250	n.a.
ranch and bacon (*Suddenly Salad*),								
½ cup	210	6.0	22.0	11.0	m.q.	n.a.	320	m.q.
tortellini Italiano (*Suddenly Salad*),								
⅕ pkg. dry	120	4.0	21.0	2.0	m.q.	n.a.	450	n.a.
tortellini Italiano (*Suddenly Salad*),								
½ cup	160	4.0	21.0	7.0	m.q.	n.a.	450	m.q.

1. *Prepared according to package directions, except as noted.*

Food and Measure	cal.	prot. (gms)	carbo. (gms)	tot. fat (gms)	sat. fat (gms)	chol. (mgs)	sod. (mgs)	fiber (gms)
SALAD NUGGET (see also "Crouton"):								
garlic'n cheese (*Flavor Tree*), ¼ cup	167	3.2	11.0	12.4	m.q.	n.a.	336	.1 c
onion (*Flavor Tree*), ¼ cup	163	3.6	11.5	11.0	m.q.	n.a.	299	.1 c
sesame (*Flavor Tree* Original Sesame), ¼ cup	160	3.4	12.9	10.9	m.q.	n.a.	435	.1 c
SALAD SEASONING:								
(*McCormick/Schilling* Salad Supreme), 1 tsp.	11	.7	.5	.1	n.a.	0	2807	m.q.
SALAD TOPPING:								
(*Tone's* American), 1 tsp.	7	.6	.5	.3	.1	1	34	.1 d
SALAMI:								
beef:								
(*Boar's Head*), 1 oz.	60	5.0	<1.0	4.0	m.q.	20	288	0
(*Hebrew National* Original Deli Style), 1 oz.	80	7.0	<1.0	7.0	m.q.	15	230	0
(*Hormel* Perma-Fresh), 2 slices ..	50	3.0	0	5.0	m.q.	m.q.	219	0
(*Kahn's*), 1 slice	70	3.0	1.0	6.0	m.q.	m.q.	250	0
(*Kahn's* Family Pack), 1 slice	60	2.0	1.0	5.0	m.q.	m.q.	190	0
(*Oscar Mayer* Machiaeh Brand), .8-oz. slice	60	3.0	0	5.0	m.q.	15	265	0
cooked, 1 oz.	72	4.2	.7	5.7	2.4	17	328	0
cooked, 1 slice, 4″ diam. × ¼″, approx. .8 oz.	58	3.4	.6	4.6	2.0	14	266	0
cotto, see "cotto," below								
beef and pork, cooked:								
1 oz.	71	4.0	.6	5.7	2.3	18	302	0
1 slice, 4″ diam. × ¼″, approx. .8 oz.	57	3.2	.5	4.6	1.9	15	245	0
beer (see also "Beerwurst"):								
(*Eckrich*), 1-oz. slice	70	4.0	1.0	6.0	m.q.	m.q.	330	0
(*Oscar Mayer* Salami for Beer), .8-oz. slice	50	3.2	.4	4.0	1.7	15	286	0
beef (*Oscar Mayer* Salami for Beer), .8-oz. slice	63	2.9	.4	5.6	2.5	16	280	0
cooked (*Kahn's*), 1 slice	60	4.0	1.0	4.0	m.q.	m.q.	300	0
cooked (*OHSE*), 1 oz.	65	4.0	1.0	5.0	m.q.	m.q.	330	0
cotto:								
(*Eckrich*), 1-oz. slice	70	4.0	1.0	6.0	m.q.	m.q.	380	0
(*Hormel* Chub), 1 oz.	100	5.0	0	5.0	m.q.	m.q.	385	0
(*Hormel* Perma-Fresh), 2 slices ..	105	9.0	1.0	7.0	m.q.	m.q.	750	0
(*JM*), 1-oz. slice	80	4.0	2.0	6.0	m.q.	m.q.	270	0
(*Kahn's* Family Pack), 1 slice	45	3.0	1.0	3.0	m.q.	m.q.	230	0
(*Light & Lean*), 2 slices	80	6.0	0	6.0	m.q.	m.q.	m.q.	0
(*Oscar Mayer*), .8-oz. slice	52	3.1	.4	4.2	1.9	19	287	0
(*Oscar Mayer*), .5-oz. slice	34	2.0	.3	2.8	1.2	12	187	0
beef:								
(*Eckrich*), 1.3 oz.	100	5.0	2.0	8.0	m.q.	m.q.	460	0

Food and Measure	cal.	prot. (gms)	carbo. (gms)	tot. fat (gms)	sat. fat (gms)	chol. (mgs)	sod. (mgs)	fiber (gms)
(*Oscar Mayer*), .8-oz. slice	45	3.3	.4	3.4	1.6	19	296	0
(*Oscar Mayer*), .5-oz. slice	29	2.1	.3	2.2	1.0	12	193	0
dry or hard:								
(*Hickory Farms*), 1 oz.	120	6.0	0	10.0	m.q.	30	535	0
(*Hormel*), 1 oz.	110	7.0	0	10.0	m.q.	m.q.	468	0
(*Hormel* National Brand), 1 oz. ...	120	6.0	0	11.0	m.q.	m.q.	463	0
(*Hormel* Perma-Fresh), 2 slices ..	80	4.0	0	7.0	m.q.	m.q.	339	0
(*Hormel* Sliced), 1 oz.	110	6.0	0	10.0	m.q.	m.q.	483	0
(*JM*), 1-oz. slice	110	6.0	1.0	9.0	m.q.	m.q.	580	0
(*Oscar Mayer* Hard), .3-oz. slice	33	2.0	.1	2.8	1.2	8	169	0
pork:								
4-oz. pkg.	460	25.5	1.8	38.1	13.4	m.q.	2554	0
1 oz.	115	6.4	.5	9.6	3.3	m.q.	640	0
1 slice, 3⅛″ diam. × ¹⁄₁₆″,								
approx. .4 oz.	41	2.3	.2	3.4	1.2	m.q.	226	0
pork and beef:								
4-oz. pkg.	472	25.8	2.9	38.9	13.8	89	2101	0
1 oz.	119	6.5	.7	9.7	3.5	22	527	0
1 slice, 3⅛″ diam. × ¹⁄₁₆″,								
approx. .4 oz.	42	2.3	.3	3.4	1.2	8	186	0
Genoa:								
(*Hickory Farms*), 1 oz.	110	6.0	0	10.0	m.q.	20	540	0
(*Hormel*), 1 oz.	110	6.0	0	10.0	m.q.	m.q.	456	0
(*Hormel* Gran Valore), 1 oz.	110	6.0	0	10.0	m.q.	m.q.	453	0
(*Hormel* San Remo Brand), 1 oz.	118	7.0	0	10.0	m.q.	m.q.	541	0
(*Hormel DiLusso*), 1 oz.	100	6.0	0	8.0	m.q.	m.q.	443	0
(*JM*), 1-oz. slice	100	6.0	1.0	8.0	m.q.	m.q.	540	0
(*Oscar Mayer*), .3-oz. slice	34	1.9	.1	2.8	1.2	9	162	0
(*Hormel* Party), 1 oz.	90	5.0	0	8.0	m.q.	m.q.	399	0
piccolo (*Hormel* Stick), 1 oz.	120	6.0	0	11.0	m.q.	m.q.	512	0

"SALAMI," VEGETARIAN,
frozen:

Food and Measure	cal.	prot. (gms)	carbo. (gms)	tot. fat (gms)	sat. fat (gms)	chol. (mgs)	sod. (mgs)	fiber (gms)
roll (*Worthington*), 2 slices, approx. 1.5 oz.	90	8.0	3.0	5.0	1.0	0	760	m.q.
slices (*Worthington*), 2 slices, approx. 1.3 oz.	80	7.0	3.0	4.0	1.0	0	675	m.q.

SALISBURY STEAK, see "Beef
dinner, frozen" and "Beef
entree, frozen"

SALMON, ATLANTIC, meat only,
raw:

Food and Measure	cal.	prot. (gms)	carbo. (gms)	tot. fat (gms)	sat. fat (gms)	chol. (mgs)	sod. (mgs)	fiber (gms)
1 lb.	644	90.0	0	28.8	4.6	249	198	0
1 oz.	40	5.6	0	1.8	.3	16	113	0
½ fillet, approx. 7 oz., yield from 5-lb. whole fish	281	39.3	0	12.6	1.9	109	87	0

SALMON, CANNED:

Food and Measure	cal.	prot. (gms)	carbo. (gms)	tot. fat (gms)	sat. fat (gms)	chol. (mgs)	sod. (mgs)	fiber (gms)
blueback (*S&W/Nutradiet*), ½ cup ..	188	22.0	0	11.0	m.q.	m.q.	45	0

Food and Measure	cal.	prot. (gms)	carbo. (gms)	tot. fat (gms)	sat. fat (gms)	chol. (mgs)	sod. (mgs)	fiber (gms)
SALMON, CANNED *(cont.)*								
chum:								
drained, 14 oz., yield from								
No. 1 tall can	521	79.1	0	20.3	5.5	144	1797	0
drained, 4 oz.	160	24.3	0	6.2	1.7	44	552	0
keta (*Bumble Bee*), 1 cup	306	47.3	0	11.4	m.q.	m.q.	m.q.	0
pink:								
w/liquid:								
1 lb. or No. 1 tall can	631	89.8	0	27.4	7.0	m.q.	2514	0
4 oz.	158	22.4	0	6.9	1.7	m.q.	628	0
(*Del Monte*), ½ cup	160	22.0	0	7.0	m.q.	m.q.	660	0
(*Bumble Bee*), 1 cup	310	45.1	0	13.0	m.q.	m.q.	851	0
(*Featherweight*), 2 oz.	70	11.0	0	3.0	m.q.	20	45	0
(*Libby's*), 7¾ oz.	310	45.0	0	13.0	m.q.	m.q.	790	0
Alaska (*Deming's*), ½ cup	140	20.0	0	6.0	1.0	65	450	0
chunk, skinless, boneless, in								
water (*Deming's*), 3.25 oz.	120	17.0	0	5.0	m.q.	m.q.	420	0
red:								
w/liquid (*Del Monte*), ½ cup	180	23.0	0	9.0	m.q.	m.q.	660	0
blueback (*Rubinstein's*), ½ cup ...	170	20.0	0	9.0	m.q.	m.q.	450	0
red, sockeye:								
drained, 13 oz., yield from								
No. 1 tall can	566	75.5	0	27.0	6.1	161	1987	0
drained, 4 oz.	174	23.2	0	8.3	1.9	50	610	0
(*Bumble Bee*), 1 cup	376	44.7	0	20.5	m.q.	m.q.	1148	0
(*Libby's*), 7¾ oz.	380	45.0	0	21.0	m.q.	m.q.	760	0
(*S&W/Nutradiet*), ½ cup	188	22.0	0	11.0	m.q.	m.q.	47	0
Alaska (*Deming's*), ½ cup	170	20.0	0	9.0	2.0	65	450	0
Alaska, medium (*Deming's*),								
½ cup	150	21.0	0	7.0	2.0	65	450	0
blueback (*S&W* Fancy), ½ cup ...	190	25.0	0	10.0	m.q.	m.q.	590	0
SALMON, CHINOOK, meat only:								
raw:								
1 lb.	816	91.0	0	47.4	11.4	299	213	0
1 oz.	51	5.7	0	3.0	.7	19	13	0
½ fillet, approx. 7 oz., yield from								
5-lb. whole fish	356	39.7	0	20.7	5.0	131	93	0
smoked:								
4 oz.	133	20.7	0	4.9	1.1	26	889	0
1 oz.	33	5.2	0	1.2	.3	7	222	0
lox, 4 oz.	133	20.7	0	4.9	1.1	26	2268	0
lox, 1 oz.	33	5.2	0	1.2	.3	7	567	0
SALMON, CHUM, meat only, raw:								
1 lb.	544	91.3	0	17.1	3.8	336	449	0
1 oz.	34	5.7	0	1.1	.2	21	14	0
½ fillet, approx. 7 oz., yield from								
5-lb. whole fish	237	39.9	0	7.5	1.7	147	98	0

Food and Measure	cal.	prot. (gms)	carbo. (gms)	tot. fat (gms)	sat. fat (gms)	chol. (mgs)	sod. (mgs)	fiber (gms)
SALMON, COHO, meat only:								
raw:								
1 lb.	662	98.1	0	27.0	5.0	177	211	0
1 oz.	41	7.6	0	1.7	.3	11	13	0
½ fillet, approx. 7 oz., yield from								
5-lb. whole fish	289	42.8	0	11.8	2.2	77	92	0
boiled, poached, or steamed[1], 4 oz.	210	31.0	0	8.6	1.6	56	67	0
canned, Alaska (*Deming's*), ½ cup ..	140	22.0	0	5.0	m.q.	m.q.	450	0
SALMON, FROZEN:								
steaks, w/out seasoning mix								
(*SeaPak*), 8-oz. pkg.	270	46.0	0	9.0	m.q.	170	115	0
SALMON, KETA, see "Salmon, chum"								
SALMON, PINK, meat only, raw:								
1 lb.	527	90.4	0	15.6	2.5	236	302	0
1 oz.	33	5.7	0	1.0	.2	15	19	0
½ fillet, approx. 5.6 oz., yield from								
4-lb. whole fish	185	31.7	0	5.5	.9	83	106	0
SALMON, RED, see "Salmon, sockeye" and "Salmon, canned"								
SALMON, SMOKED, see "Salmon, chinook"								
"SALMON," SMOKED, IMITATION:								
(*Mox Lox*), 1.5 oz.	25	2.0	3.0	<1.0	n.a.	5	380	n.a.
SALMON, SOCKEYE, meat only:								
raw:								
1 lb.	763	96.6	0	38.8	6.8	283	211	0
1 oz.	48	6.0	0	2.4	.4	18	13	0
½ fillet, approx. 7 oz., yield from								
5-lb. whole fish	333	42.2	0	16.9	3.0	123	92	0
baked, broiled, or microwaved[1],								
4 oz.	245	31.0	0	12.4	2.2	99	75	0
SALSA, canned or in jars:								
brava (*La Victoria*), 1 tbsp.	6	<1.0	1.0	<1.0	(0)	0	100	m.q.
burrito (*Del Monte*), ¼ cup	20	0	4.0	0	0	0	355	m.q.
casera (*La Victoria*), 1 tbsp.	4	<1.0	1.0	<1.0	(0)	0	80	m.q.
green chili:								
(La Victoria), 1 tbsp.	3	<1.0	1.0	<1.0	(0)	0	44	m.q.
(*Old El Paso* Thick 'n Chunky),								
2 tbsp.	3	0	1.0	0	0	0	270	m.q.
hot (*Ortega*), 1 oz.	10	0	2.0	0	0	0	180	m.q.
mild (*Del Monte*), ¼ cup	20	0	3.0	0	0	0	590	m.q.
mild or medium (*Oretga*), 1 oz. ..	8	0	2.0	0	0	0	180	m.q.
green jalapeño (*La Victoria*), 1 tbsp.	4	<1.0	1.0	<1.0	(0)	0	105	m.q.
hot (*Hain*), ¼ cup	22	1.0	4.0	0	0	0	480	m.q.

1. *Without added ingredients.*

Food and Measure	cal.	prot. (gms)	carbo. (gms)	tot. fat (gms)	sat. fat (gms)	chol. (mgs)	sod. (mgs)	fiber (gms)
SALSA *(cont.)*								
mild:								
(*Hain*), ¼ cup	20	1.0	4.0	0	0	0	410	m.q.
medium or hot (*Old El Paso*								
Thick'n Chunky), 2 tbsp.	6	<1.0	1.0	<1.0	(0)	0	170	m.q.
or hot (*Enrico's* Chunky Style),								
2 tbsp.	8	1.0	2.0	0	0	0	34	m.q.
or hot (*Enrico's* Chunky Style No								
Salt Added), 2 tbsp.	8	1.0	2.0	0	0	0	10	m.q.
omelette (*La Victoria*), 1 tbsp.	6	<1.0	1.0	<1.0	(0)	0	95	m.q.
picante (see also "Picante sauce"):								
(*La Victoria*), 1 tbsp.	4	<1.0	1.0	<1.0	(0)	0	80	m.q.
(*Old El Paso*), 2 tbsp.	10	0	2.0	0	0	0	160	m.q.
(*Ortega*), 1 oz.	10	0	2.0	0	0	0	300	m.q.
all varieties (*Old El Paso*), 2 tbsp.	10	<1.0	2.0	<1.0	(0)	0	160	n.a.
hot (*Del Monte*), ¼ cup	20	0	4.0	0	0	0	385	m.q.
hot and chunky (*Del Monte*),								
¼ cup	15	0	3.0	0	0	0	405	m.q.
ranchera (*La Victoria*), 1 tbsp.	6	<1.0	1.0	<1.0	(0)	0	85	m.q.
ranchera (*Ortega*), 1 oz.	12	0	3.0	0	0	0	250	m.q.
red jalapeño (*La Victoria*), 1 tbsp. ..	6	<1.0	1.0	<1.0	(0)	0	95	m.q.
roja, mild (*Del Monte*), ¼ cup	20	0	4.0	0	0	0	510	m.q.
suprema (*La Victoria*), 1 tbsp.	4	<1.0	1.0	<1.0	(0)	0	95	m.q.
taco (see also "Taco sauce"):								
hot (*Ortega*), 1 oz.	10	0	2.0	0	0	0	300	m.q.
mild (*Ortega*), 1 oz.	10	0	2.0	0	0	0	290	m.q.
mild (*Rosarita*), 2 oz.	27	1.0	6.1	.1	tr.	<1	304	.1 d
Texas (*Hot Cha Cha*), 1 oz.	6	.3	2.5	0	0	0	2	.4 d
verde (*Old El Paso* Thick 'n Chunky),								
2 tbsp.	10	<1.0	2.0	<1.0	0	0	135	m.q.
Victoria (*La Victoria*), 1 tbsp.	4	<1.0	1.0	<1.0	(0)	0	80	m.q.
SALSIFY:								
raw:								
untrimmed, 1 lb.	325	13.0	73.4	.8	n.a.	0	79	7.1 c
trimmed, 1 oz.	23	.9	5.3	.1	(0)	0	6	.5 c
sliced, ½ cup	55	2.2	12.5	.1	(0)	0	13	1.2 c
boiled, drained, 4 oz.	77	3.1	17.4	.2	(0)	0	18	1.7 c
boiled, drained, sliced, ½ cup	46	1.9	10.5	.1	(0)	0	11	1.0 c
SALSIFY, BLACK:								
1 lb.	372	15.0	84.4	.1	(0)	0	91	m.q.
1 oz.	23	.9	5.3	tr.	(0)	0	6	m.q.
SALT:								
1 oz.	0	0	0	0	0	0	10,988	0
1 tbsp.	0	0	0	0	0	0	6589	0
1 tsp.	0	0	0	0	0	0	2132	0
iodized or non-iodized (*Morton*),								
1 tsp.	0	0	0	0	0	0	2300	0
kosher (*Morton*), 1 tsp.	0	0	0	0	0	0	1880	0
mixture (*Morton Lite Salt*), 1 tsp. ..	<1	0	tr.	0	0	0	1100	0

Food and Measure	cal.	prot. (gms)	carbo. (gms)	tot. fat (gms)	sat. fat (gms)	chol. (mgs)	sod. (mgs)	fiber (gms)
sea (Hain), 1 tsp.	0	0	0	0	0	0	2255	0
sea (Tone's), 1 tsp.	0	0	0	0	0	0	2132	0
SALT, SEASONED (see also specific listings), 1 tsp.:								
(Lawry's)	4	.1	.6	.1	(0)	0	1367	.1 c
(Lawry's Hot n' Spicy)	3	.1	1.5	.1	(0)	0	79	.1 c
(Lawry's Lite)	8	.3	1.7	<.1	(0)	0	357	.1 c
(McCormick/Schilling)	4	.2	.6	n.a.	(0)	0	980	n.a.
(McCormick/Schilling Salt'n Spice) ..	3	.2	.6	n.a.	(0)	0	939	n.a.
(Morton)	4	<1.0	<1.0	<.1	(0)	0	1300	n.a.
(Morton Nature's Seasons)	3	<.1	<1.0	<.1	(0)	0	1400	n.a.
SALT, SUBSTITUTE OR IMITATION:								
(Estee), ⅛ tsp.	0	0	0	0	0	0	0	0
(Lawry's Salt-Free 17), 1 tsp.	10	.3	1.8	.2	(0)	0	2	.4 c
(Morton), 1 tsp.	<1	0	.1	0	0	0	<1	n.a.
regular or seasoned (Featherweight),								
¼ tsp.	0	0	0	0	0	0	0	0
seasoned:								
(Lawry's Salt-Free), 1 tsp.	3	.1	.6	<.1	(0)	0	7	<.1 c
(Morton), 1 tsp.	2	<.1	.5	<.1	(0)	0	<1	n.a.
all purpose (Health Valley Instead of Salt), 1 tsp.	11	.5	1.5	.5	(0)	0	3	0
SALT PORK:								
raw, 1 oz.	212	1.4	0	22.8	8.3	25	404	0
SANDWICH, see specific listings								
SANDWICH SAUCE:								
(Hunt's Manwich), 2.5 oz.	40	1.0	10.0	0	0	n.a.	390	n.a.
SANDWICH SPREAD, MEAT:								
(Oscar Mayer Chub), 1 oz.	67	2.0	4.3	4.7	1.8	10	273	0
pork and beef, 1 oz.	67	2.2	3.4	4.9	1.7	11	287	0
pork and beef, 1 tbsp.	35	1.2	1.8	2.6	.9	6	152	0
SANDWICH SPREAD, MEATLESS:								
1 oz.	110	.3	6.4	9.6	1.4	22	m.q.	m.q.
1 cup	953	2.3	54.9	83.2	12.4	187	m.q.	m.q.
1 tbsp.	60	.1	3.4	5.2	.8	12	m.q.	m.q.
(Hellman's/Best Foods), 1 tbsp.	50	0	2.0	5.0	1.0	5	170	m.q.
(Kraft), 1 tbsp.	50	0	3.0	5.0	1.0	5	95	m.q.
SAPODILLA:								
untrimmed, 1 lb.	300	1.6	72.5	4.0	n.a.	0	44	19.2 d
trimmed, 1 oz.	24	.1	5.7	.3	n.a.	0	3	1.5 d
trimmed, ½ cup	100	.5	24.1	1.3	n.a.	0	15	6.4 d
1 medium, 3″ × 2½″, approx. 7.5 oz.	140	.7	33.9	1.9	n.a.	0	20	9.0 d
SAPOTE:								
untrimmed, 1 lb.	431	6.8	108.7	1.9	n.a.	0	31	6.1 c
trimmed, 1 oz.	38	.6	9.6	.2	n.a.	0	3	.5 c
1 medium, approx. 11.2 oz.	301	4.8	76.0	1.4	n.a.	0	21	4.3 c

Food and Measure	cal.	prot. (gms)	carbo. (gms)	tot. fat (gms)	sat. fat (gms)	chol. (mgs)	sod. (mgs)	fiber (gms)
SARDINE, fresh, see "Herring"								
SARDINE, CANNED:								
Atlantic, in soybean oil, drained:								
3.2 oz., yield from 3.75-oz. can ..	192	22.7	0	10.5	1.4	131	465	0
2 oz.	118	14.8	0	6.5	.9	81	286	0
2 medium, 3″ × 1″ × ½″, approx.								
.8 oz.	50	5.9	0	2.8	.4	34	121	0
brisling, w/liquid (*Underwood*),								
3.75 oz.	260	19.0	1.0	20.0	m.q.	m.q.	450	0
Norway, in sild sardine oil:								
w/liquid (*Empress*), 3.75-oz. can	460	19.0	1.0	42.0	m.q.	m.q.	m.q.	0
drained (*Empress*), 3.75-oz. can ..	260	19.0	1.0	20.0	m.q.	m.q.	m.q.	0
Norwegian brisling (*S&W*), 1.5 oz.	130	10.0	0	10.0	m.q.	m.q.	220	0
Pacific, in tomato sauce, drained:								
13 oz., yield from No. 300 can ...	658	60.5	n.a.	44.3	11.4	225	1532	<.1 c
2 oz.	101	9.3	n.a.	6.8	1.8	35	235	.1 c
1 medium, 4¾″ × 1⅛″ × ⅝″,								
approx. 1.3 oz.	68	6.2	n.a.	4.6	1.2	23	157	<.1 c
in water (*Featherweight*), 1⅛ oz. ...	95	9.0	1.0	7.0	m.q.	20	65	0
in oil (*Featherweight*), 1⅛ oz.	130	19.0	1.0	10.0	m.q.	45	65	0
in mustard sauce (*Underwood*),								
3.75 oz.	220	16.0	2.0	16.0	m.q.	m.q.	650	n.a.
in *Tabasco* sauce, drained								
(*Underwood*), 3 oz.	220	16.0	1.0	16.0	m.q.	m.q.	400	n.a.
in tomato sauce (*Del Monte*), ½ cup	360	19.0	45.0	12.0	m.q.	m.q.	540	m.q.
in tomato sauce (*Underwood*),								
3.75 oz.	220	16.0	2.0	16.0	m.q.	m.q.	500	n.a.
kippered (*Brunswick Kippered*								
Snacks), 3½ oz.	185	16.0	1.0	14.0	m.q.	m.q.	610	0
SAUCE, see specific listings								
SAUERKRAUT, canned, ½ cup,								
except as noted:								
w/liquid:								
4 oz.	22	1.0	4.9	.2	<.1	0	750	1.2 c
½ cup	22	1.0	5.1	.2	<.1	0	780	1.3 c
(*Del Monte*)	25	1.0	6.0	0	0	0	775	m.q.
(*A&P*)	20	1.0	5.0	<1.0	(0)	0	800	m.q.
(*Claussen*)	17	.6	3.2	.2	(0)	0	517	m.q.
(*Finast*)	30	1.0	6.0	0	0	0	800	m.q.
(*Pathmark*)	20	0	4.0	0	0	0	880	m.q.
(*Snow Floss*)	28	1.0	4.0	0	0	0	780	1.0 d
(*Stokely* Bavarian)	30	1.0	7.0	0	0	0	780	m.q.
(*Vlasic* Old Fashioned), 1 oz.	4	0	1.0	0	0	0	280	m.q.
shredded (*Allens*)	21	1.0	5.0	<1.0	(0)	0	880	m.q.
shredded and chopped (*Stokely*)	20	1.0	4.0	0	0	0	810	m.q.
SAUERKRAUT JUICE, canned or								
bottled:								
(*Biotta*), 6 fl. oz.	21	1.1	4.0	.1	(0)	0	1482	m.q.
(*S&W*), 5 fl. oz.	14	1.0	3.0	0	0	0	1120	m.q.

Food and Measure	cal.	prot. (gms)	carbo. (gms)	tot. fat (gms)	sat. fat (gms)	chol. (mgs)	sod. (mgs)	fiber (gms)
SAUSAGE (see also "Frankfurter," "Sausage, canned," "Sausage sticks," and specific sausage listings):								
beef (*Jones Dairy Farm* Golden Brown), 1 link	75	3.8	tr.	6.1	m.q.	18	159	0
beef and cheddar (*Hillshire Farm* Flavorseal), 2 oz.	190	8.0	1.0	15.0	m.q.	m.q.	500	0
brown and serve:								
(*Hormel*), 2 uncooked links	180	7.0	0	17.0	m.q.	m.q.	411	0
(*Hormel*), 2 links	140	6.0	0	13.0	m.q.	m.q.	430	0
(*Jones Dairy Farm* Light), 1 link ..	60	3.5	1.0	4.1	m.q.	16	150	0
(*Swift Premium* Brown 'N Serve Country Recipe), 1 patty or link	130	4.0	1.0	12.0	m.q.	m.q.	240	0
(*Swift Premium* Original Brown 'N Serve), 1 link	130	3.0	1.0	12.0	m.q.	m.q.	260	0
(*Swift Premium* Original Brown 'N Serve), 1 patty	120	4.0	1.0	12.0	m.q.	m.q.	270	0
w/bacon (*Swift Premium* Brown 'N Serve), 1 link	120	4.0	1.0	11.0	m.q.	m.q.	270	0
beef (*Swift Premium* Brown 'N Serve), 1 link	120	4.0	1.0	12.0	m.q.	m.q.	250	0
w/ham (*Swift Premium* Brown 'N Serve), 1 link	130	3.0	1.0	13.0	m.q.	m.q.	260	0
maple flavored (*Swift Premium* Brown 'N Serve), 1 link	120	3.0	1.0	12.0	m.q.	m.q.	260	0
microwave (*Swift Premium* Brown 'N Serve), 1 link	120	4.0	1.0	12.0	m.q.	m.q.	270	0
smoked flavor (*Swift Premium* Brown 'N Serve), 1 link	120	4.0	1.0	11.0	m.q.	m.q.	280	0
country (*Hillshire Farm* Country Recipe), 2 oz.	180	7.0	2.0	16.0	m.q.	m.q.	490	0
heat 'n serve (*Eckrich* Lean Supreme), 2 links	120	7.0	1.0	10.0	m.q.	m.q.	440	0
(*Hickory Farms* Safari), 1 oz.	98	5.0	1.0	9.0	m.q.	14	343	0
hot (*OHSE* Hot Links), 1 oz.	80	4.0	4.0	3.0	m.q.	m.q.	310	0
Italian, see "Italian sausage"								
minced roll (*Eckrich*), 1-oz. slice ...	80	4.0	1.0	7.0	m.q.	m.q.	300	0
pickled:								
firecracker (*Penrose*), 1 link, approx. 1.5 oz.	120	6.0	1.0	10.0	m.q.	m.q.	620	0
firecracker, giant (*Penrose*), 1 link, approx. 2.1 oz.	170	9.0	1.0	14.0	m.q.	m.q.	870	0
hot, red hot, Polish, beer, or firecracker (*Penrose*), 1 link, approx. .5 oz.	40	2.0	1.0	3.0	m.q.	m.q.	220	0
pork:								
(*Hormel* Midget Links), 2 links ...	143	7.0	0	13.0	m.q.	m.q.	327	0
(*Hormel Little Sizzlers*), 2 links ...	103	6.0	0	9.0	m.q.	m.q.	172	0

Food and Measure	cal.	prot. (gms)	carbo. (gms)	tot. fat (gms)	sat. fat (gms)	chol. (mgs)	sod. (mgs)	fiber (gms)
SAUSAGE, SMOKED, PORK *(cont.)*								
(*JM* Tasty Link), 2 raw links,								
approx. 1.8 oz.	260	6.0	1.0	26.0	m.q.	m.q.	380	0
(*JM* Tasty Link), 2 links, cooked,								
approx. 1.4 oz.	190	6.0	1.0	18.0	m.q.	m.q.	290	0
(*Jones Dairy Farm*), 1 link	140	2.9	tr.	13.7	m.q.	24	176	0
(*Jones Dairy Farm* Golden Brown								
Light), 1 link	55	3.3	.5	4.2	m.q.	16	132	0
(*Jones Dairy Farm* Light), 1 link ..	70	4.2	1.0	5.0	m.q.	21	232	0
(*Oscar Mayer Little Friers*), 8.9 oz.								
cooked, yield from 12-oz. pkg.								
raw	989	40.7	2.8	90.3	33.4	210	2641	0
(*Oscar Mayer Little Friers*), 1 link,								
cooked, yield from 1-oz. raw								
link	82	3.4	.2	7.5	2.7	17	219	0
fresh:								
raw, 1-oz. link, 4″ × ⅞″	118	3.3	.3	11.4	4.1	19	189	0
raw, 1 patty, 3⅞″ × ¼″,								
approx. 2 oz.	238	6.7	.6	23.0	8.3	39	380	0
cooked, 1 oz.	105	5.6	.3	8.8	3.1	24	367	0
cooked, 1 link, .5 oz., yield								
from 1-oz. raw link	48	2.6	.1	4.1	1.4	11	168	0
cooked, 1 patty, approx. 1 oz.,								
yield from 2-oz. raw patty ...	100	5.3	.3	8.4	2.9	22	349	0
hot (*JM*), 1-oz. raw patty	130	3.0	1.0	14.0	m.q.	m.q.	180	0
hot (*JM*), 1 patty, cooked, approx.								
.5 oz.	70	2.0	1.0	6.0	m.q.	m.q.	170	0
mild (*Jones Dairy Farm* Golden								
Brown), 1 link	100	2.6	tr.	9.8	m.q.	18	150	0
patty:								
(*JM*), 1-oz. raw patty	130	3.0	1.0	14.0	m.q.	m.q.	180	0
(*JM*), 1 patty, cooked, approx.								
.5 oz.	70	2.0	1.0	6.0	m.q.	m.q.	170	0
(*Jones Dairy Farm*), 1 patty	155	5.5	tr.	14.4	m.q.	36	281	0
(*Jones Dairy Farm* Golden								
Brown), 1 patty	155	4.6	tr.	14.7	m.q.	29	250	0
roll (*Jones Dairy Farm* Cello Roll),								
1 slice	105	3.7	tr.	9.6	m.q.	24	200	0
smoked, see "smoked," below								
spicy (*Jones Dairy Farm* Golden								
Brown), 1 link	100	2.8	tr.	9.5	m.q.	18	159	0
pork and bacon (*JM* Tasty Link),								
2 raw links, approx. 1.8 oz. ...	220	6.0	1.0	21.0	m.q.	m.q.	340	0
pork and bacon (*JM* Tasty Link),								
2 links, cooked, approx.								
1.4 oz.	100	6.0	1.0	9.0	m.q.	m.q.	240	0
pork and beef, fresh, cooked:								
1 oz.	112	3.9	.8	10.3	3.7	m.q.	228	0

Food and Measure	cal.	prot. (gms)	carbo. (gms)	tot. fat (gms)	sat. fat (gms)	chol. (mgs)	sod. (mgs)	fiber (gms)
.5-oz. link, yield from 1-oz. raw link	52	1.8	.4	4.7	1.7	m.q.	105	0
1-oz. patty, yield from 3⅞″ × ¼″ raw patty	107	3.7	.7	9.8	3.5	m.q.	217	0
smoked:								
(Eckrich Lean Supreme), 1 oz. ..	70	4.0	1.0	6.0	m.q.	m.q.	230	0
(Eckrich Skinless), 1 link	180	7.0	2.0	16.0	m.q.	m.q.	420	0
(Hillshire Farm Bun Size), 2 oz.	180	8.0	2.0	16.0	m.q.	m.q.	570	0
(Hillshire Farm Flavorseal), 2 oz.	190	7.0	1.0	17.0	m.q.	m.q.	500	0
(Hillshire Farm Links), 2 oz.	190	8.0	1.0	18.0	m.q.	m.q.	520	0
(Hillshire Farm Lite), 2 oz.	160	8.0	2.0	13.0	m.q.	m.q.	520	0
(Hormel Smokies), 2 links	160	9.0	2.0	14.0	m.q.	m.q.	597	0
(OHSE), 1 oz.	80	4.0	1.0	7.0	m.q.	m.q.	320	0
(Oscar Mayer Little Smokies), .3-oz. link	27	1.2	.1	2.5	.9	6	92	0
(Oscar Mayer Smokie Links), 1.5-oz. link	126	5.4	.6	11.3	4.2	28	426	0
(Pilgrim's Pride), 3 oz.	144	13.1	2.5	9.1	m.q.	64	890	0
beef:								
(Eckrich), 1 oz.	100	3.0	<1.0	9.0	m.q.	m.q.	270	0
(Eckrich Lean Supreme), 1 oz.	80	4.0	1.0	7.0	m.q.	m.q.	230	0
(Eckrich Smok-Y-Links), 2 links	160	6.0	2.0	14.0	m.q.	m.q.	350	0
(Hillshire Farm Bun Size), 2 oz.	180	8.0	2.0	16.0	m.q.	m.q.	570	0
(Hillshire Farm Flavorseal), 2 oz.	180	7.0	2.0	16.0	m.q.	m.q.	490	0
(Oscar Mayer Smokies), 1.5-oz. link	124	5.4	.7	11.0	4.7	27	429	0
cheese (see also "Cheddarwurst"):								
(Eckrich Smok-Y-Links), 2 links	160	6.0	2.0	14.0	m.q.	m.q.	360	0
(Hormel Smokie Cheezers), 2 links	168	9.0	1.0	15.0	m.q.	m.q.	623	0
(Oscar Mayer Smokies), 1.5-oz. link	126	5.7	.7	11.2	4.4	28	452	0
ham (Eckrich Smok-Y-Links), 2 links	160	6.0	2.0	15.0	m.q.	m.q.	500	0
hot (Eckrich Smok-Y-Links), 2 links	150	6.0	1.0	14.0	m.q.	m.q.	360	0
hot (Hillshire Farm Flavorseal), 2 oz.	180	7.0	2.0	16.0	m.q.	m.q.	510	0
maple flavored (Eckrich Smok-Y-Links), 2 links	160	6.0	2.0	14.0	m.q.	m.q.	390	0
original (Eckrich Smok-Y-Links), 2 links	160	6.0	2.0	14.0	m.q.	m.q.	340	0
pork:								
1 oz.	110	6.3	.6	9.0	3.2	19	425	0

Food and Measure	cal.	prot. (gms)	carbo. (gms)	tot. fat (gms)	sat. fat (gms)	chol. (mgs)	sod. (mgs)	fiber (gms)
SAUSAGE, PORK *(cont.)*								
1 small link, 2″ × ¾″, approx.								
.6 oz.	62	3.6	.3	5.1	1.8	11	240	0
1 link, 4 × 1⅛″, approx.								
2.4 oz.	265	15.1	1.4	21.6	7.7	46	1020	0
(*Hormel*), 3 oz.	290	12.0	1.0	27.0	m.q.	m.q.	m.q.	0
pork and beef:								
1 oz.	95	3.8	.4	8.6	3.0	20	268	0
1 oz.[1]	76	4.0	1.1	6.1	2.2	25	309	(0)
1 oz.[2]	89	3.8	.5	7.8	2.8	18	333	0
1 link, 4″ × 1⅛″, approx.								
2.4 oz.	229	9.1	1.0	20.6	7.2	48	642	0
1 link[1], 4″ × 1⅛″, approx.								
2.4 oz.	182	9.5	2.7	14.6	5.3	59	741	(0)
1 link[2], 4″ × 1⅛″, approx.								
2.4 oz.	213	9.0	1.3	18.8	6.6	44	798	0
1 small link, 2″ × ¾″, approx.								
.6 oz.	54	2.1	.2	4.9	1.7	11	151	0
1 small link[1], 2″ × ¾″, approx.								
.6 oz.	43	2.2	.6	3.4	1.3	14	174	(0)
1 small link[2], 2″ × ¾″, approx.								
.6 oz.	50	2.1	.3	4.4	1.6	10	188	0
summer, see "Summer sausage"								
SAUSAGE, CANNED (see also specific listings):								
hot (*Hormel*), 1 patty	150	7.0	0	13.0	m.q.	m.q.	549	0
mild (*Hormel*), 1 patty	150	7.0	0	13.0	m.q.	m.q.	541	0
"SAUSAGE," VEGETARIAN:								
1 oz.	73	5.3	2.8	5.1	.8	0	252	.1 d
1 link, .9 oz.	64	4.6	2.5	4.5	.7	0	222	.1 d
1 patty, 1.3 oz.	97	7.0	3.7	6.9	1.1	0	337	.2 d
canned (*Worthington Saucettes*),								
2 links, approx. 2.4 oz.	140	10.0	5.0	9.0	1.0	0	350	m.q.
frozen:								
links (*Morningstar Farms* Breakfast Links), 3 links,								
2.4 oz.	190	12.0	3.0	14.0	2.0	0	500	m.q.
links (*Worthington Prosage*),								
3 links, approx. 2.4 oz.	190	13.0	4.0	14.0	2.0	0	570	m.q.
patties (*Morningstar Farms* Breakfast Patties), 2 patties,								
approx. 2.7 oz.	190	15.0	7.0	12.0	2.0	0	710	m.q.
patties (*Worthington Prosage*),								
2 patties, approx. 2.7 oz.	210	18.0	4.0	14.0	3.0	0	780	m.q.
roll (*Worthington Prosage*),								
2 slices, ⅜″, approx. 2.5 oz. . .	180	13.0	4.0	12.0	2.0	0	570	m.q.

1. *Flour and nonfat dry milk added.*
2. *Nonfat dry milk added.*

Food and Measure	cal.	prot. (gms)	carbo. (gms)	tot. fat (gms)	sat. fat (gms)	chol. (mgs)	sod. (mgs)	fiber (gms)
SAUSAGE BREAKFAST BISCUIT:								
frozen (*Swanson Great Starts* Breakfast On a Biscuit), 4.7 oz.	410	14.0	36.0	22.0	m.q.	m.q.	1180	m.q.
frozen (*Weight Watchers* Microwave), 3 oz.	220	11.0	19.0	11.0	2.0	70	560	m.q.
refrigerated:								
(*Owens Border Breakfasts*), 2 oz.	210	6.0	14.0	14.0	m.q.	m.q.	400	m.q.
egg and cheese (*Owens Border Breakfasts*), 2.5 oz.	250	8.0	15.0	15.0	m.q.	m.q.	500	m.q.
smoked (*Owens Border Breakfasts*), 2 oz.	200	4.0	15.0	6.0	m.q.	m.q.	786	m.q.
SAUSAGE BREAKFAST TACO, refrigerated:								
(*Owens Border Breakfasts*), 2.17 oz.	190	7.0	11.0	12.0	m.q.	65	345	m.q.
SAUSAGE SEASONING:								
pork (*Tone's*), 1 tsp.	12	.4	2.7	.3	.2	0	1	.7 d
SAUSAGE STICK (see also "Beef jerky" and "Sausage"), 1 stick (*Hickory Farms* Sportsman Stick), 1 oz.	138	9.0	4.0	10.0	m.q.	40	1075	0
beef:								
pepperoni (*Pemmican*), approx. 1.64 oz.	240	13.0	3.0	20.0	m.q.	m.q.	740	0
pepperoni (*Pemmican*), approx. 1.1 oz.	170	8.0	2.0	14.0	m.q.	m.q.	500	0
Tabasco (*Pemmican*), approx. 1.64 oz.	250	11.0	4.0	21.0	m.q.	m.q.	880	0
Tabasco (*Pemmican*), approx. 1.1 oz.	120	5.0	2.0	10.0	m.q.	m.q.	410	0
teriyaki (*Pemmican*), approx. 1.64 oz.	220	12.0	7.0	16.0	m.q.	m.q.	610	0
teriyaki (*Pemmican*), approx. 1.1 oz.	150	8.0	5.0	11.0	m.q.	m.q.	410	0
smoked:								
(*Slim Jim Big Slim*), approx. .52 oz.	80	3.0	1.0	7.0	m.q.	m.q.	220	0
(*Slim Jim Giant Slim*), approx. 1.1 oz.	180	7.0	2.0	16.0	m.q.	m.q.	470	0
(*Slim Jim Jumbo Jim*), approx. 1 oz.	150	8.0	2.0	12.0	m.q.	m.q.	430	0
(*Slim Jim Super Slim/Super Slim Tabasco*), approx. .7 oz.	110	4.0	1.0	10.0	m.q.	m.q.	300	0
mild, pepperoni, spicy, or *Tabasco* (*Slim Jim* Handi-Paks), approx. .31 oz.	50	2.0	1.0	4.0	m.q.	m.q.	130	0
nacho (*Slim Jim Super Slim*), approx. .7 oz.	100	6.0	1.0	7.0	m.q.	m.q.	350	0

Food and Measure	cal.	prot. (gms)	carbo. (gms)	tot. fat (gms)	sat. fat (gms)	chol. (mgs)	sod. (mgs)	fiber (gms)
SAUSAGE STICK, SMOKED *(cont.)*								
nacho *(Slim Jim Super Slim)*,								
approx. .31 oz.	40	2.0	1.0	3.0	m.q.	m.q.	160	0
summer sausage:								
beef *(Hickory Farms)*, 1 oz.	100	5.0	1.0	8.0	m.q.	20	345	0
regular or teriyaki *(Pemmican)*,								
approx. .8 oz.	110	5.0	1.0	10.0	m.q.	m.q.	410	0
smoked *(Slim Jim)*, approx. .5 oz.	80	3.0	1.0	7.0	m.q.	m.q.	200	0
SAVORY, ground:								
1 oz.	77	1.9	19.5	1.7	n.a.	0	7	4.3 c
1 tbsp.	12	.3	3.0	.3	(0)	0	1	.7 c
1 tsp.	4	.1	1.0	.1	(0)	0	tr.	.2 c
(Spice Islands), 1 tsp.	5	.1	1.0	.1	(0)	0	<1	.2 c
summer *(Tone's)*, 1 tsp.	4	.1	1.0	.1	0	0	1	.2 d
SAVOY CABBAGE, see "Cabbage,								
savoy"								
SCALLION, see "Onion, green"								
SCALLOP, mixed species, meat								
only:								
raw:								
1 lb.	400	76.1	10.7	3.4	.4	152	730	0
1 oz.	25	4.8	.7	.2	<.1	9	46	0
2 large or 5 small, approx. 1.1 oz.	26	5.0	.7	.2	<.1	10	48	0
breaded[1], fried:								
4 oz.	244	20.5	11.5	12.4	3.0	69	526	.2 c
2 large, approx. 1.1 oz.	67	5.6	3.1	3.4	.8	19	144	.1 c
SCALLOP, FROZEN:								
fried *(Mrs. Paul's)*, 3 oz.	200	9.0	22.0	8.0	m.q.	m.q.	410	m.q.
SCALLOP, IMITATION[2]**:**								
1 lb.	447	57.9	48.2	1.9	m.q.	98	3606	0
1 oz.	28	3.6	3.0	.1	n.a.	6	225	0
"SCALLOP," VEGETARIAN,								
canned:								
(Worthington Vegetable Skallops),								
½ cup	90	15.0	4.0	2.0	m.q.	0	430	m.q.
no salt *(Worthington Vegetable*								
Skallops), ½ cup	80	13.0	4.0	1.0	n.a.	0	80	m.q.
SCALLOP AND SHRIMP								
DINNER, frozen:								
Mariner *(The Budget Gourmet)*,								
11.5 oz.	320	16.0	43.0	9.0	m.q.	70	690	m.q.
SCALLOP SQUASH:								
raw:								
untrimmed, 1 lb.	81	5.3	17.1	.9	.2	0	5	2.5 c
trimmed, 1 oz.	5	.3	1.1	.1	<.1	0	<1	.2 c
sliced, ½ cup	12	.8	2.5	.1	<.1	0	1	.4 c

1. *Recipe: 84.2% scallops, 9.3% bread crumbs, 4.6% egg, 1.4% milk, and .5% salt.*
2. *Made from surimi (see "Surimi").*

Food and Measure	cal.	prot. (gms)	carbo. (gms)	tot. fat (gms)	sat. fat (gms)	chol. (mgs)	sod. (mgs)	fiber (gms)
boiled, drained:								
4 oz.	18	1.2	3.7	.2	<.1	0	1	.5 c
sliced, ½ cup	14	.9	3.0	.2	<.1	0	1	.4 c
mashed, ½ cup	19	1.2	4.0	.2	<.1	0	1	.6 c
SCORZONERA, see "Salsify, black"								
SCOTCH KALE, see "Kale, Scotch"								
SCOTCH LIQUOR, see "Liquor"								
SCRAPPLE:								
(*Jones Dairy Farm*), 1 slice	65	2.7	4.2	3.7	m.q.	24	165	0
SCREWDRIVER[1]**:**								
1 fl. oz.	25	.2	2.6	tr.	tr.	0	tr.	n.a.
SCROD, see "Cod, Atlantic"								
SCROD ENTREE, frozen:								
baked (*Gorton's Microwave Entrees*),								
1 pkg.	320	22.0	17.0	18.0	4.0	80	420	m.q.
SCUP, meat only, raw:								
1 lb.	477	85.6	0	12.4	m.q.	m.q.	191	0
1 oz.	30	5.4	0	.8	m.q.	m.q.	12	0
1 fillet, approx. 2.25 oz., yield from								
1-lb. whole fish	67	12.1	0	1.8	m.q.	m.q.	27	0
SEA BASS, mixed species, meat only:								
raw:								
1 lb.	439	83.6	0	9.1	2.3	186	308	0
1 oz.	27	5.2	0	.6	.1	12	19	0
1 fillet, approx. 4.6 oz., yield from								
1½-lb. whole fish	125	23.8	0	2.6	.7	53	88	0
baked, broiled, or microwaved[2],								
4 oz.	141	26.8	0	2.9	.7	60	99	0
SEA TROUT, mixed species, meat only, raw:								
1 lb.	472	76.0	0	16.4	4.6	376	263	0
1 oz.	29	4.7	0	1.0	.3	24	16	0
1 fillet, approx. 8.4 oz., yield from								
3-lb. whole fish	248	39.8	0	8.6	2.4	198	138	0
SEAFOOD, see specific listings								
SEAFOOD CASSEROLE, see "Seafood entree"								
SEAFOOD DINNER, frozen:								
w/natural herbs (*Armour Classics Lite*), 10 oz.	190	13.0	29.0	2.0	m.q.	35	1020	m.q.
SEAFOOD ENTREE, frozen:								
casserole (*Pillsbury Microwave Classic*), 1 pkg.	420	15.0	37.0	24.0	m.q.	m.q.	950	m.q.
Creole, w/rice (*Swanson* Homestyle Recipe), 9 oz.	240	7.0	40.0	6.0	m.q.	m.q.	810	m.q.

1. *Recipe: 80.2% orange juice and 19.8% vodka.*
2. *Without added ingredients.*

Food and Measure	cal.	prot. (gms)	carbo. (gms)	tot. fat (gms)	sat. fat (gms)	chol. (mgs)	sod. (mgs)	fiber (gms)
SEAFOOD ENTREE *(cont.)*								
gumbo (*Cajun Cookin'*[1]), 17 oz.	330	16.0	51.0	7.0	m.q.	m.q.	1330	m.q.
Newberg (*The Budget Gourmet*),								
10 oz.	350	17.0	43.0	12.0	m.q.	70	660	m.q.
Newburg (*Healthy Choice*), 8 oz. ...	200	13.0	30.0	3.0	1.0	55	440	m.q.
SEAFOOD SAUCE (see also "Cocktail sauce" and "Tartar sauce"):								
(*Progresso* Authentic Pasta Sauces),								
½ cup	190	7.0	5.0	15.0	9.0	95	570	<1.0 d
Creole (*Great Impressions*), 1 tbsp.	21	.2	4.7	.1	n.a.	0	182	n.a.
dipping (*Great Impressions*), 1 tbsp.	17	.6	2.2	.7	n.a.	0	129	n.a.
dipping, Polynesian (*Great Impressions*), 1 tbsp.	38	<1.0	9.5	<1.0	n.a.	0	127	n.a.
mixed (*Progresso*), ½ cup	110	5.0	12.0	6.0	<1.0	11	445	2.3 d
SEAFOOD SEASONING, see "Fish seasoning and coating mix"								
SEAFOOD AND CRABMEAT SALAD:								
(*Longacre* Saladfest), 1 oz.	45	1.0	3.0	3.0	m.q.	5	130	n.a.
SEASONING AND COATING MIX (see also specific listings):								
breading (*Golden Dipt*), 1 oz.	90	3.0	20.0	0	0	0	630	m.q.
country, mild (*Shake 'n Bake*),								
¼ pouch	80	1.0	10.0	4.0	m.q.	0	500	m.q.
SEAWEED:								
agar:								
raw, 1 lb.	116	2.5	30.6	.1	<.1	0	40	2.0 c
raw, 1 oz.	7	.2	1.9	tr.	tr.	0	3	.1 c
dried, 1 oz.	87	1.8	22.9	.1	<.1	0	29	.2 c
Irish moss, raw, 1 lb.	222	6.9	55.8	.7	.2	0	303	m.q.
Irish moss, raw, 1 oz.	14	.4	3.5	<.1	tr.	0	19	m.q.
kelp, raw, 1 lb.	195	7.6	43.4	2.5	1.1	0	1056	6.0 c
kelp, raw, 1 oz.	12	.5	2.7	.2	.1	0	66	.4 c
laver, raw, 1 lb.	158	26.4	23.2	1.3	.3	0	217	1.2 c
laver, raw, 1 oz.	10	1.6	1.4	.1	<.1	0	14	.1 c
spirulina:								
raw, 1 lb.	120	26.9	11.0	1.8	.6	0	444	1.5 c
raw, 1 oz.	8	1.7	.7	.1	<.1	0	28	.1 c
dried, 1 oz.	82	16.3	6.8	2.2	.8	0	297	1.0 c
wakame, raw, 1 lb.	206	13.7	41.5	2.9	.6	0	3957	2.5 c
wakame, raw, 1 oz.	13	.9	2.6	.2	<.1	0	247	.2 c
SEMOLINA, whole grain:								
1 oz.	102	3.6	20.6	.3	<.1	0	<1	1.1 d
1 cup	602	21.2	121.6	1.8	.3	0	2	6.5 d
SESAME BUTTER:								
paste, from whole sesame seeds:								
1 oz.	169	5.1	7.2	14.5	2.0	0	3	1.6 c

Food and Measure	cal.	prot. (gms)	carbo. (gms)	tot. fat (gms)	sat. fat (gms)	chol. (mgs)	sod. (mgs)	fiber (gms)
1 tbsp.	95	2.9	4.1	8.1	1.1	0	2	.9 c
tahini (see also "Tahini mix"):								
from raw, stone-ground kernels,								
1 oz.	162	5.1	7.4	13.6	1.9	0	21	2.6 d
from raw, stone-ground kernels,								
1 tbsp.	86	2.7	3.9	7.2	1.0	0	11	1.4 d
from unroasted kernels, 1 oz. ...	173	5.1	5.1	16.0	2.2	0	tr.	2.6 d
from unroasted kernels, 1 tbsp. ...	85	2.5	2.5	7.9	1.1	0	tr.	1.3 d
from roasted and toasted kernels,								
1 oz.	169	4.8	6.0	15.3	2.1	0	33	2.6 d
from roasted and toasted kernels,								
1 tbsp.	89	2.6	3.2	8.1	1.1	0	17	1.4 d
organic (*Arrowhead Mills*), 1 oz.	170	6.0	4.0	17.0	m.q.	0	<1	2.6 d
SESAME CHIPS:								
(*Flavor Tree*), ¼ cup	163	3.2	10.6	9.2	m.q.	0	380	.1 c
SESAME FLOUR[1]:								
high fat, 1 oz.	149	8.7	7.6	10.5	1.5	0	12	1.8 c
partially defatted, 1 oz.	109	11.5	10.0	3.4	.5	0	12	1.7 c
low-fat, 1 oz.	95	14.2	10.1	.5	.1	0	11	1.4 c
SESAME MEAL[1]:								
partially defatted, 1 oz.	161	4.8	7.4	13.6	1.9	0	11	1.1 c
SESAME NUT MIX:								
dry-roasted (*Planters*), 1 oz.	160	5.0	8.0	12.0	3.0	0	330	m.q.
SESAME OIL:								
1 oz.	251	0	0	28.4	4.0	0	0	0
½ cup	964	0	0	109.0	15.5	0	0	0
1 tbsp.	120	0	0	13.6	1.9	0	0	0
(*Hain*), 1 tbsp.	120	0	0	14.0	2.0	0	0	0
SESAME PASTE, see "Sesame								
butter"								
SESAME SEASONING:								
all-purpose (*McCormick/Schilling*								
Parsley Patch), 1 tsp.	15	.6	1.0	1.0	n.a.	0	2	n.a.
SESAME SEED:								
(*Spice Islands*), 1 tsp.	9	.5	.9	.4	n.a.	0	1	.7 c
whole:								
dried:								
1 lb.	2598	80.4	106.4	225.3	31.6	0	51	20.9 c
1 oz.	162	5.0	6.6	14.1	2.0	0	3	1.3 c
1 cup	825	25.5	33.8	71.5	10.0	0	16	6.6 c
1 tbsp.	52	1.6	2.1	4.5	.6	0	1	.4 c
(*Arrowhead Mills*), 1 oz.	160	5.0	6.0	14.0	m.q.	0	4	3.1 d
roasted and toasted, 1 oz.	161	4.8	7.3	13.6	1.9	0	3	2.4 c
kernels, decorticated (hulled):								
dried:								
1 oz.	167	7.5	2.7	15.5	2.2	0	11	.8 c
1 cup	882	39.6	14.1	82.2	11.5	0	59	4.4 c

1. *Made from sesame seed kernels.*

Food and Measure	cal.	prot. (gms)	carbo. (gms)	tot. fat (gms)	sat. fat (gms)	chol. (mgs)	sod. (mgs)	fiber (gms)
SESAME SEED, KERNELS, DRIED *(cont.)*								
1 tbsp.	47	2.1	.8	4.4	.6	0	3	.2 c
1 tsp.	16	.7	.3	1.5	.2	0	1	.1 c
(Arrowhead Mills), 1 oz.	160	6.0	4.0	14.0	m.q.	0	3	3.7 d
toasted, 1 oz.	161	4.8	7.4	13.6	1.9	0	11	1.4 c
SESAME STICKS:								
(Flavor Tree), ¼ cup	133	3.1	10.6	9.1	m.q.	0	358	.1 c
(Flavor Tree) No Salt, ¼ cup	131	3.2	13.4	8.1	m.q.	0	7	.1 c
SESBANIA FLOWER:								
raw:								
untrimmed, 1 lb.	106	4.9	25.9	.2	(0)	0	59	5.8 c
trimmed, 1 oz.	8	.4	1.9	<.1	(0)	0	4	.4 c
trimmed, 1 cup	5	.3	1.4	<.1	(0)	0	3	.3 c
1 flower, 2¾″ × 1⅛″ × ⅜″,								
.1 oz.	1	<.1	.2	tr.	(0)	0	tr.	<.1 c
steamed, 4 oz.	25	1.3	5.9	.1	(0)	0	12	1.8 c
steamed, ½ cup	11	.6	2.7	<.1	(0)	0	6	.8 c
7-ELEVEN:								
Big Bite (2-oz. beef weiner), 3.4 oz.	287	10.2	20.3	18.1	7.3	27	781	1.1 d
Big Bite, super (4-oz. beef weiner),								
5.4 oz.	460	17.0	20.6	34.1	14.1	54	1322	1.1 d
burritos, 1 serving:								
bean and cheese, 10 oz.	616	23.3	84.3	23.1	7.5	46	1118	6.2 d
beef and bean:								
5 oz.	308	11.6	42.1	11.5	3.8	23	559	3.1 d
green chili, 10 oz.	617	23.3	84.3	23.1	7.5	46	1118	6.1 d
red chili, 5 oz.	308	11.6	42.1	11.5	3.8	23	559	3.1 d
red hot, 5 oz.	310	11.7	42.6	11.6	3.8	23	561	3.2 d
red hot, 10 oz.	620	23.5	85.1	23.2	7.6	47	1122	6.3 d
red hot, premium, 5.2 oz.	359	13.3	41.9	17.1	5.7	31	603	3.3 d
beef, bean, and cheese, 5.2 oz. . .	395	14.9	41.5	20.5	8.1	40	738	2.8 d
beef and potato, 5.2 oz.	394	13.2	48.0	18.4	6.3	32	607	2.4 d
chicken and rice, premium, 5 oz.	244	9.6	42.2	5.6	1.0	13	474	2.3 d
chicken, breast of, 4.8 oz.	405	17.6	48.6	15.7	m.q.	29	441	m.q.
chimichanga, beef, 5 oz.	363	15.0	42.3	14.9	m.q.	m.q.	674	.4 d
enchilada, beef and cheese, 6.5 oz.	369	18.6	27.6	21.7	10.2	55	524	3.5 d
fajitas, 5 oz.	311	13.8	40.4	11.4	3.5	32	795	1.8 d
sandito, ham and cheese, 5 oz.	347	17.7	35.9	16.0	6.9	40	1118	1.9 d
sandito, pizza, 5 oz.	345	12.8	38.0	17.0	5.1	23	711	2.0 d
tacos, soft, twin, 5.9 oz.	399	17.3	40.7	19.7	7.9	50	862	2.5 d
Deli-Shoppe microwave products,								
1 serving:								
bacon cheeseburger, 6 oz.	558	24.1	42.7	28.7	2.3	11	1217	m.q.
bagel and cream cheese, 4 oz. . . .	338	10.5	37.3	16.1	9.6	47	440	.9 d
char sandwich, large, 8.4 oz.	713	32.1	46.2	47.2	2.3	11	1478	.1 d
fish sandwich, w/cheese, 5.2 oz.	433	20.4	54.1	14.5	2.3	11	955	m.q.
sausage, red hot, large, 9.3 oz. . .	845	31.0	43.3	59.2	20.3	128	2204	2.2 d
turkey, wedge, 3.4 oz.	193	13.9	20.3	5.6	1.6	24	482	.7 d

Food and Measure	cal.	prot. (gms)	carbo. (gms)	tot. fat (gms)	sat. fat (gms)	chol. (mgs)	sod. (mgs)	fiber (gms)
SHAD, American, meat only, raw:								
1 lb.	891	76.8	0	62.5	m.q.	m.q.	233	0
1 oz.	56	4.8	0	3.9	m.q.	m.q.	14	0
1 fillet, approx. 6.5 oz., yield from								
1½-lb. whole fish	362	31.2	0	25.3	m.q.	m.q.	95	0
SHAKE, see "Milkshake"								
SHAKEY'S:								
fried chicken (3 pieces) and potatoes	947	57.0	51.0	56.0	m.q.	m.q.	2293	m.q.
fried chicken (5 pieces) and potatoes	1700	97.0	130.0	90.0	m.q.	m.q.	5327	m.q.
Hot Ham and Cheese	550	36.0	56.0	21.0	m.q.	m.q.	2135	m.q.
pizza, *Homestyle Pan Crust,* ⅟₁₀ of 12″ pie:								
cheese only	303	14.1	31.0	13.7	m.q.	21	591	m.q.
onion, green pepper, black olives,								
mushrooms	320	14.7	32.1	14.7	m.q.	21	652	m.q.
pepperoni	343	15.8	31.1	15.4	m.q.	27	740	m.q.
sausage, mushroom	343	16.4	31.4	16.9	m.q.	24	677	m.q.
sausage, pepperoni	374	17.4	31.2	19.9	m.q.	24	676	m.q.
Shakey's Special	384	17.9	31.6	20.7	m.q.	29	878	m.q.
pizza, thick crust, ⅟₁₀ of 12″ pie:								
cheese only	170	9.0	21.6	4.8	m.q.	13	421	m.q.
green pepper, black olives,								
mushrooms	162	9.1	22.2	4.1	m.q.	13	418	m.q.
pepperoni	185	10.1	21.8	6.4	m.q.	17	422	m.q.
sausage, mushrooms	179	10.2	21.8	5.6	m.q.	15	420	m.q.
sausage, pepperoni	177	11.1	21.7	8.0	m.q.	19	424	m.q.
Shakey's Special	208	13.1	22.3	8.3	m.q.	18	423	m.q.
pizza, thin crust, ⅟₁₀ of 12″ pie:								
cheese only	133	8.4	13.2	5.2	m.q.	14	323	m.q.
onion, green pepper, black olives,								
mushrooms	125	7.2	13.8	4.5	m.q.	11	313	m.q.
pepperoni	148	8.4	13.2	6.9	m.q.	14	403	m.q.
sausage, mushroom	141	8.5	13.3	6.0	m.q.	13	336	m.q.
sausage, pepperoni	166	9.4	13.2	8.4	m.q.	17	397	m.q.
Shakey's Special	171	13.3	13.5	8.7	m.q.	16	475	m.q.
potatoes, 15 pieces	950	17.0	120.0	36.0	m.q.	n.a.	3703	m.q.
Shakey's Super Hot Hero	810	36.0	67.0	44.0	m.q.	m.q.	2688	m.q.
spaghetti, w/meat sauce and garlic								
bread	940	26.0	134.0	33.0	m.q.	m.q.	1904	m.q.
SHALLOT:								
untrimmed, 1 lb.	287	10.0	67.1	.4	.1	0	48	2.8 c
trimmed, 1 oz.	20	.7	4.8	<.1	tr.	0	3	.2 c
chopped, 1 tbsp.	7	.3	1.7	<.1	tr.	0	1	.1 c
SHALLOT, FREEZE-DRIED:								
1 oz.	99	3.5	22.9	.1	<.1	0	17	1.3 c
¼ cup	13	.4	2.9	<.1	tr.	0	2	.1 c
1 tbsp.	3	.1	.7	tr.	tr.	0	1	<.1 c
SHARK, mixed species, meat only:								
raw, 1 lb.	591	95.2	0	20.5	4.2	232	360	0

Food and Measure	cal.	prot. (gms)	carbo. (gms)	tot. fat (gms)	sat. fat (gms)	chol. (mgs)	sod. (mgs)	fiber (gms)
SHARK *(cont.)*								
raw, 1 oz.	37	5.9	0	1.3	.3	14	22	0
batter-dipped[1], 4 oz.	259	21.1	7.2	15.7	3.6	67	138	.2 c
SHEANUT OIL:								
1 oz.	251	0	0	28.4	13.2	0	0	0
½ cup	964	0	0	109.0	50.8	0	0	0
1 tbsp.	120	0	0	13.6	6.3	0	0	0
SHEEPSHEAD, meat only:								
raw:								
1 lb.	490	91.7	0	10.9	2.8	m.q.	324	0
1 oz.	31	5.7	0	.7	.2	m.q.	20	0
1 fillet, approx. 8.4 oz., yield from 3-lb. whole fish	257	48.1	0	5.8	1.4	m.q.	170	0
baked, broiled, or microwaved[2]:								
4 oz.	143	29.5	0	1.8	.4	m.q.	83	0
1 fillet, approx. 6.6 oz., yield from 8.4-oz. raw fillet	234	48.4	0	3.0	.7	m.q.	136	0
SHELLFISH OF THE FOREST, see "Mushroom, oyster"								
SHELLIE BEAN, canned:								
w/liquid, 4 oz.	34	2.0	7.0	.2	<.1	0	379	.6 c
w/liquid, ½ cup	37	2.1	7.6	.2	<.1	0	408	.7 c
(Stokely), ½ cup	35	2.0	7.0	0	0	0	470	m.q.
SHELLS, STUFFED, see "Pasta dinner, frozen" and "Pasta entree, frozen"								
SHERBET (see also "Sorbet" and "Ice"):								
all flavors *(Sealtest)*, ½ cup	130	1.0	28.0	1.0	0	5	30	n.a.
orange:								
1 oz.	40	.3	8.6	.6	.3	2	13	tr.c
½ cup	135	1.1	29.4	1.9	1.2	7	44	tr.c
(Bordon), ½ cup	110	1.0	25.0	1.0	m.q.	m.q.	40	n.a.
(Darigold), ½ cup	120	1.0	26.0	1.0	m.q.	m.q.	25	n.a.
rainbow *(Baskin-Robbins)*, 1 regular scoop	160	1.0	34.0	2.0	m.q.	6	85	n.a.
SHERBET BAR, frozen, 1 bar:								
all flavors:								
(Fudgsicle Fat Free*)*	70	2.0	14.0	0	0	0	45	n.a.
(Fudgsicle Sugar Free*)*	35	2.0	6.0	1.0	n.a.	5	50	n.a.
w/cream *(Creamsicle* Sugar Free*)*	25	1.0	5.0	1.0	n.a.	n.a.	20	n.a.
chocolate *(Fudgsicle)*	70	2.0	12.0	1.0	n.a.	n.a.	70	n.a.
chocolate, w/nuts *(Fudgsicle* Sugar Free Fudge Nut Dip*)*	130	2.0	12.0	8.0	m.q.	5	40	m.q.
SHERRY, see "Wine"								
SHIITAKE MUSHROOM, see "Mushroom, shiitake"								

1. *Recipe: 75.2% fish and 24.8% batter mixture (water, flour, oil, egg, milk, baking powder, and salt).*
2. *Without added ingredients.*

Food and Measure	cal.	prot. (gms)	carbo. (gms)	tot. fat (gms)	sat. fat (gms)	chol. (mgs)	sod. (mgs)	fiber (gms)
SHIMEJI MUSHROOM, see								
"Mushroom, oyster"								
SHONEY'S:								
breakfast, kitchen ordered:								
bacon, 3 strips	109	5.8	.1	9.4	m.q.	16	303	0
biscuit, 1 piece	170	2.7	21.6	8.1	m.q.	0	364	0
country gravy, 3 oz.	114	1.2	5.7	9.8	m.q.	2	358	0
croissant, 1 piece	260	5.0	22.0	16.0	m.q.	2	260	0
egg, fried, 1 egg	159	6.1	.6	14.7	m.q.	274	69	0
grits, 3 oz.	57	.7	6.2	3.2	m.q.	0	62	0
ham, breakfast, 2 slices	59	7.2	.6	2.1	m.q.	28	526	0
hashbrowns, 3 oz.	90	1.6	14.1	3.1	m.q.	0	50	0
home fries, 3 oz.	115	2.0	18.7	3.7	m.q.	0	53	0
honey bun, 1 piece	265	4.0	32.0	14.0	m.q.	3	33	0
muffin, blueberry, 2	214	2.9	35.4	7.0	m.q.	33	2	.9
pancake, 6″ cake	91	1.8	19.9	.2	m.q.	0	522	0
sausage, 1 patty	103	3.7	.2	9.6	m.q.	17	161	0
sirloin, charbroiled, 6 oz.	357	31.9	0	24.5	m.q.	99	160	0
syrup, lo-cal, 2.2 oz.	98	0	24.4	0	0	0	0	0
toast, buttered, 2 slices	163	4.2	24.6	5.2	m.q.	0	296	1.2
soups, 6 oz. serving:								
bean	63	3.8	9.8	1.1	m.q.	4	479	1.4
beef cabbage	86	6.1	9.4	3.0	m.q.	13	503	2.3
broccoli, cream of	75	1.8	10.5	4.6	m.q.	1	415	.4
broccoli/cauliflower	124	3.8	11.9	9.2	m.q.	12	560	.5
cheddar chowder	91	3.0	14.4	2.3	m.q.	m.q.	948	n.a.
cheese Florentine ham	110	3.7	11.8	7.8	m.q.	11	890	.6
chicken, cream of	136	4.6	13.5	8.9	m.q.	11	1164	.3
chicken gumbo	60	4.0	7.0	2.0	m.q.	m.q.	1050	n.a.
chicken noodle	62	3.1	9.2	1.4	m.q.	14	127	n.a.
chicken rice	72	3.0	13.3	.5	m.q.	6	117	.5
chicken vegetable, cream	79	3.5	13.4	1.3	m.q.	m.q.	714	n.a.
clam chowder	94	1.7	9.6	5.4	m.q.	0	66	0
corn chowder	148	4.0	22.1	4.7	m.q.	n.a.	510	0
onion	29	1.1	1.5	2.0	m.q.	1	88	.1
potato	102	1.4	16.8	3.4	m.q.	0	335	1.6
tomato Florentine	63	2.3	11.0	1.1	m.q.	0	683	0
tomato vegetable	46	1.9	9.8	.3	m.q.	0	314	.4
vegetable beef	82	3.5	14.1	1.5	m.q.	5	1254	.3
entrees, 1 serving:								
beef patty, light	289	20.7	0	22.9	m.q.	82	187	0
fish, light fried	297	19.8	21.5	14.4	m.q.	65	536	.1
Italian feast	500	37.5	43.8	19.6	m.q.	74	369	1.1
shrimp, boiled	93	19.6	0	1.0	m.q.	182	210	0
shrimp sampler	412	25.5	26.1	22.7	m.q.	217	783	.1
charbroiled steak and chicken:								
chicken, charbroiled	239	39.0	1.3	7.4	m.q.	85	592	0
chicken, Hawaiian	262	39.1	7.4	7.4	m.q.	85	593	.3
Half O' Pound	435	31.1	0	34.4	m.q.	123	280	0

Food and Measure	cal.	prot. (gms)	carbo. (gms)	tot. fat (gms)	sat. fat (gms)	chol. (mgs)	sod. (mgs)	fiber (gms)
SHONEY'S, ENTREES *(cont.)*								
ribeye, 8 oz.	605	35.2	0	50.5	m.q.	141	211	0
sirloin, 6 oz.	357	31.9	0	24.5	m.q.	99	160	0
Steak N' Shrimp:								
w/charbroiled shrimp	361	36.5	1.0	22.6	m.q.	141	198	0
w/fried shrimp	507	36.5	15.0	32.7	m.q.	150	249	.1
America's Favorites:								
chicken tenders	388	34.9	16.6	20.4	m.q.	64	239	0
country fried steak	449	19.4	33.9	27.2	m.q.	27	1177	.9
lasagna	297	8.3	44.9	9.8	m.q.	26	870	2.8
liver n' onions	411	34.9	15.4	22.9	m.q.	529	321	.8
spaghetti	496	24.2	63.4	16.3	m.q.	55	387	2.2
seafood:								
baked fish	170	34.6	2.4	1.4	m.q.	83	1641	0
Fish N' Shrimp	487	28.1	36.5	25.5	m.q.	127	644	.3
Fish N' Chips, w/fries	639	32.3	50.4	34.8	n.a.	103	873	2.9
seafood platter	566	32.8	45.7	28.0	m.q.	127	893	.3
shrimp, bite-size	387	16.4	24.7	24.7	m.q.	140	1266	0
shrimp, charbroiled	138	24.7	3.0	3.0	m.q.	162	170	0
shrimper's feast	383	16.5	29.9	22.2	m.q.	125	216	.3
shrimper's feast, large	575	24.8	44.9	33.3	m.q.	188	324	.4
burgers and sandwiches:								
All-American burger	501	25.0	26.8	32.6	m.q.	86	597	.5
bacon burger	591	28.7	28.6	40.0	m.q.	86	801	.5
baked ham sandwich	290	19.2	28.2	10.3	m.q.	42	1263	1.8
chicken, charbroiled	451	43.2	28.1	17.0	m.q.	90	1002	.5
chicken fillet sandwich	464	29.7	38.9	21.2	m.q.	51	585	.5
country fried sandwich	588	24.5	67.0	25.8	m.q.	29	1501	1.4
fish sandwich	323	12.2	41.0	12.7	m.q.	21	740	.4
grilled bacon & cheese	440	18.2	27.9	28.2	m.q.	36	1200	1.3
grilled cheese	302	12.4	25.1	16.9	m.q.	36	880	1.4
ham club/whole wheat	642	37.0	45.2	35.5	m.q.	78	2105	10.5
mushroom/Swiss burger	616	31.6	28.8	41.7	m.q.	106	1135	.7
old-fashioned burger	470	25.1	25.6	28.2	m.q.	82	681	.6
patty melt	640	38.8	29.5	41.7	m.q.	121	826	6.7
Philly steak sandwich	673	31.8	37.2	44.0	m.q.	103	1242	.1
Reuben sandwich	596	32.7	31.5	34.7	m.q.	138	3873	6.3
Slim Jim sandwich	484	27.4	40.4	23.9	m.q.	57	1620	.5
Shoney burger	498	23.4	22.2	35.7	m.q.	79	782	.2
turkey club/whole wheat	635	43.5	44.1	32.7	m.q.	100	1289	10.2
side dishes, 1 serving:								
baked potato, 10 oz.	264	5.6	61.1	.3	n.a.	0	16	6.8
french fries, 3 oz.	189	2.9	28.9	7.5	m.q.	0	273	2.7
french fries, 4 oz.	252	3.9	38.6	9.9	m.q.	0	364	3.6
Grecian bread	80	2.0	13.2	2.2	m.q.	0	94	0
onion rings, 1 piece	52	.9	5.0	3.1	m.q.	2	102	.4
rice, 3.5 oz.	137	2.4	23.1	3.7	m.q.	1	765	.1
sauteed mushrooms, 3 oz.	75	1.6	4.3	6.5	m.q.	0	968	1.3
sauteed onions, 2.5 oz.	37	.8	4.3	2.1	m.q.	0	221	.5

Food and Measure	cal.	prot. (gms)	carbo. (gms)	tot. fat (gms)	sat. fat (gms)	chol. (mgs)	sod. (mgs)	fiber (gms)
salads, prepared, ¼ cup:								
ambrosia salad	75	.8	11.5	3.3	m.q.	0	167	.8
apple grape surprise	19	0	4.9	0	0	0	2	.1
beet onion salad	25	.6	3.0	1.3	m.q.	0	167	.8
broccoli/cauliflower	98	2.3	4.0	8.5	m.q.	0	478	.9
broccoli/cauliflower/carrot	53	1.1	2.7	4.4	m.q.	1	193	.9
broccoli/cauliflower/ranch	65	.9	1.6	6.4	m.q.	9	12	.9
carrot apple	99	.6	4.2	9.1	m.q.	8	10	.9
cole slaw	69	1.1	5.1	5.1	m.q.	7	106	.9
cucumber lite	12	.2	2.7	.1	n.a.	0	344	.2
Don's pasta	82	1.8	8.6	4.6	m.q.	0	223	.2
fruit delight	54	.6	10.1	1.6	m.q.	0	2	.7
Italian vegetable	11	.4	2.5	.1	n.a.	0	110	.7
kidney bean salad	55	2.6	6.8	2.1	m.q.	2	154	1.9
macaroni salad	207	4.2	17.0	13.9	m.q.	14	382	.2
mixed fruit salad	37	.4	9.3	.1	n.a.	0	3	.2
mixed squash	49	1.1	2.3	4.1	m.q.	0	230	.3
Oriental salad	79	.8	13.4	2.7	m.q.	1	31	.5
pea salad	73	2.5	3.5	5.5	m.q.	42	89	2.4
rotelli pasta	78	1.4	8.9	4.0	m.q.	0	82	.2
Seigan salad	72	2.3	8.1	3.6	m.q.	5	122	1.2
snow salad	72	.6	9.0	4.1	m.q.	0	18	.1
spaghetti salad	81	1.6	8.7	4.6	m.q.	0	20	.2
spring salad	38	.8	2.4	2.9	m.q.	0	162	.7
summer salad	114	1.1	2.2	11.6	m.q.	0	233	.9
three bean salad	96	1.4	11.9	5.1	m.q.	0	189	1.3
Waldorf	81	.9	8.5	5.2	m.q.	2	68	.8
dressings, 2 tbsp.:								
Biscayne lo-cal	62	6.0	1.0	1.0	n.a.	0	334	0
blue cheese	113	0	0	13.0	m.q.	15	109	0
honey mustard	165	2.4	2.4	17.0	m.q.	18	5	0
Italian, creamy	135	0	1.0	15.0	m.q.	0	454	0
Italian, golden	141	0	1.0	15.0	m.q.	0	302	0
Italian, W.W.	10	0	2.4	0	0	0	615	0
French	124	2.0	2.0	12.0	m.q.	12	204	0
French, Rue	122	5.0	2.0	10.0	m.q.	0	364	0
ranch	95	0	0	10.0	m.q.	15	10	0
Thousand Island	130	1.0	2.0	13.0	m.q.	12	179	0
sauces, 1 souffle cup:								
BBQ	41	.1	8.2	1.0	n.a.	0	232	0
cocktail	36	.4	8.7	.1	n.a.	0	260	0
sweet N' sour	58	0	14.7	0	0	0	5	0
tartar	84	.2	3.6	7.7	m.q.	11	177	0
desserts, 1 serving:								
apple pie a la mode	492	6.0	67.0	23.0	m.q.	35	574	n.a.
carrot cake	500	9.0	56.0	26.0	m.q.	37	476	0
hot fudge cake	522	7.4	81.9	19.7	m.q.	27	485	0
hot fudge sundae	451	7.0	60.0	22.0	m.q.	60	226	0

Food and Measure	cal.	prot. (gms)	carbo. (gms)	tot. fat (gms)	sat. fat (gms)	chol. (mgs)	sod. (mgs)	fiber (gms)
SHONEY'S*, DESSERTS *(cont.)								
strawberry pie	332	2.1	44.5	16.7	m.q.	0	247	2.3
strawberry sundae	380	6.0	47.7	19.0	m.q.	69	145	.3
walnut brownie a la mode	576	9.6	60.6	33.7	m.q.	35	435	0
SHORTENING[1], BREAD:								
1 oz.	251	0	0	28.4	6.2	0	0	0
1 cup	1812	0	0	205.0	45.1	0	0	0
1 tbsp.	113	0	0	12.8	2.8	0	0	0
SHORTENING[2], CAKE MIX:								
1 oz.	251	0	0	28.4	7.7	0	0	0
1 cup	1812	0	0	205.0	55.8	0	0	0
1 tbsp.	113	0	0	12.8	3.5	0	0	0
SHORTENING, CONFECTIONERY:								
hydrogenated coconut and/or palm kernel:								
1 oz.	251	0	0	28.4	25.9	0	0	0
1 cup	1812	0	0	205.0	187.3	0	0	0
1 tbsp.	113	0	0	12.8	11.7	0	0	0
fractionated palm:								
1 oz.	251	0	0	28.4	18.6	0	0	0
1 cup	1927	0	0	218.0	142.9	0	0	0
1 tbsp.	120	0	0	13.6	8.9	0	0	0
SHORTENING, FRYING:								
regular, hydrogenated soybean and cottonseed:								
1 oz.	251	0	0	28.4	4.4	0	0	0
1 cup	1812	0	0	205.0	31.6	0	0	0
1 tbsp.	113	0	0	12.8	2.0	0	0	0
heavy duty:								
beef tallow and cottonseed:								
1 oz.	255	0	0	28.4	12.7	m.q.	0	0
1 cup	1845	0	0	205.0	92.0	m.q.	0	0
1 tbsp.	115	0	0	12.8	5.7	m.q.	0	0
hydrogenated palm:								
1 oz.	251	0	0	28.4	13.5	0	0	0
1 cup	1812	0	0	205.0	97.4	0	0	0
1 tbsp.	113	0	0	12.8	6.1	0	0	0
soybean[3]:								
1 oz.	251	0	0	28.4	6.0	0	0	0
1 cup	1812	0	0	205.0	43.3	0	0	0
1 tbsp.	113	0	0	12.8	2.7	0	0	0
soybean[4]:								
1 oz.	251	0	0	28.4	5.2	0	0	0
1 cup	1812	0	0	205.0	37.7	0	0	0
1 tbsp.	113	0	0	12.8	2.4	0	0	0

1. *Hydrogenated soybean, and cottonseed.*
2. *Hydrogenated soybean and hydrogenated cottonseed.*
3. *Hydrogenated; less than 1% linoleic.*
4. *Hydrogenated; approx. 30% linoleic; stabilized with silicones.*

Food and Measure	cal.	prot. (gms)	carbo. (gms)	tot. fat (gms)	sat. fat (gms)	chol. (mgs)	sod. (mgs)	fiber (gms)
SHORTENING, HOUSEHOLD								
(see also specific shortening listings):								
lard and vegetable oil:								
1 oz.	255	0	0	28.4	11.4	m.q.	0	0
1 cup	1845	0	0	205.0	82.6	m.q.	0	0
1 tbsp.	115	0	0	12.8	5.2	m.q.	0	0
hydrogenated soybean and cottonseed:								
1 oz.	251	0	0	28.4	7.1	0	0	0
1 cup	1812	0	0	205.0	51.2	0	0	0
1 tbsp.	113	0	0	12.8	3.2	0	0	0
hydrogenated soybean, and palm:								
1 oz.	251	0	0	28.4	8.7	0	0	0
1 cup	1812	0	0	205.0	62.7	0	0	0
1 tbsp.	113	0	0	12.8	3.9	0	0	0
vegetable:								
(*Finast*), 1 tbsp.	110	0	0	13.0	m.q.	0	0	0
regular or butter flavor (*Crisco*), 1 tbsp.	110	0	0	12.0	3.0	0	0	0
butter flavor (*Finast*), 1 tbsp.	110	0	0	12.0	3.0	0	0	0
SHORTENING, INDUSTRIAL:								
lard and vegetable oil:								
1 oz.	255	0	0	28.4	10.1	m.q.	0	0
1 cup	1845	0	0	205.0	73.2	m.q.	0	0
1 tbsp.	115	0	0	12.8	4.6	m.q.	0	0
hydrogenated soybean, and cottonseed:								
1 oz.	251	0	0	28.4	7.3	0	0	0
1 cup	1812	0	0	205.0	52.5	0	0	0
1 tbsp.	113	0	0	12.8	3.3	0	0	0
SHOYU, see "Soy sauce"								
SHRIMP, mixed species, meat only:								
raw, 1 lb.	481	92.1	4.1	7.8	1.5	692	673	0
raw, 1 oz. or 4 large	30	5.7	.3	.5	.1	43	42	0
boiled, poached, or steamed[1]:								
4 oz.	112	23.7	m.q.	1.2	.3	221	254	0
4 large, approx. .8 oz.	22	4.6	m.q.	.2	.1	43	49	0
breaded[2], fried:								
4 oz.	274	24.3	13.0	13.9	2.4	201	390	.2 c
4 large, approx. 1.1 oz.	73	6.4	3.4	3.7	.6	53	103	<.1 c
SHRIMP, CANNED, mixed species, drained:								
4 oz.	136	26.2	1.2	2.2	.4	196	192	0
1 cup, approx. 4.5 oz.	154	29.6	1.3	2.5	.5	222	216	0
(*Louisiana Brand*), 2 oz.	58	12.0	0	1.0	m.q.	m.q.	m.q.	0
large (*ShopRite*), 2 oz.	50	10.0	0	1.0	m.q.	m.q.	720	0

1. *Without added ingredients.*
2. *Recipe: 84.2% shrimp, 9.3% bread crumbs, 4.6% egg, 1.4% milk, and .5% salt.*

Food and Measure	cal.	prot. (gms)	carbo. (gms)	tot. fat (gms)	sat. fat (gms)	chol. (mgs)	sod. (mgs)	fiber (gms)
SHRIMP, FROZEN (see also "Shrimp entree, frozen"):								
(*SeaPak* PDQ), 3.5 oz.	60	13.0	0	0	0	m.q.	250	0
butterfly (*Gorton's* Specialty), 4 oz.	160	19.0	16.0	<1.0	n.a.	m.q.	540	n.a.
SHRIMP, IMITATION[1]:								
1 lb.	458	56.2	41.4	6.7	m.q.	163	3198	0
1 oz.	29	3.5	2.6	.4	n.a.	10	200	0
SHRIMP COCKTAIL:								
(*Sau-Sea*), 4 oz.	113	7.0	19.0	1.0	m.q.	102	1020	0
SHRIMP AND CRAB SEASONING, see "Fish seasoning and coating mix"								
SHRIMP DINNER, frozen:								
baby bay (*Armour Classics Lite*), 9.75 oz.	220	12.0	31.0	6.0	m.q.	105	890	m.q.
Creole (*Armour Classics Lite*), 11.25 oz.	260	6.0	53.0	2.0	m.q.	45	900	m.q.
Creole (*Healthy Choice*), 11.25 oz. ...	210	8.0	42.0	1.0	<1.0	65	560	m.q.
marinara (*Healthy Choice*), 10.5 oz.	220	9.0	42.0	1.0	<1.0	50	320	m.q.
SHRIMP ENTREE, CANNED:								
chow mein (*La Choy* Bi-Pack), ¾ cup	50	3.0	7.0	1.0	m.q.	19	860	2.0 d
SHRIMP ENTREE, FROZEN (see also "Shrimp, frozen"):								
'n batter (*SeaPak*), 4 oz.	260	11.0	20.0	15.0	m.q.	20	470	m.q.
'n batter, w/crabmeat stuffing (*SeaPak*), 4 oz.	260	8.0	27.0	13.0	m.q.	m.q.	780	m.q.
breaded:								
butterfly (*SeaPak* Mikado), 4 oz.	160	12.0	26.0	1.0	m.q.	110	170	m.q.
butterfly/round (*SeaPak*), 4 oz. ..	150	14.0	20.0	1.0	m.q.	m.q.	m.q.	m.q.
fried (*Mrs. Paul's*), 3 oz.	200	9.0	16.0	11.0	m.q.	m.q.	430	m.q.
Cajun style (*Mrs. Paul's* Light), 9 oz.	230	9.0	37.0	5.0	1.0	60	740	m.q.
and chicken Cantonese, w/noodles (*Lean Cuisine*), 10⅛ oz.	270	22.0	25.0	9.0	1.0	100	920	m.q.
and clams, w/linguini (*Mrs. Paul's* Light), 10 oz.	240	12.0	36.0	5.0	2.0	40	750	m.q.
Creole (*Cajun Cookin'*), 12 oz.	390	17.0	55.0	11.0	m.q.	m.q.	1130	m.q.
crisps (*Gordon's* Specialty), 4 oz. ...	280	9.0	26.0	15.0	m.q.	m.q.	740	m.q.
crunchy, whole (*Gorton's* Microwave Specialty), 5 oz.	380	14.0	35.0	20.0	3.0	65	870	m.q.
etouffee (*Cajun Cookin'*), 17 oz. ...	360	19.0	52.0	9.0	m.q.	m.q.	1170	m.q.
and fettuccine (*The Budget Gourmet*), 9.5 oz.	375	10.0	38.0	20.0	m.q.	145	660	m.q.
fettuccine Alfredo (*Booth*), 10 oz. ..	260	19.0	28.0	8.0	m.q.	m.q.	620	m.q.
w/garlic butter sauce and vegetable rice, (*Booth*), 10 oz.	400	13.0	40.0	25.0	m.q.	m.q.	750	m.q.

1. *Made from surimi (see "Surimi").*

Food and Measure	cal.	prot. (gms)	carbo. (gms)	tot. fat (gms)	sat. fat (gms)	chol. (mgs)	sod. (mgs)	fiber (gms)
heat and serve (*SeaPak Super Valu*),								
4 oz.	210	12.0	30.0	4.0	m.q.	80	730	m.q.
jambalaya (*Cajun Cookin'*), 12 oz.	450	20.0	43.0	20.0	m.q.	m.q.	800	m.q.
w/lobster sauce (*La Choy Fresh &*								
Lite), 10 oz.	240	12.0	36.4	6.2	m.q.	118	946	2.8 d
New Orleans, w/wild rice (*Booth*),								
10 oz.	230	13.0	35.0	5.0	m.q.	m.q.	950	m.q.
Oriental, w/pineapple rice (*Booth*),								
10 oz.	190	11.0	30.0	3.0	m.q.	m.q.	950	m.q.
primavera:								
(*Mrs. Paul's* Light), 9½ oz.	180	11.0	28.0	3.0	1.0	125	840	m.q.
(*Right Course*), 9⅝ oz.	240	12.0	32.0	7.0	1.0	50	590	m.q.
w/fettuccine (*Booth*), 10 oz.	200	16.0	28.0	3.0	m.q.	m.q.	760	m.q.
scampi (*Gorton's Microwave Entrees*),								
1 pkg.	390	10.0	21.0	30.0	m.q.	m.q.	470	m.q.
SHRIMP SALAD:								
(*Longacre* Saladfest), 1 oz.	45	2.0	2.0	3.0	m.q.	25	150	n.a.
SHRIMP AND SEAFOOD								
SALAD:								
(*Longacre* Saladfest), 1 oz.	42	2.0	2.0	3.0	m.q.	15	160	n.a.
SHRIMP SAUCE:								
(*Tone's* Craboil), 1 tsp.	10	.3	1.2	.6	.1	1	1	.3 d
SICAMA, see "Yam bean tuber"								
SIM-SIM, see "Sesame seed"								
SISYMBRIUM SEED, whole:								
dried, 1 oz.	90	3.5	16.6	1.3	.3	0	26	8.4 c
dried, 1 cup	235	9.0	43.1	3.4	.7	0	68	22.0 c
SKIPPER'S:								
thick cut cod:								
3 piece, fries	665	27.0	68.0	32.0	m.q.	38	1054	m.q.
4 piece, fries	759	34.0	74.0	36.0	m.q.	50	1388	m.q.
5 piece, fries	853	42.0	80.0	41.0	m.q.	62	1723	m.q.
famous fish fillets:								
1 fish, fries	558	17.0	51.0	28.0	m.q.	55	408	m.q.
2 fish, fries	733	28.0	71.0	38.0	m.q.	108	765	m.q.
3 fish, fries	908	39.0	82.0	48.0	m.q.	160	1122	m.q.
seafood combos:								
clam strips, 1 fish, fries	868	25.0	81.0	54.0	m.q.	61	667	m.q.
oysters, 1 fish, fries	885	25.0	95.0	44.0	m.q.	80	809	m.q.
jumbo shrimp, 1 fish, fries	720	24.0	75.0	36.0	m.q.	91	1268	m.q.
original shrimp, 1 fish, fries	728	24.0	77.0	37.0	m.q.	105	943	m.q.
seafood baskets:								
clam strips, fries	1003	22.0	90.0	70.0	m.q.	14	569	m.q.
oysters, fries	1038	28.0	118.0	51.0	m.q.	52	853	m.q.
jumbo shrimp, fries	707	20.0	79.0	35.0	m.q.	73	911	m.q.
original shrimp, fries	723	20.0	82.0	36.0	m.q.	102	1121	m.q.
Skipper's Platter, fries	1038	32.0	97.0	63.0	m.q.	111	1202	m.q.
chicken tenderloin strips:								
5 piece, fries	793	44.0	69.0	38.0	m.q.	77	798	m.q.

Food and Measure	cal.	prot. (gms)	carbo. (gms)	tot. fat (gms)	sat. fat (gms)	chol. (mgs)	sod. (mgs)	fiber (gms)
SKIPPER'S, CHICKEN TENDERLOIN STRIPS *(cont.)*								
3 piece, 1 fish, fries	805	80.0	72.0	40.0	m.q.	100	858	m.q.
3 piece, original shrimp, fries	800	36.0	77.0	39.0	m.q.	97	1036	m.q.
salads & lite catch:								
3 chicken, small green salad	305	26.0	17.0	15.0	m.q.	58	673	m.q.
2 fish, small green salad	409	25.0	27.0	23.0	m.q.	119	937	m.q.
1 fish, 2 chicken, small green salad	399	29.0	24.0	21.0	m.q.	96	880	m.q.
small green salad	59	3.0	6.0	3.0	m.q.	13	223	m.q.
shrimp and seafood salad	167	23.0	15.0	3.0	m.q.	80	657	m.q.
Create A Catch:								
chicken sandwich	606	31.0	44.0	32.0	m.q.	82	976	m.q.
chicken strip	82	8.0	4.0	4.0	m.q.	15	150	m.q.
fish fillet	175	11.0	11.0	10.0	m.q.	53	357	m.q.
fish sandwich	524	19.0	43.0	33.0	m.q.	86	1191	m.q.
fish sandwich, double	698	30.0	54.0	73.0	m.q.	139	1548	m.q.
fries	383	6.0	50.0	18.0	m.q.	<2	51	m.q.
clam chowder cup	100	3.0	14.0	3.5	m.q.	12	525	m.q.
clam chowder pint	200	5.0	19.0	7.0	m.q.	24	1050	m.q.
coleslaw, 5 oz.	289	2.0	10.0	27.0	m.q.	50	329	m.q.
Jell-O	55	1.0	12.0	0	0	0	35	0
condiments, 1 tbsp.:								
barbeque sauce	25	0	5.0	1.0	n.a.	0	226	n.a.
cocktail sauce	20	0	5.0	0	0	0	216	n.a.
tartar sauce	65	0	0	7.0	m.q.	4	102	n.a.
salad dressing, 1 pouch:								
premium bleu cheese	222	1.0	4.0	23.0	m.q.	8	240	n.a.
gourmet Italian	140	0	2.0	15.0	m.q.	0	200	n.a.
lo-cal Italian	17	0	2.0	1.0	n.a.	0	680	n.a.
ranch house	188	1.0	2.0	20.0	m.q.	0	302	n.a.
Thousand Island	160	0	8.0	14.0	m.q.	6	415	n.a.
root beer float	302	3.0	33.0	10.0	m.q.	10	66	n.a.
SLOPPY JOE SAUCE, see "Barbecue sauce"								
SLOPPY JOE SEASONING:								
(*Lawry's* Seasoning Blends), 1 pkg.	126	2.8	27.7	.4	n.a.	0	3442	.8 c
(*Tone's*), 1 tsp.	14	.3	3.1	.1	n.a.	0	347	m.q.
mix (*French's*), ⅛ pkg.	16	0	4.0	0	0	0	390	m.q.
mix (*McCormick/Schilling*), ¼ pkg.	26	.5	6.0	.5	n.a.	0	750	m.q.
SMALL WHITE BEAN, see "White bean"								
SMELT, rainbow, meat only:								
raw, 1 lb.	440	80.0	0	11.0	2.1	318	272	0
raw, 1 oz.	27	5.0	0	.7	.1	20	17	0
baked, broiled, or microwaved[1], 4 oz.	141	25.6	0	3.5	.7	102	87	0

1. *Without added ingredients.*

Food and Measure	cal.	prot. (gms)	carbo. (gms)	tot. fat (gms)	sat. fat (gms)	chol. (mgs)	sod. (mgs)	fiber (gms)
SNACK BAR (see also "Granola and cereal bar"), 1 bar, except as noted:								
apple (*Health Valley Apple Bakes*) ...	100	2.0	16.0	3.0	m.q.	0	27	2.8 d
date (*Health Valley Date Bakes*)	100	3.0	16.0	3.0	m.q.	0	25	2.8 d
fruit (*Health Valley Fruit & Fitness*), 2 bars	200	4.0	39.0	3.0	m.q.	0	234	4.8 d
oat bran:								
almond and date (*Health Valley Oat Bran Jumbo Fruit Bars*)	170	4.0	28.0	5.0	m.q.	0	9	6.7 d
apricot (*Health Valley Oat Bran Apricot Bakes*)	100	2.0	19.0	2.0	m.q.	0	18	2.9 d
fig and nut (*Health Valley Fig & Nut Bakes*)	110	2.0	19.0	3.0	m.q.	0	18	3.1 d
fruit and nut (*Health Valley Oat Bran Jumbo Fruit Bars*)	150	4.0	29.0	4.0	m.q.	0	11	8.4 d
raisin and cinnamon (*Health Valley Oat Bran Jumbo Fruit Bars*) ...	140	3.0	32.0	2.0	m.q.	0	12	6.3 d
raisin (*Health Valley Raisin Bakes*) ..	100	2.0	16.0	3.0	m.q.	0	19	2.8 d
rice bran, almond, and date (*Health Valley Rice Bran Jumbo Fruit Bars*)	190	4.0	29.0	6.0	m.q.	0	6	5.6 d
SNACK CHIPS (see also specific chip listings), 1 pouch:								
barbecue flavor (*Great Snackers*) ...	60	1.0	8.0	3.0	m.q.	0	170	m.q.
cheddar cheese flavor (*Great Snackers*)	60	1.0	8.0	3.0	m.q.	0	170	m.q.
toasted onion flavor (*Great Snackers*)	60	1.0	8.0	3.0	m.q.	0	120	m.q.
SNACK MIX (see also specific listings):								
(*Eagle*), 1 oz.	140	4.0	18.0	6.0	m.q.	0	370	m.q.
(*Flavor Tree* Party Mix), ¼ cup	163	3.4	12.3	11.0	m.q.	0	407	.1 c
(*Flavor Tree* Party Mix No Salt), ¼ cup	163	3.9	13.2	10.8	m.q.	0	8	.1 c
(*Pepperidge Farm* Classic), 1 oz.	140	4.0	14.0	8.0	1.0	0	360	1.0 d
(*Ralston Chex* Traditional), 1 oz. or ⅔ cup	120	3.0	19.0	5.0	m.q.	0	320	m.q.
(*Super Snax*), 1 oz.	137	3.4	17.0	6.5	m.q.	0	207	m.q.
cheddar, golden (*Ralston Chex*), 1 oz. or ⅔ cup	130	3.0	19.0	5.0	m.q.	n.a.	300	m.q.
cheese, nacho (*Ralston Chex*), 1 oz. or ⅔ cup	130	3.0	19.0	5.0	m.q.	n.a.	430	m.q.
lightly smoked (*Pepperidge Farm*), 1 oz.	150	4.0	13.0	9.0	1.0	0	350	1.0 d
sour cream, cool, and onion (*Ralston Chex*), 1 oz. or ⅔ cup	130	3.0	19.0	5.0	m.q.	n.a.	300	m.q.
spicy (*Pepperidge Farm*), 1 oz.	140	4.0	14.0	8.0	2.0	<5	340	1.0 d
SNAIL, SEA, see "Whelk"								
SNAP BEAN, see "Green bean"								

Food and Measure	cal.	prot. (gms)	carbo. (gms)	tot. fat (gms)	sat. fat (gms)	chol. (mgs)	sod. (mgs)	fiber (gms)
SNAPPER, mixed species, meat only:								
raw:								
1 lb.	452	93.0	0	6.1	1.3	168	291	0
1 oz.	28	5.8	0	.4	.1	10	18	0
1 fillet, approx. 7.7 oz., yield from 3-lb. whole fish	217	44.7	0	2.9	.6	81	140	0
baked, broiled, or microwaved[1], 4 oz.	145	3.0	0	2.0	.1	53	65	0
SNOW PEAS, see "Peas, edible-podded"								
SOBA, see "Noodles, Japanese"								
SODA, see "Soft drinks and mixers"								
SOFT DRINKS AND MIXERS:								
all flavors (*Natural 90* Diet), 6 fl. oz.	2	0	<1.0	0	0	0	<10	0
berry, red (*Shasta*), 12 fl. oz.	158	0	43.0	0	0	0	20	0
berry, wild (*Health Valley*), 12 fl. oz.	142	1.0	33.0	1.0	(0)	0	27	0
blackberry (*Schweppes* Royal), 6 fl. oz.	35	0	8.0	0	0	0	<5	0
cherry, black (*Shasta*), 12 fl. oz. ...	162	0	44.0	0	0	0	29	0
cherry, wild (*Schweppes* Royal), 6 fl. oz.	35	0	8.0	0	0	0	<5	0
cherry cola:								
(*Coca-Cola*), 6 fl. oz.	76	0	20.0	0	0	0	4	0
(*Diet Coke*), 6 fl. oz.	<1	0	.2	0	0	0	4	0
(*Diet Wild Cherry Pepsi*), 12 fl. oz.	1	0	n.a.	0	0	0	2	0
(*Pepsi* Wild Cherry), 12 fl. oz. ...	163	0	43.2	0	0	0	2	0
(*Shasta*), 12 fl. oz.	140	0	38.0	0	0	0	22	0
cherry-lime (*Spree*), 12 fl. oz.	158	0	43.0	0	0	0	2	0
chocolate (*Yoo-Hoo*), 9 fl. oz.	140	3.0	27.0	1.0	(0)	(0)	130	0
citrus, tropical (*Schweppes* Royal), 6 fl. oz.	35	0	8.0	0	0	0	<5	0
citrus mist (*Shasta*), 12 fl. oz.	170	0	46.0	0	0	0	19	0
club soda:								
(*Schweppes*), 6 fl. oz.	0	0	0	0	0	0	25	0
(*Shasta*), 12 fl. oz.	0	0	0	0	0	0	46	0
cola:								
(*Coca-Cola* Regular/Caffeine-free), 6 fl. oz.	77	0	20.0	0	0	0	4	0
(*Coca-Cola* Classic), 6 fl. oz.	72	0	19.0	0	0	0	7	0
(*Diet Coke* Regular/Caffeine-free), 6 fl. oz.	<1	0	.2	0	0	0	4	0
(*Diet Pepsi* Regular/Caffeine-free), 12 fl. oz.	<1	0	.2	0	0	0	2	0
(*Jolt*), 6 fl. oz.	85	0	20.7	0	0	0	10	0
(*Pathmark* No Frills Sugar Free), 8 fl. oz.	0	0	tr.	0	0	0	m.q.	0

1. *Without added ingredients.*

Food and Measure	cal.	prot. (gms)	carbo. (gms)	tot. fat (gms)	sat. fat (gms)	chol. (mgs)	sod. (mgs)	fiber (gms)
(*Pepsi* Regular/Caffeine-free),								
12 fl. oz.	160	0	39.6	0	0	0	2	0
(*Pepsi Light*), 12 fl. oz.	<1	0	.1	0	0	0	2	0
(*Shasta*), 12 fl. oz.	147	0	40.0	0	0	0	3	0
(*Shasta* Free), 12 fl. oz.	151	0	41.0	0	0	0	2	0
(*Spree*), 12 fl. oz.	147	0	40.0	0	0	0	1	0
(*Tab* Regular/Caffeine-free),								
6 fl. oz.	<1	0	.2	0	0	0	4	0
cherry, see "cherry cola," above								
collins mixer:								
(*Canada Dry*), 8 fl. oz.	80	0	20.0	0	0	0	17	0
(*Schweppes*), 6 fl. oz.	75	0	18.0	0	0	0	51	0
(*Shasta*), 12 fl. oz.	118	0	32.0	0	0	0	23	0
cream:								
(*A&W*), 1 fl. oz.	14	.1	3.6	tr.	0	0	2	0
(*A&W* Diet), 1 fl. oz.	<1	.1	0	<.1	0	0	4	0
(*Shasta* Creme), 12 fl. oz.	154	0	42.0	0	0	0	23	0
(*Dr. Diablo*), 12 fl. oz.	140	0	38.0	0	0	0	14	0
(*Dr Pepper* Regular/Caffeine-free),								
12 fl. oz.	150	0	38.4	0	0	0	18	0
(*Dr Pepper* Diet Regular/Caffeine-								
free), 12 fl. oz.	3	0	.2	0	0	0	18	0
(*Fresca*), 6 fl. oz.	2	0	.2	0	0	0	tr.	0
fruit punch (*Shasta*), 12 fl. oz.	173	0	47.0	0	0	0	32	0
ginger ale:								
(*Canada Dry*), 8 fl. oz.	90	0	21.0	0	0	0	7	0
(*Canada Dry* Golden), 8 fl. oz. . . .	100	0	24.0	0	0	0	24	0
(*Fanta*), 6 fl. oz.	63	0	16.0	0	0	0	14	0
(*Health Valley*), 12 fl. oz.	153	1.0	35.0	1.0	0	0	30	0
(*Schweppes*), 6 fl. oz.	65	0	16.0	0	0	0	10	0
(*Schweppes* Sugar Free), 6 fl. oz.	2	0	<1.0	0	0	0	39	0
(*Shasta*), 12 fl. oz.	120	0	33.0	0	0	0	23	0
(*Spree*), 12 fl. oz.	120	0	33.0	0	0	0	1	0
raspberry (*Schweppes*), 6 fl. oz. . .	65	0	16.0	0	0	0	10	0
raspberry (*Schweppes* Diet),								
6 fl. oz.	2	0	<1.0	0	0	0	55	0
ginger beer (*Schweppes*), 6 fl. oz. . . .	70	0	17.0	0	0	0	30	0
grape:								
(*Canada Dry* Concord), 8 fl. oz. . .	130	0	32.0	0	0	0	21	0
(*Fanta*), 6 fl. oz.	86	0	22.0	0	0	0	7	0
(*Schweppes*), 6 fl. oz.	95	0	23.0	0	0	0	15	0
(*Shasta*), 12 fl. oz.	177	0	48.0	0	0	0	34	0
grapefruit:								
(*Schweppes*), 6 fl. oz.	80	0	20.0	0	0	0	28	0
(*Spree*), 12 fl. oz.	154	0	42.0	0	0	0	1	0
(*Wink*), 8 fl. oz.	120	0	30.0	0	0	0	19	0
half & half (*Canada Dry*), 8 fl. oz. . .	110	0	26.0	0	0	0	17	0
kiwi-passion fruit (*Schweppes* Royal),								
6 fl. oz.	35	0	8.0	0	0	0	<5	0

Food and Measure	cal.	prot. (gms)	carbo. (gms)	tot. fat (gms)	sat. fat (gms)	chol. (mgs)	sod. (mgs)	fiber (gms)
SOFT DRINKS AND MIXERS *(cont.)*								
lemon, bitter (*Schweppes*), 6 fl. oz.	82	0	20.0	0	0	0	13	0
lemon, sour (*Schweppes*), 6 fl. oz. ..	79	0	19.0	0	0	0	12	0
lemon-lime:								
(*Diet Slice*), 12 fl. oz.	16	0	2.4	0	0	0	<69	0
(*Schweppes*), 6 fl. oz.	72	0	18.0	0	0	0	30	0
(*Shasta*), 12 fl. oz.	146	0	39.0	0	0	0	19	0
(*Slice*), 12 fl. oz.	150	0	38.4	0	0	0	<69	0
(*Spree*), 12 fl. oz.	154	0	42.0	0	0	0	1	0
lemon-tangerine (*Spree*), 12 fl. oz. ..	165	0	45.0	0	0	0	1	0
lime, Mandarin (*Spree*), 12 fl. oz. ...	154	0	42.0	0	0	0	1	0
(*Mello Yello*), 6 fl. oz.	87	0	22.0	0	0	0	14	0
(*Mello Yello* Diet), 6 fl. oz.	3	0	.2	0	0	0	<1	0
(*Mountain Dew*), 12 fl. oz.	179	0	44.4	0	0	0	31	0
(*Mountain Dew* Diet), 12 fl. oz.	4	0	.7	0	0	0	<1	0
(*Mr. Pibb*), 6 fl. oz.	71	0	19.0	0	0	0	10	0
orange:								
(*Diet Slice*), 12 fl. oz.	12	0	2.3	0	0	0	2	0
(*Fanta*), 6 fl. oz.	88	0	23.0	0	0	0	7	0
(*Minute Maid*), 6 fl. oz.	87	0	22.0	0	0	0	tr.	0
(*Minute Maid* Diet), 6 fl. oz.	3	0	.4	0	0	0	tr.	0
(*Shasta*), 12 fl. oz.	177	0	48.0	0	0	0	28	0
Mandarin (*Slice*), 12 fl. oz.	193	0	50.4	0	0	0	<1	0
sparkling (*Schweppes*), 6 fl. oz. ...	88	0	22.0	0	0	0	17	0
peaches 'n cream (*Schweppes* Royal),								
6 fl. oz.	35	0	8.0	0	0	0	<5	0
pop, red (*Shasta*), 12 fl. oz.	158	0	43.0	0	0	0	20	0
raspberry, wild (*Schweppes* Royal),								
6 fl. oz.	35	0	8.0	0	0	0	<5	0
root beer:								
(*A&W*), 1 fl. oz.	15	<.1	3.5	<.1	0	0	5	0
(*A&W* Diet), 1 fl. oz.	<1	.1	0	tr.	0	0	4	0
(*Diet Mug*), 12 fl. oz.	4	0	1.2	0	0	0	39	0
(*Fanta*), 6 fl. oz.	78	0	20.0	0	0	0	10	0
(*Health Valley* Old Fashioned),								
12 fl. oz.	120	1.0	26.0	1.0	0	0	12	0
(*Mug*), 12 fl. oz.	168	0	42.0	0	0	0	39	0
(*Ramblin'*), 6 fl. oz.	88	0	23.0	0	0	0	17	0
(*Schweppes*), 6 fl. oz.	76	0	19.0	0	0	0	17	0
(*Shasta*), 12 fl. oz.	154	0	42.0	0	0	0	31	0
(*Spree*), 12 fl. oz.	154	0	42.0	0	0	0	2	0
sarsaparilla root beer (*Health Valley*),								
12 fl. oz.	153	1.0	35.0	1.0	0	0	27	0
seltzer:								
(*Schweppes* Low Sodium), 6 fl. oz.	0	0	0	0	0	0	7	0
(*Schweppes* Sodium-free), 6 fl. oz.	0	0	0	0	0	0	<5	0
flavored, all flavors (*Schweppes*),								
6 fl. oz.	0	0	0	0	0	0	<5	0

Food and Measure	cal.	prot. (gms)	carbo. (gms)	tot. fat (gms)	sat. fat (gms)	chol. (mgs)	sod. (mgs)	fiber (gms)
(7•Up), 12 fl. oz.	144	0	36.2	0	0	0	32	0
(7•Up Cherry), 12 fl. oz.	148	0	38.7	0	0	0	32	0
(7•Up Diet), 12 fl. oz.	4	0	0	0	0	0	32	0
(7•Up Diet Cherry), 12 fl. oz.	4	0	tr.	0	0	0	32	0
(Sprite), 6 fl. oz.	71	0	18.0	0	0	0	23	0
(Sprite Diet), 6 fl. oz.	2	0	0	0	0	0	tr.	0
strawberry (Shasta), 12 fl. oz.	147	0	40.0	0	0	0	36	0
strawberry-banana (Schweppes								
Royal), 6 fl. oz.	35	0	8.0	0	0	0	<5	0
sugar free, see specific flavors								
tonic:								
(Canada Dry), 8 fl. oz.	90	0	22.0	0	0	0	7	0
(Schweppes), 6 fl. oz.	64	0	16.0	0	0	0	8	0
(Schweppes Diet), 6 fl. oz.	2	0	<1.0	0	0	0	45	0
(Shasta), 12 fl. oz.	121	0	33.0	0	0	0	17	0
tropical blend (Spree), 12 fl. oz.	146	0	41.0	0	0	0	2	0
vanilla bean (Schweppes Royal),								
6 fl. oz.	35	0	8.0	0	0	0	<5	0
vichy water (Schweppes), 6 fl. oz. ...	0	0	0	0	0	0	76	0
whiskey sour mixer (Canada Dry),								
8 fl. oz.	90	0	22.0	0	0	0	17	0
SOLE, see "Flatfish"								
SOLE, FROZEN:								
(Gorton's Fishmarket Fresh), 5 oz. ..	110	24.0	1.0	1.0	m.q.	m.q.	140	0
Atlantic (Booth), 4 oz.	90	19.0	0	1.0	m.q.	m.q.	180	0
fillets (SeaPak), 4 oz.	90	20.0	0	1.0	m.q.	m.q.	135	0
fillets (Van de Kamp's Natural), 4 oz.	100	22.0	0	2.0	1.0	35	105	0
SOLE DINNER, frozen:								
au gratin (Healthy Choice), 11 oz. ...	270	16.0	40.0	5.0	3.0	55	470	m.q.
SOLE ENTREE, frozen:								
in lemon butter (Gorton's Microwave								
Entrees), 1 pkg.	380	25.0	17.0	24.0	11.0	120	560	m.q.
w/lemon butter sauce (Healthy								
Choice), 8.25 oz.	230	16.0	33.0	4.0	2.0	45	390	m.q.
fillets, breaded (Mrs. Paul's Light),								
1 piece	240	16.0	20.0	10.0	m.q.	50	450	m.q.
fillets, breaded (Van de Kamp's								
Light), 1 piece	250	17.0	18.0	12.0	2.0	45	480	m.q.
SOMEN, see "Noodles, Japanese"								
SORBET (see also "Sherbet" and								
"Ice"):								
orange, Mandarin (Dole), 4 oz.	110	.5	28.0	.1	(0)	0	9	n.a.
peach (Dole), 4 oz.	120	.6	28.0	.6	n.a.	0	11	n.a.
pineapple (Dole), 4 oz.	120	.5	28.0	.1	(0)	0	11	n.a.
raspberry:								
(Dole), 4 oz.	110	.4	28.0	<.1	n.a.	0	12	n.a.
(Frusen Glädjé), ½ cup	140	0	36.0	0	0	0	10	n.a.

Food and Measure	cal.	prot. (gms)	carbo. (gms)	tot. fat (gms)	sat. fat (gms)	chol. (mgs)	sod. (mgs)	fiber (gms)
SORBET, RASPBERRY *(cont.)*								
red (*Baskin-Robbins*), 1 regular								
scoop	140	0	34.0	0	0	0	25	n.a.
strawberry (*Dole*), 4 oz.	110	.5	28.0	.1	(0)	0	1	n.a.
and vanilla ice cream:								
blueberry (*Häagen-Dazs*), ½ cup	190	3.0	25.0	8.0	m.q.	m.q.	35	n.a.
Key lime (*Häagen-Dazs*), ½ cup	200	2.0	29.0	7.0	m.q.	m.q.	30	n.a.
orange (*Häagen-Dazs*), ½ cup ...	190	3.0	27.0	8.0	m.q.	m.q.	35	n.a.
raspberry (*Häagen-Dazs*), ½ cup	180	2.0	23.0	8.0	m.q.	m.q.	35	n.a.
SORGHUM, whole grain:								
1 oz.	96	3.2	21.2	.9	.1	0	n.a.	.7 c
1 cup	650	21.7	143.3	6.3	.9	0	n.a.	4.6 c
SORGHUM SYRUP:								
½ cup	424	0	112.2	0	0	0	n.a.	0
1 tbsp.	53	0	14.0	0	0	0	n.a.	0
SORREL, see "Dock"								
SOUP, CANNED, READY-TO-SERVE:								
bean (*Grandma Brown's*), 1 cup	190	9.0	30.9	3.4	m.q.	<1	700	9.8 d
bean, black (*Health Valley*), 7½ oz.	160	7.0	24.0	3.0	m.q.	0	285	17.0 d
bean, black (*Health Valley* No Salt								
Added), 7½ oz.	160	7.0	24.0	3.0	m.q.	0	20	17.0 d
bean w/bacon and ham (*Campbell's*								
Microwave), 7½ oz.	230	8.0	38.0	5.0	m.q.	m.q.	830	m.q.
bean w/ham:								
(*Campbell's* Home Cookin'),								
10¾-oz. can	210	14.0	29.0	4.0	m.q.	m.q.	1000	m.q.
(*Campbell's* Home Cookin'),								
9½ oz.	180	12.0	25.0	4.0	m.q.	m.q.	890	m.q.
chowder (*Hormel Micro-Cup*								
Hearty Soups), 1 cont.	191	10.0	31.0	3.0	m.q.	30	664	m.q.
chunky:								
1 can, 19¼ oz.	519	28.3	60.9	19.1	7.5	49	2184	m.q.
1 cup	231	12.6	27.1	8.5	3.3	22	972	m.q.
(*Campbell's* Chunky Old								
Fashioned), 11-oz. can	290	14.0	38.0	9.0	m.q.	n.a.	1110	m.q.
(*Campbell's* Chunky Old								
Fashioned), 9⅝ oz.	250	12.0	33.0	8.0	m.q.	n.a.	960	m.q.
beef:								
(*Progresso*), 10½-oz. can	180	15.0	17.0	6.0	m.q.	35	840	m.q.
(*Progresso*), 9½ oz.	160	13.0	15.0	5.0	m.q.	35	760	m.q.
chunky:								
1 can, 19 oz.	383	26.3	43.9	11.6	5.7	32	1947	1.6 c
1 cup	171	11.7	19.6	5.1	2.6	14	867	.7 c
(*Campbell's* Chunky), 10¾ oz.	200	15.0	24.0	5.0	m.q.	m.q.	1100	m.q.
(*Campbell's* Chunky), 9½ oz. ..	170	13.0	21.0	4.0	m.q.	m.q.	970	m.q.
hearty (*Progresso*), 9½ oz.	160	15.0	15.0	4.0	2.0	35	820	m.q.
beef, Stroganoff style (*Campbell's*								
Chunky), 10¾-oz. can	320	15.0	28.0	16.0	m.q.	m.q.	1230	m.q.

(handwritten note at left margin): 21.33c →
p/o2

Food and Measure	cal.	prot. (gms)	carbo. (gms)	tot. fat (gms)	sat. fat (gms)	chol. (mgs)	sod. (mgs)	fiber (gms)
beef barley (*Progresso*), 10½-oz. can	150	13.0	16.0	5.0	m.q.	30	870	3.0 d
beef barley (*Progresso*), 9½ oz.	140	12.0	16.0	4.0	m.q.	30	780	3.0 d
beef broth:								
(*College Inn*), 1 cup	18	2.0	1.0	0	0	m.q.	1280	0
(*Health Valley*), 7½ oz.	17	1.0	2.0	1.0	n.a.	1	420	0
(*Health Valley* No Salt Added),								
7½ oz.	17	1.0	2.0	1.0	n.a.	1	0	0
(*Swanson*), 7¼ oz.	18	2.0	0	1.0	n.a.	m.q.	750	0
or bouillon, 14-oz. can	27	4.5	.2	.9	.4	1	1294	tr.c
or bouillon, 1 cup	16	2.7	.1	.5	.3	tr.	782	tr.c
seasoned (*Progresso*), 4 oz.	10	2.0	<1.0	<1.0	n.a.	0	380	0
beef minestrone (*Progresso*),								
10½-oz. can	180	15.0	18.0	6.0	m.q.	35	1000	m.q.
beef minestrone (*Progresso*), 9½ oz.	170	13.0	16.0	5.0	m.q.	30	910	m.q.
beef noodle (*Progresso*), 9½ oz.	170	15.0	18.0	4.0	m.q.	40	1030	m.q.
beef w/vegetables and pasta:								
(*Campbell's* Home Cookin'),								
10¾ oz.	140	12.0	18.0	2.0	m.q.	m.q.	1060	m.q.
(*Campbell's* Home Cookin'),								
9½ oz.	120	10.0	16.0	2.0	m.q.	m.q.	940	m.q.
beef vegetable:								
(*Hormel Micro-Cup* Hearty								
Soups), 1 cont.	71	5.0	12.0	1.0	m.q.	9	811	m.q.
(*Lipton Hearty Ones*), 11-oz. cont.	229	10.4	40.0	3.0	m.q.	29	921	m.q.
(*Progresso*), 10½-oz. can	170	17.0	18.0	3.0	m.q.	40	880	m.q.
(*Progresso*), 9½ oz.	150	15.0	16.0	3.0	m.q.	35	790	m.q.
berry fruit, three (*Great*								
Impressions), 6 oz.	107	.5	25.8	.2	n.a.	0	90	m.q.
blueberry fruit (*Great Impressions*),								
6 oz.	95	.4	22.5	.3	n.a.	0	92	m.q.
borscht:								
(*Gold's*), 8 oz.	100	4.0	21.0	0	0	0	1280	m.q.
(*Rokeach*), 1 cup	96	.8	23.0	.3	(0)	0	985	.3 c
(*Rokeach* Unsalted), 1 cup	103	.8	23.0	.3	(0)	0	50	.5 c
(*Rokeach Diet*), 1 cup	29	.8	5.8	.2	(0)	0	897	.8 c
w/beets (*Manischewitz*), 1 cup ...	80	1.0	20.0	0	0	0	660	m.q.
low calorie (*Gold's*), 8 oz.	20	1.0	5.0	<1.0	0	0	1160	m.q.
low calorie (*Manischewitz*), 1 cup	20	1.0	4.0	0	0	0	725	m.q.
broth, see specific listings								
cherry fruit (*Great Impression*),								
6 oz.	123	.6	29.6	.2	n.a.	0	88	m.q.
chickarina (*Progresso*), 9½ oz.	130	8.0	13.0	5.0	m.q.	20	820	m.q.
chicken:								
(*Progresso* Homestyle), 9½ oz. ..	110	11.0	12.0	3.0	m.q.	20	740	n.a.
chunky:								
1 can, 10¾ oz.	216	15.4	21.0	8.1	2.4	37	1078	.3 c
1 cup	178	12.7	17.3	6.6	2.0	30	887	.3 c
(*Campbell's* Chunky Old								
Fashioned), 10¾-oz. can	180	12.0	21.0	5.0	m.q.	m.q.	1220	n.a.

Food and Measure	cal.	prot. (gms)	carbo. (gms)	tot. fat (gms)	sat. fat (gms)	chol. (mgs)	sod. (mgs)	fiber (gms)
SOUP, CANNED, READY-TO-SERVE, CHICKEN *(cont.)*								
(*Campbell's* Chunky Old								
Fashioned), 9½ oz.	150	10.0	18.0	4.0	m.q.	m.q.	1070	n.a.
hearty (*Progresso*), 10½-oz. can	130	14.0	9.0	4.0	m.q.	30	960	n.a.
hearty (*Progresso*), 9½ oz.	130	13.0	11.0	4.0	m.q.	25	900	n.a.
chicken, cream of (*Progresso*),								
9½ oz.	190	10.0	12.0	11.0	m.q.	35	970	m.q.
chicken barley (*Progresso*), 9¼ oz.	100	10.0	12.0	2.0	m.q.	20	740	3.5 d
chicken broth:								
(*Campbell's* Low Sodium),								
10½ oz.	30	3.0	2.0	1.0	n.a.	m.q.	85	0
(*College Inn*), 1 cup	35	1.0	0	3.0	m.q.	m.q.	1320	0
(*Hain*), 8¾ oz.	70	2.0	0	6.0	m.q.	5	870	0
(*Hain* No Salt Added), 8¾ oz. ...	60	3.0	0	5.0	m.q.	5	75	0
(*Health Valley*), 7½ oz.	35	4.0	1.0	2.0	m.q.	2	410	0
(*Health Valley* No Salt Added),								
7½ oz.	35	4.0	1.0	2.0	m.q.	2	0	0
(*Progresso*), 4 oz.	8	2.0	0	0	0	<5	360	0
(*Swanson*), 7¼ oz.	30	2.0	2.0	2.0	m.q.	m.q.	900	0
(*Swanson* Natural Goodness),								
7¼ oz.	20	2.0	1.0	1.0	n.a.	m.q.	580	0
chicken corn chowder (*Campbell's*								
Chunky), 10¾ oz.	340	14.0	23.0	21.0	m.q.	m.q.	1200	m.q.
chicken corn chowder (*Campbell's*								
Chunky), 9½ oz.	300	12.0	21.0	19.0	m.q.	m.q.	1060	m.q.
chicken gumbo, w/sausage								
(*Campbell's* Home Cookin'),								
10¾ oz.	140	11.0	15.0	4.0	m.q.	m.q.	1090	m.q.
chicken gumbo, w/sausage								
(*Campbell's* Home Cookin'),								
9½ oz.	120	9.0	13.0	3.0	m.q.	m.q.	960	m.q.
chicken minestrone:								
(*Campbell's* Home Cookin'),								
10¾ oz.	180	15.0	17.0	6.0	m.q.	m.q.	950	m.q.
(*Campbell's* Home Cookin'),								
9½ oz.	160	13.0	15.0	5.0	m.q.	m.q.	840	m.q.
(*Progresso*), 10½-oz. can	140	12.0	14.0	4.0	m.q.	20	1060	m.q.
(*Progresso*), 9½ oz.	130	12.0	12.0	3.0	m.q.	20	870	m.q.
chicken mushroom, creamy								
(*Campbell's* Chunky),								
10½-oz. can	270	12.0	13.0	19.0	m.q.	m.q.	1280	m.q.
chicken mushroom, creamy								
(*Campbell's* Chunky), 9⅜ oz. ...	240	10.0	12.0	17.0	m.q.	m.q.	1140	m.q.
chicken w/noodles:								
(*Campbell's* Home Cookin'),								
10¾-oz. can	140	13.0	12.0	4.0	m.q.	m.q.	1150	m.q.
(*Campbell's* Home Cookin'),								
9½ oz.	110	11.0	10.0	3.0	m.q.	m.q.	1020	m.q.

Food and Measure	cal.	prot. (gms)	carbo. (gms)	tot. fat (gms)	sat. fat (gms)	chol. (mgs)	sod. (mgs)	fiber (gms)
(*Campbell's* Low Sodium),								
10¾ oz.	170	13.0	17.0	5.0	m.q.	m.q.	90	m.q.
chicken noodle:								
(*Campbell's* Chunky), 10¾-oz.								
can	200	14.0	20.0	7.0	m.q.	m.q.	1140	m.q.
(*Campbell's* Chunky), 9½ oz.	180	12.0	18.0	7.0	m.q.	m.q.	1000	m.q.
(*Campbell's* Microwave), 7½ oz. . .	100	5.0	11.0	4.0	m.q.	m.q.	870	m.q.
(*Hain*), 9½ oz.	120	9.0	11.0	4.0	m.q.	20	980	m.q.
(*Hain* No Salt Added), 9½ oz. . . .	120	9.0	12.0	4.0	m.q.	25	90	m.q.
(*Hormel Micro-Cup* Hearty								
Soups), 1 cont.	108	7.0	14.0	3.0	m.q.	22	686	m.q.
(*Lipton Hearty Ones* Homestyle),								
11-oz. cont.	227	10.1	37.4	4.0	m.q.	37	989	m.q.
(*Progresso*), 10½-oz. can	120	12.0	8.0	4.0	m.q.	40	970	m.q.
(*Progresso*), 9½ oz.	120	11.0	10.0	4.0	m.q.	40	920	m.q.
(*Weight Watchers*), 10½ oz.	80	6.0	9.0	2.0	m.q.	m.q.	1230	m.q.
w/meatballs, 1 can, 20 oz.	227	18.5	19.1	8.2	2.4	23	2376	1.3 c
w/meatballs, 1 cup	99	8.1	8.4	3.6	1.1	10	1039	.6 c
chicken nuggets, w/vegetables and								
noodles (*Campbell's* Chunky),								
10¾-oz. can	190	11.0	24.0	6.0	m.q.	m.q.	1060	m.q.
chicken nuggets, w/vegetables and								
noodles (*Campbell's* Chunky),								
9½ oz.	170	9.0	21.0	6.0	m.q.	m.q.	940	m.q.
chicken w/rice (*Campbell's* Chunky),								
9½ oz.	140	10.0	16.0	4.0	m.q.	30	1060	m.q.
chicken w/rice (*Campbell's*								
Microwave), 7½ oz.	100	3.0	14.0	4.0	m.q.	m.q.	820	m.q.
chicken rice:								
(*Campbell's* Home Cookin'),								
10¾ oz.	150	14.0	10.0	6.0	m.q.	m.q.	1090	m.q.
(*Campbell's* Home Cookin'),								
9½ oz.	130	12.0	9.0	5.0	m.q.	m.q.	960	m.q.
(*Progresso*), 10½-oz. can	120	9.0	12.0	4.0	m.q.	25	990	m.q.
(*Progresso*), 9½ oz.	130	9.0	16.0	3.0	m.q.	25	750	m.q.
chunky, 1 can, 20 oz.	286	27.5	29.2	7.3	2.1	27	1994	m.q.
chunky, 1 cup	127	12.3	13.0	3.2	1.0	12	888	m.q.
chicken vegetable:								
(*Progresso*), 9½ oz.	140	9.0	17.0	4.0	m.q.	25	800	m.q.
chunky:								
1 can, 19 oz.	374	27.7	42.4	10.9	3.2	38	2399	m.q.
1 cup	167	12.3	18.9	4.8	1.4	17	1068	m.q.
(*Campbell's* Chunky), 9½ oz. . .	170	10.0	19.0	6.0	m.q.	25	1080	m.q.
(*Campbell's* Chunky Low								
Sodium), 10¾ oz.	240	15.0	21.0	11.0	m.q.	10	95	m.q.
(*Health Valley*), 7½ oz.	125	7.0	20.0	2.0	m.q.	11	425	4.0 d
(*Health Valley* No Salt Added),								
7½ oz.	125	7.0	20.0	2.0	m.q.	11	60	4.0 d

Food and Measure	cal.	prot. (gms)	carbo. (gms)	tot. fat (gms)	sat. fat (gms)	chol. (mgs)	sod. (mgs)	fiber (gms)
SOUP, CANNED, READY-TO-SERVE, CHICKEN VEGETABLE *(cont.)*								
and rice (*Hormel Micro-Cup*								
Hearty Soups), 1 cont.	114	5.0	16.0	3.0	m.q.	7	1025	m.q.
chili beef:								
(*Campbell's* Chunky), 11-oz. can	290	21.0	37.0	7.0	m.q.	m.q.	1120	m.q.
(*Campbell's* Chunky), 9¾ oz.	260	18.0	33.0	6.0	m.q.	m.q.	990	m.q.
(*Campbell's* Microwave), 7½ oz.	190	7.0	32.0	4.0	m.q.	m.q.	870	m.q.
clam chowder, Manhattan:								
(*Health Valley*), 7½ oz.	110	6.0	15.0	2.0	m.q.	15	510	13.4 d
(*Health Valley* No Salt Added),								
7½ oz.	110	6.0	15.0	2.0	m.q.	15	60	13.4 d
(*Progresso*), 9½ oz.	120	13.0	13.0	2.0	m.q.	10	800	m.q.
chunky:								
1 can, 19 oz.	299	16.3	42.3	7.6	4.7	32	2245	1.1 c
1 cup	133	7.3	18.8	3.4	2.1	14	1000	.5 c
(*Campbell's* Chunky),								
10¾-oz. can	160	7.0	24.0	4.0	m.q.	m.q.	1110	m.q.
(*Campbell's* Chunky), 9½ oz. ..	150	7.0	21.0	4.0	m.q.	m.q.	980	m.q.
clam chowder, New England:								
(*Campbell's* Chunky), 10¾-oz. can	290	9.0	26.0	·17.0	m.q.	m.q.	1200	m.q.
(*Campbell's* Chunky), 9½ oz.	260	8.0	23.0	15.0	m.q.	m.q.	1060	m.q.
(*Hain*), 9¼ oz.	180	8.0	26.0	4.0	.m.q.	25	780	m.q.
(*Hormel Micro-Cup* Hearty								
Soups), 1 cont.	118	5.0	15.0	5.0	m.q.	30	882	m.q.
(*Progresso*), 10½-oz. can	220	7.0	21.0	12.0	m.q.	20	1050	m.q.
(*Progresso*), 9¼ oz.	220	8.0	20.0	12.0	m.q.	m.q.	950	m.q.
corn chowder (*Progresso*), 9¼ oz. ..	200	5.0	22.0	10.0	m.q.	10	840	m.q.
crab, 1 can, 13 oz.	114	8.3	15.6	2.3	.6	15	1866	.8 c
crab, 1 cup	76	5.5	10.3	1.5	.4	10	1234	.5 c
Creole style (*Campbell's* Chunky),								
10¾ oz.	240	11.0	31.0	8.0	m.q.	n.a.	910	n.a.
Creole style (*Campbell's* Chunky),								
9½ oz.	220	10.0	28.0	7.0	m.q.	n.a.	800	n.a.
escarole:								
1 can, 19½ oz.	61	3.4	4.0	4.0	1.2	6	8618	1.7 c
1 cup	27	1.5	1.8	1.8	.5	2	3865	.7 c
in chicken broth (*Progresso*),								
9¼ oz.	30	2.0	2.0	1.0	n.a.	<5	1100	m.q.
gazpacho, 1 can, 13 oz.	87	13.1	1.2	3.4	.4	0	1790	1.2 c
gazpacho, 1 cup	57	8.7	.8	2.2	.3	0	1183	.8 c
ham and bean (*Progresso*), 9½ oz. ..	140	11.0	28.0	2.0	m.q.	10	950	8.0 d
ham and butter bean (*Campbell's*								
Chunky), 10¾-oz. can	280	12.0	34.0	10.0	m.q.	m.q.	1180	m.q.
lemon fruit (*Great Impressions*), 6 oz.	90	.2	22.1	<1.0	n.a.	0	109	m.q.
lentil:								
(*Health Valley*), 7½ oz.	170	9.0	28.0	2.0	m.q.	0	435	17.0 d
(*Health Valley* No Salt Added),								
7½ oz.	170	9.0	28.0	2.0	m.q.	0	25	17.0 d
(*Progresso*), 10½-oz. can	140	10.0	24.0	4.0	m.q.	0	1000	6.5 d

Food and Measure	cal.	prot. (gms)	carbo. (gms)	tot. fat (gms)	sat. fat (gms)	chol. (mgs)	sod. (mgs)	fiber (gms)
(*Progresso*), 9½ oz.	140	10.0	25.0	4.0	m.q.	0	840	6.5 d
hearty (*Campbell's* Home Cookin'),								
10¾-oz. can	170	11.0	28.0	2.0	m.q.	n.a.	930	m.q.
hearty (*Campbell's* Home Cookin'),								
9½ oz.	140	9.0	24.0	1.0	n.a.	n.a.	820	m.q.
vegetarian (*Hain*), 9½ oz.	160	9.0	25.0	3.0	m.q.	5	690	m.q.
vegetarian (*Hain* No Salt Added),								
9½ oz.	160	9.0	24.0	3.0	m.q.	5	65	m.q.
lentil, w/ham, 1 can, 20 oz.	320	21.2	46.3	6.4	2.6	17	3014	3.2 c
lentil, w/ham, 1 cup	140	9.3	20.2	2.8	1.1	7	1318	1.4 c
lentil, w/sausage (*Progresso*), 9½ oz.	170	8.0	21.0	8.0	m.q.	20	840	5.0 d
macaroni and bean (*Progresso*),								
10½-oz. can	150	9.0	27.0	4.0	m.q.	0	1020	8.0 d
macaroni and bean (*Progresso*),								
9½ oz.	140	8.0	25.0	5.0	m.q.	0	920	m.q.
minestrone:								
(*Campbell's* Home Cookin'),								
10¾-oz. can	140	4.0	22.0	3.0	m.q.	n.a.	1220	m.q.
(*Campbell's* Home Cookin'),								
9½ oz.	120	4.0	20.0	3.0	m.q.	n.a.	1080	m.q.
(*Hain*), 9½ oz.	170	8.0	27.0	2.0	m.q.	0	1060	m.q.
(*Hain* No Salt Added), 9½ oz. . . .	160	7.0	28.0	4.0	m.q.	0	35	m.q.
(*Health Valley*), 7½ oz.	130	6.0	19.0	3.0	m.q.	0	637	12.5 d
(*Health Valley* No Salt Added),								
7½ oz.	130	6.0	19.0	3.0	m.q.	0	80	12.5 d
(*Hormel Micro-Cup* Hearty								
Soups), 1 cont.	104	7.0	15.0	2.0	m.q.	10	903	m.q.
(*Lipton Hearty Ones*), 11-oz. cont.	189	8.0	36.1	3.2	m.q.	6	821	m.q.
(*Progresso*), 10½-oz. can	120	7.0	25.0	3.0	m.q.	0	930	7.0 d
(*Progresso*), 9½ oz.	130	7.0	22.0	4.0	m.q.	0	1010	6.0 d
chunky:								
1 can, 19 oz.	285	11.5	46.6	6.3	3.3	11	1940	m.q.
1 cup	127	5.1	20.7	2.8	1.5	5	864	m.q.
(*Campbell's* Chunky), 9½ oz. . .	160	6.0	24.0	4.0	m.q.	0	870	m.q.
hearty (*Progresso*), 9¼ oz.	110	7.0	16.0	2.0	m.q.	<5	740	m.q.
zesty (*Progresso*), 9½ oz.	150	7.0	19.0	8.0	m.q.	10	1130	4.0 d
mushroom:								
cream of:								
(*Campbell's* Low Sodium),								
10½ oz.	210	3.0	18.0	14.0	m.q.	m.q.	55	m.q.
(*Progresso*), 9¼ oz.	160	4.0	14.0	10.0	m.q.	15	1120	m.q.
(*Weight Watchers*), 10½ oz.	90	3.0	14.0	2.0	m.q.	n.a.	1250	m.q.
creamy:								
(*Hain*), 9¼ oz.	110	4.0	16.0	4.0	m.q.	15	740	m.q.
mushroom barley:								
(*Hain*), 9½ oz.	100	4.0	17.0	2.0	m.q.	10	600	m.q.
(*Health Valley*), 7½ oz.	100	5.0	16.0	2.0	m.q.	0	394	8.5 d
(*Health Valley* No Salt Added),								
7½ oz.	100	5.0	16.0	2.0	m.q.	0	20	8.5 d

Food and Measure	cal.	prot. (gms)	carbo. (gms)	tot. fat (gms)	sat. fat (gms)	chol. (mgs)	sod. (mgs)	fiber (gms)
SOUP, CANNED, READY-TO-SERVE *(cont.)*								
pea, split:								
(*Campbell's* Low Sodium),								
10¾ oz.	230	12.0	37.0	4.0	m.q.	m.q.	30	m.q.
(*Grandma Brown's*), 1 cup	208	11.7	31.0	4.1	m.q.	<1	522	5.8 d
(*Hain*), 9½ oz.	170	11.0	28.0	1.0	n.a.	0	970	m.q.
(*Hain* No Salt Added),								
9½ oz.	170	11.0	29.0	1.0	n.a.	0	40	m.q.
green:								
(*Health Valley*), 7½ oz.	190	11.0	34.0	.3	n.a.	0	276	14.7 d
(*Health Valley* No Salt Added),								
7½ oz.	190	11.0	34.0	.3	n.a.	0	25	14.7 d
(*Progresso*), 10½-oz. can	201	12.0	31.0	3.0	m.q.	n.a.	920	m.q.
(*Progresso*), 9½ oz.	160	11.0	27.0	3.0	m.q.	<5	1050	4.5 d
vegetarian (*Hain*), 9½ oz.	170	11.0	28.0	1.0	n.a.	0	970	m.q.
vegetarian (*Hain* No Salt Added),								
9½ oz.	170	130	27.0	1.0	n.a.	0	70	m.q.
pea, split, w/ham:								
(*Campbell's* Chunky), 10¾-oz.								
can	230	12.0	33.0	6.0	m.q.	m.q.	1080	m.q.
(*Campbell's* Chunky),								
9½ oz.	210	11.0	30.0	5.0	m.q.	m.q.	950	m.q.
(*Campbell's* Home Cookin'),								
10¾-oz. can	230	16.0	38.0	1.0	n.a.	m.q.	1310	m.q.
(*Campbell's* Home Cookin'),								
9½ oz.	200	14.0	34.0	1.0	n.a.	m.q.	1150	m.q.
(*Progresso*), 10½-oz. can	160	11.0	24.0	5.0	m.q.	15	980	6.0 d
(*Progresso*), 9½ oz.	150	11.0	23.0	5.0	m.q.	15	880	5.0 d
pepper steak (*Campbell's* Chunky),								
10¾-oz. can	180	14.0	24.0	3.0	m.q.	m.q.	1050	m.q.
pepper steak (*Campbell's* Chunky),								
9½ oz.	160	12.0	21.0	3.0	m.q.	m.q.	920	m.q.
potato leek (*Health Valley*),								
7½ oz.	130	4.0	23.0	2.0	m.q.	0	360	7.4 d
potato leek (*Health Valley* No Salt								
Added), 7½ oz.	130	4.0	23.0	2.0	m.q.	0	20	7.4 d
schav (*Gold's*), 8 oz.	25	2.0	4.0	0	0	15	1380	n.a.
sirloin burger (*Campbell's* Chunky),								
10¾-oz. can	220	12.0	23.0	9.0	m.q.	m.q.	1240	n.a.
sirloin burger (*Campbell's* Chunky),								
9½ oz.	200	11.0	20.0	8.0	m.q.	m.q.	1090	n.a.
steak and potato (*Campbell's*								
Chunky), 10¾-oz. can	200	14.0	24.0	5.0	m.q.	m.q.	1140	m.q.
steak and potato (*Campbell's*								
Chunky), 9½ oz.	170	12.0	21.0	4.0	m.q.	m.q.	1000	m.q.
tomato:								
(*Health Valley*), 7½ oz.	100	2.0	17.0	3.0	m.q.	0	450	1.2 d

Food and Measure	cal.	prot. (gms)	carbo. (gms)	tot. fat (gms)	sat. fat (gms)	chol. (mgs)	sod. (mgs)	fiber (gms)
(*Health Valley* No Salt Added),								
7½ oz.	100	2.0	17.0	3.0	m.q.	0	40	1.2 d
(*Progresso*), 9½ oz.	120	4.0	20.0	3.0	m.q.	0	1100	m.q.
garden (*Campbell's* Home								
Cookin'), 10¾-oz. can	150	2.0	29.0	3.0	m.q.	n.a.	930	m.q.
garden (*Campbell's* Home								
Cookin'), 9½ oz.	130	2.0	25.0	2.0	m.q.	n.a.	820	m.q.
w/tomato pieces (*Campbell's* Low								
Sodium), 10½ oz.	190	4.0	30.0	6.0	m.q.	m.q.	45	m.q.
w/tortellini (*Progresso*), 9¼ oz. ..	130	5.0	16.0	5.0	m.q.	10	1040	m.q.
tomato beef, w/rotini (*Progresso*),								
9½ oz.	170	12.0	18.0	6.0	m.q.	30	930	m.q.
tortellini (*Progresso*), 9½ oz.	90	5.0	11.0	3.0	m.q.	10	930	m.q.
tortellini, creamy (*Progresso*), 9¼ oz.	240	5.0	17.0	16.0	8.5	35	910	m.q.
turkey rice (*Hain*), 9½ oz.	100	8.0	10.0	3.0	m.q.	20	970	m.q.
turkey rice (*Hain* No Salt Added),								
9½ oz.	120	7.0	13.0	4.0	m.q.	15	85	m.q.
turkey vegetable (*Campbell's*								
Chunky), 9⅜ oz.	150	9.0	16.0	6.0	m.q.	m.q.	1060	m.q.
turkey vegetable (*Weight Watchers*),								
10½ oz.	70	4.0	10.0	2.0	m.q.	m.q.	1020	m.q.
vegetable:								
(*Health Valley*), 7½ oz.	110	4.0	20.0	1.0	n.a.	0	296	4.0 d
(*Health Valley* No Salt Added),								
7½ oz.	110	4.0	20.0	1.0	n.a.	0	40	4.0 d
(*Progresso*), 9½ oz.	80	4.0	15.0	2.0	m.q.	<5	1190	3.5 d
w/beef stock (*Weight Watchers*),								
10½ oz.	90	4.0	13.0	2.0	m.q.	m.q.	1370	m.q.
chunky:								
1 can, 19 oz.	274	7.9	42.7	8.3	1.2	0	2269	2.7 c
1 cup	122	3.5	19.0	3.7	.6	0	1010	1.2 c
(*Campbell's* Chunky), 10¾-oz.								
can	160	4.0	28.0	4.0	m.q.	0	1100	m.q.
(*Campbell's* Chunky), 9½ oz. ...	150	4.0	25.0	4.0	m.q.	0	970	m.q.
country:								
(*Campbell's* Home Cookin'),								
10¾ oz.	120	4.0	20.0	2.0	m.q.	n.a.	1070	m.q.
(*Campbell's* Home Cookin'),								
9½ oz.	100	3.0	18.0	2.0	m.q.	n.a.	940	m.q.
Hormel Micro-Cup Hearty								
Soups), 1 cont.	89	5.0	13.0	2.0	m.q.	1	865	m.q.
five bean, chunky (*Health Valley*),								
7½ oz.	110	4.0	21.0	2.0	m.q.	0	448	10.6 d
five bean, chunky (*Health Valley* No								
Salt Added), 7½ oz.	110	4.0	21.0	2.0	m.q.	0	56	10.6 d
Mediterranean (*Campbell's*								
Chunky), 9½ oz.	170	4.0	24.0	6.0	m.q.	n.a.	1010	m.q.

Food and Measure	cal.	prot. (gms)	carbo. (gms)	tot. fat (gms)	sat. fat (gms)	chol. (mgs)	sod. (mgs)	fiber (gms)
SOUP, CANNED, READY-TO-SERVE, VEGETABLE *(cont.)*								
vegetarian:								
(*Hain*), 9½ oz.	140	4.0	22.0	4.0	m.q.	0	920	m.q.
(*Hain* No Salt Added), 9½ oz.	150	5.0	23.0	5.0	m.q.	0	45	m.q.
chunky (*Weight Watchers*),								
10½ oz.	100	3.0	18.0	2.0	m.q.	0	1250	m.q.
vegetable beef:								
(*Campbell's* Chunky Low Sodium),								
10¾ oz.	180	14.0	19.0	5.0	m.q.	m.q.	90	m.q.
(*Campbell's* Chunky Old								
Fashioned), 10¾-oz. can	190	13.0	20.0	6.0	m.q.	25	1100	m.q.
(*Campbell's* Chunky Old								
Fashioned), 9½ oz.	160	12.0	17.0	5.0	m.q.	25	970	m.q.
(*Campbell's* Home Cookin'),								
10¾-oz. can	140	13.0	17.0	3.0	m.q.	m.q.	1160	m.q.
(*Campbell's* Home Cookin'),								
9½ oz.	120	11.0	15.0	2.0	m.q.	m.q.	1020	m.q.
(*Campbell's* Microwave), 7½ oz.	100	5.0	16.0	2.0	m.q.	m.q.	830	m.q.
vegetable broth (*Hain*), 9½ oz.	45	1.0	10.0	0	0	0	1180	n.a.
vegetable broth (*Hain* Low Sodium),								
9½ oz.	40	1.0	8.0	<1.0	n.a.	0	85	n.a.
vegetable chicken (*Hain*), 9½ oz. ..	120	8.0	14.0	4.0	m.q.	15	930	m.q.
vegetable chicken (*Hain* No Salt								
Added), 9½ oz.	130	8.0	14.0	4.0	m.q.	20	100	m.q.
vegetable pasta, Italian (*Hain*),								
9½ oz.	160	4.0	25.0	5.0	m.q.	20	910	m.q.
vegetable pasta, Italian (*Hain* Low								
Sodium), 9½ oz.	140	4.0	22.0	6.0	m.q.	20	90	m.q.
SOUP, CANNED, CONDENSED[1]:								
asparagus, cream of:								
undiluted, 1 can, 10¾ oz.	210	5.6	26.0	9.9	2.5	12	2385	1.8 c
1 cup	87	2.3	10.7	4.1	1.0	5	981	.7 c
1 cup[2]	161	6.3	16.4	8.2	3.3	22	1041	.7 c
(*Campbell's*), 8 oz.	80	2.0	10.0	4.0	m.q.	5	820	m.q.
barley and mushroom (*Rokeach*),								
1 cup	85	3.4	17.3	.2	n.a.	n.a.	904	m.q.
bean (*Campbell's* Homestyle), 8 oz.	130	6.0	25.0	1.0	m.q.	n.a.	700	m.q.
bean, black:								
undiluted, 1 can, 11 oz.	285	15.1	48.1	4.1	1.1	0	3026	m.q.
1 cup	116	5.6	19.8	1.5	.4	0	1198	1.3 c
bean w/bacon:								
undiluted, 1 can, 11½ oz.	420	19.2	55.3	14.4	3.7	6	2311	4.2 c
1 cup	173	7.9	22.8	5.9	1.5	3	952	1.5 c
(*Campbell's*), 8 oz.	140	6.0	21.0	4.0	m.q.	5	840	m.q.
(*Campbell's Special Request*								
⅓ Less Salt), 8 oz.	140	6.0	21.0	4.0	m.q.	5	470	m.q.

1. *Prepared according to package directions, with water, except as noted.*
2. *Prepared with whole milk.*

Food and Measure	cal.	prot. (gms)	carbo. (gms)	tot. fat (gms)	sat. fat (gms)	chol. (mgs)	sod. (mgs)	fiber (gms)
bean w/frankfurters:								
undiluted, 1 can, 11¼ oz.	454	24.2	53.4	16.9	5.1	29	2651	4.2 c
1 cup	187	10.0	22.0	7.0	2.1	12	1092	1.5 c
beef (*Campbell's*), 8 oz.	80	5.0	10.0	2.0	m.q.	10	830	m.q.
beef broth or bouillon (*Campbell's*),								
8 oz.	16	3.0	1.0	0	0	0	820	n.a.
beef noodle:								
undiluted, 1 can, 10¾ oz.	204	11.7	21.8	7.5	2.8	12	2313	.3 c
1 cup	84	4.8	9.0	3.1	1.2	5	952	tr.
(*Campbell's*), 8 oz.	70	4.0	7.0	3.0	m.q.	15	830	m.q.
(*Campbell's* Homestyle), 8 oz. . . .	80	5.0	7.0	4.0	m.q.	20	810	m.q.
broccoli, cream of (*Campbell's*), 8 oz.	80	1.0	8.0	5.0	m.q.	n.a.	790	m.q.
broccoli, cream of (*Campbell's*),								
8 oz.[1]	140	5.0	14.0	7.0	m.q.	m.q.	850	m.q.
celery, cream of:								
undiluted, 1 can, 10¾ oz.	219	4.0	21.5	13.6	3.4	34	2308	.9 c
1 cup	90	1.7	8.8	5.6	1.4	15	949	.4 c
1 cup[1]	165	5.7	14.5	9.7	4.0	32	1010	.4 c
(*Campbell's*), 8 oz.	100	2.0	8.0	7.0	m.q.	<5	820	m.q.
cheese:								
undiluted, 1 can, 11 oz.	377	13.2	25.6	25.4	16.2	72	2331	n.a.
1 cup	155	5.4	10.5	10.5	6.7	30	959	n.a.
1 cup[1]	230	9.5	16.2	14.6	9.1	48	1020	n.a.
cheddar (*Campbell's*), 8 oz.	110	4.0	10.0	6.0	m.q.	10	810	n.a.
nacho (*Campbell's*), 8 oz.	110	4.0	8.0	8.0	m.q.	n.a.	740	n.a.
nacho (*Campbell's*), 8 oz.[1]	180	8.0	13.0	12.0	m.q.	m.q.	800	n.a.
chicken alphabet (*Campbell's*), 8 oz.	80	3.0	10.0	3.0	m.q.	10	800	m.q.
chicken barley (*Campbell's*), 8 oz. . .	70	3.0	10.0	2.0	m.q.	m.q.	850	m.q.
chicken broth:								
undiluted, 1 can, 10¾ oz.	94	13.5	2.3	3.2	1.0	3	1909	tr.c
1 cup	39	4.9	.9	1.4	.4	1	776	tr.c
(*Campbell's*), 8 oz.	30	1.0	2.0	2.0	m.q.	0	710	n.a.
and noodles (*Campbell's*), 8 oz. . .	45	1.0	8.0	1.0	m.q.	10	860	m.q.
chicken, cream of:								
undiluted, 1 can, 10¾ oz.	283	8.3	22.5	17.9	5.1	24	2397	.3 c
1 cup	116	3.4	9.3	7.4	2.1	10	986	.1 c
1 cup[1]	191	7.5	15.0	11.5	4.6	27	1046	.1 c
(*Campbell's*), 8 oz.	110	2.0	9.0	7.0	m.q.	10	810	n.a.
(*Campbell's Special Request*								
⅓ Less Salt), 8 oz.	110	3.0	9.0	7.0	m.q.	10	490	n.a.
chicken and dumplings:								
undiluted, 1 can, 10½ oz.	236	13.7	14.7	13.4	3.2	80	2093	m.q.
1 cup	97	5.6	6.0	5.2	1.3	34	861	m.q.
(*Campbell's* Chicken 'n								
Dumplings), 8 oz.	80	4.0	9.0	3.0	m.q.	25	960	m.q.

1. *Prepared with whole milk.*

Food and Measure	cal.	prot. (gms)	carbo. (gms)	tot. fat (gms)	sat. fat (gms)	chol. (mgs)	sod. (mgs)	fiber (gms)
SOUP, CANNED, CONDENSED *(cont.)*								
chicken gumbo:								
undiluted, 1 can, 10¾ oz.	137	6.4	20.3	3.5	.8	9	2321	.6 c
1 cup	56	2.6	8.4	1.4	.3	5	955	.2 c
(*Campbell's*), 8 oz.	60	2.0	8.0	2.0	m.q.	5	900	m.q.
chicken mushroom, creamy								
(*Campbell's*), 8 oz.	120	3.0	8.0	8.0	m.q.	15	920	m.q.
chicken noodle:								
undiluted, 1 can, 10½ oz.	182	9.6	22.7	5.5	1.5	15	2257	.3 c
1 cup	75	4.0	9.4	2.5	.7	7	1107	.2 c
(*Campbell's*), 8 oz.	60	3.0	8.0	2.0	m.q.	15	900	m.q.
(*Campbell's* Homestyle), 8 oz. . . .	70	3.0	8.0	3.0	m.q.	15	880	m.q.
(*Campbell's* Noodle-O's), 8 oz. . . .	70	3.0	9.0	2.0	m.q.	20	820	m.q.
(*Campbell's Special Request*								
⅓ Less Salt), 8 oz.	60	3.0	8.0	2.0	m.q.	15	440	m.q.
chicken rice:								
undiluted, 1 can, 10½ oz.	146	8.6	17.4	4.7	1.1	15	1980	.3 c
1 cup	60	3.5	7.2	1.9	.5	7	814	tr.c
(*Campbell's*), 8 oz.	60	2.0	7.0	3.0	m.q.	10	790	m.q.
(*Campbell's Special Request*								
⅓ Less Salt), 8 oz.	60	2.0	7.0	3.0	m.q.	10	480	m.q.
chicken and stars (*Campbell's*), 8 oz.	60	3.0	7.0	2.0	m.q.	10	870	m.q.
chicken vegetable:								
undiluted, 1 can, 10½ oz.	181	8.8	20.9	6.9	1.7	17	2297	.3 c
1 cup	74	3.6	8.6	2.8	.9	10	944	.1 c
(*Campbell's*), 8 oz.	70	3.0	8.0	3.0	m.q.	10	850	m.q.
chili beef:								
undiluted, 1 can, 11¼ oz.	411	16.2	52.1	16.0	7.8	32	2513	3.5 c
1 cup	169	6.7	21.5	6.6	3.3	12	1035	1.5 c
(*Campbell's*), 8 oz.	140	5.0	20.0	5.0	m.q.	10	840	m.q.
clam chowder, Manhattan:								
undiluted, 1 can, 10¾ oz.	187	5.3	29.7	5.4	.9	6	2446	1.1 c
1 cup	77	2.2	12.2	2.2	.4	3	1029	.5 c
(*Campbell's*), 8 oz.	70	2.0	10.0	2.0	m.q.	0	820	m.q.
(*Doxsee*), 7.5 oz.	70	3.0	11.0	2.0	m.q.	m.q.	780	m.q.
(*Snow's*), 7.5 oz.	70	3.0	11.0	2.0	m.q.	m.q.	780	m.q.
clam chowder, New England:								
undiluted, 1 can, 10¾ oz.	214	13.2	26.5	6.1	.9	12	2266	m.q.
1 cup	95	4.8	12.4	2.9	.4	5	914	.3 c
1 cup[1]	163	9.5	16.6	6.6	3.0	22	992	m.q.
(*Campbell's*), 8 oz.	80	3.0	12.0	3.0	m.q.	5	870	m.q.
(*Campbell's*), 8 oz.[1]	150	7.0	17.0	7.0	m.q.	m.q.	930	m.q.
(*Gorton's*), ¼ can[1]	140	7.0	17.0	5.0	m.q.	15	740	m.q.
(*Snow's*), 7.5 oz.[1]	140	8.0	13.0	6.0	m.q.	m.q.	670	m.q.
consommè, w/gelatin:								
undiluted, 1 can, 10½ oz.	71	13.0	4.3	0	0	0	1550	n.a.
1 cup	29	5.4	1.8	0	0	0	637	n.a.

1. *Prepared with whole milk.*

Food and Measure	cal.	prot. (gms)	carbo. (gms)	tot. fat (gms)	sat. fat (gms)	chol. (mgs)	sod. (mgs)	fiber (gms)
beef (*Campbell's*), 8 oz.	25	4.0	2.0	0	0	0	750	n.a.
corn chowder (*Snow's*), 7.5 oz.[1]	150	5.0	18.0	6.0	m.q.	m.q.	640	m.q.
fish chowder (*Snow's*), 7.5 oz.[1]	130	9.0	11.0	6.0	m.q.	m.q.	620	m.q.
minestrone:								
undiluted, 1 can, 10½ oz.	202	10.4	27.3	6.1	1.3	3	2217	1.2 c
1 cup	83	4.3	11.2	2.5	.5	2	911	.7 c
(*Campbell's*), 8 oz.	80	3.0	13.0	2.0	m.q.	0	900	m.q.
mushroom, w/beef stock:								
undiluted, 1 can, 10¾ oz.	208	7.7	22.6	9.8	3.8	18	2358	m.q.
1 cup	85	3.2	9.3	4.0	1.6	7	970	m.q.
mushroom, beefy (*Campbell's*),								
8 oz.	60	4.0	5.0	3.0	m.q.	10	960	m.q.
mushroom, cream of:								
undiluted, 1 can, 10¾ oz.	313	4.9	22.6	23.1	6.3	3	2469	.6 c
1 cup	129	2.3	9.3	9.0	2.4	1	1031	.5 c
1 cup[1]	203	6.1	15.0	13.6	5.1	20	1076	.3 c
(*Campbell's*), 8 oz.	100	2.0	8.0	7.0	m.q.	0	820	m.q.
(*Campbell's Special Request*								
⅓ Less Salt), 8 oz.	100	2.0	8.0	7.0	m.q.	<5	480	m.q.
mushroom, golden (*Campbell's*),								
8 oz.	70	2.0	9.0	3.0	m.q.	<5	870	m.q.
noodle:								
and ground beef (*Campbell's*),								
8 oz.	90	4.0	10.0	4.0	m.q.	25	820	m.q.
curly, w/chicken (*Campbell's*),								
8 oz.	80	3.0	11.0	3.0	m.q.	15	800	m.q.
onion:								
undiluted, 1 can, 10½ oz.	138	9.1	19.9	4.2	.6	0	2563	1.2 c
1 cup	57	3.8	8.2	1.7	.3	0	1053	.5 c
cream of (*Campbell's*), 8 oz.	100	2.0	12.0	5.0	m.q.	15	830	m.q.
cream of (*Campbell's*), 8 oz.[2]	140	4.0	15.0	7.0	m.q.	m.q.	860	m.q.
French (*Campbell's*), 8 oz.	60	2.0	9.0	2.0	m.q.	<5	900	m.q.
oyster stew:								
undiluted, 1 can, 10½ oz.	144	5.1	9.9	9.3	6.1	33	2384	m.q.
1 cup	59	2.1	4.1	3.8	2.5	14	980	m.q.
1 cup[1]	134	6.1	9.8	7.9	5.1	32	1040	m.q.
(*Campbell's*), 8 oz.	70	2.0	5.0	5.0	m.q.	25	840	m.q.
(*Campbell's*), 8 oz.[1]	140	6.0	10.0	9.0	m.q.	m.q.	890	m.q.
pea, green:								
undiluted, 1 can, 11¼ oz.	398	20.9	64.4	7.1	3.4	0	2397	1.6 c
1 cup	164	8.6	26.5	2.9	1.4	0	987	.7 c
1 cup[1]	239	12.6	32.2	7.0	4.0	18	1048	.7 c
(*Campbell's*), 8 oz.	160	8.0	25.0	3.0	m.q.	5	820	m.q.
pea, split, w/egg barley (*Rokeach*),								
1 cup	132	8.2	23.6	.5	n.a.	n.a.	757	m.q.
pea, split, w/ham:								
undiluted, 1 can, 11½ oz.	459	25.0	67.8	10.7	4.3	20	2446	1.6 c

1. *Prepared with whole milk.*
2. *Prepared with 4 oz. soup, 2 oz. water, and 2 oz. whole milk.*

Food and Measure	cal.	prot. (gms)	carbo. (gms)	tot. fat (gms)	sat. fat (gms)	chol. (mgs)	sod. (mgs)	fiber (gms)
SOUP, CANNED, CONDENSED, PEA, SPLIT, W/HAM *(cont.)*								
1 cup	189	10.3	28.0	4.4	1.8	8	1008	.7 c
and bacon (*Campbell's*), 8 oz.	160	9.0	24.0	4.0	m.q.	5	780	m.q.
pepper pot:								
undiluted, 1 can, 10½ oz.	251	15.5	22.8	11.3	5.0	24	2360	1.2 c
1 cup	103	6.4	9.4	4.6	2.1	10	970	.5 c
(*Campbell's*), 8 oz.	90	5.0	9.0	4.0	m.q.	40	970	m.q.
potato, cream of:								
undiluted, 1 can, 10¾ oz.	178	4.2	27.9	5.7	3.0	15	2431	m.q.
1 cup	73	1.7	11.5	2.4	1.2	5	1000	m.q.
1 cup[1]	148	5.8	17.2	6.5	3.8	22	1060	m.q.
(*Campbell's*), 8 oz.	80	1.0	12.0	3.0	m.q.	5	870	m.q.
(*Campbell's*), 8 oz.[2]	120	3.0	15.0	4.0	m.q.	m.q.	900	m.q.
Scotch broth:								
undiluted, 1 can, 10½ oz.	195	12.1	23.0	6.4	2.7	12	2461	n.a.
1 cup	80	5.0	9.5	2.6	1.1	5	1012	n.a.
(*Campbell's*), 8 oz.	80	4.0	9.0	3.0	m.q.	10	870	n.a.
seafood chowder (*Snow's*), 7.5 oz.[1]	140	8.0	14.0	6.0	m.q.	m.q.	670	n.a.
shrimp, cream of:								
undiluted, 1 can, 10¾ cup	219	6.8	19.9	12.6	7.9	40	2373	n.a.
1 cup	90	2.8	8.2	5.2	3.2	17	976	n.a.
1 cup[1]	165	6.8	13.9	9.3	5.8	35	1036	n.a.
(*Campbell's*), 8 oz.	90	2.0	8.0	6.0	m.q.	20	810	n.a.
(*Campbell's*), 8 oz.[1]	160	5.0	13.0	10.0	m.q.	m.q.	860	n.a.
stockpot:								
undiluted, 1 can, 11 oz.	242	11.8	27.9	9.5	2.1	9	2546	1.3 c
1 cup	100	4.9	11.5	3.9	.9	5	1048	.5 c
tomato:								
undiluted, 1 can, 10¾ oz.	208	5.0	40.3	4.7	.9	0	2120	1.2 c
1 cup	86	2.1	16.6	1.9	.4	0	872	.5 c
1 cup[1]	160	6.1	22.3	6.0	2.9	17	932	.5 c
(*Campbell's*), 8 oz.	90	1.0	17.0	2.0	m.q.	0	680	m.q.
(*Campbell's*), 8 oz.[1]	150	5.0	22.0	4.0	m.q.	m.q.	740	m.q.
(*Campbell's Special Request* ⅓ Less Salt), 8 oz.	90	1.0	17.0	2.0	m.q.	0	430	m.q.
(*Campbell's Special Request* ⅓ Less Salt), 8 oz.[1]	150	5.0	22.0	4.0	m.q.	10	490	m.q.
zesty (*Campbell's*), 8 oz.	100	1.0	20.0	2.0	n.a.	n.a.	760	m.q.
tomato, cream of (*Campbell's Homestyle*), 8 oz.	110	1.0	20.0	3.0	m.q.	<5	810	m.q.
tomato, cream of (*Campbell's Homestyle*), 8 oz.[1]	180	5.0	25.0	7.0	m.q.	m.q.	860	m.q.
tomato beef w/noodle:								
undiluted, 1 can, 10¾ oz.	341	10.8	51.5	10.4	3.9	9	2230	m.q.
1 cup	140	4.5	21.2	4.3	1.6	5	917	m.q.
tomato bisque:								
undiluted, 1 can, 11 oz.	300	5.5	57.6	6.1	1.3	11	2546	m.q.

1. *Prepared with whole milk.*
2. *Prepared with 4 oz. soup, 2 oz. water, and 2 oz. whole milk.*

Food and Measure	cal.	prot. (gms)	carbo. (gms)	tot. fat (gms)	sat. fat (gms)	chol. (mgs)	sod. (mgs)	fiber (gms)
1 cup	123	2.3	23.7	2.5	.5	4	1048	m.q.
1 cup[1]	198	6.3	29.4	6.6	3.1	22	1180	m.q.
(*Campbell's*), 8 oz.	120	2.0	22.0	3.0	m.q.	<5	820	m.q.
tomato rice:								
undiluted, 1 can, 11 oz.	291	5.1	53.3	6.6	1.3	3	1981	1.6 c
1 cup	120	2.1	21.9	2.7	.5	2	815	.6 c
(*Campbell's* Old Fashioned), 8 oz.	110	1.0	22.0	2.0	m.q.	0	730	m.q.
turkey noodle:								
undiluted, 1 can, 10¾ oz.	168	9.5	21.0	4.8	1.4	12	1983	.3 c
1 cup	69	3.9	8.6	2.0	.6	5	815	.2 c
(*Campbell's*), 8 oz.	70	3.0	9.0	2.0	m.q.	15	880	m.q.
turkey vegetable:								
undiluted, 1 can, 10½ oz.	179	7.5	21.0	7.4	2.2	3	2202	m.q.
1 cup	74	3.1	8.6	3.0	.9	2	905	m.q.
(*Campbell's*), 8 oz.	70	2.0	8.0	3.0	m.q.	10	710	m.q.
vegetable:								
(*Campbell's*), 8 oz.	90	3.0	14.0	2.0	m.q.	0	830	m.q.
(*Campbell's* Homestyle), 8 oz. ...	60	2.0	9.0	2.0	m.q.	0	880	m.q.
(*Campbell's* Old Fashioned), 8 oz.	60	2.0	9.0	2.0	m.q.	0	880	m.q.
w/beef stock (*Campbell's Special*								
Request ⅓ Less Salt), 8 oz. ...	90	3.0	14.0	2.0	m.q.	<5	500	m.q.
vegetable beef:								
undiluted, 1 can, 10¾ oz.	192	13.6	24.7	4.6	2.1	12	2326	.8 c
1 cup	79	5.6	10.2	1.9	.9	5	957	.3 c
(*Campbell's*), 8 oz.	70	4.0	10.0	2.0	m.q.	10	780	m.q.
(*Campbell's Special Request*								
⅓ Less Salt), 8 oz.	70	4.0	10.0	2.0	m.q.	10	470	m.q.
vegetable w/beef broth:								
undiluted, 1 can, 10½ oz.	197	7.2	31.9	4.6	1.1	6	1969	1.5 c
1 cup	81	3.0	13.1	1.9	.4	2	810	.7 c
vegetable, vegetarian:								
undiluted, 1 can, 10½ oz.	176	5.1	29.1	4.7	.7	0	2001	1.2 c
1 cup	72	2.1	12.0	1.9	.3	0	823	.5 c
(*Campbell's*), 8 oz.	80	2.0	13.0	2.0	m.q.	0	790	m.q.
won ton (*Campbell's*), 8 oz.	40	2.0	5.0	1.0	n.a.	10	850	m.q.
SOUP, FROZEN, 6 fl. oz., except								
as noted:								
asparagus, cream of (*Kettle Ready*) ..	62	.8	5.1	4.3	1.5	n.a.	406	m.q.
asparagus, cream of (*Myers*),								
9.75 oz.	152	11.0	10.0	8.0	m.q.	n.a.	992	m.q.
barley and bean (*Tabatchnick*),								
7.5 oz.	130	6.0	22.0	2.0	m.q.	0	217	m.q.
bean:								
black w/ham (*Kettle Ready*)	154	8.1	23.0	6.2	1.3	m.q.	613	m.q.
northern (*Tabatchnick*) 7.5 oz. ...	164	8.0	29.0	2.0	m.q.	0	240	m.q.
savory, w/ham (*Kettle Ready*)	113	6.8	20.2	3.6	1.0	m.q.	459	m.q.
beef, hearty, vegetable (*Kettle Ready*)	85	4.2	10.7	3.0	.6	m.q.	448	m.q.

1. *Prepared with whole milk.*

Food and Measure	cal.	prot. (gms)	carbo. (gms)	tot. fat (gms)	sat. fat (gms)	chol. (mgs)	sod. (mgs)	fiber (gms)
SOUP, FROZEN *(cont.)*								
broccoli, cream of:								
(*Kettle Ready*)	94	.9	6.4	7.2	2.6	n.a.	417	m.q.
(*Myers*), 9.75 oz.	174	8.0	11.0	11.0	m.q.	n.a.	905	m.q.
(*Tabatchnick*), 7.5 oz.	90	4.0	10.0	4.0	m.q.	4	285	m.q.
cabbage (*Tabatchnick*), 7.5 oz.	110	2.0	21.0	2.0	m.q.	0	185	m.q.
cauliflower, cream of (*Kettle Ready*)	93	2.3	5.5	7.0	3.1	n.a.	445	m.q.
cheddar cheese:								
cream of (*Kettle Ready*)	158	4.1	7.3	12.5	6.1	n.a.	616	.1 c
and broccoli, cream of (*Kettle*								
Ready)	137	4.0	4.7	11.3	5.2	n.a.	533	n.a.
cheese and broccoli (*Myers*),								
9.75 oz.	325	12.0	19.0	23.0	m.q.	n.a.	1257	m.q.
chicken:								
(*Tabatchnick*), 7.5 oz.	65	2.0	10.0	2.0	m.q.	0	255	n.a.
cream of (*Kettle Ready*)	98	5.7	5.0	6.2	2.3	m.q.	668	n.a.
gumbo (*Kettle Ready*)	94	3.5	12.1	3.5	.7	m.q.	473	m.q.
noodle (*Kettle Ready*)	94	5.0	12.0	3.0	.6	m.q.	569	m.q.
noodle (*Myers*), 9.75 oz.	87	8.0	5.0	5.0	m.q.	m.q.	1046	m.q.
chili, jalapeño (*Kettle Ready*)	173	11.0	14.7	8.0	2.1	n.a.	531	m.q.
chili, traditional (*Kettle Ready*)	161	11.7	14.0	6.5	2.0	n.a.	454	m.q.
clam chowder:								
Boston (*Kettle Ready*)	131	3.5	13.0	7.3	1.5	m.q.	417	m.q.
Manhattan (*Kettle Ready*)	69	3.6	8.0	2.6	.5	m.q.	549	m.q.
New England:								
(*Kettle Ready*)	116	3.0	11.4	6.5	2.4	m.q.	373	m.q.
(*Myers*), 9.75 oz.	152	7.0	21.0	5.0	m.q.	m.q.	910	m.q.
(*Stouffer's*), 8 oz.	180	8.0	16.0	9.0	m.q.	m.q.	790	m.q.
corn and broccoli chowder (*Kettle*								
Ready)	102	1.4	13.0	5.0	1.8	n.a.	323	m.q.
lentil (*Tabatchnick*), 7.5 oz.	170	11.0	27.0	2.0	m.q.	0	240	m.q.
minestrone (*Tabatchnick*), 7.5 oz. . .	137	8.0	24.0	2.0	m.q.	0	265	m.q.
minestrone, hearty (*Kettle Ready*) . .	104	3.3	15.2	4.4	1.1	n.a.	577	m.q.
mushroom, cream of (*Kettle Ready*)	85	.6	6.2	6.4	2.4	n.a.	371	m.q.
mushroom, cream of (*Tabatchnick*),								
6 oz.	75	3.0	11.0	2.0	m.q.	3	325	m.q.
mushroom barley (*Tabatchnick*),								
7.5 oz.	92	2.0	16.0	2.0	m.q.	0	234	m.q.
mushroom barley (*Tabatchnick* No								
Salt), 7.5 oz.	97	4.0	18.0	1.0	n.a.	0	77	m.q.
New England chowder (*Tabatchnick*),								
7.5 oz.	98	6.0	14.0	2.0	m.q.	0	255	m.q.
onion, French (*Kettle Ready*)	42	.7	5.0	2.2	.4	n.a.	562	m.q.
pea:								
(*Tabatchnick*), 7.5 oz.	175	10.0	31.0	1.0	n.a.	0	290	m.q.
(*Tabatchnick* No Salt), 7.5 oz. . . .	175	10.0	31.0	1.0	n.a.	0	79	m.q.
split, w/ham (*Kettle Ready*)	155	11.1	25.3	4.4	1.3	m.q.	483	m.q.
tortellini, in tomato (*Kettle Ready*)	122	3.5	15.0	5.4	1.3	n.a.	447	m.q.
seafood bisque (*Myers*), 9.75 oz. . . .	163	9.0	13.0	8.0	m.q.	m.q.	1393	n.a.

Food and Measure	cal.	prot. (gms)	carbo. (gms)	tot. fat (gms)	sat. fat (gms)	chol. (mgs)	sod. (mgs)	fiber (gms)
spinach, cream of:								
(Myers), 9.75 oz.	174	9.0	10.0	11.0	m.q.	n.a.	905	m.q.
(Stouffer's), 8 oz.	210	7.0	12.0	15.0	m.q.	n.a.	1020	m.q.
(Tabatchnick), 7.5 oz.	85	5.0	12.0	2.0	m.q.	4	200	m.q.
tomato rice (Tabatchnick), 6 oz.	73	2.0	14.0	1.0	n.a.	0	300	m.q.
vegetable:								
(Tabatchnick), 7.5 oz.	97	4.0	18.0	1.0	n.a.	0	190	m.q.
(Tabatchnick No Salt), 7.5 oz. ...	92	2.0	16.0	2.0	m.q.	0	77	m.q.
vegetable, garden (Kettle Ready) ...	85	2.6	12.3	3.0	.5	n.a.	296	m.q.
vegetable beef (Myers), 9.75 oz. ...	120	9.0	8.0	6.0	m.q.	m.q.	1030	m.q.
zucchini (Tabatchnick), 6 oz.	80	3.0	12.0	2.0	m.q.	3	285	m.q.
SOUP BASE:								
beef (Tone's), 1 tsp.	11	.2	1.2	.6	n.a.	n.a.	1	n.a.
SOUP MIX[1], 6 fl. oz., except as noted:								
asparagus, cream of, 1 cup	59	2.2	9.0	1.7	.3	tr.	801	.1 c
bean with bacon, 1 cup	105	5.5	16.4	2.2	1.0	3	928	1.5 c
beef or beef flavor:								
(Lipton Cup-A-Soup)	44	1.7	7.6	.7	n.a.	n.a.	746	n.a.
broth or bouillon, 1 cup	19	1.3	1.9	.7	.3	1	1368	<.1 c
hearty, and noodles (Lipton), 7 fl. oz.	107	3.5	20.2	1.4	n.a.	n.a.	698	.2 c
noodle:								
1 cup[2]	41	2.2	6.0	.8	.3	2	1041	.1 c
(Campbell's Cup Microwave), 1.35-oz. cont.	130	6.0	23.0	2.0	m.q.	m.q.	1270	m.q.
(Campbell's Ramen Noodle), 8 fl. oz.	190	5.0	26.0	8.0	m.q.	n.a.	1010	m.q.
(Campbell's Ramen Noodle Low Fat Block), 8 fl. oz.	160	5.0	32.0	1.0	n.a.	n.a.	890	m.q.
(Estee), 6 oz.	20	1.0	3.0	<1.0	<1.0	<1	140	m.q.
w/vegetables (Campbell's Cup-A-Ramen), 8 fl. oz.	270	6.0	38.0	10.0	m.q.	n.a.	1530	m.q.
w/vegetables (Campbell's Cup-A-Ramen Low Fat), 8 fl. oz.	220	7.0	44.0	2.0	m.q.	n.a.	1600	m.q.
broccoli:								
creamy (Lipton Cup-A-Soup)	62	1.1	9.1	2.4	m.q.	n.a.	610	.3 c
creamy (Lipton Cup-A-Soup Food Service)	62	1.7	8.9	2.3	m.q.	n.a.	658	m.q.
creamy, and cheese (Lipton Cup-A-Soup)	70	1.7	9.8	3.4	m.q.	n.a.	595	m.q.
golden (Lipton Cup-A-Soup Lite)	42	1.3	6.3	1.2	n.a.	1	427	m.q.
cauliflower, 1 cup	68	2.9	10.7	1.7	.3	tr.	843	.2 c
celery, cream of, 1 cup	63	2.6	9.8	1.6	.2	1	839	.2 c
cheddar, creamy, w/noodles (Fantastic Noodles), 7 oz.	178	7.0	21.0	8.0	m.q.	n.a.	578	m.q.

1. *Prepared according to package directions, with water, except as noted.*
2. *Includes beef and macaroni and beef-flavor noodle.*

Food and Measure	cal.	prot. (gms)	carbo. (gms)	tot. fat (gms)	sat. fat (gms)	chol. (mgs)	sod. (mgs)	fiber (gms)
SOUP MIX *(cont.)*								
cheese (*Hain* Savory Soup & Sauce Mix)	250	6.0	20.0	16.0	m.q.	n.a.	890	n.a.
cheese and broccoli (*Hain* Soup & Recipe Mix)	310	7.0	19.0	22.0	m.q.	n.a.	980	m.q.
chicken or chicken flavor:								
broth or bouillon, 1 cup	21	1.3	1.4	1.1	.3	tr.	1484	<.1 c
broth (*Lipton Cup-A-Soup*)	20	.4	3.3	.6	n.a.	1	605	n.a.
cream of:								
1 cup	107	1.8	13.4	5.3	3.4	3	1184	1.2 c
(*Lipton Cup-A-Soup*)	84	1.4	9.7	4.4	m.q.	n.a.	757	n.a.
(*Lipton Cup-A-Soup* Food Service)	84	1.7	9.4	4.4	m.q.	n.a.	840	n.a.
creamy, w/vegetables (*Lipton Cup-A-Soup*)	93	1.7	14.4	3.1	m.q.	n.a.	708	m.q.
creamy, w/white meat (*Campbell's* Cup 2 Minute Soup)	90	3.0	12.0	4.0	m.q.	m.q.	1020	n.a.
w/sweet corn (*Lipton Cup-A-Soup* Country Style)	133	3.3	17.5	5.5	m.q.	n.a.	704	.2 c
Florentine (*Lipton Cup-A-Soup* Lite)	42	10.0	7.6	.5	n.a.	6	481	n.a.
hearty (*Lipton Cup-A-Soup* Country Style)	69	3.8	11.1	1.1	n.a.	n.a.	688	n.a.
hearty, supreme (*Lipton Cup-A-Soup*)	107	2.0	11.4	5.9	m.q.	n.a.	848	n.a.
lemon (*Lipton Cup-A-Soup* Lite)	48	2.0	9.1	.4	n.a.	4	419	n.a.
noodle:								
1 cup[1]	53	2.9	7.4	1.2	.3	3	1284	.1 c
(*Campbell's* Cup Microwave), 1.35-oz. cont.	140	7.0	22.0	3.0	m.q.	n.a.	1340	m.q.
(*Campbell's* Quality Soup & Recipe), 1 cup	100	5.0	16.0	2.0	m.q.	n.a.	710	m.q.
(*Campbell's* Ramen Noodle), 1 cup	190	5.0	26.0	8.0	m.q.	n.a.	970	m.q.
(*Campbell's* Ramen Noodle Low Fat Block), 1 cup	160	5.0	32.0	1.0	n.a.	n.a.	940	m.q.
(*Estee Instant*), 6 oz.	25	1.0	4.0	<1.0	<1.0	<1	135	m.q.
(*Lipton*), 1 cup	81	4.3	12.0	1.8	n.a.	n.a.	792	m.q.
(*Lipton Cup-A-Soup*)	48	3.0	6.6	1.1	n.a.	n.a.	635	m.q.
(*Mrs. Grass* Chickeny Rich), ¼ pkg.	70	2.0	10.0	2.0	m.q.	n.a.	900	m.q.
hearty (*Lipton*), 1 cup	83	4.4	13.3	1.3	n.a.	n.a.	753	m.q.
hearty (*Lipton Lots-A-Noodles Cup-A-Soup*), 7 fl. oz.	110	4.0	20.0	1.6	n.a.	n.a.	587	m.q.
hearty (*Lipton Lots-A-Noodles Cup-A-Soup,* Food Service), 7 fl. oz.	118	4.8	21.2	1.5	n.a.	n.a.	655	m.q.

1. *Includes chicken broth with noodles.*

Food and Measure	cal.	prot. (gms)	carbo. (gms)	tot. fat (gms)	sat. fat (gms)	chol. (mgs)	sod. (mgs)	fiber (gms)
hearty, creamy (*Lipton Lots-A-Noodles Cup-A-Soup*),								
7 fl. oz.	179	5.1	21.4	8.2	m.q.	n.a.	639	m.q.
w/meat (*Lipton Cup-A-Soup*) . .	46	2.6	6.6	1.0	n.a.	m.q.	660	m.q.
w/meat (*Lipton Cup-A-Soup* Value pack)	46	2.6	6.6	1.0	n.a.	m.q.	660	m.q.
w/white meat (*Campbell's* Cup 2 Minute Soup)	90	6.0	12.0	2.0	m.q.	m.q.	770	m.q.
w/white meat, diced (*Lipton*), 1 cup	81	4.3	12.1	1.8	m.q.	m.q.	795	m.q.
w/vegetables (*Campbell's* Cup-A-Ramen), 1 cup	270	6.0	38.0	10.0	m.q.	n.a.	1470	m.q.
w/vegetables (*Campbell's* Cup-A-Ramen Low Fat), 1 cup . . .	220	7.0	44.0	2.0	m.q.	n.a.	1500	m.q.
w/vegetables, hearty (*Lipton*), 1 cup	75	3.0	12.3	1.6	n.a.	n.a.	687	m.q.
rice, 1 cup	60	2.4	9.3	1.4	.3	tr.	980	m.q.
'n rice (*Lipton Cup-A-Soup*)	47	2.2	7.7	.8	n.a.	n.a.	667	m.q.
supreme (*Lipton Cup-A-Soup* Country Style)	107	1.7	11.8	5.9	m.q.	n.a.	757	m.q.
vegetable, 1 cup	49	2.7	7.8	.8	.2	3	808	m.q.
vegetable, (*Lipton Cup-A-Soup*) . .	47	2.5	7.8	.6	n.a.	8	566	.2 c
clam chowder, Manhattan (*Golden Dipt*), ¼ pkg.	80	2.0	13.0	2.0	1.0	3	700	m.q.
clam chowder, New England (*Golden Dipt*), ¼ pkg.	70	2.0	12.0	2.0	1.0	2	680	m.q.
consomme w/gelatin, 1 cup	17	2.2	2.1	<.1	tr.	0	3299	<.1 c
leek, 1 cup	71	2.1	11.4	2.1	1.0	3	966	.3 c
lentil (*Hain* Savory Soup Mix)	130	4.0	20.0	2.0	m.q.	n.a.	810	m.q.
lobster bisque (*Golden Dipt*), ¼ pkg.	30	1.0	5.0	1.0	n.a.	2	560	n.a.
minestrone:								
1 cup	79	4.4	11.9	1.7	.8	3	1026	.4 c
(*Hain* Savory Soup Mix)	110	4.0	20.0	1.0	n.a.	n.a.	870	m.q.
(*Manischewitz*)	50	3.0	9.0	<1.0	n.a.	n.a.	160	m.q.
mushroom:								
1 cup	96	2.2	11.1	4.9	.8	1	1019	.1 c
(*Estee Instant*), 6 oz.	40	1.0	3.0	2.0	1.0	10	115	m.q.
(*Hain* Savory Soup & Recipe Mix)	210	4.0	11.0	15.0	m.q.	n.a.	710	m.q.
(*Hain* Savory Soup & Recipe Mix No Salt Added)	250	5.0	15.0	20.0	m.q.	n.a.	180	m.q.
beef flavor (*Lipton*), 1 cup	38	1.7	6.7	.5	n.a.	n.a.	763	m.q.
cream of (*Lipton Cup-A-Soup*) . . .	71	1.3	9.1	3.2	m.q.	n.a.	756	m.q.
noodle:								
Campbell's Quality Soup & Recipe), 1 cup	110	5.0	19.0	2.0	m.q.	n.a.	700	m.q.
(*Lipton Cup-A-Soup* Ring Noodle)	47	2.7	7.6	.7	n.a.	n.a.	650	m.q.
beef (*Cup O'Noodles*), 1 cup	290	8.0	33.0	14.0	m.q.	n.a.	1490	m.q.
beef flavor (*Oodles of Noodles/Top Ramen*), 1 cup	390	9.0	49.0	18.0	m.q.	n.a.	1810	m.q.

Food and Measure	cal.	prot. (gms)	carbo. (gms)	tot. fat (gms)	sat. fat (gms)	chol. (mgs)	sod. (mgs)	fiber (gms)
SOUP MIX, NOODLE (cont.)								
beefy, hearty, w/vegetables								
(*Lipton*), 1 cup	85	2.5	16.7	.9	n.a.	n.a.	810	m.q.
chicken or chicken flavor:								
(*Cup O'Noodles*), 1 cup	300	9.0	32.0	16.0	m.q.	n.a.	1790	m.q.
(*Oodles of Noodles/Top Ramen*),								
1 cup	400	10.0	48.0	18.0	m.q.	n.a.	1910	m.q.
country (*Cup O'Noodles*								
Hearty), 1 cup	300	8.0	35.0	14.0	m.q.	n.a.	1210	m.q.
w/chicken broth:								
(*Campbell's* Cup Microwave),								
1.35-oz. cont.	130	6.0	23.0	2.0	m.q.	n.a.	1360	m.q.
(*Campbell's* Cup 2 Minute								
Soup)	90	4.0	15.0	2.0	m.q.	n.a.	910	m.q.
(*Lipton Giggle Noodle*), 1 cup	77	2.9	11.4	2.1	m.q.	n.a.	784	m.q.
(*Lipton Ring-O-Noodle*), 1 cup	71	2.7	10.4	2.0	m.q.	n.a.	784	m.q.
hearty (*Campbell's* Quality Soup &								
Recipe), 1 cup	90	4.0	15.0	1.0	n.a.	n.a.	840	m.q.
hearty, w/vegetables (*Lipton*),								
1 cup	75	3.0	12.3	1.6	n.a.	n.a.	687	m.q.
Oriental:								
(*Campbell's* Ramen Noodle),								
1 cup	190	5.0	26.0	8.0	m.q.	n.a.	930	m.q.
(*Campbell's* Ramen Noodle Low								
Fat Block), 1 cup	150	5.0	31.0	1.0	n.a.	n.a.	940	m.q.
(*Oodles of Noodles/Top Ramen*),								
1 cup	390	10.0	49.0	18.0	m.q.	n.a.	1660	m.q.
w/vegetables (*Campbell's* Cup-								
A-Ramen), 1 cup	270	6.0	38.0	10.0	m.q.	n.a.	1210	m.q.
w/vegetables (*Campbell's* Cup-								
A-Ramen Low Fat), 1 cup ...	220	7.0	44.0	2.0	m.q.	n.a.	1400	m.q.
pork flavor:								
(*Campbell's* Ramen Noodle),								
1 cup	200	5.0	26.0	8.0	m.q.	n.a.	860	m.q.
(*Campbell's* Ramen Noodle Low								
Fat Block), 1 cup	150	4.0	31.0	1.0	n.a.	n.a.	1140	m.q.
(*Oodles of Noodles/Top Ramen*),								
1 cup	390	10.0	51.0	20.0	m.q.	n.a.	2060	m.q.
seafood, savory (*Cup O'Noodles*								
Hearty), 1 cup	300	7.0	34.0	15.0	m.q.	n.a.	1170	m.q.
shrimp (*Cup O'Noodles*), 1 cup ...	300	10.0	32.0	14.0	m.q.	n.a.	1480	m.q.
w/vegetables, hearty (*Campbell's*								
Cup Microwave), 1.7-oz. cont.	180	7.0	32.0	2.0	m.q.	n.a.	1320	m.q.
vegetable, old fashioned (*Cup*								
O'Noodles Hearty), 1 cup	290	6.0	34.0	15.0	m.q.	n.a.	1250	m.q.
vegetable beef (*Cup O'Noodles*								
Hearty), 1 cup	290	8.0	36.0	15.0	m.q.	n.a.	1150	m.q.
onion:								
1 cup[1]	28	1.1	5.1	.6	.1	0	848	.2 c

1. *Includes French onion.*

Food and Measure	cal.	prot. (gms)	carbo. (gms)	tot. fat (gms)	sat. fat (gms)	chol. (mgs)	sod. (mgs)	fiber (gms)
(*Campbell's* Quality Soup & Recipe), 1 cup	30	1.0	7.0	0	0	0	700	m.q.
(*Estee*), 6 oz.	25	1.0	4.0	<1.0	<1.0	0	140	m.q.
(*Hain* Savory Soup, Dip & Recipe Mix)	50	2.0	6.0	2.0	m.q.	n.a.	900	m.q.
(*Hain* Savory Soup, Dip & Recipe Mix No Salt Added)	50	1.0	9.0	1.0	n.a.	n.a.	470	m.q.
(*Lipton*), 1 cup	20	.7	4.3	.2	n.a.	n.a.	632	m.q.
(*Lipton Cup-A-Soup*)	27	.9	4.7	.5	n.a.	n.a.	665	.1 c
(*Mrs. Grass* Soup & Dip Mix), ¼ pkg.	35	1.0	6.0	<1.0	n.a.	0	1070	m.q.
beefy (*Lipton*), 1 cup	29	.8	4.2	1.0	n.a.	n.a.	803	m.q.
creamy (*Lipton Cup-A-Soup*)	70	1.2	9.5	3.2	m.q.	n.a.	678	.2 c
golden, w/chicken broth (*Lipton*), 1 cup	62	1.1	11.0	1.5	n.a.	n.a.	716	m.q.
mushroom (*Lipton*), 1 cup	41	1.4	6.8	.9	n.a.	n.a.	684	m.q.
Oriental (*Lipton Cup-A-Soup* Lite) ..	45	1.5	5.8	1.7	n.a.	3	457	n.a.
oxtail, 1 cup	71	2.8	9.0	2.6	1.3	3	1210	.1 c
pea:								
green:								
(*Lipton Cup-A-Soup*)	113	4.2	14.4	4.2	m.q.	n.a.	553	.2 c
(*Lipton Cup-A-Soup* Food Service)	115	3.5	15.1	4.5	m.q.	n.a.	635	.7 c
green or split[1], 1 cup	133	7.7	22.7	1.6	.4	3	1220	.7 c
split (*Hain* Savory Soup Mix)	310	4.0	16.0	10.0	m.q.	n.a.	940	m.q.
split (*Manischewitz*)	45	3.0	9.0	<1.0	n.a.	0	320	m.q.
Virginia (*Lipton Cup-A-Soup* Country Style)	148	5.3	17.3	6.4	m.q.	n.a.	828	.8 c
Virginia (*Lipton Cup-A-Soup* Country Style Food Service) ..	113	4.7	14.6	4.1	m.q.	<1	664	.4 c
potato leek (*Hain* Savory Soup Mix)	260	4.0	20.0	18.0	m.q.	n.a.	690	m.q.
seafood chowder (*Golden Dipt*), ¼ pkg. dry	70	2.0	12.0	2.0	1.0	2	730	n.a.
shrimp bisque (*Golden Dipt*), ¼ pkg. dry	30	1.0	5.0	1.0	n.a.	2	570	n.a.
shrimp flavor, w/vegetables (*Campbell's* Cup-A-Ramen), 1 cup	280	6.0	40.0	10.0	m.q.	n.a.	1190	m.q.
shrimp flavor, w/vegetables (*Campbell's* Cup-A-Ramen Low Fat), 1 cup	230	7.0	45.0	2.0	m.q.	n.a.	1290	m.q.
tomato:								
1 cup[2]	102	2.5	19.4	2.4	1.1	1	943	.4 c
(*Estee* Instant), 6 oz.	40	1.0	5.0	<1.0	<1.0	0	95	m.q.
(*Hain* Savory Soup & Recipe Mix)	220	3.0	19.0	14.0	m.q.	n.a.	770	m.q.
(*Lipton Cup-A-Soup*)	103	2.5	21.2	.9	n.a.	n.a.	524	m.q.

1. *Includes peas with ham.*
2. *Includes cream of tomato.*

Food and Measure	cal.	prot. (gms)	carbo. (gms)	tot. fat (gms)	sat. fat (gms)	chol. (mgs)	sod. (mgs)	fiber (gms)
SOUP MIX, TOMATO *(cont.)*								
(*Lipton Cup-A-Soup* Food Service)	100	2.8	20.1	.9	n.a.	n.a.	563	m.q.
creamy, and herb (*Lipton Cup-A-Soup* Lite)	66	1.6	14.1	.3	n.a.	2	305	m.q.
vegetable [1], 1 cup	55	2.0	10.2	.9	.4	tr.	1146	.5 c
vegetable:								
(*Campbell's* Quality Soup & Recipe), 1 cup	40	1.0	8.0	0	0	0	710	m.q.
(*Hain* Savory Soup Mix)	80	2.0	13.0	1.0	n.a.	n.a.	730	m.q.
(*Hain* Savory Soup Mix No Salt Added)	80	2.0	13.0	1.0	n.a.	n.a.	330	m.q.
(*Lipton*), 1 cup	39	1.6	6.9	.5	n.a.	n.a.	640	.4 c
(*Manischewitz*)	50	3.0	9.0	<1.0	n.a.	0	65	m.q.
country (*Lipton*), 1 cup	80	2.6	15.7	.7	n.a.	n.a.	803	m.q.
cream of, 1 cup	105	1.9	12.3	5.7	1.4	0	1171	.1 c
curry, w/noodles (*Fantastic Noodles*), 7 oz.	150	5.0	18.0	7.0	m.q.	n.a.	472	m.q.
garden (*Lipton Lots-A-Noodles Cup-A-Soup*), 7 fl. oz.	123	4.3	23.1	1.5	n.a.	n.a.	720	m.q.
harvest (*Lipton Cup-A-Soup Country Style*)	91	1.7	18.8	1.2	n.a.	n.a.	459	.5 c
harvest (*Lipton Cup-A-Soup Country Style, Food Service*) ..	95	2.0	18.9	1.2	n.a.	n.a.	569	.5 c
miso, w/noodles (*Fantastic Noodles*), 7 oz.	152	5.0	19.0	7.0	m.q.	n.a.	434	m.q.
noodle, w/meatballs, (*Lipton Cup-A-Soup Country Style*)	95	4.9	15.4	1.6	n.a.	n.a.	764	.5 c
spring (*Lipton Cup-A-Soup*)	33	1.1	5.9	.8	n.a.	6	746	.3 c
tomato, w/noodles (*Fantastic Noodles*), 7 oz.	158	5.0	20.0	8.0	m.q.	n.a.	434	m.q.
vegetable beef, 1 cup	53	2.9	8.0	1.1	.6	1	1000	.2 c
SOUR CREAM, see "Cream, sour"								
SOUR CREAM SAUCE MIX:								
1.24-oz. pkt.	180	5.5	17.0	11.1	5.5	28	444	n.a.
½ cup [2]	255	9.5	22.7	15.1	8.1	46	504	n.a.
(*McCormick/Schilling*), ¼ pkg.	44	1.3	4.0	2.8	m.q.	n.a.	272	n.a.
SOUR CREAM AND CHIVE TOPPING:								
(*Tone's*), 1 tsp.	16	.3	1.1	1.2	.4	1	57	tr.d
SOUR CREAM AND ONION SNACK STICKS:								
(*Flavor Tree*), ¼ cup	127	3.0	12.5	8.3	m.q.	n.a.	360	.1 c
SOUR DRINK MIX, see "Whiskey sour mix"								

1. *Includes Italian vegetable and spring vegetable.*
2. *Prepared according to package directions, with whole milk.*

Food and Measure	cal.	prot. (gms)	carbo. (gms)	tot. fat (gms)	sat. fat (gms)	chol. (mgs)	sod. (mgs)	fiber (gms)
SOURSOP:								
untrimmed, 1 lb.	202	3.0	51.2	.9	n.a.	0	42	3.3 c
trimmed, 1 oz.	19	.3	4.8	.1	n.a.	0	4	.3 c
trimmed, ½ cup	75	1.1	18.9	.3	n.a.	0	16	1.2 c
1 medium, approx. 2.1 lb.	416	6.3	105.3	1.9	n.a.	0	87	6.9 c
SOUSE LOAF:								
(*Kahn's*), 1 slice	90	4.0	1.0	7.0	m.q.	m.q.	190	0
SOY BEVERAGE (see also "Soy milk" and specific listings):								
(*Soy Moo*), 8 fl. oz.	125	9.0	11.0	5.0	m.q.	0	55	0
flavored, 6 fl. oz.:								
almond malted (*Westbrae Natural*)	250	7.0	31.0	11.0	m.q.	0	140	m.q.
carob (*Ah Soy*)	160	4.0	30.0	3.0	m.q.	0	120	m.q.
carob malted (*Westbrae Natural*) ..	270	7.0	37.0	11.0	m.q.	0	120	m.q.
chocolate (*Ah Soy*)	160	4.0	29.0	3.0	m.q.	0	120	m.q.
java malted (*Westbrae Natural*) ...	270	7.0	37.0	11.0	m.q.	0	140	m.q.
vanilla (*Ah Soy*)	160	5.0	23.0	5.0	m.q.	0	140	m.q.
vanilla malted (*Westbrae Natural*)	250	7.0	31.0	11.0	m.q.	0	140	m.q.
SOY FLOUR:								
(*Arrowhead Mills*), 2 oz.	250	20.0	18.0	11.0	m.q.	0	1	8.1 d
full-fat:								
raw, 1 oz.	124	9.8	10.0	5.9	.8	0	4	1.3 c
raw, 1 cup, stirred	371	29.4	29.9	17.6	2.5	0	11	4.0 c
roasted, 1 oz.	125	9.9	9.5	6.2	.9	0	3	.6 c
roasted, 1 cup, stirred	375	29.6	28.6	18.6	2.7	0	11	1.9 c
defatted, 1 oz.	93	13.3	10.9	.3	<.1	0	6	1.2 c
defatted, 1 cup, stirred	329	47.0	38.4	1.2	.1	0	20	4.3 c
low-fat, 1 oz.	92	13.2	10.8	1.9	.3	0	5	1.2 c
low-fat, 1 cup, stirred	287	40.9	33.4	2.4	.9	0	16	3.7 c
SOY MEAL, defatted, raw:								
1 oz.	96	12.7	11.4	.7	.1	0	1	3.3 d
1 cup...........................	414	54.8	49.0	2.9	.3	0	3	14.0 d
SOY MILK (see also "Soy beverage"):								
fluid, 1 oz.	9	.8	.5	.5	.1	0	3	.3 d
fluid, 8 fl. oz.	79	6.6	4.3	4.6	.5	0	30	2.6 d
powder (*Soyamel*), 8 fl. oz.[1]	130	7.0	10.0	7.0	1.0	0	210	n.a.
SOY PROTEIN:								
concentrate, w/alcohol, 1 oz.	94	16.5	8.8	.1	.1	0	1	1.1 c
concentrate, acid/water wash, 1 oz.	94	16.5	8.8	.1	.1	0	255	1.1 c
isolate, w/potassium, 1 oz.	96	22.9	.2	1.0	.1	0	14	.1 c
isolate, w/sodium, 1 oz.	96	22.9	.2	1.0	.1	0	281	.1 c
SOY SAUCE:								
from soy (tamari):								
1 oz.	17	3.0	1.6	<.1	tr.	0	1584	0
1 tbsp.	11	1.9	1.0	<.1	tr.	0	1005	0
¼ cup	35	6.1	3.2	.1	tr.	0	3240	0

1. *Prepared according to package directions.*

Food and Measure	cal.	prot. (gms)	carbo. (gms)	tot. fat (gms)	sat. fat (gms)	chol. (mgs)	sod. (mgs)	fiber (gms)
SOY SAUCE *(cont.)*								
from soy and wheat (shoyu):								
1 oz.	15	1.5	2.4	<.1	tr.	0	1620	0
1 tbsp.	9	.9	1.5	tr.	tr.	0	3314	0
¼ cup	30	3.0	4.9	.1	tr.	0	3314	0
low-sodium:								
1 oz.	15	1.5	2.4	<.1	tr.	0	945	0
1 tbsp.	9	.9	1.5	tr.	tr.	0	600	0
¼ cup	30	3.0	4.9	.1	tr.	0	1933	0
from vegetable protein:								
1 oz.	12	.7	2.2	tr.	tr.	0	1613	0
1 tbsp.	7	.4	1.4	tr.	tr.	0	1024	0
¼ cup	24	1.4	4.5	.1	tr.	0	3300	0
(Kikkoman), 1 tbsp.	10	n.a.	.9	tr.	(0)	0	892	0
(Kikkoman Lite), 1 tbsp.	11	n.a.	1.3	tr.	(0)	0	600	0
(La Choy), 1 tsp.	<1	.2	.3	0	0	0	429	0
(La Choy Lite), 1 tsp.	<1	.2	.3	0	0	0	220	0
SOYBEAN, green:								
raw:								
in pods, 1 lb.	353	31.1	26.6	16.4	1.8	0	n.a.	4.0 c
shelled, 1 oz.	42	3.7	3.1	1.9	.2	0	n.a.	.6 c
shelled, ½ cup	188	16.6	14.1	8.7	.9	0	n.a.	2.6 c
boiled, drained, 4 oz.	160	14.0	12.5	7.3	.8	0	n.a.	2.1 c
boiled, drained, ½ cup	127	11.1	10.0	5.8	.6	0	n.a.	1.7 c
SOYBEAN, DRIED:								
raw:								
1 oz.	118	10.3	8.6	5.7	.8	0	1	3.5 d
½ cup	387	33.9	28.1	18.5	2.7	0	2	11.6 d
(Arrowhead Mills), 2 oz.	230	19.0	19.0	10.0	n.a.	0	2	13.2 d
boiled, 4 oz.	196	18.9	11.2	10.2	1.5	0	1	2.3 c
boiled, ½ cup	149	14.3	8.5	7.7	1.1	0	1	1.8 c
dry-roasted, 1 oz.	128	11.2	9.3	6.1	.9	0	1	1.5 c
dry-roasted, ½ cup	387	34.0	28.1	18.6	2.7	0	2	4.6 c
roasted, 1 oz.	134	10.0	9.5	7.2	1.0	0	46	1.3 c
roasted, ½ cup	405	30.3	28.9	21.8	3.2	0	140	4.0 c
SOYBEAN, FERMENTED OR PASTE, see "Miso" and "Natto"								
SOYBEAN, SPROUTED, mature seeds:								
raw:								
1 lb.	580	59.4	50.7	30.4	3.3	0	62	10.4 c
1 oz.	36	3.7	3.2	1.9	.2	0	4	.7 c
½ cup	45	4.6	3.9	2.3	.3	0	5	.8 c
10 sprouts, approx. .4 oz.	12	1.2	1.1	.6	.1	0	1	.2 c
steamed, 4 oz.	92	9.6	7.4	5.0	.5	0	11	2.2 c
steamed, ½ cup	38	4.0	3.1	2.1	.2	0	5	.9 c
stir-fried in vegetable oil, 4 oz.	142	14.9	10.7	8.1	m.q.	0	m.q.	2.8 c

Food and Measure	cal.	prot. (gms)	carbo. (gms)	tot. fat (gms)	sat. fat (gms)	chol. (mgs)	sod. (mgs)	fiber (gms)
SOYBEAN CAKE OR CURD, see "Tofu"								
SOYBEAN FLAKES:								
(*Arrowhead Mills*), 2 oz.	250	20.0	18.0	11.0	m.q.	0	2	8.1 d
SOYBEAN FLOUR, see "Soy flour"								
SOYBEAN KERNELS, roasted and toasted:								
1 oz., approx. 95 kernels	129	10.5	8.7	6.8	.9	0	1	1.0 c
whole kernels, 1 cup	490	40.0	33.0	25.9	3.4	0	4	3.8 c
salted, 1 oz.	129	10.5	8.7	6.8	.9	0	46	1.0 c
salted, whole kernels, 1 cup	490	40.0	33.0	25.9	3.4	0	176	3.8 c
SOYBEAN OIL:								
1 oz.	251	0	0	28.4	4.1	0	0	0
½ cup	964	0	0	109.0	15.7	0	0	0
1 tbsp.	120	0	0	13.6	0	0	0	
(*Hain*), 1 tbsp.	120	0	0	14.0	2.0	0	0	0
(*IGA*), 1 tbsp.	120	0	0	14.0	2.0	0	0	0
hydrogenated:								
1 oz.	251	0	0	28.4	4.2	0	0	0
½ cup	964	0	0	109.0	16.3	0	0	0
1 tbsp.	120	0	0	13.6	2.0	0	0	0
SOYBEAN PRODUCTS, see specific listings								
SOYBEAN AND COTTONSEED OIL, hydrogenated:								
1 oz.	251	0	0	28.4	5.1	0	0	0
½ cup	964	0	0	109.0	19.6	0	0	0
1 tbsp.	120	0	0	13.6	2.4	0	0	0
SOYBEAN LECITHIN OIL:								
1 oz.	251	0	0	28.4	4.3	0	0	0
½ cup	964	0	0	109.0	16.7	0	0	0
1 tbsp.	120	0	0	13.6	2.1	0	0	0
SPAGHETTI, see "Pasta"								
SPAGHETTI DINNER, FROZEN:								
w/meat sauce (*Kid Cuisine*), 9.25 oz.	310	9.0	43.0	12.0	m.q.	35	690	m.q.
and meatballs:								
(*Banquet*), 10 oz.	290	11.0	44.0	10.0	m.q.	30	580	m.q.
(*Morton*), 10 oz.	200	6.0	39.0	3.0	m.q.	10	1090	m.q.
(*Swanson*), 12.5 oz.	390	14.0	46.0	17.0	m.q.	m.q.	1100	m.q.
SPAGHETTI DISHES, MIX[1]:								
(*Kraft* Mild American Dinner), 1 cup	300	10.0	50.0	7.0	2.0	0	630	m.q.
w/condensed meat sauce (*Chef Boyardee* Dinner), 3.25 oz.	250	12.0	37.0	6.0	m.q.	m.q.	595	m.q.
w/meat sauce (*Chef Boyardee* Dinner), 7.9 oz.	240	12.0	42.0	3.0	m.q.	m.q.	1155	m.q.

1. *Prepared according to package directions.*

Food and Measure	cal.	prot. (gms)	carbo. (gms)	tot. fat (gms)	sat. fat (gms)	chol. (mgs)	sod. (mgs)	fiber (gms)
SPAGHETTI DISHES, MIX *(cont.)*								
w/meat sauce (*Kraft* Dinner), 1 cup	360	12.0	47.0	14.0	4.0	15	880	m.q.
w/mushroom sauce (*Chef Boyardee* Dinner), 7.9 oz.	210	11.0	41.0	1.0	n.a.	n.a.	1085	m.q.
tangy (*Kraft* Italian Style Dinner), 1 cup	310	11.0	49.0	8.0	2.0	5	670	m.q.
SPAGHETTI ENTREE, CANNED:								
and beef (*Chef Boyardee* Beef-O-Getti), 7.5 oz.	220	7.0	27.0	9.0	m.q.	m.q.	1240	m.q.
and beef, in tomato sauce (*Chef Boyardee*), 7.5 oz.	240	7.0	30.0	9.0	m.q.	m.q.	1120	m.q.
w/franks (*Van Camp's Spaghettee Weenee*), 1 cup	243	9.4	34.7	7.4	m.q.	m.q.	1128	.5 c
w/franks, sliced, in tomato sauce (*Franco-American* SpaghettiOs), 7.5 oz.	220	8.0	26.0	9.0	m.q.	m.q.	1000	m.q.
and meatballs:								
(*Chef Boyardee* Microwave), 7.5 oz.	230	7.0	29.0	10.0	m.q.	20	1060	m.q.
(*Estee*), 7½ oz.	240	9.0	19.0	14.0	6.0	30	130	m.q.
(*Featherweight*), 7.5 oz.	160	12.0	23.0	3.0	m.q.	20	400	m.q.
(*Nalley's*), 7.5 oz.	190	10.0	29.0	4.0	m.q.	m.q.	950	m.q.
in sauce (*Buitoni*), 7.5 oz.	190	9.0	21.0	8.0	6.0	20	940	m.q.
w/meatballs, in tomato sauce:								
(*Chef Boyardee*), 7.5 oz.	230	8.0	30.0	9.0	m.q.	m.q.	970	m.q.
(*Franco-American*), 7⅜ oz.	220	10.0	28.0	8.0	m.q.	m.q.	870	m.q.
(*Franco-American* SpaghettiOs), 7⅜ oz.	220	9.0	25.0	9.0	m.q.	m.q.	950	m.q.
(*Pathmark* No Frills), 7.5 oz.	200	9.0	22.0	8.0	m.q.	m.q.	860	m.q.
in tomato sauce, w/cheese (*Franco-American*), 7⅜ oz.	180	5.0	36.0	2.0	m.q.	n.a.	840	m.q.
in tomato and cheese sauce (*Franco-American* SpaghettiOs), 7.5 oz.	170	5.0	33.0	2.0	m.q.	n.a.	860	m.q.
rings, in tomato sauce (*Finast*), 7.5 oz.	150	4.0	31.0	1.0	n.a.	n.a.	480	m.q.
SPAGHETTI ENTREE, FREEZE-DRIED[1]**:**								
w/meat and sauce (*Mountain House*), 1 cup	260	12.0	41.0	5.0	m.q.	m.q.	m.q.	m.q.
SPAGHETTI ENTREE, FROZEN:								
w/beef (*Dining Lite*), 9 oz.	220	12.0	25.0	8.0	m.q.	20	440	m.q.
w/beef, and mushroom sauce (*Lean Cuisine*), 11.5 oz.	280	16.0	38.0	7.0	2.0	25	940	m.q.
w/beef sauce and mushrooms (*Le Menu* LightStyle), 9 oz.	280	12.0	45.0	6.0	1.0	15	450	m.q.
w/Italian style meatballs (*Swanson* Homestyle Recipe), 13 oz.	490	23.0	60.0	18.0	m.q.	m.q.	940	m.q.

1. *Prepared according to package directions.*

Food and Measure	cal.	prot. (gms)	carbo. (gms)	tot. fat (gms)	sat. fat (gms)	chol. (mgs)	sod. (mgs)	fiber (gms)
w/meat sauce:								
(*Banquet* Casserole), 8 oz.	270	14.0	35.0	8.0	m.q.	m.q.	1250	m.q.
(*Freezer Queen* Single Serve),								
10 oz.	350	14.0	47.0	12.0	m.q.	m.q.	610	m.q.
(*Healthy Choice*), 10 oz.	310	16.0	48.0	6.0	2.0	15	440	m.q.
(*Stouffer's*), 12⅞ oz.	370	18.0	49.0	11.0	m.q.	m.q.	1510	m.q.
(*Weight Watchers*), 10.5 oz.	280	20.0	32.0	7.0	3.0	25	610	m.q.
w/meatballs (*Stouffer's*), 12⅝ oz. ...	380	20.0	42.0	15.0	m.q.	m.q.	1510	m.q.
SPAGHETTI MIX, see "Spaghetti dishes, mix"								
SPAGHETTI SAUCE, see "Pasta sauce"								
SPAGHETTI SEASONING:								
(*Tone's*), 1 tsp.	11	.2	2.5	<.1	tr.	tr.	469	.1 d
SPAGHETTI SQUASH:								
raw:								
untrimmed, 1 lb.	106	2.1	22.3	1.8	.4	0	55	4.5 c
trimmed, 1 oz.	9	.2	2.0	.2	<.1	0	5	.4 c
cubed, ½ cup	17	.3	3.5	.3	.1	0	9	.7 c
baked or boiled, drained, 4 oz.	33	.7	7.3	.3	.1	0	20	1.6 c
baked or boiled, drained, ½ cup	23	.5	5.0	.2	<.1	0	14	1.1 c
SPAGHETTINI ENTREE, packaged:								
(*Hormel Top Shelf*), 1 serving	240	13.0	35.0	5.0	m.q.	5	1020	m.q.
SPARERIBS, see "Pork" and "Pork entree, frozen or refrigerated"								
SPICE LOAF:								
(*Kahn's* Family Pack), 1 slice	70	3.0	1.0	6.0	m.q.	m.q.	180	0
beef (*Kahn's* Family Pack), 1 slice ..	60	2.0	1.0	5.0	m.q.	m.q.	200	0
SPINACH:								
raw:								
untrimmed, 1 lb.	73	9.3	11.4	1.1	.2	0	257	8.5 d
partially trimmed, 10-oz. pkg. ...	46	5.8	7.1	.7	.1	0	160	7.4 d
trimmed, 1 oz. or ½ cup chopped	6	.8	1.0	.1	<.1	0	22	.7 d
boiled, drained, 4 oz.	26	3.4	4.3	.3	<.1	0	79	2.5 d
boiled, drained, ½ cup	21	2.7	3.4	.2	<.1	0	63	2.0 d
SPINACH, CANNED, ½ cup, except as noted:								
w/liquid:								
4 oz.	22	2.4	3.3	.4	.1	0	362	1.0 d
½ cup	22	2.5	3.4	.4	.1	0	373	1.1 d
low-sodium, 4 oz.	22	2.4	3.3	.4	.1	0	85	1.0 d
low-sodium	22	2.5	3.4	.4	.1	0	88	1.1 d
drained, no salt added, 4 oz.	26	3.2	3.9	.6	.1	0	31	3.2 d
drained, no salt added	25	3.0	3.6	.5	.1	0	29	3.0 d
(*A&P*)	20	2.0	3.0	<1.0	(0)	0	350	m.q.
(*Allens* Low Sodium)	28	2.0	3.0	<1.0	(0)	0	35	m.q.
(*Finast*)	25	3.0	4.0	0	0	0	360	m.q.
(*Finast* No Salt Added)	25	3.0	4.0	0	0	0	110	m.q.

Food and Measure	cal.	prot. (gms)	carbo. (gms)	tot. fat (gms)	sat. fat (gms)	chol. (mgs)	sod. (mgs)	fiber (gms)
SPINACH, CANNED *(cont.)*								
(*Pathmark* No Salt Added)	30	2.0	4.0	1.0	(0)	0	35	m.q.
(*S&W* Premium Northwest)	25	2.0	3.0	0	0	0	395	m.q.
(*Stokely*)	30	2.0	3.0	0	0	0	420	m.q.
leaf:								
(*Featherweight*)	35	2.0	4.0	1.0	(0)	0	30	m.q.
(*Pathmark* No Frills), 1 cup	45	5.0	8.0	1.0	(0)	0	700	m.q.
whole:								
(*Pathmark*)	30	2.0	4.0	1.0	(0)	0	370	m.q.
or chopped, w/liquid (*Del*								
Monte)	25	2.0	4.0	0	0	0	355	m.q.
w/liquid (*Del Monte* No Salt								
Added)	25	2.0	4.0	0	0	0	35	m.q.
sliced or chopped, curly (*Allens*)	28	2.0	3.0	<1.0	(0)	0	330	m.q.
SPINACH, FROZEN:								
10-oz. pkg.	68	8.3	11.4	.9	.1	0	211	6.0 d
boiled, drained, 4 oz.	32	3.6	6.1	.2	<.1	0	98	2.4 d
boiled, drained, leaf, ½ cup	27	3.0	5.1	.2	<.1	0	82	2.0 d
(*Green Giant* Polybag), ½ cup	25	3.0	6.0	0	0	0	100	5.0 d
(*Green Giant Harvest Fresh*), ½ cup	25	4.0	5.0	0	0	0	170	3.0 d
leaf:								
(*A&P*), 3.3 oz.	25	3.0	4.0	<1.0	(0)	0	100	m.q.
(*Birds Eye* Portion Pack), 3.2 oz.	20	3.0	3.0	0	0	0	70	2.0 d
(*Finast*), 3.3 oz.	20	3.0	4.0	0	0	0	75	m.q.
(*Frosty Acres*), 3.3 oz.	20	3.0	4.0	0	0	0	75	1.0 c
whole (*Birds Eye*), 3.3 oz.	20	3.0	4.0	0	0	0	90	3.0 d
whole (*Southern*), 3.5 oz.	25	2.9	3.6	.3	(0)	0	100	m.q.
cut (*Seabrook*), 3.3 oz.	20	3.0	4.0	0	0	0	77	1.0 c
chopped:								
(*A&P*), 3.3 oz.	20	3.0	4.0	<1.0	(0)	0	90	m.q.
(*Birds Eye*), 3.3 oz.	20	3.0	3.0	0	0	0	90	3.0 d
(*Finast*), 3.3 oz.	20	3.0	3.0	0	0	0	70	m.q.
(*Frosty Acres*), 3.3 oz.	20	3.0	3.0	0	0	0	70	1.0 c
(*Seabrook*), 3.3 oz.	20	3.0	3.0	0	0	0	70	1.0 c
(*Southern*), 3.5 oz.	25	3.0	3.5	.3	(0)	0	100	m.q.
creamed:								
(*Birds Eye* Combinations), 3 oz. ..	60	2.0	5.0	4.0	m.q.	0	310	1.0 d
(*Green Giant*), ½ cup	70	3.0	10.0	3.0	<1.0	2	480	m.q.
(*Stouffer's*), 4.5 oz.	170	4.0	7.0	14.0	m.q.	n.a.	380	m.q.
in butter sauce, cut (*Green Giant*),								
½ cup	40	3.0	6.0	2.0	<1.0	5	380	3.5 d
SPINACH, MUSTARD, see								
"Mustard spinach"								
SPINACH, NEW ZEALAND, see								
"New Zealand spinach"								
SPINACH AU GRATIN, frozen:								
(*The Budget Gourmet*), 6 oz.	120	5.0	14.0	5.0	m.q.	40	410	m.q.
SPINACH PASTA, see "Pasta"								

Food and Measure	cal.	prot. (gms)	carbo. (gms)	tot. fat (gms)	sat. fat (gms)	chol. (mgs)	sod. (mgs)	fiber (gms)
SPINACH SOUFFLÉ[1]**:**								
4 oz.	183	9.2	2.4	15.3	6.0	153	636	.7 c
½ cup	109	5.5	1.4	9.2	3.6	92	382	.4 c
SPINACH SOUFFLÉ, FROZEN:								
(*Stouffer's*), 4 oz.	140	6.0	8.0	9.0	m.q.	n.a.	500	m.q.
SPINY LOBSTER, mixed species,								
meat only, raw:								
1 lb.	506	93.4	11.0	6.9	1.1	318	803	0
1 oz.	32	5.8	.7	.4	.1	20	50	0
7.4 oz., yield from 2-lb. whole								
lobster	233	43.1	5.1	3.2	.5	146	370	0
SPIRULINA, see "Seaweed"								
SPLEEN[2]**:**								
beef:								
raw, 1 oz.	30	5.2	0	.9	m.q.	75	24	0
braised, 10.9 oz., yield from								
1 lb. raw	447	77.3	0	12.9	m.q.	1069	176	0
braised, 4 oz.	164	28.5	0	4.8	m.q.	393	65	0
lamb:								
raw, 1 oz.	29	4.9	0	.9	m.q.	71	24	0
braised, 10.4 oz., yield from								
1 lb. raw	460	78.0	0	14.1	m.q.	1134	171	0
braised, 4 oz.	177	23.2	0	5.4	m.q.	437	66	0
pork:								
raw, 1 oz.	28	5.1	0	.7	.2	103	m.q.	0
braised, 10.6 oz., yield from								
1 lb. raw	446	84.3	0	9.6	3.2	1506	m.q.	0
braised, 4 oz.	169	32.0	0	3.6	1.2	572	m.q.	0
veal:								
raw, 1 oz.	28	5.2	0	.6	m.q.	97	28	0
braised, 12.2 oz., yield from								
1 lb. raw	444	83.0	0	10.0	m.q.	1542	198	0
braised, 4 oz.	146	27.3	0	3.3	m.q.	507	66	0
SPLIT PEAS:								
raw:								
1 oz.	97	7.0	17.1	.3	<.1	0	4	1.6 d
½ cup	334	24.1	59.2	1.1	.2	0	15	5.5 d
green (*Arrowhead Mills*), 2 oz. ..	200	14.0	35.0	1.0	n.a.	0	14	7.5 d
boiled:								
4 oz.	134	9.5	23.9	.4	.1	0	2	2.6 d
½ cup	116	8.2	20.7	.4	.1	0	2	2.3 d
(*A&P*), 1 cup	220	16.0	40.0	<1.0	(0)	0	15	m.q.
SPONGE GOURD:								
raw, trimmed, 1 oz.	6	.2	1.4	.1	tr.	0	n.a.	.1 c
SPOT, meat only, raw:								
1 lb.	559	84.0	0	22.2	6.7	m.q.	130	0
1 oz.	35	5.2	0	1.4	.4	m.q.	8	0

1. *Recipe: 29% whole milk, 26% spinach, 13% egg white, 13% cheddar cheese, 7% egg yolk, 7% butter, 4% flour, 1% salt, and pepper.*
2. *Cooked meats are prepared without added ingredients.*

Food and Measure	cal.	prot. (gms)	carbo. (gms)	tot. fat (gms)	sat. fat (gms)	chol. (mgs)	sod. (mgs)	fiber (gms)
SPOT *(cont.)*								
1 fillet, approx. 2.25 oz., yield from								
1-lb. whole fish	79	11.9	0	3.1	.9	m.q.	18	0
SPRING ONION, see "Onion,								
green"								
SPROUTS, SPROUTED SEEDS,								
see specific bean listings								
SQUAB, fresh, raw:								
meat w/skin:								
1 squab, 7 oz., yield from 9.1 oz.								
w/bone	584	36.8	0	47.4	16.8	m.q.	m.q.	0
1 lb.	1334	83.8	0	108.0	38.2	m.q.	m.q.	0
1 oz.	83	5.2	0	6.7	2.4	m.q.	m.q.	0
meat only:								
1 squab, 5.9 oz., yield from								
9.1 oz. w/bone and skin	239	29.4	0	12.6	3.3	m.q.	m.q.	0
1 lb.	644	79.4	0	34.0	8.9	m.q.	m.q.	0
1 oz.	40	5.0	0	2.1	.6	m.q.	m.q.	0
breast, meat only, 1 breast, approx.								
3.6 oz.	135	22.0	0	4.6	1.2	91	m.q.	0
breast, meat only, 1 oz.	38	6.2	0	1.3	.3	26	m.q.	0
SQUASH, fresh, see specific listings								
SQUASH, FROZEN (see also								
specific squash listings):								
cooked (*Frosty Acres*), 3.3 oz.	18	1.0	4.0	0	0	0	1	1.0 c
SQUASH, SUMMER, all varieties								
(see also specific listings):								
raw:								
w/ends, 1 lb.	87	5.1	18.7	.9	.2	0	8	5.2 d
trimmed, 1 oz.	6	.3	1.2	.1	<.1	0	1	.3 d
sliced, ½ cup	13	.8	2.8	.1	<.1	0	1	.8 d
boiled, drained, 4 oz.	23	1.0	4.9	.4	.1	0	1	1.6 d
boiled, drained, sliced, ½ cup	18	.8	3.9	.3	.1	0	1	1.3 d
SQUASH, WINTER, all varieties								
(see also specific squash								
listings):								
raw:								
untrimmed, 1 lb.	119	4.7	28.4	.7	.1	0	12	5.8 d
trimmed, 1 oz.	11	.4	2.5	.1	<.1	0	1	.5 d
cubed, ½ cup	21	.8	5.1	.1	<.1	0	2	1.0 d
baked, 4 oz.	44	1.0	9.9	.7	.1	0	1	3.2 d
baked, cubed, ½ cup	39	.9	8.9	.6	.1	0	1	2.9 d
SQUASH, WINTER, FROZEN:								
cooked (*Birds Eye*), 4 oz.	45	1.0	11.0	0	0	0	0	2.0 d
cooked (*Seabrook*), 4 oz.	45	1.0	11.0	0	0	0	2	1.0 c
SQUASH SEED, see "Pumpkin								
seed"								
SQUID, mixed species, meat only:								
raw, 1 lb.	416	70.7	14.0	6.3	1.6	1059	199	0

Food and Measure	cal.	prot. (gms)	carbo. (gms)	tot. fat (gms)	sat. fat (gms)	chol. (mgs)	sod. (mgs)	fiber (gms)
raw, 1 oz.	26	4.4	.9	.4	.1	66	12	0
dried, 1 oz.	86	17.7	m.q.	1.2	m.q.	m.q.	m.q.	0
fried[1], 4 oz.	198	20.3	8.8	8.5	2.1	295	347	.1 c
SQUIRREL, meat only:								
raw, 1 oz.	34	6.0	0	.9	.1	24	29	0
roasted[2]:								
14 oz., yield from 1 lb. raw								
boneless	543	96.3	0	14.6	1.7	378	374	0
4 oz.	154	27.4	0	4.1	.5	108	107	0
diced, 1 cup, approx. 4.9 oz.	190	33.8	0	5.1	.6	133	132	0
STAR APPLE, see "Caimit"								
STAR FRUIT, see "Carambola"								
STEAK, see specific listings								
STEAK SAUCE (see also specific listings):								
(*A•1*), 1 tbsp.	12	0	3.0	0	0	0	280	n.a.
(*Estee*), 1 tbsp.	15	<1.0	3.0	<1.0	<1.0	0	10	n.a.
(*French's*), 1 tbsp.	25	0	6.0	0	0	0	150	n.a.
(*Heinz 57*), 1 tbsp.	17	.3	3.6	.2	(0)	0	199	.1 c
(*Lea & Perrins*), 1 oz.	40	<1.0	10.0	<1.0	(0)	0	220	n.a.
(*Life* All Natural), 1 tbsp.	11	<1.0	3.0	tr.	(0)	0	<10	n.a.
(*Steak Supreme*), 1 tbsp.	20	0	5.0	0	0	0	25	n.a.
traditional (*Heinz*), 1 tbsp.	12	.2	2.6	0	0	0	200	n.a.
STEAK SEASONING:								
blackened (*Tone's*), 1 tsp.	9	.4	1.6	.3	(0)	0	486	n.a.
broiled (*McCormick/Schilling* Spice Blends), ¼ tsp.	1	.1	.1	(0)	(0)	0	273	n.a.
STIR-FRY SAUCE:								
(*Kikkoman*), 1 tsp.	6	.3	2.3	tr.	(0)	0	120	tr.d
(*Lawry's*), ¼ cup	120	1.9	19.6	3.8	m.q.	n.a.	1128	.2 c
STOMACH:								
pork, raw, 1 oz.	44	4.7	0	2.7	m.q.	55	15	0
STRAIGHTNECK SQUASH, see "Crookneck squash"								
STRAWBERRY, fresh:								
untrimmed, 1 lb.	130	2.6	30.0	1.6	.1	0	5	11.1 d
untrimmed, 1 pint, approx. 12 oz. ...	97	2.0	22.5	1.2	.1	0	4	8.3 d
trimmed, 1 oz.	9	.2	2.0	.1	tr.	0	<1	.7 d
trimmed, ½ cup	23	.5	5.2	.3	<.1	0	1	1.9 d
STRAWBERRY, CANNED:								
in heavy syrup, 4 oz.	104	.6	26.7	.3	<.1	0	5	m.q.
in heavy syrup, ½ cup	117	.7	29.9	.3	<.1	0	5	m.q.
STRAWBERRY, FREEZE-DRIED:								
(*Mountain House*), ¼ cup [3]	45	1.0	12.0	0	0	0	<1	m.q.

1. *Recipe: 94.6% squid, 4.9% flour, and .6% salt.*
2. *Without added ingredients.*
3. *Prepared according to package directions.*

Food and Measure	cal.	prot. (gms)	carbo. (gms)	tot. fat (gms)	sat. fat (gms)	chol. (mgs)	sod. (mgs)	fiber (gms)
STRAWBERRY, FROZEN:								
unsweetened:								
20-oz. pkg.	200	2.4	51.8	.6	<.1	0	11	4.5 c
4 oz.	40	.5	10.4	.1	tr.	0	2	.9 c
½ cup	26	.3	6.8	.1	tr.	0	2	.6 c
sweetened:								
whole:								
10-oz. pkg.	223	1.5	59.6	.4	<.1	0	3	1.7 c
4 oz.	88	.6	23.8	.2	tr.	0	1	.7 c
½ cup	100	.7	26.8	.2	tr.	0	2	.8 c
sliced:								
10-oz. pkg.	273	1.5	73.6	.4	<.1	0	9	1.8 c
4 oz.	109	.6	29.4	.1	tr.	0	3	.7 c
½ cup	123	.7	33.0	.2	tr.	0	4	.8 c
(*Finast*), 3.3 oz.	125	1.0	30.0	0	0	0	5	m.q.
in lite syrup, whole (*Birds Eye*),								
4 oz.	80	1.0	20.0	0	0	0	0	2.0 d
in lite syrup, halves (*Birds Eye* Quick								
Thaw Pouch), 5 oz.	90	1.0	22.0	0	0	0	5	1.0 d
in syrup, halves (*Birds Eye* Quick								
Thaw Pouch), 5 oz.	120	1.0	30.0	0	0	0	0	2.0 d
STRAWBERRY COBBLER, see								
"Cobbler, frozen"								
STRAWBERRY DANISH, see								
"Danish pastry"								
STRAWBERRY FLAVOR DRINK,								
canned:								
(*Frostee*), 8 fl. oz.	180	2.0	27.0	7.0	m.q.	n.a.	150	(0)
(*Sego* Lite), 10 fl. oz.	150	11.0	17.0	4.0	m.q.	5	390	(0)
(*Sego* Very Strawberry), 10 fl. oz. ..	225	11.0	34.0	5.0	m.q.	5	360	(0)
STRAWBERRY FLAVOR DRINK								
MIX[1]**, 8 fl. oz.:**								
(*Kool-Aid*)	100	0	25.0	0	0	0	25	(0)
(*Kool-Aid* Presweetened)	80	0	20.0	0	0	0	0	(0)
wild (*Wyler's Crystals*)	85	0	20.7	.3	n.a.	0	43	(0)
STRAWBERRY FLAVOR MILK								
DRINK MIX:								
powder:								
1 oz.	110	<.1	28.1	.1	n.a.	0	11	<.1 c
2–3 heaping tsp. or .8 oz. dry ...	84	tr.	21.4	tr.	n.a.	0	8	tr.c
(*Carnation* Instant Breakfast),								
1 pouch	130	6.0	25.0	.2	.1	3	210	.1 d
(*Carnation* Instant Breakfast No								
Sugar Added), 1 pouch	70	6.0	10.0	.3	.2	3	120	.1 d
(*Nestlé Quik*), ¾ oz., approx.								
2½ heaping tsp.	80	0	21.0	0	0	0	m.q.	m.q.

1. *Prepared according to package directions.*

Food and Measure	cal.	prot. (gms)	carbo. (gms)	tot. fat (gms)	sat. fat (gms)	chol. (mgs)	sod. (mgs)	fiber (gms)
(*Pillsbury* Instant Breakfast),								
1 pouch	130	5.0	27.0	0	0	0	180	m.q.
beverage:								
w/whole milk:								
1 cup milk and 2–3 heaping tsp.								
powder	234	8.1	32.8	8.2	5.1	33	128	(0)
(*Nestlé Quick*), 1 cup milk and								
approx. 2½ heaping tsp.								
powder	220	8.0	32.0	8.0	m.q.	m.q.	120	(0)
(*Pillsbury* Instant Breakfast),								
8 fl. oz.	290	14.0	39.0	9.0	m.q.	m.q.	300	(0)
w/lowfat 2% milk:								
1 cup milk and 2–3 heaping tsp.								
powder	205	8.1	33.1	4.7	m.q.	18	130	(0)
(*Nestlé Quik*), 1 cup milk and								
approx. 2½ heaping tsp.								
powder	200	8.0	32.0	5.0	m.q.	m.q.	120	(0)
1 cup lowfat 1% milk and 2–3								
heaping tsp. powder	186	8.1	33.1	2.6	m.q.	10	131	(0)
w/skim milk:								
1 cup milk and 2–3 heaping tsp.								
powder	170	8.4	33.3	.5	n.a.	4	134	(0)
(*Nestlé Quik*), 1 cup milk and								
approx. 2½ heaping tsp.								
powder	160	8.0	32.0	0	0	n.a.	125	(0)
STRAWBERRY FRUIT ROLL, see								
"Fruit snack"								
STRAWBERRY JUICE DRINK:								
(*Tang* Fruit Box), 8.45 fl. oz.	120	0	32.0	0	0	0	10	(0)
(*Wylers* Fruit Slush), 4 fl. oz.	157	0	39.3	0	0	0	10	(0)
STRAWBERRY NECTAR:								
(*Libby's*), 6 fl. oz.	110	0	27.0	0	0	0	0	m.q.
STRAWBERRY SYRUP:								
w/saccharin (*S&W*), 1 tsp.	4	0	1.0	0	0	0	25	n.a.
STRAWBERRY TOPPING:								
(*Kraft*), 1 tbsp.	50	0	14.0	0	0	0	5	n.a.
(*Smucker's*), 2 tbsp.	120	0	30.0	0	0	0	0	n.a.
STRING BEAN, see "Green Bean"								
STROGANOFF DINNER, see								
"Beef dinner, frozen"								
STROGANOFF ENTREE, see								
"Beef entree, frozen"								
STROGANOFF ENTREE MIX,								
VEGETARIAN:								
creamy (*Tofu Classics*), ½ cup[1]	94	7.0	11.0	3.0	m.q.	0	264	m.q.
creamy (*Tofu Classics*), ½ cup[2]	127	7.0	11.0	7.0	m.q.	m.q.	310	m.q.

1. *Prepared according to package directions, with tofu.*
2. *Prepared according to package directions, with tofu and 2 tbsp. salted butter.*

Food and Measure	cal.	prot. (gms)	carbo. (gms)	tot. fat (gms)	sat. fat (gms)	chol. (mgs)	sod. (mgs)	fiber (gms)
STROGANOFF SAUCE MIX:								
1.6-oz. pkg.	161	5.6	26.5	4.4	2.9	12	1863	.6 c
½ cup [1]	136	5.9	17.0	5.4	3.4	19	915	.3 c
(Lawry's), 1 pkg.	123	4.5	25.5	.3	n.a.	n.a.	2814	.8 c
(Natural Touch), 4 oz. [2]	90	4.0	10.0	3.0	m.q.	n.a.	n.a.	n.a.
STUFFED CABBAGE, see "Cabbage entree"								
STUFFING, 1 oz.:								
apple and raisin (Pepperidge Farm Distinctive Stuffing)	110	3.0	21.0	1.0	n.a.	n.a.	410	m.q.
chicken, classic (Pepperidge Farm Distinctive Stuffing)	110	4.0	20.0	1.0	n.a.	n.a.	410	m.q.
corn (Brownberry)	103	3.7	20.6	1.6	n.a.	0	350	1.5 d
corn bread (Pepperidge Farm)	110	3.0	22.0	1.0	n.a.	n.a.	320	m.q.
country style (Pepperidge Farm)	100	4.0	21.0	1.0	n.a.	n.a.	400	m.q.
cube (Pepperidge Farm)	110	3.0	22.0	1.0	n.a.	n.a.	400	m.q.
herb:								
(Brownberry)	100	3.6	20.7	1.3	n.a.	0	297	1.6 d
country garden (Pepperidge Farm Distinctive Stuffing)	120	4.0	18.0	4.0	m.q.	n.a.	300	m.q.
seasoned (Pepperidge Farm)	110	3.0	22.0	1.0	n.a.	n.a.	380	m.q.
vegetable, harvest, and almond (Pepperidge Farm Distinctive Stuffing)	110	4.0	19.0	3.0	m.q.	n.a.	250	m.q.
wild rice and mushroom (Pepperidge Farm Distinctive Stuffing)	130	4.0	17.0	5.0	m.q.	n.a.	310	m.q.
STUFFING, FROZEN, ½ cup:								
chicken (Green Giant Stuffing Originals)	170	4.0	21.0	7.0	m.q.	n.a.	670	m.q.
cornbread (Green Giant Stuffing Originals)	170	3.0	25.0	6.0	m.q.	n.a.	660	m.q.
mushroom (Green Giant Stuffing Originals)	150	4.0	19.0	7.0	m.q.	n.a.	780	m.q.
wild rice (Green Giant Stuffing Originals)	160	3.0	21.0	7.0	m.q.	n.a.	540	m.q.
STUFFING MIX:								
dry:								
(Croutettes), .7 oz.	70	3.0	14.0	0	0	0	260	0
Cajun style (Golden Dipt), ¼ cup	40	1.0	9.0	0	0	0	590	n.a.
cheddar and French (Golden Dipt), ½ cup	80	4.0	9.0	3.0	2.0	14.0	580	n.a.
chicken (Betty Crocker), ⅙ pkg. ..	110	4.0	21.0	1.0	n.a.	n.a.	530	n.a.
chicken (Golden Grain), 1 oz. ...	106	3.9	20.0	1.2	.3	<1	637	1.2 d
cornbread (Golden Grain), 1 oz.	105	3.3	20.9	1.0	.1	<1	774	1.2 d
herb, garden (Golden Dipt), ¼ cup	40	1.0	9.0	0	0	0	330	n.a.

1. *Prepared according to package directions, with whole milk and water.*
2. *Prepared according to package directions.*

Food and Measure	cal.	prot. (gms)	carbo. (gms)	tot. fat (gms)	sat. fat (gms)	chol. (mgs)	sod. (mgs)	fiber (gms)
herb, traditional (*Betty Crocker*),								
⅙ pkg.	110	4.0	22.0	1.0	n.a.	n.a.	550	n.a.
herb and butter (*Golden Grain*),								
1 oz.	104	3.7	19.7	1.1	.2	<1	713	1.4 d
w/wild rice (*Golden Grain*), 1 oz.	108	3.6	20.9	1.1	.2	<1	611	1.3 d
prepared[1], ½ cup:								
beef (*Stove Top*)	180	4.0	21.0	9.0	m.q.	20	590	m.q.
broccoli and cheese (*Stove Top*								
Microwave)	170	4.0	20.0	8.0	m.q.	15	580	m.q.
chicken flavor:								
(*Betty Crocker*)[2]	180	4.0	21.0	9.0	m.q.	n.a.	620	m.q.
(*Stove Top*)	180	4.0	20.0	9.0	m.q.	20	570	m.q.
(*Stove Top* Flexible Serving) ...	170	4.0	20.0	9.0	m.q.	15	580	m.q.
(*Stove Top* Microwave)	160	4.0	20.0	7.0	m.q.	10	480	m.q.
cornbread:								
(*Stove Top*)	170	3.0	21.0	9.0	m.q.	20	570	m.q.
(*Stove Top* Flexible Serving) ...	180	4.0	22.0	9.0	m.q.	15	600	m.q.
homestyle (*Stove Top*								
Microwave)	160	3.0	20.0	7.0	m.q.	10	450	m.q.
herb:								
homestyle (*Stove Top* Flexible								
Serving)	170	4.0	20.0	9.0	m.q.	15	520	m.q.
savory (*Stove Top*)	170	4.0	20.0	9.0	m.q.	20	590	m.q.
traditional (*Betty Crocker*)[2]	190	4.0	22.0	9.0	m.q.	n.a.	640	m.q.
long grain and wild rice (*Stove Top*)	180	4.0	22.0	9.0	m.q.	20	560	m.q.
mushroom and onion (*Stove Top*)	180	4.0	20.0	9.0	m.q.	20	490	m.q.
mushroom and onion (*Stove Top*								
Microwave)	170	4.0	21.0	7.0	m.q.	10	510	m.q.
pork (*Stove Top*)	170	4.0	20.0	9.0	m.q.	20	570	m.q.
pork (*Stove Top* Flexible Serving)	170	4.0	20.0	9.0	m.q.	15	630	m.q.
w/rice (*Stove Top*)	180	4.0	22.0	9.0	m.q.	20	570	m.q.
San Francisco style (*Stove Top*								
Americana*)	170	4.0	20.0	9.0	m.q.	20	650	m.q.
turkey (*Stove Top*)	170	4.0	20.0	9.0	m.q.	20	640	m.q.
STURGEON, mixed species, meat								
only:								
raw, 1 lb.	478	73.2	0	18.3	4.2	m.q.	m.q.	0
raw, 1 oz.	30	4.6	0	1.1	.3	m.q.	m.q.	0
baked, broiled, or microwaved[3],								
4 oz.	153	23.5	0	5.9	1.3	m.q.	m.q.	0
smoked, 4 oz.	196	35.4	0	5.0	1.2	m.q.	m.q.	0
smoked, 1 oz.	49	8.8	0	1.2	.3	m.q.	m.q.	0
STURGEON ROE, see "Caviar"								
SUCCOTASH:								
raw, 1 lb.	451	22.8	88.9	4.6	.9	0	19	11.8 d
raw, 1 oz.	28	1.4	5.6	.3	.1	0	1	.7 d

1. *Prepared according to package directions, with salted butter, except as noted.*
2. *Prepared with butter or margarine.*
3. *Without added ingredients.*

Food and Measure	cal.	prot. (gms)	carbo. (gms)	tot. fat (gms)	sat. fat (gms)	chol. (mgs)	sod. (mgs)	fiber (gms)
SUCCOTASH *(cont.)*								
boiled, drained, 4 oz.	130	5.7	27.6	.9	.2	0	19	1.5 c
boiled, drained, ½ cup	111	4.9	23.4	.8	.1	0	16	1.3 c
SUCCOTASH, CANNED:								
w/cream-style corn, 4 oz.	87	3.0	20.0	.6	.1	0	278	1.5 c
w/cream-style corn, ½ cup	102	3.5	23.4	.7	.1	0	325	1.7 c
w/whole kernel corn, w/liquid, 4 oz.	71	2.9	15.9	.6	.1	0	251	.7 c
w/whole kernel corn, w/liquid,								
½ cup	81	3.3	17.9	.6	.1	0	283	.8 c
(*S&W* Country Style), ½ cup	80	4.0	16.0	1.0	(0)	0	250	m.q.
(*Stokely*), ½ cup	90	3.0	20.0	0	0	0	300	m.q.
SUCCOTASH, FROZEN:								
10-oz. pkg.	265	12.2	56.6	2.5	.5	0	128	2.9 c
boiled, drained, 4 oz.	105	4.9	22.6	1.0	.2	0	51	1.2 c
boiled, drained, ½ cup	79	3.7	17.0	.8	.1	0	38	.9 c
(*Frosty Acres*), 3.3 oz.	100	4.0	19.0	0	0	0	47	1.0 c
(*Seabrook*), 3.3 oz.	100	4.0	19.0	0	0	0	47	1.0 c
SUCKER, white, meat only, raw:								
1 lb.	419	76.0	0	10.5	2.1	187	181	0
1 oz.	26	4.8	0	.7	.1	12	11	0
1 fillet, approx. 5.6 oz., yield from								
2-lb. whole fish	147	26.6	0	3.7	.7	66	64	0
SUET, beef:								
raw, 1 oz.	242	.4	0	26.7	14.8	19	(0)	0
SUGAR, BEET OR CANE (see also "Sugar cane baton"):								
brown:								
1 oz.	106	0	27.3	0	0	0	1	0
1 cup, not packed	541	0	139.8	0	0	0	44	0
1 cup, packed	821	0	212.1	0	0	0	66	0
granulated:								
1 oz.	109	0	28.2	0	0	0	<1	0
1 cup	770	0	199.0	0	0	0	<1	0
1 tbsp.	46	0	11.9	0	0	0	tr.	0
1 tsp.	15	0	4.0	0	0	0	tr.	0
1 lump, 1⅛″ × ¾″ × ⁵⁄₁₆″ or								
2 cubes, ½″	19	0	5.0	0	0	0	tr.	0
1 packet, approx. .2 oz.	23	0	6.0	0	0	0	tr.	0
(*Crystal*), 1 tsp.	16	0	4.0	0	0	0	0	0
juice, organic (*Sucanat*), 1 tsp. ...	12	0	3.0	0	0	0	0	n.a.
powdered or confectioner's:								
1 oz.	109	0	28.2	0	0	0	<1	0
1 cup, unsifted	462	0	119.4	0	0	0	1	0
1 tbsp., unsifted	31	0	8.0	0	0	0	tr.	0
1 cup, sifted	385	0	99.5	0	0	0	1	0
SUGAR, DEXTROUS:								
anhydrous, 1 oz.	104	0	28.2	0	0	0	tr.	0
crystallized, 1 oz.	95	0	25.8	0	0	0	tr.	0

Food and Measure	cal.	prot. (gms)	carbo. (gms)	tot. fat (gms)	sat. fat (gms)	chol. (mgs)	sod. (mgs)	fiber (gms)
SUGAR, MAPLE:								
1-oz. piece, 1¾″ × 1¼″ × ½″	99	(0)	25.5	0	0	0	4	0
SUGAR, SUBSTITUTE:								
(*Equal*), 1 pkg.	4	0	<1.0	0	0	0	0	0
(*Sprinkle Sweet*), 1 tsp.	2	0	.5	0	0	0	1	0
(*Sweet 'n Low*), 1 pkt.	4	0	1.0	0	0	0	0	0
(*Sweet* 10*), ⅛ tsp.	0	0	0	0	0	0	2	0
(*Weight Watchers* Sweet'ner), 1 pkt.	4	0	1.0	0	0	0	30	0
liquid (*Featherweight*), 3 drops	0	0	0	0	0	0	0	0
liquid table (*S&W/Nutradiet*), ⅛ tsp.	0	0	0	0	0	0	0	0
saccharin (*Featherweight*), ¼-grain tablet	0	0	0	0	0	0	2	0
SUGAR, TURBINADO:								
(*Hain*), 1 tbsp.	50	0	12.0	0	0	0	0	0
SUGAR APPLE:								
untrimmed, 1 lb.	236	5.1	59.0	.7	(0)	0	24	3.7 c
trimmed, 1 oz.	27	.6	6.7	.1	(0)	0	3	.4 c
trimmed, ½ cup	118	2.6	29.6	.4	(0)	0	12	1.8 c
1 medium, 2⅞″ × 3¼″, approx. 9.9 oz.	146	3.2	36.6	.5	(0)	0	15	2.3 c
SUGAR CANE BATON:								
(*Frieda* of California), 1 oz.	21	<.1	49.9	.1	(0)	0	n.a.	(0)
SUGAR CANE JUICE:								
1 oz.	21	.1	5.1	tr.	0	0	n.a.	tr.c
SUGAR SNAP PEAS, see "Peas, edible-podded"								
SUMMER SAUSAGE (see also "Thuringer cervelat" and "Sausage stick"):								
(*Eckrich*), 1-oz. slice	80	4.0	1.0	7.0	m.q.	m.q.	320	0
(*Hillshire Farm*), 2 oz.	180	9.0	1.0	16.0	m.q.	m.q.	670	0
(*Hormel* Perma-Fresh), 2 slices	140	10.0	0	11.0	m.q.	m.q.	706	0
(*Hormel* Tangy, Chub), 1 oz.	90	5.0	0	7.0	m.q.	m.q.	317	0
(*Hormel* Thuringer), 1 oz.	90	4.0	0	9.0	m.q.	m.q.	332	0
(*Lean & Lite*), 1 oz.	43	6.1	1.0	2.3	m.q.	18	m.q.	0
(*Light & Lean*), 2 slices	100	6.0	0	8.0	m.q.	m.q.	m.q.	0
(*OHSE*), 1 oz.	75	5.0	2.0	5.0	m.q.	m.q.	340	0
(*Oscar Mayer*), .8-oz. slice	69	3.5	.2	6.1	2.7	19	331	0
beef:								
(*Hillshire Farm*), 2 oz.	190	9.0	1.0	17.0	m.q.	m.q.	m.q.	0
(*Hormel* Beefy), 1 oz.	100	5.0	0	9.0	m.q.	m.q.	313	0
(*OHSE*), 1 oz.	80	5.0	1.0	6.0	m.q.	m.q.	330	0
(*Oscar Mayer*), .8-oz. slice	70	3.5	.3	6.2	2.7	18	325	0
w/cheese (*Hillshire Farm*), 2 oz. ...	200	9.0	1.0	18.0	m.q.	m.q.	m.q.	0
SUNCHOKE, see "Jerusalem artichoke"								

Food and Measure	cal.	prot. (gms)	carbo. (gms)	tot. fat (gms)	sat. fat (gms)	chol. (mgs)	sod. (mgs)	fiber (gms)
SUNFISH, pumpkinseed, meat only, raw:								
1 lb.	404	88.0	0	3.2	.6	304	3 3	0
1 oz.	25	5.5	0	.2	<.1	19	23	0
1 fillet, approx. 1.7 oz., yield from ¾-lb. whole fish	43	9.3	0	.3	.1	32	38	0
SUNFLOWER OIL:								
(*Hain*), 1 tbsp.	120	0	0	14.0	2.0	0	0	0
(*IGA*), 1 tbsp.	120	0	0	14.0	2.0	0	0	0
(*Pathmark*), 1 tbsp.	130	0	0	14.0	2.0	0	0	0
(*Wesson*), 1 tbsp.	120	0	0	14.0	2.0	0	0	0
linoleic:								
1 oz.	251	0	0	28.4	2.9	0	0	0
½ cup	964	0	0	109.0	11.3	0	0	0
1 tbsp.	120	0	0	13.6	1.4	0	0	0
hydrogenated:								
1 oz.	251	0	0	28.4	3.7	0	0	0
½ cup	964	0	0	109.0	14.2	0	0	0
1 tbsp.	120	0	0	13.6	1.8	0	0	0
SUNFLOWER SEED:								
dried:								
in hull, 1 lb.	1397	55.8	46.0	121.4	12.7	0	8	10.2 c
kernels:								
1 oz.	162	6.5	5.3	14.1	1.5	0	1	1.2 c
1 cup	821	32.8	27.0	71.4	7.5	0	4	6.0 c
(*Arrowhead Mills*), 1 oz.	160	7.0	6.0	13.0	m.q.	0	3	4.4 d
dry-roasted, kernels:								
1 oz.	165	5.5	6.8	14.1	1.5	0	1	.5 c
1 cup	745	24.8	30.8	63.7	6.7	0	4	2.3 c
salted, 1 oz.	165	5.5	6.8	14.1	1.5	0	221	.5 c
salted, 1 cup	745	24.8	30.8	63.7	6.7	0	998	2.3 c
(*Flavor House*), 1 oz.	180	8.0	4.0	15.0	m.q.	0	200	m.q.
shelled (*Pathmark*), 1 oz.	180	5.0	7.0	14.0	m.q.	0	150	m.q.
oil-roasted, kernels:								
1 oz.	175	6.1	4.2	16.3	1.7	0	1	1.9 d
1 cup	830	28.8	19.9	77.6	8.1	0	4	9.2 d
salted, 1 oz.	175	6.1	4.2	16.3	1.7	0	171	1.9 d
salted, 1 cup	830	28.8	19.9	77.6	8.1	0	814	9.2 d
toasted, kernels:								
1 oz.	176	4.9	5.9	16.1	1.7	0	1	.5 c
1 cup	829	23.1	27.6	76.1	8.0	0	4	2.4 c
salted, 1 oz.	176	4.9	5.9	16.1	1.7	0	174	.5 c
salted, 1 cup	829	23.1	27.6	76.1	8.0	0	821	2.4 c
SUNFLOWER SEED BUTTER:								
1 oz.	165	5.6	7.8	13.6	1.4	0	1	1.4 d
1 tbsp.	93	3.2	4.4	7.6	.8	0	1	.8 d
salted, 1 oz.	165	5.6	7.8	13.6	1.4	0	147	1.4 d
salted, 1 tbsp.	93	3.2	4.4	7.6	.8	0	83	.8 d

Food and Measure	cal.	prot. (gms)	carbo. (gms)	tot. fat (gms)	sat. fat (gms)	chol. (mgs)	sod. (mgs)	fiber (gms)
SUNFLOWER SEED FLOUR,								
partially defatted:								
1 oz.	92	13.6	10.2	.5	<.1	0	1	1.5 c
1 cup	261	38.5	28.7	1.3	.1	0	2	4.2 c
1 tbsp.	16	2.4	1.8	.1	tr.	0	tr.	.3 c
SURIMI[1]:								
1 lb.	449	68.9	31.1	4.1	m.q.	135	649	0
1 oz.	28	4.3	1.9	.3	n.a.	9	41	0
SURINAM CHERRY, see "Pitanga"								
SWAMP CABBAGE:								
raw:								
untrimmed, 1 lb.	67	9.1	11.0	.7	(0)	0	395	3.8 c
trimmed, 1 oz. or ½ cup chopped	6	.7	.9	.1	(0)	0	32	.3 c
1 shoot, approx. .6 oz.	2	.3	.4	<.1	(0)	0	15	.1 c
boiled, drained, 4 oz.	23	2.4	4.2	.3	(0)	0	138	1.0 c
boiled, drained, chopped, ½ cup	10	1.0	1.8	.1	(0)	0	60	.4 c
SWEDE, see "Turnip"								
SWEDISH MEATBALLS, see								
"Meatball entree, frozen"								
SWEDISH SAUSAGE:								
(*Hickory Farms*), 1 oz.	100	5.0	0	9.0	m.q.	20	380	0
SWEET POTATO:								
raw:								
untrimmed, 1 lb.	343	5.4	79.3	1.0	.2	0	44	9.8 d
trimmed, 1 oz.	30	.5	6.9	.1	<.1	0	4	.9 d
1 medium, 5″ × 2″ diam., approx.								
6.3 oz.	136	2.1	31.6	.4	.1	0	17	3.9 d
cubed, ½ cup	72	1.1	16.6	.2	<.1	0	9	2.0 d
baked in skin, pulp only:								
4 oz.	117	2.0	27.5	.1	<.1	0	11	3.4 d
1 sweet potato, 5″ × 2″ diam.,								
approx. 5.1 oz.	118	2.0	27.7	.1	<.1	0	12	3.4 d
mashed, ½ cup	103	1.7	24.3	.1	<.1	0	10	3.0 d
boiled w/out skin, 4 oz.	119	1.9	27.5	.3	.1	0	15	1.0 c
boiled w/out skin, mashed, ½ cup	172	2.7	39.8	.5	.1	0	21	1.4 c
candied[2]:								
w/butter, 4 oz.	155	1.0	31.6	3.7	1.5	9	79	.4 c
w/butter, 1 piece, 2½″ × 2″,								
3.7 oz.	144	.9	29.3	3.4	1.4	8	73	.4 c
w/margarine, 4 oz.	155	1.0	31.6	3.7	1.5	0	79	.4 c
w/margarine, 1 piece, 2½″ × 2″,								
3.7 oz.	144	.9	29.3	3.4	1.4	0	73	.4 c
SWEET POTATO, CANNED,								
½ cup, except as noted:								
in water, cut (*Allens*)	70	1.0	16.0	<1.0	(0)	0	20	m.q.
in light syrup (*Finast*)	110	2.0	25.0	<1.0	(0)	0	45	m.q.

1. *Processed from walleye (Alaska) pollock.*
2. *Recipe: 82% canned sweet potatoes and syrup, 14% brown sugar, 4% butter or margarine, and salt.*

Food and Measure	cal.	prot. (gms)	carbo. (gms)	tot. fat (gms)	sat. fat (gms)	chol. (mgs)	sod. (mgs)	fiber (gms)
SWEET POTATO, CANNED *(cont.)*								
in light syrup (*Joan of Arc/Princella/*								
Royal Prince)	110	1.0	28.0	0	0	0	25	m.q.
in syrup:								
w/liquid, 4 oz. or ½ cup	101	1.1	23.9	.2	<.1	0	50	.5 c
drained, 4 oz.	122	1.5	28.8	.4	.1	0	44	2.0 d
drained	106	1.3	24.9	.3	.1	0	38	1.8 d
(*Pathmark* No Frills)	105	1.0	25.0	0	0	0	33	m.q.
(*Pathmark* Southern), 1 cup......	230	2.0	55.0	0	0	0	100	m.q.
whole (*Allens*)	90	2.0	20.0	<1.0	(0)	0	40	m.q.
whole and cut (*Taylor's Brand*),								
1 cup	240	3.0	58.0	0	0	0	56	m.q.
cut (*Allens*)	90	2.0	20.0	<1.0	(0)	0	20	m.q.
cut (*Kohl's*)	110	1.0	31.0	<1.0	(0)	0	30	m.q.
in heavy syrup (*Joan of Arc/Princella/*								
Royal Prince)	130	1.0	34.0	0	0	0	35	m.q.
in extra heavy syrup (*S&W*								
Southern)	139	1.0	31.0	1.0	(0)	0	27	m.q.
in pineapple-orange sauce (*Joan of*								
Arc/Princella/Royal Prince)	210	1.0	54.0	0	0	0	35	m.q.
candied (*Joan of Arc/Princella/Royal*								
Prince)	240	1.0	60.0	0	0	0	15	m.q.
candied (*S&W*)	180	1.0	44.0	0	0	0	355	m.q.
mashed:								
4 oz.	115	2.2	26.3	.2	<.1	0	85	m.q.
½ cup	129	2.5	29.6	.3	.1	0	96	m.q.
(*Joan of Arc/Princella/Royal*								
Prince)	90	1.0	24.0	0	0	0	45	m.q.
vacuum pack:								
4 oz.	103	1.9	24.0	.2	<.1	0	60	.8 c
pieces	92	1.7	21.1	.2	<.1	0	54	.7 c
mashed	117	2.1	26.9	.3	.1	0	68	.9 c
whole (*Taylor's Brand*), 1 cup	210	4.0	55.0	0	0	0	56	m.q.
SWEET POTATO, FROZEN:								
10 oz.	272	4.8	63.0	.5	.1	0	17	4.8 d
baked, 4 oz.	113	1.9	26.5	.1	<.1	0	9	1.7 d
baked, cubed, ½ cup	88	1.5	20.6	.1	<.1	0	7	1.3 d
candied (*Mrs. Paul's*), 4 oz.	170	1.0	42.0	0	0	0	40	m.q.
candied, w/apples (*Mrs. Paul's*								
Sweets 'n Apples), 4 oz.	160	1.0	38.0	0	0	0	60	m.q.
SWEET POTATO LEAF:								
raw:								
untrimmed, 1 lb.	149	17.1	27.2	1.3	.3	0	38	5.1 c
trimmed, 1 oz.	10	1.1	1.8	.1	<.1	0	3	.3 c
1 leaf, 12¼" long, approx. .6 oz.	6	.6	1.0	.1	<.1	0	1	.2 c
chopped, ½ cup	6	.7	1.1	.1	<.1	0	2	.2 c
steamed, 4 oz.	39	2.6	8.3	.3	.1	0	15	1.5 c
steamed, ½ cup	11	.7	2.3	.1	<.1	0	4	.4 c

Food and Measure	cal.	prot. (gms)	carbo. (gms)	tot. fat (gms)	sat. fat (gms)	chol. (mgs)	sod. (mgs)	fiber (gms)
SWEET AND SOUR DRINK MIX:								
liquid (*Holland House*), 1 fl. oz.	34	0	8.0	0	0	0	107	n.a.
SWEET AND SOUR SAUCE:								
(*Kikkoman*), 1 tbsp.	18	n.a.	4.0	0	0	0	63	n.a.
(*La Choy*), 1 tbsp.	30	n.a.	7.0	n.a.	n.a.	0	320	n.a.
(*Lawry's*), ¼ cup	549	3.4	11.7	7.5	m.q.	n.a.	4056	.4 c
(*Sauceworks*), 1 tbsp.	25	0	5.0	0	0	0	50	n.a.
duck sauce (*La Choy*), 1 tbsp.	26	<.1	6.9	tr.	0	0	59	0
regular or hot (*Great Impressions*),								
2 tbsp.	102	0	25.5	0	0	0	<1	n.a.
regular (*Hickory Farms*), 2 tbsp. ...	102	0	25.5	0	0	0	<1	n.a.
Hawaiian (*Great Impressions*),								
2 tbsp.	102	0	25.5	0	0	0	<1	n.a.
Hawaiian ((*Hickory Farms*), 2 tbsp.	102	0	25.5	0	0	0	2	n.a.
mix, 2-oz. pkt.	220	.6	54.5	.1	<.1	0	584	n.a.
mix, prepared w/water and vinegar,								
½ cup	147	.4	36.3	<.1	tr.	0	390	n.a.
SWEETBREADS, see "Pancreas"								
and "Thymus"								
SWEETSOP, see "Sugar apple"								
SWISS CHARD:								
raw:								
untrimmed, 1 lb.	81	7.5	15.6	.8	(0)	0	888	3.3 c
trimmed, 1 oz.	5	.5	1.1	.1	(0)	0	60	.2 c
1 leaf, approx. 1.7 oz.	9	.9	1.8	.1	(0)	0	102	.4 c
chopped, ½ cup	3	.3	.7	<.1	(0)	0	38	.1 c
boiled, drained, 4 oz.	23	2.1	4.7	.1	(0)	0	203	1.1 c
boiled, drained, chopped, ½ cup ...	18	1.7	3.6	.1	(0)	0	158	.8 c
SWISS STEAK, see "Beef dinner"								
SWORDFISH, meat only;								
raw:								
1 lb.	548	89.8	0	18.2	5.0	178	408	0
1 oz.	34	5.6	0	1.1	.3	11	26	0
1 steak, 4½" × 2⅛" × ⅞",								
approx. 4.8 oz.	164	26.9	0	5.5	1.5	54	122	0
baked, broiled, or microwaved[1],								
4 oz.	176	28.8	0	5.8	1.6	57	130	0
SWORDFISH, FROZEN:								
steaks, w/out seasoning mix								
(*SeaPak*), 6-oz. pkg.	210	34.0	0	7.0	m.q.	70	155	0
SYRUP (see also specific listings):								
(*Weight Watchers* Reduced Calorie),								
1 tbsp.	25	0	7.0	0	0	0	40	0
SZECHWAN SAUCE:								
hot and spicy (*La Choy*), 1 oz.	48	.1	12.0	.2	0	0	141	0

1. *Without added ingredients.*

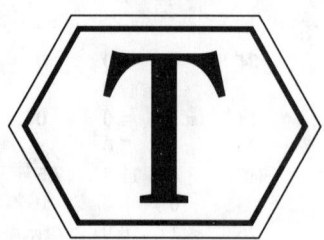

Food and Measure	cal.	prot. (gms)	carbo. (gms)	tot. fat (gms)	sat. fat (gms)	chol. (mgs)	sod. (mgs)	fiber (gms)
TABBOULEH MIX:								
(*Fantastic Foods*), ½ cup[1]	161	2.0	17.0	10.0	m.q.	0	250	m.q.
(*Near East*), ½ cup[2]	170	3.0	20.0	9.0	m.q.	0	290	m.q.
salad (*Casbah*), 1 oz. dry	126	4.0	28.0	1.0	n.a.	0	m.q.	m.q.
TABLE QUEEN SQUASH, see "Acorn squash"								
TABOULI, see "Tabbouleh mix"								
TACO BELL:								
burrito:								
bean, 7.3 oz.	447	15.0	63.0	14.0	4.0	9	1148	m.q.
beef, 7.3 oz.	493	25.0	48.0	21.0	8.0	57	1311	m.q.
chicken, 6 oz.	334	17.0	38.0	12.0	4.0	52	880	m.q.
combination, 7 oz.	407	18.0	46.0	16.0	5.0	33	1136	m.q.
Supreme, 9 oz.	503	20.0	55.0	22.0	8.0	33	1181	m.q.
taco:								
regular, 2.75 oz.	183	10.0	11.0	11.0	5.0	32	276	m.q.
regular, soft, 3.25 oz.	225	12.0	18.0	12.0	5.0	32	554	m.q.
Bellgrande, 5.7 oz.	335	18.0	18.0	23.0	11.0	56	472	m.q.
chicken, 3 oz.	171	12.0	11.0	9.0	3.0	52	337	m.q.
chicken, soft, 3.8 oz.	213	14.0	19.0	10.0	4.0	52	615	m.q.
steak, soft, 3.5 oz.	218	14.0	18.0	11.0	5.0	30	456	m.q.
Supreme, 3.25 oz.	230	11.0	12.0	15.0	8.0	32	276	m.q.
Supreme, soft, 4.4 oz.	272	13.0	19.0	16.0	8.0	32	554	m.q.
tostada, w/red sauce, 5.5 oz.	243	9.0	27.0	11.0	4.0	16	596	m.q.
tostada, chicken, w/red sauce, 5.8 oz.	264	12.0	20.0	15.0	7.0	37	454	m.q.
specialty items:								
chilito, 5.5 oz.	383	18.0	36.0	18.0	8.0	47	893	m.q.
cinnamon twists, 1.2 oz.	171	2.0	24.0	8.0	3.0	0	234	m.q.
Enchirito, w/ red sauce, 7.5 oz. ..	382	20.0	31.0	20.0	9.0	54	1243	m.q.

1. *Prepared according to package directions, with oil and tomatoes.*
2. *Prepared according to package directions.*

Food and Measure	cal.	prot. (gms)	carbo. (gms)	tot. fat (gms)	sat. fat (gms)	chol. (mgs)	sod. (mgs)	fiber (gms)
Meximelt, 3.7 oz.	266	13.0	19.0	15.0	8.0	38	689	m.q.
Meximelt, chicken, 3.8 oz.	257	14.0	19.0	15.0	7.0	48	779	m.q.
nachos, 3.7 oz.	346	7.0	37.0	18.0	6.0	9	399	m.q.
nachos *Bellgrande*, 10.1 oz.	649	22.0	61.0	35.0	12.0	36	997	m.q.
nachos *Supreme*, 5.1 oz.	367	12.0	41.0	27.0	5.0	18	471	m.q.
pintos and cheese, w/red sauce,								
4.5 oz.	190	9.0	19.0	9.0	4.0	16	642	m.q.
pizza, Mexican, 7.9 oz.	575	21.0	40.0	37.0	11.0	52	1031	m.q.
taco salad, 21 oz.	905	34.0	55.0	61.0	19.0	80	910	m.q.
taco salad, w/out shell, 18.3 oz. ...	484	28.0	22.0	31.0	14.0	80	680	m.q.
side orders and condiments:								
green sauce, 1 oz.	4	0	1.0	0	0	0	136	n.a.
guacamole, .75 oz.	34	1.0	3.0	2.0	0	0	113	m.q.
jalapeño peppers, 3.5 oz.	20	1.0	4.0	0	0	0	1370	m.q.
nacho cheese, 2 oz.	103	4.0	5.0	8.0	3.0	9	393	0
pico de gallo, .7 oz.	6	0	1.0	0	0	0	66	n.a.
ranch dressing, 2.6 oz.	236	2.0	1.0	25.0	5.0	35	571	n.q.
red sauce, 1 oz.	10	0	2.0	0	0	0	261	n.a.
salsa, .34 oz.	18	1.0	4.0	0	0	0	376	n.a.
sour cream, .75 oz.	46	1.0	1.0	4.0	2.0	31	0	0
taco sauce, 1 pkt.	2	0	0	0	0	0	126	n.a.
taco sauce, hot, 1 pkt.	3	0	0	0	0	0	82	n.a.
TACO DIP:								
(*Wise*), 2 tbsp.	12	0	3.0	0	0	0	115	n.a.
and sauce (*Hain*), 4 tbsp.	25	1.0	5.0	1.0	n.a.	5	350	n.a.
TACO JOHN'S:								
apple grande, 3 oz.	257	5.0	44.0	8.0	m.q.	n.a.	231	m.q.
beans, refried, 9.5 oz.	331	19.0	79.0	6.0	m.q.	n.a.	1195	m.q.
burrito:								
bean, 5 oz.	249	10.0	36.0	6.0	m.q.	n.a.	636	m.q.
beef, 5 oz.	355	16.0	25.0	18.0	m.q.	m.a.	666	m.q.
combo, 5 oz.	302	11.0	30.0	12.0	m.q.	m.a.	651	m.q.
smothered, w/green chili,								
12.3 oz.	405	18.0	38.0	24.0	m.q.	n.a.	995	m.q.
smothered, w/Texas chili,								
12.3 oz.	518	23.0	48.0	24.0	m.q.	n.a.	746	m.q.
super, 8.3 oz.	434	17.0	66.0	11.0	m.q.	n.a.	1022	m.q.
chili, Texas, 9.5 oz.	430	23.0	35.0	22.0	m.q.	m.q.	1580	m.q.
chimi, 12 oz.	487	16.0	54.0	19.0	m.q.	m.q.	1226	m.q.
churro, 1.2 oz.	122	1.7	12.0	7.0	m.q.	n.a.	153	n.a.
enchilada, 7 oz.	379	19.0	33.0	18.0	m.q.	m.q.	431	m.q.
nachos, 4 oz.	407	11.0	42.0	19.0	m.q.	m.q.	307	m.q.
nachos, super, 11.25 oz.	657	23.0	57.0	34.0	m.q.	m.q.	857	m.q.
Potato Ole Large, 6 oz.	414	6.0	96.0	6.0	m.q.	n.a.	1595	m.q.
taco:								
Bravo, super, 8 oz.	485	18.0	51.0	20.0	m.q.	m.q.	1006	m.q.
burger, 6 oz.	332	14.0	31.0	14.0	m.q.	m.q.	660	m.q.
regular, 4.3 oz.	228	11.0	15.0	13.0	m.q.	m.q.	347	m.q.
soft shell, 5 oz.	276	13.0	23.0	13.0	m.q.	m.q.	505	m.q.

Food and Measure	cal.	prot. (gms)	carbo. (gms)	tot. fat (gms)	sat. fat (gms)	chol. (mgs)	sod. (mgs)	fiber (gms)
TACO JOHN'S (cont.)								
taco salad, super, 12.3 oz.	450	16.0	48.0	18.0	m.q.	n.a.	880	m.q.
tostada, 4.3 oz.	228	11.0	15.0	13.0	m.q.	n.a.	347	m.q.
TACO MIX:								
(*Old El Paso*), 1 taco[1]	67	2.0	8.0	3.0	m.q.	n.a.	423	m.q.
(*Tio Sancho* Dinner Kit):								
taco sauce, 2 oz.	62	1.6	13.4	.2	n.a.	n.a.	750	.5 c
taco seasoning, 1.25 oz.	104	2.1	20.9	1.4	n.a.	n.a.	2500	1.7 c
taco shell	64	1.1	8.1	3.1	m.q.	n.a.	1	.5 c
vegetarian (*Natural Touch*), 2 tbsp.	90	10.0	6.0	2.0	m.q.	0	m.q.	m.q.
TACO SALAD SEASONING:								
(*Lawry's* Seasoning Blends), 1 pkg.	124	4.0	24.7	.9	n.a.	0	1451	1.6 c
TACO SALAD SHELL:								
flour (*Azteca*), 1 piece	200	3.0	18.0	12.0	m.q.	n.a.	130	m.q.
TACO SAUCE (see also "Salsa" and specific listings):								
(*Estee*), 2 tbsp.	14	<1.0	3.0	0	0	0	25	m.q.
(*Lawry's* Sauce'n Seasoner), ¼ cup	40	.7	7.6	.6	(0)	0	636	0
(*Old El Paso*), 2 tbsp.	15	1.0	3.0	0	0	0	300	1.0 d
chunky (*Lawry's*), ¼ cup	22	.9	4.0	.4	(0)	0	549	.4 c
green (*La Victoria*), 1 tbsp.	4	<1.0	1.0	<1.0	(0)	0	85	m.q.
hot (*Del Monte*), ¼ cup	15	0	4.0	0	0	0	440	m.q.
hot (*Ortega*), 1 oz.	12	0	3.0	0	0	0	210	m.q.
mild:								
(*Del Monte*), ¼ cup	15	0	4.0	0	0	0	480	m.q.
(*Enrico's* No Salt Added), 2 tbsp.	14	1.0	3.0	0	0	0	25	m.q.
(*Ortega*), 1 oz.	12	0	3.0	0	0	0	220	m.q.
or medium (*Heinz*), 1 tbsp.	6	0	1.0	0	0	0	m.q.	m.q.
medium or hot (*Old El Paso,* Jars), 2 tbsp.	10	<1.0	2.0	<1.0	n.a.	0	130	m.q.
red (*La Victoria*), 1 tbsp.	6	<1.0	1.0	<1.0	(0)	0	85	m.q.
red, mild (*El Molino*), 2 tbsp.	10	0	2.0	0	0	0	170	m.q.
western style (*Ortega*), 1 oz.	8	0	2.0	0	0	0	180	m.q.
TACO SEASONING:								
(*Old El Paso*), 1 pkg.	100	1.0	21.0	1.0	n.a.	n.a.	3570	m.q.
mix:								
(*Hain*), ⅒ pkg.	10	1.0	2.0	0	0	0	200	m.q.
(*Lawry's* Seasoning Blends), 1 pkg.	118	3.4	23.6	1.1	n.a.	0	1441	1.0 c
(*McCormick/Schilling*), ¼ pkg. ..	31	1.0	6.0	.5	n.a.	0	675	m.q.
(*Old El Paso*), ¹⁄₁₂ pkg.	8	<1.0	2.0	<1.0	n.a.	0	298	m.q.
(*Tio Sancho*), 1.51 oz.	132	2.9	26.0	1.7	n.a.	0	2623	2.0 c
meat (*Ortega*), 1 oz.	90	2.0	18.0	1.0	0	0	1970	m.q.
meat (*Ortega*), 1 oz.[1]	60	4.0	1.0	4.0	2.0	20	105	m.q.
TACO SHELL, 1 piece, except as noted:								
(*Gebhardt*)	30	0	4.0	2.0	m.q.	0	0	m.q.

1. *Prepared according to package directions.*

Food and Measure	cal.	prot. (gms)	carbo. (gms)	tot. fat (gms)	sat. fat (gms)	chol. (mgs)	sod. (mgs)	fiber (gms)
(*Lawry's*)	50	.8	8.0	2.1	m.q.	0	123	.2 c
(*Lawry's* Super)	86	1.4	13.0	3.6	m.q.	0	210	.4 c
(*Old El Paso*)	55	0	6.0	3.0	m.q.	0	50	.5 d
(*Old El Paso* Super Size)	100	1.0	11.0	6.0	m.q.	0	95	1.5 d
(*Ortega*)	50	0	8.0	2.0	m.q.	0	5	m.q.
(*Rosarita*)	45	1.0	6.0	2.0	m.q.	0	0	m.q.
(*Tio Sancho*)	64	1.1	8.1	3.1	m.q.	0	1	.5 c
(*Tio Sancho* Super)	94	1.6	11.3	4.7	m.q.	0	2	.7 c
corn (*Azteca*)	60	1.0	7.0	3.0	m.q.	0	65	m.q.
miniature (*Old El Paso*), 3 pieces	70	1.0	7.0	4.0	m.q.	0	60	1.0 d
TACO STARTER:								
(*Del Monte*), 8 oz.	140	3.0	28.0	1.0	n.a.	n.a.	2180	n.a.
TAHINI, see "Sesame butter"								
TAHINI MIX:								
(*Casbah*), 1 oz. dry	25	2.0	2.0	5.0	m.q.	0	m.q.	m.q.
TALLOW, see "Beef tallow" and								
"Mustard tallow"								
TAMALE, CANNED:								
(*Old El Paso*), 2 pieces	190	5.0	16.0	12.0	m.q.	20	380	m.q.
(*Wolf* Brand), scant cup, 7.75 oz.	328	8.3	24.9	24.5	m.q.	m.q.	1181	1.5 c
beef:								
(*Gebhardt*), 4 oz.	230	4.0	15.0	17.0	m.q.	m.q.	620	m.q.
(*Hormel*), 2 pieces	140	4.0	8.0	10.0	m.q.	m.q.	550	m.q.
(*Hormel* Hot'N Spicy), 2 pieces	140	4.0	9.0	10.0	m.q.	m.q.	612	m.q.
w/sauce (*Van Camp's*), 1 cup	293	8.3	28.6	16.2	m.q.	m.q.	1132	2.2 c
TAMALE, FROZEN:								
beef (*Hormel*), 1 piece	140	6.0	13.0	7.0	m.q.	m.q.	555	m.q.
TAMALE DINNER, frozen:								
(*Patio*), 13 oz.	470	12.0	58.0	21.0	m.q.	35	1850	m.q.
TAMALITO, canned:								
in chili gravy (*Dennison's*), 7.5 oz.	310	6.0	37.0	16.0	m.q.	m.q.	1395	m.q.
TAMARI, see "Soy sauce"								
TAMARIND:								
untrimmed, 1 lb.	369	4.3	96.4	.9	.4	0	43	7.9 c
trimmed, 1 oz.	68	.8	17.7	.2	.1	0	8	1.4 c
1 tamarind, 3″ × 1″, .2 oz.	5	.1	1.3	<.1	tr.	0	1	.1 c
½ cup	144	1.7	37.5	.4	.2	0	17	3.1 c
(*Frieda* of California Tamarindos),								
3½ oz.	239	2.8	62.5	.6	m.q.	0	51	m.q.
TANGERINE:								
untrimmed, 1 lb.	144	2.1	36.6	.6	.1	0	4	1.1 c
peeled and seeded, 1 oz.	12	.2	3.2	.1	tr.	0	<1	.1 c
1 medium, 2⅜″ diam., 4.1 oz.	37	.5	9.4	.2	<.1	0	1	.3 c
sections w/out membrane, ½ cup	43	.6	10.9	.2	<.1	0	2	.3 c
TANGERINE, CANNED:								
(*Del Monte* Mandarin Orange), 5½ oz.	100	0	25.0	0	0	0	<10	m.q.

Food and Measure	cal.	prot. (gms)	carbo. (gms)	tot. fat (gms)	sat. fat (gms)	chol. (mgs)	sod. (mgs)	fiber (gms)
TANGERINE, CANNED *(cont.)*								
(*S&W* Natural Style), ½ cup	60	0	15.0	0	0	0	10	m.q.
in water (*Featherweight* Mandarin								
Orange), ½ cup	35	0	8.0	0	0	0	<10	m.q.
in juice, 4 oz.	42	.7	10.9	<.1	tr.	0	6	.1 c
in juice, ½ cup	46	.8	11.9	<.1	tr.	0	7	.1 c
in light syrup:								
4 oz.	69	.5	18.4	.1	<.1	0	7	.1 c
½ cup	76	.6	20.4	.1	<.1	0	8	.2 c
(*A&P*), ½ cup	80	<1.0	20.0	<1.0	(0)	0	0	m.q.
(*Dole*), ½ cup	76	.6	20.0	.1	(0)	0	0	m.q.
(*Empress*), 5½ oz.	100	0	25.0	0	0	0	<10	m.q.
segments (*Finast*), 5½ oz.	100	0	25.0	0	0	0	n.a.	m.q.
in heavy syrup (*S&W*), ½ cup	76	0	20.0	0	0	0	10	m.q.
unsweetened (*S&W/Nutradiet*),								
½ cup	28	0	7.0	0	0	0	10	m.q.
TANGERINE JUICE:								
fresh, 1 fl. oz.	13	.2	3.1	.1	tr.	0	tr.	<.1 c
fresh, 6 fl. oz.	80	.9	18.7	.4	<.1	0	2	.2 c
canned, sweetened, 1 fl. oz.	16	.2	3.7	.1	tr.	0	tr.	<.1 c
canned, sweetened, 6 fl. oz.	94	.9	22.4	.4	<.1	0	2	.2 c
chilled (*Dole Pure & Light* Mandarin								
Tangerine), 6 fl. oz.	97	.6	25.0	.1	(0)	0	20	m.q.
chilled or frozen[1] (*Minute Maid*),								
6 fl. oz.	91	.9	21.9	.2	(0)	0	19	m.q.
frozen[2], sweetened:								
undiluted, 6-fl.-oz. cont.	344	3.2	83.1	.8	.1	0	7	m.q.
1 fl. oz.	14	.1	3.3	<.1	tr.	0	tr.	m.q.
6 fl. oz.	83	.8	20.0	.2	<.1	0	2	m.q.
TANGLE, see "Seaweed, kelp"								
TAPIOCA, pearl, dry:								
1 oz.	97	<.1	25.1	tr.	(0)	0	tr.	.3 d
1 cup	519	.3	134.8	<.1	(0)	0	1	1.7 d
TARO:								
raw:								
untrimmed, 1 lb.	419	5.9	103.2	.8	.2	0	43	3.1 c
trimmed, 1 oz.	30	.4	7.5	.1	<.1	0	3	.2 c
sliced, ½ cup	56	.8	13.8	.1	<.1	0	6	.4 c
cooked, 4 oz.	161	.6	39.2	.1	<.1	0	11	1.0 c
cooked, sliced, ½ cup	94	.3	22.8	.1	<.1	0	10	.6 c
TARO, TAHITIAN:								
raw, trimmed:								
1 lb.	181	12.7	31.3	4.4	.9	0	227	7.9 c
1 oz.	11	.8	2.0	.3	.1	0	14	.5 c
sliced, ½ cup	25	1.7	4.3	.6	.1	0	31	1.1 c

1. *Diluted according to package directions.*
2. *Diluted according to package directions, except as noted.*

Food and Measure	cal.	prot. (gms)	carbo. (gms)	tot. fat (gms)	sat. fat (gms)	chol. (mgs)	sod. (mgs)	fiber (gms)
cooked, 4 oz.	50	4.7	7.8	.8	.2	0	61	2.6 c
cooked, sliced, ½ cup	30	2.8	4.7	.5	.1	0	37	1.6 c
TARO CHIPS:								
1 oz.	135	.6	19.1	7.2	2.2	0	105	.3 c
½ cup	57	.3	8.1	3.1	.9	0	44	.1 c
10 chips, approx. .8 oz.	110	.5	15.5	5.9	1.8	0	85	.3 c
snack (*Ray's*), 1 oz.	139	1.4	20.0	6.0	m.q.	0	167	m.q.
TARO LEAF:								
raw:								
untrimmed, 1 lb.	115	13.5	18.3	2.0	.4	0	8	5.5 c
trimmed, 1 oz.	12	1.4	1.9	.2	<.1	0	1	.6 c
1 leaf, 11″ × 6½″, approx. .6 oz.	4	.5	.7	.1	<.1	0	tr.	.2 c
½ cup	6	.7	.9	.1	<.1	0	1	.3 c
steamed, 4 oz.	27	3.1	4.6	.5	.1	0	2	.6 c
steamed, ½ cup	18	2.0	3.0	.3	.1	0	2	.4 c
TARO SHOOTS:								
raw:								
untrimmed, 1 lb.	45	3.7	9.3	.4	.1	0	4	2.3 c
trimmed, 1 oz.	3	.3	.7	<.1	tr.	0	<1	.2 c
1 shoot, 15½″ × 1⅛″ diam.,								
approx. 3.3 oz.	9	.8	1.9	.1	<.1	0	1	.5 c
sliced, ½ cup	5	.4	1.0	<.1	tr.	0	<1	.3 c
cooked, 4 oz.	16	.8	3.6	.1	<.1	0	2	.6 c
cooked, sliced, ½ cup	10	.5	2.2	.1	<.1	0	1	.4 c
TARPON, Atlantic, meat only, raw:								
1 lb.	422	94.8	0	1.8	m.q.	m.q.	m.q.	0
1 oz.	26	5.0	0	.1	m.q.	m.q.	m.q.	0
TARRAGON, ground:								
1 oz.	84	6.5	14.2	2.1	m.q.	0	18	2.1 c
1 tbsp.	14	1.1	2.4	.4	n.a.	0	3	.4 c
1 tsp.	5	.4	.8	.1	n.a.	0	1	.1 c
(*Spice Islands*), 1 tsp.	5	.3	.7.	.1	n.a.	0	1	.1 c
TART SHELL (see also "Puff pastry"):								
frozen (*Pet-Ritz*), 3″ shell	150	3.0	12.0	10.0	m.q.	7	150	m.q.
TARTAR SAUCE: 1 tbsp.:								
(*Golden Dipt*)	70	0	2.0	7.0	1.0	10	100	n.a.
(*Golden Dipt Lite*)	50	0	4.0	4.0	1.0	5	40	n.a.
(*Great Impressions*)	86	.2	1.2	9.0	m.q.	10	76	n.a.
(*Heinz*)	71	0	2.1	7.2	m.q.	m.q.	124	.1 c
(*Hellmann's/Best Foods*)	70	0	0	8.0	1.0	5	220	n.a.
(*Sauceworks*)	50	0	2.0	5.0	1.0	5	85	n.a.
(*Weight Watchers*)	35	0	3.0	3.0	1.0	5	80	n.a.
egg-free (*Life* All Natural)	38	<1.0	<1.0	4.0	m.q.	0	<2	n.a.
natural lemon and herb flavor								
(*Sauceworks*)	70	0	0	8.0	1.0	5	85	n.a.
TEA, brewed:								
6 fl. oz.	2	0	0	tr.	tr.	0	5	0
(*Nestea*), 6 fl. oz.	0	0	0	0	0	0	0	0

Food and Measure	cal.	prot. (gms)	carbo. (gms)	tot. fat (gms)	sat. fat (gms)	chol. (mgs)	sod. (mgs)	fiber (gms)
TEA, *(cont.)*								
caffeine-free (*Celestial Seasonings*),								
8 fl. oz.	4	tr.	.8	tr.	(0)	0	5	tr.d
instant, regular or decaffeinated								
(*Lipton*), 6 fl. oz.	0	0	0	0	0	0	0	0
instant, lemon flavor (*Lipton*),								
6 fl. oz.	3	.1	.6	0	0	0	1	0
TEA, FLAVORED OR SPECIAL								
BLEND (see also "Tea,								
herbal"):								
Amaretto (*Celestial Seasonings*								
Amaretto Nights), 8 fl. oz.	3	tr.	.6	tr.	(0)	0	1	tr.d
apple spice (*Celestial Seasonings*								
Fruit & Tea), 8 fl. oz.	<3	<.1	.2	tr.	(0)	0	1	tr.d
(*Bigelow Chinese Fortune*),								
5¼ fl. oz.	1	<.1	.1	tr.	(0)	0	<1	0
(*Bigelow Constant Comment*),								
5¼ fl. oz.	1	<.1	.1	tr.	(0)	0	<1	0
(*Bigelow English Teatime*), 5¼ fl. oz.	1	<.1	.1	tr.	(0)	0	tr.	0
(*Celestial Seasonings Classic English*								
Breakfast), 8 fl. oz.	3	tr.	.4	tr.	(0)	0	<1	tr.d
(*Celestial Seasonings Morning*								
Thunder), 8 fl. oz.	3	tr.	.4	tr.	(0)	0	<1	tr.d
chocolate orange (*Celestial*								
Seasonings Bavarian Chocolate								
Orange), 8 fl. oz.	7	tr.	1.6	tr.	(0)	0	5	tr.d
cinnamon (*Bigelow Cinnamon Stick*),								
5¼ fl. oz.	1	<.1	.1	tr.	(0)	0	<1	0
cinnamon (*Celestial Seasonings*								
Cinnamon Vienna), 8 fl. oz. . . .	2	tr.	.4	tr.	(0)	0	2	tr.d
darjeeling (*Bigelow*), 5¼ fl. oz.	1	<.1	.1	tr.	(0)	0	<1	0
darjeeling (*Celestial Seasonings*								
Darjeeling Gardens), 8 fl. oz. . .	3	tr.	.5	tr.	(0)	0	<1	tr.d
Earl Grey (*Bigelow*), 5¼ fl. oz.	1	<.1	.1	tr.	(0)	0	1	0
Earl Grey (*Celestial Seasonings*								
Extraordinary Earl Grey),								
8 fl. oz.	3	tr.	.5	tr.	(0)	0	<1	tr.d
Irish cream (*Celestial Seasonings*								
Irish Cream Mist), 8 fl. oz.	3	tr.	.6	tr.	(0)	0	1	tr.d
lemon (*Bigelow Lemon Lift*),								
5¼ fl. oz.	1	<.1	.2	tr.	(0)	0	<1	0
lemon (*Celestial Seasonings* Fruit &								
Tea), 8 fl. oz.	<3	tr.	.5	tr.	(0)	0	<1	tr.d
mint (*Bigelow Plantation Mint*),								
5¼ fl. oz.	1	<.1	.1	tr.	(0)	0	1	0
mint, Swiss (*Celestial Seasonings*),								
8 fl. oz.	<3	tr.	.4	tr.	(0)	0	<1	tr.d
orange spice (*Celestial Seasonings*								
Fruit & Tea), 8 fl. oz.	<3	tr.	.4	tr.	(0)	0	<1	tr.d

Food and Measure	cal.	prot. (gms)	carbo. (gms)	tot. fat (gms)	sat. fat (gms)	chol. (mgs)	sod. (mgs)	fiber (gms)
raspberry (*Bigelow Raspberry Royale*), 5¼ fl. oz.	1	<.1	.1	tr.	(0)	0	<1	0
raspberry (*Celestial Seasonings* Fruit & Tea), 8 fl. oz.	2	tr.	.5	tr.	(0)	0	<1	tr.d
TEA, HERBAL, brewed:								
6 fl. oz.	1	.1	.3	tr.	tr.	0	2	tr.c
almond:								
(*Celestial Seasonings Almond Sunset*), 8 fl. oz.	3	tr.	1.1	tr.	(0)	0	2	tr.d
(*Lipton Almond Pleasure*), 8 fl. oz.	4	0	1.0	0	0	0	0	0
orange (*Bigelow*), 5 fl. oz.	<1	<.1	<.1	tr.	(0)	0	<1	0
apple (*Bigelow Apple Orchard*), 5¼ fl. oz.	5	<.1	1.2	tr.	(0)	0	1	0
apple spice (*Bigelow*), 5 fl. oz.	<1	tr.	<.1	tr.	(0)	0	1	0
(*Bigelow Sweet Dreams*), 5¼ fl. oz.	1	<.1	.1	tr.	(0)	0	1	0
(*Bigelow Take-A-Break*), 5¼ fl. oz.	1	<.1	.6	tr.	(0)	0	1	0
blackberry (*Celestial Seasonings Wild Forest Blackberry*), 8 fl. oz.	2	tr.	1.8	tr.	(0)	0	1	tr.d
(*Celestial Seasonings Emperor's Choice*), 8 fl. oz.	4	<.1	.9	<.1	(0)	0	2	<.1 d
(*Celestial Seasonings Mo's 24*), 8 fl. oz.	2	<.1	.2	tr.	(0)	0	4	tr.d
(*Celestial Seasonings Red Zinger*), 8 fl. oz.	4	tr.	1.1	tr.	(0)	0	2	<.1 d
(*Celestial Seasonings Roastaroma*), 8 fl. oz.	11	<.1	2.0	<.1	(0)	0	4	<.1 d
(*Celestial Seasonings Sleepytime*), 8 fl. oz.	5	tr.	1.1	tr.	(0)	0	2	<.1 d
(*Celestial Seasonings Sunburst C*), 8 fl. oz.	3	tr.	1.1	tr.	(0)	0	6	<.1 d
chamomile:								
(*Bigelow*), 5 fl. oz.	<1	<.1	tr.	tr.	(0)	0	2	0
(*Celestial Seasonings*), 8 fl. oz. . . .	2	tr.	.5	tr.	(0)	0	5	tr.d
(*Lipton*), 8 fl. oz.	4	0	1.0	0	0	0	0	0
mint (*Bigelow*), 5 fl. oz.	<1	tr.	tr.	tr.	(0)	0	1	0
cinnamon:								
(*Celestial Seasonings Cinnamon Rose*), 8 fl. oz.	2	tr.	1.1	tr.	(0)	0	1	tr.d
apple (*Lipton*), 8 fl. oz.	2	0	<1.0	0	0	0	0	0
apple spice (*Celestial Seasonings Cinnamon Apple Spice*), 8 fl. oz.	3	tr.	.4	tr.	(0)	0	1	tr.d
orange (*Bigelow*), 5 fl. oz.	<1	<.1	.1	tr.	(0)	0	<1	0
citrus (*Lipton Citrus Sunset*), 8 fl. oz.	4	0	1.0	0	0	0	0	0
cranberry (*Celestial Seasonings Cranberry Cove*), 8 fl. oz.	3	tr.	.7	tr.	(0)	0	1	tr.d
cranberry apple (*Bigelow*), 5 fl. oz.	1	.1	.3	tr.	(0)	0	1	0

Food and Measure	cal.	prot. (gms)	carbo. (gms)	tot. fat (gms)	sat. fat (gms)	chol. (mgs)	sod. (mgs)	fiber (gms)
TEA, HERBAL *(cont.)*								
fruit and almond (*Bigelow Fruit &*								
Almond), 5¼ fl. oz.	1	<.1	<.1	tr.	(0)	0	<1	0
ginseng (*Celestial Seasonings*								
Ginseng Plus), 8 fl. oz.	3	tr.	<.5	tr.	(0)	0	4	tr.d
grains, roasted, w/carob (*Bigelow*),								
5 fl. oz.	3	<.1	.6	tr.	(0)	0	1	0
hibiscus and rose hips (*Bigelow*),								
5 fl. oz.	1	<.1	.2	tr.	(0)	0	1	0
lemon:								
(*Bigelow I Love Lemon*),								
5¼ fl. oz.	1	<.1	<.1	tr.	(0)	0	<1	0
(*Bigelow Lemon & C*), 5 fl. oz. . . .	<1	tr.	<.1	tr.	(0)	0	<1	0
(*Celestial Seasonings Lemon Mist*),								
8 fl. oz.	2	tr.	<.5	tr.	(0)	0	3	tr.d
(*Celestial Seasonings Lemon*								
Zinger), 8 fl. oz.	4	<.1	.7	tr.	(0)	0	1	tr.d
(*Lipton Lemon Soother*), 8 fl. oz.	4	0	1.0	0	0	0	0	0
mint:								
(*Bigelow Mint Blend*), 5 fl. oz. . . .	<1	<.1	.2	tr.	(0)	0	3	0
(*Bigelow Mint Medley*), 5¼ fl. oz.	1	<.1	.2	tr.	(0)	0	<1	0
(*Celestial Seasonings Grandma's*								
Tummy Mint), 8 fl. oz.	2	tr.	<.3	tr.	(0)	0	7	tr.d
(*Celestial Seasonings Mellow*								
Mint), 8 fl. oz.	2	tr.	.4	tr.	(0)	0	4	tr.d
(*Celestial Seasonings Mint Magic*),								
8 fl. oz.	1	tr.	.4	tr.	(0)	0	3	tr.d
orange:								
(*Bigelow Orange & C*), 5 fl. oz. . .	<1	tr.	<.1	tr.	(0)	0	<1	0
(*Celestial Seasonings Orange*								
Zinger), 8 fl. oz.	5	tr.	1.2	tr.	(0)	0	1	tr.d
(*Lipton Gentle/Tangy Orange*),								
8 fl. oz.	4	0	1.0	0	0	0	0	0
and spice (*Bigelow Orange &*								
Spice), 5¼ fl. oz.	1	<.1	<.1	tr.	(0)	0	1	0
spice (*Celestial Seasonings*								
Mandarin Orange Spice),								
8 fl. oz.	5	tr.	1.1	tr.	(0)	0	2	tr.d
peace spice (*Celestial Seasonings*								
Country Peach Spice), 8 fl. oz.	3	tr.	.7	tr.	(0)	0	3	tr.d
peppermint (*Bigelow*), 5 fl. oz.	<1	<.1	<.1	<.1	(0)	0	2	0
peppermint (*Celestial Seasonings*),								
8 fl. oz.	2	tr.	1.1	tr.	(0)	0	8	tr.d
raspberry (*Celestial Seasonings*								
Raspberry Patch), 8 fl. oz.	4	tr.	1.1	tr.	(0)	0	1	tr.d
raspberry, red (*Bigelow*), 5 fl. oz. . .	1	.1	.2	tr.	(0)	0	<1	0
spearmint (*Bigelow*), 5 fl. oz.	<1	<.1	<.1	tr.	(0)	0	1	0
spearmint (*Celestial Seasonings*),								
8 fl. oz.	5	<.1	.2	<.1	(0)	0	6	<.1 d

Food and Measure	cal.	prot. (gms)	carbo. (gms)	tot. fat (gms)	sat. fat (gms)	chol. (mgs)	sod. (mgs)	fiber (gms)
spice (*Lipton Toasty Spice*), 8 fl. oz.	6	0	1.0	0	0	0	0	0
strawberry (*Bigelow Specially Strawberry*), 5 fl. oz.	1	.1	.2	tr.	(0)	0	<1	0
strawberry (*Celestial Seasonings Strawberry Fields*), 8 fl. oz. ...	4	tr.	.8	tr.	(0)	0	1	tr.d
TEA, ICED:								
canned, bottled, or chilled:								
(*Shasta*), 12 fl. oz.	124	0	34.0	0	0	0	28	0
w/lemon:								
(*Lipton* Presweetened), 8 fl. oz.	83	0	20.2	0	0	0	11	0
(*Lipton* Sugar Free), 8 fl. oz. ..	<1	0	.1	0	0	0	10	0
(*Nestea* Sugar Free), 8 fl. oz. ..	2	0	1.0	0	0	0	0	0
(*Nestea* Sugar Sweetened), 8 fl. oz.	70	0	17.0	0	0	0	0	0
(*Veryfine*), 8 fl. oz.	80	<1.0	16.0	0	0	0	<10	0
natural lemon flavor (*Lipton* Aseptic), 8.45 oz.	96	1.6	24.0	.3	(0)	0	20	0
flavored (*Wylers* Fruit Tea Punch), 12 oz.	118	0	29.6	0	0	0	1	0
instant or mix[1]:								
1 tsp. powder	2	.1	.4	0	0	0	8	0
(*Crystal Light* Sugar Free Decaffeinated)	4	0	0	0	0	0	0	0
(*Lipton* Sugar Free)	1	0	.3	0	0	0	6	0
(*Nestea* 100%), 1 scant tsp. tea ..	2	0	0	0	0	0	0	0
(*Pathmark* No Frills), ¾-oz. mix	70	0	21.0	0	0	0	75	0
decaffeinated (*Lipton* Sugar Free)	1	0	.3	0	0	0	5	0
decaffeinated (*Nestea* 100%)	0	0	0	0	0	0	0	0
flavored, all flavors (*Nestea* Ice Teasers)	6	0	1.0	0	0	0	0	0
lemon flavor:								
1 rounded tsp.	4	.1	1.1	tr.	tr.	0	7	0
sugar sweetened, 1 rounded tsp.	29	<.1	7.4	<.1	tr.	0	n.a.	0
(*Lipton*), 6 fl. oz.	55	0	14.3	0	0	0	1	0
(*Nestea*), 8 fl. oz.	6	0	1.0	0	0	0	0	0
(*Nestea* Presweetened), w/1 tbsp. mix, 8 fl. oz.	70	0	19.0	0	0	0	0	0
(*Nestea* Sugar Free), 8 fl. oz. ..	4	0	1.0	0	0	0	0	0
(*Pathmark*), 1 rounded tsp. ...	6	0	1.0	0	0	0	0	0
decaffeinated (*Lipton*), 6 fl. oz.	55	0	14.2	0	0	0	<1	0
decaffeinated (*Nestea* Sugar Free), 2 tsp.	6	0	1.0	0	0	0	0	0
decaffeinated, natural lemon flavor (*Pathmark* Sugar Sweetened), 2 tbsp.	80	0	20.0	0	0	0	0	0

1. *Prepared with 8 fl. oz. water.*

Food and Measure	cal.	prot. (gms)	carbo. (gms)	tot. fat (gms)	sat. fat (gms)	chol. (mgs)	sod. (mgs)	fiber (gms)
TEA, ICED, MIX, LEMON FLAVOR *(cont.)*								
artificially sweetened, lemon flavor								
(see also specific brands):								
(*Pathmark*), 1 level tsp.	4	0	1.0	0	0	0	20	0
w/*Nutrasweet* (*Lipton*), 8 fl. oz.	5	.1	1.2	0	0	0	2	0
w/saccharin, 2 tsp.	5	.1	1.3	tr.	tr.	0	17	0
low-calorie, regular or								
decaffeinated, natural lemon								
flavor (*Pathmark*), 8 fl. oz.	4	0	1.0	0	0	0	0	0
TEASEED OIL:								
1 oz.	251	0	0	28.4	6.0	0	0	0
½ cup	964	0	0	109.0	23.1	0	0	0
1 tbsp.	120	0	0	13.6	2.9	0	0	0
TEFF FLOUR:								
whole grain (*Arrowhead Mills*), 2 oz.	200	7.0	41.0	1.0	n.a.	0	6	7.7 d
TEFF SEED:								
(*Arrowhead Mills*), 2 oz.	200	7.0	41.0	1.0	n.a.	0	6	7.7 d
TEMPEH:								
1 oz.	56	5.4	4.8	2.2	.3	0	2	.8 c
½ cup	165	15.7	14.1	6.4	.9	0	5	2.5 c
TEMPURA BATTER MIX:								
(*Golden Dipt*), 1 oz.	100	3.0	22.0	0	0	0	130	m.q.
TENDERGREEN, see "Mustard								
spinach"								
TEQUILA, see "Liquor"								
TEQUILA SUNRISE[1]:								
1 fl. oz.	34	.1	2.7	tr.	tr.	0	1	n.a.
TERIYAKI SAUCE (see also								
specific listings):								
1 tbsp.	15	1.1	2.9	0	0	0	690	n.a.
(*Kikkoman*), 1 tbsp.	15	n.a.	2.7	tr.	(0)	tr.	630	n.a.
(*Kikkoman* Baste & Glaze), 1 tbsp.	27	n.a.	6.0	tr.	(0)	0	420	n.a.
(*La Choy* Sauce and Marinade),								
1 oz.	30	1.0	5.0	0	0	n.a.	1640	n.a.
barbecue marinade (*Lawry's*), ¼ cup	164	8.2	27.4	2.3	m.q.	n.a.	12,330	.2 c
ginger marinade (*Golden Dipt*),								
1 fl. oz.	120	1.0	12.0	7.0	1.0	0	920	n.a.
w/pineapple juice (*Lawry's*), ¼ cup	72	6.4	11.0	.4	(0)	n.a.	7100	<.1 c
thick and rich (*La Choy*), 1 oz.	41	.7	9.4	.1	<.1	<1	509	<.1 d
mix, dry, 1.6-oz. pkg.	130	4.1	27.6	.9	.1	0	4784	n.a.
mix[2], ½ cup	66	2.1	13.8	.5	.1	0	2396	n.a.
THIRST QUENCHER DRINK,								
bottled:								
1 fl. oz.	7	tr.	1.9	tr.	0	0	12	0
1 cup	60	tr.	15.2	tr.	0	0	96	0

1. *Recipe: 54.4% orange juice, 32.6% tequila, 9.0% lime juice, and 4.0% grenadine.*
2. *Prepared according to package directions, with water.*

Food and Measure	cal.	prot. (gms)	carbo. (gms)	tot. fat (gms)	sat. fat (gms)	chol. (mgs)	sod. (mgs)	fiber (gms)
THREE-GRAIN PILAF MIX:								
w/herbs (*Quick Pilaf*), ½ cup[1]	110	3.0	24.0	.6	n.a.	0	278	m.q.
w/herbs (*Quick Pilaf*), ½ cup[2]	142	3.0	24.0	4.0	m.q.	m.q.	324	m.q.
THURINGER CERVELAT (see								
also "Summer sausage"):								
(*Hillshire Farm*), 2 oz.	180	9.0	1.0	15.0	m.q.	m.q.	650	0
(*Hormel* Viking Club Cervelat), 1 oz.	90	5.0	0	8.0	m.q.	m.q.	325	0
(*Hormel Old Smokehouse*), 1 oz.	90	4.0	1.0	8.0	m.q.	m.q.	328	0
(*Hormel Old Smokehouse* Chub),								
1 oz.	100	5.0	0	9.0	m.q.	m.q.	332	0
(*Hormel Old Smokehouse* Sliced),								
1 oz.	100	5.0	0	9.0	m.q.	m.q.	321	0
(*JM* Cervalot), 1-oz. slice	70	4.0	1.0	6.0	m.q.	m.q.	260	0
beef:								
(*JM* Thuringer), 1-oz. slice	80	5.0	1.0	7.0	m.q.	m.q.	340	0
and pork, 1 oz.	98	4.6	.7	8.5	3.4	19	412	0
and pork, 1 slice, 4⅛″ × ¼″,								
approx. .8 oz.	80	3.7	.5	6.9	2.8	16	334	0
THYME, ground:								
1 oz.	78	2.6	18.1	2.1	.8	0	16	5.3 c
1 tbsp.	12	.4	2.6	.3	.1	0	2	.8 c
1 tsp.	4	.1	.9	.1	<.1	0	1	.3 c
(*Spice Islands*), 1 tsp.	5	.1	1.0	.1	(0)	0	1	.4 c
THYMUS[3]:								
beef:								
raw, 1 oz.	67	3.5	0	5.8	m.q.	63	27	0
braised, 13.4 oz., yield from								
1 lb. raw	1214	83.3	0	95.2	m.q.	1119	442	0
braised, 4 oz.	362	24.8	0	28.3	m.q.	333	132	0
veal:								
raw, 1 oz.	28	5.1	0	.7	m.q.	76	24	0
braised, 9.1 oz., yield from								
1 lb. raw	449	81.7	0	11.1	m.q.	1214	169	0
braised, 4 oz.	197	35.8	0	4.9	m.q.	532	75	0
TILEFISH, meat only:								
raw:								
1 lb.	433	79.4	0	10.5	2.0	m.q.	239	0
1 oz.	27	5.0	0	.7	.1	m.q.	15	0
½ fillet, approx. 6.8 oz., yield								
from 5-lb. whole fish	184	33.8	0	4.5	.9	m.q.	102	0
baked, broiled, or microwaved[4],								
4 oz.	167	27.8	0	5.3	1.0	m.q.	67	0
TOASTER MUFFINS AND								
PASTRIES, 1 piece:								
apple, Dutch, frosted (*Kellogg's Pop-*								
Tarts), 1.8 oz.	210	2.0	37.0	6.0	m.q.	0	200	0

1. *Prepared according to package directions, without butter.*
2. *Prepared according to package directions, with 2 tbsp. salted butter.*
3. *Cooked meats are prepared without added ingredients.*
4. *Without added ingredients.*

Food and Measure	cal.	prot. (gms)	carbo. (gms)	tot. fat (gms)	sat. fat (gms)	chol. (mgs)	sod. (mgs)	fiber (gms)
TOASTER MUFFINS AND PASTRIES *(cont.)*								
apple cinnamon (*Pepperidge Farm*								
Croissant Toaster Tarts)	170	3.0	25.0	7.0	2.0	0	120	m.q.
apple spice (*Toaster Muffins*)	130	2.0	21.0	5.0	m.q.	n.a.	100	m.q.
banana nut:								
(*Thomas' Toast-r-Cakes*)	111	1.7	16.7	4.4	m.q.	10	192	.6 d
(*Toaster Muffins*)	130	2.0	19.0	6.0	m.q.	n.a.	85	m.q.
(*Toaster Strudel* Breakfast								
Pastries)	190	2.0	28.0	8.0	m.q.	n.a.	190	m.q.
blueberry:								
(*Kellogg's Pop-Tarts*), 1.8 oz.	210	2.0	37.0	6.0	m.q.	0	210	0
(*Thomas' Toast-r-Cakes*)	108	1.6	18.0	3.3	m.q.	n.a.	158	m.q.
(*Toaster Strudel* Breakfast								
Pastries)	190	2.0	28.0	8.0	m.q.	n.a.	200	m.q.
frosted (*Kellogg's Pop-Tarts*),								
1.8 oz.	210	2.0	37.0	6.0	m.q.	0	210	0
wild Maine (*Toaster Muffins*)	120	2.0	23.0	3.0	m.q.	n.a.	135	m.q.
bran (*Thomas' Toast-r-Cakes*)	103	1.7	17.6	2.9	m.q.	n.a.	163	m.q.
brown sugar cinnamon (*Kellogg's Pop-*								
Tarts), 1.8 oz.	210	3.0	33.0	8.0	m.q.	0	210	0
brown sugar cinnamon, frosted								
(*Kellogg's Pop-Tarts*), 1.8 oz. ..	210	3.0	34.0	7.0	m.q.	0	180	0
cheese (*Pepperidge Farm* Croissant								
Toaster Tarts)	190	5.0	22.0	10.0	3.0	10	180	m.q.
cherry:								
(*Kellogg's Pop-Tarts*), 1.8 oz.	210	2.0	37.0	6.0	m.q.	0	220	0
(*Toaster Strudel* Breakfast								
Pastries)	190	2.0	26.0	9.0	m.q.	n.a.	200	m.q.
frosted (*Kellogg's Pop-Tarts*),								
1.8 oz.	200	2.0	37.0	5.0	m.q.	0	220	0
chocolate fudge, frosted (*Kellogg's*								
Pop-Tarts), 1.8 oz.	200	3.0	37.0	5.0	m.q.	0	220	0
chocolate-vanilla creme, frosted								
(*Kellogg's Pop-Tarts*), 1.8 oz. ..	200	3.0	37.0	5.0	m.q.	0	230	0
cinnamon (*Toaster Strudel* Breakfast								
Pastries)	190	2.0	26.0	8.0	m.q.	n.a.	200	m.q.
corn (*Thomas' Toast-r-Cakes*)	120	1.8	19.2	4.0	m.q.	n.a.	142	m.q.
corn, old fashioned (*Toaster Muffins*)	120	2.0	17.0	5.0	m.q.	n.a.	200	m.q.
grape, frosted (*Kellogg's Pop-Tarts*),								
1.8 oz.	200	2.0	37.0	5.0	m.q.	0	200	0
oat bran, w/raisins (*Awrey's*								
Toastums)	130	3.0	17.0	5.0	1.0	0	310	1.0 d
raisin bran (*Toaster Muffins*)	120	3.0	16.0	5.0	m.q.	n.a.	220	m.q.
raspberry (*Toaster Strudel* Breakfast								
Pastries)	190	2.0	27.0	8.0	m.q.	n.a.	200	m.q.
raspberry, frosted (*Kellogg's Pop-*								
Tarts), 1.8 oz.	200	2.0	37.0	5.0	m.q.	0	210	0
strawberry:								
(*Kellogg's Pop-Tarts*), 1.8 oz.	210	2.0	37.0	6.0	m.q.	0	200	0

Food and Measure	cal.	prot. (gms)	carbo. (gms)	tot. fat (gms)	sat. fat (gms)	chol. (mgs)	sod. (mgs)	fiber (gms)
(*Pepperidge Farm* Croissant Toaster Tarts)	190	3.0	28.0	7.0	2.0	0	120	m.q.
(*Toaster Strudel* Breakfast Pastries)	190	2.0	27.0	8.0	m.q.	n.a.	200	m.q.
frosted (*Kellogg's Pop-Tarts*), 1.8 oz.	200	2.0	37.0	5.0	m.q.	0	190	0
TOFU:								
raw:								
1 oz.	22	2.3	.5	1.4	.2	0	2	.3 d
¼ block, 2¼″ × 1¾″ × 1½″, approx. 4.1 oz.	88	9.4	2.2	5.6	.8	0	8	1.4 d
½ cup	94	10.0	2.3	5.9	.9	0	9	1.5 d
firm, 1 oz.	41	4.5	1.2	2.5	.4	0	4	<.1 c
firm, ½ cup	183	19.9	5.4	11.0	1.6	0	17	.2 c
pasturized (*Frieda* of California), approx. 4.2 oz.	86	9.6	2.9	m.q.	.8	0	8	m.q.
dried-frozen (koyadofu), 1 oz.	136	13.6	4.1	8.6	1.2	0	2	<.1 c
dried-frozen (koyadofu), 1 piece, .6 oz.	82	8.2	2.5	5.2	.7	0	1	<.1 c
flavored:								
Chinese 5-spice (*Nasoya*), 5 oz.	150	15.0	2.0	8.0	m.q.	0	15	m.q.
French country herb (*Nasoya*), 5 oz.	150	15.0	2.0	8.0	m.q.	0	15	m.q.
fried, 1 oz.	77	4.9	3.0	5.7	.8	0	5	<.1 c
grilled (yakidofu), 1 oz.	25	2.2	.3	1.7	m.q.	0	5	m.q.
okara, 1 oz.	22	.9	3.6	.5	.1	0	3	1.2 c
okara, ½ cup	47	2.0	7.7	1.1	.1	0	6	2.5 c
salted and fermented (fuyu), 1 oz.	33	2.3	1.5	2.3	.3	0	814	.1 c

TOFU BURGER MIX, see
" 'Burger,' vegetarian"

TOFU CHOCOLATE, see "Candy"

TOFU DINNER, see specific
listings

TOFU ENTREE, see specific
listings

TOFU PATTY, frozen:

Food and Measure	cal.	prot. (gms)	carbo. (gms)	tot. fat (gms)	sat. fat (gms)	chol. (mgs)	sod. (mgs)	fiber (gms)
garden (*Natural Touch*), 2.5-oz. patty	90	10.0	3.0	4.0	1.0	0	260	m.q.
okara (*Natural Touch Okara*), 2.25-oz. patty	160	11.0	7.0	10.0	1.0	0	420	m.q.

TOFU SPREAD, canned:

Food and Measure	cal.	prot. (gms)	carbo. (gms)	tot. fat (gms)	sat. fat (gms)	chol. (mgs)	sod. (mgs)	fiber (gms)
green chili (*Natural Touch Tofu Topper*), 2 tbsp.	50	2.0	2.0	4.0	m.q.	0	m.q.	m.q.
herb and spice (*Natural Touch Tofu Topper*), 2 tbsp.	50	2.0	2.0	4.0	m.q.	0	m.q.	m.q.
Mexican (*Natural Touch Tofu Topper*), 2 tbsp.	60	2.0	2.0	5.0	m.q.	0	m.q.	m.q.

Food and Measure	cal.	prot. (gms)	carbo. (gms)	tot. fat (gms)	sat. fat (gms)	chol. (mgs)	sod. (mgs)	fiber (gms)
TOM COLLINS[1]:								
1 fl. oz.	16	tr.	.4	tr.	tr.	0	5	n.a.
TOM COLLINS MIX:								
bottled (*Holland House*), 1 fl. oz.	47	0	11.0	0	0	0	96	n.a.
instant (*Holland House*), .56 oz.	65	0	16.0	0	0	0	14	n.a.
TOMATILLO, fresh:								
(*Frieda* of California), 3½ oz.	25	1.4	4.2	.5	n.a.	0	n.a.	m.q.
TOMATILLO ENTERO:								
(*La Victoria*), 1 tbsp.	4	<1.0	1.0	<1.0	n.a.	n.a.	102	n.a.
TOMATO, red, ripe:								
raw:								
untrimmed, 1 lb.	88	3.5	19.2	1.4	.2	0	36	5.4 d
trimmed, 1 oz.	6	.2	1.3	.1	<.1	0	3	.4 d
1 tomato, approx. 2⅗" diam.,								
4.75 oz.	26	1.0	5.7	.4	.1	0	11	1.6 d
chopped, ½ cup	19	.8	4.2	.3	<.1	0	8	1.2 d
boiled, 4 oz.	31	1.2	6.6	.5	.1	0	12	.9 c
boiled, ½ cup	32	1.3	7.0	.5	.1	0	13	1.0 c
stewed[2], 4 oz.	90	2.2	14.8	3.0	.6	0	516	.9 c
stewed[2], ½ cup	40	1.0	6.6	1.4	.3	0	230	.4 c
TOMATO, CANNED, ½ cup,								
except as noted:								
(*A&P*)	25	1.0	6.0	<1.0	(0)	0	220	m.q.
(*Featherweight*)	20	1.0	4.0	0	0	0	<1.0	m.q.
(*Pathmark* No Frills), 1 cup	50	2.0	11.0	0	0	0	440	m.q.
whole:								
½ cup	24	1.1	5.2	.3	<.1	0	195	.8 d
4 oz.	23	1.1	4.9	.3	<.1	0	185	.8 d
low-sodium	24	1.1	5.2	.3	<.1	0	16	.8 d
low-sodium, 4 oz.	23	1.1	4.9	.3	<.1	0	15	.8 d
(*Hunt's*), 4 oz.	20	1.0	5.0	0	0	0	415	m.q.
(*Hunt's* No Salt Added), 4 oz. ...	20	1.0	5.0	0	0	0	20	m.q.
(*S&W/Nutradiet*)	25	1.0	5.0	0	0	0	20	m.q.
(*Stokely*)	25	1.0	5.0	0	0	0	190	m.q.
whole, peeled:								
(*Contadina*)	25	1.0	5.0	<1.0	(0)	0	260	m.q.
(*Finast*)	25	1.0	6.0	0	0	0	195	m.q.
(*Pathmark* No Salt Added)	25	1.0	6.0	0	0	0	20	m.q.
(*S&W*)	25	1.0	6.0	0	0	0	220	m.q.
Italian style pear, w/basil (*S&W*)	25	1.0	5.0	0	0	0	200	m.q.
w/liquid (*Del Monte*)	25	1.0	5.0	0	0	0	220	m.q.
w/tomato juice (*Pathmark*)	25	1.0	6.0	0	0	0	220	m.q.
crushed:								
(*Hunt's*), 4 oz.	25	1.1	5.2	.2	(0)	0	297	m.q.
(*Pathmark*)	40	1.0	9.0	0	0	0	210	m.q.
(*Pathmark* No Frills), 1 cup	90	3.0	20.0	0	0	0	510	m.q.

1. Recipe: 73.3% club soda, 18.9% gin, 6.9% lemon juice, and .9% sugar.
2. Recipe: 86% tomatoes, 7% bread crumbs, 2% margarine, 2% sugar, 2% onions, 1% salt, and pepper.

Food and Measure	cal.	prot. (gms)	carbo. (gms)	tot. fat (gms)	sat. fat (gms)	chol. (mgs)	sod. (mgs)	fiber (gms)
in puree (*Contadina*)	30	1.0	6.0	<1.0	(0)	0	350	m.q.
cut, peeled (*S&W* Ready-Cut)	25	1.0	6.0	0	0	0	220	m.q.
diced, in rich puree (*S&W*)	35	1.0	8.0	0	0	0	290	m.q.
wedges:								
in tomato juice	34	1.0	8.3	.2	<.1	0	285	.6 c
in tomato juice, 4 oz.	29	.9	7.2	.2	<.1	0	246	.5 c
w/liquid (*Del Monte*)	30	1.0	8.0	0	0	0	355	m.q.
aspic, supreme (*S&W*)	60	1.0	16.0	0	0	0	860	m.q.
w/green chilies	18	.8	4.3	.1	<.1	0	481	.4 c
w/green chilies (*Old El Paso*), ¼ cup	14	0	3.0	0	0	0	480	m.q.
w/jalapeños (*Ortega*), 1 oz.	8	0	1.0	0	0	0	120	m.q.
Italian style, pear (*Contadina*)	25	1.0	5.0	<1.0	(0)	0	220	m.q.
stewed:								
½ cup	34	1.2	8.3	.2	<.1	0	325	.5 c
4 oz.	29	1.1	7.3	.2	<.1	0	288	.5 c
(*Contadina*)	35	1.0	8.0	<1.0	(0)	0	350	m.q.
(*Del Monte*)	35	1.0	8.0	0	0	0	355	m.q.
(*Del Monte* No Salt Added)	35	1.0	8.0	0	0	0	45	m.q.
(*Hunt's*), 4 oz.	35	1.0	8.0	0	0	0	460	m.q.
(*Hunt's* No Salt Added), 4 oz. . . .	35	1.0	8.0	0	0	0	20	m.q.
(*S&W* 50% Salt Reduced)	35	1.0	9.0	0	0	0	180	m.q.
(*Stokely*)	35	1.0	8.0	0	0	0	220	m.q.
sliced:								
(*A&P*)	35	1.0	8.0	<1.0	(0)	0	350	m.q.
(*Finast*)	35	1.0	9.0	0	0	0	355	m.q.
(*Pathmark*)	35	1.0	9.0	0	0	0	360	m.q.
(*S&W*)	35	1.0	9.0	0	0	0	355	m.q.
Italian, sliced (*S&W*)	35	1.0	9.0	0	0	0	355	m.q.
Italian style (*Contadina*)	35	1.0	8.0	<1.0	(0)	0	250	m.q.
w/jalapeños (*Contadina*)	35	1.0	8.0	<1.0	(0)	0	250	m.q.
Mexican style (*S&W*)	40	1.0	8.0	0	0	0	360	m.q.
no salt added, see specific brands								
TOMATO, GREEN:								
untrimmed, 1 lb.	99	5.0	21.1	.8	.1	0	55	2.1 c
trimmed, 1 oz.	7	.3	1.4	.1	tr.	0	4	.1 c
1 medium, approx. 2⅗″ diam.,								
4.75 oz.	30	1.5	6.3	.3	<.1	0	16	.6 c
TOMATO, PICKLED, in jars:								
kosher (*Claussen*), 1 oz.	5	.2	1.0	<1.0	(0)	0	330	m.q.
kosher (*Claussen*), 1 piece, approx.								
1.7 oz.	9	.4	1.8	tr.	(0)	0	571	m.q.
TOMATO JUICE, 6 fl. oz., except								
as noted:								
6 fl. oz.	32	1.4	7.7	.1	<.1	0	658	.7 c
½ cup	21	.9	5.2	.1	<.1	0	441	.5 c
low-sodium	32	1.4	7.7	.1	<.1	0	18	.7 c
low-sodium, ½ cup	21	.9	5.2	.1	<.1	0	12	.5 c
(*A&P*)	30	1.0	7.0	0	0	0	550	m.q.
(*Biotta*)	28	1.3	5.8	.1	(0)	0	277	m.q.

Food and Measure	cal.	prot. (gms)	carbo. (gms)	tot. fat (gms)	sat. fat (gms)	chol. (mgs)	sod. (mgs)	fiber (gms)
TOMATO JUICE *(cont.)*								
(Campbell's)	40	1.0	8.0	0	0	0	540	m.q.
(Featherweight)	35	1.0	8.0	0	0	0	10	m.q.
(Hunt's)	30	1.0	7.0	0	0	0	640	m.q.
(Hunt's No Salt Added)	45	2.0	11.0	0	0	0	30	m.q.
(Pathmark)	30	1.0	6.0	0	0	0	510	m.q.
(S&W California), 5½ fl. oz.	35	1.0	8.0	0	0	0	550	m.q.
(S&W California)	35	1.0	8.0	0	0	0	600	m.q.
(S&W/Nutradiet)	35	1.0	8.0	0	0	0	20	m.q.
(Stokely), 4 fl. oz.	20	1.0	4.0	0	0	0	330	m.q.
(Welch's)	35	1.0	7.0	0	0	0	550	0
from concentrate *(Pathmark)*	35	1.0	8.0	0	0	0	450	m.q.
TOMATO PASTE, canned:								
1 oz.	24	1.1	5.3	.3	<.1	0	224	1.2 d
½ cup	110	5.0	24.7	1.2	.2	0	1035	5.6 d
no salt added (see also specific brands):								
1 oz.	24	1.1	5.3	.3	<.1	0	18	1.2 d
½ cup	110	5.0	24.7	1.2	.2	0	86	5.6 d
(A&P), 6 oz.	150	6.0	35.0	<1.0	(0)	0	100	m.q.
(Contadina), 2 oz. or approx. ¼ cup	50	2.0	11.0	<1.0	(0)	0	40	m.q.
(Del Monte), ¾ cup	150	6.0	34.0	1.0	(0)	0	110	m.q.
(Del Monte No Salt Added), 6 oz. ...	150	6.0	34.0	1.0	(0)	0	110	m.q.
(Finast No Salt Added), ¼ cup	50	2.0	11.0	0	0	0	35	m.q.
(Hunt's), 2 oz.	45	2.0	11.0	0	0	0	140	m.q.
(Hunt's No Salt Added), 2 oz.	45	2.0	11.0	0	0	0	30	m.q.
(Pathmark California), ⅔ cup	150	6.0	35.0	0	0	0	100	m.q.
(S&W), 6 oz.	150	6.0	35.0	0	0	0	100	m.q.
Italian *(Contadina)*, 2 oz. or approx. ¼ cup	65	2.0	12.0	1.0	(0)	0	520	m.q.
Italian style *(Hunt's)*, 2 oz.	50	2.0	11.0	0	0	0	470	m.q.
TOMATO POWDER:								
1 oz.	86	3.7	21.2	.1	<.1	0	38	1.9 c
TOMATO PUREE, canned, ½ cup, except as noted:								
4 oz.	46	1.9	11.4	.1	<.1	0	452	2.6 d
½ cup	51	2.1	12.5	.1	<.1	0	499	2.9 d
no salt added (see also specific brands):								
4 oz.	46	1.9	11.4	.1	<.1	0	23	2.6 d
½ cup	51	2.1	12.5	.1	<.1	0	25	2.9 d
(A&P)	60	2.0	14.0	<1.0	(0)	0	30	m.q.
(Contadina)	40	2.0	8.0	<1.0	(0)	0	35	m.q.
(Finast No Salt Added)	45	2.0	10.0	0	0	0	35	m.q.
(Hunt's), 4 oz.	45	2.0	10.0	.2	(0)	0	170	m.q.
(Pathmark)	45	2.0	10.0	0	0	0	35	m.q.
(S&W)	60	2.0	14.0	0	0	0	35	m.q.
heavy *(Pathmark* California)	60	2.0	14.0	0	0	0	35	m.q.

Food and Measure	cal.	prot. (gms)	carbo. (gms)	tot. fat (gms)	sat. fat (gms)	chol. (mgs)	sod. (mgs)	fiber (gms)
TOMATO SAUCE, canned (see also "Pasta sauce"):								
4 oz.	34	1.5	8.1	.2	<.1	0	686	1.7 d
½ cup	37	1.6	8.8	.2	<.1	0	738	1.8 d
(A&P), ½ cup	45	2.0	9.0	<1.0	(0)	0	600	m.q.
(Contadina), ½ cup	30	1.0	7.0	<1.0	(0)	0	580	m.q.
(Contadina Thick and Zesty), ½ cup	40	2.0	8.0	<1.0	(0)	0	650	m.q.
(Del Monte), 1 cup	70	3.0	16.0	1.0	(0)	0	1330	m.q.
(Del Monte No Salt Added), 1 cup	70	3.0	16.0	1.0	(0)	0	50	m.q.
(Finast), ½ cup	45	2.0	9.0	0	0	0	650	m.q.
(Finast No Salt Added), 8 oz.	90	4.0	18.0	0	0	0	10	m.q.
(Health Valley), 1 cup	70	2.4	13.0	.5	(0)	0	460	.3 d
(Health Valley No Salt Added), 1 cup	70	2.4	13.0	.5	(0)	0	43	.3 d
(Hunt's), 4 oz.	30	1.0	7.0	0	0	0	730	m.q.
(Hunt's No Salt Added), 4 oz.	35	1.0	8.0	0	0	0	25	m.q.
(Hunt's Special), 4 oz.	35	1.0	8.0	0	0	0	320	m.q.
(Pathmark), ½ cup	40	2.0	9.0	0	0	0	620	m.q.
(Pathmark No Salt Added), ½ cup	45	2.0	9.0	0	0	0	25	m.q.
(Rokeach Low Sodium), 3 oz.	50	1.0	8.0	2.0	n.a.	0	124	m.q.
(S&W), ½ cup	40	2.0	9.0	0	0	0	620	m.q.
(Stokely), ½ cup	30	2.0	7.0	0	0	0	810	m.q.
w/green chilies (Old El Paso), ¼ cup	14	<1.0	3.0	<1.0	n.a.	0	480	m.q.
w/herbs and cheese, 4 oz.	67	2.4	11.6	2.2	.7	n.a.	m.q.	m.q.
w/herbs and cheese, ½ cup	72	2.6	12.5	2.4	.8	n.a.	m.q.	m.q.
Italian style:								
(Contadina), ½ cup	30	1.0	7.0	<1.0	(0)	0	670	m.q.
(Hunt's), 4 oz.	60	2.0	11.0	2.0	m.q.	n.a.	520	m.q.
Rokeach), 3 oz.	60	1.0	8.0	2.0	m.q.	0	243	m.q.
w/jalapeños (Old El Paso), ¼ cup	11	1.0	2.0	1.0	0	0	150	m.q.
marinara:								
15½ oz.	300	7.0	44.7	14.7	2.1	0	2760	2.9 c
4 oz.	77	1.8	11.5	3.8	.5	0	713	.7 c
½ cup	86	2.0	12.7	4.2	.6	0	786	.8 c
(Buitoni), ½ cup	70	1.0	11.0	3.0	<1.0	0	570	m.q.
(Pathmark No Frills), ½ cup	80	1.0	12.0	3.0	m.q.	0	620	m.q.
(Rokeach), 3 oz.	60	1.0	9.0	2.0	m.q.	0	257	m.q.
w/mushrooms, 4 oz.	40	1.6	9.6	.1	<.1	0	513	1.0 c
w/mushrooms, ½ cup	42	1.8	10.3	.2	<.1	0	552	1.0 c
no salt added, see specific brands								
w/onions:								
4 oz.	48	1.8	11.3	.2	<.1	0	625	.9 c
½ cup	52	1.9	12.1	.2	<.1	0	672	1.0 c
(Del Monte), 1 cup	100	3.0	23.0	1.0	n.a.	0	1150	m.q.
w/onions, green peppers, and celery, 4 oz.	46	1.1	9.9	.8	.2	0	n.a.	m.q.
w/onions, green peppers, and celery, ½ cup	50	1.2	10.7	.9	.2	0	n.a.	m.q.
Spanish style, 4 oz.	37	1.6	8.2	.3	<.1	0	535	m.q.
Spanish style, ½ cup	40	1.8	8.8	.3	<.1	0	576	m.q.

Food and Measure	cal.	prot. (gms)	carbo. (gms)	tot. fat (gms)	sat. fat (gms)	chol. (mgs)	sod. (mgs)	fiber (gms)
TOMATO SAUCE *(cont.)*								
w/tomato tidbits, low sodium, 4 oz.	36	1.5	8.0	.4	.1	0	17	1.2 c
w/tomato tidbits, low sodium, ½ cup	39	1.6	8.7	.5	.1	0	18	1.3 c
TOMATO SAUCE, REFRIGERATED, 7.5 oz.:								
marinara (*Contadina Fresh*)	100	4.0	12.0	4.0	m.q.	0	700	m.q.
plum, w/basil (*Contadina Fresh*)	100	3.0	14.0	4.0	m.q.	5	700	m.q.
TOMATO-BEEF COCKTAIL:								
6 fl. oz.	66	1.2	15.6	.2	.1	n.a.	240	.2 c
(*Beefamato*), 6 fl. oz.	80	1.0	19.0	0	0	n.a.	240	m.q.
TOMATO-CHILE COCKTAIL:								
(*Snap-E-Tom*), 6 fl. oz.	40	2.0	7.0	0	0	0	980	m.q.
TOMATO-CLAM JUICE COCKTAIL:								
1 fl. oz.	14	.2	3.3	tr.	tr.	n.a.	121	tr.c
(*Clamato*), 6 fl. oz.	96	1.0	23.0	0	0	n.a.	815	m.q.
TOMATOSEED OIL:								
1 oz.	251	0	0	28.4	5.6	0	0	0
½ cup	964	0	0	109.0	21.5	0	0	0
1 tbsp.	120	0	0	13.6	2.7	0	0	0
TONGUE[1]:								
beef:								
raw, 1 oz.	63	4.2	1.0	4.6	2.0	25	20	0
simmered, 9.1 oz., yield from 1 lb. raw	732	57.3	.9	53.7	23.1	278	155	0
simmered, 4 oz.	321	25.1	.4	23.5	10.1	121	68	0
lamb:								
raw, 1 oz.	63	4.5	0	4.9	1.9	44	22	0
braised, 9 oz., yield from 1 lb. raw untrimmed	702	55.1	0	51.8	20.0	484	170	0
braised, 4 oz.	312	24.5	0	23.0	8.9	214	76	0
pork:								
raw, 1 oz.	64	4.6	0	4.9	1.7	29	31	0
braised, 4 oz.	307	27.3	0	21.1	7.3	166	124	0
braised, 8.2 oz., yield from 1 lb. raw untrimmed	626	55.7	0	43.0	14.9	337	252	0
cured, canned (*Hormel*, 8 lb.), 3 oz.	190	17.0	0	13.0	m.q.	m.q.	966	0
veal:								
raw, 1 oz.	37	4.9	.2	1.6	m.q.	m.q.	23	0
braised, 9 oz. (yield from 1 lb. raw untrimmed)	515	66.0	0	25.8	m.q.	m.q.	163	0
braised, 4 oz.	229	29.3	0	11.5	m.q.	m.q.	73	0
TONIC WATER, see "Soft drinks and mixers"								

1. *Cooked meats are prepared without added ingredients.*

Food and Measure	cal.	prot. (gms)	carbo. (gms)	tot. fat (gms)	sat. fat (gms)	chol. (mgs)	sod. (mgs)	fiber (gms)
TOPPING, see specific listings								
TORTELLINI, FROZEN (see also "Tortellini dishes, frozen"):								
meatless (*Tofutti*), 2 oz.	220	12.0	38.0	2.0	m.q.	0	110	m.q.
nondairy, regular or spinach (*Tofutti*), 2 oz.	210	12.0	32.0	4.0	m.q.	0	158	m.q.
TORTELLINI, REFRIGERATED, 4.5 oz.:								
egg:								
w/cheese (*Contadina Fresh*)	380	21.0	60.0	6.0	m.q.	70	570	m.q.
w/chicken and prosciutto (*Contadina Fresh*)	370	24.0	53.0	7.0	m.q.	75	560	m.q.
w/meat (*Contadina Fresh*)	380	22.0	60.0	6.0	m.q.	75	580	m.q.
spinach:								
w/cheese (*Contadina Fresh*)	380	21.0	60.0	6.0	m.q.	70	590	m.q.
w/chicken and prosciutto (*Contadina Fresh*)	340	24.0	53.0	7.0	m.q.	75	580	m.q.
w/meat (*Contadina Fresh*)	380	22.0	60.0	6.0	m.q.	75	610	m.q.
TORTELLINI DINNER, frozen:								
w/meat (*Dinner Classics Lite*), 10 oz.	250	9.0	8.0	10.0	m.q.	m.q.	850	m.q.
TORTELLINI DISHES, FROZEN:								
beef, w/marinara sauce (*Stouffer's*), 10 oz.	360	18.0	45.0	12.0	m.q.	m.q.	780	m.q.
cheese:								
(*The Budget Gourmet* Side Dish), 5.5 oz.	180	7.0	25.0	9.0	m.q.	15	400	m.q.
(*Weight Watchers*), 9 oz.	310	14.0	50.0	6.0	1.0	15	570	m.q.
in Alfredo sauce (*Stouffer's*), 8⅞ oz.	600	28.0	32.0	40.0	m.q.	m.q.	930	m.q.
marinara (*Green Giant* One Serving), 5.5 oz.	260	8.0	37.0	9.0	3.0	25	660	m.q.
meat sauce and (*Le Menu* LightStyle), 8 oz.	250	11.0	34.0	8.0	1.0	15	480	m.q.
in tomato sauce (*Birds Eye For One*), 5.5 oz.	210	11.0	31.0	5.0	m.q.	30	500	0
w/tomato sauce (*Stouffer's*), 9⅝ oz.	360	18.0	37.0	16.0	m.q.	m.q.	860	fiber.q.
w/vinaigrette dressing (*Stouffer's*), 6⅞ oz.	400	15.0	24.0	27.0	m.q.	m.q.	540	m.q.
Provencale (*Green Giant* Microwave Garden Gourmet), 1 pkg.	260	10.0	44.0	6.0	2.0	15	840	3.0 d
veal, in Alfredo sauce (*Stouffer's*), 8⅝ oz.	500	25.0	32.0	30.0	m.q.	m.q.	860	m.q.
TORTELLINI DISHES, MIX, see "Salad mix"								

Food and Measure	cal.	prot. (gms)	carbo. (gms)	tot. fat (gms)	sat. fat (gms)	chol. (mgs)	sod. (mgs)	fiber (gms)
TORTELLINI DISHES, PACKAGED:								
cheese, w/shrimp and seafood								
(*Hormel Top Shelf*), 10 oz.	278	16.0	36.0	8.0	m.q.	89	1341	m.q.
in marinara sauce (*Hormel Top Shelf*),								
10 oz.	211	10.0	37.0	3.0	m.q.	35	663	m.q.
TORTELLONI, see "Tortellini"								
TORTILLA, 1 piece:								
corn (*Azteca*)	45	1.0	9.0	0	0	0	10	0
corn (*Old El Paso*)	60	1.0	10.0	1.0	n.a.	0	170	n.a.
flour:								
(*Azteca*), 9" diam.	130	3.0	23.0	3.0	m.q.	0	180	0
(*Azteca*), 7" diam.	80	2.0	14.0	2.0	m.q.	0	110	0
(*Old El Paso*)	150	4.0	27.0	3.0	m.q.	0	360	n.a.
TORTILLA CHIPS, see "Corn chips, puffs, and similar snacks"								
TORTILLA ENTREE, frozen:								
(*Stouffer's* Grande), 9⅝ oz.	530	24.0	34.0	33.0	m.q.	n.a.	910	m.q.
TORTILLA MIX, see "Corn flour, masa" and "wheat flour"								
TOSTACO SHELL:								
(*Old El Paso*), 1 piece	100	1.0	11.0	5.0	m.q.	0	10	1.0 d
TOSTADA SHELL:								
(*Lawry's*), 1 piece	73	1.2	9.5	3.5	m.q.	0	147	.4 c
(*Old El Paso*), 1 piece	55	<1.0	6.0	3.0	m.q.	0	65	.5 d
(*Ortega*), 1 piece	50	0	8.0	2.0	m.q.	0	5	m.q.
(*Tio Sancho*), 1 piece	67	1.2	8.4	3.2	m.q.	0	1	.5 c
TOWEL GOURD, see "Gourd, dishcloth"								
TREE FERN, cooked:								
4 oz.	45	.3	12.5	.1	(0)	0	6	.7 c
1 frond, 6½" long, ⅝" diam., 1.1 oz.	12	.1	3.4	<.1	(0)	0	2	.2 c
chopped, ½ cup	28	.2	7.8	.1	(0)	0	3	.4 c
TREE OYSTER MUSHROOM, see "Mushroom, oyster"								
TRIPE (see also "Stomach"):								
beef, raw, 1 oz.	28	4.1	0	1.1	.6	27	13	0
TRITICALE, whole grain:								
1 oz.	95	3.7	20.4	.6	.1	0	1	5.1 d
1 cup	646	25.1	138.5	4.0	.7	0	10	34.8 d
TRITICALE FLOUR, whole grain:								
1 oz.	96	3.7	20.7	.5	.1	0	<1	4.1 d
1 cup	440	17.1	95.1	2.4	.4	0	3	19.0 d
TROPICAL FRUIT SALAD, see "Fruit salad, tropical"								
TROPICAL PUNCH, see "Fruit punch"								

Food and Measure	cal.	prot. (gms)	carbo. (gms)	tot. fat (gms)	sat. fat (gms)	chol. (mgs)	sod. (mgs)	fiber (gms)
TROUT, mixed species, meat only,								
raw:								
1 lb.	673	94.2	0	30.0	5.2	264	236	0
1 oz.	42	5.9	0	1.9	.3	16	15	0
1 fillet, approx. 2.8 oz. yield from								
1-lb. whole fish	117	16.4	0	5.2	.9	46	44	0
TROUT, RAINBOW, meat only:								
raw:								
1 lb.	535	93.2	0	15.2	2.9	257	122	0
1 oz.	33	5.8	0	1.0	.2	16	8	0
1 fillet, approx. 2.8 oz., yield from								
1-lb. whole fish	93	16.2	0	2.7	.5	45	21	0
baked, broiled, or microwaved[1],								
4 oz.	171	29.9	0	4.9	.9	83	39	0
TROUT, SEA, see "Sea trout"								
TUNA, BLUEFIN, meat only:								
raw, 1 lb.	652	105.8	0	22.2	5.7	173	177	0
raw, 1 oz.	41	6.6	0	1.4	.4	11	11	0
baked, broiled, or microwaved[1],								
4 oz.	209	33.9	0	7.1	1.8	56	57	0
TUNA, CANNED, 2 oz., except as								
noted:								
light, in vegetable (soybean) oil,								
drained:								
1 oz.	56	8.3	0	2.3	.4	5	100	0
6 oz.	339	49.8	0	14.1	2.6	30	606	0
no salt added, 1 oz.	56	8.3	0	2.3	.4	5	14	0
no salt added, 6 oz.	339	49.8	0	14.1	2.6	30	86	0
(A&P)	150	13.0	<1.0	13.0	m.q.	m.q.	310	0
chunk:								
(Bumble Bee)	110	12.0	0	12.0	3.0	30	310	0
(Finast)	150	13.0	<1.0	13.0	m.q.	m.q.	310	0
(S&W Fancy)	140	13.0	0	10.0	m.q.	m.q.	450	0
(Star-Kist)	150	13.0	<1.0	13.0	1.0	25	310	0
solid (Star-Kist Prime Catch)	150	13.0	<1.0	13.0	1.0	25	310	0
solid (Progresso), ⅓ cup	150	13.0	<1.0	13.0	m.q.	m.q.	400	0
light, in water, drained:								
1 oz.	37	8.4	0	.1	<.1	m.q.	101	0
6.3 oz., yield from No. ½ can ...	216	48.8	0	.8	.3	m.q.	588	0
no salt added, 1 oz.	37	8.4	0	.1	<.1	m.q.	14	0
no salt added, 6.3 oz., yield from								
No. ½ can	216	48.8	0	.8	.3	m.q.	83	0
(A&P)	60	13.0	<1.0	<1.0	m.q.	m.q.	310	0
(Empress)	60	12.0	0	1.0	m.q.	m.q.	310	0
chunk:								
(Bumble Bee)	50	12.0	0	1.0	.5	30	310	0
(Featherweight)	60	13.0	0	1.0	m.q.	30	30	0

1. *Without added ingredients.*

Food and Measure	cal.	prot. (gms)	carbo. (gms)	tot. fat (gms)	sat. fat (gms)	chol. (mgs)	sod. (mgs)	fiber (gms)
TUNA, CANNED, LIGHT, CHUNK, IN WATER *(cont.)*								
(*Finast*)	60	13.0	<1.0	<1.0	m.q.	m.q.	310	0
(*Pathmark*)	70	15.0	0	2.0	m.q.	m.q.	310	0
(*S&W* Fancy)	60	13.0	0	1.0	m.q.	m.q.	500	0
in spring water (*Star-Kist*)	60	13.0	<1.0	<1.0	.2	25	310	0
in spring water (*Star-Kist* Select—60% Less Salt)	65	14.0	<1.0	1.0	.2	25	120	0
in spring water (*Weight Watchers* No Salt Added)	60	14.0	<1.0	<1.0	.2	25	210	0
diet, in distilled water (*Star-Kist*)	65	14.0	<1.0	<1.0	.2	25	35	0
solid, in spring water (*Star-Kist/ Star-Kist* Prime Catch)	60	14.0	<1.0	<1.0	.2	25	310	0
white, in vegetable (soybean) oil, drained:								
1 oz.	53	7.5	0	2.3	m.q.	9	112	0
6.3 oz., yield from No. ½ can ...	331	47.2	0	14.4	m.q.	55	704	0
no salt added, 1 oz.	53	7.5	0	2.3	m.q.	0	14	0
no salt added, 6.3 oz., yield from No. ½ can	331	47.2	0	14.4	m.q.	55	89	0
(*A&P*)	150	13.0	<1.0	10.0	m.q.	m.q.	310	0
chunk (*Bumble Bee*)	110	12.0	0	12.0	3.0	30	310	0
chunk (*Star-Kist*)	140	14.0	<1.0	10.0	1.0	25	310	0
solid, albacore:								
(*Bumble Bee*)	100	14.0	0	8.0	2.0	30	310	0
(*Finast*)	145	14.0	<1.0	10.0	m.q.	m.q.	320	0
(*S&W* Fancy)	160	13.0	0	12.0	m.q.	m.q.	450	0
(*Star-Kist*)	140	14.0	<1.0	10.0	1.0	25	310	0
white, in water, drained:								
1 oz.	39	7.6	0	.7	.2	12	111	0
6.1 oz., yield from No. ½ can ...	234	45.9	0	4.2	1.1	72	673	0
no salt added, 1 oz.	39	7.6	0	.7	.2	12	14	0
no salt added, 6.1 oz., yield from No. ½ can	234	45.9	0	4.2	1.1	72	86	0
chunk:								
(*A&P*)	100	12.0	<1.0	5.0	m.q.	m.q.	310	0
(*Bumble Bee*)	60	12.0	0	2.0	1.0	30	310	0
in spring water (*Star-Kist* Select—60% Less Salt)	70	15.0	<1.0	<1.0	.2	25	120	0
diet, in distilled water (*Star-Kist*)	70	15.0	<1.0	1.0	.2	25	30	0
solid, albacore:								
(*A&P*)	70	15.0	<1.0	<1.0	m.q.	m.q.	310	0
(*Bumble Bee*)	60	14.0	0	2.0	1.0	30	310	0
(*Finast*)	70	15.0	<1.0	1.0	m.q.	m.q.	310	0
(*Pathmark*)	70	15.0	0	2.0	m.q.	m.q.	310	0
in spring water (*Star-Kist*)	70	15.0	<1.0	1.0	.2	25	310	0
in spring water (*Weight Watchers* No Salt Added)	70	15.0	<1.0	1.0	.2	25	210	0

Food and Measure	cal.	prot. (gms)	carbo. (gms)	tot. fat (gms)	sat. fat (gms)	chol. (mgs)	sod. (mgs)	fiber (gms)
TUNA, FROZEN:								
steak, w/out seasoning mix (*SeaPak*),								
6-oz. pkg.	180	40.0	0	2.0	m.q.	75	65	0
TUNA, SKIPJACK, meat only, raw:								
1 lb.	468	99.8	0	4.6	1.5	213	167	0
1 oz.	29	6.2	0	.3	.1	13	10	0
½ fillet, approx. 7 oz., yield from								
5-lb. whole fish	204	43.6	0	2.0	.6	93	73	0
"TUNA," VEGETARIAN, frozen:								
(*Worthington Tuno*), 2 oz.	100	5.0	3.0	7.0	1.0	0	310	m.q.
TUNA, YELLOWFIN, meat only,								
raw:								
1 lb.	492	106.0	0	4.3	1.1	203	168	0
1 oz.	31	6.6	0	.3	.1	13	10	0
TUNA ENTREE, FROZEN:								
noodle casserole (*Stouffer's*), 10 oz.	310	17.0	31.0	13.0	m.q.	m.q.	1340	m.q.
pie (*Banquet*), 7 oz.	540	17.0	44.0	33.0	m.q.	30	810	m.q.
TUNA ENTREE MIX[1]:								
au gratin (*Tuna Helper*), ⅕ pkg. dry	180	6.0	27.0	5.0	m.q.	n.a.	800	m.q.
au gratin (*Tuna Helper*), 6 oz.	280	16.0	30.0	11.0	m.q.	m.q.	980	m.q.
fettucini Alfredo (*Tuna Helper*),								
⅕ pkg. dry	160	6.0	28.0	3.0	m.q.	n.a.	760	m.q.
fettucini Alfredo (*Tuna Helper*), 7 oz.	300	16.0	30.0	13.0	m.q.	m.q.	1000	m.q.
mushroom, creamy (*Tuna Helper*),								
⅕ pkg. dry	140	5.0	28.0	1.0	n.a.	n.a.	580	m.q.
mushroom, creamy (*Tuna Helper*),								
7 oz.	220	14.0	28.0	6.0	m.q.	m.q.	740	m.q.
noodle:								
cheesy (*Tuna Helper*), ⅕ pkg. dry	160	5.0	27.0	4.0	m.q.	n.a.	810	m.q.
cheesy (*Tuna Helper*), 7.75 oz. . . .	250	15.0	28.0	9.0	m.q.	m.q.	980	m.q.
creamy (*Tuna Helper*), ⅕ pkg. dry	210	5.0	29.0	8.0	m.q.	n.a.	790	m.q.
creamy (*Tuna Helper*), 8 oz.	300	14.0	30.0	14.0	m.q.	m.q.	960	m.q.
pot pie (*Tuna Helper*), ⅙ pkg.	290	4.0	31.0	17.0	m.q.	n.a.	730	m.q.
pot pie (*Tuna Helper*), 5.1 oz.	420	13.0	31.0	27.0	m.q.	m.q.	890	m.q.
rice, buttery (*Tuna Helper*), ⅕ pkg.								
dry	160	4.0	32.0	2.0	m.q	n.a.	830	m.q.
rice, buttery (*Tuna Helper*), 6 oz. . . .	280	13.0	32.0	11.0	m.q.	m.q.	1040	m.q.
salad (*Tuna Helper*), ⅕ pkg.	140	5.0	28.0	1.0	n.a.	n.a.	580	m.q.
salad (*Tuna Helper*), 5.5 oz.	420	14.0	29.0	27.0	m.q.	m.q.	870	m.q.
tetrazzini (*Tuna Helper*), ⅕ pkg. dry	160	6.0	26.0	3.0	m.q.	n.a.	620	m.q.
tetrazzini (*Tuna Helper*), 6 oz.	240	15.0	27.0	8.0	m.q.	m.q.	780	m.q.
TUNA NOODLE CASSEROLE,								
see "Tuna entree, frozen"								
TUNA PIE, see "Tuna entree,								
frozen"								

1. *Prepared according to package directions, with water-packed tuna, except as noted.*

Food and Measure	cal.	prot. (gms)	carbo. (gms)	tot. fat (gms)	sat. fat (gms)	chol. (mgs)	sod. (mgs)	fiber (gms)
TUNA SALAD:								
homemade[1], 4 oz.	212	18.2	10.7	10.5	1.8	15	456	.6 c
homemade [1], 1 cup	383	32.9	19.3	19.0	3.2	27	824	1.1 c
(*Longacre*), 1 oz.	58	2.0	3.0	4.0	m.q.	10	130	n.a.
(*Longacre* Saladfest), 1 oz.	52	3.0	2.0	4.0	m.q.	10	180	n.a.
TURBOT, DOMESTIC, see "Halibut, Greenland"								
TURBOT, EUROPEAN, meat only, raw:								
1 lb.	432	72.8	0	13.4	m.q.	m.q.	678	0
1 oz.	27	4.6	0	.8	m.q.	m.q.	43	0
½ fillet, approx. 7.2 oz., yield from 5-lb. whole fish	194	32.7	0	6.0	m.q.	m.q.	305	0
TURKEY, ALL CLASSES[2], fresh:								
raw:								
meat w/skin:								
½ turkey, 5.6 lbs., yield from 7.1 lbs. w/bone	4092	523.9	0	205.7	58.0	1753	1662	0
1 lb.	726	92.6	0	36.4	10.3	308	295	0
1 oz.	45	5.8	0	2.3	.6	19	18	0
meat only:								
½ turkey, 4.8 lbs., yield from 7.1 lbs w/bone and skin	2581	473.2	0	62.1	20.6	1403	1512	0
1 lb.	540	98.7	0	13.0	4.3	295	318	0
1 oz.	34	6.2	0	.8	.3	18	20	0
skin only, 1 oz.	110	3.6	0	10.5	2.7	26	10	0
dark meat:								
w/skin, 1 lb.	726	85.8	0	39.9	11.7	327	322	0
w/skin, 1 oz.	45	5.4	0	2.5	.7	20	20	0
meat only, 1 lb.	567	91.0	0	19.9	6.7	313	349	0
meat only, 1 oz.	35	5.7	0	1.2	.4	20	22	0
light meat:								
w/skin, 1 lb.	721	98.2	0	33.4	9.1	295	268	0
w/skin, 1 oz.	45	6.1	0	2.1	.6	18	17	0
meat only, 1 lb.	522	106.9	0	7.1	2.3	272	286	0
meat only, 1 oz.	33	6.7	0	.4	.1	17	18	0
back, meat w/skin, 1 oz.	56	5.1	0	3.7	1.0	21	19	0
breast, meat w/skin, 1 oz.	45	6.2	0	2.0	.5	18	17	0
leg, meat w/skin, 1 oz.	41	5.5	0	1.9	.6	20	21	0
neck, meat only, 1 oz.	38	5.7	0	1.5	.5	22	26	0
wing, meat w/skin, 1 oz.	56	5.7	0	3.5	.9	20	16	0
roasted:								
meat w/skin, ½ turkey, 4.1 lbs., yield from 5.1 lbs. w/bone	3857	521.8	0	180.5	52.7	1514	1269	0
meat w/skin, 4 oz.	236	31.9	0	11.0	3.2	93	77	0
meat only, 4 oz.	193	33.2	0	5.6	1.9	86	79	0

1. *Recipe: 53.8% light tuna in oil, 14.7% pickle relish, 14.1% salad dressing, 10.2% onion, and 7.2% celery.*
2. *Cooked poultry is prepared without added ingredients.*

Food and Measure	cal.	prot. (gms)	carbo. (gms)	tot. fat (gms)	sat. fat (gms)	chol. (mgs)	sod. (mgs)	fiber (gms)
meat only, chopped or diced,								
1 cup not packed	238	41.0	0	7.0	2.3	107	99	0
skin only, 1 oz.	125	5.6	0	11.2	2.9	32	15	0
dark meat:								
w/skin, 4 oz.	251	31.2	0	13.1	4.0	101	86	0
meat only, 4 oz.	212	32.4	0	8.2	2.7	96	90	0
meat only, chopped or diced,								
1 cup not packed	262	40.0	0	10.1	3.4	119	110	0
light meat:								
w/skin, 4 oz.	223	32.4	0	9.4	2.7	86	71	0
meat only, 4 oz.	178	33.9	0	3.7	1.2	78	73	0
meat only, chopped or diced,								
1 cup not packed	219	41.9	0	4.5	1.4	97	89	0
back, meat w/skin, 4 oz.	276	30.2	0	16.3	4.7	103	83	0
breast, meat w/skin, ½ breast,								
1.9 lbs., yield from 4.2 lbs.								
w/bone	1637	248.1	0	64.1	18.1	643	541	0
breast, meat w/skin, 4 oz.	214	32.6	0	8.4	2.4	84	71	0
leg, meat w/skin, 1 leg, 1.2 lbs.,								
yield from 1.5 lbs. w/bone	1133	152.2	0	53.6	16.7	466	420	0
leg, meat w/skin, 4 oz.	236	31.6	0	11.1	3.5	96	87	0
wing, meat w/skin, 1 wing, 6.6								
oz., yield from 9.9 oz. w/bone	426	50.9	0	23.1	6.3	150	114	0
wing, meat w/skin, 4 oz.	260	31.0	0	14.1	3.8	92	69	0
simmered:								
neck, meat only, 1 neck, 5.4 oz.,								
yield from 9 oz. w/bone and								
skin	274	40.8	0	11.0	3.7	186	84	0
neck meat only, 4 oz.	204	30.4	0	8.2	2.8	138	64	0
TURKEY, FRYER-ROASTER[1],								
fresh:								
raw:								
meat w/skin:								
½ turkey, 2.4 lbs., yield from								
3.2 lbs. w/bone	1463	244.5	0	46.5	13.2	888	631	0
1 lb.	608	101.5	0	19.3	5.5	367	263	0
1 oz.	38	6.3	0	1.2	.3	23	16	0
meat only:								
½ turkey, 2.1 lbs., yield from								
3.2 lbs. w/bone and skin	1052	214.3	0	15.2	5.1	704	584	0
1 lb.	499	101.2	0	7.2	2.4	331	277	0
1 oz.	31	6.3	0	.4	.2	21	17	0
skin only, 1 oz.	80	4.7	0	6.7	1.7	39	10	0
dark meat:								
w/skin, 1 lb.	585	91.0	0	21.7	6.5	395	299	0
w/skin, 1 oz.	37	5.7	0	1.4	.4	25	19	0
meat only, 1 lb.	503	92.8	0	12.1	4.1	367	313	0

1. *Cooked poultry is prepared without added ingredients.*

Food and Measure	cal.	prot. (gms)	carbo. (gms)	tot. fat (gms)	sat. fat (gms)	chol. (mgs)	sod. (mgs)	fiber (gms)
TURKEY, FRYER-ROASTER, RAW, DARK MEAT *(cont.)*								
meat only, 1 oz.	31	5.8	0	.8	.3	23	20	0
light meat:								
w/skin, 1 lb.	603	104.7	0	17.3	4.6	345	227	0
w/skin, 1 oz.	38	6.5	0	1.1	.3	22	14	0
meat only, 1 lb.	490	109.7	0	2.2	.7	299	236	0
meat only, 1 oz.	31	6.9	0	.1	<.1	19	15	0
back, meat w/skin, 1 oz.	43	5.6	0	2.1	.6	24	17	0
back, meat only, 1 oz.	34	5.9	0	1.0	.3	21	18	0
breast, meat w/skin, 1 oz.	35	6.7	0	.8	.2	20	14	0
breast, meat only, 1 oz.	31	7.0	0	.2	.1	18	14	0
leg, meat w/skin, 1 oz.	33	5.7	0	1.0	.3	25	20	0
leg, meat only, 1 oz.	31	5.8	0	.7	.2	24	20	0
wing, meat w/skin, 1 oz.	45	5.9	0	2.2	.6	28	16	0
wing, meat only, 1 oz.	30	6.4	0	.3	.1	23	18	0
roasted:								
meat w/skin, ½ turkey, 1.8 lbs.,								
yield from 2.4 lbs. w/bone	1392	228.4	0	46.2	13.3	849	532	0
meat w/skin, 4 oz.	195	32.0	0	6.5	1.9	119	75	0
meat only, 4 oz.	170	33.5	0	3.0	1.0	111	76	0
meat only, chopped or diced,								
1 cup not packed	210	41.4	0	3.7	1.2	138	94	0
1 oz.	85	5.9	0	6.6	1.7	41	17	0
dark meat:								
w/skin, 4 oz.	206	31.4	0	8.0	2.4	133	86	0
meat only, 4 oz.	184	32.7	0	4.9	1.6	127	90	0
meat only, chopped or diced,								
1 cup not packed	227	40.4	0	6.0	2.0	157	110	0
light meat:								
w/skin, 4 oz.	186	32.6	0	5.2	1.4	108	65	0
meat only, 4 oz.	159	34.2	0	1.3	.4	98	64	0
meat only, chopped or diced,								
1 cup not packed	195	42.3	0	1.7	.5	121	79	0
back, meat w/skin, 4 oz.	231	29.7	0	11.6	3.4	122	79	0
back, meat only, 4 oz.	193	31.8	0	6.4	2.1	108	83	0
breast:								
meat w/skin, ½ breast,								
12.1 oz., yield from 1.7 lbs.								
w/bone	526	100.0	0	11.0	3.0	310	182	0
meat w/skin, 4 oz.	174	33.0	0	3.6	1.0	102	60	0
meat only, ½ breast, 10.8 oz.,								
yield from 1.7 lbs. w/bone								
and skin	413	92.0	0	2.3	.7	255	159	0
meat only, 4 oz.	153	34.1	0	.8	.3	94	59	0
leg:								
meat w/skin, 1 leg, 8.6 oz.,								
yield from 11.4 oz. w/bone . .	418	69.8	0	13.3	4.1	171	195	0
meat w/skin, 4 oz.	193	32.3	0	6.1	1.9	79	91	0

Food and Measure	cal.	prot. (gms)	carbo. (gms)	tot. fat (gms)	sat. fat (gms)	chol. (mgs)	sod. (mgs)	fiber (gms)
meat only, 1 leg, 7.9 oz., yield from 11.4 oz. w/bone and skin	355	65.4	0	8.5	2.8	267	182	0
meat only, 4 oz.	180	33.1	0	4.3	1.4	135	92	0
wing:								
meat w/skin, 1 wing, 3.2 oz., yield from 5.2 oz. w/bone . . .	186	24.9	0	8.9	2.4	104	65	0
meat w/skin, 4 oz.	235	31.4	0	11.2	3.1	130	83	0
meat only, 1 wing, 2.1 oz., yield from 5.2 oz. w/bone and skin	98	18.5	0	2.1	.7	61	47	0
meat only, 4 oz.	185	35.0	0	3.9	1.2	116	88	0
TURKEY, YOUNG HEN[1], fresh:								
raw:								
meat w/skin:								
½ turkey, 4.5 lbs., yield from 5.75 lbs. w/bone	3451	414.2	0	186.6	52.5	1293	1259	0
1 lb.	762	91.5	0	41.2	11.6	286	277	0
1 oz.	48	5.7	0	2.6	.7	18	17	0
meat only:								
½ turkey, 3.8 lbs., yield from 5.75 lbs. w/bone and skin . . .	2105	376.7	0	55.1	18.2	1034	1144	0
1 lb.	553	98.7	0	14.4	4.8	272	299	0
1 oz.	35	6.2	0	.9	.3	17	19	0
dark meat:								
w/skin, 1 lb.	780	84.6	0	46.5	13.6	295	304	0
w/skin, 1 oz.	49	5.3	0	2.9	.8	18	19	0
meat only, 1 lb.	590	91.0	0	22.1	7.4	281	336	0
meat only, 1 oz.	37	5.7	0	1.4	.5	18	21	0
light meat:								
w/skin, 1 lb.	748	97.6	0	36.7	9.9	281	249	0
w/skin, 1 oz.	47	6.1	0	2.3	.6	18	16	0
meat only, 1 lb.	526	107.2	0	7.5	2.4	263	272	0
meat only, 1 oz.	33	6.7	0	.5	.2	16	17	0
back, meat w/skin, 1 oz.	62	5.0	0	4.5	1.3	19	17	0
breast, meat w/skin, 1 oz.	47	6.1	0	2.4	.6	18	16	0
leg, meat w/skin, 1 oz.	43	5.5	0	2.1	.6	18	20	0
wing, meat w/skin, 1 oz.	60	5.7	0	3.9	1.0	18	14	0
roasted:								
meat w/skin, ½ turkey, 3.4 lbs., yield from 4.2 lbs. w/bone	3323	428.1	0	165.8	48.4	1190	977	0
meat w/skin, 4 oz.	247	31.9	0	12.3	3.6	88	73	0
meat only, 4 oz.	198	33.2	0	6.2	2.1	83	76	0
meat only, chopped or diced, 1 cup not packed	244	41.0	0	7.7	2.5	102	93	0
skin only, 1 oz.	137	5.4	0	12.6	3.3	30	12	0
dark meat:								
w/skin, 4 oz.	263	31.0	0	14.5	4.4	95	82	0

1. *Cooked poultry is prepared without added ingredients.*

Food and Measure	cal.	prot. (gms)	carbo. (gms)	tot. fat (gms)	sat. fat (gms)	chol. (mgs)	sod. (mgs)	fiber (gms)
TURKEY, YOUNG HEN, ROASTED, DARK MEAT *(cont.)*								
meat only, 4 oz.	218	32.2	0	8.8	3.0	91	85	0
meat only, chopped or diced,								
1 cup not packed	268	39.8	0	10.9	3.7	111	105	0
light meat:								
w/skin, 4 oz.	235	32.5	0	10.7	3.0	84	66	0
meat only, 4 oz.	183	33.9	0	4.2	1.3	77	68	0
meat only, chopped or diced,								
1 cup not packed	226	41.9	0	5.2	1.7	95	84	0
back, meat w/skin, 4 oz.	288	29.9	0	17.7	5.1	96	78	0
breast, meat w/skin, 4 oz.	220	32.7	0	8.9	2.6	82	66	0
breast, meat w/skin, ½ breast,								
1.5 lbs., yield from 3.3 lbs.								
w/bone	1330	197.5	0	53.9	15.4	492	401	0
leg, meat w/skin, 4 oz.	242	31.4	0	11.9	3.7	93	83	0
leg, meat w/skin, 1 leg, 15.8 oz.,								
yield from 1.2 lbs. w/bone	955	124.2	0	47.1	14.7	365	326	0
wing, meat w/skin, 4 oz.	270	31.0	0	15.3	4.2	87	64	0
wing, meat w/skin, 1 wing, 6.1								
oz., yield from 8.9 oz. w/bone	414	47.5	0	23.4	6.4	134	98	0
TURKEY, YOUNG TOM[1], fresh:								
raw:								
meat w/skin:								
½ turkey, 8.6 lbs., yield from								
10.6 lbs. w/bone	6013	796.7	0	289.4	81.7	2796	2665	0
1 lb.	699	92.8	0	33.7	9.5	327	308	0
1 oz.	44	5.8	0	2.1	.6	20	19	0
meat only:								
½ turkey, 7.3 lbs., yield from								
10.6 lbs. w/bone and skin . . .	3867	717.2	0	89.2	29.5	2240	2422	0
1 lb.	531	98.5	0	12.2	4.0	308	331	0
1 oz.	33	6.2	0	.8	.3	19	21	0
skin only, 1 oz.	104	3.8	0	9.8	2.6	27	11	0
dark meat:								
w/skin, 1 lb.	689	86.4	0	35.8	10.5	349	340	0
w/skin, 1 oz.	43	5.4	0	2.2	.7	22	21	0
meat only, 1 lb.	558	90.9	0	18.6	6.3	340	363	0
meat only, 1 oz.	35	5.7	0	1.2	.4	21	23	0
light meat:								
w/skin, 1 lb.	708	98.1	0	31.9	8.7	304	286	0
w/skin, 1 oz.	44	6.1	0	2.0	.5	19	18	0
meat only, 1 lb.	517	106.3	0	7.1	2.3	281	304	0
meat only, 1 oz.	32	6.6	0	.4	.1	18	19	0
back, meat w/skin, 1 oz.	51	5.2	0	3.2	.9	22	20	0
breast, meat w/skin, 1 oz.	43	6.2	0	1.8	.5	7	18	0
leg, meat w/skin, 1 oz.	40	5.5	0	1.8	.5	22	22	0
wing, meat w/skin, 1 oz.	53	5.8	0	3.2	.8	20	17	0

1. *Cooked poultry is prepared without added ingredients.*

Food and Measure	cal.	prot. (gms)	carbo. (gms)	tot. fat (gms)	sat. fat (gms)	chol. (mgs)	sod. (mgs)	fiber (gms)
roasted:								
meat w/skin, ½ turkey, 6.1 lbs.,								
yield from 7.6 lbs. w/bone	5545	772.5	0	249.0	72.6	2265	1993	0
meat w/skin, 4 oz.	229	31.9	0	10.3	3.0	93	82	0
meat only, 4 oz.	191	33.3	0	5.3	1.7	87	84	0
meat only, chopped or diced,								
1 cup not packed	235	41.1	0	5.6	2.2	108	104	0
skin only, 1 oz.	120	5.7	0	10.6	2.8	33	17	0
dark meat:								
w/skin, 4 oz.	245	31.3	0	12.3	3.7	103	91	0
meat only, 4 oz.	210	32.5	0	7.9	2.7	100	93	0
meat only, chopped or diced,								
1 cup not packed	260	40.2	0	9.8	3.3	123	115	0
light meat:								
w/skin, 4 oz.	217	32.3	0	8.7	2.4	85	76	0
meat only, 4 oz.	175	33.9	0	3.3	1.1	78	77	0
meat only, chopped or diced,								
1 cup not packed	215	41.8	0	4.1	1.3	97	95	0
back, meat w/skin, 4 oz.	270	30.4	0	15.5	4.5	107	87	0
breast, meat w/skin, 4 oz.	214	32.4	0	8.4	2.4	85	76	0
breast, meat w/skin, ½ breast,								
2.9 lbs., yield from 6.4 lbs.								
w/bone	2510	380.3	0	98.3	27.6	1002	892	0
leg, meat w/skin, 4 oz.	234	31.7	0	10.9	3.4	102	91	0
leg, meat w/skin, 1 leg, 1.8 lbs.,								
yield from 2.2 lbs. w/bone	1660	224.9	0	77.5	24.1	727	648	0
wing, meat w/skin, 4 oz.	251	31.1	0	13.0	3.5	92	75	0
wing, meat w/skin, 1 wing, 8.4								
oz., yield from 13.3 oz. w/bone	524	65.1	0	27.3	7.4	192	157	0
TURKEY, BONELESS AND								
LUNCHEON MEAT, cooked								
(see also "Turkey, frozen and								
refrigerated"), 1 oz., except as								
noted:								
bologna, see "Turkey bologna"								
breast:								
1 oz.	31	6.4	0	.4	.1	12	406	0
1 slice, 3½" square, 8 slices per								
6-oz. pkg.	23	4.7	0	.3	.1	9	301	0
(*Butterball* Cold Cuts)	30	5.0	1.0	1.0	m.q.	m.q.	230	0
(*Butterball Deli* No Salt Added) ..	45	7.0	0	2.0	m.q.	m.q.	15	0
(*Butterball Slice 'n Serve*)	35	5.0	<1.0	1.0	m.q.	m.q.	230	0
(*Healthy Deli* Gourmet)	28	4.9	.5	.6	m.q.	9	170	0
(*Healthy Deli* Lessalt)	25	4.5	.4	.5	m.q.	9	140	0
(*Hormel* Perma-Fresh), 2 slices ..	60	9.0	0	2.0	m.q.	m.q.	484	0
(*Light & Lean*), 2 slices	60	8.0	0	2.0	m.q.	m.q.	m.q.	0
(*Longacre* Catering)	35	6.0	<1.0	1.0	m.q.	15	280	0
(*Longacre* Gourmet)	35	5.0	1.0	1.0	m.q.	15	300	0
(*Longacre* Gourmet Low Salt) ...	30	6.0	1.0	<1.0	m.q.	10	150	0

Food and Measure	cal.	prot. (gms)	carbo. (gms)	tot. fat (gms)	sat. fat (gms)	chol. (mgs)	sod. (mgs)	fiber (gms)
TURKEY, BONELESS AND LUNCHEON MEAT, BREAST *(cont.)*								
(*Longacre* Premium)	30	4.0	1.0	1.0	m.q.	10	250	0
(*Longacre* Salt Watchers)	32	7.0	0	<1.0	m.q.	15	10	0
(*Mr. Turkey*)	31	5.8	.3	.7	m.q.	10	233	0
barbecue seasoned (*Butterball*								
Slice 'n Serve BBQ)	40	5.0	1.0	2.0	m.q.	m.q.	210	0
browned:								
glazed (*Longacre* Gourmet) ...	35	5.0	1.0	1.0	m.q.	15	240	0
glazed (*Longacre* Premium) ...	30	4.0	1.0	1.0	m.q.	10	300	0
roasted (*Longacre* Gourmet) ..	35	5.0	1.0	1.0	m.q.	15	260	0
roasted (*Longacre* Premium) ..	30	4.0	1.0	1.0	m.q.	10	300	0
honey (*Healthy Deli*)	28	4.9	.5	.5	m.q.	9	170	0
honey-roasted (*Louis Rich*)	32	4.9	1.2	.8	.3	11	315	0
golden (*Boar's Head*)	35	6.0	<1.0	1.0	m.q.	20	200	0
golden, skinless (*Boar's Head*) ...	30	6.0	<1.0	<1.0	m.q.	10	m.q.	0
lean lite:								
(*Longacre* Deli)	35	6.0	0	1.0	m.q.	15	160	0
skinless (*Longacre* Deli)	35	6.0	0	<1.0	m.q.	15	160	0
smoked (*Longacre* Deli)	35	6.0	0	1.0	m.q.	15	160	0
loaf, 6-oz. pkg.	187	38.3	0	2.7	.8	69	2433	0
loaf, 2 slices or 1.5 oz.	47	9.6	0	.7	.2	17	608	0
oven cooked (*Healthy Deli*)	26	4.7	.4	.2	m.q.	8	180	0
oven roasted:								
(*Hillshire Farm* Deli Select) ...	31	6.0	<1.0	.2	m.q.	m.q.	340	0
(*Louis Rich*)	31	4.8	1.1	.8	.3	11	323	0
(*Louis Rich* Thin Sliced), .4-oz.								
slice	12	1.9	.4	.3	.1	4	127	0
(*Oscar Mayer*), .75-oz. slice ...	23	4.2	.5	.5	.1	9	290	0
roast (*Oscar Mayer* Thin Sliced),								
.4-oz slice	12	2.2	.3	.2	.1	5	151	0
w/skin:								
(*Norbest* Blue Label)	28	5.1	.2	.7	m.q.	m.q.	239	0
(*Norbest* Orange Label)	28	5.7	.1	.3	m.q.	m.q.	232	0
(*Norbest* Yellow Label)	26	5.1	.1	.4	m.q.	m.q.	271	0
(*Norbest Norfresh* Orange Label)	26	5.3	.1	.3	m.q.	m.q.	256	0
(*Norbest Norfresh* Yellow Label)	25	4.8	.1	.5	m.q.	m.q.	244	0
prebrowned (*Norbest* Orange								
Label)	29	5.1	.2	.8	m.q.	m.q.	259	0
salt-free (*Norbest* Blue Label) ..	35	7.5	.2	.5	m.q.	m.q.	13	0
smoked (*Norbest* Orange Label)	30	5.3	.9	.5	m.q.	m.q.	284	0
skinless:								
(*Longacre* Catering)	35	6.0	<1.0	<1.0	m.q.	15	280	0
(*Longacre* Gourmet)	30	5.0	1.0	<1.0	m.q.	15	260	0
(*Longacre* Premium)	30	4.0	1.0	<1.0	m.q.	10	250	0
(*Norbest* Blue Label)	26	5.1	.4	.4	m.q.	m.q.	252	0
(*Norbest* Orange Label)	26	5.1	.5	.2	m.q.	m.q.	239	0
(*Norbest* Tan Label)	24	4.3	.5	.5	m.q.	m.q.	354	0
(*Norbest* Yellow Label)	26	4.3	.8	.5	m.q.	m.q.	272	0
(*Norbest Norfresh*)	27	5.2	.5	.3	m.q.	m.q.	269	0

Food and Measure	cal.	prot. (gms)	carbo. (gms)	tot. fat (gms)	sat. fat (gms)	chol. (mgs)	sod. (mgs)	fiber (gms)
(*Norbest Norfresh* Blue Label) ..	24	4.4	.7	.3	m.q.	m.q.	253	0
(*Norbest Norfresh* Yellow Label)	24	4.4	.4	.5	m.q.	m.q.	284	0
salt-free (*Norbest* Blue Label) ..	33	7.7	<.1	.3	m.q.	m.q.	13	0
sliced (*Longacre*)	30	5.0	1.0	1.0	m.q.	10	280	0
smoked:								
(*Butterball* Cold Cuts)	35	5.0	0	1.0	m.q.	m.q.	190	0
(*Healthy Deli*, 3 lb.)	29	4.8	.5	.5	m.q.	8	180	0
(*Healthy Deli* Gourmet)	31	5.8	.4	.5	m.q.	11	170	0
(*Hillshire Farm* Deli Select) ...	31	6.0	<1.0	.2	m.q.	m.q.	290	0
(*Hormel* Perma-Fresh), 2 slices	60	10.0	0	2.0	m.q.	m.q.	540	0
(*Longacre*)	35	6.0	0	1.0	m.q.	15	240	0
(*Louis Rich*), .74-oz. slice	21	4.5	.2	.3	.1	9	211	0
(*Louis Rich* Thin Sliced), .4-oz.								
slice	11	2.3	.1	.1	tr.	5	111	0
(*Mr. Turkey*)	31	5.9	.3	.7	m.q.	10	332	0
(*Norbest* Gold Label)	29	6.4	.1	<.6	m.q.	m.q.	270	0
(*OHSE*)	30	5.0	1.0	1.0	m.q.	m.q.	340	0
(*Oscar Mayer*), .75-oz. slice ...	20	4.3	.2	.2	.1	9	300	0
hickory (*Butterball Slice 'n*								
Serve)	35	5.0	1.0	1.0	m.q.	m.q.	250	0
sliced (*Longacre*)	26	5.0	1.0	<1.0	m.q.	10	260	0
breast and white:								
(*Longacre Deli Chef*)	35	5.0	1.0	1.0	m.q.	15	240	0
browned and roasted (*Longacre*								
Deli Chef)	40	5.0	1.0	2.0	m.q.	15	240	0
skinless (*Longacre Deli Chef*)	40	4.0	1.0	2.0	m.q.	15	240	0
breast and thigh (*Norbest* Blue								
Label)	31	5.8	.2	.9	m.q.	m.q.	238	0
diced, white and dark meat,								
seasoned	39	5.3	.3	1.7	.5	m.q.	241	0
diced, white meat (*Norbest*)	31	4.4	1.0	.9	m.q.	m.q.	318	0
ham, see "Turkey ham"								
ham flavor, hickory smoked, dark								
meat (*Norbest* Gourmet Cured)	39	4.6	.1	2.2	m.q.	m.q.	335	0
loaf (*Louis Rich*)	45	4.6	.4	2.8	.8	16	270	0
luncheon loaf, spiced (*Mr. Turkey*) ..	51	4.2	.5	3.6	m.q.	11	292	0
oven cooked (*OHSE*)	30	5.0	1.0	1.0	m.q.	m.q.	190	0
pastrami, see "Turkey pastrami"								
roll:								
light meat, 2 oz. or 2 slices	83	10.6	.3	4.1	1.1	24	277	0
light meat	42	5.3	.2	2.1	.6	12	139	0
light and dark meat, 2 oz. or								
2 slices	84	10.3	1.2	4.0	1.2	31	332	0
light and dark meat	42	5.1	.6	2.0	.6	16	166	0
white meat (*Norbest* Orange								
Label)	29	4.1	.5	.9	m.q.	m.q.	299	0
white and dark meat (*Norbest*								
Orange Label)	36	4.0	.3	2.0	m.q.	m.q.	314	0
salami, see "Turkey salami"								

Food and Measure	cal.	prot. (gms)	carbo. (gms)	tot. fat (gms)	sat. fat (gms)	chol. (mgs)	sod. (mgs)	fiber (gms)
TURKEY, BONELESS AND LUNCHEON MEAT *(cont.)*								
sausage, see "Turkey sausage"								
smoked:								
(*Butterball* Cold Cuts)	35	5.0	1.0	1.0	m.q.	m.q.	220	0
(*Butterball Turkey Variety Pak*),								
¾ oz.	25	4.0	1.0	1.0	m.q.	m.q.	160	0
(*Louis Rich*)	32	5.4	.4	1.0	.4	14	284	0
summer sausage, see "Turkey								
summer sausage"								
TURKEY, CANNED:								
boned, w/broth, 5-oz. can	231	33.6	0	9.7	2.8	m.q.	663	0
boned, w/broth, 1 oz.	46	6.7	0	1.9	.6	m.q.	132	0
chunk (*Hormel*), 6¾ oz.	230	37.0	0	10.0	m.q.	m.q.	1278	0
white (*Swanson*), 2½ oz.	80	17.0	1.0	1.0	n.a.	m.q.	260	0
TURKEY, FROZEN AND								
REFRIGERATED:								
breast, raw:								
(*Longacre* Cook-N-Bag), 1 oz. ...	27	6.0	<1.0	<1.0	m.q.	10	120	0
(*Longacre* Ready-to-Cook), 1 oz.	39	8.0	0	<1.0	m.q.	m.q.	150	0
w/gravy (*Norbest*), 4 oz.	115	20.7	1.1	2.4	m.q.	m.q.	492	0
steaks, cubed (*Norbest*), 4-oz.								
steak	135	27.8	<.1	<2.0	m.q.	m.q.	81	0
strips and tips (*Norbest Tasti-*								
Lean), 4 oz.	135	27.8	<.1	<2.0	m.q.	m.q.	81	0
tenderloin (*Norbest Tasti-Lean*								
Tenders), 4 oz.	135	27.8	<.1	<2.0	m.q.	m.q.	81	0
breast, cooked:								
(*Land O'Lakes*), 3 oz.	100	20.0	0	1.0	<1.0	50	55	0
(*Longacre* Cook-N-Bag), 1 oz. ...	38	8.0	<1.0	<1.0	m.q.	15	85	0
(*Louis Rich*), 1 oz.	47	8.1	.1	1.5	.6	21	21	0
w/skin, roasted[1], 4 oz.	143	25.1	0	3.9	1.1	48	450	0
w/skin, roasted[1], ½ breast, 1.9								
lbs., yield from 4.2 lbs. w/bone	1087	191.5	0	29.9	8.5	359	3434	0
barbecue (*Louis Rich*), 1 oz.	33	5.3	.9	1.0	.3	12	315	0
barbecue, quarter (*Mr. Turkey*								
Chub), 1 oz.	34	5.4	1.0	1.0	m.q.	11	251	0
hen, w/out wing (*Louis Rich*),								
1 oz.	50	7.9	.1	2.0	.4	19	19	0
hickory smoked (*Louis Rich*),								
1 oz.	33	5.4	.8	1.0	.3	13	346	0
honey roasted (*Louis Rich*), 1 oz.	33	5.3	1.1	.8	.3	12	318	0
oven prepared, quarter (*Mr.*								
Turkey Chub), 1 oz.	34	5.8	.4	1.0	m.q.	12	266	0
oven roasted (*Louis Rich*), 1 oz.	31	5.3	.4	.9	.2	13	296	0
roast (*Louis Rich*), 1 oz.	42	8.3	.2	.8	.3	19	20	0
slices (*Louis Rich*), 1 oz.	39	8.4	.1	.5	.1	17	24	0
smoked (*Louis Rich*), 1 oz.	33	5.7	.2	1.0	.4	11	268	0

1. *Prebasted with broth.*

Food and Measure	cal.	prot. (gms)	carbo. (gms)	tot. fat (gms)	sat. fat (gms)	chol. (mgs)	sod. (mgs)	fiber (gms)
smoked, quarter (*Mr. Turkey*								
Chub), 1 oz.	35	6.1	.3	1.0	m.q.	10	263	0
steaks (*Louis Rich*), 1 oz.	39	8.4	.1	.5	.1	17	24	0
tenderloins (*Louis Rich*), 1 oz.	39	8.5	.2	.5	.2	18	24	0
cutlets, raw (*Norbest Tasti-Lean*),								
4 oz.	135	27.8	<.1	<2.0	m.q.	m.q.	81	0
dark meat, skinless, roasted (*Swift*								
Butterball), 3.5 oz., 2 slices,								
approx. 5″ × 3″ × ¼″	195	25.0	n.a.	10.0	m.q.	130	90	0
drumsticks (*Land O'Lakes*), 3 oz. ..	120	17.0	0	5.0	2.0	m.q.	85	0
drumsticks (*Louis Rich*), 1 oz.								
cooked	56	7.9	.1	2.6	.9	27	22	0
w/gravy, raw (*Norbest*), 4 oz.	115	20.3	1.1	2.7	m.q.	m.q.	600	0
ground, see "Turkey, ground"								
hindquarter roast (*Land O'Lakes*),								
3 oz.	140	17.0	0	8.0	3.0	m.q.	80	0
thigh:								
(*Land O'Lakes*), 3 oz.	150	17.0	0	10.0	4.0	m.q.	75	0
(*Louis Rich*), 1 oz. cooked	64	7.5	.1	3.7	1.0	27	20	0
w/skin, roasted,[1] 4 oz.	178	21.3	0	9.7	3.0	70	496	0
w/skin, roasted,[1] 1 thigh, 11.1								
oz., yield from 12.7 oz. w/bone	494	59.0	0	26.8	8.3	194	1371	0
white meat, skinless, roasted (*Swift*								
Butterball), 3.5 oz., 2 slices,								
approx. 5″ × 3″ × ¼″	160	30.0	n.a.	4.0	m.q.	80	130	0
white and dark meat, roasted,								
seasoned:								
raw, 1 lb.	544	79.8	29.0	10.0	m.q.	m.q.	3075	n.a.
raw, 1 oz.	34	5.0	1.8	.6	m.q.	m.q.	192	n.a.
roasted, 4 oz.	176	24.2	3.5	6.6	m.q.	m.q.	771	n.a.
white and dark meat w/skin, roasted								
(*Swift Butterball*), 3.5 oz., 2								
slices, approx. 5″ × 3″ × ¼″	195	27.0	n.a.	10.0	m.q.	100	115	0
whole, cooked:								
boneless (*Norbest*), 1 oz.	42	6.2	.3	1.5	m.q.	m.q.	105	0
boneless, smoked (*Norbest*), 1 oz.	42	6.4	.3	1.6	m.q.	m.q.	218	0
w/out giblets (*Louis Rich*), 1 oz.	52	7.7	.1	2.3	.7	22	23	0
wings:								
(*Land O'Lakes*), 3 oz.	120	18.0	0	5.0	2.0	m.q.	65	0
(*Louis Rich*), 1 oz. cooked	54	7.2	.1	2.7	.8	31	20	0
(*Louis Rich* Drumettes), 1 oz.								
cooked	51	7.8	.1	2.2	.7	29	20	0
portions (*Louis Rich*), 1 oz.								
cooked	54	6.9	.1	2.9	.7	29	17	0
young:								
(*Land O'Lakes*), 3 oz.	130	17.0	<1.0	7.0	2.0	65	55	0
butter basted (*Land O'Lakes*),								
3 oz.	140	17.0	<1.0	8.0	3.0	85	135	0

1. *Prebasted with broth.*

Food and Measure	cal.	prot. (gms)	carbo. (gms)	tot. fat (gms)	sat. fat (gms)	chol. (mgs)	sod. (mgs)	fiber (gms)
TURKEY, FROZEN AND REFRIGERATED, YOUNG *(cont.)*								
self-basting, broth (*Land O'Lakes*), 3 oz.	120	18.0	<1.0	5.0	2.0	77	145	0
TURKEY, GROUND (see also "Turkey sausage"):								
raw, 1 oz.	40	4.9	0	2.1	.6	21	27	0
raw (*Norbest*), 1 oz.	45	5.2	.1	2.6	m.q.	m.q.	34	0
cooked[1]:								
11.6 oz., yield from 1 lb. raw	754	80.4	0	45.5	12.4	227	273	0
4 oz.	260	27.7	0	15.6	4.3	78	94	0
1 patty, 2.9 oz., yield from 4-oz. raw patty	188	20.1	0	11.4	3.1	57	68	0
(*Louis Rich*), 1 oz.	60	6.8	.2	3.6	1.1	25	28	0
(*Louis Rich*), 1 oz.	52	6.7	.2	2.1	.7	25	32	0
(*Hudson's*), 1 oz.	55	5.0	0	3.7	m.q.	m.q.	35	0
(*Longacre*), 1 oz.	60	5.0	0	4.0	m.q.	30	20	0
w/natural flavoring (*Louis Rich*), 1 oz.	50	7.5	0	2.2	.7	24	33	0
(*Mr. Turkey*), 1 oz.	54	4.5	0	4.0	m.q.	20	27	0
"TURKEY," VEGETARIAN:								
canned (*Worthington* Turkee Slices), 2 slices, approx. 2.2 oz.	130	9.0	3.0	9.0	m.q.	0	430	m.q.
canned, drained (*Worthington 209*), 2 slices	120	8.0	3.0	8.0	m.q.	0	m.q.	m.q.
frozen, smoked, roll or slices (*Worthington*), 4 slices, approx. 2.7 oz.	180	13.0	5.0	12.0	m.q.	0	820	m.q.
TURKEY BACON, see "Bacon, substitute"								
TURKEY BOLOGNA, 1 oz., except as noted:								
1-oz. slice	57	3.9	.3	4.3	m.q.	28	249	0
(*Butterball* Cold Cuts)	70	4.0	2.0	6.0	m.q.	m.q.	370	0
(*Butterball Deli/Slice 'n Serve*)	70	4.0	2.0	6.0	m.q.	m.q.	370	0
(*Butterball Turkey Variety Pak*), ¾ oz.	50	3.0	1.0	4.0	m.q.	m.q.	280	0
(*Louis Rich*)	61	3.4	.6	5.0	1.5	22	244	0
(*Norbest* Blue Label, 2–2.5 lb.)	68	3.5	.5	5.6	m.q.	m.q.	331	0
(*Norbest* Blue Label, 5 lb.)	57	3.8	.3	4.4	m.q.	m.q.	339	0
(*OHSE*)	70	3.0	2.0	6.0	m.q.	m.q.	300	0
mild (*Louis Rich*)	59	3.8	.7	4.5	1.5	18	298	0
sliced (*Longacre*)	61	4.0	0	5.0	m.q.	25	270	0
TURKEY CASSEROLE, see "Turkey entree, frozen"								
TURKEY AND CORNED BEEF:								
(*Healthy Deli* Doubledecker), 1 oz.	30	5.1	.6	.7	m.q.	12	195	0

1. *Without added ingredients.*

Food and Measure	cal.	prot. (gms)	carbo. (gms)	tot. fat (gms)	sat. fat (gms)	chol. (mgs)	sod. (mgs)	fiber (gms)
TURKEY DINNER, frozen:								
(*Banquet*), 10.5 oz.	390	18.0	35.0	20.0	m.q.	40	1110	m.q.
(*Banquet Extra Helping*), 19 oz.	750	29.0	68.0	42.0	m.q.	65	1980	m.q.
(*Morton*), 10 oz.	230	15.0	28.0	6.0	m.q.	45	1300	m.q.
(*Swanson*), 11.5 oz.	350	21.0	42.0	11.0	m.q.	m.q.	1090	m.q.
(*Swanson Hungry Man*), 17 oz.	550	36.0	61.0	18.0	m.q.	m.q.	1810	m.q.
breast:								
(*Healthy Choice*), 10.5 oz.	290	21.0	39.0	5.0	2.0	45	420	m.q.
Dijon (*The Budget Gourmet*),								
11.2 oz.	340	20.0	37.0	12.0	m.q.	65	860	m.q.
roast (*Stouffer's Dinner Supreme*),								
10.75 oz.	300	22.0	38.0	7.0	m.q.	m.q.	1290	m.q.
sliced:								
(*The Budget Gourmet*), 11.1 oz.	290	16.0	36.0	9.0	m.q.	45	1200	m.q.
w/mushroom gravy (*Le Menu*),								
10.5 oz.	300	22.0	38.0	7.0	m.q.	m.q.	1020	m.q.
in mushroom sauce (*Lean*								
Cuisine), 8 oz.	240	23.0	20.0	7.0	2.0	50	790	m.q.
Divan (*Le Menu* LightStyle), 10 oz.	260	25.0	23.0	7.0	m.q.	60	420	m.q.
w/dressing and gravy (*Armour*								
Classics), 11.5 oz.	320	19.0	34.0	12.0	m.q.	50	1280	m.q.
sliced (*Freezer Queen*), 10 oz.	280	16.0	36.0	8.0	m.q.	m.q.	1210	m.q.
sliced (*Le Menu* LightStyle), 10 oz.	210	21.0	21.0	5.0	m.q.	30	540	m.q.
TURKEY ENTREE, FREEZE-								
DRIED[1]:								
tetrazzini (*Mountain House*), 1 cup	200	13.0	20.0	8.0	m.q.	m.q.	m.q.	m.q.
TURKEY ENTREE, FROZEN:								
(*Tyson Gourmet Selection*), 11.5 oz.	380	19.0	51.0	11.0	m.q.	m.q.	1350	m.q.
a la king, w/rice (*The Budget*								
Gourmet), 10 oz.	390	20.0	36.0	18.0	m.q.	75	740	m.q.
breast, stuffed (*Weight Watchers*),								
8.5 oz.	260	20.0	24.0	10.0	4.0	80	910	m.q.
casserole (*Pillsbury Microwave*								
Classic), 1 pkg.	430	20.0	31.0	25.0	m.q.	m.q.	880	m.q.
casserole, w/gravy and dressing								
(*Stouffer's*), 9.75 oz.	360	23.0	29.0	17.0	m.q.	m.q.	1090	m.q.
croquettes, breaded, gravy and								
(*Freezer Queen Family Suppers*),								
7 oz.	250	13.0	19.0	13.0	m.q.	m.q.	940	m.q.
Dijon (*Lean Cuisine*), 9.5 oz.	270	24.0	22.0	10.0	3.0	60	900	m.q.
w/dressing and potatoes (*Swanson*								
Homestyle Recipe), 9 oz.	290	18.0	30.0	11.0	m.q.	m.q.	1010	m.q.
glazed (*The Budget Gourmet* Slim								
Selects), 9 oz.	270	17.0	39.0	5.0	m.q.	50	760	m.q.
glazed (*Le Menu* LightStyle),								
8.25 oz.	260	18.0	34.0	6.0	m.q.	35	720	m.q.
gravy and, 5-oz. pkg.	95	8.4	6.6	3.7	1.2	m.q.	786	.4 c
gravy and, 1 cup	160	14.1	11.1	6.3	2.0	m.q.	1328	.7 c

1. *Prepared according to package directions.*

Food and Measure	cal.	prot. (gms)	carbo. (gms)	tot. fat (gms)	sat. fat (gms)	chol. (mgs)	sod. (mgs)	fiber (gms)
TURKEY ENTREE, FROZEN *(cont.)*								
and gravy, w/dressing *(Freezer Queen Deluxe Family Suppers)*, 7 oz. ...	160	12.0	18.0	5.0	m.q.	m.q.	1130	m.q.
pie:								
(Banquet), 7 oz.	510	16.0	39.0	31.0	m.q.	40	860	m.q.
(Banquet Supreme Microwave), 7 oz.	430	15.0	30.0	27.0	m.q.	35	740	m.q.
(Morton), 7 oz.	420	14.0	27.0	28.0	m.q.	40	740	m.q.
(Stouffer's), 10 oz.	540	20.0	35.0	36.0	m.q.	m.q.	1300	m.q.
(Swanson Pot Pie), 7 oz.	380	11.0	36.0	21.0	m.q.	m.q.	720	m.q.
(Swanson Hungry Man), 16 oz. ...	650	24.0	57.0	36.0	m.q.	m.q.	1470	m.q.
sliced:								
gravy and:								
(Banquet Cookin' Bags), 5 oz.	100	7.0	5.0	6.0	m.q.	m.q.	m.q.	n.a.
(Banquet Family Entrees), 8 oz.	150	12.0	8.0	8.0	m.q.	m.q.	m.q.	n.a.
(Freezer Queen Cook-In-Pouch), 5 oz.	70	7.0	6.0	2.0	m.q.	m.q.	880	n.a.
(Freezer Queen Family Suppers), 7 oz.	110	9.0	8.0	5.0	m.q.	m.q.	1160	n.a.
and gravy, w/dressing *(Freezer Queen* Single Serve), 9 oz.	230	17.0	32.0	5.0	m.q.	m.q.	1130	m.q.
in mild curry sauce, w/rice pilaf *(Right Course)*, 8.75 oz.	320	23.0	40.0	8.0	2.0	50	570	m.q.
tetrazzini *(Stouffer's)*, 10 oz.	380	22.0	28.0	20.0	m.q.	m.q.	1170	m.q.
white meat, w/gravy and stuffing *(Le Menu* LightStyle Traditional), 8 oz.	200	19.0	19.0	5.0	1.0	25	610	m.q.
TURKEY FAT:								
1 oz.	255	0	0	28.3	8.3	29	0	0
½ cup	923	0	0	102.3	30.1	105	0	0
1 tbsp.	115	0	0	12.8	3.8	13	0	0
TURKEY FRANKFURTER:								
1 oz.	64	4.1	.4	5.0	m.q.	30	404	0
1 link, approx. 1.6 oz., 10 links per 1-lb. pkg.	102	6.4	.7	8.0	m.q.	48	642	0
(Butterball), 1 link	140	7.0	2.0	11.0	m.q.	m.q.	610	0
(Health Valley Weiners), 1 link	96	5.0	1.0	8.0	m.q.	35	112	0
(Longacre), 1 oz.	66	4.0	0	6.0	m.q.	30	260	0
(Louis Rich), 1.6-oz. link	101	5.7	1.2	8.2	2.7	42	505	0
(Louis Rich Bun Length), 2-oz. link	128	7.2	1.5	10.4	3.4	53	640	0
(Mr. Turkey), 1.6 oz., 10/lb.	106	5.5	.9	8.9	m.q.	31	440	0
cheese *(Louis Rich)*, 1.6-oz. link ...	109	6.1	1.3	8.9	2.9	44	523	0
cheese *(Mr. Turkey)*, 1.6 oz.	109	5.9	.9	9.1	m.q.	29	526	0
TURKEY GIBLETS:								
raw, 1 oz.	37	5.5	.6	1.2	.4	80	25	0
raw, 8.6 oz.[1]	314	47.2	5.1	10.3	3.1	688	213	0

1. *Includes 1 gizzard, 1 heart, and 1 liver from raw whole 15.5-½ turkey.*

Food and Measure	cal.	prot. (gms)	carbo. (gms)	tot. fat (gms)	sat. fat (gms)	chol. (mgs)	sod. (mgs)	fiber (gms)
simmered[1]:								
4 oz.	189	30.1	2.4	5.8	1.7	474	67	0
5.6 oz.[2]	264	42.0	3.3	8.0	2.4	660	93	0
chopped or diced, 1 cup	243	38.5	3.0	7.4	2.2	606	85	0
TURKEY GIZZARD:								
raw, 1 oz.	33	5.4	.2	1.0	.3	45	23	0
raw, 4 oz.[3]	133	21.6	.7	4.2	1.2	178	90	0
simmered[1] :								
4 oz.	185	33.4	.7	4.4	1.3	263	61	0
2.4 oz.[4]	109	19.7	.4	2.6	.7	155	36	0
chopped or diced, 1 cup	236	42.7	.9	5.6	1.6	336	79	0
TURKEY GRAVY:								
canned:								
¼ cup	31	1.6	3.0	1.3	.4	1	n.a.	n.a.
(Franco-American), 2 oz.	30	0	3.0	2.0	n.a.	n.a.	290	n.a.
(Heinz HomeStyle), 2 oz. or ¼ cup	25	1.0	3.0	1.0	n.a.	m.q.	370	n.a.
w/chunky turkey (Hormel Great								
Beginnings), 5 oz.	138	11.0	7.0	8.0	m.q.	m.q.	585	n.a.
mix:[5]								
1 oz. dry	99	3.4	17.2	2.1	.6	2	1715	.1 c
¼ cup	22	.7	3.8	.5	.1	1	375	<.1 c
(Lawry's), 1 cup	102	2.6	13.4	4.1	m.q.	n.a.	1400	.1 c
(McCormick/Schilling), ¼ cup . .	22	.5	4.0	.5	n.a.	n.a.	353	n.a.
TURKEY HAM, 1 oz., except as								
noted:								
(Butterball Cold Cuts)	35	5.0	1.0	1.0	m.q.	m.q.	390	0
(Butterball Slice 'n Serve)	35	5.0	1.0	2.0	m.q.	m.q.	340	0
(Louis Rich Round)	34	5.4	.4	1.2	.5	19	300	0
(Louis Rich Square), .75-oz. slice . .	24	4.1	.3	.7	.3	14	213	0
(Louis Rich Thin Sliced) .4-oz. slice	12	2.2	.1	.4	.1	7	111	0
(Louis Rich Water Added)	33	4.9	.4	1.4	.4	19	294	0
(OHSE)	30	4.0	2.0	1.0	m.q.	m.q.	370	0
breakfast, smoked (Mr. Turkey)	33	5.0	.4	1.3	m.q.	16	306	0
buffet style, smoked (Mr. Turkey) . .	32	4.7	.4	1.3	m.q.	17	340	0
chopped (Louis Rich)	46	5.2	.2	2.8	.7	19	289	0
chopped (Mr. Turkey)	37	5.4	.3	1.6	m.q.	17	301	0
chunk (Longacre)	37	5.0	0	2.0	m.q.	25	360	0
cured thigh meat:								
8-oz. pkg.	291	43.0	.9	11.5	3.9	m.q.	2260	0
2 slices or 2 oz.	73	10.7	.2	2.9	1.0	m.q.	565	0
1 oz.	36	5.4	.1	1.4	.5	m.q.	282	0
(Norbest Gold Label)	27	6.1	.3	.7	m.q.	m.q.	297	0
(Norbest Tavern, 2–2.5 lb. Half) . .	29	4.7	.6	.8	m.q.	m.q.	312	0
(Norbest Tavern, 5–6 lb. Whole) . .	27	5.4	.3	.8	m.q.	m.q.	311	0

1. *Without added ingredients.*
2. *Includes 1 gizzard, 1 heart, and 1 liver from roasted whole 11.2-lb. turkey.*
3. *Gizzard from raw whole 15.5-lb. turkey.*
4. *Gizzard from roasted whole 11.2-lb. turkey.*
5. *Prepared with water, except as noted.*

Food and Measure	cal.	prot. (gms)	carbo. (gms)	tot. fat (gms)	sat. fat (gms)	chol. (mgs)	sod. (mgs)	fiber (gms)
TURKEY HAM, CURED DARK MEAT *(cont.)*								
Canadian style (*Norbest*)	35	5.1	.3	1.4	m.q.	m.q.	331	0
honey cured:								
(*Butterball* Cold Cuts)	35	5.0	1.0	1.0	m.q.	m.q.	380	0
(*Butterball Slice 'n Serve*)	40	5.0	1.0	2.0	m.q.	m.q.	370	0
(*Louis Rich*), .74-oz. slice	25	4.2	.6	.7	.2	14	217	0
chopped (*Butterball* Cold Cuts) . .	35	5.0	2.0	1.0	m.q.	m.q.	290	0
lean lite (*Longacre* Deli)	37	6.0	0	2.0	m.q.	25	150	0
roll (*Norbest*)	31	4.6	.5	1.1	m.q.	m.q.	346	0
sliced (*Butterball* Deli Thin)	35	5.0	1.0	1.0	m.q.	m.q.	390	0
sliced (*Longacre*)	33	6.0	0	1.0	m.q.	20	310	0
smoked (*Mr. Turkey*)	32	5.4	.3	1.0	m.q.	18	286	0
smoked (*Mr. Turkey* Chub)	32	4.7	.4	1.3	m.q.	17	340	0
TURKEY AND HAM:								
(*Healthy Deli* Doubledecker), 1 oz.	30	4.8	.8	.9	m.q.	11	185	0
TURKEY HAM SALAD:								
(*Longacre*), 1 oz.	53	2.0	3.0	4.0	m.q.	10	190	n.a.
(*Longacre* Saladfest), 1 oz.	58	2.0	2.0	4.0	m.q.	10	270	n.a.
TURKEY HEART, see "Heart"								
TURKEY KIELBASA, see "Turkey sausage"								
TURKEY LIVER, see "Liver"								
TURKEY LUNCHEON MEAT, see "Turkey, boneless and luncheon meat"								
TURKEY NUGGETS, breaded:								
cooked[1] (*Louis Rich*), .7-oz. piece . .	62	3.1	3.5	3.9	.8	9	155	m.q.
TURKEY PASTRAMI, 1 oz., except as noted:								
8-oz. pkg.	320	41.7	3.8	14.1	4.1	m.q.	2372	0
2 slices or 2 oz.	80	10.4	.9	3.5	1.0	m.q.	593	0
(*Butterball* Cold Cuts)	30	5.0	0	1.0	m.q.	m.q.	290	0
(*Butterball Slice 'n Serve*)	35	5.0	1.0	1.0	m.q.	m.q.	320	0
(*Louis Rich* Round)	32	5.2	.3	1.1	.4	18	288	0
(*Louis Rich* Square), .8-oz. slice . . .	24	4.2	.1	.7	.1	14	262	0
(*Louis Rich* Thin Sliced), .4-oz. slice	11	2.0	.1	.4	.2	7	125	0
(*Mr. Turkey*)	28	4.8	.1	.9	m.q.	17	383	0
(*Norbest*, 3 lb.)	29	4.8	.3	.8	m.q.	m.q.	302	0
(*Norbest*, 5–6 lb. Slab)	29	5.1	.5	.6	m.q.	m.q.	305	0
sliced (*Longacre*)	32	5.0	0	1.0	m.q.	20	260	0
TURKEY PATTY:								
breaded, battered, fried:								
1 oz.	80	4.0	4.5	5.1	m.q.	m.q.	227	m.q.
2.3-oz. patty	181	9.0	10.1	11.5	m.q.	m.q.	512	m.q.
3.3-oz. patty	266	13.2	14.8	16.9	m.q.	m.q.	752	m.q.
cooked[1] (*Louis Rich*), 2.8-oz. patty	209	11.5	13.0	12.3	2.4	32	557	m.q.

1. *Prepared according to package directions.*

Food and Measure	cal.	prot. (gms)	carbo. (gms)	tot. fat (gms)	sat. fat (gms)	chol. (mgs)	sod. (mgs)	fiber (gms)
TURKEY PIE, see "Turkey entree, frozen"								
TURKEY POCKET SANDWICH, frozen:								
w/ham and cheese (*Hot Pockets*), 5 oz.	320	17.0	37.0	11.0	m.q.	m.q.	780	m.q.
TURKEY ROLL OR LOAF, see "Turkey, boneless and luncheon meat"								
TURKEY SALAD:								
(*Longacre*), 1 oz.	70	3.0	3.0	5.0	m.q.	10	200	n.a.
(*Longacre* Saladfest), 1 oz.	68	3.0	2.0	5.0	m.q.	15	180	n.a.
TURKEY SALAMI, 1 oz., except as noted:								
(*Butterball* Cold Cuts)	50	4.0	1.0	4.0	m.q.	m.q.	350	0
(*Butterball* Deli/Slice 'n Serve)	50	4.0	1.0	4.0	m.q.	m.q.	350	0
(*Butterball* Turkey Variety Pak), ¾ oz.	40	3.0	1.0	3.0	m.q.	m.q.	260	0
(*Louis Rich*)	54	4.4	.2	4.0	1.1	20	263	0
(*Norbest* Blue Label, 2–2.5 lb.)	45	4.2	.9	2.6	m.q.	m.q.	314	0
(*Norbest* Blue Label, 5 lb.)	46	4.3	.5	2.9	m.q.	m.q.	270	0
(*OHSE*)	50	4.0	1.0	3.0	m.q.	m.q.	260	0
cooked, 8-oz. pkg.	446	37.2	1.2	31.3	m.q.	186	2278	0
cooked	56	4.6	.2	3.9	m.q.	23	285	0
cotto (*Louis Rich*)	53	4.4	.3	3.8	1.1	21	271	0
cotto (*Mr. Turkey*)	45	4.3	.4	2.9	m.q.	16	369	0
sliced (*Longacre*)	52	4.0	1.0	4.0	m.q.	20	290	0
TURKEY SANDWICH, see "Turkey pocket sandwich"								
TURKEY SAUSAGE, 1 oz, except as noted:								
(*Butterball*)	50	4.0	<1.0	4.0	m.q.	m.q.	250	0
(*Norbest* Tasti-Lean, Chub or Links)	53	4.6	.3	2.8	m.q.	m.q.	179	0
breakfast:								
(*Mr. Turkey*)	58	4.6	.4	4.3	m.q.	16	181	0
ground (*Hudson's*)	65	4.3	0	5.3	m.q.	m.q.	180	0
ground, cooked (*Louis Rich*)	56	5.9	.2	3.5	1.5	22	215	0
links, cooked (*Louis Rich*), 1 link ...	46	5.4	.1	2.7	1.5	18	234	0
Polish (*Louis Rich* Polska Kielbasa)	40	4.6	.4	2.2	.7	19	247	0
Polish (*Mr. Turkey* Polska Kielbasa)	59	4.4	.5	4.4	m.q.	15	264	0
smoked:								
(*Louis Rich*)	43	4.5	.7	2.4	.6	19	249	0
(*Mr. Turkey*)	47	4.5	.5	3.4	m.q.	19	230	0
w/cheese (*Louis Rich*)	47	4.7	.7	2.8	.8	18	269	0
TURKEY SPREAD:								
chunky (*Underwood* Light), 2⅛ oz.	75	11.0	2.0	2.0	<1.0	25	330	n.a.
TURKEY STICKS:								
breaded, battered, fried:								
1 oz.	79	4.0	4.8	4.8	m.q.	m.q.	238	m.q.
1 stick, 2.3 oz.	178	9.1	10.9	10.8	m.q.	m.q.	536	m.q.

Food and Measure	cal.	prot. (gms)	carbo. (gms)	tot. fat (gms)	sat. fat (gms)	chol. (mgs)	sod. (mgs)	fiber (gms)
TURKEY STICKS *(cont.)*								
cooked[1] (*Louis Rich*), 1 stick,								
approx. 1 oz.	81	4.1	4.8	5.0	1.0	12	197	m.q.
TURKEY SUMMER SAUSAGE:								
(*Louis Rich*), 1-oz. slice	55	4.7	.4	3.9	1.2	21	326	0
TUMERIC, ground:								
1 oz.	100	2.2	18.4	2.8	m.q.	0	11	1.9 c
1 tbsp.	24	.5	4.4	.7	n.a.	0	3	.5 c
1 tsp.	8	.2	1.4	.2	n.a.	0	1	.2 c
(*Spice Islands*), 1 tsp.	7	.2	1.3	.2	n.a.	0	<1	.1 c
TURNIP:								
raw:								
untrimmed, 1 lb.	100	3.3	22.9	.4	<.1	0	248	6.6 d
trimmed, 1 oz.	8	.3	1.8	<.1	tr.	0	19	.5 d
cubed, ½ cup	18	.6	4.1	.1	<.1	0	44	1.2 d
boiled, drained:								
4 oz.	20	.8	5.6	.1	tr.	0	57	2.3 d
cubed, ½ cup	14	.6	3.8	.1	tr.	0	39	1.6 d
mashed, ½ cup	21	.8	5.6	.1	tr.	0	58	2.3 d
TURNIP, CANNED:								
(*Stokely*), ½ cup	20	2.0	3.0	0	0	0	350	m.q.
diced (*Allens*), ½ cup	16	2.0	2.0	<1.0	(0)	0	25	m.q.
TURNIP, FROZEN:								
boiled, drained, 4 oz.	26	1.7	4.9	.3	<.1	0	41	.8 c
mashed, 10-oz. pkg.	44	3.0	8.4	.5	<.1	0	71	1.3 c
diced (*Southern*), 3.5 oz.	17	1.0	2.9	.2	(0)	0	50	m.q.
TURNIP GREENS, fresh:								
raw, untrimmed, 1 lb.	85	4.8	18.2	1.0	.2	0	126	7.6 d
raw, trimmed, 1 oz. or ½ cup								
chopped	7	.4	1.6	.1	<.1	0	11	.7 d
boiled, drained, 4 oz.	23	1.3	4.9	.3	.1	0	33	3.5 d
boiled, drained, chopped, ½ cup ...	15	.8	3.1	.2	<.1	0	21	2.2 d
TURNIP GREENS, CANNED,								
½ cup, except as noted:								
w/liquid, 4 oz.	16	1.5	2.7	.3	.1	0	314	.7 c
w/liquid	17	1.6	2.8	.4	.1	0	325	.7 c
chopped (*Allens*)	21	2.0	3.0	<1.0	(0)	0	15	m.q.
chopped, w/diced turnips (*Allens*) ..	19	2.0	1.0	<1.0	(0)	0	15	m.q.
w/diced turnips (*Stokely*)	20	2.0	0	0	0	0	340	m.q.
TURNIP GREENS, FROZEN:								
boiled, drained, 4 oz.	34	3.8	5.6	.5	.1	0	17	1.2 c
boiled, drained, ½ cup	24	2.8	4.1	.4	.1	0	12	.9 c
chopped:								
10-oz. pkg.	62	7.0	10.4	.9	.2	0	33	2.2 c
(*Frosty Acres*), 3.3 oz.	20	2.0	4.0	0	0	0	10	1.0 c
(*Seabrook*), 3.3 oz.	20	2.0	4.0	0	0	0	11	1.0 c
(*Southern*), 3.5 oz.	25	2.5	3.6	.3	(0)	0	70	m.q.

1. *Prepared according to package directions.*

Food and Measure	cal.	prot. (gms)	carbo. (gms)	tot. fat (gms)	sat. fat (gms)	chol. (mgs)	sod. (mgs)	fiber (gms)
w/turnips:								
10-oz. pkg.	59	7.0	9.7	.5	.1	0	52	1.7 c
boiled, drained, 4 oz.	19	2.4	3.3	.2	<.1	0	17	.6 c
diced turnips (*Seabrook*), 3.3 oz.	20	3.0	3.0	0	0	0	n.a.	m.q.
TURNIP-ROOTED CELERY, see "Celeriac"								
TURNOVER, FROZEN, 1 piece:								
apple (*Pepperidge Farm*)	300	3.0	34.0	17.0	m.q.	n.a.	210	m.q.
blueberry (*Pepperidge Farm*)	310	3.0	32.0	19.0	m.q.	n.a.	230	m.q.
cherry (*Pepperidge Farm*)	310	3.0	32.0	19.0	m.q.	n.a.	280	m.q.
peach (*Pepperidge Farm*)	310	3.0	34.0	18.0	m.q.	n.a.	260	m.q.
raspberry (*Pepperidge Farm*)	310	4.0	36.0	17.0	m.q.	n.a.	260	m.q.
TURNOVER, REFRIGERATED:								
apple (*Pillsbury*), 1 piece	170	2.0	23.0	8.0	2.0	0	320	m.q.
cherry (*Pillsbury*), 1 piece	170	2.0	23.0	8.0	2.0	0	320	m.q.

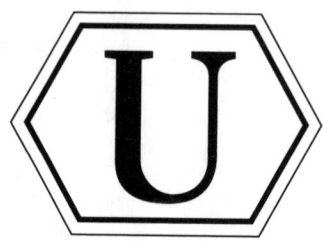

Food and Measure	cal.	prot. (gms)	carbo. (gms)	tot. fat (gms)	sat. fat (gms)	chol. (mgs)	sod. (mgs)	fiber (gms)
UCUHUBA BUTTER OIL:								
½ cup	964	0	0	109.0	92.9	0	0	0
1 tbsp.	120	0	0	13.6	11.6	0	0	0
1 oz.	251	0	0	28.4	24.2	0	0	0
UDON, see "Noodle, Japanese"								

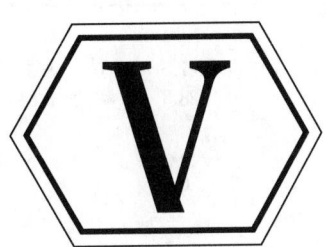

Food and Measure	cal.	prot. (gms)	carbo. (gms)	tot. fat (gms)	sat. fat (gms)	chol. (mgs)	sod. (mgs)	fiber (gms)
VANILLA, MILK, BAKING								
CHIPS, see "Chocolate,								
baking"								
VANILLA EXTRACT:								
pure (*Virginia Dare*), 1 tsp.	10	0	.3	0	0	0	0	0
VANILLA FLAVOR DRINK,								
CANNED:								
(*Sego* Very Vanilla), 10 fl. oz.	225	11.0	34.0	5.0	m.q.	5	360	n.a.
plain or French (*Sego* Lite), 10 fl. oz.	150	11.0	17.0	4.0	m.q.	5	390	n.a.
VANILLA FLAVOR DRINK MIX:								
(*Carnation* Instant Breakfast),								
1 pouch	130	6.0	25.0	.2	.1	3	135	.1 d
(*Carnation* Instant Breakfast No								
Sugar Added), 1 pouch	70	6.0	10.0	.2	.1	3	120	.1 d
(*Pillsbury* Instant Breakfast),								
1 pouch	140	6.0	29.0	0	0	n.a.	210	m.q.
(*Pillsbury* Instant Breakfast),								
8 fl. oz.[1]	300	14.0	41.0	9.0	m.q.	m.q.	330	n.a.
VEAL[2], meat only:								
cubed for stew (leg and shoulder),								
separable lean only:								
raw, 1 oz.	31	5.8	0	.7	.2	24	24	0
braised or stewed, 9.3 oz., yield								
from 1 lb. raw	495	91.9	0	11.3	3.4	382	246	0
braised or stewed, 4 oz.	213	39.6	0	4.9	1.5	164	105	0
ground:								
raw, 1 oz.	41	5.5	0	1.9	.8	23	23	0
raw, 1 cup, approx. 8 oz.	325	43.7	0	15.3	6.3	185	185	0
broiled:								
10.5 oz., yield from 1 lb. raw ..	516	73.0	0	22.6	9.1	307	248	0
5.4 oz., yield from 1 cup raw ..	265	37.5	0	11.6	4.7	159	128	0

1. *Prepared according to package directions, with whole milk.*
2. *Cooked meats are prepared without added ingredients, except as noted.*

Food and Measure	cal.	prot. (gms)	carbo. (gms)	tot. fat (gms)	sat. fat (gms)	chol. (mgs)	sod. (mgs)	fiber (gms)
VEAL, GROUND, BROILED *(cont.)*								
4 oz.	195	27.6	0	8.6	3.4	117	94	0
1 cup, approx. 4.1 oz.	200	28.3	0	8.8	3.5	119	96	0
leg (top round), separable lean and fat:								
raw, 1 oz.	33	6.0	0	.9	.3	22	18	0
braised or stewed:								
9.6 oz., yield from 1 lb. raw								
boneless	576	98.4	0	17.2	6.9	365	183	0
4 oz.	239	41.0	0	7.2	2.9	152	76	0
1 slice, 4½″ × 2½″ × ¼″, approx. 1.5 oz.	89	15.2	0	2.7	1.1	56	28	0
diced, 1 cup, approx. 4.9 oz. ...	295	50.6	0	8.9	3.5	188	94	0
pan-fried in vegetable oil:								
10.7 oz., yield from 1 lb. raw								
boneless	641	96.5	0	25.4	9.6	319	230	0
4 oz.	239	36.0	0	9.5	3.6	119	86	0
1 slice, 4½″ × 2½″ × ¼″, approx. 1.5 oz.	89	13.3	0	3.5	1.3	44	32	0
pan-fried, breaded[1]:								
10.4 oz., yield from 1 lb. raw								
boneless	673	80.5	29.0	27.1	9.0	329	1339	.4 c
4 oz.	259	30.9	11.2	10.4	3.5	127	515	.1 c
1 slice, 4½″ × 2½″ × ¼″, approx. 1.5 oz.	96	11.5	4.1	3.9	1.3	47	191	<.1 c
roasted:								
12.6 oz., yield from 1 lb. raw								
boneless	574	99.3	0	16.7	6.6	368	243	0
4 oz.	181	31.4	0	5.3	2.1	117	77	0
1 slice, 4½″ × 2½″ × ¼″, approx. 1.5 oz.	67	11.6	0	2.0	.8	43	29	0
diced, 1 cup, approx. 4.9 oz. ...	224	38.8	0	6.5	2.6	144	95	0
leg (top round), separable lean only:								
raw, 1 oz.	30	6.0	0	.5	.2	22	18	0
braised or stewed:								
9.4 oz., yield from 1 lb. raw								
w/fat	541	97.9	0	13.6	5.1	361	180	0
4 oz.	230	41.6	0	5.8	2.2	159	76	0
1 slice, 4½″ × 2½″ × ¼″, approx. 1.5 oz.	85	15.4	0	2.1	.8	57	28	0
diced, 1 cup, approx. 4.9 oz. ...	284	51.4	0	7.1	2.7	189	94	0
pan-fried in vegetable oil:								
10.2 oz., yield from 1 lb. raw								
w/fat	529	95.8	0	13.4	3.7	308	222	0
4 oz.	208	37.6	0	5.2	1.5	121	87	0
1 slice, 4½″ × 2½″ × ¼″, approx. 1.5 oz.	77	13.9	0	1.9	.5	45	32	0

1. *Recipe: 83.5% veal, 9.2% breadcrumbs, 4.6% egg, 2.2% oil, and .5% salt.*

Food and Measure	cal.	prot. (gms)	carbo. (gms)	tot. fat (gms)	sat. fat (gms)	chol. (mgs)	sod. (mgs)	fiber (gms)
pan-fried, breaded[1]:								
10.2 oz., yield from 1 lb. raw								
w/fat	609	83.8	28.9	18.5	4.7	334	1342	.4 c
4 oz.	234	32.2	11.1	7.1	1.8	128	516	.1 c
1 slice, 4½″ × 2½″ × ¼″,								
approx. 1.5 oz.	87	11.9	4.1	2.6	.7	47	191	<.1 c
roasted:								
12.4 oz., yield from 1 lb. raw								
w/fat	528	98.6	0	11.9	4.3	363	239	0
4 oz.	170	31.8	0	3.8	1.4	177	77	0
1 slice, 4½″ × 2½″ × ¼″,								
approx. 1.5 oz.	63	11.8	0	1.4	.5	43	29	0
diced, 1 cup, approx. 4.9 oz. ..	210	39.3	0	4.7	1.7	144	95	0
loin, separable lean and fat:								
raw, 1 oz.	46	5.4	0	2.6	1.1	23	24	0
braised or stewed, 1 chop, 2.8 oz.,								
yield from 6.9-oz. raw chop								
w/bone	227	24.2	0	13.8	5.4	94	64	0
braised or stewed, 4 oz.	322	34.2	0	19.5	7.6	134	91	0
roasted, 8.1 oz., yield from 1 lb.								
raw w/bone	498	56.9	0	28.3	12.1	236	212	0
roasted, 4 oz.	246	28.1	0	14.0	6.0	117	105	0
loin, separable lean only:								
raw, 1 oz.	33	5.7	0	1.0	.3	23	26	0
braised or stewed, 1 chop, 2.4 oz.,								
yield from 6.9-oz. raw chop								
w/bone and fat	155	23.1	0	6.3	1.8	86	58	0
braised or stewed, 4 oz.	256	38.1	0	10.4	2.9	142	95	0
roasted, 8.5 oz., yield from 1 lb.								
raw w/bone and fat	364	54.7	0	14.4	5.4	220	200	0
roasted, 4 oz.	198	29.8	0	7.9	2.9	120	109	0
rib, separable lean and fat:								
raw, 1 oz.	46	5.4	0	2.6	1.1	23	25	0
braised or stewed, 6.2 oz., yield								
from 1 lb. raw w/bone	446	57.5	0	22.2	8.9	246	169	0
braised or stewed, 4 oz.	285	36.8	0	14.2	5.6	158	108	0
roasted, 8.5 oz., yield from 1 lb.								
raw w/bone	548	57.5	0	33.5	13.0	264	221	0
roasted, 4 oz.	259	27.2	0	15.8	6.1	125	104	0
rib, separable lean only:								
raw, 1 oz.	34	5.7	0	1.1	.3	24	27	0
braised or stewed, 5.75 oz., yield								
from 1 lb. raw w/bone and fat ..	355	56.2	0	12.7	4.2	235	161	0
braised or stewed, 4 oz.	247	39.1	0	8.9	2.9	163	112	0
roasted, 7.6 oz., yield from 1 lb.								
raw w/bone and fat	381	55.4	0	16.0	4.5	246	208	0
roasted, 4 oz.	201	29.2	0	8.4	2.4	130	110	0

1. *Recipe: 83.5% veal, 9.2% breadcrumbs, 4.6% egg, 2.2% oil, and .5% salt.*

Food and Measure	cal.	prot. (gms)	carbo. (gms)	tot. fat (gms)	sat. fat (gms)	chol. (mgs)	sod. (mgs)	fiber (gms)
VEAL *(cont.)*								
shoulder, whole, separable lean and fat:								
raw, 1 oz.	37	5.5	0	1.5	.6	25	26	0
braised or stewed:								
6.7 oz., yield from 1 lb. raw								
w/bone	436	61.2	0	19.4	7.2	241	181	0
4 oz.	259	36.4	0	11.5	4.3	143	108	0
1 slice, 4½″ × 2½″ × ¼″,								
approx. 1.5 oz.	96	13.5	0	4.3	1.6	53	40	0
diced, 1 cup, approx. 4.9 oz. ...	319	44.9	0	14.2	5.3	176	133	0
roasted:								
9.1 oz., yield from 1 lb. raw								
w/bone	475	65.3	0	21.7	8.8	291	247	0
4 oz.	209	28.7	0	9.5	3.9	128	109	0
1 slice, 4½″ × 2½″ × ¼″,								
approx. 1.5 oz.	77	10.6	0	3.5	1.4	47	40	0
diced, 1 cup, approx. 4.9 oz. ...	258	35.4	0	11.8	4.8	158	134	0
shoulder, whole, separable lean only:								
raw, 1 oz.	32	5.6	0	.9	.3	25	26	0
braised or stewed:								
6.4 oz., yield from 1 lb. raw								
w/bone and fat	362	61.3	0	11.1	3.1	236	177	0
4 oz.	226	38.2	0	6.9	1.9	147	110	0
1 slice, 4½″ × 2½″ × ¼″,								
approx. 1.5 oz.	84	14.1	0	2.6	.7	55	41	0
diced, 1 cup, approx. 4.9 oz. ...	279	47.2	0	8.5	2.4	182	136	0
roasted:								
8.8 oz., yield from 1 lb. raw								
w/bone and fat	426	64.7	0	16.6	6.3	286	243	0
4 oz.	193	29.3	0	7.5	2.8	129	110	0
1 slice, 4½″ × 2½″ × ¼″,								
approx. 1.5 oz.	71	10.8	0	2.8	1.1	48	41	0
diced, 1 cup, approx. 4.9 oz. ...	238	36.1	0	9.3	3.5	160	136	0
shoulder, arm, separable lean and fat:								
raw, 1 oz.	37	5.5	0	1.6	.6	23	24	0
braised, 1 steak, 6.1 oz., yield from 13.6-oz. raw steak								
w/bone	409	58.2	0	17.7	6.9	257	151	0
braised, 4 oz.	268	38.1	0	11.6	4.5	168	99	0
roasted, 10 oz., yield from 13.6-oz. raw steak w/bone	518	72.1	0	23.3	9.9	306	253	0
roasted, 4 oz.	208	28.9	0	9.4	4.0	122	102	0
shoulder, arm, separable lean only:								
raw, 1 oz.	30	5.7	0	.6	.2	24	24	0
braised, 1 steak, 5.6 oz., yield from 13.6-oz. raw steak w/bone and fat	321	57.1	0	8.5	2.4	248	143	0

Food and Measure	cal.	prot. (gms)	carbo. (gms)	tot. fat (gms)	sat. fat (gms)	chol. (mgs)	sod. (mgs)	fiber (gms)
braised, 4 oz.	228	40.5	0	6.0	1.7	176	102	0
roasted, 1 steak, 9.6 oz., yield from 13.6-oz. raw steak w/bone and fat	447	71.2	0	15.8	6.3	298	248	0
roasted, 4 oz.	186	29.6	0	6.6	2.6	124	103	0
shoulder, blade, separable lean and fat:								
raw, 1 oz.	37	5.5	0	1.5	.6	25	27	0
braised or stewed:								
5.25 oz., yield from 1 lb. raw w/bone	417	58.1	0	18.7	6.8	285	183	0
4 oz.	255	35.4	0	11.4	4.1	174	111	0
1 slice, 4½″ × 2½″ × ¼″, approx. 1.5 oz.	95	13.1	0	4.2	1.5	64	41	0
diced, 1 cup, approx. 4.9 oz. ...	315	43.8	0	14.1	5.1	214	137	0
roasted:								
8.6 oz., yield from 1 lb. raw w/bone	452	61.3	0	21.1	8.4	286	245	0
4 oz.	211	28.5	0	9.8	3.9	133	113	0
1 slice, 4½″ × 2½″ × ¼″, approx. 1.5 oz.	78	10.6	0	3.6	1.5	49	42	0
diced, 1 cup, approx. 4.9 oz. ...	260	35.2	0	12.1	4.8	164	140	0
shoulder, blade, separable lean only:								
raw, 1 oz.	32	5.6	0	.9	.3	26	27	0
braised or stewed:								
6.1 oz., yield from 1 lb. raw w/bone and fat	345	56.9	0	11.3	3.2	276	176	0
4 oz.	224	37.0	0	7.3	2.1	179	115	0
1 slice, 4½″ × 2½″ × ¼″, approx. 1.5 oz.	83	13.7	0	2.7	.7	66	42	0
diced, 1 cup, approx. 4.9 oz. ...	277	45.7	0	9.1	2.5	221	141	0
roasted:								
8.3 oz., yield from 1 lb. raw w/bone and fat	406	60.6	0	16.3	6.1	281	241	0
4 oz.	194	29.1	0	7.8	2.9	135	116	0
1 slice, 4½″ × 2½″ × ¼″, approx. 1.5 oz.	72	10.8	0	2.9	1.1	50	43	0
diced, 1 cup, approx. 4.9 oz. ...	239	35.9	0	9.6	3.6	167	143	0
sirloin, separable lean and fat:								
raw, 1 oz.	43	5.4	0	2.2	1.0	22	22	0
braised or stewed:								
7.25 oz., yield from 1 lb. raw w/bone	516	64.0	0	26.9	10.6	222	161	0
4 oz.	286	35.4	0	14.9	5.9	122	90	0
1 slice, 4½″ × 2½″ × ¼″, approx. 1.5 oz.	106	13.1	0	5.5	2.2	45	33	0
diced, 1 cup, approx. 4.9 oz. ...	353	43.8	0	18.4	7.3	151	111	0

Food and Measure	cal.	prot. (gms)	carbo. (gms)	tot. fat (gms)	sat. fat (gms)	chol. (mgs)	sod. (mgs)	fiber (gms)
VEAL, SIRLOIN, LEAN AND FAT, ROASTED *(cont.)*								
roasted:								
9.5 oz., yield from 1 lb. raw								
w/bone	542	67.6	0	28.1	12.1	275	223	0
4 oz.	229	28.5	0	11.9	5.1	116	94	0
1 slice, 4½″ × 2½″ × ¼″,								
approx. 1.5 oz.	85	10.6	0	4.4	1.9	43	35	0
diced, 1 cup, approx. 4.9 oz.	283	35.2	0	14.6	6.3	143	116	0
sirloin, separable lean only:								
raw, 1 oz.	31	5.7	0	.7	.2	22	23	0
braised or stewed:								
6.5 oz., yield from 1 lb. raw								
w/bone and fat	372	62.0	0	11.9	3.3	206	149	0
4 oz.	231	38.5	0	7.4	2.1	128	92	0
1 slice, 4½″ × 2½″ × ¼″,								
approx. 1.5 oz.	86	14.3	0	2.7	.8	47	34	0
diced, 1 cup, approx. 4.9 oz.	286	47.5	0	9.1	2.5	158	113	0
roasted:								
8.9 oz., yield from 1 lb. raw								
w/bone and fat	423	66.0	0	15.6	6.0	262	213	0
4 oz.	191	29.8	0	7.1	2.7	118	96	0
1 slice, 4½″ × 2½″ × ¼″,								
approx. 1.5 oz.	71	11.1	0	2.6	1.0	44	36	0
diced, 1 cup, approx. 4.9 oz.	235	36.8	0	8.7	3.4	146	119	0
top round, see "leg"								
VEAL, VARIETY MEATS, see								
specific listings								
VEAL DINNER, frozen:								
marsala (*Le Menu* LightStyle),								
10 oz.	230	22.0	28.0	3.0	m.q.	75	700	m.q.
parmigiana:								
(*Armour Classics*), 11.25 oz.	400	18.0	34.0	22.0	m.q.	55	1320	m.q.
(*Le Menu*), 11.5 oz.	390	24.0	36.0	17.0	m.q.	m.q.	840	m.q.
(*Morton*), 10 oz.	260	10.0	35.0	8.0	m.q.	35	1510	m.q.
(*Stouffer's Dinner Supreme*),								
11.25 oz.	350	27.0	30.0	13.0	m.q.	m.q.	1090	m.q.
(*Swanson*), 12.25 oz.	430	20.0	42.0	20.0	m.q.	m.q.	1010	m.q.
(*Swanson Hungry Man*),								
18¼ oz.	590	32.0	57.0	26.0	m.q.	m.q.	1840	m.q.
breaded (*Freezer Queen*), 5 oz.	220	11.0	17.0	12.0	m.q.	m.q.	560	m.q.
platter (*Freezer Queen*), 10 oz.	400	22.0	32.0	20.0	m.q.	m.q.	870	m.q.
VEAL ENTREE, frozen:								
parmigiana:								
(*Swanson* Homestyle Recipe),								
10 oz.	330	19.0	33.0	13.0	m.q.	m.q.	960	m.q.
breaded:								
(*Banquet Cookin' Bags*), 4 oz.	230	10.0	20.0	11.0	m.q.	m.q.	m.q.	m.q.
(*Freezer Queen Cook-In-Pouch*),								
5 oz.	220	11.0	17.0	12.0	m.q.	m.q.	560	m.q.

Food and Measure	cal.	prot. (gms)	carbo. (gms)	tot. fat (gms)	sat. fat (gms)	chol. (mgs)	sod. (mgs)	fiber (gms)
(*Freezer Queen Deluxe Family Suppers*), 7 oz.	300	17.0	22.0	15.0	m.q.	m.q.	820	m.q.
patty (*Banquet Family Entrees*), 8 oz.	370	18.0	33.0	18.0	m.q.	m.q.	m.q.	m.q.
patty (*Weight Watchers*), 8.44 oz.	190	23.0	12.0	6.0	3.0	55	650	m.q.
primavera (*Lean Cuisine*), 9⅛ oz. ..	250	23.0	19.0	9.0	m.q.	80	790	m.q.
steak (*Hormel*), 4 oz.	130	22.0	2.0	4.0	m.q.	m.q.	m.q.	n.a.
steak, breaded (*Hormel*), 4 oz.	240	17.0	13.0	13.0	m.q.	m.q.	m.q.	m.q.
VEGETABLE ENTREE, CANNED:								
chow mein, meatless (*La Choy*), ¾ cup	35	2.0	6.0	.4	n.a.	0	820	2.2 d
stew (*Dinty Moore*), 8 oz.	170	5.0	20.0	8.0	m.q.	n.a.	1047	m.q.
VEGETABLE ENTREE, FREEZE-DRIED, 1 cup[1]:								
stew, w/beef (*Mountain House*)	230	11.0	27.0	7.0	m.q.	m.q.	77	m.q.
VEGETABLE ENTREE, FROZEN (see also specific listings):								
and pasta mornay, w/ham (*Lean Cuisine*), 9⅜ oz.	280	15.0	29.0	11.0	3.0	35	970	m.q.
VEGETABLE FLAKES, dehydrated:								
(*French's*), 1 tbsp.	12	0	3.0	0	0	0	20	m.q.
VEGETABLE JUICE:								
(*Biotta Breuss Juice*), 6 fl. oz.	67	1.9	13.2	.1	(0)	0	147	m.q.
(*Biotta Cocktail*), 6 fl. oz.	50	1.7	10.1	.1	(0)	0	497	m.q.
("*V-8*"), 6 fl. oz.	35	1.0	8.0	0	0	0	560	m.q.
("*V-8*" No Salt Added), 6 fl. oz.	35	1.0	8.0	0	0	0	45	m.q.
(*Veryfine* 100%), 6 fl. oz.	32	1.6	6.0	0	0	0	<600	m.q.
hearty (*Smucker's*), 8 fl. oz.	58	.6	13.0	<.1	(0)	0	714	m.q.
hot and spicy (*Smucker's*), 8 fl. oz.	58	.6	13.0	<.1	(0)	0	650	m.q.
spicy hot ("*V-8*"), 6 fl. oz.	35	1.0	8.0	0	0	0	650	m.q.
VEGETABLE JUICE COCKTAIL, canned:								
6 fl. oz.	34	1.1	8.3	.2	<.1	0	664	.4 c
½ cup	22	.8	5.5	.1	<.1	0	442	.3 c
VEGETABLE OIL (see also specific listings), 1 tbsp., except as noted:								
(*Crisco*)	120	0	0	14.0	2.0	0	0	0
(*Crisco-Puritan*)	120	0	0	14.0	1.0	0	0	0
(*Finast*)	120	0	0	14.0	2.0	0	0	0
(*Hain* All Blend)	120	0	0	14.0	2.0	0	0	0
(*Pathmark*)	120	0	0	14.0	2.0	0	0	0
(*Pathmark* No Frills)	130	0	0	14.0	2.0	0	0	0
(*Wesson*)	120	0	0	14.0	2.0	0	0	0
w/garlic (*Hain* Garlic & Oil)	120	0	0	14.0	3.0	0	0	0

1. *Prepared according to package directions.*

Food and Measure	cal.	prot. (gms)	carbo. (gms)	tot. fat (gms)	sat. fat (gms)	chol. (mgs)	sod. (mgs)	fiber (gms)
VEGETABLE OIL *(cont.)*								
spray (*Weight Watchers* Cooking Spray), 1 second spray	2	0	0	1.0	n.a.	0	0	0
spray, butter flavor (*Weight Watchers* Buttery Spray), 1 second spray	2	0	0	<1.0	n.a.	0	0	0
VEGETABLE OYSTER, see "Salsify"								
VEGETABLE SPREAD, see "Margarine"								
VEGETABLE STEW, see "Vegetable entree, canned"								
VEGETABLE STICKS, breaded, frozen:								
(*Farm Rich*), 4 oz.	240	4.0	34.0	10.0	m.q.	n.a.	980	m.q.
(*Stilwell Quickkrisp*), 3 oz.	240	3.0	40.0	8.0	m.q.	<1	670	m.q.
VEGETABLES, see specific listings								
VEGETABLES, MIXED, CANNED, ½ cup, except as noted:								
w/liquid:								
4 oz.	41	1.6	8.1	.3	.1	0	254	1.3 c
½ cup	44	1.7	8.7	.3	.1	0	273	1.5 c
(*Del Monte*)	40	2.0	7.0	0	0	0	355	m.q.
drained, 4 oz.	53	2.9	10.5	.3	.1	0	169	2.7 d
drained	39	2.1	7.6	.2	<.1	0	122	2.0 d
(*A&P* Eastern)	45	2.0	8.0	<1.0	(0)	0	330	m.q.
(*A&P* No Salt Added)	40	1.0	9.0	<1.0	(0)	0	20	m.q.
(*A&P* Western)	40	1.0	9.0	<1.0	(0)	0	380	m.q.
(*Featherweight*)	40	2.0	8.0	0	0	0	25	m.q.
(*Finast*)	40	1.0	8.0	0	0	0	390	m.q.
(*Finast* No Salt Added)	40	2.0	8.0	0	0	0	25	m.q.
(*Green Giant* Garden Medley)	40	1.0	9.0	<1.0	0	0	290	1.0 d
(*Green Giant Pantry Express*)	35	1.0	8.0	<1.0	0	0	300	1.0 d
(*P&Q* Chunky Eastern)	40	2.0	8.0	<1.0	(0)	0	330	m.q.
(*P&Q* Chunky Western)	40	1.0	9.0	<1.0	(0)	0	380	m.q.
(*Pathmark*)	35	2.0	8.0	0	0	0	320	m.q.
(*Pathmark* No Salt Added)	35	2.0	7.0	0	0	0	25	m.q.
(*S&W* Old Fashioned Harvest)	35	1.0	6.0	0	0	0	380	m.q.
(*Stokely*)	40	2.0	8.0	0	0	0	300	m.q.
(*Stokely* No Salt or Sugar Added)	40	2.0	8.0	0	0	0	25	m.q.
Chinese (*La Choy*)	12	1.0	2.0	.1	(0)	0	30	1.1 d
chop suey (*La Choy*)	9	.7	2.0	.1	(0)	0	330	1.0 d
no salt added, see specific brands								
VEGETABLES, MIXED, FROZEN:								
10-oz. pkg.	182	9.5	38.2	1.5	.3	0	132	3.3 c
boiled, drained, 4 oz.	67	3.2	14.8	.2	<.1	0	40	4.3 d
boiled, drained, ½ cup	54	2.6	11.9	.1	<.1	0	32	3.5 d

Food and Measure	cal.	prot. (gms)	carbo. (gms)	tot. fat (gms)	sat. fat (gms)	chol. (mgs)	sod. (mgs)	fiber (gms)
(A&P), 3.3 oz.	65	3.0	13.0	<1.0	(0)	0	55	m.q.
(Birds Eye), 3.3 oz.	60	3.0	13.0	0	0	0	40	2.0 d
(Birds Eye Portion Pack), 3 oz.	50	2.0	12.0	0	0	0	35	2.0 d
(Frosty Acres), 3.3 oz.	65	3.0	13.0	0	0	0	50	1.0 c
(Green Giant), ½ cup	40	2.0	9.0	0	0	0	40	2.0 d
(Green Giant Harvest Fresh), ½ cup	40	2.0	9.0	0	0	0	125	2.0 d
(Health Valley), ½ cup	68	3.0	14.0	0	0	0	39	1.9 d
(Seabrook), 3.3 oz.	65	3.0	13.0	0	0	0	50	1.0 c
(Southern), 3.5 oz.	69	3.2	13.9	0	0	0	60	m.q.
(Stokely Singles), 3 oz.	60	3.0	12.0	1.0	(0)	0	40	m.q.
California blend (A&P), 3.3 oz.	25	2.0	5.0	<1.0	(0)	0	25	m.q.
California style (Green Giant American Mixtures), ½ cup ...	25	2.0	6.0	0	0	0	40	2.0 d
Chinese style (Birds Eye Stir-Fry), 3.3 oz.	35	2.0	8.0	0	0	0	540	2.0 d
chow mein, in Oriental sauce (Birds Eye Custom Cuisine), 4.6 oz.[1]	80	3.0	14.0	2.0	m.q.	0	570	1.0 d
chow mein style, w/seasoned sauce (Birds Eye International Recipes), 3.3 oz.	90	2.0	12.0	4.0	m.q.	0	370	1.0 d
Dutch style (Frosty Acres), 3.2 oz. ..	30	2.0	5.0	0	0	0	30	m.q.
heartland (Green Giant American Mixtures), ½ cup	25	1.0	6.0	0	0	0	35	2.0 d
Italian style:								
(Frosty Acres), 3.2 oz.	40	3.0	8.0	0	0	0	20	m.q.
blend (A&P), 3.3 oz.	40	2.0	8.0	<1.0	(0)	0	35	m.q.
w/seasoned sauce (Birds Eye International Recipes), 3.3 oz.	100	2.0	11.0	5.0	m.q.	0	490	2.0 d
Japanese style:								
(Birds Eye Stir-Fry), 3.3 oz.	30	2.0	7.0	0	0	0	510	2.0 d
w/seasoned sauce (Birds Eye International Recipes), 3.3 oz.	90	2.0	10.0	5.0	m.q.	0	420	2.0 d
New England (Green Giant American Mixtures), ½ cup	70	3.0	14.0	1.0	n.a.	0	75	4.0 d
New England style, w/seasoned sauce (Birds Eye International Recipes), 3.3 oz.	130	3.0	14.0	7.0	m.q.	0	430	2.0 d
Oriental style:								
(Frosty Acres), 3.2 oz.	25	2.0	5.0	0	0	0	15	m.q.
w/authentic Oriental sauce for beef (Birds Eye Custom Cuisine), 4.6 oz.[1]	90	6.0	11.0	4.0	m.q.	0	350	2.0 d
w/seasoned sauce (Birds Eye International Recipes), 3.3 oz.	70	2.0	8.0	4.0	m.q.	0	300	1.0 d
blend (A&P), 3.3 oz.	25	2.0	5.0	<1.0	(0)	0	15	m.q.

1. *Without added meat.*

Food and Measure	cal.	prot. (gms)	carbo. (gms)	tot. fat (gms)	sat. fat (gms)	chol. (mgs)	sod. (mgs)	fiber (gms)
VEGETABLES, MIXED, FROZEN *(cont.)*								
pasta primavera style, w/seasoned sauce (*Birds Eye* International Recipes), 3.3 oz.	120	5.0	14.0	5.0	m.q.	5	340	2.0 d
San Francisco style, w/seasoned sauce (*Birds Eye* International Recipes), 3.3 oz.	100	2.0	11.0	5.0	m.q.	0	400	1.0 d
San Francisco style (*Green Giant* American Mixtures), ½ cup . . .	25	1.0	7.0	0	0	0	35	2.0 d
Santa Fe (*Green Giant* American Mixtures), ½ cup	70	2.0	16.0	1.0	n.a.	0	0	2.0 d
Seattle (*Green Giant* American Mixtures), ½ cup	25	2.0	7.0	0	0	0	35	2.0 d
in butter sauce (*Finast*), 3.3 oz. . . .	70	4.0	15.0	4.0	m.q.	n.a.	340	m.q.
in butter sauce (*Green Giant*), ½ cup	60	2.0	11.0	2.0	<1.0	5	300	2.0 d
w/herb sauce, for chicken or shrimp, (*Birds Eye Custom Cuisine*), 4.6 oz.[1]	90	3.0	8.0	5.0	m.q.	0	460	2.0 d
w/mushroom sauce, creamy, for beef (*Birds Eye Custom Cuisine*), 4.6 oz.[2]	60	3.0	9.0	2.0	m.q.	5	450	2.0 d
w/mustard sauce, Dijon, for chicken or fish (*Birds Eye Custom Cuisine*), 4.6 oz.[3]	70	4.0	9.0	3.0	m.q.	5	310	1.0 d
w/tomato basil sauce, for chicken (*Birds Eye Custom Cuisine*), 4.6 oz.[2]	110	5.0	17.0	3.0	m.q.	0	360	1.0 d
'n rice, in teriyaki sauce (*Stokely Singles*), 4 oz.	100	3.0	24.0	0	0	0	580	m.q.
'n rotini, in cheddar cheese sauce (*Stokely Singles*), 4 oz.	100	4.0	15.0	3.0	m.q.	10	380	m.q.
'n shells, in Italian style sauce (*Stokely Singles*), 4 oz.	170	3.0	5.0	15.0	m.q.	5	270	m.q.
soup mix (*Frosty Acres*), 3 oz.	45	4.0	11.0	0	0	0	35	m.q.
stew:								
(*A&P*), 4 oz.	60	1.0	13.0	<1.0	(0)	0	30	m.q.
(*Frosty Acres*), 3 oz.	42	3.0	10.0	0	0	0	21	m.q.
(*Kohl's*), 3.3 oz.	50	1.0	10.0	<1.0	(0)	0	30	m.q.
(*Ore-Ida*), 3 oz.	60	1.0	12.0	<1.0	(0)	0	40	m.q.
'n white and wild rice pilaf (*Stokely Singles*), 4 oz.	80	3.0	17.0	0	0	5	290	m.q.
w/wild rice, in white wine sauce, for chicken (*Birds Eye Custom Cuisine*), 4.6 oz.[2]	100	3.0	19.0	0	0	0	510	1.0 d
winter blend (*A&P*), 3.3 oz.	24	2.0	6.0	<1.0	(0)	0	190	m.q.

1. *Without added meat or shrimp.*
2. *Without added meat.*
3. *Without added meat or fish.*

Food and Measure	cal.	prot. (gms)	carbo. (gms)	tot. fat (gms)	sat. fat (gms)	chol. (mgs)	sod. (mgs)	fiber (gms)
VEGETARIAN BREAKFAST, see								
" 'Egg' breakfast, vegetarian"								
VEGETARIAN BURGER, see								
"Burger, vegetarian"								
VEGETARIAN ENTREE, frozen								
(see also specific listings):								
(*Natural Touch* Dinner Entree), 3-oz.								
patty	230	20.0	6.0	14.0	2.0	0	300	m.q.
VEGETARIAN FOODS, see								
specific listings								
VENISON, meat only:								
raw, 1 oz.	34	6.5	0	.7	.3	24	15	0
roasted[1]:								
12 oz., yield from 1 lb. raw								
boneless	537	102.8	0	10.8	4.2	379	183	0
4 oz.	179	34.3	0	3.6	1.4	127	61	0
diced, 1 cup, approx. 4.9 oz.	221	42.3	0	4.5	1.8	157	76	0
ground, 1 cup, approx. 4.1 oz. ...	183	35.0	0	3.7	1.5	130	63	0
VERMOUTH, see "Wine"								
VIENNA SAUSAGE, canned:								
in barbecue sauce (*Libby's*), 2½ oz.	180	8.0	2.0	15.0	m.q.	m.q.	420	0
in beef broth (*Libby's*, 9 oz.), 1.8 oz.								
or 3½ links	160	6.0	1.0	14.0	m.q.	m.q.	300	0
in beef broth (*Libby's*, 5 oz.), 2 oz. or								
3½ links	160	6.0	1.0	15.0	m.q.	m.q.	330	0
beef and pork, 1 oz.	79	2.9	.6	7.1	2.6	15	270	0
beef and pork, 1 link, 2″ × ⅞″,								
approx. .6 oz.	45	1.7	.3	4.0	1.5	8	152	0
no broth (*Hormel*), 4 links	200	7.0	1.0	18.0	m.q.	m.q.	479	0
VINE SPINACH:								
raw, 1 lb.	86	8.2	15.4	1.4	m.q.	0	m.q.	3.2 c
VINEGAR:								
raw, 1 oz.	5	.5	1.0	.1	0	0	(0)	.2 c
apple cider:								
(*Hain*), 1 tbsp.	2	0	4.0	0	0	0	1	0
(*Heinz*), 1 tbsp.	2	0	1.0	0	0	0	1	0
(*Indian Summer*), 1 cup	40	<1.0	14.0	<1.0	0	0	5	0
colored or white, distilled (*White*								
House), 1 fl. oz. or 2 tbsp.	4	0	2.0	0	0	0	5	0
pure (*Lucky Leaf/Musselman's*),								
1 fl. oz.	4	0	2.0	0	0	0	0	0
white:								
(*Indian Summer*), 1 cup	30	<1.0	12.0	<1.0	0	0	5	0
distilled (*Heinz*), 1 tbsp.	2	0	0	0	0	0	1	0
distilled (*Lucky Leaf/Musselman's*),								
1 fl. oz.	4	0	2.0	0	0	0	0	0

1. *Without added ingredients.*

Food and Measure	cal.	prot. (gms)	carbo. (gms)	tot. fat (gms)	sat. fat (gms)	chol. (mgs)	sod. (mgs)	fiber (gms)
VINEGAR *(cont.)*								
wine:								
all varieties *(Regina)*, 1 fl. oz.	4	0	0	0	0	0	0	0
basil *(Great Impressions)*, 1 tbsp.	7	0	.6	0	0	0	<1	0
garlic *(Great Impressions)*, 1 tbsp.	7	0	.9	0	0	0	<1	0
hot paprika *(Great Impressions)*, 1 tbsp.	6	0	.6	0	0	0	<1	0
raspberry *(Great Impressions)*, 1 tbsp.	7	0	1.0	0	0	0	<1	0
red *(Great Impressions)*, 1 tbsp. . . .	6	0	.6	0	0	0	<1	0
red *(Lucky Leaf/Musselman's)*, 1 fl. oz.	0	0	0	0	0	0	0	0
VODKA, see "Liquor"								

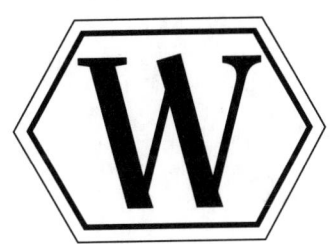

Food and Measure	cal.	prot. (gms)	carbo. (gms)	tot. fat (gms)	sat. fat (gms)	chol. (mgs)	sod. (mgs)	fiber (gms)
WAFFLE, FROZEN:								
(*Aunt Jemima* Original), 2.5-oz.								
piece	173	4.3	27.8	5.6	1.4	6	591	1.5 d
(*Downyflake*), 2 pieces	120	3.0	20.0	3.0	1.0	0	420	m.q.
(*Downyflake* Hot-N-Buttery),								
2 pieces	180	4.0	27.0	6.0	m.q.	n.a.	620	m.q.
(*Downyflake* Jumbo), 2 pieces	170	4.0	30.0	4.0	1.0	0	570	m.q.
(*Eggo* Homestyle), 1 piece	120	3.0	16.0	5.0	m.q.	10	250	m.q.
(*Eggo Nutri-Grain*), 1 piece	130	3.0	18.0	5.0	m.q.	0	250	2.0 d
(*Roman Meal*), 2 pieces	280	5.0	33.0	14.0	m.q.	4	680	3.0 d
apple cinnamon (*Aunt Jemima*),								
2.5-oz. piece	176	4.5	28.8	5.6	1.3	6	616	2.0 d
apple cinnamon (*Eggo*), 1 piece	130	3.0	18.0	5.0	m.q.	n.a.	250	m.q.
Belgian (*Weight Watchers* Microwave),								
½ pkg. or 1.5 oz.	120	4.0	17.0	4.0	2.0	5	220	m.q.
blueberry:								
(*Aunt Jemima*), 2.5-oz. piece	175	4.2	29.2	5.2	1.3	5	684	1.3 d
(*Downyflake*), 2 pieces	180	4.0	32.0	4.0	m.q.	0	570	m.q.
(*Eggo*), 1 piece	130	3.0	18.0	5.0	m.q.	n.a.	250	m.q.
buttermilk:								
(*Aunt Jemima*), 2.5-oz. piece	179	4.4	28.7	5.8	1.4	7	615	1.3 d
(*Downyflake*), 2 pieces	190	5.0	32.0	5.0	m.q.	0	750	m.q.
(*Eggo*), 1 piece	120	3.0	16.0	5.0	m.q.	10	250	m.q.
multigrain (*Downyflake*), 2 pieces ...	250	6.0	28.0	4.0	m.q.	0	500	3.5 d
oat bran:								
(*Aunt Jemima*), 2.5 oz.	154	5.9	29.4	2.8	m.q.	n.a.	676	3.0 d
(*Downyflake*), 2 pieces	260	6.0	30.0	13.0	m.q.	0	650	3.0 d
(*Eggo Common Sense*), 1 piece ..	110	3.0	16.0	4.0	m.q.	0	220	2.0 d
w/fruit and nut (*Eggo Common*								
Sense), 1 piece	120	3.0	17.0	5.0	m.q.	0	220	2.0 d
raisin and bran (*Eggo Nutri-Grain*),								
1 piece	130	3.0	18.0	5.0	m.q.	0	250	2.0 d

Food and Measure	cal.	prot. (gms)	carbo. (gms)	tot. fat (gms)	sat. fat (gms)	chol. (mgs)	sod. (mgs)	fiber (gms)
WAFFLE, FROZEN *(cont.)*								
rice bran (*Downyflake*), 2 pieces ...	210	5.0	25.0	11.0	m.q.	0	230	3.5 d
strawberry (*Eggo*), 1 piece	130	3.0	18.0	5.0	m.q.	n.a.	250	m.q.
whole grain wheat (*Aunt Jemima*),								
2.5-oz. piece	154	5.9	29.4	2.8	m.q.	n.a.	676	3.0 d
WAFFLE BREAKFAST, frozen:								
w/bacon (*Swanson Great Starts*),								
2.2 oz.	230	7.0	19.0	14.0	m.q.	m.q.	710	m.q.
Belgian, and sausage (*Swanson Great*								
Starts), 2.85 oz	280	7.0	21.0	19.0	m.q.	m.q.	420	m.q.
Belgian, w/strawberries and								
sausages (*Swanson Great*								
Starts), 3.5 oz.	210	3.0	31.0	8.0	m.q.	m.q.	240	m.q.
WAFFLE MIX (see also "Pancake								
and waffle mix"):								
(*Bisquick Shake 'n Pour* Complete								
Waffle Mix), 2 pieces	280	6.0	51.0	6.0	m.q.	0	930	m.q.
WAKAME, see "Seaweed"								
WALNUT, BLACK,[1] dried:								
in shell, 1 lb.	661	26.5	13.2	61.6	3.9	0	2	5.4 d
1 oz.	172	6.9	3.4	16.1	1.0	0	tr.	1.4 d
chopped, 1 cup	759	30.4	15.1	70.7	4.5	0	2	6.3 d
finely ground, 1 cup	486	19.5	9.7	45.3	2.9	0	1	4.0 d
(*Planters*), 1 oz.	180	7.0	3.0	17.0	1.0	0	0	m.q.
WALNUT, ENGLISH OR								
PERSIAN[1], dried:								
in shell, 1 lb.	1310	29.2	37.4	126.3	11.4	0	21	9.8 d
1 oz., approx. 14 halves	182	4.1	5.2	17.6	1.6	0	3	1.4 d
pieces or chips, 1 cup	770	17.2	22.0	74.2	6.7	0	12	5.8 d
halves, 1 cup	642	14.3	18.3	61.9	5.6	0	10	4.8 d
(*Diamond*), 1 oz.	192	5.0	4.0	19.0	m.q.	0	n.a.	m.q.
whole, halves or pieces (*Planters*),								
1 oz.	190	4.0	3.0	20.0	2.0	0	0	m.q.
WALNUT OIL:								
(*Hain*), 1 tbsp.	120	0	0	14.0	2.0	0	0	0
WALNUT TOPPING:								
in syrup (*Smucker's*), 2 tbsp.	130	2.0	27.0	1.0	n.a.	0	0	m.q.
WASABI:								
powder, ¼ oz.	24	.8	4.9	<.1	0	0	2	n.a.
WASABI SNACK CHIPS:								
(*Eden*), 1 oz.	130	1.0	22.0	4.0	m.q.	0	200	m.q.
WATER, MINERAL, see "Soft								
drinks and mixers"								
WATER BUFFALO, meat only:								
raw, 1 oz.	28	5.8	0	.4	.1	13	15	0
roasted[2]:								
12 oz., yield from 1 lb. boneless	445	91.3	0	6.1	2.1	206	191	0

1. *Shelled, except as noted.*
2. *Without added ingredients.*

Food and Measure	cal.	prot. (gms)	carbo. (gms)	tot. fat (gms)	sat. fat (gms)	chol. (mgs)	sod. (mgs)	fiber (gms)
4 oz.	149	30.4	0	2.0	.7	69	64	0
diced, 1 cup, approx. 4.9 oz.	183	37.6	0	2.5	.8	85	78	0
WATER CONVULVOLUS, see "Swamp cabbage"								
WATERCHESTNUT, Chinese:								
untrimmed, 1 lb.	369	4.9	83.6	.4	n.a.	0	50	2.8 c
trimmed, 1 oz.	30	.4	6.8	<.1	(0)	0	4	.2 c
4 medium, 1¼"–2" diam., approx.								
1.7 oz.	38	.5	8.6	<.1	(0)	0	5	.3 c
sliced, ½ cup	66	.9	14.8	.1	(0)	0	9	.5 c
WATERCHESTNUT, CANNED, Chinese:								
w/liquid, 4 oz.	57	1.0	14.1	.1	(0)	0	9	.7 c
w/liquid, sliced, ½ cup	35	.6	8.7	<.1	(0)	0	6	.4 c
4 medium, approx. 1 oz.	14	.3	3.5	<.1	(0)	0	2	.2 c
(*La Choy*), 1.28 oz.	18	.3	4.5	<.1	(0)	0	3	m.q.
WATERCRESS:								
untrimmed, 1 lb.	46	9.6	5.4	.4	.1	0	170	9.6 d
trimmed, 1 oz.	3	.7	.4	<.1	tr.	0	12	.7 d
10 sprigs, 11¼" long, approx. .9 oz.	3	.6	.3	<.1	<.1	0	10	.6 d
chopped, ½ cup	2	.4	.2	<.1	tr.	0	7	.4 d
WATERMELON:								
untrimmed, 1 lb.	74	1.5	16.9	1.0	n.a.	0	5	.9 d
trimmed, 1 oz.	9	.2	2.0	.1	(0)	0	1	.1 d
¹⁄₁₆ of 10"-diam. melon, 1"-thick slice	152	3.0	34.6	2.0	(0)	0	10	1.9 d
diced, ½ cup	25	.5	5.7	.3	(0)	0	2	.3 d
WATERMELON SEED, dried:								
in hard coat, 1 lb.	935	47.5	25.7	79.5	16.4	0	166	5.1 c
kernels, 1 oz.	158	8.1	4.4	13.5	2.8	0	28	.9 c
kernels, 1 cup	602	30.6	16.5	51.2	10.6	0	107	3.3 c
WAX BEAN, fresh, see "Green bean"								
WAX BEAN, CANNED:								
(*Allens*), ½ cup	15	1.0	3.0	<1.0	(0)	0	260	m.q.
(*Stokely*), ½ cup	20	1.0	4.0	0	0	0	360	m.q.
(*Stokely* No Salt or Sugar), ½ cup ..	20	1.0	4.0	0	0	0	5	m.q.
golden, cut or French style (*Del Monte*), ½ cup	20	0	4.0	0	0	0	355	m.q.
WAX BEAN, FROZEN:								
(*Frosty Acres*), 3 oz.	25	2.0	5.0	0	0	0	1	1.0 c
cut (*Seabrook*), 3 oz.	25	2.0	5.0	0	0	0	1	1.0 c
WAX GOURD:								
raw:								
untrimmed, 1 lb.	42	1.3	9.7	.6	.1	0	358	1.9 d
trimmed, 1 oz.	4	.1	.9	.1	tr.	0	31	.2 d
1 gourd, 17.7 lbs.	741	22.8	171.0	11.4	.9	0	6327	34.2 d
cubed, ½ cup	9	.3	2.0	.1	<.1	0	74	.4 d
boiled, drained, 4 oz.	15	.5	3.4	.2	<.1	0	121	.6 c
boiled, drained, cubed, ½ cup	11	.4	2.6	.2	<.1	0	93	.4 c

Food and Measure	cal.	prot. (gms)	carbo. (gms)	tot. fat (gms)	sat. fat (gms)	chol. (mgs)	sod. (mgs)	fiber (gms)
WELSH ONION, see "Onion, Welsh"								
WELSH RAREBIT (see also "Cheese sauce"):								
canned (*Snow's*), ½ cup	170	9.0	10.0	11.0	m.q.	m.q.	460	n.a.
frozen (*Stouffer's*), 10 oz.	350	13.0	8.0	30.0	m.q.	m.q.	680	n.a.
WENDY'S:								
sandwiches, 1 serving:								
chicken, 6.9 oz.	440	26.0	43.0	19.0	2.6	60	725	m.q.
chicken, grilled, 6.2 oz.	340	24.0	37.0	13.0	2.2	60	815	m.q.
chicken club, 7.2 oz.	506	30.0	43.0	25.0	4.8	70	930	m.q.
fish fillet, 6 oz.	460	18.0	42.0	25.0	4.7	50	780	m.q.
hamburger, single, plain, 4.4 oz.	340	24.0	30.0	15.0	5.5	65	500	m.q.
hamburger, single, w/everything, 7.4 oz.	420	25.0	35.0	21.0	5.5	70	890	m.q.
Jr. cheeseburger, 4.4 oz.	310	18.0	34.0	13.0	3.0	35	770	m.q.
Jr. bacon cheeseburger, 5.5 oz. ..	430	22.0	33.0	25.0	5.2	50	840	m.q.
Jr. Swiss deluxe, 5.8 oz.	360	18.0	35.0	18.0	3.0	40	765	m.q.
Kids' Meal cheeseburger, 4.1 oz.	300	18.0	33.0	13.0	3.0	35	770	m.q.
Kid's Meal hamburger, 3.7 oz. ...	260	15.0	33.0	9.0	3.0	35	570	m.q.
steak, country fried, 5.1 oz.	440	14.0	45.0	25.0	5.7	35	870	m.q.
Wendy's Big Classic, 9.2 oz.	570	27.0	47.0	33.0	5.6	80	1085	m.q.
chicken nuggets, crispy, 6 pieces ..	280	14.0	12.0	20.0	4.5	50	600	m.q.
chicken nugget sauces:								
barbecue, 1 oz.	50	<1.0	11.0	<1.0	tr.	0	100	n.a.
honey, .5 oz.	45	<1.0	12.0	<1.0	tr.	0	tr.	0
sweet & sour, 1 oz.	45	<1.0	11.0	<1.0	tr.	0	55	n.a.
sweet mustard, 1 oz.	50	<1.0	9.0	1.0	<1.0	0	140	m.q.
chili and chili condiments:								
chili, regular, 9 oz.	220	21.0	23.0	7.0	2.6	45	750	m.q.
cheddar cheese, shredded, 1 oz.	110	7.0	1.0	10.0	6.0	30	175	0
sour cream, 1 oz.	60	1.0	1.0	6.0	3.6	10	15	0
potatoes:								
baked, plain, 8.8 oz.	270	6.0	63.0	<1.0	tr.	0	20	m.q.
baked, hot stuffed:								
bacon and cheese, 12.8 oz. ...	520	20.0	70.0	18.0	5.1	20	1460	m.q.
broccoli and cheese, 12.3 oz. ..	400	8.0	58.0	16.0	2.9	tr.	455	m.q.
cheese, 11.2 oz.	420	8.0	66.0	15.0	4.0	10	310	m.q.
chili and cheese, 14.2 oz.	500	15.0	71.0	18.0	4.0	25	630	m.q.
sour cream and chives, 11.4 oz.	500	8.0	67.0	23.0	9.3	25	135	m.q.
french fries, small, 3.2 oz.	240	3.0	33.0	12.0	2.5	0	145	m.q.
salads, prepared:								
chef, 9.1 oz.	130	14.0	8.0	5.0	1.2	40	460	m.q.
garden, 8.1 oz.	70	4.0	9.0	2.0	0	0	60	m.q.
taco, 17.3 oz.	530	27.0	55.0	23.0	m.q.	35	825	m.q.
salad dressing, 1 tbsp.:								
bacon and tomato, reduced calorie	45	<1.0	3.0	4.0	.6	<1	190	n.a.
blue cheese	90	<1.0	<1.0	10.0	1.9	10	105	0

Food and Measure	cal.	prot. (gms)	carbo. (gms)	tot. fat (gms)	sat. fat (gms)	chol. (mgs)	sod. (mgs)	fiber (gms)
celery seed	70	<1.0	3.0	6.0	.9	5	65	n.a.
French	60	<1.0	4.0	6.0	.9	0	178	n.a.
French, sweet red	70	<1.0	5.0	6.0	.8	0	125	n.a.
Hidden Valley Ranch	50	<1.0	<1.0	6.0	1.0	5	95	n.a.
Italian, golden	45	<1.0	3.0	4.0	.5	0	250	n.a.
Italian, reduced calorie	25	<1.0	2.0	2.0	.3	0	185	n.a.
Italian Caesar	80	<1.0	<1.0	9.0	1.4	5	140	n.a.
Thousand Island	70	<1.0	2.0	7.0	1.1	5	105	n.a.
SuperBar, Mexican Fiesta:								
cheese sauce, 2 oz.	39	1.0	5.0	2.0	1.0	tr.	305	0
picante sauce, 2 oz.	18	<1.0	4.0	<1.0	<1.0	n.a.	5	n.a.
refried beans, 2 oz.	70	4.0	10.0	3.0	.9	tr.	215	m.q.
rice, Spanish, 2 oz.	70	2.0	13.0	1.0	.2	tr.	440	m.q.
sour topping, imitation, 1 oz.	58	<1.0	2.0	5.0	5.0	0	30	0
taco chips, 1.4 oz.	260	4.0	40.0	10.0	.7	0	20	m.q.
taco meat, 2 oz.	110	10.0	4.0	7.0	1.7	25	300	n.a.
taco sauce, 1 oz.	16	<1.0	3.0	<1.0	tr.	tr.	140	n.a.
taco shells, .4-oz. shell	45	<1.0	6.0	3.0	.7	0	45	m.q.
tortilla, flour, 1.3-oz. shell	110	3.0	19.0	3.0	.4	n.a.	220	m.q.
SuperBar, pasta:								
Alfredo sauce, 2 oz.	35	1.0	5.0	1.0	.8	tr.	300	n.a.
cheese ravioli in spaghetti sauce,								
2 oz.	45	1.0	8.0	1.0	.3	5	290	m.q.
cheese tortellini in spaghetti								
sauce, 2 oz.	60	2.0	12.0	1.0	.3	5	280	m.q.
fettuccini, 2 oz.	190	4.0	27.0	3.0	.6	10	3	m.q.
garlic toast, .6-oz. piece	70	2.0	9.0	3.0	.6	tr.	65	m.q.
pasta medley, 2 oz.	60	2.0	9.0	2.0	.3	tr.	5	m.q.
rotini, 2 oz.	90	3.0	15.0	2.0	.3	tr.	tr.	m.q.
spaghetti sauce, 2 oz.	28	<1.0	7.0	<1.0	tr.	tr.	345	m.q.
spaghetti meat sauce, 2 oz.	60	4.0	8.0	2.0	.7	10	315	m.q.
dessert:								
chocolate chip cookie, 2.25 oz. ..	275	3.0	40.0	13.0	4.2	15	256	m.q.
frosty, dairy, small, 8.6 oz.	340	9.0	57.0	10.0	5.0	40	200	(0)
WEST INDIAN CHERRY, see "Acerola"								
WESTERN DINNER, frozen:								
(*Banquet*), 11 oz.	630	28.0	40.0	41.0	m.q.	90	720	m.q.
(*Morton*), 10 oz.	290	14.0	29.0	14.0	m.q.	35	1450	m.q.
style (*Swanson*), 11½ oz.	430	22.0	43.0	19.0	m.q.	m.q.	1060	m.q.
WHEAT, whole grain:								
durum, 1 oz.	96	3.9	20.2	.7	.1	0	<1	m.q.
durum, 1 cup	650	26.3	136.6	4.7	.9	0	3	m.q.
hard red:								
spring:								
1 oz.	93	4.4	19.3	.5	.1	0	<1	.6 c
1 cup	631	29.6	130.6	3.7	.6	0	4	4.4 c
or winter (*Arrowhead Mills*),								
2 oz.	190	8.0	41.0	1.0	n.a.	0	1	8.3 d

Food and Measure	cal.	prot. (gms)	carbo. (gms)	tot. fat (gms)	sat. fat (gms)	chol. (mgs)	sod. (mgs)	fiber (gms)
WHEAT, HARD RED *(cont.)*								
winter, 1 oz.	93	3.6	20.2	.4	.1	0	<1	.6 c
winter, 1 cup	628	24.2	136.7	3.0	.5	0	4	4.4 c
soft red:								
for pastry (*Arrowhead Mills*),								
2 oz.	190	8.0	41.0	1.0	n.a.	0	1	8.3 d
winter, 1 oz.	94	2.9	21.0	.4	.1	0	<1	.5 c
winter, 1 cup	556	17.4	124.7	2.6	.5	0	4	2.9 c
hard white, 1 oz.	97	3.2	21.5	.5	.1	0	n.a.	m.q.
hard white, 1 cup	656	21.7	145.7	3.3	.5	0	n.a.	m.q.
soft white, 1 oz.	96	3.0	21.4	.6	.1	0	n.a.	m.q.
soft white, 1 cup	571	18.0	126.6	3.3	.6	0	n.a.	m.q.
WHEAT, PARBOILED, see								
"Bulgur"								
WHEAT, SPROUTED:								
1 oz.	56	2.1	12.1	.4	.1	0	5	m.q.
1 cup	214	8.1	45.9	1.4	.2	0	18	m.q.
WHEAT BRAN:								
crude:								
1 oz.	61	4.4	18.3	1.2	.2	0	<1	12.0 d
1 cup	130	9.3	38.7	2.6	.4	0	2	25.4 d
2 tbsp.	15	1.1	4.5	.3	<.1	0	tr.	3.0 d
(*Arrowhead Mills*), 2 oz.	50	10.0	30.0	2.0	m.q.	0	3	24.4 d
toasted (*Kretschmer*), 1 oz., approx.								
⅓ cup	57	5.7	14.8	2.3	.2	0	2	11.4 d
unprocessed (*Quaker*), 2 tbsp.,								
¼ oz.	8	1.0	3.8	.2	0	0	0	3.3 d
WHEAT CAKE:								
(*Quaker* Grain Cakes), .32-oz. piece	34	1.4	6.7	.3	.1	0	52	.8 d
WHEAT FLAKES:								
(*Arrowhead Mills*), 2 oz.	210	8.0	42.0	1.0	n.a.	0	1	6.7 d
WHEAT FLOUR:								
whole-grain:								
1 oz.	96	3.9	20.6	.5	.1	0	1	3.6 d
1 cup	407	16.4	87.1	2.2	.4	0	1	15.1 d
(*Ceresota/Heckers*), 4 oz., approx.								
1 cup	400	15.0	80.0	2.0	m.q.	0	0	m.q.
(*Gold Medal*), 4 oz. or 1 cup	350	16.0	78.0	2.0	m.q.	0	0	10.0 d
(*Pillsbury's Best*), 1 cup	400	15.0	80.0	2.0	m.q.	0	10	m.q.
blend (*Gold Medal*), 4 oz. or 1 cup	380	14.0	84.0	2.0	m.q.	0	0	8.0 d
pastry (*Arrowhead Mills*), 2 oz. ..	180	6.0	41.0	1.0	m.q.	0	1	6.8 d
stone ground (*Arrowhead Mills*),								
2 oz.	200	8.0	40.0	1.0	m.q.	0	1	6.7 d
white:								
(*Drifted Snow*), 4 oz. or 1 cup ...	400	11.0	87.0	1.0	m.q.	0	0	m.q.
(*Softasilk*), 1 oz. or ¼ cup	100	2.0	23.0	0	0	0	0	m.q.
(*Wondra*), 4 oz. or 1 cup	400	11.0	87.0	1.0	m.q.	0	0	m.q.
all-purpose:								
1 oz.	103	2.9	21.6	.3	<.1	0	<1	.8 d

Food and Measure	cal.	prot. (gms)	carbo. (gms)	tot. fat (gms)	sat. fat (gms)	chol. (mgs)	sod. (mgs)	fiber (gms)
1 cup	455	12.9	95.4	1.2	.2	0	2	3.4 d
(Ballard/Pillsbury's Best),								
1 cup	400	11.0	87.0	1.0	m.q.	0	0	m.q.
(Ceresota/Heckers), 4 oz.	390	12.5	82.5	1.0	m.q.	0	0	m.q.
(Gold Medal), 4 oz. or 1 cup ...	400	11.0	87.0	1.0	m.q.	0	0	m.q.
(Red Band), 4 oz. or 1 cup	390	10.0	85.0	1.0	m.q.	0	0	m.q.
(Robin Hood), 4 oz. or 1 cup ...	400	13.0	85.0	1.0	m.q.	0	0	m.q.
(White Deer), 4 oz. or 1 cup ...	400	11.0	87.0	1.0	m.q.	0	0	m.q.
unbleached (Gold Medal), 4 oz.								
or 1 cup	400	11.0	87.0	1.0	m.q.	0	0	m.q.
unbleached (Pillsbury's Best),								
1 cup	400	12.0	86.0	1.0	m.q.	0	0	m.q.
unbleached (Robin Hood), 4 oz.								
or 1 cup	400	13.0	85.0	1.0	m.q.	0	0	m.q.
bread:								
1 oz.	102	3.4	20.6	.5	.1	0	<1	m.q.
1 cup	495	16.4	99.4	2.3	.3	0	2	m.q.
(Gold Medal Better for Bread),								
4 oz. or 1 cup	400	14.0	83.0	1.0	m.q.	0	0	m.q.
(Pillsbury's Best), 1 cup	400	14.0	83.0	2.0	m.q.	0	0	m.q.
cake, 1 oz.	103	2.3	22.1	.2	<.1	0	<1	m.q.
cake, 1 cup	395	8.9	85.1	.9	.1	0	2	m.q.
self-rising:								
1 oz.	100	2.8	21.0	.3	<.1	0	360	<.1 c
1 cup	442	12.4	92.8	1.2	.2	0	1587	.3 c
(Ballard/Pillsbury's Best),								
1 cup	380	9.0	84.0	1.0	m.q.	0	1290	m.q.
(Gold Medal), 4 oz. or 1 cup ...	380	10.0	83.0	1.0	m.q.	0	1520	m.q.
(Red Band), 4 oz. or 1 cup	380	9.0	83.0	1.0	m.q.	0	1520	m.q.
(Robin Hood), 4 oz. or 1 cup ...	380	10.0	83.0	1.0	m.q.	0	1520	m.q.
enriched (Aunt Jemima), 1 oz.,								
approx. ¼ cup	109	3.0	23.6	.3	n.a.	0	368	.1 c
tortilla mix, 1 oz.	115	2.7	19.0	3.0	1.2	0	192	<.1 c
tortilla mix, 1 cup	449	10.7	74.5	11.8	4.6	0	751	.2 c
unbleached (Arrowhead Mills),								
2 oz.	200	7.0	53.0	1.0	m.q.	0	1	m.q.
WHEAT GERM:								
(Kretschmer), 1 oz., approx. ¼ cup	103	9.3	12.3	3.4	.5	0	2	3.3 d
crude, 1 oz.	102	6.6	14.7	2.8	.5	0	3	4.3 d
crude, 1 cup	414	26.6	59.6	11.2	1.9	0	14	17.3 d
honey crunch (Kretschmer), 1 oz.,								
approx. ¼ cup	105	7.6	15.2	2.8	.4	0	2	3.0 d
raw (Arrowhead Mills), 2 oz.	210	15.0	26.0	6.0	m.q.	0	1	6.5 d
toasted, 1 oz., approx. ¼ cup	108	8.3	14.1	3.0	.5	0	1	3.7 d
toasted, 1 cup	431	32.9	56.1	12.1	2.1	0	4	14.6 d
WHEAT GLUTEN:								
vital (Arrowhead Mills), 1 oz.	100	15.0	9.0	1.0	n.a.	0	1	.9 d
WHEAT "NUTS":								
unflavored, 1 oz.	177	3.9	6.7	16.4	2.5	0	143	.2 c

Food and Measure	cal.	prot. (gms)	carbo. (gms)	tot. fat (gms)	sat. fat (gms)	chol. (mgs)	sod. (mgs)	fiber (gms)
WHEAT "NUTS" *(cont.)*								
macadamia flavored, 1 oz.	176	3.2	7.9	16.1	2.4	0	13	.2 c
all other flavors, 1 oz.	184	3.7	5.9	17.7	2.7	0	26	.3 c
WHEAT PILAF MIX:								
(*Casbah*), 1 oz. dry or ½ cup								
cooked	100	3.0	20.0	0	0	0	m.q.	m.q.
WHELK, unspecified, meat only:								
raw, 1 lb.	623	108.1	35.2	1.8	.1	294	934	0
raw, 1 oz.	39	6.8	2.2	.1	<.1	18	54	0
WHEY:								
acid:								
fluid, 1 oz.	7	.2	1.5	<.1	<.1	(0)	14	0
fluid, 1 cup, approx. 8.7 oz.	59	1.9	12.6	.2	.1	(0)	118	0
dry:								
1 oz.	96	3.3	20.8	.2	.1	(0)	274	0
1 cup, approx. 2 oz.	193	6.7	41.9	.3	.2	(0)	552	0
1 tbsp.	10	.3	2.1	<.1	<.1	(0)	28	0
sweet:								
fluid, 1 oz.	8	.2	1.5	.1	<.1	<1	15	0
fluid, 1 cup, approx. 8.7 oz.	66	2.1	12.6	.9	.6	5	132	0
dry:								
1 oz.	100	3.7	21.1	.3	.2	2	306	0
1 cup, approx. 5.1 oz.	512	18.8	108.0	1.6	1.0	9	1565	0
1 tbsp.	26	1.0	5.6	.1	.1	tr.	80	0
WHIPPED TOPPING, see "Cream								
topping"								
WHISKEY, see "Liquor"								
WHISKEY SOUR[1]:								
1 fl. oz.	41	.1	1.7	tr.	tr.	0	3	(0)
WHISKEY SOUR MIX:								
bottled:								
1 fl. oz.	27	tr.	6.9	tr.	tr.	0	m.q.	.1 d
1 fl. oz.[2]	45	tr.	4.0	tr.	tr.	0	m.q.	<.1 d
(*Holland House*), 1 fl. oz.	37	0	9.0	0	0	0	105	n.a.
powdered:								
.6-oz. pkt.	64	.1	16.2	tr.	tr.	0	m.q.	.1 d
1 fl. oz.[2]	48	tr.	4.7	tr.	tr.	0	m.q.	<.1 d
instant (*Bar-Tender's*), 3½ fl. oz.[2]	177	0	18.0	0	0	0	50	0
instant (*Holland House*), .56 oz.								
dry	64	0	16.0	0	0	0	16	n.a.
WHITE BEAN:								
raw:								
1 oz.	94	6.6	17.1	.2	.1	0	5	1.7 c
½ cup	337	23.6	60.9	.9	.2	0	16	6.0 c
small, 1 oz.	95	6.0	17.6	.3	.1	0	3	2.9 d
small, ½ cup	363	22.8	67.2	1.3	.3	0	13	11.1 d

1. *Recipe: 51% lemon juice, 46.8% whiskey, and 2.2% sugar.*
2. *Prepared according to package directions, with whiskey.*

Food and Measure	cal.	prot. (gms)	carbo. (gms)	tot. fat (gms)	sat. fat (gms)	chol. (mgs)	sod. (mgs)	fiber (gms)
boiled:								
4 oz.	158	11.0	28.5	.4	.1	0	7	2.8 c
½ cup	125	8.6	22.5	.3	.1	0	6	2.2 c
small, 4 oz.	161	10.2	29.3	.7	.2	0	2	5.0 d
small, ½ cup	127	8.1	23.2	.6	.1	0	2	3.7 d
WHITE BEAN, CANNED:								
w/liquid, 4 oz.	133	8.2	24.9	.3	.1	0	515	.8 c
w/liquid, ½ cup	153	9.5	28.7	.4	.1	0	595	.9 c
WHITE CASTLE:								
sandwiches, 1 serving:								
cheeseburger, 2.3 oz.	200	7.8	15.5	11.2	m.q.	m.q.	361	2.7 d
chicken sandwich, 2.25 oz.	186	12.5	32.1	11.7	m.q.	m.q.	497	1.7 d
fish sandwich, w/out tartar sauce,								
2.1 oz.	155	5.8	20.9	5.0	m.q.	m.q.	201	1.4 d
hamburger, 2.1 oz.	161	5.9	15.4	7.9	m.q.	m.q.	266	2.1 d
sausage sandwich, 1.7 oz.	196	6.7	13.3	12.3	m.q.	m.q.	488	2.0 d
sausage and egg sandwich,								
3.4 oz.	322	12.6	16.1	22.0	m.q.	m.q.	698	3.0 d
side dishes, 1 serving:								
french fries, 3.4 oz.	301	2.5	37.7	14.7	m.q.	n.a.	193	4.6 d
onion chips, 3.3 oz.	329	3.7	38.8	16.6	m.q.	n.a.	823	3.5 d
onion rings, 2.1 oz.	245	2.9	26.6	13.4	m.q.	n.a.	566	2.6 d
condiments:								
bun, .9 oz.	74	2.2	13.9	.9	n.a.	0	<1	.5 d
cheese, .3 oz.	31	1.5	2.3	1.6	m.q.	n.a.	154	.2 d
WHITE-FLOWERED GOURD,								
see "Gourd, white-flowered"								
WHITE SAUCE MIX:								
1.75-oz. pkt. dry	230	5.4	25.1	13.2	3.3	tr.	1691	.1 c
½ cup[1]	121	5.1	10.7	6.7	3.2	17	398	<.1 c
WHITEFISH, mixed species, meat only:								
raw:								
1 lb.	610	86.6	0	26.6	4.1	272	232	0
1 oz.	38	5.4	0	1.7	.3	17	14	0
1 fillet, approx. 7 oz., yield from								
2½-lb. whole fish	266	37.8	0	11.6	1.8	119	101	0
smoked, 4 oz.	122	26.5	0	1.1	.3	37	1156	0
smoked, 1 oz.	31	6.6	0	.3	<.1	9	289	0
WHITING, mixed species, meat only:								
raw:								
1 lb.	408	83.1	0	6.0	1.1	303	326	0
1 oz.	26	5.2	0	.4	<.1	19	20	0
1 fillet, approx. 3.2 oz., yield from								
1½-lb. whole fish	83	16.9	0	1.2	.2	61	66	0

1. *Prepared according to package directions, with whole milk.*

Food and Measure	cal.	prot. (gms)	carbo. (gms)	tot. fat (gms)	sat. fat (gms)	chol. (mgs)	sod. (mgs)	fiber (gms)
WHITING *(cont.)*								
baked, broiled, or microwaved[1],								
4 oz.	130	26.6	0	1.9	.4	95	150	0
WHITING, FROZEN:								
(*Booth*), 4 oz.	100	19.0	0	1.0	m.q.	m.q.	90	0
(*Booth* Individually Wrapped), 4 oz.	80	19.0	0	1.0	m.q.	m.q.	85	0
WIENER, see "Frankfurter"								
WILD RICE:								
raw, 1 oz.	101	4.2	21.2	.3	<.1	0	2	1.5 d
raw, 1 cup	571	23.6	119.8	1.7	.2	0	12	8.3 d
cooked:								
4 oz.	115	4.5	24.2	.4	.1	0	3	.4 c
1 cup	166	6.5	35.0	.6	.1	0	6	.5 c
(*Fantastic Foods*), ½ cup	83	3.0	18.0	0	0	0	0	m.q.
WILD RICE DISHES, see "Rice dishes, frozen" and "Rice dishes, mix"								
WINE, 4 fl. oz., except as noted:								
barbera, white (*Colony*)	91	0	3.5	0	0	0	4	0
burgundy:								
(*Bravo*)	91	0	1.7	0	0	0	4	0
(*Carlo Rossi*)	92	0	1.6	0	0	0	n.a.	0
(*Colony* Classic)	90	0	1.2	0	0	0	4	0
(*Gallo*)	88	0	.8	0	0	0	n.a.	0
(*Gallo* Hearty)	92	0	1.6	0	0	0	n.a.	0
(*Gambarelli & Davitto Parma*)	91	0	1.7	0	0	0	4	0
(*Petri*)	91	0	1.7	0	0	0	4	0
white (*Colony* Classic)	80	0	.8	0	0	0	4	0
Cabernet Sauvignon (*Colony*)	88	0	.7	0	0	0	4	0
Cabernet Sauvignon (*Gallo*)	88	0	0	0	0	0	n.a.	0
carbonated:								
almond (*Jacques Bonet*)	104	0	7.7	0	0	0	4	0
apricot or peach (*Jacques Bonet*)	111	0	9.5	0	0	0	4	0
raspberry or cherry (*Jacques Bonet*)	106	0	8.3	0	0	0	4	0
(*Carlo Rossi* Paisano)	92	0	1.6	0	0	0	n.a.	0
chablis:								
(*Bravo*)	86	0	1.7	0	0	0	4	0
(*Carlo Rossi*)	84	0	2.0	0	0	0	n.a.	0
(*Colony* Classic)	84	0	1.8	0	0	0	4	0
(*Gallo* Blanc)	80	0	.6	0	0	0	n.a.	0
(*Gambarelli & Davitto Parma*)	86	0	1.7	0	0	0	4	0
(*Petri* Chablis Blanc)	86	0	1.7	0	0	0	4	0
emerald (*Colony*)	102	0	5.3	0	0	0	4	0
gold (*Colony*)	97	0	4.3	0	0	0	4	0
pink:								
(*Carlo Rossi*)	92	0	3.6	0	0	0	n.a.	0
(*Colony*)	98	0	4.5	0	0	0	4	0

1. *Without added ingredients.*

Food and Measure	cal.	prot. (gms)	carbo. (gms)	tot. fat (gms)	sat. fat (gms)	chol. (mgs)	sod. (mgs)	fiber (gms)
(*Gallo*)	80	0	4.0	0	0	0	n.a.	0
(*Petri*)	98	0	4.5	0	0	0	4	0
ruby (*Colony*)	104	0	5.9	0	0	0	4	0
champagne:								
brut (*Jacques Bonet*)	92	0	2.1	0	0	0	4	0
brut (*Lejon*)	92	0	3.4	0	0	0	4	0
extra dry (*Jacques Bonet*)	97	0	3.4	0	0	0	4	0
extra dry (*Lejon*)	97	0	2.1	0	0	0	4	0
pink (*Jacques Bonet*)	98	0	3.7	0	0	0	4	0
pink (*Lejon*)	98	0	3.7	0	0	0	4	0
Chardonnay (*Gallo*)	88	0	n.a.	0	0	0	n.a.	0
chenin blanc (*Colony*)	86	0	2.4	0	0	0	4	0
chenin blanc (*Gallo*)	88	0	1.6	0	0	0	n.a.	0
Chianti (*Carlo Rossi* Light)	92	0	2.4	0	0	0	n.a.	0
Chianti (*Petri*)	91	0	1.7	0	0	0	4	0
cold duck (*Jacques Bonet*)	108	0	5.9	0	0	0	4	0
cold duck (*Lejon*)	108	0	5.9	0	0	0	4	0
French colombard (*Colony*)	84	0	1.8	0	0	0	4	0
French colombard (*Gallo*)	88	0	2.0	0	0	0	n.a.	0
Gewurztraminer (*Gallo*)	88	0	1.6	0	0	0	n.a.	0
Marsala (*Gambarelli & Davitto*)	77	0	4.0	0	0	0	4	0
(*Mission Bell* Arriba), 2 fl. oz.	95	0	6.8	0	0	0	4	0
(*Mission Bell* Diamond Red),								
2 fl. oz.	95	0	6.8	0	0	0	4	0
(*Mission Bell* Silver Satin), 2 fl. oz.	83	0	5.4	0	0	0	4	0
(*Mission Bell* Silver Satin Bitter								
Lemon), 2 fl. oz.	83	0	5.5	0	0	0	4	0
(*Mission Bell* Swiss Up), 2 fl. oz. ...	84	0	5.6	0	0	0	4	0
Moselle (*Colony* Rhineskeller)	97	0	4.3	0	0	0	4	0
muscatel (*Italian Swiss Colony*),								
2 fl. oz.	122	0	5.9	0	0	0	4	0
pastoso (*Petri*)	92	0	1.8	0	0	0	4	0
port, 2 fl. oz.:								
(*Gallo*)	64	0	2.0	0	0	0	n.a.	0
(*Italian Swiss Colony*)	85	0	5.7	0	0	0	4	0
tawny (*Livingston Cellars*)	86	0	6.4	0	0	0	n.a.	0
white (*Gallo*)	86	0	5.6	0	0	0	n.a.	0
white (*Italian Swiss Colony*)	86	0	6.3	0	0	0	4	0
Rhine:								
(*Bravo*)	97	0	4.3	0	0	0	4	0
(*Carlo Rossi*)	84	0	4.4	0	0	0	n.a.	0
(*Colony* Classic)	89	0	3.8	0	0	0	4	0
(*Gallo*)	80	0	4.0	0	0	0	n.a.	0
(*Gambarelli & Davitto* Parma) ...	92	0	1.2	0	0	0	4	0
(*Petri*)	97	0	4.3	0	0	0	4	0
Riesling (*Gallo* Johannisberg)	84	0	1.6	0	0	0	n.a.	0
rosé:								
(*Bravo*)	92	0	3.1	0	0	0	4	0
(*Carlo Rossi* Vin Rose)	88	0	2.8	0	0	0	n.a.	0

Food and Measure	cal.	prot. (gms)	carbo. (gms)	tot. fat (gms)	sat. fat (gms)	chol. (mgs)	sod. (mgs)	fiber (gms)
WINE, ROSÉ *(cont.)*								
(*Colony* Classic)	89	0	3.0	0	0	0	4	0
(*Gallo* Grenache)	88	0	2.4	0	0	0	n.a.	0
(*Gallo* Red Rose)	112	0	6.4	0	0	0	n.a.	0
(*Gallo* Vin Rose)	88	0	2.8	0	0	0	n.a.	0
(*Gambarelli & Davitto Parma*) ...	92	0	3.1	0	0	0	4	0
(*Petri*)	92	0	3.1	0	0	0	4	0
sauvignon blanc (*Gallo*)	80	0	.8	0	0	0	n.a.	0
sherry, 2 fl. oz.:								
(*Gallo*)	64	0	2.0	0	0	0	n.a.	0
cream (*Italian Swiss Colony*)	85	0	6.8	0	0	0	4	0
cream (*Livingston Cellars*)	78	0	5.6	0	0	0	n.a.	0
dry (*Italian Swiss Colony*)	63	0	1.2	0	0	0	4	0
dry (*Livingston Cellars* Very Dry)	60	0	1.0	0	0	0	n.a.	0
straight (*Italian Swiss Colony*) ...	67	0	2.1	0	0	0	4	0
Tokay (*Italian Swiss Colony*),								
2 fl. oz.	82	0	5.1	0	0	0	4	0
vermouth, 2 fl. oz.:								
dry:								
(*Gallo*)	56	0	.8	0	0	0	n.a.	0
(*Gambarelli & Davitto*)	64	0	1.5	0	0	0	4	0
(*Lejon*)	64	0	1.5	0	0	0	4	0
sweet:								
(*Gallo*)	90	0	9.4	0	0	0	n.a.	0
(*Gambarelli & Davitto*)	77	0	8.4	0	0	0	4	0
(*Lejon*)	77	0	8.4	0	0	0	4	0
Zinfandel:								
(*Colony*)	91	0	.7	0	0	0	4	0
(*Gallo*)	92	0	0	0	0	0	n.a.	0
white (*Colony*)	82	0	2.7	0	0	0	4	0
WINE, COOKING:								
burgundy (*Regina*), ¼ cup	2	<1.0	<1.0	<1.0	(0)	0	365	0
marsala (*Holland House*), 1 fl. oz. ..	9	0	2.3	0	0	0	186	0
red (*Holland House*), 1 fl. oz.	6	0	1.5	0	0	0	186	0
sauterne (*Regina*), ¼ cup	2	<1.0	<1.0	<1.0	(0)	0	365	0
sherry (*Holland House*), 1 fl. oz. ...	5	0	1.2	0	0	0	186	0
sherry (*Regina*), ¼ cup	20	<1.0	5.0	<1.0	(0)	0	70	0
vermouth or white (*Holland House*),								
1 fl. oz.	2	0	<1.0	0	0	0	186	0
WINE VINEGAR, see "Vinegar"								
WINGED BEAN:								
raw:								
untrimmed, 1 lb.	218	30.9	19.2	3.9	1.1	0	17	11.4 c
trimmed, 1 oz.	14	2.0	1.2	.2	.1	0	1	.7 c
1 pod, .6 oz.	8	1.1	.7	.1	<.1	0	1	.4 c
sliced, ½ cup	11	1.5	1.0	.2	.1	0	1	.6 c
boiled, drained, 4 oz.	43	6.0	3.6	.7	.2	0	5	1.6 c
boiled, drained, ½ cup	12	1.6	1.0	.2	.1	0	1	.4 c

Food and Measure	cal.	prot. (gms)	carbo. (gms)	tot. fat (gms)	sat. fat (gms)	chol. (mgs)	sod. (mgs)	fiber (gms)
WINGED BEAN, DRIED:								
raw, 1 oz.	116	8.4	11.8	4.6	.7	0	11	4.4 d
raw, ½ cup	372	27.0	38.0	14.9	2.1	0	35	14.1 d
boiled, 4 oz.	167	12.0	16.9	6.6	.9	0	15	2.8 c
boiled, ½ cup	126	9.1	12.8	5.0	.7	0	11	2.1 c
WINGED BEAN LEAVES, trimmed:								
1 lb.	336	26.5	64.0	5.0	1.2	0	n.a.	11.3 c
1 oz.	21	1.7	4.0	.3	.1	0	n.a.	.7 c
WINGED BEAN TUBER, trimmed:								
1 lb.	268	52.6	127.5	4.1	1.0	0	n.a.	33.6 c
1 oz.	45	3.3	8.0	.3	.1	0	n.a.	2.1 c
WINTER RADISH, see "Radish, black"								
WINTER SQUASH, see "Squash, winter" and specific listings								
WOLF FISH, Atlantic, meat only, raw:								
1 lb.	437	79.4	0	10.8	1.7	209	386	0
1 oz.	27	5.0	0	.7	.1	13	24	0
½ fillet, approx. 5.4 oz., yield from 5-lb. whole fish	147	26.8	0	3.7	.6	70	130	0
WONTON SKIN:								
(*Nasoya*), 1 piece	23	1.0	4.5	0	0	0	19	m.q.
WORCESTERSHIRE SAUCE:								
(*Lea & Perrins*), 1 tsp.	5	<1.0	1.0	<1.0	n.a.	0	55	(0)
(*Life* All Natural), ¼ fl. oz. or ½ tbsp.	5	<1.0	1.0	<1.0	n.a.	0	2	(0)
regular or smoky (*French's*), 1 tbsp.	10	0	2.0	0	0	0	160	(0)
white wine (*Lea & Perrins*), 1 tsp. ...	3	<1.0	1.0	<1.0	n.a.	0	42	(0)

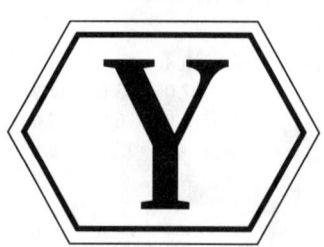

Food and Measure	cal.	prot. (gms)	carbo. (gms)	tot. fat (gms)	sat. fat (gms)	chol. (mgs)	sod. (mgs)	fiber (gms)
YAKIDOFU, see "Tofu, grilled"								
YAM:								
raw:								
untrimmed, 1 lb.	460	6.0	108.8	.7	.1	0	37	m.q.
trimmed, 1 oz.	33	.4	7.9	<.1	<.1	0	3	m.q.
cubed, ½ cup	89	1.1	20.9	.1	<.1	0	7	m.q.
baked or boiled, drained, 4 oz.	132	1.7	31.2	.2	<.1	0	9	m.q.
baked or boiled, drained, ½ cup	79	1.0	18.8	.1	<.1	0	6	m.q.
YAM, CANNED OR FROZEN, see "Sweet potato"								
YAM, MOUNTAIN, Hawaiian:								
raw:								
untrimmed, 1 lb.	253	5.0	61.4	.4	.1	0	49	1.7 c
trimmed, 1 oz.	19	.4	4.6	<.1	0	tr.	4	.1 c
1 medium, 8¼″ × 2½″ diam.,								
approx. 1.1 lb.	282	5.6	68.5	.4	.1	0	55	1.9 c
cubed, ½ cup	46	.9	11.1	.1	<.1	0	9	.3 c
steamed, 4 oz.	93	2.0	22.7	.1	<.1	0	14	.6 c
steamed, cubed, ½ cup	59	1.2	14.4	.1	<.1	0	9	.4 c
YAM BEAN TUBER:								
raw:								
untrimmed, 1 lb.	170	5.8	36.5	.3	n.a.	0	26	2.9 c
trimmed:								
1 oz.	12	.4	2.5	.1	(0)	0	2	.2 c
sliced, ½ cup	25	.8	5.3	.1	(0)	0	4	.4 c
1 slice, ⅛″ thick, 4⅞″ diam.	2	.1	.5	<.1	(0)	0	tr.	<.1 c
(*Frieda* of California), 1 lb.	204	5.4	48.1	.5	n.a.	0	m.q.	m.q.
(*Frieda* of California), 1 oz.	13	.3	3.0	<.1	(0)	0	n.a.	m.q.
boiled, drained, 4 oz.	52	1.3	11.8	.1	(0)	0	7	1.3 c

Food and Measure	cal.	prot. (gms)	carbo. (gms)	tot. fat (gms)	sat. fat (gms)	chol. (mgs)	sod. (mgs)	fiber (gms)
YARDLONG BEAN, fresh:								
raw:								
untrimmed, 1 lb.	203	12.1	36.0	1.7	.5	0	17	m.q.
trimmed, 1 oz.	13	.8	2.4	.1	<.1	0	1	m.q.
1 pod, 13¼″ × ¼″ diam., .5 oz.	6	.3	1.0	.1	<.1	0	tr.	m.q.
sliced, ½ cup	22	1.3	3.8	.2	<.1	0	2	m.q.
boiled, drained:								
4 oz.	53	2.9	10.4	.1	<.1	0	5	1.7 c
1 pod, 13¼″ × ¼″ diam., approx.								
.5 oz.	7	.4	1.3	<.1	tr.	0	1	.2 c
sliced, ½ cup	25	1.3	4.8	.1	<.1	0	2	.8 c
YARDLONG BEAN, dried:								
raw, 1 oz.	98	6.9	17.6	.4	.1	0	5	1.4 c
raw, ½ cup	292	20.4	52.0	1.1	.3	0	14	4.0 c
boiled, 4 oz.	134	9.4	23.9	.5	.1	0	6	1.8 c
boiled, ½ cup	102	7.1	18.1	.4	.1	0	4	1.4 c
YEAST:								
(*Fleischmann's* Active Dry/								
RapidRise), ¼ oz.	20	3.0	3.0	0	0	0	10	m.q.
(*Red Star* Active Dry), ¼ oz.	20	3.0	2.7	.3	(0)	0	4	1.2 c
fresh or household (*Fleischmann's*),								
.6 oz.	15	2.0	2.0	0	0	0	5	m.q.
YELLOW BEAN, dried:								
raw, 1 oz.	98	6.2	17.2	.7	.2	0	3	.8 c
raw, ½ cup	338	21.6	59.5	2.6	.7	0	12	2.7 c
boiled, 4 oz.	163	10.4	28.7	1.2	.3	0	6	1.3 c
boiled, ½ cup	126	8.1	22.2	1.0	.2	0	4	1.0 c
YELLOW EYE BEAN, canned:								
baked style (*B&M*), 8 oz.	326	15.0	50.0	7.0	m.q.	4	770	15.0 d
YELLOW SQUASH, see								
"Crookneck or straightneck								
squash"								
YELLOW OR WAX BEAN, see								
"Green bean"								
YELLOWTAIL, mixed species,								
meat only, raw:								
1 lb.	662	105.0	0	23.8	m.q.	m.q.	177	0
1 oz.	41	6.6	0	1.5	m.q.	m.q.	11	0
½ fillet, approx. 6.6 oz., yield from								
5-lb. whole fish	273	43.3	0	9.8	m.q.	m.q.	73	0
YOGURT (see also "Yogurt,								
frozen"):								
plain:								
whole milk, 8 oz.	139	7.9	10.6	7.4	4.8	29	105	0
lowfat, 8 oz.	144	11.9	16.0	3.5	2.3	14	159	0
skim milk, 8 oz.	127	13.0	17.4	.4	.3	4	174	0
(*Bison* Lowfat), 1 cup	150	12.0	17.0	4.0	m.q.	10	180	0
(*Bison* Nonfat), 1 cup	120	12.0	16.0	0	0	0	170	0
(*Breyers* Lowfat), 8 oz.	140	12.0	16.0	3.0	2.0	20	170	0

Food and Measure	cal.	prot. (gms)	carbo. (gms)	tot. fat (gms)	sat. fat (gms)	chol. (mgs)	sod. (mgs)	fiber (gms)
YOGURT, PLAIN *(cont.)*								
(Colombo), 8 oz.	160	9.0	13.0	8.0	m.q.	m.q.	160	0
(Colombo Nonfat Lite), 8 oz.	110	11.0	17.0	<1.0	n.a.	5	160	0
(Crowley), 1 cup	160	10.0	14.0	8.0	m.q.	30	150	0
(Crowley Lowfat), 1 cup	140	12.0	17.0	2.0	m.q.	10	180	0
(Crowley Nonfat), 1 cup	120	13.0	17.0	<1.0	0	<1	180	0
(Dannon Lowfat), 8 oz.	140	10.0	16.0	4.0	m.q.	15	160	0
(Dannon Nonfat), 8 oz.	110	11.0	16.0	0	0	5	160	0
(Friendship Lowfat 1.5%), 1 cup	150	12.0	17.0	3.0	m.q.	14	190	0
(Knudsen), 8 oz.	200	12.0	16.0	9.0	5.0	35	170	0
(Knudsen Lowfat), 8 oz.	160	12.0	17.0	5.0	1.0	25	180	0
(Lite-Line Swiss Style 1.5%), 1 cup	140	12.0	18.0	2.0	m.q.	m.q.	150	0
(Meadow Gold Lowfat 2%), 1 cup	160	12.0	16.0	5.0	m.q.	m.q.	160	0
(Mountain High), 1 cup	200	12.0	16.0	9.0	m.q.	m.q.	140	0
(Weight Watchers Nonfat), 1 cup ..	90	10.0	13.0	<1.0	0	5	135	0
(Yoplait), 6 oz.	130	10.0	15.0	3.0	m.q.	15	140	0
(Yoplait Nonfat), 8 oz.	120	13.0	18.0	0	0	5	160	0
all flavors *(Weight Watchers Ultimate 90)*, 1 cup	90	10.0	13.0	0	0	5	120	n.a.
all flavors, except strawberry fruit cup *(Light n' Lively Free)*, 4.4 oz.	50	4.0	8.0	0	0	0	60	m.q.
all fruit flavors:								
(Colombo Fruit on the Bottom), 8 oz.	230	7.0	36.0	6.0	m.q.	m.q.	140	m.q.
(Colombo Nonfat Fruit on the Bottom), 8 oz.	190	8.0	38.0	<1.0	n.a.	5	140	m.q.
(Colombo Nonfat Lite Minipack), 4.4 oz.	100	5.0	20.0	0	0	m.q.	70	m.q.
(Crowley Nonfat), 1 cup[1]	100	8.0	17.0	<1.0	n.a.	<1	135	m.q.
(Crowley Swiss Style), 1 cup	240	8.0	48.0	2.0	m.q.	10	150	m.q.
(Crowley Sundae Style), 1 cup ...	250	9.0	47.0	2.0	m.q.	10	170	m.q.
(Dannon Extra Smooth), 4.4 oz.	130	5.0	24.0	2.0	m.q.	10	80	m.q.
(Dannon Fruit-on-the-Bottom), 8 oz.	240	9.0	43.0	3.0	m.q.	10	120	m.q.
(Dannon Fruit-on-the-Bottom), 4.4 oz.	130	5.0	23.0	2.0	m.q.	5	65	m.q.
(Dannon Hearty Nuts & Raisins), 8 oz.	260	11.0	48.0	3.0	m.q.	10	120	m.q.
(Ripple 70), 6 oz.	70	5.0	13.0	0	0	5	85	m.q.
(Yoplait), 6 oz.	190	8.0	32.0	3.0	m.q.	10	110	m.q.
(Yoplait), 4 oz.	120	5.0	21.0	2.0	m.q.	10	75	m.q.
(Yoplait Fat Free), 6 oz.	150	7.0	31.0	0	0	5	95	m.q.
(Yoplait Light), 6 oz.	90	7.0	14.0	0	0	<5	100	m.q.
(Yoplait Light), 4 oz.	60	5.0	9.0	0	0	<5	65	m.q.
(Yoplait Custard Style), 4 oz.	130	5.0	21.0	3.0	m.q.	15	60	m.q.

1. *Aspartame sweetened.*

Food and Measure	cal.	prot. (gms)	carbo. (gms)	tot. fat (gms)	sat. fat (gms)	chol. (mgs)	sod. (mgs)	fiber (gms)
except lemon (*Dannon* Fresh Flavors), 8 oz.	200	10.0	34.0	4.0	m.q.	10	160	m.q.
except strawberry (*Knudsen* Lowfat), 8 oz.	240	11.0	43.0	4.0	2.0	15	135	m.q.
except cherry and mixed berries (*Yoplait Custard Style*), 6 oz. . .	190	7.0	32.0	4.0	m.q.	20	95	m.q.
apple crisp (*New Country* Lowfat), 6 oz.	150	5.0	30.0	2.0	m.q.	m.q.	85	m.q.
berries, mixed:								
(*Breyers* Lowfat), 8 oz.	250	9.0	48.0	2.0	1.0	10	120	m.q.
(*New Country* Lowfat), 6 oz.	150	5.0	31.0	2.0	m.q.	m.q.	85	m.q.
(*Yoplait Breakfast Yogurt*), 6 oz. . .	210	8.0	40.0	3.0	1.0	10	95	2.0 d
(*Yoplait Custard Style*), 6 oz.	180	7.0	30.0	4.0	m.q.	20	95	m.q.
blueberry:								
(*Breyers* Lowfat), 8 oz.	250	9.0	48.0	2.0	1.0	10	120	m.q.
(*Knudsen Cal 70*), 6 oz.	70	6.0	11.0	0	0	5	80	m.q.
(*Light n' Lively*), 8 oz.	240	8.0	46.0	2.0	1.0	10	130	m.q.
(*Light n' Lively*), 4.4 oz.	130	5.0	26.0	1.0	1.0	5	70	m.q.
(*Light n' Lively 100*), 8 oz.	90	8.0	15.0	0	0	0	110	m.q.
(*New Country* Supreme), 6 oz. . . .	150	5.0	31.0	2.0	m.q.	m.q.	90	m.q.
w/other natural flavors (*Mountain High*), 1 cup	220	10.0	31.0	6.0	m.q.	m.q.	140	m.q.
cherry:								
(*New Country* Supreme), 6 oz. . . .	150	5.0	32.0	2.0	m.q.	m.q.	90	m.q.
(*Light n' Lively*), 4.4 oz.	140	5.0	27.0	.1.0	1.0	5	70	m.q.
(*Yoplait Custard Style*), 6 oz.	180	7.0	30.0	4.0	m.q.	20	95	m.q.
black:								
(*Breyers* Lowfat), 8 oz.	260	9.0	49.0	3.0	1.0	10	120	m.q.
(*Knudsen Cal 70*), 6 oz.	70	5.0	12.0	0	0	5	75	m.q.
(*Light n' Lively*), 8 oz.	230	9.0	44.0	2.0	1.0	15	125	m.q.
(*Light n' Lively 100*), 8 oz.	100	8.0	17.0	0	0	0	100	m.q.
cherry, w/almonds (*Yoplait Breakfast Yogurt*), 6 oz.	200'	8.0	38.0	3.0	2.0	10	90	2.0 d
cherry-vanilla (*Lite-Line* Swiss Style 1%), 1 cup	240	10.0	45.0	2.0	m.q.	m.q.	150	m.q.
coffee:								
lowfat, 8 oz.	194	11.2	31.3	2.8	1.8	11	149	0
(*Bison* Lowfat), 1 cup	210	11.0	33.0	4.0	m.q.	10	160	0
(*Dannon* Fresh Flavors), 8 oz. . . .	200	10.0	34.0	3.0	m.q.	10	140	0
(*Friendship* Lowfat), 1 cup	210	11.0	35.0	3.0	m.q.	14	170	0
fruit:								
crunch (*New Country* Lowfat), 6 oz.	150	5.0	30.0	2.0	m.q.	m.q.	90	m.q.
tropical (*Ripple 70*), 6 oz.	70	5.0	13.0	0	0	5	85	m.q.
tropical (*Yoplait Breakfast Yogurt*), 6 oz.	210	7.0	39.0	4.0	2.0	10	90	2.0 d
grape (*Light n' Lively*), 4.4 oz.	130	6.0	24.0	1.0	1.0	10	70	m.q.
Hawaiian salad (*New Country* Lowfat), 6 oz.	150	5.0	31.0	2.0	m.q.	m.q.	90	m.q.

Food and Measure	cal.	prot. (gms)	carbo. (gms)	tot. fat (gms)	sat. fat (gms)	chol. (mgs)	sod. (mgs)	fiber (gms)
YOGURT *(cont.)*								
lemon:								
(*Bison* Lowfat), 1 cup	210	11.0	33.0	4.0	m.q.	10	160	n.a.
(*Dannon* Fresh Flavors), 8 oz.	200	10.0	34.0	3.0	m.q.	10	140	n.a.
(*Knudsen Cal 70*), 6 oz.	70	6.0	12.0	0	0	0	125	n.a.
(*Light n' Lively 100*), 8 oz.	100	9.0	16.0	0	0	5	150	n.a.
(*New Country* Supreme), 6 oz.	150	5.0	31.0	2.0	m.q.	m.q.	90	n.a.
orange (*New Country* Supreme),								
6 oz.	150	5.0	31.0	2.0	m.q.	m.q.	90	n.a.
peach:								
(*Breyers* Lowfat), 8 oz.	250	9.0	48.0	2.0	1.0	10	120	m.q.
(*Knudsen Cal 70*), 6 oz.	70	6.0	11.0	0	0	0	95	m.q.
(*Light n' Lively*), 8 oz.	240	9.0	46.0	2.0	1.0	15	120	m.q.
(*Light n' Lively*), 4.4 oz.	130	5.0	26.0	1.0	1.0	10	65	m.q.
(*Light n' Lively 100*), 8 oz.	100	9.0	16.0	0	0	5	115	m.q.
(*Lite-Line* Swiss Style 1%), 1 cup	230	10.0	42.0	2.0	m.q.	m.q.	150	m.q.
peaches 'n cream (*New Country*								
Lowfat), 6 oz.	150	5.0	31.0	2.0	m.q.	m.q.	90	m.q.
piña colada or pineapple (*Yoplait*),								
6 oz.	190	8.0	32.0	3.0	m.q.	10	110	m.q.
pineapple:								
(*Breyers* Lowfat), 8 oz.	250	9.0	50.0	2.0	1.0	10	120	m.q.
(*Knudsen Cal 70*), 6 oz.	70	6.0	12.0	0	0	0	125	m.q.
(*Light n' Lively*), 8 oz.	230	9.0	47.0	2.0	1.0	10	120	m.q.
(*Light n' Lively*), 4.4 oz.	130	5.0	26.0	1.0	1.0	5	65	m.q.
raspberry, red:								
(*Breyers* Lowfat), 8 oz.	250	9.0	48.0	2.0	1.0	10	120	m.q.
(*Knudsen Cal 70*), 6 oz.	70	6.0	11.0	0	0	5	80	m.q.
(*Light n' Lively*), 8 oz.	230	9.0	43.0	2.0	1.0	10	130	m.q.
(*Light n' Lively*), 4.4 oz.	130	5.0	24.0	1.0	1.0	5	70	m.q.
(*Light n' Lively Free*), 4.4 oz.	50	4.0	8.0	0	0	0	60	m.q.
(*Light n' Lively 100*), 8 oz.	90	8.0	15.0	0	0	0	105	m.q.
(*Meadow Gold* Lowfat 1.5%),								
1 cup	250	10.0	42.0	4.0	m.q.	m.q.	160	m.q.
(*New Country* Supreme), 6 oz.	150	5.0	31.0	2.0	m.q.	m.q.	90	m.q.
strawberry:								
(*Breyers* Lowfat), 8 oz.	250	9.0	48.0	2.0	1.0	10	120	m.q.
(*Colombo*), 8 oz.	210	8.0	29.0	7.0	m.q.	m.q.	140	m.q.
(*Crowley* Nonfat), 1 cup	190	12.0	35.0	<1.0	n.a.	<1	190	m.q.
(*Knudsen* Lowfat), 8 oz.	250	10.0	45.0	4.0	2.0	15	135	m.q.
(*Knudsen Cal 70*), 6 oz.	70	6.0	11.0	0	0	0	85	m.q.
(*Light n' Lively*), 8 oz.	240	9.0	45.0	2.0	2.0	15	130	m.q.
(*Light n' Lively*), 4.4 oz.	130	5.0	25.0	1.0	1.0	10	70	m.q.
(*Light n' Lively Free*), 4.4 oz.	50	4.0	8.0	0	0	0	60	m.q.
(*Light n' Lively 100*), 8 oz.	90	8.0	15.0	0	0	5	105	m.q.
(*Lite-Line* Lowfat 1%), 1 cup	240	10.0	46.0	2.0	m.q.	m.q.	150	m.q.
(*New Country* Supreme), 6 oz.	150	5.0	30.0	2.0	m.q.	m.q.	90	m.q.
fruit basket (*Knudsen Cal 70*),								
6 oz.	70	6.0	11.0	0	0	5	75	m.q.

Food and Measure	cal.	prot. (gms)	carbo. (gms)	tot. fat (gms)	sat. fat (gms)	chol. (mgs)	sod. (mgs)	fiber (gms)
fruit cup:								
(*Light n' Lively*), 8 oz.	240	9.0	47.0	2.0	1.0	15	120	m.q.
(*Light n' Lively*), 4.4 oz.	130	5.0	26.0	1.0	1.0	10	65	m.q.
(*Light n' Lively Free*), 4.4 oz. ..	50	4.0	8.0	0	0	0	55	m.q.
(*Light n' Lively 100*), 8 oz. ..	90	8.0	15.0	0	0	0	100	m.q.
(*New Country* Lowfat), 6 oz. ..	150	5.0	30.0	2.0	m.q.	m.q.	85	m.q.
strawberry-almond (*Yoplait Breakfast*								
Yogurt), 6 oz.	200	8.0	38.0	3.0	2.0	10	90	2.0 d
strawberry-banana:								
(*Breyers* Lowfat), 8 oz.	250	9.0	50.0	2.0	1.0	10	120	m.q.
(*Knudsen Cal 70*), 6 oz.	70	6.0	12.0	0	0	0	80	m.q.
(*Light n' Lively*), 8 oz.	260	9.0	52.0	2.0	1.0	10	120	m.q.
(*Light n' Lively*), 4.4 oz.	140	5.0	29.0	1.0	1.0	5	65	m.q.
(*New Country*), 6 oz.	150	5.0	31.0	2.0	m.q.	m.q.	85	m.q.
(*Yoplait Breakfast Yogurt*), 6 oz. ..	220	8.0	42.0	3.0	1.0	10	90	2.0 d
strawberry-rhubarb (*Yoplait*), 6 oz.	190	8.0	32.0	3.0	m.q.	10	110	m.q.
vanilla:								
lowfat, 8 oz.	194	11.2	31.3	2.8	1.8	11	149	0
(*Bison* Lowfat), 1 cup	210	11.0	33.0	4.0	m.q.	10	160	0
(*Colombo* Nonfat Lite), 8 oz.	160	10.0	30.0	<1.0	n.a.	5	140	0
(*Crowley* Lowfat), 1 cup	200	12.0	33.0	2.0	m.q.	10	170	0
(*Dannon* Fresh Flavors), 8 oz. ...	200	10.0	34.0	3.0	m.q.	10	140	0
(*Dannon* Fresh Flavors), 4.4 oz.	110	5.0	20.0	2.0	m.q.	5	90	0
(*Friendship* Lowfat), 1 cup	210	11.0	35.0	3.0	m.q.	14	170	0
(*Knudsen* Lowfat), 8 oz.	240	11.0	43.0	4.0	2.0	15	135	0
(*Knudsen Cal 70*), 6 oz.	70	6.0	11.0	0	0	0	90	0
(*Yoplait*), 6 oz.	180	9.0	29.0	3.0	m.q.	15	120	0
(*Yoplait* Fat Free), 6 oz.	150	8.0	28.0	0	0	<5	110	0
(*Yoplait* Nonfat), 8 oz.	180	11.0	35.0	0	0	5	140	0
(*Yoplait Custard Style*), 6 oz.	180	7.0	30.0	4.0	m.q.	20	110	0
(*Yoplait Custard Style*), 4 oz.	130	5.0	20.0	3.0	m.q.	15	70	0
bean (*Breyers* Lowfat), 8 oz.	230	11.0	41.0	3.0	2.0	20	150	0
French (*Colombo*), 8 oz.	215	8.0	30.0	7.0	m.q.	m.q.	140	0
French (*New Country* Lowfat),								
6 oz.	150	5.0	31.0	2.0	m.q.	m.q.	90	0
w/wheat, nuts and raisins (*Dannon*								
Hearty Nuts & Raisins), 8 oz.	270	9.0	48.0	5.0	m.q.	10	120	m.q.
YOGURT, FROZEN (see also								
"Yogurt, frozen, soft-serve"):								
all flavors, except raspberry (*Dannon*								
Nonfat), 4 fl. oz.	90	3.0	22.0	0	0	0	65	(0)
blueberry (*Dreyer's Inspirations*),								
3 oz.	80	2.0	15.0	1.0	m.q.	5	40	(0)
caramel-pecan chunk (*Colombo*								
Gourmet), 3 fl. oz.	120	4.0	19.0	3.0	m.q.	10	150	(0)
cheesecake, wild raspberry								
(*Colombo* Gourmet), 3 fl. oz. ..	100	2.0	18.0	2.0	m.q.	5	40	(0)
cherry:								
(*Crowley*), 3 fl. oz.	80	2.0	16.0	1.0	m.q.	5	40	(0)

Food and Measure	cal.	prot. (gms)	carbo. (gms)	tot. fat (gms)	sat. fat (gms)	chol. (mgs)	sod. (mgs)	fiber (gms)
YOGURT, FROZEN, CHERRY *(cont.)*								
(Dreyer's Inspirations), 3 oz.	80	2.0	15.0	1.0	m.q.	5	40	(0)
black *(Breyers)*, ½ cup	120	3.0	24.0	1.0	m.q.	10	50	(0)
black, nonfat *(Sealtest Free)*,								
½ cup	110	2.0	24.0	0	0	0	50	(0)
chocolate:								
(Bison), 3½ fl. oz.	94	3.0	18.0	2.0	m.q.	5	50	(0)
(Breyers), ½ cup	120	3.0	24.0	1.0	m.q.	10	65	(0)
(Crowley), 3 fl. oz.	80	2.0	15.0	2.0	m.q.	10	40	(0)
(Dreyer's Inspirations), 3 oz.	80	2.0	15.0	1.0	m.q.	5	40	(0)
(Häagen-Dazs), 3 fl. oz.	130	6.0	21.0	3.0	2.0	25	40	(0)
chunk, Bavarian *(Colombo*								
Gourmet)*, 3 fl. oz.	120	3.0	18.0	4.0	m.q.	10	40	(0)
nonfat *(Sealtest Free)*, ½ cup	110	3.0	24.0	0	0	0	55	(0)
chocolate almond *(Elan)*, ½ cup ...	160	5.0	23.0	7.0	m.q.	m.q.	65	(0)
Heath bar crunch *(Colombo*								
Gourmet)*, 3 fl. oz.	130	3.0	19.0	5.0	m.q.	15	75	(0)
mocha Swiss almond *(Colombo*								
Gourmet)*, 3 fl. oz.	120	3.0	17.0	5.0	m.q.	10	45	(0)
peach:								
(Breyers), ½ cup	110	3.0	22.0	1.0	m.q.	10	50	(0)
(Crowley), 3 fl. oz.	80	2.0	16.0	1.0	m.q.	5	40	(0)
(Dreyer's Inspirations Perfectly								
Peach)*, 3 oz.	80	2.0	15.0	1.0	m.q.	5	40	(0)
(Häagen-Dazs), 3 fl. oz.	120	4.0	20.0	3.0	1.5	31	30	(0)
nonfat *(Sealtest Free)*, ½ cup	100	2.0	23.0	0	0	0	35	(0)
peanut butter cup *(Colombo*								
Gourmet)*, 3 fl. oz.	140	4.0	16.0	7.0	m.q.	5	90	(0)
raspberry:								
(Crowley), 3 fl. oz.	80	2.0	16.0	1.0	m.q.	5	40	(0)
(Dreyer's Inspirations), 3 oz.	80	2.0	15.0	1.0	m.q.	5	40	(0)
red *(Breyers)*, ½ cup	120	3.0	23.0	1.0	m.q.	10	50	(0)
red *(Dannon* Nonfat), 4 fl. oz. ...	90	3.0	21.0	0	0	0	65	(0)
red, nonfat *(Sealtest Free)*, ½ cup	100	2.0	23.0	0	0	0	40	(0)
strawberry:								
(Breyers), ½ cup	110	3.0	22.0	1.0	m.q.	10	45	(0)
(Crowley), 3 fl. oz.	80	2.0	16.0	1.0	m.q.	5	40	(0)
(Dreyer's Inspirations), 3 oz.	80	2.0	15.0	1.0	m.q.	5	40	(0)
(Häagen-Dazs), 3 fl. oz.	120	4.0	21.0	3.0	1.6	29	30	(0)
nonfat *(Sealtest Free)*, ½ cup	100	2.0	22.0	0	0	0	35	(0)
passion *(Colombo* Gourmet),								
3 fl. oz.	100	1.0	18.0	2.0	m.q.	5	40	(0)
strawberry-banana *(Breyers)*, ½ cup	110	3.0	22.0	1.0	m.q.	10	45	(0)
strawberry-banana *(Dreyer's*								
Inspirations)*, 3 oz.	80	2.0	15.0	1.0	m.q.	5	40	(0)
vanilla:								
(Breyers), ½ cup	120	3.0	23.0	1.0	m.q.	15	55	0
(Crowley), 3 fl. oz.	80	2.0	15.0	2.0	m.q.	10	40	0

Food and Measure	cal.	prot. (gms)	carbo. (gms)	tot. fat (gms)	sat. fat (gms)	chol. (mgs)	sod. (mgs)	fiber (gms)
(*Dreyer's Inspirations*), 3 oz.	80	2.0	15.0	1.0	m.q.	5	50	0
(*Häagen-Dazs*), 3 fl. oz.	130	5.0	20.0	3.0	1.7	36	40	0
dream (*Colombo* Gourmet), 3 fl. oz.	90	3.0	16.0	2.0	m.q.	10	45	0
nonfat (*Sealtest Free*), ½ cup	100	2.0	23.0	0	0	0	45	0
vanilla almond crunch (*Häagen-Dazs*), 3 fl. oz.	150	5.0	22.0	5.0	1.5	33	65	(0)
vanilla-raspberry swirl (*Dreyer's Inspirations*), 3 oz.	80	2.0	15.0	1.0	m.q.	5	45	(0)
YOGURT, FROZEN, SOFT-SERVE, ½ cup, except as noted:								
plain (*Crowley* Peaks of Perfection), 3.5 fl. oz.	90	2.0	20.0	1.0	m.q.	5	40	0
all flavors (*Bresler's* Gourmet), 1 oz.	29	.9	5.5	.5	n.a.	2	15	(0)
all flavors (*Bresler's* Lite), 1 oz.	27	1.1	6.0	0	0	0	11	(0)
banana (*Crowley* Peaks of Perfection), 3.5 fl. oz.	100	3.0	19.0	2.0	m.q.	5	50	(0)
blueberry (*Dannon*)	100	3.0	18.0	2.0	m.q.	5	50	(0)
butter pecan (*Dannon*)	100	3.0	18.0	2.0	m.q.	5	55	(0)
cappuccino (*Dannon*)	100	3.0	18.0	2.0	m.q.	5	55	0
cheesecake (*Dannon*)	100	4.0	18.0	2.0	m.q.	5	55	0
chocolate (*Crowley* Peaks of Perfection), 3.5 fl. oz.	100	4.0	19.0	2.0	m.q.	5	60	(0)
chocolate (*Dannon*)	120	5.0	23.0	2.0	m.q.	5	65	(0)
lemon (*Crowley* Peaks of Perfection), 3.5 fl. oz.	100	3.0	19.0	2.0	m.q.	5	50	(0)
lemon meringue (*Dannon*)	100	4.0	18.0	2.0	m.q.	5	55	(0)
peach (*Dannon*)	100	4.0	18.0	2.0	m.q.	5	55	(0)
piña colada (*Dannon*)	100	4.0	18.0	2.0	m.q.	5	55	(0)
raspberry:								
(*Crowley* Peaks of Perfection), 3.5 fl. oz.	100	3.0	19.0	2.0	m.q.	5	50	(0)
(*Dannon*)	100	3.0	18.0	2.0	m.q.	5	50	(0)
red (*Dannon* Nonfat)	90	3.0	21.0	0	0	0	65	(0)
strawberry (*Crowley* Peaks of Perfection), 3.5 fl. oz.	100	3.0	19.0	2.0	m.q.	5	50	(0)
strawberry (*Dannon*)	100	3.0	18.0	2.0	m.q.	5	50	(0)
strawberry-banana (*Dannon*)	100	3.0	18.0	2.0	m.q.	5	50	(0)
vanilla (*Crowley* Peaks of Perfection), 3.5 fl. oz.	100	3.0	19.0	2.0	m.q.	5	50	0
YOGURT DESSERT:								
strawberry (*Sara Lee Free & Light*), ¹⁄₁₀ pkg.	120	2.0	26.0	1.0	n.a.	0	90	n.a.
YOGURT DRINK:								
all flavors (*Dan'up*), 8 oz.	190	6.0	32.0	4.0	m.q.	10	110	(0)

Food and Measure	cal.	prot. (gms)	carbo. (gms)	tot. fat (gms)	sat. fat (gms)	chol. (mgs)	sod. (mgs)	fiber (gms)
YOGURT AND FRUIT BAR, see "Fruit bar, frozen"								
YOKAN:								
1 oz.	74	.9	17.2	<.1	(0)	0	24	.4 c
1 slice, ¼″ thick, approx. .5 oz.	36	.5	8.5	<.1	(0)	0	12	.2 c

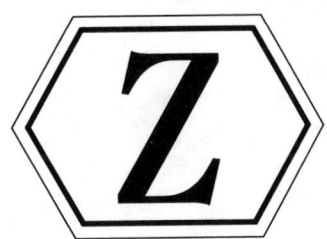

Food and Measure	cal.	prot. (gms)	carbo. (gms)	tot. fat (gms)	sat. fat (gms)	chol. (mgs)	sod. (mgs)	fiber (gms)
ZANTE CURRANT, see "Currant, Zante"								
ZINFANDEL, see "Wine"								
ZITI, see "Pasta"								
ZITI, FROZEN:								
in marinara sauce (*The Budget Gourmet* Side Dish), 6.25 oz. . .	220	9.0	25.0	9.0	m.q.	15	380	m.q.
ZUCCHINI:								
raw:								
w/ends, 1 lb.	62	5.0	12.5	.6	.1	0	11	2.2 d
trimmed, 1 oz.	4	.3	.8	<.1	tr.	0	1	.1 d
sliced, ½ cup	9	.8	1.9	.1	<.1	0	2	.3 d
boiled, drained:								
4 oz.	18	.7	4.5	.1	<.1	0	3	.6 c
sliced, ½ cup	14	.6	3.5	.1	tr.	0	2	.5 c
mashed, ½ cup	19	.8	4.7	.1	<.1	0	3	.6 c
ZUCCHINI, CANNED:								
Italian style (*Progresso*), ½ cup	50	1.0	8.0	2.0	<1.0	<1	540	2.0 d
in tomato juice, 4 oz. or ½ cup	33	1.2	7.8	.1	<.1	0	424	.6 c
in tomato sauce (*Del Monte*), ½ cup	30	1.0	8.0	0	0	0	485	m.q.
ZUCCHINI, FROZEN:								
10-oz. pkg.	48	3.3	10.2	.4	.1	0	7	2.6 d
boiled, drained, 4 oz. or ½ cup	19	1.3	4.0	.1	<.1	0	2	.6 c
(*Seabrook*), 3.3 oz.	16	1.0	3.0	0	0	0	2	1.0 c
(*Southern*), 3.5 oz.	18	1.2	3.6	.1	(0)	0	20	m.q.
breaded (*Stilwell Quickkrisp*), 3.3 oz.	200	4.0	24.0	10.0	m.q.	15	410	m.q.
ZUCCHINI COMBINATIONS, frozen:								
carrots, pearl onions and mushrooms (*Birds Eye* Farm Fresh), 4 oz. ..	30	1.0	7.0	0	0	0	15	1.0 d
ZUCCHINI LASAGNA, see "Lasagna entree, frozen"								

VITAMINS
AND MINERALS

Vitamins and Minerals

The more nutrition conscious we become, the more importance we must place on vitamins and minerals and their vital role in forming and maintaining our overall good health. Indeed, any discussion of nutrients and nutrition would be incomplete without including these life-sustaining substances . . . which is why I have added this section to my *Encyclopedia*.

I have divided this special section into two parts: *Vitamins* (starting on page 695) and *Minerals* (page 799). Within each part is a brief description of the major vitamins and minerals, their main functions and sources, recommended dosages and toxicity. Following this are listings that give the vitamin and mineral content for several hundred foods. The listings will be especially valuable if you, like me, prefer getting these dietary nutrients from natural sources.

Because of space limitations, I could not cover all the vitamins and minerals currently recognized. To determine which nutrients to omit, I used this criteria: when a substance, as in the case of pantothenic acid and Vitamin K, was plentiful and deficiencies extremely rare; when the natural sources of a substance, as with Vitamin D and iodine, were so limited that I was able to cover them within the descriptive text; and when I did not find the data plentiful enough or reliable enough to be of use to the reader. If a vitamin or a mineral is not included, this does not mean it is unimportant. *All* vitamins and minerals are *essential*, even those whose functions and requirements have not yet been well defined. They all are interrelated and work together to maintain good health—a deficiency in one substance can disrupt the body's entire balance.

My primary source of data for this section is the federal government; however, I have used data from individual food producers and distributors when government information was unavailable.

As with all nutrients, the values in this section can vary according to seasonal and regional differences. In the case of vitamins, values may vary greatly depending on when a food is harvested and how it is stored and shipped. Mineral values will vary according to the soil in which the food is grown (this affects animal feed and thereby includes foods of animal origin).

A word about recommended dosages: RDAs (Recommended Dietary Allowances) for several vitamins and minerals have been established by the National Research Council of the Food and Nutrition Board, National Academy of Sciences. Based on these standards, similar recommendations (called USRDAs) have been established by the Food and Drug Administration.

These RDAs are guidelines only, given to help define the safe and adequate intake of specific nutrients needed for optimal health in most individuals. While they are meant to offset nutritional deficiencies, RDAs are not meant as a cure or treatment for physical disorders. Bear in mind that individual requirements may differ and that RDAs do not cover special nutritional needs resulting from physical disorders or the use of specific medications.

For vitamins and minerals that have a designated RDA, I have given the latest information available; for those that do not have an "official" RDA at this time, I have given the dosage generally recommended by health professionals.

It's important to note that the RDAs are periodically revised. This is because scientific knowledge of our nutritional requirements is not yet complete and many questions related to our health remain to be solved. The world of nutrition is still being explored, and new essential nutrients may be found as research progresses. These facts emphasize the importance of a balanced and varied diet.

VITAMINS

Vitamins are organic substances found in all living things. With a few exceptions, our bodies cannot manufacture an adequate supply of vitamins, and we must obtain them from dietary sources—in the form either of food or dietary supplements. We need only minute quantities to sustain life, but a deficiency in even one vitamin can endanger the entire body.

At this time there are thirteen recognized vitamins, and they are generally distinguished as being *fat-soluble* or *water-soluble*.

Fat-soluble vitamins (which include vitamin A, D, E, and K) are absorbed into the body with the aid of fats in the diet or bile produced by the liver. These vitamins are stored in body fat, and if you are getting adequate amounts it's generally not necessary to consume them daily. On the other hand, because they are stored in the body, they can build up to toxic levels if too many are consumed.

Water-soluble vitamins (including the B-complex group and vitamin C) do not need fat or bile to be absorbed, and generally are not stored in the body. What the body does not use is excreted through urination and perspiration, so they should be replaced daily. These vitamins are fragile and can be destroyed during food processing, storage, or preparation.

The following is an overview of the major vitamins.

Vitamin A

Fat-soluble. Comes in two forms: *preformed vitamin A* or *retinol,* which is found only in foods of animal origin; and *provitamin A* or *carotene,* found in foods of both plant and animal origin. While retinol is absorbed almost instantly, the body must convert carotene into retinol-like vitamin A before it can be utilized. One well-known indicator of a deficiency of this vitamin is night blindness.

Main Functions: aids in the treatment of many eye disorders; promotes bone growth, healthy hair, skin, and teeth; helps protect mucous membranes and boosts resistance to respiratory and other infections; fights acne.

Best Natural Sources: retinol: liver and fish-liver oil; carotene: yellow and dark green fruits and vegetables (carrots, apricots, cantaloupe, sweet potatoes, spinach, kale, broccoli, mustard greens), cheese, butter, fortified margarine.

Recommended Daily Dosage: 4000 to 5000 International Units, for adults. These amounts increase during illness, trauma, pregnancy, and lactation. Requirements may be higher for people who smoke or who live in areas of high air pollution.

Toxicity: because the body stores vitamin A, daily dosages of over 50,000 International Units may be toxic if there is no deficiency. Symptoms of prolonged excessive intake include blurred vision, hair loss, nausea and vomiting, diarrhea and skin rash. Symptoms usually disappear in a short time if vitamin A intake is discontinued.

Thiamine (vitamin B_1)

Water-soluble; part of the B-complex group, which works together. Vulnerable to heat, air, and water in cooking. Thiamine is sometimes called the "nerve vitamin" or "morale vitamin" because of its beneficial effect on the nervous system and mental attitude.

Main Functions: maintains muscle tissue and a healthy nervous system and heart; promotes growth; aids in digestion, particularly of carbohydrates.

Best Natural Sources: pork, liver, brewer's yeast, bran, whole grains, enriched breads, cereals, and pasta.

Recommended Daily Dosage: 1 to 1.5 milligrams for adults. Need increases during illness, stress, pregnancy, and lactation.

Toxicity: nontoxic. However, very large doses may contribute to an imbalance of B complex. This group of vitamins is interrelated and an excess in one might result in a deficiency of other B vitamins.

Riboflavin (Vitamin B_2)

Water-soluble; part of the B-complex group. Easily absorbed and not vulnerable to heat or air, but can be destroyed by exposure to sunlight.

Main Functions: acts with other substances to utilize carbohydrates, fats, and proteins; helps maintain mucous membranes and cell respiration; promotes good vision and healthy skin, hair, and nails.

Best Natural Sources: liver and other organ meats, poultry, milk, eggs, brewer's yeast, whole grains, enriched bread, cereal and pasta, almonds, dried beans and peas, dark green vegetables.

Recommended Daily Dosage: 1.2 to 1.7 milligrams for adults, slightly higher for pregnant and lactating women.

Toxicity: nontoxic. However, as with all B vitamins, it is important to maintain a proper balance within this group (see thiamine).

Niacin (Vitamin B₃)

Water-soluble, part of the B-complex group. Very resistant to heat, light, and air. With the amino acid *tryptophan,* the body can manufacture its own niacin, assuming there is no deficiency in the other B vitamins. There are also three synthetic forms: niacinamide, nicotinic acid, and nicotinamide.

Main Functions: promotes a healthy nervous and digestive system and maintains healthy skin and hair; aids circulation and assists in breakdown of carbohydrates, fats, and proteins.

Best Natural Sources: tuna, liver, lean meat, poultry, fish, whole grains, enriched wheat products, and nuts.

Recommended Daily Dosage: 13 to 19 milligrams for adults.

Toxicity: basically nontoxic, but doses over 100 milligrams may cause temporary burning, tingling, or itching of the skin. These side effects are not present in niacinamide, but excessive doses of this substance have been known to cause depression in some individuals.

Pantothenic Acid (Vitamin B₅)

Water-soluble, part of the B-complex group. Occurs in all living cells, but can be destroyed with overprocessing.

Main Functions: aids cell building, healing, and the formation and maintenance of adrenal hormones; helps in metabolism of carbohydrates, fats, and proteins.

Best Natural Sources: all plants and foods of animal origin, particularly liver and other organ meats, poultry, egg yolks, whole grains, nuts, dark-green vegetables, and brewer's yeast.

Recommended Daily Dosage: 10 milligrams for adults. Need may increase with illness, stress, or use of antibiotics.

Toxicity: nontoxic (see thiamine).

Pyridoxine, Pyridoxal, and Pyridoxamine (Vitamin B$_6$)

Water-soluble, part of the B-complex group. Helps maintain the body's sodium-potassium balance; useful in preventing various nerve and skin disorders.

Main Functions: aids in formation of red blood cells and metabolism of proteins and fats; helps regulate body fluids and nervous system; alleviates nausea.

Best Natural Sources: whole grains, liver, beef, avocado, cantaloupe, bananas, nuts, dark green leafy vegetables.

Recommended Daily Dosage: 1.5 to 2 milligrams for adults. Higher doses are suggested for pregnant and lactating women, and for those on a high-protein diet.

Toxicity: nontoxic (see thiamine).

Cobalamin (Vitamin B$_{12}$)

Water-soluble, part of the B-complex group; the only vitamin that contains essential mineral elements. Highly effective in very small doses, B$_{12}$ needs calcium for proper absorption.

Main Functions: forms and regulates red blood cells and prevents anemia; helps maintain a healthy nervous system; alleviates irritability and increases energy.

Best Natural Sources: found only in foods of animal origin, particularly liver, kidneys, beef, pork, fish, eggs, milk, cheese. (*Note:* Strict vegetarians may require supplements.)

Recommended Daily Dosage: 2 micrograms for adults, higher during pregnancy and lactation.

Toxicity: nontoxic (see thiamine).

Folicin (Folic Acid)

Water-soluble, part of the B-complex group. Easily destroyed by heat, light, and air. Although the body can store folicin, it is one of the vitamins most deficient in our diets.

Main Functions: aids in formation of red blood cells; helps maintain healthy nervous system and promotes mental health; essential for reproduction of all cells.

Best Natural Sources: dark green leafy vegetables, brewer's yeast, liver, kidneys, dried beans and peas, broccoli, carrots, asparagus.

Recommended Daily Dosage: 400 micrograms; 800 micrograms during pregnancy and 500 micrograms during lactation. Need increases with use of alcohol or oral contraceptives and during periods of stress or illness.

Toxicity: nontoxic, but temporary skin rash might occur in some individuals, and an overabundance may mask a deficiency in B_{12} (see thiamine).

Ascorbic Acid (Vitamin C)
Water-soluble. Very sensitive to oxygen; its potency can be lost through exposure to air, light, and heat. Vitamin C has been—and continues to be—the subject of a wide range of studies, and has been touted as a cure-all for everything from the common cold to cancer. While most animals synthesize their own supply, man, apes, and a few other animals must rely on dietary sources.

Main Functions: aids production of collagen and red blood cells; maintains healthy blood vessels, bones, teeth, and gums; helps body absorb iron; promotes healing.

Best Natural Sources: fresh fruits and vegetables, especially citrus fruits, leafy green vegetables, tomatoes, strawberries, melon, green peppers, broccoli, Brussels sprouts, cabbage, potatoes.

Recommended Daily Dosage: 60 milligrams for adults, with increased dosage during illness, stress, pregnancy, or lactation. Smokers require higher doses, and it is believed that the need for vitamin C increases with age. (*Note:* supplements are best taken in frequent small doses, because the body can absorb only so much at once.)

Toxicity: basically nontoxic, but excessive doses may cause diarrhea, skin rashes, or other temporary side effects in some individuals.

Cholecalciferol (Vitamin D)
Fat-soluble. Called the "sunshine vitamin" because it can be acquired by exposure to the sun's ultraviolet rays. Best utilized when combined with vitamin A.

Main Functions: aids in formation and maintenance of bones and teeth; helps body absorb and utilize calcium and phosphorus; in adults it also helps maintain the nervous system, heart action, and blood clotting.

Best Natural Sources: sunlight, but pigmentation is a determining factor: the darker the skin—whether natural or tanned—the less vitamin D produced. Adequate absorption can be inhibited by air pollution, clouds, and clothing. Other sources are cod-liver oil and fortified milk and dairy products.

Recommended Daily Dosage: 400 International Units, or 5 to 10 micrograms for adults.

Toxicity: excessive doses (over 5000 International Units daily) over an extended period can produce temporary toxic effects, such as frequent urination, nausea and vomiting, dizziness, and muscular weakness.

Tocopherol (Vitamin E)

Fat-soluble. Composed of eight tocopherols (named for letters in the Greek alphabet), with alpha-tocopherol the most potent and effective form. Like vitamin C, E has been the subject of numerous studies and health claims. Vitamin E deficiencies are extremely rare in humans.

Main Functions: supplies oxygen to the body; aids in formation of red blood cells; helps maintain muscles and other tissues; protects Vitamin A and fatty acids from oxidation; promotes healing and is effective in preventing raised scar tissue.

Best Natural Sources: cold-pressed vegetable oils, wheat germ, whole grains, liver, raw seeds, and margarine.

Recommended Daily Dosage: 8 to 10 milligrams for adults. Need increases with a diet high in polyunsaturated fats and exposure to air pollution. (*Note:* Many health professionals consider the official RDA exceedingly low and have recommended dosages of 600 International Units, and even higher.)

Toxicity: basically nontoxic (excessive doses are extracted in the urine); but may have an adverse effect on individuals with high blood pressure or chronic heart disorders.

Vitamin K

Fat-soluble. There are three K vitamins: two (K_1 and K_2) can be produced in the body by intestinal bacteria; the third (K_3) is a synthetic used when a supplement is needed for a specific purpose, such as during surgery, or when the body is unable to manufacture its own supply.

Main Functions: promotes proper blood clotting and helps prevent internal bleeding; aids normal liver functioning; enhances vitality.

Best Natural Sources: dark green leafy vegetables, kelp, Brussels sprouts, cabbage, cauliflower, peas, liver, fish liver oils.

Recommended Daily Dosage: 55 to 80 micrograms for adults.

Toxicity: basically nontoxic, but possibly toxic when large doses of synthetic (K_3) are mixed with anticoagulants; supplements can also build up in the blood and result in symptoms such as flushing and sweating.

THE
VITAMIN CONTENT
OF FOOD

VITAMIN A
◆
VITAMIN C
◆
THIAMINE
◆
RIBOFLAVIN
◆
NIACIN
◆
VITAMIN B_6
◆
FOLIC ACID
◆
VITAMIN B_{12}

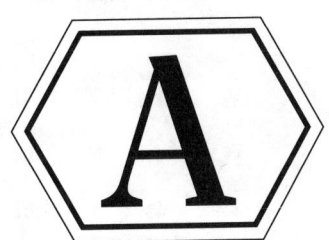

Food and Measure	A I.U.	C mg.	Thi mg.	Rib mg.	Nia mg.	B6 mg.	Fol mcg.	B12 mcg.
Acerola, trimmed, ½ cup	376	822	.01	.03	.20	<.01	n.a.	0
Acerola juice, fresh, 6 fl. oz.	924	2,899	.04	.11	.73	.01	n.a.	0
Acorn squash, ½ cup:								
raw, cubed	238	8	.10	.01	.49	.11	11.7	0
boiled, drained, cubed	437	11	.17	.01	.90	.20	19.1	0
boiled, drained, mashed	315	8	.12	.01	.65	.14	13.8	0
Aduzi beans, boiled, ½ cup	7	0	.13	.07	.83	n.a.	m.q.	0
Allspice, ground, 1 tsp.	10	1	<.01	<.01	.01	n.a.	n.a.	0
Almond, shelled, 1 oz.:								
dried, unblanched	0	<1	.06	.22	.96	.03	16.7	0
dried, blanched	0	<1	.05	.19	.90	.03	10.9	0
dry-roasted, unblanched	0	<1	.04	.17	.80	.02	18.1	0
oil-roasted, unblanched	0	<1	.04	.28	.99	.02	18.1	0
oil-roasted, blanched	0	<1	.02	.08	1.11	.03	18.0	0
toasted, unblanched	0	<1	.04	.17	.80	.02	18.2	0
Almond butter, 1 tbsp.:								
plain	0	<1	.02	.10	.46	.01	10.4	0
honey and cinnamon	0	<1	.02	.10	.46	.01	10.3	0
Almond paste, 1 oz.	0	<1	.06	.21	.82	.03	15.8	0
Amaranth, ½ cup:								
raw	408	6	<.01	.02	.09	tr.	11.9	0
boiled, drained	1828	27	.01	.09	.37	tr.	m.q.	0
Amaranth, whole grain, 1 cup	n.a.	8	.16	.41	2.51	.44	95.0	0
Amaranth dinner, canned, w/ garden vegetables (*Health Valley Fast Menu*), 7½ oz.	254	5	.17	.23	1.60	.11	9.6	0
Anchovy, meat only, European, raw, 1 oz.	m.q.	(0)	.02	.07	3.97	.04	m.q.	.18
Anchovy, canned, in oil, 5 medium	m.q.	(0)	.02	.07	3.98	.04	m.q.	.18

Food and Measure	A I.U.	C mg.	Thi mg.	Rib mg.	Nia mg.	B_6 mg.	Fol mcg.	B_{12} mcg.
Apple, ½ cup, except as noted:								
fresh, cored, unpeeled:								
raw, sliced	30	3	.01	.01	.04	.03	1.6	0
raw, 1 medium, 2¾″ diam.,								
approx. 3 per lb.	74	8	.02	.02	.11	.07	3.9	0
fresh, cored, peeled:								
raw, sliced	24	2	.01	.01	.05	.03	.2	0
raw, 1 medium, 2¾″ diam.,								
approx. 3 per lb.	56	5	.02	.01	.12	.06	.5	0
boiled, sliced	38	<1	.01	.01	.08	.04	.5	0
microwaved, sliced	34	<1	.01	.01	.05	.04	.5	0
canned, sweetened, sliced:								
unheated	52	<1	.01	.01	.07	.05	.3	0
heated	57	<1	.01	.01	.08	.05	.1	0
dehydrated, sulfured:								
uncooked	24	1	.01	.04	.20	.08	.3	0
cooked	18	1	.01	.03	.14	.05	.1	0
dried, sulfured:								
uncooked	0	2	0	.07	.40	.05	n.a.	0
cooked, unsweetened	22	1	.01	.02	.17	.06	0	0
cooked, sweetened	22	1	.01	.03	.17	.07	n.a.	0
frozen, unsweetened, sliced:								
unheated	29	<1	.01	.01	.04	.03	.6	0
heated	21	<1	.01	.01	.04	.03	.6	0
Apple juice[1], 6 fl. oz.:								
canned or bottled	2	2	.04	.03	.19	.05	0	0
frozen[2]	m.q.	1	.01	.02	.07	.06	.6	0
Applesauce, canned, ½ cup:								
unsweetened[1]	35	2	.02	.03	.23	.03	.7	0
sweetened	14	2	.02	.04	.24	.03	.7	0
Apricot, ½ cup, except as noted:								
fresh, pitted, halves	2024	8	.02	.03	.47	.04	6.7	0
fresh, 3 medium, approx. 4 oz.	2769	11	.03	.04	.64	.06	9.1	0
canned, unpeeled, halves:								
in water	1571	4	.03	.03	.48	.07	2.1	0
in juice	2098	6	.02	.02	.43	m.q.	m.q.	0
in light syrup	1672	4	.02	.03	.38	.07	2.2	0
in heavy syrup	1587	4	.03	.03	.49	.07	2.2	0
canned, peeled, whole:								
in water	2055	2	.02	.03	.50	.06	2.0	0
in heavy syrup	1600	4	.02	.03	.54	.07	2.2	0
in extra heavy syrup	1809	3	.02	.03	.42	.07	2.0	0
dehydrated, sulfured:								
uncooked	7601	6	.03	.09	2.10	.31	2.7	0
cooked	5465	9	.02	.08	2.00	.20	1.9	0

1. *Without added ascorbic acid.*
2. *Diluted according to package directions.*

Food and Measure	A I.U.	C mg.	Thi mg.	Rib mg.	Nia mg.	B₆ mg.	Fol mcg.	B₁₂ mcg.
dried, sulfured, halves:								
uncooked	4706	2	.01	.10	1.94	.10	4.5	0
cooked, unsweetened	2955	2	.01	.04	1.18	.14	0	0
cooked, sweetened	2888	2	.01	.04	1.15	.14	0	0
frozen, sweetened	2033	11	.02	.05	.97	.07	m.q.	0
Apricot nectar[1], canned,								
6 fl. oz.	2478	1	.02	.02	.49	m.q.	2.4	0
Arrowroot flour, 1 cup	0	0	<.01	0	0	.01	9.0	0
Artichoke, globe, boiled, drained:								
1 medium, approx. 10.6 oz.	212	12	.08	.08	.41	.13	61.0	0
hearts, ½ cup	149	8	.06	.06	.84	.09	42.0	0
frozen, ⅓ of 9-oz. pkg.	131	4	.05	.13	.73	.07	95.0	0
Asparagus, boiled, drained:								
fresh, 4 spears, ½"-diam. base	498	16	.06	.07	.63	.09	58.8	0
fresh, cuts and spears, ½ cup	746	18	.09	.11	.95	.13	88.2	0
canned w/liquid, ½ cup	578	20	.07	.11	1.04	.12	104.1	0
frozen, 4 spears	491	15	.04	.06	.62	.01	80.8	0
Avocado:								
California, 1 medium, approx.								
8 oz.	1059	14	.19	.21	3.32	.48	113.3	0
California, pureed, ½ cup	704	9	.12	.14	2.20	.32	75.4	0
Florida, 1 medium, approx. 1 lb. ...	1860	24	.33	.37	5.80	.85	161.9	0
Florida, pureed, ½ cup	704	9	.12	.14	2.20	.32	61.3	0

1. *Without added ascorbic acid.*

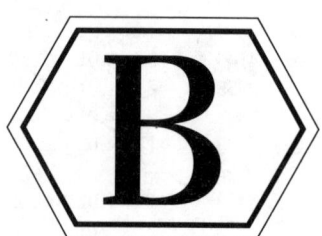

Food and Measure	A I.U.	C mg.	Thi mg.	Rib mg.	Nia mg.	B₆ mg.	Fol mcg.	B₁₂ mcg.
Bacon[1], cooked, 3 medium slices,								
20 per lb.	0	6	.13	.05	1.39	.05	1.0	.33
Bacon, Canadian-style[1]:								
unheated, 1-oz. slice	0	6	.21	.05	1.77	.44	4.5	.76
grilled, 2 slices, yield from								
2 unheated 1-oz. slices	0	10	.38	.09	3.22	.21	2.0	.36
Bacon, substitute:								
beef[2], heated, 3 strips or 1.2 oz.	0	12	.03	.09	2.20	.11	m.q.	1.17
pork[1], cured, heated, 3 strips,								
15 per 12-oz. pkg.	0	15	.25	.13	2.58	.12	1.0	.60
Bagel:								
plain or water, 3½″ diam.	0	0	.26	.20	2.40	m.q.	m.q.	0
egg, 3½″ diam.	22	0	.26	.20	2.40	m.q.	m.q.	m.q.
Baked beans, canned, ½ cup:								
plain or vegetarian	217	m.q.	.19	.08	.54	.17	30.4	0
(*Van Camp's*), 1 cup	0	0	.12	.14	1.20	m.q.	m.q.	n.a.
(*Van Camp's* Deluxe), 1 cup	0	0	.30	.10	.80	m.q.	m.q.	n.a.
(*Van Camp's* Vegetarian), 1 cup	179	2	.13	.12	1.00	m.q.	m.q.	n.a.
Boston (*Health Valley*), 4 oz.	304	<1	.70	.72	10.20	.16	4.5	0
w/beef	283	2	.07	.60	1.25	.12	m.q.	.33
w/franks	197	3	.07	.07	1.15	.06	38.4	.44
w/pork	225	3	.07	.05	.56	.08	45.8	.03
w/pork and sweet sauce	144	4	.06	.08	.44	.11	47.1	.03
w/pork and tomato sauce	156	4	.07	.06	.63	.09	28.3	.02
Baking powder, all types, 1 tsp. ...	0	0	0	0	0	n.a.	n.a.	n.a.
Balsam pear, boiled, drained:								
leafy tips, ½ cup	503	16	.04	.08	.29	.22	25.4	0
pods, ½″ pieces, ½ cup	70	21	.03	.03	.17	n.a.	n.a.	0
Bamboo shoots, fresh, ½ cup:								
raw, ½″ slices	15	3	.11	.05	.46	m.q.	m.q.	0

1. *With added ascorbic acid or sodium ascorbate; Vitamin C value for product without additives would be negligible.*
2. *With added sodium ascorbate.*

Food and Measure	A I.U.	C mg.	Thi mg.	Rib mg.	Nia mg.	B$_6$ mg.	Fol mcg.	B$_{12}$ mcg.
boiled, drained, ½" slices	0	0	.01	.03	.18	m.q.	m.q.	0
Banana:								
fresh, peeled, mashed, ½ cup	91	10	.05	.11	.61	.65	21.5	0
fresh, 1 medium, 8¾" × 1¹³⁄₃₂",								
approx. 6.2 oz.	92	10	.05	.11	.62	.66	21.8	0
dehydrated or powdered, 1 oz.	87	2	.05	.07	.79	m.q.	m.q.	0
Barbecue loaf[1], pork and beef,								
1 oz.	n.a.	5	.10	.07	.64	.07	m.q.	.48
Barbecue sauce, 1 tbsp.	139	1	.01	<.01	.14	.01	m.q.	0
Barley:								
raw, 1 cup	n.a.	0	1.19	.53	n.a.	.59	35.0	0
pearled, raw, 1 cup	44	0	.38	.23	9.21	.52	46.0	0
pearled, cooked, 1 cup	n.a.	0	.13	.10	3.24	.18	26.0	0
Basil, ground, 1 tsp.	131	1	<.01	<.01	.10	n.a.	n.a.	0
Bay leaf, crumbled, 1 tsp.	37	<1	tr.	<.01	.01	n.a.	n.a.	0
Beef[2], retail trim[3], meat only, 4 oz.:								
brisket, whole, all grades, braised:								
lean and fat[4]	0	0	.07	.20	3.40	.27	6.8	2.59
lean and fat[5]	0	0	.08	.23	3.82	.31	7.9	2.78
lean only[6]	0	0	.08	.25	4.21	.33	9.1	2.95
brisket, flat half, all grades, braised:								
lean and fat[4]	0	0	.07	.20	3.56	.29	6.8	2.63
lean and fat[5]	0	0	.08	.24	4.24	.34	9.1	2.93
lean only[6]	0	0	.08	.25	4.38	.35	9.1	2.98
brisket, point half, all grades, braised:								
lean and fat[4]	0	0	.07	.20	3.27	.26	6.8	2.55
lean and fat[5]	0	0	.07	.22	3.45	.27	7.9	2.64
lean only[6]	0	0	.08	.26	4.05	.32	9.1	2.93
chuck, arm pot roast, choice grade, braised:								
lean and fat[4]	0	0	.08	.27	3.55	.32	10.2	3.31
lean and fat[5]	0	0	.08	.29	3.82	.34	11.3	3.54
lean only[6]	0	0	.09	.33	4.22	.37	12.5	3.85
chuck, arm pot roast, select grade, braised:								
lean and fat[4]	0	0	.08	.27	3.65	.33	10.2	3.39
lean and fat[5]	0	0	.08	.29	3.90	.35	11.3	3.59
lean only[6]	0	0	.09	.33	4.22	.37	12.5	3.86
chuck, blade roast, choice grade, braised:								
lean and fat[4]	0	0	.08	.27	2.72	.28	5.7	2.57
lean and fat[5]	0	0	.08	.28	2.77	.29	5.7	2.61
lean only[6]	0	0	.09	.32	3.03	.33	6.8	2.80

1. *With added sodium ascorbate; vitamin C value for product without added sodium ascorbate would be negligible.*
2. *Prepared without added ingredients, except as noted.*
3. *Meat trimmed to 0" or ¼" fat refers to the amount of fat present during cooking. For "lean only" listings, all visible fat is trimmed after cooking. (Bear in mind that a small amount of fat is always present, even in meat trimmed to 0" fat before cooking.)*
4. *Trimmed to ¼" fat.*
5. *Trimmed to 0" fat.*
6. *Trimmed to ¼" or 0" fat.*

Food and Measure	A I.U.	C mg.	Thi mg.	Rib mg.	Nia mg.	B_6 mg.	Fol mcg.	B_{12} mcg.
Beef *(cont.)*								
chuck, blade roast, select grade, braised:								
lean and fat[1]	0	0	.08	.28	2.77	.29	5.7	2.61
lean and fat[2]	0	0	.08	.28	2.81	.29	5.7	2.64
lean only[3]	0	0	.09	.32	3.03	.33	6.8	2.80
flank, choice grade[2]:								
braised, lean and fat	0	0	.16	.20	5.01	.40	10.2	3.74
braised, lean only	0	0	.16	.22	5.22	.41	10.2	3.87
broiled, lean and fat	0	0	.11	.20	5.56	.39	9.1	3.62
broiled, lean only	0	0	.12	.22	5.70	.39	9.1	3.69
ground, extra lean:								
baked, medium	0	0	.05	.27	4.72	.25	10.2	1.96
baked, well-done	0	0	.06	.35	6.13	.33	12.5	2.11
broiled, medium	0	0	.07	.31	5.62	.31	10.2	2.46
broiled, well-done	0	0	.08	.36	6.63	.36	12.5	2.90
pan-fried, medium	0	0	.07	.29	5.34	.31	10.2	2.27
pan-fried, well-done	0	0	.08	.34	6.17	.35	11.3	2.63
ground, lean:								
baked, medium	0	0	.06	.22	4.85	.23	10.2	2.01
baked, well-done	0	0	.08	.27	6.19	.29	13.6	2.56
broiled, medium	0	0	.06	.24	5.85	.29	10.2	2.66
broiled, well-done	0	0	.07	.27	6.77	.34	12.5	3.08
pan-fried, medium	0	0	.06	.25	5.43	.32	10.2	2.57
pan-fried, well-done	0	0	.07	.27	6.18	.36	11.3	2.93
ground, regular:								
baked, medium	0	0	.03	.18	5.39	.26	10.2	2.65
baked, well-done	0	0	.05	.23	6.68	.33	12.5	3.29
broiled, medium	0	0	.03	.22	6.54	.31	10.2	3.32
broiled, well-done	0	0	.05	.24	7.34	.34	11.3	3.72
pan-fried, medium	0	0	.03	.23	6.61	.27	10.2	3.07
pan-fried, well-done	0	0	.05	.24	7.33	.31	11.3	3.40
ground, frozen, patties, broiled, medium	0	0	.06	.23	5.98	.29	10.2	2.80
Porterhouse steak (short loin), choice grade, broiled[1]:								
lean and fat	0	0	.11	.25	4.59	.40	7.9	2.44
lean only	0	0	.12	.28	5.25	.45	9.1	2.57
rib, whole (ribs 6–12), choice grade[1]:								
broiled, lean and fat	0	0	.09	.19	3.64	.31	6.8	3.22
broiled, lean only	0	0	.10	.23	4.35	.36	7.9	3.76
roasted, lean and fat	0	0	.08	.19	3.81	.26	7.9	2.86
roasted, lean only	0	0	.09	.24	4.72	.31	9.1	3.30

1. *Trimmed to ¼″ fat.*
2. *Trimmed to 0″ fat.*
3. *Trimmed to ¼″ or 0″ fat.*

Food and Measure	A I.U.	C mg.	Thi mg.	Rib mg.	Nia mg.	B6 mg.	Fol mcg.	B12 mcg.
rib, whole (ribs 6–12), prime grade[1]:								
broiled, lean and fat	0	0	.09	.19	3.57	.33	6.8	3.20
broiled, lean only	0	0	.10	.24	4.29	.40	7.9	3.72
roasted, lean and fat	0	0	.08	.19	3.79	.29	7.9	2.87
roasted, lean only	0	0	.09	.24	4.66	.34	10.2	3.31
rib, whole (ribs 6–12), select grade[1]:								
broiled, lean and fat	0	0	.09	.19	3.73	.31	6.8	3.29
broiled, lean only	0	0	.10	.23	4.35	.36	7.9	3.76
roasted, lean and fat	0	0	.08	.20	3.93	.26	7.9	2.91
roasted, lean only	0	0	.09	.24	4.72	.31	9.1	3.29
rib, large end (ribs 6–9), choice grade:								
broiled, lean and fat[1]	0	0	.08	.18	3.07	.26	6.8	3.20
broiled, lean only[1]	0	0	.09	.22	3.61	.29	7.9	3.75
roasted, lean and fat[1]	0	0	.08	.20	4.03	.25	7.9	2.61
roasted, lean and fat[2]	0	0	.08	.22	4.13	.26	7.9	2.64
roasted, lean only[3]	0	0	.10	.25	5.05	.29	10.2	2.96
rib, large end (ribs 6–9), prime grade[1]:								
broiled, lean and fat	0	0	.08	.19	2.95	.29	6.8	3.12
broiled, lean only	0	0	.10	.23	3.48	.36	7.9	3.70
roasted, lean and fat	0	0	.08	.20	4.06	.25	7.9	2.62
roasted, lean only	0	0	.10	.25	5.05	.29	10.2	2.96
rib, large end (ribs 6–9), select grade:								
broiled, lean and fat[1]	0	0	.08	.18	3.15	.26	6.8	3.28
broiled, lean only[1]	0	0	.09	.22	3.61	.29	7.9	3.75
roasted, lean and fat[1]	0	0	.08	.22	4.20	.26	7.9	2.66
roasted, lean and fat[2]	0	0	.08	.22	4.25	.26	9.1	2.69
roasted, lean only[3]	0	0	.10	.25	5.05	.29	10.2	2.96
rib, shortrib, choice grade:								
braised, lean and fat	0	0	.06	.17	2.78	.25	5.7	2.97
braised, lean only	0	0	.07	.23	3.64	.32	7.9	3.92
rib, small end (ribs 10–12), choice grade:								
broiled, lean and fat[1]	0	0	.10	.20	4.49	.37	7.9	3.27
broiled, lean and fat[2]	0	0	.10	.22	4.74	.40	7.9	3.40
broiled, lean only[3]	0	0	.11	.25	5.44	.45	9.1	3.76
roasted, lean and fat[1]	0	0	.07	.18	3.50	.27	6.8	3.20
roasted, lean only[1]	0	0	.08	.22	4.24	.32	9.1	3.78
rib, small end (ribs 10–12), prime grade[1]:								
broiled, lean and fat	0	0	.10	.22	4.56	.39	7.9	3.30
broiled, lean only	0	0	.11	.25	5.44	.45	9.1	3.76
roasted, lean and fat	0	0	.07	.18	3.41	.34	6.8	3.22
roasted, lean only	0	0	.09	.22	4.12	.42	9.1	3.82

1. *Trimmed to 1/4" fat.*
2. *Trimmed to 0" fat.*
3. *Trimmed to 1/4" or 0" fat.*

Food and Measure	A I.U.	C mg.	Thi mg.	Rib mg.	Nia mg.	B6 mg.	Fol mcg.	B12 mcg.
Beef *(cont.)*								
rib, small end (ribs 10–12), select grade:								
broiled, lean and fat[1]	0	0	.10	.22	4.56	.39	7.9	3.30
broiled, lean and fat[2]	0	0	.10	.22	4.79	.40	7.9	3.41
broiled, lean only[3]	0	0	.11	.25	5.44	.45	9.1	3.76
roasted, lean and fat[1]	0	0	.07	.18	3.57	.27	6.8	3.25
roasted, lean only[1]	0	0	.08	.22	4.24	.32	9.1	3.78
rib eye, small end (ribs 10–12), choice grade, broiled[2]:								
lean and fat	0	0	.10	.22	4.79	.40	7.9	3.41
lean only	0	0	.11	.25	5.44	.45	9.1	3.76
round, full cut, choice grade[1]:								
broiled, lean and fat	0	0	.10	.24	4.52	.43	10.2	3.41
broiled, lean only	0	0	.11	.25	4.83	.45	11.3	3.59
round, full cut, select grade[1]:								
broiled, lean and fat	0	0	.10	.24	4.54	.43	10.2	3.42
broiled, lean only	0	0	.11	.25	4.84	.46	11.3	3.59
round, bottom, choice grade:								
braised, lean and fat[1]	0	0	.08	.27	4.23	.37	11.3	2.66
braised, lean and fat[2]	0	0	.08	.28	4.55	.40	12.5	2.77
braised, lean only[3]	0	0	.08	.29	4.63	.41	12.5	2.80
roasted, lean and fat[1]	0	0	.09	.25	4.25	.39	12.5	2.90
roasted, lean and fat[2]	0	0	.09	.27	4.56	.42	13.6	3.04
roasted, lean only[3]	0	0	.09	.27	4.62	.42	13.6	3.06
round, bottom, select grade:								
braised, lean and fat[1]	0	0	.08	.27	4.25	.37	11.3	2.68
braised, lean and fat[2]	0	0	.08	.29	4.57	.41	12.5	2.78
braised, lean only[3]	0	0	.08	.29	4.63	.41	12.5	2.80
roasted, lean and fat[1]	0	0	.09	.26	4.31	.40	12.5	2.93
roasted, lean and fat[2]	0	0	.09	.27	4.59	.42	13.6	3.05
roasted, lean only[3]	0	0	.09	.27	4.62	.42	13.6	3.06
round, eye of, choice grade, roasted:								
lean and fat[1]	0	0	.09	.18	3.93	.40	6.8	2.38
lean and fat[2]	0	0	.10	.19	4.23	.43	7.9	2.45
lean only[3]	0	0	.10	.19	4.25	.43	7.9	2.46
round, eye of, select grade, roasted:								
lean and fat[1]	0	0	.09	.18	3.98	.40	7.9	2.39
lean and fat[2]	0	0	.10	.19	4.23	.43	7.9	2.45
lean only[3]	0	0	.10	.19	4.25	.43	7.9	2.46
round, tip, choice grade, roasted:								
lean and fat[1]	0	0	.10	.28	3.95	.42	7.9	3.11
lean and fat[2]	0	0	.11	.29	4.14	.44	9.1	3.22
lean only[3]	0	0	.11	.31	4.24	.45	9.1	3.28
round, tip, prime grade[1], roasted:								
lean and fat	0	0	.10	.27	3.92	.42	7.9	3.08
lean only	0	0	.11	.31	4.24	.45	9.1	3.28

1. *Trimmed to ¼" fat.*
2. *Trimmed to 0" fat.*
3. *Trimmed to ¼" or 0" fat.*

Food and Measure	A I.U.	C mg.	Thi mg.	Rib mg.	Nia mg.	B$_6$ mg.	Fol mcg.	B$_{12}$ mcg.
round, tip, select grade, roasted:								
lean and fat[1]	0	0	.10	.28	4.01	.43	9.1	3.15
lean and fat[2]	0	0	.11	.29	4.16	.44	9.1	3.23
lean only[3]	0	0	.11	.31	4.24	.45	9.1	3.28
round, top, choice grade:								
braised, lean and fat[1]	0	0	.08	.27	4.06	.31	10.2	2.94
braised, lean and fat[2]	0	0	.08	.28	4.26	.32	10.2	3.04
braised, lean only[3]	0	0	.08	.28	4.32	.32	10.2	3.06
broiled, lean and fat[1]	0	0	.12	.29	6.48	.60	12.5	2.74
broiled, lean only[1]	0	0	.14	.31	6.85	.64	13.6	2.81
pan-fried in vegetable oil, lean and fat[1]	0	0	.11	.29	5.73	.64	13.6	3.66
pan-fried in vegetable oil, lean only[1]	0	0	.12	.32	6.21	.69	14.7	3.89
round, top, prime grade[1]:								
broiled, lean and fat	0	0	.14	.29	6.69	.62	13.6	2.78
broiled, lean only	0	0	.14	.31	6.85	.64	13.6	2.81
round, top, select grade:								
braised, lean and fat[1]	0	0	.08	.27	4.12	.31	10.2	2.96
braised, lean and fat[2]	0	0	.08	.28	4.26	.32	10.2	3.04
braised, lean only[3]	0	0	.08	.28	4.32	.32	10.2	3.06
broiled, lean and fat[1]	0	0	.12	.29	6.48	.60	12.5	2.74
broiled, lean only[1]	0	0	.14	.31	6.85	.64	13.6	2.81
shank, crosscuts, choice grade[1]:								
simmered, lean and fat	0	0	.14	.23	6.04	.39	10.2	3.98
simmered, lean only	0	0	.16	.24	6.68	.42	11.3	4.30
short loin, see "Porterhouse steak," "T-bone steak," and "top loin"								
sirloin, top, choice grade:								
broiled, lean and fat[1]	0	0	.12	.31	4.42	.46	10.2	3.04
broiled, lean and fat[2]	0	0	.14	.32	4.67	.49	11.3	3.15
broiled, lean only[3]	0	0	.15	.33	4.85	.51	11.3	3.23
pan-fried in vegetable oil, lean and fat[1]	0	0	.14	.32	4.25	.49	10.2	3.72
pan-fried in vegetable oil, lean only[1]	0	0	.16	.37	4.88	.57	11.3	4.18
sirloin, top, select grade, broiled:								
lean and fat[1]	0	0	.12	.31	4.48	.46	10.2	3.06
lean and fat[2]	0	0	.14	.33	4.76	.50	11.3	3.19
lean only[3]	0	0	.15	.33	4.85	.51	11.3	3.23
T-bone steak (short loin), choice grade[1]:								
broiled, lean and fat	0	0	.11	.25	4.63	.39	7.9	2.44
broiled, lean only	0	0	.12	.28	5.25	.44	9.1	2.57

1. *Trimmed to ¼" fat.*
2. *Trimmed to 0" fat.*
3. *Trimmed to ¼" or 0" fat.*

Food and Measure	A I.U.	C mg.	Thi mg.	Rib mg.	Nia mg.	B$_6$ mg.	Fol mcg.	B$_{12}$ mcg.
Beef *(cont.)*								
tenderloin, choice grade:								
broiled, lean and fat[1]	0	0	.12	.29	3.97	.44	6.8	2.72
broiled, lean and fat[2]	0	0	.14	.32	4.26	.48	7.9	2.84
broiled, lean only[3]	0	0	.15	.34	4.45	.50	7.9	2.91
roasted, lean and fat[1]	0	0	.17	.31	4.34	.53	9.1	3.78
roasted, lean only[1]	0	0	.20	.37	5.16	.65	10.2	4.39
tenderloin, prime grade[1]:								
broiled, lean and fat	0	0	.12	.29	3.93	.43	6.8	2.71
broiled, lean only	0	0	.15	.34	4.45	.50	7.9	2.91
roasted, lean and fat	0	0	.10	.31	3.37	.37	7.9	2.85
roasted, lean only	0	0	.11	.36	3.84	.43	9.1	3.14
tenderloin, select grade:								
broiled, lean and fat[1]	0	0	.14	.31	4.05	.44	6.8	2.76
broiled, lean and fat[2]	0	0	.14	.33	4.29	.48	7.9	2.85
broiled, lean only[3]	0	0	.15	.34	4.45	.50	7.9	2.91
roasted, lean and fat[1]	0	0	.09	.29	3.37	.28	7.9	2.78
roasted, lean only[1]	0	0	.11	.35	3.87	.33	10.2	3.07
top loin (short loin), choice grade, broiled:								
lean and fat[1]	0	0	.09	.20	5.28	.42	7.9	2.19
lean and fat[2]	0	0	.10	.22	5.89	.46	9.1	2.25
lean only[3]	0	0	.10	.23	6.06	.48	9.1	2.27
top loin (short loin), prime grade[1]:								
broiled, lean and fat	0	0	.09	.20	5.28	.42	7.9	2.19
broiled, lean only	0	0	.10	.23	6.06	.48	9.1	2.27
top loin (short loin), select grade, broiled:								
lean and fat[1]	0	0	.09	.20	5.41	.43	7.9	2.20
lean and fat[2]	0	0	.10	.22	5.93	.46	9.1	2.26
lean only[3]	0	0	.10	.23	6.06	.48	9.1	2.27
Beef, corned:								
brisket, cured[4], cooked, 4 oz.	0	18	.03	.19	3.44	.26	m.q.	1.85
loaf, jellied, 1-oz. slice[5]	0	2	<.01	.03	.46	.04	m.q.	.33
Beef gravy, canned, ¼ cup	0	0	.02	.02	.38	.01	m.q.	.06
Beef luncheon meat[5]:								
loaf, 1-oz. slice	0	4	.03	.06	1.04	.05	m.q.	1.10
thin sliced, 5 slices, approx. ¾ oz.	0	3	.02	.04	1.11	.07	m.q.	.54
Beef stew, canned (*Wolf* Brand),								
scant cup	8090	m.q.	.02	.30	3.49	.17	13.0	2.00
Beer, 12 fl. oz.:								
regular	0	0	.02	.09	1.60	.18	21.4	.06
light	0	0	.03	.11	1.40	.12	14.7	.02
Beet, sliced, ½ cup:								
fresh, raw	14	8	.03	.01	.27	.03	63.0	0

1. *Trimmed to ¼" fat.*
2. *Trimmed to 0" fat.*
3. *Trimmed to ¼" or 0" fat.*
4. *Contains added sodium ascorbate.*
5. *With added ascorbic acid or sodium ascorbate; vitamin C value for product without additives would be negligible.*

Food and Measure	A I.U.	C mg.	Thi mg.	Rib mg.	Nia mg.	B₆ mg.	Fol mcg.	B₁₂ mcg.
fresh, boiled, drained	11	5	.03	.01	.23	.03	45.2	0
canned, w/liquid	14	5	.01	.05	.19	.07	35.7	0
Harvard, canned, w/liquid	m.q.	3	n.a.	.06	.10	m.q.	m.q.	0
pickled, canned, w/liquid	7	3	.03	.06	.29	m.q.	m.q.	0
Beet greens, ½ cup:								
raw, 1″ pieces	1159	6	.02	.04	.08	.02	m.q.	0
boiled, drained, 1″ pieces	3672	18	.08	.21	.36	.10	m.q.	0
Berliner[1]**,** pork and beef, 1 oz. . . .	0	2	.11	.06	.88	.06	m.q.	.76
Biscuit, baking powder:								
mix[2], 1-oz. piece, 2″ diam.	20	tr.	.12	.11	.80	n.a.	m.q.	n.a.
refrigerated, 2″-diam. piece	0	0	.08	.05	.70	n.a.	m.q.	n.a.
Black bean, boiled, ½ cup	5	0	.21	.05	.43	.06	127.9	0
Black bean dinner, canned, western, w/garden vegetables (*Health Valley Fast Menu*),								
7½ oz.	4184	<1	.23	.23	1.30	.17	87.8	0
Black turtle soup bean, ½ cup:								
boiled	5	0	.21	.52	.49	.07	78.7	0
canned w/liquid	5	3	.17	.14	.74	.07	73.0	0
Blackberry, ½ cup:								
fresh, trimmed	119	15	.02	.03	.29	.04	n.a.	0
canned, in heavy syrup	280	4	.04	.05	.37	.05	33.9	0
frozen, unsweetened	86	2	.02	.03	.31	.05	25.7	0
Blueberry, ½ cup:								
fresh, trimmed	73	10	.04	.04	.26	.03	4.7	0
canned, in heavy syrup	82	1	.04	.07	.15	.05	2.1	0
frozen, unsweetened	63	2	.03	.03	.40	.05	5.2	0
frozen, sweetened	51	1	.02	.06	.29	.07	7.8	0
Bluefish, meat only, raw, 1 oz. . . .	113	(0)	.02	.02	1.69	.11	.5	1.53
Bologna[1]**:**								
beef, 1-oz. slice	0	5	.02	.04	.75	.05	1.0	.40
beef and pork, 1-oz. slice	0	6	.05	.04	.73	.05	1.0	.38
Lebanon, beef, 1 oz.	0	10	.02	.06	1.33	.07	1.0	.79
pork, 1-oz. slice	0	10	.15	.05	1.11	.08	1.0	.26
Boysenberry, ½ cup:								
fresh, see "Blackberry"								
canned, in heavy syrup	51	8	.03	.04	.29	.05	44.1	0
frozen, unsweetened	45	4	.08	.02	.51	.04	41.8	0
Brains[3]**,** 4 oz.:								
beef, pan-fried in vegetable oil	0	4	.15	.29	4.29	.44	6.8	17.24
beef, simmered	0	1	.09	.19	2.47	.27	7.9	9.75
lamb, braised	0	14	.12	.27	2.80	.12	5.7	10.49
lamb, pan-fried in vegetable oil	0	26	.19	.42	5.16	.26	7.9	27.33
pork, braised	0	16	.09	.25	3.78	.16	m.q.	1.61
veal, braised	0	15	.09	.23	2.76	.19	3.4	10.94
veal, pan-fried in vegetable oil	0	17	.17	.41	6.37	.37	6.8	24.15

1. *With added ascorbic acid or sodium ascorbate; vitamin C value for product without additives would be negligible.*
2. *Prepared according to package directions.*
3. *Prepared without added ingredients, except as noted.*

Food and Measure	A I.U.	C mg.	Thi mg.	Rib mg.	Nia mg.	B6 mg.	Fol mcg.	B12 mcg.
Bran, unprocessed (*Quaker*),								
2 tbsp.	0	0	.04	.03	1.54	.04	9.0	n.a.
Bratwurst, 1 oz.:								
pork, cooked	n.a.	0	.14	.05	.91	.06	m.q.	.27
pork and beef[1, 2]	n.a.	8	.07	.06	.94	.04	m.q.	.58
Braunschweiger, pork, 1 oz.[1] . . .	3984	3	.07	.43	2.37	.09	m.q.	5.69
Brazil nut, shelled, dried, 1 oz.	0	<1	.28	.04	.46	.07	1.1	0
Bread, 1 slice or piece:								
Boston brown[3], canned, 1.6 oz.	0	0	.06	.04	.70	n.a.	n.a.	n.a.
Boston brown[4], canned, 1.6 oz.	32	0	.06	.04	.70	n.a.	n.a.	n.a.
French, enriched, 1.2 oz.	tr.	tr.	.16	.12	1.40	m.q.	m.q.	0
Italian, enriched, 1.1 oz.	0	0	.12	.07	1.00	n.a.	m.q.	0
mixed grain, enriched, 18 slices/lb.	tr.	tr.	.10	.10	1.10	m.q.	m.q.	0
oatmeal, 18 slices/lb.	0	0	.12	.07	.90	n.a.	m.q.	0
pita, enriched, 6½″ diam.	0	0	.27	.12	2.20	m.q.	m.q.	0
pumpernickel, 1.1 oz.	0	0	.11	.17	1.10	m.q.	n.a.	0
raisin, enriched, 18 slices/lb.	tr.	tr.	.08	.15	1.00	n.a.	m.q.	0
rye, light, .9 oz.	0	0	.10	.08	.80	m.q.	m.q.	0
Vienna, enriched, .9 oz.	tr.	tr.	.12	.09	1.00	m.q.	m.q.	0
wheat:								
cracked, 18 slices/lb.	tr.	tr.	.10	.09	.80	m.q.	m.q.	0
enriched, 18 slices/lb.	tr.	tr.	.12	.08	1.20	m.q.	m.q.	0
whole, 16 slices/lb.	tr.	tr.	.10	.06	1.10	m.q.	m.q.	0
white, enriched:								
18 slices/lb.	tr.	tr.	.12	.08	.90	m.q.	m.q.	(0)
22 slices/lb.	tr.	tr.	.09	.06	.70	m.q.	m.q.	(0)
Bread, sweet, mix[5], cornbread,								
2½″ × 2½″ sq. piece	130	tr.	.10	.10	.80	n.a.	n.a.	n.a.
Bread cubes, white, 1 cup	tr.	tr.	.14	.09	1.10	m.q.	m.q.	(0)
Breadcrumbs, enriched, 1 cup:								
dry, grated	0	0	.35	.35	4.80	n.a.	n.a.	n.a.
soft	tr.	tr.	.21	.14	1.70	n.a.	n.a.	n.a.
Breadfruit, trimmed, ½ cup	44	32	.12	.03	.99	n.a.	n.a.	0
Breadsticks:								
regular, 7¾″ long, 10 pieces	tr.	tr.	.03	.04	.50	n.a.	m.q.	0
Vienna, 6½″ × 1¼″, 1 piece	tr.	tr.	.02	.03	.30	n.a.	m.q.	0
Breakfast bar, all flavors								
(*Carnation*), 1 bar	1750	28	.30	.03	5.00	.40	100.0	.63
Broadbean, dried, ½ cup:								
boiled	13	<1	.08	.08	.60	.06	88.5	0
canned, w/liquid	13	2	.03	.06	1.23	.06	41.9	0
Broccoli:								
fresh:								
raw, 1 spear, 5.3 oz.	2328	141	.10	.18	.96	.24	107.2	0
boiled, drained, 1 spear, 6.3 oz.	2498	134	.10	.20	1.03	.26	89.0	0

1. *With added ascorbic acid and sodium ascorbate; vitamin C value for product without these additives would be negligible.*
2. *Nonfat dry milk added.*
3. *Made with white cornmeal.*
4. *Made with yellow cornmeal.*
5. *Prepared according to package directions, with eggs and milk.*

Food and Measure	A I.U.	C mg.	Thi mg.	Rib mg.	Nia mg.	B6 mg.	Fol mcg.	B12 mcg.
boiled, drained, chopped, ½ cup	1082	58	.04	.09	.45	.11	39.0	0
frozen, boiled, drained, ½ cup	1741	37	.05	.75	.42	.12	51.9	0
Brownie, 1 piece:								
w/nuts, .9 oz.	70	tr.	.08	.07	.30	n.a.	m.q.	n.a.
frozen, w/chocolate icing, .9 oz. ...	50	tr.	.02	.02	.10	n.a.	m.q.	n.a.
mix[1], 7 oz.	20	tr.	.03	.02	.10	n.a.	m.q.	n.a.
Brussels sprouts, boiled, drained:								
fresh, 1 sprout, .75 oz.	151	13	.02	.02	.13	.04	12.6	0
fresh, ½ cup	561	48	.08	.06	.47	.14	46.8	0
frozen, ½ cup	459	36	.08	.09	.42	.23	79.0	0
Buckwheat, whole grain, 1 cup ...	(0)	0	.17	.72	11.93	.36	51.0	0
Buckwheat flour, 1 cup	(0)	0	.50	.23	7.38	.70	64.0	0
Buckwheat groats, roasted:								
dry, 1 oz.	(0)	0	.06	.08	1.46	.10	11.9	0
cooked, 1 cup	(0)	0	.08	.08	1.86	.15	27.0	0
Bulgur:								
dry, 1 oz.	(0)	0	.07	.03	1.45	.10	7.7	0
cooked, 1 cup	(0)	0	.10	.05	1.82	.15	33.0	0
Butter:								
regular, 1 stick	3468	0	.01	.04	.05	<.01	3.0	(0)
regular, 1 tbsp.	434	0	tr.	<.01	.01	tr.	.4	(0)
whipped, 1 stick	2312	0	<.01	.03	.03	<.01	2.0	(0)
whipped, 1 tbsp.	287	0	tr.	tr.	tr.	tr.	.3	(0)
Butterbeans (*Van Camp's*), 1 cup	0	0	.09	.08	.53	n.a.	n.a.	n.a.
Butternut squash, ½ cup:								
fresh, raw, cubed	5460	15	.07	.01	.84	.11	18.7	0
fresh, boiled, drained, cubed	7141	15	.07	.02	.99	.13	19.6	0
frozen, boiled, mashed	4007	4	.06	.05	.56	.08	m.q.	0

1. *Prepared according to package directions, with eggs, water, and nuts.*

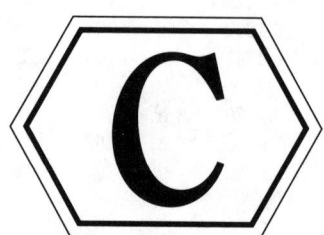

Food and Measure	A I.U.	C mg.	Thi mg.	Rib mg.	Nia mg.	B₆ mg.	Fol mcg.	B₁₂ mcg.
Cabbage:								
raw, 5⅜″-diam. head	1143	429	.45	.27	2.72	.86	514.8	0
raw, shredded, ½ cup	44	17	.02	.01	.05	.03	19.8	0
boiled, drained, shredded, ½ cup . .	64	18	.04	.04	.17	.05	15.2	0
Cabbage, Chinese, shredded, ½ cup:								
bok-choy, raw	1050	16	.01	.03	.18	m.q.	m.q.	0
bok-choy, boiled, drained	2183	22	.03	.05	.36	m.q.	m.q.	0
pe-tsai, raw	456	10	.02	.02	.15	.09	29.9	0
pe-tsai, boiled, drained	576	9	.03	.03	.30	.11	63.5	0
Cabbage, red, ½ cup:								
raw, shredded	14	20	.02	.01	.11	.07	7.3	0
boiled, drained, shredded	20	26	.03	.02	.15	.11	9.4	0
Cabbage, savoy, ½ cup:								
raw, shredded	350	11	.03	.01	.11	.07	m.q.	0
boiled, drained, shredded	649	12	.04	.02	.02	.11	m.q.	0
Cake:								
cheesecake, ¹⁄₁₂ of 9″-diam. cake . . .	230	5	.03	.12	.40	m.q.	m.q.	m.q.
pound, 1-oz. slice	160	0	.06	.06	.50	n.a.	m.q.	m.q.
white, w/white frosting, 2 layer, 2.5-oz. slice	40	0	.20	.13	1.70	m.q.	n.a.	n.a.
yellow, w/chocolate frosting, 2 layer, 2.4-oz. slice	120	0	.05	.14	.60	n.a.	n.a.	n.a.
Cake, frozen, devil's food:								
w/chocolate frosting, ⅙ of 7½″-diam. cake	370	tr.	.02	.07	.20	m.q.	m.q.	m.q.
w/whipped cream filling and chocolate frosting, 2 layer, ⅙ of 7¼″-diam. cake	230	tr.	.02	.07	.20	m.q.	m.q.	m.q.
Cake, snack, 1 piece:								
devil's food, w/creme filling, 1 oz. . .	20	0	.06	.09	.70	n.a.	m.q.	n.a.

Food and Measure	A I.U.	C mg.	Thi mg.	Rib mg.	Nia mg.	B₆ mg.	Fol mcg.	B₁₂ mcg.
sponge, w/creme filling, 1.5 oz.	30	0	.07	.06	.60	n.a.	m.q.	n.a.
Cake mix[1], 1 piece:								
angel food, ¹⁄₁₂ of 9¾″ tube	0	0	.32	1.27	1.60	n.a.	m.q.	n.a.
brownie, see "Brownie"								
coffee cake, crumb, 2.5 oz	120	tr.	.14	.15	1.30	n.a.	m.q.	n.a.
devil's food, w/chocolate frosting,								
2 layer, 2.4 oz.	100	tr.	.07	.10	.60	m.q.	m.q.	m.q.
gingerbread, ⅑ of 8″ square	0	tr.	.09	.11	.80	m.q.	m.q.	n.a.
yellow, w/chocolate frosting, 2 layer,								
2.4 oz.	100	tr.	.08	.10	.70	n.a.	n.a.	n.a.
Candy, 1 oz., except as noted:								
almond, chocolate coated	tr.	tr.	.03	.15	.50	m.q.	m.q.	n.a.
almond, sugar coated	0	0	.01	.08	.30	m.q.	m.q.	n.a.
(*Bar None*), 1.5-oz. bar	21	n.a.	.03	.11	.67	n.a.	n.a.	n.a.
butterscotch	40	0	0	tr.	tr.	n.a.	m.q.	n.a.
candy corn	0	0	tr.	tr.	tr.	n.a.	n.a.	n.a.
caramel:								
plain or chocolate	tr.	tr.	.01	.05	.10	n.a.	m.q.	n.a.
plain or chocolate, w/nuts	10	tr.	.03	.05	.10	n.a.	m.q.	n.a.
chocolate coated (*Rolo*), 1.93 oz.	33	n.a.	.03	.14	.05	n.a.	m.q.	n.a.
(*Caramello*), 1.6-oz. bar	n.a.	n.a.	.02	.18	.52	n.a.	n.a.	n.a.
cherry (*Y&S Nibs*), 1 oz.	6	n.a.	<.01	.01	.03	n.a.	n.a.	n.a.
chocolate, milk:								
1 oz.	30	tr.	.02	.10	.10	n.a.	m.q.	n.a.
(*Hershey's*), 1.55-oz. bar	26	n.a.	.04	.16	.16	n.a.	m.q.	n.a.
(*Hershey's Kisses*), 1.46 oz. or								
9 pieces	25	n.a.	.03	.14	.15	n.a.	m.q.	n.a.
(*Symphony*), 1.4-oz. bar	28	n.a.	.04	.15	.13	n.a.	m.q.	n.a.
w/almonds	30	tr.	.02	.12	.20	m.q.	m.q.	n.a.
w/almonds (*Hershey's*),								
1.45-oz. bar	37	n.a.	.01	.12	.16	n.a.	m.q.	n.a.
w/crisps	30	tr.	.01	.08	.10	n.a.	m.q.	n.a.
w/crisps (*Krackel*), 1.55-oz. bar ..	31	n.a.	.02	.16	.24	n.a.	m.q.	n.a.
w/peanuts	30	tr.	.07	.07	1.40	m.q.	m.q.	n.a.
w/peanuts (*Mr. Goodbar*),								
1.75-oz. bar	20	n.a.	.02	.13	2.34	m.q.	m.q.	n.a.
chocolate, semisweet (*Hershey's*								
Special Dark), 1.45-oz. bar	8	n.a.	.01	.10	.28	n.a.	m.q.	n.a.
chocolate chips, see "Chocolate,								
baking"								
chocolate disk, sugar coated	30	tr.	.02	.06	.10	n.a.	n.a.	n.a.
chocolate flavored roll, 1 medium,								
2½″ long	tr.	tr.	tr.	.01	tr.	n.a.	n.a.	n.a.
coconut, chocolate coated:								
1 oz.	0	0	.01	.02	.10	m.q.	m.q.	n.a.
(*Mounds*), 1.9-oz. bar	0	(0)	.02	.04	.02	m.q.	m.q.	n.a.

1. *Prepared according to package directions.*

Food and Measure	A I.U.	C mg.	Thi mg.	Rib mg.	Nia mg.	B$_6$ mg.	Fol mcg.	B$_{12}$ mcg.
Candy, coconut, chocolate coated *(cont.)*								
w/almonds (*Almond Joy*),								
1.75-oz. bar	n.a.	n.a.	.01	.07	.23	m.q.	m.q.	n.a.
(*5th Avenue*), 2.1-oz. bar	18	n.a.	.01	.13	1.95	n.a.	n.a.	n.a.
fondant, mint	0	0	tr.	tr.	tr.	n.a.	n.a.	n.a.
fudge:								
chocolate or chocolate w/nuts ...	tr.	tr.	.01	.03	.10	n.a.	m.q.	n.a.
vanilla or vanilla w/nuts	tr.	tr.	.01	.04	tr.	n.a.	n.a.	n.a.
fudge, chocolate coated:								
chocolate	tr.	.01	.04	.10	0	n.a.	m.q.	n.a.
chocolate, w/nuts	tr.	.02	.04	.10	tr.	n.a.	m.q.	n.a.
w/caramel and peanuts	tr.	tr.	.05	.06	.50	n.a.	m.q.	n.a.
w/peanuts and caramel	tr.	tr.	.07	.04	1.00	n.a.	m.q.	n.a.
(*Golden Almond*), 1.6-oz. bar	27	n.a.	.03	.24	.48	m.q.	m.q.	n.a.
(*Golden III*), 1.6-oz. bar	41	n.a.	.03	.13	.07	n.a.	n.a.	n.a.
gumdrops	0	0	0	tr.	tr.	n.a.	n.a.	n.a.
hard	0	0	.10	0	0	n.a.	n.a.	n.a.
honeycomb, w/peanut butter,								
chocolate coated	tr.	tr.	.01	.03	.80	m.q.	m.q.	n.a.
jelly beans	0	0	0	tr.	tr.	n.a.	n.a.	n.a.
(*Kit Kat*), 1.625-oz. bar	32	n.a.	.02	.13	.16	n.a.	n.a.	n.a.
marshmallow, all sizes	0	0	0	tr.	tr.	n.a.	n.a.	n.a.
nougat and caramel, chocolate								
coated	10	tr.	.02	.05	.10	n.a.	m.q.	n.a.
peanut, chocolate coated	tr.	tr.	.10	.05	2.10	m.q.	m.q.	n.a.
peanut bar	0	0	.12	.02	2.70	m.q.	m.q.	n.a.
peanut brittle	0	0	.05	.01	1.00	m.q.	m.q.	n.a.
peanut butter, candy coated (*Reese's*								
Pieces), 1.85 oz. or 8 pieces ...	10	n.a.	.03	.13	2.99	m.q.	m.q.	n.a.
peanut butter, chocolate coated								
(*Reese's* Peanut Butter Cups)								
1.8 oz	10	n.a.	.02	.11	2.02	m.q.	m.q.	n.a.
peppermint, chocolate coated (*York*								
Peppermint Pattie), 1.5 oz.	n.a.	n.a.	.01	.04	.36	n.a.	n.a.	n.a.
raisin, chocolate coated	40	tr.	.02	.06	.10	m.q.	m.q.	n.a.
(*Solitaires*), 1.6 oz. or ½ pkg.	23	n.a.	.03	.23	.49	n.a.	n.a.	n.a.
toffee (*Skor*), 1.4-oz. bar	111	n.a.	.01	.13	.04	n.a.	m.q.	n.a.
vanilla creme, chocolate coated	tr.	tr.	.01	.02	tr.	n.a.	n.a.	n.a.
(*Whatchamacallit*), 1.8-oz. bar	36	n.a.	.31	.14	1.06	n.a.	m.q.	n.a.
Cantaloupe:								
½ of 5″-diam. melon	8608	113	.10	.06	1.53	.31	45.5	0
pulp, cubed, ½ cup	2579	34	.03	.02	.46	.09	13.7	0
Carambola, trimmed, cubed,								
½ cup	338	15	.02	.02	.28	n.a.	n.a.	0
Caraway seed, 1 tsp.	8	n.a.	.01	.01	.08	n.a.	n.a.	0
Cardamom, ground, 1 tsp.	0	n.a.	<.01	.01	.02	n.a.	n.a.	0
Carissa, trimmed, sliced, ½ cup. ...	30	29	.03	.05	.15	n.a.	n.a.	0
Carob flour, 1 cup	15	<1	.06	.48	1.95	.38	29.9	0

Food and Measure	A I.U.	C mg.	Thi mg.	Rib mg.	Nia mg.	B6 mg.	Fol mcg.	B12 mcg.
Carp, meat only:								
raw, 1 oz.	8	<1	(0)	(0)	m.q.	.05	m.q.	.18
baked, broiled, or microwaved[1],								
4 oz.	36	2	(0)	(0)	m.q.	.25	m.q.	1.67
Carrot, ½ cup, except as noted:								
fresh:								
raw, 7½"-long carrot, approx.								
2.5 oz.	20,253	7	.07	.04	.67	.11	10.1	0
raw, shredded	15,471	5	.05	.03	.51	.08	7.7	0
boiled, drained, sliced	19,152	2	.03	.04	.40	.19	10.8	0
canned, w/liquid, sliced	16,196	3	.02	.03	.52	.14	10.0	0
canned, drained, sliced	10,055	2	.01	.02	.40	.08	6.7	0
frozen, boiled, drained, sliced	12,922	2	.02	.03	.32	.09	7.9	0
Carrot juice, canned, 6 fl. oz.	47,381	16	.17	.10	.71	.40	7.0	0
Casaba, pulp, cubed, ½ cup	26	14	.05	.02	.34	n.a.	n.a.	0
Cashew, 1 oz.:								
dry-roasted	0	0	.06	.06	.40	.07	19.7	0
oil-roasted	0	0	.12	.05	.51	.07	19.2	0
Cashew butter, 1 tbsp.	0	0	.09	.05	.45	.07	19.4	0
Catfish, channel, meat only, raw,								
1 oz.	n.a.	(0)	.05	.12	2.43	m.q.	m.q.	m.q.
Catsup, 1 tbsp.	152	2	.01	.01	.21	.03	2.0	0
Cauliflower:								
fresh:								
raw, 3 flowerets, 5 oz.	9	40	.04	.03	.35	.13	37.0	0
raw, 1" pieces, ½ cup	8	36	.04	.03	.32	.12	33.1	0
boiled, drained, 3 flowerets	8	30	.03	.03	.30	.11	27.6	0
boiled, drained, 1" pieces, ½ cup	9	34	.04	.03	.34	.13	31.7	0
frozen, boiled, drained, 1" pieces,								
½ cup	20	28	.03	.05	.28	.08	36.9	0
Celery:								
raw, 7½"-long stalk, 1.6 oz.	54	3	.02	.02	.13	.04	11.0	0
raw, diced, ½ cup	80	4	.03	.03	.19	.05	17.0	0
boiled, drained, diced, ½ cup.	99	5	.03	.04	.24	.07	16.0	0
Cereal, ready to eat, 1 oz., except								
as noted:								
amaranth:								
(*Health Valley Amaranth Flakes*),								
½ cup	26	1	.02	.03	.74	.02	3.1	0
w/bananas (*Health Valley*),								
½ cup	160	1	.09	.14	1.60	.02	4.2	0
w/raisins (*Health Valley Amaranth*								
Crunch), ¼ cup.	7	<1	.09	.07	.40	.03	13.1	0
bran (see also "oat bran," "rice								
bran," and "wheat bran,"								
below):								
(*All Bran*)	750	15	.38	.43	5.00	.50	.1	n.a.

1. *Without added ingredients.*

Food and Measure	A I.U.	C mg.	Thi mg.	Rib mg.	Nia mg.	B6 mg.	Fol mcg.	B12 mcg.
Cereal, ready to eat, bran *(cont.)*								
(*All Bran* Extra Fiber)	750	15	.38	.43	5.00	.50	.1	2.00
(*Bran Buds*)	750	15	.38	.43	5.00	.50	.1	n.a.
(*40+ Bran Flakes*)	750	tr.	.38	.43	5.00	.50	.1	2.00
(*Fruitful Bran*), 1 oz. cereal								
w/.3 oz. fruit	750	tr.	.38	.43	5.00	.50	.1	2.00
(*Kellogg's* Raisin Bran), 1 oz.								
cereal w/.4 oz. fruit	750	tr.	.38	.43	5.00	.50	.1	2.00
(*Quaker Crunchy Bran*)	0	0	.23	.31	6.30	.50	177.0	.96
w/apples and cinnamon (*Health*								
Valley 100% Natural), ¼ cup ...	<1	1	.09	.04	1.20	.03	10.7	0
w/raisins (*Health Valley* Flakes),								
½ cup	<1	1	.15	.03	2.60	.13	31.8	0
w/raisins (*Health Valley* 100%								
Natural), ¼ cup	0	1	.03	.34	4.00	.08	18.0	0
corn:								
(*Corn Pops*)	750	15	.38	.43	5.00	.50	.1	n.a.
(*Health Valley Fruit Lites*), ½ cup	40	<1	.05	.01	.17	.03	2.0	0
(*Health Valley Lites* Puffed Corn),								
½ cup	73	<1	.03	.01	.27	.03	3.4	0
(*Kellogg's Corn Flakes*)	750	15	.38	.43	5.00	.50	.1	n.a.
(*Kellogg's Frosted Flakes*)	750	15	.38	.43	5.00	.50	.1	n.a.
(*Nut & Honey Crunch*)	750	15	.38	.43	5.00	.50	.1	n.a.
(*Nut & Honey Crunch* Biscuits) ..	n.a.	tr.	.38	.43	5.00	.50	.1	2.00
(*Nutri•Grain* Corn)	n.a.	15	.38	.43	5.00	.50	.1	2.00
blue (*Health Valley* Corn Flakes),								
½ cup	203	0	.15	.02	1.20	.01	<.1	0
granola, see "mixed grain," below								
mixed grain:								
(*Apple Jacks*)	750	15	.38	.43	5.00	.50	.1	n.a.
(*Cap'n Crunch*)	0	0	.36	.28	5.15	.51	157.0	1.37
(*Cap'n Crunch's Crunchberries*) ..	0	0	.44	.28	5.08	.54	147.0	1.33
(*Cap'n Crunch's Peanut Butter*								
Crunch)	0	0	.38	.29	6.22	.64	146.0	1.12
(*Crispix*)	750	15	.38	.43	5.00	.50	.1	n.a.
(*Crunchy Nut Oh!s*)	0	0	.55	.37	7.42	.65	190.0	1.72
(*Health Valley Fiber 7* Flakes),								
½ cup	73	1	.03	.04	1.70	.04	16.8	0
(*Honey Graham Oh!s*)	0	0	.52	.40	7.59	.73	193.0	1.43
(*King Vitaman*)	1500	24	.60	.68	8.00	.60	160.0	2.40
(*Müeslix* Bran), 1 oz. cereal								
w/.4 oz. fruit and nuts	1250	tr.	.38	.43	5.00	.50	.1	1.00
(*Müeslix Five Grain*), 1 oz. cereal								
w/.45 oz. fruit and nuts	206	0	.39	.44	5.00	.52	.1	1.50
(*Nutri•Grain* Nuggets)	n.a.	15	.38	.43	5.00	.50	.1	2.00
(*Nutrific*), 1 oz. cereal w/.5 oz.								
fruit and nuts	1250	tr.	.38	.43	5.00	.50	.1	2.00

Food and Measure	A I.U.	C mg.	Thi mg.	Rib mg.	Nia mg.	B₆ mg.	Fol mcg.	B₁₂ mcg.
(*Product 19*)	750	60	1.50	1.70	20.00	2.00	.4	6.00
(*Quaker* 100% Natural)	0	0	.08	.07	.40	.05	12.0	.26
(*Special K*)	750	15	.53	.60	7.00	.70	.1	n.a.
w/almonds (*Sun Country* 100% Natural Granola)	0	0	.08	.05	.24	.03	9.0	0
almond date (*Health Valley Healthy Crunch*), ¼ cup	1	3	.07	.15	2.80	.03	18.2	0
almond raisin (*Nutri•Grain*), 1 oz. cereal and .4 oz. fruit and nuts	n.a.	tr.	.38	.43	5.00	.50	.1	2.00
apple cinnamon (*Health Valley Healthy Crunch*), ¼ cup	<1	3	.07	.08	2.60	.03	16.7	0
apple and cinnamon (*Quaker* 100% Natural)	38	0	.09	.11	.39	.03	4.0	.05
w/apple and raisins (*Apple Raisin Crisp*), 1 oz. cereal w/.3 oz. fruit	750	tr.	.38	.43	5.00	.50	.1	2.00
w/bananas and Hawaiian fruit (*Health Valley Sprouts 7*), ¼ cup	212	1	.12	.17	1.60	.03	3.6	0
w/fiber nuggets or fruit and nuts (*Just Right*)	750	tr.	1.50	1.70	20.00	2.00	.4	6.00
w/raisins (*Health Valley Sprouts 7*), ¼ cup	<1	1	.06	.07	2.00	.03	4.4	0
w/raisins (*Sun Country* Granola)	0	0	.08	.05	.21	.03	8.0	.05
raisin and date (*Quaker* 100% Natural)	0	0	.07	.05	.38	.04	10.0	0
w/raisins and dates (*Sun Country* Granola)	0	0	.07	.05	.21	.03	8.0	.05
oat:								
(*Life*)	0	0	.46	.45	5.58	.04	19.0	n.a.
(*Quaker Oat Squares*)	1616	0	.41	.34	6.89	.69	156.0	2.31
cinnamon (*Life*)	0	0	.50	.51	6.84	.05	19.0	n.a.
oat bran:								
(*Common Sense*)	750	tr.	.38	.43	5.00	.50	.1	2.00
(*Cracklin' Oat Bran*)	750	tr.	.38	.43	5.00	.50	.1	2.00
(*Health Valley* Flakes), ½ cup	5	<1	.15	.11	1.90	.03	12.8	0
(*Oat Bran O's*), ¾ cup	10	3	.10	.07	.63	.26	22.9	0
almond crunch (*Real*), ¼ cup	277	2	.12	.22	3.30	.05	19.5	0
w/almonds and dates (*Health Valley* Flakes), ½ cup	8	<1	.09	.07	.40	.04	n.a.	0
fruit, Hawaiian (*Real*), ¼ cup	494	2	.13	.09	.38	.01	21.6	0
fruit and nut (*Oat Bran O's*), ¾ cup	837	1	.12	.08	.85	.05	21.4	0
w/raisins (*Common Sense*), 1 oz. cereal w/.3 oz. raisins	750	tr.	.38	.43	5.00	.50	.1	2.00
w/raisins (*Health Valley* Flakes), ½ cup	8	<1	.09	.06	.38	.03	11.6	0

Food and Measure	A I.U.	C mg.	Thi mg.	Rib mg.	Nia mg.	B$_6$ mg.	Fol mcg.	B$_{12}$ mcg.
Cereal, ready to eat, oat bran *(cont.)*								
raisin nut (*Real*), ¼ cup	144	2	.13	.83	.17	.06	19.7	0
rice:								
(*Cocoa/Frosted Krispies*)	750	15	.53	.60	7.00	.70	.1	n.a.
(*Health Valley Fruit Lites*), ½ cup	1	1	.04	.01	.28	.01	.23	0
(*Health Valley Lites* Puffed Rice),								
½ cup	0	1	.03	0	.40	0	0	0
(*Quaker* Puffed Rice), .5 oz	0	0	.05	.01	.80	.01	1.0	n.a.
(*Rice Krispies*)	750	15	.53	.60	7.00	.70	.1	n.a.
rice bran (*Rice Bran O's*), ¾ cup . . .	8	1	.18	.04	2.30	.02	.2	0
rice bran, w/almonds and dates								
(*Health Valley*), ½ cup	4	2	.37	.8	3.00	.03	.6	0
wheat:								
(*Apple Cinnamon Squares*)	0	tr.	.38	.43	5.00	.50	.1	2.00
(*Blueberry Squares*)	n.a.	tr.	.38	.43	5.00	.50	.1	1.50
(*Frosted Mini Wheats* Regular/Bite								
Size)	n.a.	tr.	.38	.43	5.00	.50	.1	2.00
(*Health Valley Fruit Lites*), ½ cup	1	<1	.07	.01	.30	.04	5.2	0
(*Health Valley Lites* Puffed Wheat),								
½ cup	0	1	.05	.01	.40	.04	7.7	0
(*Honey Smacks*)	750	15	.38	.43	5.00	.50	.1	n.a.
(*Nutri•Grain* Biscuits)	n.a.	tr.	.38	.43	5.00	.50	.1	2.00
(*Nutri•Grain* Wheat)	n.a.	15	.38	.43	5.00	.50	.1	2.00
(*Nutri•Grain* Wheat & Raisins),								
1 oz. cereal and .4 oz. fruit								
and nuts	n.a.	tr.	.38	.43	5.00	.50	.1	2.00
(*Quaker* Puffed Wheat), 5 oz.	0	0	.07	.03	1.61	.02	4.0	.05
(*Quaker* Shredded Wheat),								
2 biscuits	0	0	.08	.04	1.70	.09	18.0	n.a.
(*Raisin Squares*)	n.a.	tr.	.38	.43	5.00	.50	.1	2.00
(*S.W. Graham*)	n.a.	tr.	.38	.43	5.00	.50	.1	2.00
(*S.W. Graham* Cinnamon)	n.a.	n.a.	.38	.43	5.00	.50	.1	2.00
(*Strawberry Squares*)	n.a.	tr.	.38	.43	5.00	.50	.1	2.00
wheat bran, toasted (*Kretschmer*) . .	0	0	.28	.08	5.29	.17	49.0	.06
Cereal, cooking, uncooked, 1 pkt.,								
except as noted:								
corn grits, yellow, enriched, regular								
or quick[1]	125	n.a.	.18	.11	1.41	.04	1.4	n.a.
oat and oatmeal:								
(*Instant Quaker*)	1237	0	.44	.21	3.64	.47	122.0	n.a.
(*Quaker* Quick/Old Fashioned),								
⅓ cup or ⅔ cup cooked	26	0	.14	.03	.22	.03	7.0	n.a.
(*Quaker Extra*)	5115	60	1.50	1.70	21.57	2.00	400.0	6.00
apple and cinnamon (*Instant*								
Quaker)	1233	<1	.37	.21	3.69	.43	113.0	0
apples and spice (*Quaker Extra*)	5001	60	1.50	1.70	20.00	2.00	400.0	6.00

1. *White corn grits contain only a trace of vitamin A.*

Food and Measure	A I.U.	C mg.	Thi mg.	Rib mg.	Nia mg.	B_6 mg.	Fol mcg.	B_{12} mcg.
cinnamon and spice (*Instant*								
Quaker)	1309	0	.39	.23	3.72	.46	120.0	n.a.
maple and brown sugar (*Instant*								
Quaker)	1380	0	.40	.23	3.77	.44	116.0	n.a.
peaches and cream (*Instant*								
Quaker)	1245	0	.33	.22	3.65	.41	121.0	n.a.
raisin and cinnamon (*Quaker*								
Extra)	5001	60	1.50	1.70	20.00	2.00	400.0	6.00
raisin, date and walnut (*Instant*								
Quaker)	988	0	.30	.20	3.14	.37	95.0	n.a.
raisins and spice (*Instant Quaker*)	1298	0	.36	.23	3.68	.44	103.0	.08
strawberries and cream (*Instant*								
Quaker)	1186	0	.31	.21	3.25	.37	118.0	n.a.
oat bran:								
(*Quaker/Mother's*), ⅓ cup or								
⅔ cup cooked	26	0	.27	.08	.28	.04	14.0	n.a.
apples and cinnamon or raisins and								
spice (*Health Valley* Natural),								
¼ cup	<1	1	.06	.06	1.20	.08	24.1	0
wheat, farina, enriched	n.a.	n.a.	.16	.10	1.15	.02	6.8	n.a.
wheat, whole (*Quaker/Mother's*								
Natural), ⅓ cup or ⅔ cup								
cooked	26	0	.09	.03	1.30	.04	13.0	n.a.
Chayote:								
raw, 1 medium, approx. 7.2 oz.	114	22	.06	.08	1.02	n.a.	n.a.	0
boiled, drained, 1″ pieces, ½ cup ...	37	6	.02	.03	.34	n.a.	n.a.	0
Cheese, 1 oz., except as noted:								
American, pasturized process	343	0	.01	.10	.02	.02	2.0	.20
blue	204	0	.01	.11	.29	.05	10.0	.35
brick	307	0	<.01	.10	.03	.02	6.0	.36
brie	189	0	.02	.15	.11	.07	18.0	.47
Camembert	262	0	.01	.14	.18	.06	18.0	.37
cheddar	300	0	.01	.11	.02	.02	5.0	.23
colby	293	0	<.01	.11	.03	.02	m.q.	.23
cottage, ½ cup not packed:								
creamed, large curd	183	tr.	.02	.18	.14	.08	13.5	.70
creamed, small curd	171	tr.	.02	.17	.13	.07	12.6	.65
creamed, w/fruit	139	tr.	.02	.15	.11	.06	11.0	.56
dry curd	22	0	.02	.10	.11	.06	10.9	.60
lowfat 2%	79	tr.	.03	.21	.16	.09	15.0	.81
lowfat 1%	42	tr.	.02	.19	.15	.08	14.0	.72
cream	405	0	.01	.06	.03	.01	4.0	.12
Edam	260	0	.01	.11	.02	.02	5.0	.44
fontina	333	0	.01	.06	.04	n.a.	m.q.	m.q.
Gouda	183	0	.01	.10	.02	.02	6.0	m.q.
Gruyère	346	0	.02	.08	.03	.02	3.0	.45
Limburger	363	0	.02	.14	.05	.02	16.0	.30

Food and Measure	A I.U.	C mg.	Thi mg.	Rib mg.	Nia mg.	B_6 mg.	Fol mcg.	B_{12} mcg.
Cheese *(cont.)*								
mozzarella:								
whole milk	225	0	<.01	.07	.02	.02	2.0	.19
low-moisture	256	0	.01	.08	.03	.02	2.0	.21
part skim	166	0	.01	.09	.03	.02	2.0	.23
part skim, low-moisture	178	0	.01	.10	.03	.02	3.0	.26
Muenster	318	0	<.01	.09	.03	.02	3.0	.42
Neufchâtel	321	0	<.01	.06	.04	.01	3.0	.08
Parmesan:								
grated	199	0	.01	.11	.09	.03	2.0	m.q.
grated, 1 tbsp.	35	0	<.01	.02	.02	.01	tr.	m.q.
hard	171	0	.01	.09	.08	.03	2.0	m.q.
pimiento, pasteurized process	358	0	.01	.10	.02	.02	2.0	.20
Port du Salut	378	0	0	.07	.02	.02	5.0	.43
provolone	231	0	.01	.09	.04	.02	3.0	.42
ricotta, whole milk, ½ cup	608	0	.02	.24	.13	.05	m.q.	.41
ricotta, part skim, ½ cup	536	0	.03	.23	.10	.03	m.q.	.36
Romano	162	0	n.a.	.11	.02	n.a.	2.0	m.q.
Roquefort	297	0	.01	.17	.21	.04	14.0	.18
Swiss	240	0	.01	.10	.03	.02	2.0	.48
Swiss, pasteurized process	229	0	<.01	.08	.01	.01	m.q.	.35
Tilsit, whole milk	296	0	.02	.10	.06	n.a.	m.q.	.60
Cheese food, 1 oz.:								
American, cold pack	200	0	.01	.13	.02	.04	2.0	.36
American, pasteurized process	259	0	.01	.13	.04	n.a.	m.q.	.32
Swiss, pasteurized process	243	0	<.01	.11	.03	n.a.	m.q.	.65
Cheese spread, American,								
pasteurized process, 1 oz.	223	0	.01	.12	.04	.03	2.0	.11
Cheese stick or straw, 5″ long, 10								
pieces or 2.1 oz.	230	0	.01	.10	.20	n.a.	n.a.	n.a.
Cherimoya, trimmed, 1 oz.	3	3	.03	.03	.37	n.a.	n.a.	0
Cherry, ½ cup, except as noted:								
fresh:								
sour, red, trimmed	995	8	.02	.03	.31	.03	5.8	0
sour, red, w/pits	661	5	.02	.02	.21	.02	3.9	0
sweet, trimmed	155	5	.04	.04	.29	.03	3.1	0
sweet, 10 medium, approx.								
2.6 oz.	146	5	.03	.04	.27	.02	2.8	0
canned, sour, red:								
in water	920	3	.02	.05	.22	.05	9.8	0
in light syrup	914	3	.02	.05	.21	.06	9.7	0
in heavy syrup	914	3	.02	.05	.22	.06	9.7	0
canned, sweet:								
in water	198	3	.03	.05	.51	.04	m.q.	0
in juice	156	3	.02	.03	.51	m.q.	m.q.	0
in light syrup	197	5	.03	.05	.51	.04	m.q.	0
in heavy syrup	199	5	.03	.05	.51	.04	m.q.	0
frozen, sour, red, unsweetened	675	1	.03	.03	.11	.05	3.5	0
frozen, sweet, sweetened	245	1	.04	.06	.23	m.q.	m.q.	0

Food and Measure	A I.U.	C mg.	Thi mg.	Rib mg.	Nia mg.	B6 mg.	Fol mcg.	B12 mcg.
Chestnut, Chinese, shelled, 1 oz.:								
raw	57	10	.05	.05	.23	m.q.	m.q.	0
roasted	1	m.q.	.04	.03	.43	m.q.	m.q.	0
Chestnut, European, shelled, 1 oz.:								
raw, unpeeled	8	12	.07	.05	.34	.11	17.6	0
dried, unpeeled	0	4	.08	.10	.24	.19	31.0	0
roasted	7	7	.07	.05	.38	.14	19.9	0
Chestnut, Japanese, shelled, 1 oz.:								
raw	10	8	.10	.05	.43	m.q.	m.q.	0
boiled or steamed	4	3	.04	.02	.15	m.q.	m.q.	0
dried	24	17	.23	.11	.99	.m.q.	m.q.	0
roasted	21	8	.13	.07	.20	m.q.	m.q.	0
Chicken[1], fresh, 4 oz., except as noted:								
broiler-fryer, fried, flour coated, meat w/skin:								
4 oz.	101	0	.10	.22	10.20	.46	6.8	.35
dark meat	118	0	.11	.27	7.76	.36	9.1	.34
light meat	77	0	.09	.15	13.65	.61	4.5	.37
back meat	139	0	.12	.27	8.27	.34	9.1	.32
breast meat	57	0	.09	.15	15.58	.66	4.5	.39
drumstick, 1.7 oz. (2.6-oz. raw drumstick w/bone)	41	0	.04	.11	2.96	.17	4.0	.16
leg, 4 oz. (5.5-oz. raw leg w/bone)	103	0	.10	.26	7.33	.38	9.0	.35
thigh, 2.2 oz. (2.9-oz. raw thigh w/bone)	61	0	.06	.15	4.31	.21	5.0	.19
wing, 1.1 oz. (2.2-oz. raw wing w/bone)	40	0	.02	.04	2.14	.13	1.0	.09
broiler-fryer, roasted:								
meat w/skin	183	0	.07	.19	9.62	.45	5.7	.34
meat only	60	0	.08	.20	10.40	.53	6.8	.37
skin only, 1 oz.	74	0	.01	.04	1.58	.03	.6	.06
dark meat w/skin	228	0	.07	.23	7.21	.35	7.9	.33
dark meat only	82	0	.08	.26	7.43	.41	9.1	.36
light meat w/skin	125	0	.07	.13	12.63	.59	3.4	.36
light meat only	33	0	.07	.13	14.09	.68	4.5	.39
roaster, roasted:								
meat w/skin	94	0	.06	.16	8.41	.40	5.7	.31
meat only	46	0	.07	.17	8.94	.46	5.7	.32
dark meat only	61	0	.07	.22	6.50	.35	7.9	.31
light meat only	28	0	.07	.11	11.87	.61	3.4	.35
stewing, stewed:								
meat w/skin	149	0	.11	.27	6.57	.28	5.7	.26
meat only	127	0	.13	.31	7.27	.35	6.8	.29

1. *Prepared without added ingredients, except as noted.*

Food and Measure	A I.U.	C mg.	Thi mg.	Rib mg.	Nia mg.	B₆ mg.	Fol mcg.	B₁₂ mcg.
Chicken, stewing, stewed *(cont.)*								
dark meat only	164	0	.15	.39	5.17	.27	9.1	.28
light meat only	83	0	.11	.22	9.68	.44	4.5	.31
capon, roasted, meat w/skin	77	0	.08	.19	10.15	.49	6.8	.37
Chicken, canned, boned, w/broth,								
5-oz. can	m.q.	3	.02	.18	8.99	.50	m.q.	.42
Chicken giblets, simmered[1], 4 oz.	8427	9	.10	1.08	4.65	.39	426.4	11.50
Chicken gizzard, simmered[1],								
4 oz.	213	2	.03	.28	4.51	.14	60.1	2.20
Chicken gravy, canned, ¼ cup ...	220	0	.01	.03	.26	.01	m.q.	m.q.
Chicken heart, see "Heart"								
Chicken liver, see "Liver"								
Chick-pea, ½ cup:								
boiled	22	1	.10	.05	.43	.11	141.0	0
canned, w/liquid	29	5	.04	.04	.17	.57	80.1	0
Chicory, witloof, raw, 5–7″ head,								
approx. 2.1 oz.	0	5	.04	.07	.27	.02	n.a.	0
Chicory greens, raw, chopped,								
½ cup	3600	22	.05	.09	.45	n.a.	n.a.	0
Chicory root, raw, 1″ pieces,								
½ cup	3	2	.02	.01	.18	n.a.	n.a.	0
Chili, canned:								
w/beans:								
½ cup	432	2	.06	.13	.46	.17	m.q.	.01
(*Wolf* Brand), 1 cup	3940	m.q.	.09	.82	2.68	.25	32.0	0
extra spicy (*Wolf* Brand), scant								
cup	3690	m.q.	.08	.77	2.51	.23	30.0	0
vegetarian, mild (*Health Valley*),								
4 oz.	750	1	.09	.18	1.20	.11	2.9	0
vegetarian, spicy (*Health Valley*),								
4 oz.	750	1	.09	.18	1.20	.10	2.9	0
w/out beans (*Wolf* Brand), 1 cup ...	4770	m.q.	.11	1.27	3.86	.10	25.0	1.00
w/out beans, extra spicy (*Wolf*								
Brand), scant cup	4470	m.q.	.10	1.19	3.62	.09	23.0	1.00
w/lentils, vegetarian, mild (*Health*								
Valley), 4 oz.	750	1	.06	.14	1.60	.10	6.8	0
w/macaroni (*Wolf* Brand Chili Mac),								
scant cup	2450	m.q.	.08	.53	3.51	.13	40.0	2.00
Chili beans, Mexican-style (*Van*								
Camp's), 1 cup	1595	1	.12	.14	.89	n.a.	n.a.	n.a.
Chili powder, 1 tsp.	908	2	.01	.02	.21	n.a.	n.a.	0
Chili sauce, hot dog (*Wolf* Brand),								
approx. ⅙ cup	410	m.q.	.06	.10	.35	.05	9.0	0
Chitterlings, pork, simmered[1],								
4 oz.	0	0	0	.09	.11	m.q.	m.q.	m.q.
Chives, raw, chopped, 1 tbsp.	192	2	<.01	.01	.02	.01	m.q.	0
Chocolate, see "Candy"								

1. *Without added ingredients.*

Food and Measure	A I.U.	C mg.	Thi mg.	Rib mg.	Nia mg.	B₆ mg.	Fol mcg.	B₁₂ mcg.
Chocolate, baking:								
chips, semisweet, ¼ cup	8	tr.	.03	.04	.23	n.a.	n.a.	n.a.
unsweetened, 1 oz.	10	0	.01	.07	.40	n.a.	n.a.	0
Chocolate flavor drink mix,								
powder:								
2–3 heaping tsp. or ¾ oz.	4	<1	.01	.03	.11	<.01	n.a.	0
(*Carnation* Instant Breakfast),								
1 pkt.	1750	27	.30	.17	5.00	.40	100.0	.60
malt (*Carnation* Instant Breakfast),								
1 pkt.	1750	27	.30	.10	5.00	.40	100.0	.60
Chocolate milk, 1 cup:								
whole	302	2	.09	.41	.31	.10	12.0	.84
lowfat 2%[1]	500	2	.09	.41	.32	.10	12.0	.85
lowfat 1%[1]	500	2	.10	.42	.32	.10	12.0	.86
Chocolate syrup:								
w/out added nutrients, 2 tbsp. or								
1 fl. oz.	11	<1	<.01	.02	.12	<.01	1.5	0
w/added nutrients, 1 tbsp.	817	<1	<.01	.16	6.31	<.01	m.q.	0
Cinnamon, ground, 1 tsp.	6	1	<.01	<.01	.03	n.a.	n.a.	0
Cisco, smoked, 4 oz.	1069	tr.	.05	.18	2.62	.30	2.4	4.83
Citrus fruit juice drink, frozen[2],								
6 fl. oz.	78	50	.03	n.a.	.33	.04	3.7	0
Clam, mixed species, meat only:								
raw, 1 oz.	85	tr.	n.a.	.06	.50	m.q.	m.q.	14.01
raw, 9 large or 20 small, approx.								
6.3 oz.	540	tr.	n.a.	.38	3.18	m.q.	m.q.	89.00
Clam, canned, drained, 4 oz.	646	tr.	n.a.	.48	3.80	m.q.	m.q.	112.14
Clove, ground, 1 tsp.	11	2	<.01	.01	.03	n.a.	n.a.	0
Cocoa mix, powder:								
w/out added nutrients, 1-oz. pkt. or								
3–4 heaping tsp.	4	1	.03	.16	.17	.03	0	.38
w/added nutrients, 1.1-oz. pkt.	500	6	.15	.17	2.00	n.a.	n.a.	n.a.
(*Carnation* 70 Calorie), 1 pkt.	3	<1	.03	.11	.07	.03	4.0	.30
chocolate:								
fudge (*Carnation*), 1 pkt.	5	<1	.03	.11	.12	<.01	3.2	.12
milk (*Carnation*), 1 pkt. or								
4 heaping tsp.	3	<1	.04	.15	.12	.04	2.0	.23
rich (*Carnation*), 1 pkt. or								
4 heaping tsp.	3	<1	.04	.15	.12	.04	1.0	.17
w/marshmallows (*Carnation*), 1 pkt.								
or 4 heaping tsp.	3	<1	.03	.14	.12	.04	1.0	.16
reduced calorie[3], 53-oz. pkt.	n.a.	0	.04	.21	.16	.05	2.2	n.a.
Coconut:								
raw, 1 piece, 2" × 2" × ½", approx.								
1.6 oz.	0	2	.03	.01	.24	.02	11.9	0

1. *Vitamin A added.*
2. *Diluted according to package directions.*
3. *Aspartame sweetened.*

Food and Measure	A I.U.	C mg.	Thi mg.	Rib mg.	Nia mg.	B₆ mg.	Fol mcg.	B₁₂ mcg.
Coconut *(cont.)*								
dried, unsweetened, 1 oz.	0	<1	.02	.03	.17	.09	2.6	0
dried, sweetened, shredded,								
1 oz.	0	<1	.01	.01	.13	m.q.	m.q.	0
Cod, Atlantic, meat only:								
raw, 1 oz.	11	<1	.02	.02	.58	.07	m.q.	.26
baked, broiled, or microwaved[1],								
4 oz.	52	1	.10	.09	2.85	.32	m.q.	1.19
dried, salted, 1 oz.	40	1	.08	.07	2.10	.24	m.q.	2.80
Cod, canned, Atlantic, w/liquid,								
4 oz.	52	1	.10	.09	2.84	.32	m.q.	1.19
Coffee, brewed, 6 fl. oz.	0	0	0	0	.39	0	.3	0
Coffee, flavored, instant[2]:								
cappuccino flavor, 6 fl. oz.	0	0	.02	.01	.32	0	0	0
mocha flavor, 6 fl. oz.	0	0	<.01	<.01	.26	0	0	0
Coffee flavor drink mix								
(*Carnation* Instant Breakfast),								
1 pkt.	1750	27	.30	.17	5.00	.40	100.00	.60
Collards, chopped, ½ cup:								
fresh, raw	599	4	.01	.01	.07	.01	2.0	0
fresh, boiled, drained	1745	8	.01	.03	.19	.03	4.0	0
frozen, boiled, drained	5084	23	.04	.10	.54	.10	64.7	0
Cookie:								
almond date (*Health Valley Fruit*								
Jumbos), 1 piece	1	3	.06	.03	1.20	.03	4.3	0
amaranth (*Health Valley*), 1 piece ...	88	3	.09	.03	.40	.03	4.3	0
animal crackers, 10 pieces or .9 oz.	30	tr.	.01	.03	.10	n.a.	m.q.	n.a.
animal crackers, oat bran (*Health*								
Valley), 7 pieces	2	3	.13	.04	.70	.07	10.1	0
apricot-almond (*Health Valley Fancy*								
Fruit Chunks), 2 pieces	217	3	.07	.03	.40	.04	6.2	0
butter, thin, rich, 10 pieces or								
1.8 oz.	330	0	.02	.03	.20	n.a.	m.q.	n.a.
chocolate chip, 4 pieces or 1.5 oz. ...	50	tr.	.10	.23	1.00	n.a.	m.q.	n.a.
coconut bar, 10 pieces or 3.2 oz.	140	0	.04	.05	.40	m.q.	m.q.	n.a.
date pecan (*Health Valley Fancy Fruit*								
Chunks), 2 pieces	6	3	.08	.03	.40	.04	6.2	0
fig bar, square, 4 pieces or 2 oz. ...	60	tr.	.08	.07	.70	m.q.	m.q.	n.a.
fruit:								
(*Health Valley Fruit & Fitness*),								
5 pieces	257	n.a.	.14	.16	1.30	.12	20.0	0
tropical (*Health Valley Fancy Fruit*								
Chunks), 2 pieces	216	3	.08	.03	.40	.05	7.6	0
tropical (*Health Valley Fruit*								
Jumbos), 1 piece	51	3	.09	.03	.40	.02	4.2	0
gingersnap, 10 pieces or 2.5 oz. ...	50	tr.	.03	.04	.30	n.a.	m.q.	n.a.

1. *Without added ingredients.*
2. *Prepared according to package directions.*

Food and Measure	A I.U.	C mg.	Thi mg.	Rib mg.	Nia mg.	B₆ mg.	Fol mcg.	B₁₂ mcg.
graham cracker:								
plain, 1 square piece	0	0	.02	.03	.60	m.q.	m.q.	n.a.
amaranth (*Health Valley Amaranth Graham Crackers*), 7 pieces ...	0	5	.36	.20	.96	.06	11.1	0
chocolate coated, 1 piece, 2½″ × 2″	10	(0)	.01	.04	.20	m.q.	m.q.	n.a.
honey, fancy (*Health Valley*), 7 pieces	1	4	.23	.24	2.90	.03	9.2	0
oat bran (*Health Valley*), 7 pieces	1	4	.01	.04	.59	.07	12.4	0
sugar honey, 2 square pieces	m.q.	(0)	tr.	.02	.10	m.q.	m.q.	n.a.
honey:								
cinnamon (*Health Valley Honey Jumbos*), 1 piece	3	3	.06	.03	.80	.02	4.0	0
oat bran, fancy (*Health Valley Honey Jumbos*), 1 piece	1	<1	.08	.15	.25	.01	13.3	0
peanut butter crisp (*Health Valley Honey Jumbos*), 1 piece	<1	2	.01	.11	.34	.02	5.2	0
ladyfinger, 4 pieces or 1.6 oz.	290	0	.03	.06	.10	n.a.	m.q.	n.a.
macaroon, 2 pieces or 1.3 oz.	0	0	.02	.06	.20	n.a.	m.q.	n.a.
molasses, 1 piece or 1.1 oz.	30	0	.01	.02	.20	n.a.	m.q.	n.a.
oat bran (*Health Valley Fruit Jumbos*), 1 piece	8	<1	.12	.07	.40	.03	5.0	0
oat bran fruit and nut (*Health Valley*), 2 pieces	3	3	.11	.05	.50	.06	9.5	0
oatmeal raisin, 4 pieces or 1.8 oz. ..	40	0	.09	.08	1.00	m.q.	m.q.	n.a.
peanut (*Health Valley Fancy Peanut Chunks*), 2 pieces	4	3	.02	.12	.55	.04	8.3	0
raisin nut (*Health Valley Fruit Jumbos*), 1 piece	1	3	.09	.03	.40	.03	4.3	0
raisin oat bran (*Health Valley Fancy Fruit Chunks*), 2 pieces	4	2	.07	.03	.30	.04	5.3	0
sandwich, chocolate or vanilla, 4 pieces or 1.4 oz.	0	0	.09	.07	.80	n.a.	m.q.	n.a.
shortbread, 4 small or 1.1. oz.	30	0	.10	.09	.90	n.a.	m.q.	n.a.
tofu (*The Great Tofu Cookie*), 2 pieces	99	3	.04	.05	.46	0	1.1	0
vanilla wafer, 10 pieces or 1.4 oz. ..	50	0	.07	.10	1.00	n.a.	m.q.	n.a.
vanilla wafer, brown-edge, 10 pieces or 2 oz.	80	0	.01	.04	.20	n.a.	m.q.	n.a.
wheat-free (*The Great Wheat Free Cookie*), 4 pieces	3	4	.07	.08	.39	0	1.3	0
Cookie, refrigerated:								
chocolate chip, 4 pieces or 1.7 oz. ...	30	0	.06	.10	.90	n.a.	m.q.	n.a.
sugar, 4 pieces or 1.7 oz.	40	0	.09	.06	1.10	m.q.	m.q.	n.a.
Coriander, raw, 9 plants, approx. .8 oz.	553	2	.02	.02	.15	m.q.	m.q.	0
Coriander seed, 1 tsp.	tr.	tr.	<.01	.01	.04	m.q.	m.q.	0

Food and Measure	A I.U.	C mg.	Thi mg.	Rib mg.	Nia mg.	B6 mg.	Fol mcg.	B12 mcg.
Corn:								
fresh:								
raw, 3.2-oz. ear	253	6	.18	.05	1.53	.05	41.2	0
boiled, drained, 3.2-oz. ear	167	5	.17	.06	1.24	.05	35.7	0
boiled, drained, ½ cup	178	5	.18	.06	1.32	.05	38.1	0
canned:								
w/liquid, ½ cup	153	9	.03	.08	1.20	.05	48.8	0
cream style, ½ cup	124	6	.03	.07	1.23	.08	57.3	0
vacuum pack, ½ cup	253	9	.04	.08	1.23	.06	51.8	0
frozen, boiled, 4-oz. ear	133	3	.11	.04	.96	.14	19.2	0
frozen, boiled, drained, ½ cup	204	2	.06	.06	1.05	.08	18.7	0
Corn, whole-grain, 1 cup	n.a.	0	.64	.33	6.02	1.03	n.a.	0
Corn bran, crude, 1 cup	54	0	.01	.08	2.08	.12	3.0	0
Corn chips and similar snacks, 1 oz.:								
(*Health Valley* Regular/No Salt Added)	97	2	.06	.02	.36	.03	4.6	0
w/cheddar cheese (*Health Valley*)....	114	2	.06	.02	.36	.03	4.9	.01
tortilla (*Buenitos* Regular/No Salt Added)	109	2	.08	.02	.42	.05	5.2	0
Corn flour, 1 cup:								
whole grain	n.a.	0	.29	.09	2.22	n.a.	30.0	0
masa, enriched	n.a.	0	1.63	.86	11.22	.42	28.0	0
Corn grits, cooked, 1 cup:								
white, enriched	tr.	n.a.	.24	.15	1.96	.06	1.0	0
yellow, enriched	145	n.a.	.24	.15	1.96	.06	1.0	0
Cornbread, see "Bread, sweet, mix"								
Cornmeal, 1 cup:								
whole grain, white	tr.	0	.47	.25	4.43	.37	n.a.	0
whole grain, yellow	573	0	.47	.25	4.43	.37	n.a.	0
degermed, enriched, white	tr.	0	.99	.56	6.95	.35	66.0	0
degermed, enriched, yellow	570	0	.99	.56	6.95	.35	66.0	0
self-rising, enriched:								
bolted	n.a.	0	.81	.49	6.46	.66	70.0	0
bolted, w/wheat flour, white[1]	tr.	0	1.21	.74	8.84	.65	112.0	0
bolted, w/wheat flour, yellow[1] ...	488	0	1.21	.74	8.84	.65	112.0	0
degermed[1]	n.a.	0	.94	.54	6.30	.54	43.0	0
Cornstarch, stirred, 1 tbsp.	(0)	(0)	(0)	(0)	(0)	n.a.	n.a.	n.a.
Cottonseed flour, lowfat, 1 oz. ...	123	1	.59	.11	1.15	.22	n.a.	0
Couscous, cooked, 1 cup	n.a.	0	.11	.05	1.76	.09	26.1	0
Cowpea, ½ cup:								
raw	588	2	.08	.10	1.04	.05	121.0	0
boiled, drained	648	2	.08	.12	1.15	.05	104.0	0
frozen, boiled, drained	64	2	.22	.05	.62	.08	120.1	0
Cowpea, dried, ½ cup:								
boiled	13	<1	.17	.05	.43	.09	178.8	0

1. *With added nutrients.*

Food and Measure	A I.U.	C mg.	Thi mg.	Rib mg.	Nia mg.	B$_6$ mg.	Fol mcg.	B$_{12}$ mcg.
canned, w/liquid	16	3	.09	.09	.43	.05	61.5	0
canned, w/pork	0	<1	.08	.06	.52	m.q.	m.q.	.02
Crab, Alaska king, meat only:								
raw, 1 oz.	7	(0)	.12	.12	.31	m.q.	m.q.	m.q.
boiled or steamed[1], 4 oz.	33	(0)	.06	.06	1.52	m.q.	m.q.	m.q.
Crabapple, w/skin, sliced, ½ cup	22	4	.02	.01	.06	m.q.	m.q.	0
Cracker:								
butter, 10 round or 1.2 oz.	70	(0)	tr.	.01	.30	n.a.	n.a.	n.a.
cheese, plain, 1″ square, 10 pieces ..	20	0	.05	.04	.40	n.a.	m.q.	n.a.
cheese-peanut butter sandwich,								
.3-oz. piece	tr.	0	.04	.03	.60	n.a.	m.q.	n.a.
graham, see "Cookie"								
melba toast, plain, .2-oz. piece	0	0	.01	.01	.10	n.a.	n.a.	n.a.
rice bran (*Health Valley*), 7 pieces ..	15	2	.18	.05	1.90	.01	.5	0
rye wafer, whole-grain, 2 pieces or								
.5 oz.	0	0	.06	.03	.50	n.a.	m.q.	n.a.
saltine, 10 pieces or 1 oz.	(0)	(0)	tr.	.01	.30	n.a.	m.q.	n.a.
snack type, 1 round or .1 oz.	tr.	0	.01	.01	.10	n.a.	n.a.	n.a.
soda biscuit, 10 pieces or 1.8 oz. ...	(0)	(0)	.01	.03	.50	n.a.	m.q.	n.a.
soup or oyster, 10 pieces	(0)	(0)	tr.	tr.	.10	n.a.	m.q.	n.a.
wheat:								
(*Health Valley* Stoned Wheat								
Regular/No Salt Added),								
13 pieces	0	3	.02	.03	1.10	.07	16.9	0
herbed (*Health Valley* Stoned								
Wheat), 13 pieces	107	3	.03	.03	1.20	.07	15.9	0
herbed (*Health Valley* Stoned								
Wheat No Salt Added),								
13 pieces	380	3	.03	.03	1.20	.07	16.2	0
sesame (*Health Valley* Stoned								
Wheat), 13 pieces	128	3	.14	.03	1.90	.08	16.9	0
sesame (*Health Valley* Stoned								
Wheat No Salt Added),								
13 pieces	128	3	.14	.03	1.90	.08	17.2	0
thin, 4 pieces or .3 oz.	tr.	0	.04	.03	.40	m.q.	m.q.	0
vegetable, seven grain (*Health								
Valley* Stoned Wheat), 13 pieces	126	2	.09	.04	.80	.08	17.7	0
whole, 2 pieces or .3 oz.	0	0	.02	.03	.40	m.q.	m.q.	0
Cranberry, fresh, ½ cup:								
whole	22	6	.01	.01	.05	.03	.8	0
chopped	25	7	.02	.01	.06	.04	1.0	0
Cranberry bean, boiled, ½ cup ..	0	0	.19	.06	.45	.07	181.9	0
Cranberry juice cocktail[2]:								
bottled, 6 fl. oz.	7	68	.02	.02	.07	.04	.5	0
frozen[3], 6 fl. oz.	18	18	.01	.02	.02	.03	0	0

1. *Without added ingredients.*
2. *With added ascorbic acid.*
3. *Diluted according to package directions.*

Food and Measure	A I.U.	C mg.	Thi mg.	Rib mg.	Nia mg.	B$_6$ mg.	Fol mcg.	B$_{12}$ mcg.
Cranberry sauce, canned,								
sweetened, ½ cup	28	3	.02	.03	.14	.02	n.a.	0
Cranberry-apple juice drink[1],								
bottled, 6 fl. oz.	n.a.	59	.01	.04	.11	n.a.	n.a.	0
Cranberry-apricot juice drink,								
bottled, 6 fl. oz.	n.a.	0	.01	.02	.22	n.a.	n.a.	0
Cranberry-grape juice drink[1],								
bottled, 6 fl. oz.	n.a.	59	.02	.03	.22	n.a.	n.a.	0
Cranberry-orange relish, canned,								
½ cup	97	25	.04	.03	.14	n.a.	n.a.	0
Crayfish, mixed species, meat only:								
raw, 1 oz.	n.a.	1	m.q.	.02	.68	m.q.	m.q.	.77
boiled or steamed[2], 4 oz.	n.a.	4	m.q.	.09	3.31	m.q.	m.q.	3.93
Cream:								
half and half, 1 cup	1050	2	.09	.36	.19	.09	6.0	.80
half and half, 1 tbsp.	65	<1	.01	.02	.01	.01	tr.	.05
light, coffee or table, 1 cup	1728	2	.08	.36	.14	.08	6.0	.53
light, coffee or table, 1 tbsp.	108	<1	.01	.02	.01	.01	tr.	.03
medium (25% fat), 1 cup	2251	2	.07	.33	.12	.07	6.0	.52
medium, (25% fat), 1 tbsp.	141	<1	<1	.02	.01	.01	tr.	.03
whipping:								
light, 1 cup, approx. 2 cups								
whipped	2694	2	.06	.30	.10	.07	9.0	.47
light, 1 tbsp.	169	<1	<.01	.02	.01	<.01	1.0	.03
heavy, 1 cup, approx. 2 cups								
whipped	3499	1	.05	.26	.09	.06	9.0	.43
heavy, 1 tbsp.	220	<1	<.01	.02	.01	<.01	1.0	.03
whipped topping, pressurized, 1 cup	548	0	.02	.03	.04	.03	m.q.	.18
whipped topping, pressurized,								
1 tbsp.	27	0	<.01	<.01	<.01	<.01	m.q.	.01
Cream, sour, cultured:								
1 cup	1817	2	.08	.34	.15	.04	25.0	.69
1 tbsp.	95	<1	<.01	.02	.01	<.01	1.0	.04
half and half, 1 tbsp.	68	<1	.01	.02	.01	<.01	2.0	.05
Cream, sour, nondairy, 1 oz. ...	0	0	0	0	0	0	0	0
Cream topping, nondairy:								
frozen, semisolid, 1 tbsp.	34	0	0	0	0	0	0	0
powdered[3], 1½ oz. dry	458	0	0	0	0	0	0	0
powdered[3], prepared w/whole milk,								
1 tbsp.	14	<1	<.01	.01	<.01	<.01	tr.	.01
pressurized, 1 tbsp.	19	0	0	0	0	0	0	0
Creamer, nondairy:								
liquid (*Coffee-mate*), ½ fl. oz.	18	0	0	0	0	0	0	0
liquid,[3] frozen, 1 tbsp.	13	0	0	0	0	0	0	0
powdered,[3] 1 tsp.	4	0	0	0	0	0	0	0
Cress, garden, raw, ½ cup	2325	17	.02	.07	.25	.06	n.a.	0

1. *With added ascorbic acid.*
2. *Without added ingredients.*
3. *Includes vitamin A contributed from beta-carotene used for coloring.*

Food and Measure	A I.U.	C mg.	Thi mg.	Rib mg.	Nia mg.	B$_6$ mg.	Fol mcg.	B$_{12}$ mcg.
Croissant, 2-oz. piece	50	0	.17	.13	1.30	n.a.	n.a.	n.a.
Crookneck squash, ½ cup:								
fresh, raw, sliced	220	5	.03	.03	.30	.07	14.9	0
fresh, boiled, drained, sliced	259	5	.04	.04	.46	.09	18.1	0
canned, drained, sliced	130	3	.02	.03	.45	.05	11.3	0
frozen, boiled, drained, sliced	187	7	.04	.05	.42	.10	12.2	0
Cucumber, w/peel:								
1 medium, 8¼" long, 10.9 oz.	135	14	.09	.06	.90	.16	41.8	0
sliced ½ cup	23	2	.02	.01	.16	.03	7.2	0
Cumin seed, 1 tsp.	27	<1	.01	.01	.10	n.a.	n.a.	0
Cupcake mix[1], devil's food,								
w/chocolate frosting,								
2½"-diam. piece	50	tr.	.04	.05	.30	n.a.	n.a.	n.a.
Currant, ½ cup:								
black European, fresh, trimmed	129	101	.03	.03	.17	.04	n.a.	0
red or white, fresh, trimmed[2]	67	23	.02	.03	.06	.04	n.a.	0
Zante, dried	52	3	.12	.10	1.16	.21	7.3	0
Curry powder, 1 tsp.	20	<1	.01	.01	.07	n.a.	n.a.	0
Custard apple, trimmed, 1 oz. ...	n.a.	5	.02	.03	.14	.06	n.a.	0
Cuttlefish, mixed species, meat								
only, raw, 1 oz.	n.a.	2	<.01	.26	.34	n.a.	m.q.	.85

1. *Prepared according to package directions.*
2. *Vitamin A figure applies to red currant only.*

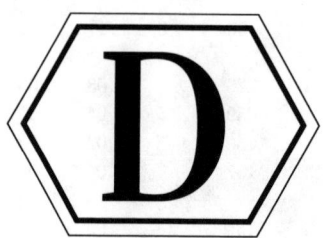

Food and Measure	A I.U.	C mg.	Thi mg.	Rib mg.	Nia mg.	B₆ mg.	Fol mcg.	B₁₂ mcg.
Danish pastry:								
plain, 2-oz. round piece	60	tr.	.16	.17	1.40	n.a.	m.q.	n.a.
w/fruit, 2.3-oz. round piece	40	tr.	.16	.14	1.40	n.a.	m.q.	n.a.
Date, domestic, natural and dry:								
pitted, 10 dates, 2.9 oz.	42	0	.08	.08	1.83	.16	10.4	0
pitted, chopped, ½ cup	45	0	.08	.09	1.96	.17	11.1	0
Dill, 1 tsp.:								
seed	1	n.a.	.01	.01	.06	n.a.	n.a.	0
weed, dried	tr.	n.a.	<.01	<.01	.03	n.a.	n.a.	0
Donut, 1 piece:								
cake type, plain, 1.8 oz.	20	tr.	.12	.12	1.10	n.a.	m.q.	n.a.
yeast type, glazed, 3¾″ diam.	tr.	0	.28	.12	1.80	n.a.	m.q.	n.a.
Duck[1]:								
domesticated, roasted, meat w/skin,								
4 oz.	238	0	.20	.31	5.47	.20	6.8	.34
domesticated, roasted, meat only,								
4 oz.	87	0	.29	.53	5.78	.28	11.3	.45
wild, raw, meat w/skin, 1 oz.	m.q.	1	.10	.08	.94	.15	m.q.	.18
Dutch brand loaf, pork and beef,								
1-oz. slice[2]	0	5	.09	.08	.68	.06	m.q.	.37

1. *Cooked meats are prepared without added ingredients.*
2. *With added ascorbic acid or sodium ascorbate; vitamin C value for product without additives would be negligible.*

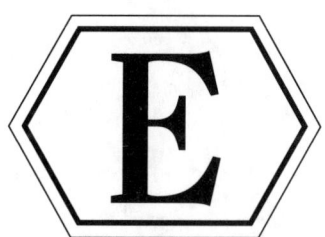

Food and Measure	A I.U.	C mg.	Thi mg.	Rib mg.	Nia mg.	B6 mg.	Fol mcg.	B12 mcg.
Eel, mixed species, meat only:								
raw, 1 oz.	985	(0)	.04	.01	.99	.02	m.q.	.85
baked, broiled, or microwaved[1], 4 oz.	4294	(0)	.21	.06	5.09	.09	m.q.	3.27
Egg, chicken:								
raw:								
whole, fresh or frozen, 1 large,								
approx. 1.75 oz.	317	0	.03	.25	.04	.07	23.0	.50
white, fresh or frozen, from								
1 large egg	n.a.	0	<.01	.15	.03	<.01	1.0	.07
yolk, fresh, from 1 large egg	323	0	.03	.11	<.01	.07	24.0	.52
yolk, frozen[2], 1 oz.	465	0	.04	.17	.01	.09	34.9	.74
yolk, frozen, sugared, 1 oz.	404	0	.05	.10	.01	.06	30.9	.76
cooked, 1 large egg:								
fried[3]	394	0	.03	.24	.04	.07	18.0	.42
hard boiled	280	0	.03	.26	.03	.06	22.0	.56
omelet[4]	399	0	.03	.24	.04	.07	18.0	.43
poached	316	0	.03	.22	.03	.06	18.0	.40
scrambled[5]	416	<1	.03	.27	.05	.07	18.0	.47
dried, 1 oz.:								
whole	553	0	.09	.33	.07	.11	52.2	2.84
whole, stabilized[6]	581	0	.09	.35	.07	.12	54.7	2.98
white, stabilized[6], flakes	0	0	.01	.61	.19	.01	25.2	.14
white, stabilized[6], powder	0	0	.01	.66	.20	.01	27.2	.15
yolk	970	0	.12	.23	.04	.16	60.4	2.01

1. *Without added ingredients.*
2. *Includes approximately 17% white.*
3. *Recipe: 95% egg. 5% margarine, and salt.*
4. *Recipe: 74% egg, 22% water, 4% margarine, and salt.*
5. *Recipe: 74% egg, 22% whole milk, 4% margarine, and salt.*
6. *Glucose reduced.*

Food and Measure	A I.U.	C mg.	Thi mg.	Rib mg.	Nia mg.	B6 mg.	Fol mcg.	B12 mcg.
Egg, chicken, substitute or imitation, 1 oz.:								
frozen[1]	383	n.a.	.03	.11	n.a.	.04	m.q.	n.a.
liquid[1]	612	0	.03	.09	.03	n.a.	m.q.	.08
Egg, duck, fresh, whole, raw,								
1 egg, approx. 2.5 oz.	930	0	.11	.28	.14	.18	56.0	3.78
Egg, quail, fresh, whole, raw,								
1 egg, approx. .3 oz.	27	0	.01	.07	.01	.01	m.q.	m.q.
Eggnog, dairy, 1 cup	894	4	.09	.48	.27	.13	2.0	1.14
Eggplant, ½ cup:								
raw, 1″ pieces	29	1	.04	.01	.25	.04	7.2	0
boiled, drained, cubes	31	1	.04	.01	.29	.04	6.9	0
Elderberry, ½ cup	435	26	.05	.04	.36	.17	n.a.	0
Endive:								
1 head, approx. 1.3 lbs.	10,517	33	.41	.39	2.05	.10	728.5	0
chopped, ½ cup	513	2	.02	.02	.10	.01	35.5	0

1. *Vitamin A contributed largely from beta-carotene used for coloring.*

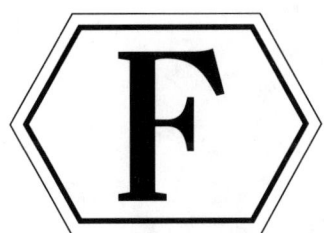

Food and Measure	A I.U.	C mg.	Thi mg.	Rib mg.	Nia mg.	B₆ mg.	Fol mcg.	B₁₂ mcg.
Farina, whole grain, enriched,								
cooked, 1 cup	0	0	.19	.12	1.28	.02	6.0	0
Fast foods, unspecified:								
breakfast:								
biscuit, plain, 2.6 oz.	98	0	.26	.17	1.62	.03	6.0	.10
biscuit, w/egg, 4.8 oz.	649	0	.34	.33	.71	.08	29.0	.75
and bacon, 5.3 oz.	191	3	.13	.22	2.41	.13	29.0	1.03
and ham, 6.8 oz.	874	<1	.68	.60	2.00	.26	32.0	1.20
and sausage, 6.3 oz.	635	<1	.50	.46	3.60	.20	40.0	1.37
and steak, 5.2 oz.	704	<1	.36	.53	3.06	.18	28.0	1.41
cheese and bacon, 5.1 oz.	648	2	.30	.43	2.30	.11	37.0	1.05
biscuit, w/ham, 4 oz.	133	<1	.51	.31	3.48	.14	8.0	.03
biscuit, w/sausage, 4.4 oz.	56	<1	.40	.28	3.28	.12	9.0	.51
biscuit, w/steak, 5 oz.	65	<1	.35	.40	4.16	.16	11.0	.95
croissant, w/egg and cheese:								
4.5 oz.	1000	<1	.19	.38	1.51	.10	36.0	.78
and bacon, 4.6 oz.	472	2	.35	.34	2.19	.12	35.0	.86
and ham, 5.4 oz.	451	11	.52	.30	3.19	.23	36.0	1.01
and sausage, 5.6 oz.	422	<1	.99	.32	4.00	.12	38.0	.90
danish pastry:								
cheese, 3.2 oz.	155	3	.27	.21	2.55	.06	15.0	.23
cinnamon, 3.1 oz.	18	3	.26	.19	2.20	.06	14.0	.22
fruit, 3.3 oz.	86	2	.29	.21	1.79	.06	15.0	.23
eggs, scrambled, 2 eggs	835	3	.08	.49	.19	.18	52.0	.95
English muffin:								
w/butter, 2.2 oz.	136	1	.25	.32	2.61	.04	17.0	.02
w/cheese and sausage, 4.1 oz.	379	1	.70	.25	4.14	.15	18.0	.68
w/egg, cheese, and Canadian								
bacon, 5.1 oz.	594	1	.49	.53	3.93	.16	44.0	.80
w/egg, cheese, and sausage,								
5.8 oz.	660	1	.84	.49	4.45	.20	54.0	1.37

Food and Measure	A I.U.	C mg.	Thi mg.	Rib mg.	Nia mg.	B$_6$ mg.	Fol mcg.	B$_{12}$ mcg.
Fast foods, breakfast *(cont.)*								
French toast, w/butter, 2 slices,								
4.8 oz.	472	<1	.58	.50	3.91	.05	30.0	.36
French toast sticks, 5 sticks,								
5 oz.	45	0	.23	.25	2.96	.26	134.0	.06
pancakes, w/butter and syrup,								
3 cakes, 8.2 oz.	281	3	.40	.56	3.39	.12	34.0	.22
potatoes, hashed brown, ½ cup ..	18	6	.08	.01	1.07	.17	8.0	.02
sausage, 1-oz. patty	tr.	0	.20	.07	1.22	.09	m.q.	.47
sausage, .5-oz. link	tr.	0	.10	.03	.59	.04	m.q.	.22
entrees:								
chicken, breaded, fried:								
dark meat, 5.2 oz. or 1 thigh								
and 1 drumstick	222	0	.14	.43	7.21	.33	10.0	.83
light meat, 5.7 oz. or								
combination of 2 pieces	192	0	.14	.30	11.98	.57	9.0	.67
chicken, breaded, fried, boneless,								
6 pieces:								
plain, 3.6 oz.	102	<1	.09	.15	6.86	.31	11.0	.30
w/barbecue sauce, 4.6 oz.	342	1	.10	.16	7.02	.33	28.0	.30
w/honey, 4.1 oz.	101	<1	.09	.15	6.81	.31	11.0	.30
w/mustard sauce, 4.6 oz.	110	<1	.11	.15	6.94	.32	12.0	.32
w/sweet and sour sauce,								
4.6 oz.	242	1	.10	.20	6.86	.32	12.0	.36
chili con carne, 1 cup	1663	2	.14	1.13	2.49	.32	30.0	1.15
clams, breaded, fried, ¾ cup	122	0	.20	.27	2.87	.04	9.0	1.11
crab, baked, 2.1-oz. cake	43	2	.15	.09	2.47	.25	11.0	8.67
crab, soft shell, fried, 4.4-oz. crab	15	1	.10	.08	1.75	.15	20.0	4.47
crab cake, 3.8-oz. cake	568	<1	.10	.14	2.12	.27	17.0	7.99
fish, battered or breaded, fried,								
3.2-oz. fillet	35	0	.10	.10	1.91	.09	51.0	1.01
oysters, battered or breaded,								
fried, 6 pieces, 4.9 oz.	363	4	.31	.35	4.42	.03	13.0	1.01
pizza, ⅛ of 12″ pie:								
w/cheese	297	1	.14	.13	1.93	.03	46.0	.26
w/cheese, meat, vegetables ...	431	1	.18	.14	1.61	.08	22.0	.30
w/pepperoni	210	1	.10	.17	2.28	.04	39.0	.14
scallops, breaded, fried, 6 pieces,								
5.1 oz.	139	0	.20	.85	0	.07	40.0	.43
shrimp, breaded, fried, 6–8								
pieces, 5.8 oz.	119	0	.21	.90	0	.06	48.0	.15
Mexican foods:								
burrito, w/beans, 2 pieces:								
7.7 oz.	332	2	.62	.62	4.06	.31	118.0	1.09
and cheese, 6.6 oz.	1250	2	.22	.71	3.57	.25	81.0	.90
and chilies, 7.2 oz.	205	1	.45	.71	4.38	.29	118.0	1.16
and meat, 8.1 oz.	636	2	.53	.83	5.41	.37	73.0	1.74
cheese and beef, 7.2 oz.	799	5	.30	.71	3.86	.23	61.0	1.10
cheese and chilies, 11.9 oz. ...	1596	7	.55	1.20	7.71	.41	146.0	1.99

Food and Measure	A I.U.	C mg.	Thi mg.	Rib mg.	Nia mg.	B6 mg.	Fol mcg.	B12 mcg.
burrito, w/beef, 2 pieces:								
7.8 oz.	277	1	.23	.92	6.45	.32	39.0	1.97
and chilies, 7.1 oz.	463	2	.39	.80	5.08	.29	37.0	1.30
cheese and chilies, 10.7 oz. ...	972	4	.62	1.24	8.34	.38	58.0	2.07
chimichanga, w/beef, 1 piece:								
6.1 oz.	147	5	.48	.64	5.77	.27	31.0	1.52
and cheese, 6.5 oz.	540	3	.39	.85	4.68	.22	34.0	1.31
and red chilies, 6.7 oz.	262	<1	.29	.66	5.34	.24	34.0	1.09
cheese and red chilies, 6.3 oz.	702	2	.24	.96	3.46	.16	33.0	1.28
enchilada, w/cheese, 1 piece:								
5.7 oz.	1160	1	.09	.42	1.91	.39	34.0	.74
and beef, 6.8 oz.	1135	1	.11	.40	2.51	.26	192.0	1.02
enchirito, w/cheese, beef and								
beans, 1 piece, 6.8 oz.	1015	5	.18	.69	2.99	.21	254.0	1.63
frijoles, w/cheese, 1 cup	457	2	.14	.33	1.48	.19	111.0	.68
nachos, w/cheese, 6–8 pieces:								
4 oz.	559	1	.19	.37	1.53	.20	10.0	.82
and jalapeños, 7.2 oz.	4061	1	.13	.49	2.84	.38	19.0	1.02
beans, ground beef, and								
peppers, 9 oz.	3401	5	.24	.69	3.35	.41	39.0	1.01
taco, 1 small, 6 oz.	855	2	.15	.45	3.22	.24	23.0	1.04
taco, 1 large, 9.3 oz.	1315	3	.23	.69	4.96	.36	36.0	1.61
taco salad[1], 1½ cup	589	4	.10	.35	2.46	.21	40.0	.64
taco salad, w/chili[2], 1½ cup	1573	3	.16	.49	2.54	.53	64.0	.73
tostada, 1 piece:								
w/beans and cheese, 5.1 oz. ..	622	1	.10	.33	1.33	.17	75.0	.68
w/beans, beef, and cheese,								
7.9 oz.	1275	4	.09	.50	2.85	.26	97.0	1.13
w/beef and cheese, 5.7 oz.	713	3	.10	.55	3.14	.22	15.0	1.17
w/guacamole, 2.3 oz.	876	2	.07	.30	1.00	.13	55.0	.49
sandwiches, 1 piece:								
cheeseburger, single meat patty:								
plain, 3.6 oz.	153	0	.40	.40	3.70	.10	26.0	.97
w/condiments[3], 4 oz.	462	2	.25	.23	3.72	.12	18.0	.94
w/condiments and vegetables[4],								
5.4 oz.	431	2	.32	.23	6.38	.15	22.0	1.23
cheeseburger, double meat patty:								
plain, 5.5 oz.	332	0	.25	.37	6.01	.25	29.0	2.31
w/condiments and vegetables[4],								
5.9 oz.	398	2	.35	.28	8.05	.18	23.0	1.93
double-decker bun, plain,								
5.6 oz.	276	0	.33	.38	6.02	.22	36.0	1.92
double-decker bun,								
w/condiments and								
vegetables[4], 8 oz.	371	3	.57	.44	8.34	.26	34.0	2.07

1. *Recipe: lettuce, tomato, chili sauce, ground beef, cheese, and taco shell.*
2. *Recipe: chili con carne, lettuce, tomato, cheese, and taco shell.*
3. *Condiments include catsup, mustard, pickles, and onions.*
4. *Condiments and vegetables include catsup, mustard, mayonnaise-style dressing, pickles, onions, lettuce, and tomatoes.*

Food and Measure	A I.U.	C mg.	Thi mg.	Rib mg.	Nia mg.	B_6 mg.	Fol mcg.	B_{12} mcg.
Fast foods, sandwiches *(cont.)*								
cheeseburger, large, single meat patty:								
plain, 6.5 oz.	615	32	.48	.57	11.17	.28	38.0	2.53
w/bacon and condiments[1], 6.9 oz.	406	2	.32	.42	6.63	.31	33.0	2.34
w/condiments and vegetables[2], 7.7 oz.	614	8	.40	.46	7.37	.29	28.0	2.56
w/ham, condiments and vegetables[2], 9 oz.	505	7	.54	.56	9.18	.39	50.0	2.88
cheeseburger, large, double meat patty, w/condiments and vegetables[2], 9.1 oz.	348	1	.37	.50	7.24	.41	48.0	3.40
chicken fillet sandwich:								
plain, 6.4 oz.	100	9	.34	.24	6.80	.19	28.0	.38
w/cheese, 8 oz.	620	3	.42	.46	9.08	.41	46.0	.46
fish sandwich, w/tartar sauce:								
5.6 oz.	110	3	.33	.22	3.40	.11	44.0	1.07
and cheese, 6.5 oz.	432	3	.45	.42	4.23	.12	32.0	1.08
hamburger, single meat patty:								
plain, 3.2 oz.	0	0	.33	.27	3.72	.06	25.0	.89
w/condiments[1], 3.8 oz.	126	3	.26	.32	4.70	.12	17.0	.84
w/condiments and vegetables[2], 3.9 oz.	82	2	.23	.20	3.68	.12	18.0	.89
hamburger, double meat patty:								
plain, 6.2 oz.	0	0	.33	.37	8.26	.32	38.0	2.92
w/condiments[1], 7.6 oz.	53	1	.35	.42	6.73	.37	45.0	3.33
hamburger, large, single meat patty:								
plain, 4.8 oz.	0	0	.28	.29	6.24	.23	32.0	2.05
w/condiments and vegetables[2], 7.7 oz.	311	3	.42	.38	7.28	.33	36.0	2.38
hamburger, large, double meat patty, w/condiments and vegetables[2], 8 oz.	102	1	.36	.39	7.57	.54	27.0	4.07
ham and cheese, 5.1 oz.	319	3	.31	.49	2.69	.20	71.0	.54
ham, egg, and cheese, 5 oz.	561	3	.43	.56	4.21	.16	43.0	1.24
hot dog:								
plain, 3.5 oz.	0	<1	.24	.27	3.65	.05	30.0	.51
w/chili, 4 oz.	58	3	.21	.40	3.74	.05	50.0	.29
coated (corn dog), 6.2 oz.	207	0	.29	.71	4.16	.10	60.0	.44
roast beef, plain, 4.9 oz.	210	2	.38	.31	5.86	.27	40.0	1.22
roast beef, w/cheese, 6.2 oz.	193	0	.38	.46	5.90	.34	41.0	2.05
steak, chopped, w/lettuce, tomato, mayonnaise, 7.2 oz.	367	6	.40	.37	7.30	.37	89.0	1.57

1. *Condiments include catsup, mustard, pickles, and onions.*
2. *Condiments and vegetables include catsup, mustard, mayonnaise-style dressing, pickles, onions, lettuce, and tomatoes.*

Food and Measure	A I.U.	C mg.	Thi mg.	Rib mg.	Nia mg.	B6 mg.	Fol mcg.	B12 mcg.
submarine:								
w/cold cuts[1], 8 oz.	425	12	1.00	.80	5.50	.13	54.0	1.09
w/roast beef[2], 7.6 oz.	412	6	.42	.42	5.97	.32	45.0	1.82
w/tuna salad[3], 9 oz.	188	4	.46	.35	11.33	.23	58.0	1.61
salad, w/out dressing, 1½ cup:								
plain[4]	2352	48	.06	.10	1.15	.16	77.0	0
w/added cheese and eggs[5]	822	10	.10	.17	.98	.11	85.0	.31
w/added chicken[6]	935	17	.11	.13	5.89	.43	67.0	.20
w/added pasta and seafood[7]	6245	38	.30	.21	3.56	.35	100.0	1.73
w/added shrimp[8]	791	9	.12	.16	1.17	.15	87.0	3.78
chef, w/added turkey, ham, and								
cheese[9]	1053	17	.41	.39	5.97	.43	100.0	.84
side dishes:								
coleslaw, ¾ cup	337	8	.04	.03	.08	.11	39.0	.18
corn on cob, w/butter, 1 ear	391	7	.25	.10	2.17	.32	44.0	0
hush puppies, 5 pieces, 2.8 oz. ..	94	0	0	.02	2.03	.10	21.0	.18
onion rings, 8–9 rings, 2.9 oz. ...	8	1	.09	.10	.92	.06	11.0	.12
potato, baked, 1 potato:								
topped w/cheese sauce:								
10.4 oz.	834	26	.22	.22	3.35	.72	28.0	.18
and bacon, 10.5 oz.	627	29	.28	.24	3.96	.74	28.0	.33
and broccoli, 12 oz.	1695	49	.26	.26	3.58	.80	61.0	.33
and chili, 13.9 oz.	768	32	.30	.34	4.17	.94	50.0	.22
topped w/sour cream and								
chives, 10.1 oz.	1346	34	.27	.18	3.70	.79	32.0	.20
potato, french fried:								
regular, 2.7 oz.	22	4	.10	.03	1.72	.20	25.0	.09
large, 4.1 oz.	33	6	.16	.04	2.60	.30	38.0	.14
potato, mashed, w/milk and								
margarine, ⅓ cup	33	<1	.07	.04	.96	.19	7.0	.04
potato chips, 1 oz.	0	12	.04	.01	1.19	.14	12.8	0
potato salad, ⅓ cup	95	1	.06	.11	.26	.14	24.0	.12
desserts:								
animal crackers, 2.4-oz. box	27	1	.25	.24	2.46	.02	22.0	.05
brownie, 1 piece, 2.1 oz.	10	3	.07	.13	.58	.03	4.0	.15
chocolate chip cookies, 1.9-oz.								
box	52	1	.09	.19	1.39	.03	16.0	.11
fruit pie[10], fried, 3-oz. pie	148	1	.10	.08	.98	.03	4.0	.08
ice milk cone, vanilla, soft-serve,								
3.6 oz.	211	1	.05	.26	.31	.06	5.0	.21

1. *Recipe: bread, lettuce, cheese, salami, ham, tomato, onion, and oil.*
2. *Recipe: bread, beef, tomato, lettuce, and mayonnaise.*
3. *Recipe: tuna salad, bread, lettuce, oil.*
4. *Recipe: lettuce, cabbage, cucumber, green pepper, tomato, radish, and carrot.*
5. *Recipe: lettuce, tomato, egg, cheese, celery, cucumber, and radish.*
6. *Recipe: lettuce, chicken, celery, tomato, green pepper, and carrot.*
7. *Recipe: lettuce, macaroni, salad dressing, pollock, sweet pepper, carrot, celery, crab, turbot, olives, and onion.*
8. *Recipe: lettuce, shrimp, celery, tomato, green pepper, and carrot.*
9. *Recipe: lettuce, tomato, turkey, ham, cheese, egg, celery, cucumber, radish, and carrots.*
10. *Apple, cherry, or lemon.*

Food and Measure	A I.U.	C mg.	Thi mg.	Rib mg.	Nia mg.	B_6 mg.	Fol mcg.	B_{12} mcg.
Fast foods, desserts *(cont.)*								
sundae:								
caramel, 5.5 oz.	263	3	.06	.29	.95	.05	12.0	.60
hot fudge, 5.6 oz.	221	2	.06	.30	1.07	.13	9.0	.65
strawberry, 5.4 oz.	222	2	.06	.28	.91	.07	18.0	.64
beverages:								
beer, regular, 12 fl. oz.	0	0	.02	.09	1.61	.18	21.4	.06
beer, light, 12 fl. oz.	0	0	.03	.11	1.39	.12	14.7	.02
coffee, brewed, 6 fl. oz.	0	0	0	0	.07	0	0	0
coffee, instant, decaffeinated,								
6 fl. oz.	0	0	.03	.51	<.01	0	0	0
hot chocolate, 6 fl. oz.	4	1	.03	.16	.17	.03	0	.37
juice, 6 fl. oz.:								
grapefruit	17	62	.08	.04	.40	.08	6.7	0
orange	146	73	.15	.03	.38	.08	81.7	0
tomato	1012	33	.09	.06	1.23	.20	36.1	0
lemonade, 8 fl. oz.	53	10	.02	.05	.04	.02	5.5	0
milk, whole, 8 fl. oz.	307	2	.09	.40	.21	.10	12.0	.87
milk, lowfat 2%, 8 fl. oz.	500	2	.10	.40	.21	.11	12.0	.89
orange drink, 6 fl. oz.	33	64	.01	.01	.06	.02	n.a.	0
shake, 10 fl. oz.:								
chocolate	263	1	.16	.69	.46	.14	9.9	.97
strawberry	340	2	.13	.55	.50	.13	8.5	.88
vanilla	368	2	.13	.52	.52	.15	9.2	1.01
soda, 12-fl.-oz. can:								
cola, pepper type, ginger ale,								
or root beer	0	0	0	0	0	0	0	0
cola, low-calorie[1]	0	0	.02	.08	0	0	0	0
lemon-lime	0	0	0	0	.06	0	0	0
orange	0	0	0	0	n.a.	0	0	0
tea, brewed, 6 fl. oz.	0	0	0	.03	0	0	9.2	0
tea, iced, instant, sugar								
sweetened, lemon flavor,								
12 fl. oz.	0	0	0	.07	.14	0	14.4	0
Fat, see specific listings								
Fennel seed, 1 tsp.	3	n.a.	.01	.01	.12	n.a.	n.a.	0
Fenugreek seed, 1 tsp.	n.a.	<1	.01	.01	.06	n.a.	2.1	0
Fig, ½ cup, except as noted:								
fresh, 1 medium, approx. 1.8 oz. ...	71	1	.03	.03	.20	.06	n.a.	0
canned:								
in water or heavy syrup	48	1	.03	.05	.55	n.a.	n.a.	0
in light or extra heavy syrup	47	1	.03	.05	.55	n.a.	n.a.	0
dried:								
uncooked, 10 figs, approx. 6.6 oz.	248	2	.13	.17	1.30	.42	14.1	0
uncooked	132	1	.07	.09	.69	.22	7.5	0
cooked	207	6	.01	.14	.83	.17	1.3	0
Filberts, dried, unblanched, 1 oz.	19	<1	.14	.03	.32	.17	20.4	0

1. *Aspartame sweetened.*

Food and Measure	A I.U.	C mg.	Thi mg.	Rib mg.	Nia mg.	B6 mg.	Fol mcg.	B12 mcg.
Fish, see specific listings								
Fish fillet, breaded, fried, frozen,								
2-oz. piece, 4″ × 2″ × ½″	60	m.q.	.07	.10	1.21	.03	10.4	1.02
Fish stick, breaded, fried, frozen,								
1-oz. stick, 4″ × 1″ × ½″	30	m.q.	.04	.05	.60	.02	5.1	.50
Flatfish, meat only:								
raw, 1 oz.	9	tr.	.03	.02	.82	.06	m.q.	.43
baked, broiled, or microwaved[1],								
4 oz.	43	tr.	.09	.13	2.47	.27	m.q.	2.85
Flounder, see "Flatfish"								
Flour, see "Wheat flour" and								
specific listings								
Frankfurter[2]:								
beef, 1 link, 5″ long × ⅞″, approx.								
2 oz.	n.a.	11	.02	.05	1.14	.05	2.0	.74
beef and pork, 1 link, 5″ long × ⅞″,								
approx. 2 oz.	n.a.	12	.09	.05	1.19	.06	2.0	.58
cheese (cheesefurter or cheese								
smokie), 1 oz.	n.a.	6	.07	.05	.82	.04	m.q.	.49
French toast, frozen, 3 oz.:								
(*Aunt Jemima* Original)	145	0	.27	.25	2.83	.37	n.a.	1.35
cinnamon swirl (*Aunt Jemima*)	163	0	.24	.24	2.71	.34	n.a.	1.36
Frosting mix[3], fudge, prepared,								
1 cup:								
chocolate	840	0	.03	.12	.60	n.a.	n.a.	n.a.
creamy[4]	tr.	tr.	.05	.20	.70	n.a.	n.a.	n.a.
creamy[5]	960	tr.	.05	.17	.70	n.a.	n.a.	n.a.
Fruit, see specific listings								
Fruit, mixed:								
canned, in heavy syrup, ½ cup[6]	248	88	.02	.05	.77	n.a.	m.q.	0
dried, pitted, 1 oz.	692	1	.01	.04	.55	.05	m.q.	0
frozen, sweetened, ½ cup[6]	403	94	.02	.04	.50	n.a.	m.q.	0
Fruit cocktail, canned, ½ cup:								
in water	305	3	.02	.01	.44	.06	m.q.	0
in juice	378	3	.02	.02	.50	n.a.	m.q.	0
in light or heavy syrup	262	2	.02	.02	.48	.06	m.q.	0
Fruit punch drink[6], 1 cup:								
canned	32	74	.06	.06	.06	0	3.2	0
frozen[7]	27	108	.03	.03	.05	.02	2.3	0
Fruit punch flavor drink mix[6],								
2 rounded tsp.	1	31	<.01	.01	<.01	0	.2	0
Fruit punch juice drink, frozen[7],								
1 cup	15	14	<.01	.16	.15	.03	0	0

1. *Without added ingredients.*
2. *With added sodium ascorbate; vitamin C value for product without additive would be negligible.*
3. *Prepared according to package directions.*
4. *Prepared with water.*
5. *Prepared with water and vegetable table fat.*
6. *With added ascorbic acid.*
7. *Diluted according to package directions.*

Food and Measure	A I.U.	C mg.	Thi mg.	Rib mg.	Nia mg.	B_6 mg.	Fol mcg.	B_{12} mcg.
Fruit salad, canned, ½ cup:								
in water	536	2	.02	.03	.46	.04	m.q.	0
in juice	744	4	.01	.02	.44	n.a.	m.q.	0
in light syrup	541	3	.02	.03	.46	.04	m.q.	0
in heavy syrup	646	3	.02	.03	.44	.04	m.q.	0
tropical, in heavy syrup[1]	162	22	.07	.06	.72	n.a.	m.q.	0

5. *With added ascorbic acid.*

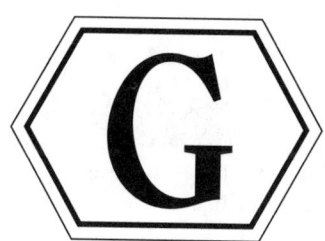

Food and Measure	A I.U.	C mg.	Thi mg.	Rib mg.	Nia mg.	B₆ mg.	Fol mcg.	B₁₂ mcg.
Garlic, raw, 1 clove	0	1	.01	<.01	.02	(0)	.1	0
Garlic powder, 1 tsp.	tr.	tr.	.01	<.01	.02	n.a.	n.a.	0
Gefilte fish, in jars, sweet,								
w/broth, 1.5-oz. piece	37	n.a.	.03	.03	m.q.	m.q.	1.2	.35
Gelatin, unflavored, powder dry,								
.2-oz. pkt.	0	0	0	0	0	n.a.	n.a.	0
Ginger, ground, 1 tsp.	3	tr.	<.01	<.01	.09	n.a.	n.a.	0
Ginger root, raw, sliced, ¼ cup. . .	0	1	.01	.01	.17	.05	m.q.	0
Ginkgo nuts, 1 oz.:								
raw	158	4	.06	.03	1.70	n.a.	n.a.	0
dried	310	8	.12	.05	3.33	n.a.	n.a.	0
Goose[1]**,** domesticated, 4 oz:								
roasted, meat w/skin	79	0	.09	.37	4.73	.42	2.3	m.q.
roasted, meat only	n.a.	0	.10	.44	4.63	.53	m.q.	m.q.
Gooseberry, ½ cup:								
fresh, trimmed	218	21	.03	.02	.22	.06	m.q.	0
canned, in light syrup	174	13	.03	.07	.19	.02	4.0	0
Gourd, dishcloth, boiled, drained,								
1″ slices, ½ cup	463	10	.08	.08	.46	n.a.	m.q.	0
Granola and cereal bars, 1 bar:								
caramel nut (*Quaker Granola Dipps*)	0	0	.02	.06	.35	.01	10.0	.15
chocolate chip (*Quaker Chewy*)	0	0	.05	.05	.24	.03	6.0	.04
chocolate chip (*Quaker Granola*								
Dipps)	0	0	.02	.05	.15	.03	7.0	.15
chocolate fudge (*Quaker Granola*								
Dipps)	48	<1	.03	.07	.14	.01	2.0	.01
honey and oats (*Quaker Chewy*)	0	0	.07	.05	.26	.03	6.0	.10
nut and raisin, chunky (*Quaker*								
Chewy)	0	0	.05	.05	.67	.03	8.0	.06
peanut butter:								
(*Quaker Chewy*)	0	0	.05	.05	.81	.03	8.0	.05

1. *Prepared without added ingredients.*

Food and Measure	A I.U.	C mg.	Thi mg.	Rib mg.	Nia mg.	B6 mg.	Fol mcg.	B12 mcg.
Granola and cereal bars, peanut butter (cont.)								
(*Quaker Granola Dipps*)	29	<1	.03	.06	1.47	.01	2.0	.01
chocolate chip (*Quaker Chewy*) ...	0	0	.03	.03	.80	.03	8.0	.11
chocolate chip (*Quaker Granola Dipps*)	30	<1	.03	.06	.79	.01	2.0	.01
raisin and cinnamon (*Quaker Chewy*)	0	0	.05	.06	.28	.03	5.0	.05
S'mores (*Quaker Chewy*)	0	0	.04	.04	.26	.01	5.0	n.a.
Grape:								
fresh:								
American type, 10 medium, approx. 1.4 oz.	24	1	.02	.01	.07	.27	.9	0
American type, peeled and seeded, ½ cup	46	2	.04	.03	.14	.05	1.8	0
European type, seedless or seeded, 10 medium, ⅝" × ⅞", approx. 1.75 oz.	36	5	.05	.03	.15	.06	2.0	0
European type, seedless or seeded, ½ cup	59	9	.07	.05	.24	.09	3.2	0
canned, Thompson seedless, in water or heavy syrup, ½ cup ..	81	1	.04	.03	.16	n.a.	m.q.	0
Grape drink[1], canned, 1 fl. oz. ...	tr.	11	<.01	<.01	.01	<.01	.1	0
Grape juice, 6 fl. oz.:								
canned or bottled	12	<1	.05	.07	.50	.13	4.8	0
frozen[2]	12	45	.03	.05	.23	.08	2.4	0
Grape juice drink[1], canned, 1 fl. oz.	1	5	<.01	<.01	.03	.01	.3	0
Grapefruit:								
fresh, pink and red, all areas:								
½ of 3¾"-diam. fruit, approx. 8.5 oz.[3]	318	47	.04	.03	.24	.05	15.0	0
sections w/juice, ½ cup[4]	298	44	.04	.02	.22	.05	14.1	0
fresh, white, all areas:								
½ of 3¾"-diam. fruit, approx. 8.5 oz.	12	39	.04	.02	.32	.05	11.8	0
sections w/juice, ½ cup	12	38	.04	.02	.31	.05	11.5	0
canned or in jars, ½ cup:								
in water	0	27	.05	.03	.30	.02	10.7	0
in juice	0	42	.04	.02	m.q.	m.q.	m.q.	0
in light syrup	0	27	.05	.03	.31	.03	10.8	0
Grapefruit juice, 6 fl. oz.:								
fresh	n.a.	70	.07	.04	.37	m.q.	m.q.	0
canned, unsweetened	12	54	.08	.04	.43	.04	19.2	0
canned, sweetened	0	50	.07	.04	.60	.04	19.2	0
frozen[2]	18	62	.08	.04	.40	.08	6.6	0
Great northern beans, ½ cup:								
boiled	1	1	.14	.05	.60	.10	89.9	0

1. *With added ascorbic acid.*
2. *Diluted according to package directions.*
3. *Vitamin A for Texas red grapefruit is 743 IU, ½ of 3¾"-diam. fruit.*
4. *Vitamin A for Texas red grapefruit is 695 IU.*

Food and Measure	A I.U.	C mg.	Thi mg.	Rib mg.	Nia mg.	B₆ mg.	Fol mcg.	B₁₂ mcg.
canned, w/liquid	1	2	.19	.08	.60	.36	106.5	0
Green bean, ½ cup:								
fresh, raw	368	9	.05	.06	.41	.04	20.1	0
fresh, boiled, drained	413	6	.05	.06	.38	.04	20.6	0
canned, drained	237	3	.01	.04	.14	m.q.	21.6	0
frozen, boiled, drained	359	6	.03	.05	.28	.04	m.q.	0
Ground cherry, trimmed, ½ cup	504	8	.08	.03	1.96	m.q.	m.q.	0
Grouper, meat only:								
raw, 1 oz.	n.a.	(0)	.03	<.01	.90	n.a.	m.q.	.17
baked, broiled, or microwaved[1],								
4 oz.	n.a.	(0)	.09	.01	.43	n.a.	m.q.	.78
Guava, trimmed, ½ cup:								
common	654	151	.04	.04	.99	.12	n.a.	0
strawberry	110	45	.04	.04	.73	m.q.	n.a.	0
Guava sauce, cooked, ½ cup	337	174	.03	.02	.50	n.a.	n.a.	0

1. *Without added ingredients.*

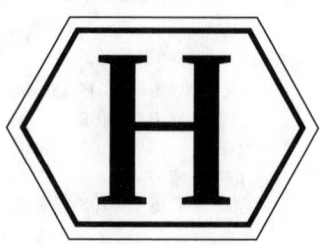

Food and Measure	A I.U.	C mg.	Thi mg.	Rib mg.	Nia mg.	B₆ mg.	Fol mcg.	B₁₂ mcg.
Haddock, meat only:								
raw, 1 oz.	16	(0)	.01	.01	1.08	.08	m.q.	.34
baked, broiled, or microwaved[1],								
4 oz.	71	(0)	.05	.05	5.25	.39	m.q.	1.57
smoked, 4 oz.	83	(0)	.05	.06	5.75	.45	m.q.	1.82
Halibut, meat only:								
Atlantic and Pacific, raw, 1 oz.	44	(0)	.02	.02	1.66	.10	m.q.	.34
Atlantic and Pacific, baked, broiled,								
or microwaved[1], 4 oz.	203	(0)	.08	.10	8.08	.45	m.q.	1.55
Greenland, raw, 1 oz.	16	(0)	.02	.02	.43	m.q.	.28	.33
Ham, fresh, roasted[1], 4 oz. (see								
also "Ham, cured"):								
whole leg, lean and fat	9	<1	.72	.35	5.18	.44	11.3	.79
whole leg, lean only	8	<1	.78	.40	5.60	.51	13.6	.82
rump half, lean and fat	11	<1	.81	.37	5.38	.31	6.8	.81
rump half, lean only	10	<1	.86	.40	5.69	.34	6.8	.83
shank half, lean and fat	9	<1	.65	.34	5.05	.44	5.7	.78
shank half, lean only	8	<1	.72	.39	5.54	.52	6.8	.81
Ham, cured, whole[2]:								
lean and fat, unheated, 1 oz.	n.a.	n.a.	.22	.05	1.27	.12	1.0	.21
lean and fat, roasted, 4 oz.	n.a.	n.a.	.68	.25	5.06	.43	3.4	.73
lean only, unheated, 1 oz.	n.a.	n.a.	.26	.06	1.49	.15	1.0	.25
lean only, roasted, 4 oz.	n.a.	n.a.	.77	.29	5.69	.53	4.5	.79
Ham, canned[2, 3]:								
regular (approx. 13% fat):								
unheated, 1 oz.	0	6	.27	.07	.91	.14	2.0	.22
roasted, 4 oz.	0	16	.93	.29	6.01	.34	5.7	1.20
extra lean and regular:								
unheated, 1 oz.	0	7	.25	.07	1.30	.13	2.0	.23
roasted, 4 oz.	0	26	1.09	.28	5.71	.45	5.7	.94

1. *Without added ingredients.*
2. *Roasted meats are prepared without added ingredients.*
3. *With added ascorbic acid or sodium ascorbate; vitamin C value for product without additives would be negligible.*

Food and Measure	A I.U.	C mg.	Thi mg.	Rib mg.	Nia mg.	B₆ mg.	Fol mcg.	B₁₂ mcg.
extra lean (approx. 4% fat):								
unheated, 1 oz.	0	8	.24	.07	1.50	.13	2.0	.23
roasted, 4 oz.	0	32	1.17	.28	5.55	.51	5.7	.81
chopped, 1 oz.	0	0	.15	.05	.91	.09	n.a.	.20
Ham, cured, boneless[1,2]:								
regular (approx. 11% fat):								
unheated, 1-oz. slice	0	8	.25	.07	1.49	.10	1.0	.23
roasted, 4 oz.	0	26	.83	.37	6.97	.35	m.q.	.79
extra lean and regular:								
unheated, 1-oz. slice	0	8	.25	.07	1.44	.11	1.0	.23
roasted, 4 oz.	0	25	.84	.32	6.04	.40	3.4	.77
extra lean (approx. 5% fat):								
unheated, 1-oz. slice	0	7	.26	.06	1.37	.13	1.0	.21
roasted, 4 oz.	0	24	.86	.23	4.56	.45	3.4	.74
steak, extra lean, unheated, 1 oz. ..	0	9	.23	.06	1.44	.10	1.0	.22
Ham luncheon meat[1]:								
chopped, 1-oz. slice	0	6	.18	.06	1.10	.10	0	.26
cooked, sliced, extra lean (5% fat),								
1-oz. slice	0	7	.26	.06	1.37	.13	1.0	.21
cooked, sliced, regular (11% fat),								
1-oz. slice	0	8	.25	.07	1.49	.10	1.0	.23
minced, 1 oz.	0	8	.20	.05	1.18	.07	m.q.	.27
Ham patty[2], grilled, 4 oz.	0	0	.40	.21	3.68	.18	m.q.	.79
Ham salad spread[1], 1 tbsp.	n.a.	1	.07	.02	.31	.02	m.q.	.11
Ham and cheese loaf or roll[1],								
1-oz. slice	n.a.	7	.17	.05	.98	.07	m.q.	.23
Ham and cheese spread[1], 1 tbsp.	n.a.	1	.05	.03	.32	.02	m.q.	.11
Hazelnut, see "Filberts"								
Head cheese[1], pork, 1-oz. slice ...	n.a.	6	.01	.05	.32	.05	1.0	3.0
Heart[3], 4 oz.:								
beef, simmered	0	2	.16	1.75	4.62	.24	2.3	16.22
chicken, simmered	32	2	.08	.84	3.18	.36	90.7	8.27
lamb, braised	0	8	.19	1.35	4.94	.34	2.3	12.70
pork, braised	25	2	.63	1.93	6.86	.44	4.5	4.30
turkey, simmered	32	2	.08	1.00	3.69	.36	89.6	8.10
veal, braised	0	11	.40	1.05	5.53	m.q.	m.q.	n.a.
Herring, Atlantic, meat only, 4 oz.,								
except as noted:								
raw, 1 oz.	27	<1	.02	.07	.91	.09	m.q.	3.87
baked, broiled, or microwaved[3]	116	1	.13	.34	4.68	.39	m.q.	14.90
kippered	145	1	.14	.36	4.99	.47	m.q.	21.21
pickled	1153	(0)	.04	.16	m.q.	m.q.	2.7	4.84
Hominy, canned, ½ cup:								
white	0	0	<.01	.01	.03	<.01	1.0	0
yellow	88	0	<.01	.01	.03	<.01	1.0	0
Hominy grits, see "Corn grits"								

1. *With added ascorbic acid or sodium ascorbate; vitamin C value for product without additives would be negligible.*
2. *Fully cooked as purchased.*
3. *Prepared without added ingredients.*

Food and Measure	A I.U.	C mg.	Thi mg.	Rib mg.	Nia mg.	B$_6$ mg.	Fol mcg.	B$_{12}$ mcg.
Honey, 1 tbsp.	0	tr.	tr.	.01	.10	n.a.	n.a.	0
Honey loaf[1], pork and beef,								
1-oz. slice	n.a.	6	.14	.07	.89	.09	m.q.	.31
Honey roll sausage[1], beef, 1 oz.	n.a.	5	.02	.05	1.18	.08	m.q.	.67
Honeydew:								
1/10 of 7″-diam. melon, 2″ slice,								
approx. 8 oz.	52	32	.10	.02	.77	.08	m.q.	0
pulp, cubed, 1/2 cup	34	21	.07	.02	.51	.05	m.q.	0
Hubbard squash, 1/2 cup:								
raw, cubed	3132	6	.04	.02	.29	.09	9.5	0
boiled, drained, cubed	6156	10	.08	.05	.57	.18	16.5	0
boiled, drained, mashed	4726	8	.05	.03	.39	.12	11.5	0
Hyacinth bean, fresh, 1/2 cup:								
raw	44	5	.03	.04	.21	n.a.	m.q.	0
boiled, drained	62	2	.03	.04	.21	n.a.	m.q.	0
Hyacinth bean, dried, boiled,								
1/2 cup	n.a.	0	.26	.04	.40	n.a.	m.q.	0

1. *With added ascorbic acid or sodium ascorbate; vitamin C value for product without additives would be negligible.*

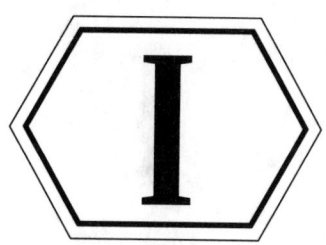

Food and Measure	A I.U.	C mg.	Thi mg.	Rib mg.	Nia mg.	B₆ mg.	Fol mcg.	B₁₂ mcg.
Ice cream, vanilla, ½ cup, except as noted:								
hardened, 10% fat	272	<1	.03	.16	.07	.03	2.0	.31
hardened, 16% fat	449	<1	.02	.14	.06	.03	1.0	.27
French, soft-serve	397	<1	.04	.22	.09	.05	5.0	.50
nuggets, chocolate coated:								
dark chocolate (*Carnation Bon Bons*), 5 pieces	160	<1	.02	.08	.05	m.q.	m.q.	.16
milk chocolate (*Carnation Bon Bons*), 5 pieces	170	<1	.02	.10	.07	m.q.	m.q.	.23
Ice milk, vanilla, hardened, ½ cup	107	<1	.04	.17	.06	.04	2.0	.44

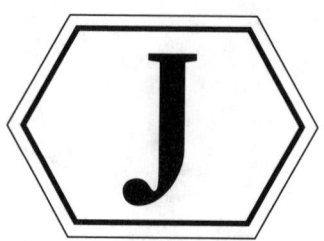

Food and Measure	A I.U.	C mg.	Thi mg.	Rib mg.	Nia mg.	B₆ mg.	Fol mcg.	B₁₂ mcg.
Jackfruit, trimmed, 1 oz.	84	2	.01	n.a.	.11	.03	n.a.	0
Jam and preserves, 1 tbsp.:								
all flavors except cherry and								
strawberry	tr.	tr.	tr.	.01	tr.	n.a.	n.a.	n.a.
cherry and strawberry	tr.	3	tr.	.01	tr.	n.a.	n.a.	n.a.
Java plum, seeded, ½ cup	3	10	<.01	.01	.18	.03	n.a.	0
Jelly, 1 tbsp:								
all flavors except guava	tr.	1	tr.	.01	tr.	n.a.	n.a.	n.a.
guava	tr.	7	tr.	.01	tr.	n.a.	n.a.	n.a.
Jerusalem artichoke, raw, sliced,								
½ cup	15	3	.15	.05	.98	n.a.	n.a.	0
Jujube, fresh, seeded, 1 oz.	11	20	.01	.01	.26	.02	n.a.	0

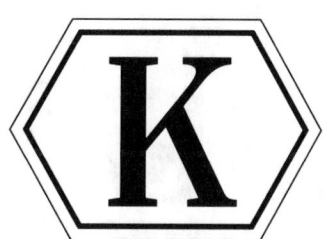

Food and Measure	A I.U.	C mg.	Thi mg.	Rib mg.	Nia mg.	B₆ mg.	Fol mcg.	B₁₂ mcg.
Kale, ½ cup:								
fresh, raw, chopped	3026	41	.04	.04	.34	.09	10.0	0
fresh, boiled, drained, chopped	4810	27	.03	.05	.33	.09	8.6	0
frozen, boiled, drained, chopped ...	4130	16	.03	.07	.44	.06	9.3	0
Kale, Scotch, ½ cup:								
raw, chopped	1054	44	.02	.02	.44	.08	m.q.	0
boiled, drained, chopped	1296	34	.03	.03	.52	.09	8.6	0
Kidney beans, red, ½ cup:								
boiled	0	1	.14	.05	.51	.11	114.1	0
canned, w/liquid	0	2	.13	.11	.58	.03	64.7	0
Kidneys[1], 4 oz.:								
beef, simmered	1407	1	.22	4.60	6.83	.59	111.1	58.17
lamb, braised	516	14	.40	2.35	6.79	.14	91.9	89.47
pork, braised	295	12	.45	1.80	6.56	.52	46.5	8.83
veal, braised	759	9	.22	2.26	5.25	.20	23.8	41.84
Kielbasa[2,3], pork and beef, 1 oz. ..	(0)	6	.07	.06	.82	.05	n.a.	.46
Kiwifruit, 1 medium, approx.								
3.1 oz.	133	75	.02	.04	.38	n.a.	n.a.	0
Knockwurst[2,3] pork and beef, 1 oz.	(0)	8	.10	.04	.78	.05	m.q.	.33
Kohlrabi, ½ cup:								
raw, sliced	25	43	.04	.01	.28	.11	m.q.	0
boiled, drained, sliced	29	44	.03	.02	.32	m.q.	m.q.	0
Kumquat, seeded, 1 oz.	86	11	.02	.03	m.q.	m.q.	n.a.	0

1. *Prepared without added ingredients.*
2. *With added ascorbic acid or sodium ascorbate; vitamin C value for product without additives would be negligible.*
3. *Nonfat dry milk added.*

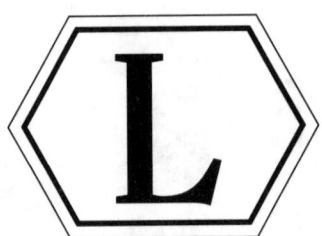

Food and Measure	A I.U.	C mg.	Thi mg.	Rib mg.	Nia mg.	B$_6$ mg.	Fol mcg.	B$_{12}$ mcg.
Lamb[1], domestic, meat only, 4 oz.:								
cubed, for stew or kabob, leg and								
shoulder:								
braised, lean only	0	0	.08	.27	6.75	.14	23.8	3.10
broiled, lean only	0	0	.12	.34	7.50	.16	26.1	3.44
foreshank, braised:								
lean w/fat	0	0	.06	.22	6.19	.11	19.3	2.59
lean only	0	0	.05	.22	5.75	.12	21.5	2.56
ground, broiled	0	0	.11	.28	7.60	.16	21.5	2.96
leg, roasted:								
whole, lean w/fat	0	0	.11	.31	7.47	.17	22.7	2.94
whole, lean only	0	0	.12	.33	7.19	.19	26.1	2.99
shank half, lean w/fat	0	0	.11	.31	7.43	.18	24.9	3.03
shank half, lean only	0	0	.12	.32	7.25	.19	27.2	3.07
sirloin, lean w/fat	0	0	.12	.32	7.51	.16	19.3	2.87
sirloin, lean only	0	0	.14	.35	7.11	.19	23.8	2.93
loin:								
broiled, lean w/fat	0	0	.11	.28	8.05	.15	20.4	2.80
broiled, lean only	0	0	.12	.32	7.77	.18	27.2	2.86
roasted, lean w/fat	0	0	.11	.27	8.05	.12	21.5	2.51
roasted, lean only	0	0	.11	.31	7.75	.18	28.4	2.45
rib:								
broiled, lean w/fat	0	0	.10	.25	7.94	.12	15.9	2.88
broiled, lean only	0	0	.11	.28	7.43	.17	23.8	2.99
roasted, lean w/fat	0	0	.10	.24	7.65	.12	17.0	2.53
roasted, lean only	0	0	.10	.26	6.99	.17	24.9	2.45
shoulder, whole:								
braised, lean w/fat	0	0	.08	.25	7.18	.11	19.3	3.18
braised, lean only	0	0	.07	.26	6.76	.14	23.8	3.30

1. *Prepared without added ingredients.*

Food and Measure	A I.U.	C mg.	Thi mg.	Rib mg.	Nia mg.	B₆ mg.	Fol mcg.	B₁₂ mcg.
broiled, lean w/fat	0	0	.10	.29	7.31	.14	21.5	3.37
broiled, lean only	0	0	.11	.32	6.97	.16	26.1	3.53
roasted, lean w/fat	0	0	.10	.27	6.97	.15	23.8	2.99
roasted, lean only	0	0	.10	.29	6.53	.17	28.4	3.06
shoulder, arm:								
braised, lean w/fat	0	0	.08	.28	7.55	.12	20.4	2.93
braised, lean only	0	0	.08	.31	7.18	.15	24.9	3.01
broiled, lean w/fat	0	0	.11	.31	7.96	.14	20.4	3.24
broiled, lean only	0	0	.11	.33	7.72	.16	26.1	3.40
roasted, lean w/fat	0	0	.10	.28	7.55	.14	22.7	2.89
roasted, lean only	0	0	.11	.31	7.19	.16	28.4	2.96
shoulder, blade:								
braised, lean w/fat	0	0	.07	.24	6.85	.12	20.4	3.21
braised, lean only	0	0	.07	.25	6.38	.14	23.8	3.33
broiled, lean w/fat	0	0	.10	.28	7.23	.17	20.4	3.10
broiled, lean only	0	0	.11	.29	6.88	.19	23.8	3.19
roasted, lean w/fat	0	0	.10	.26	6.70	.12	23.8	3.03
roasted, lean only	0	0	.10	.28	6.20	.17	28.4	3.11
Leek:								
raw, 1 medium, approx. 9.9 oz.	118	15	.07	.04	.50	n.a.	79.5	0
boiled, drained, chopped, ½ cup ...	24	2	.01	.01	.10	n.a.	12.6	0
Lemon:								
w/peel, 1 medium, 2⅛″ diam.,								
3.9 oz.	32	83	.05	.04	.22	.12	n.a.	0
w/peel, 1-oz. wedge, ¼ medium ...	8	21	.01	.01	.05	.03	n.a.	0
w/out peel, 1 medium, 2⅛″ diam.,								
3.9 oz.	17	31	.02	.01	.06	.05	6.2	0
Lemon juice, 1 fl. oz.:								
fresh	6	14	.01	<.01	.03	.02	3.9	0
canned or bottled	5	8	.01	<.01	.06	.01	3.1	0
frozen, single strength	4	10	.02	<.01	.04	.02	2.9	0
Lemon peel, fresh, 1 tsp.	1	3	<.01	<.01	.01	<.01	n.a.	0
Lemonade:								
frozen[1], 1 cup	53	10[2]	<.01	.01	.01	.02	5.5	0
mix[3], 2 tbsp. or 1 scoop	0	9	<.01	n.a.	.04	.01	3.5	0
Lemonade flavor drink mix,								
powder[3], 2 tbsp. or ½ scoop	0	34	<.01	<.01	0	0	0	0
Lentil dinner, canned, hearty,								
w/garden vegetables (*Health*								
Valley Fast Menu), 7½ oz.	5519	4	.17	.19	1.40	.24	22.7	0
Lentils, sprouted, raw ½ cup	17	6	.09	.05	.43	.07	38.0	0
Lentils, dried, boiled, ½ cup	8	2	.17	.07	1.05	.18	178.9	0
Lettuce:								
bibb, Boston, or butterhead,								
5″-diam. head, 7.75 oz.	1581	13	.10	.10	.49	n.a.	118.7	0

1. *Diluted according to package directions.*
2. *Average value.*
3. *With added ascorbic acid.*

Food and Measure	A I.U.	C mg.	Thi mg.	Rib mg.	Nia mg.	B6 mg.	Fol mcg.	B12 mcg.
Lettuce (cont.)								
cos or romaine, shredded, ½ cup,								
approx. 1 oz.	728	7	.03	.03	.14	n.a.	38.0	0
iceberg, 6″-diam. head, 1.25 lbs.	1779	21	.25	.16	1.01	.22	301.8	0
iceberg, 1 leaf, approx. .7 oz.	66	1	.01	.01	.04	.01	11.2	0
looseleaf, shredded, 1 oz. or ½ cup	532	5	.01	.02	.11	.02	m.q.	0
Lima bean, ½ cup:								
fresh, boiled, drained	315	9	.12	.08	.88	.16	m.q.	0
canned, w/liquid	214	11	.04	.05	.66	.12	m.q.	0
frozen, baby, boiled, drained	150	5	.06	.05	.16	.10	m.q.	0
frozen, Fordhook, boiled, drained	162	11	.06	.05	.91	.10	m.q.	0
Lima bean, dried, ½ cup:								
large, boiled	0	0	.15	.05	.40	.15	78.1	0
large, canned, w/liquid	0	0	.07	.04	.31	.11	60.5	0
baby, boiled	0	0	.15	.05	.60	.07	136.4	0
Lime, 1 medium, 2″ diam.,								
approx. 2.8 oz.	7	20	.02	.01	.13	n.a.	5.5	0
Lime juice, 1 fl. oz.:								
fresh	3	9	.01	<.01	.03	.01	m.q.	0
canned or bottled	5	2	.01	tr.	.05	.01	2.4	0
Ling, meat only, raw, 1 oz.	28	(0)	.03	.05	.65	.09	m.q.	.16
Litchee:								
fresh, shelled and seeded, ½ cup	0	68	.01	.06	.57	n.a.	m.q.	0
dried, 1 oz.	0	52	<.01	.16	.88	n.a.	m.q.	0
Liver[1], 4 oz.:								
beef, braised	40,460	26	.23	4.65	12.16	1.03	246.1	80.51
beef, pan-fried in vegetable oil	40,943	26	.24	4.69	16.37	1.62	249.5	126.78
chicken, simmered	18,569	18	.17	1.98	5.05	.66	873.2	21.99
lamb, braised	28,288	5	.26	4.57	13.78	.56	82.8	86.75
lamb, pan-fried in vegetable oil	29,482	15	.40	5.21	18.92	1.08	453.6	97.18
pork, braised	20,409	27	.29	2.49	9.57	.65	184.8	21.17
turkey, simmered	14,267	2	.06	1.61	6.74	.59	755.2	53.90
veal (calf), braised	30,485	35	.15	2.20	9.62	.56	860.7	41.39
veal (calf), pan-fried in vegetable oil	21,317	25	.28	3.81	19.19	.98	362.9	72.52
Liver cheese, pork, 1 oz.	4958	1	.06	.63	3.34	.13	m.q.	6.96
Liver pâté, see "Pâté"								
Liverwurst, pork, 1 oz.	m.q.	(0)	.08	.29	m.q.	.05	8.0	3.82
Lobster, northern, meat only,								
boiled or steamed[2], 4 oz.	99	(0)	.01	.07	1.21	.09	12.6	3.53
Loganberry:								
fresh, trimmed, 1 cup	290	35	.04	.06	.60	m.q.	m.q.	0
frozen, ½ cup	26	11	.04	.03	.62	.05	18.9	0
Loquat, peeled and seeded, 1 oz.	433	<1	.01	.01	.05	n.a.	m.q.	0
Luncheon meat[3]:								
pork and beef, 1-oz. slice	0	4	.09	.04	.80	.06	2.0	.36

1. *Prepared without added ingredients, except as noted.*
2. *Without added ingredients.*
3. *With added ascorbic acid or sodium ascorbate; vitamin C value for product without additives would be negligible.*

Food and Measure	A I.U.	C mg.	Thi mg.	Rib mg.	Nia mg.	B₆ mg.	Fol mcg.	B₁₂ mcg.
pork and beef, sausage, 1 oz.	0	5	.06	.06	1.00	.06	m.q.	.56
canned, pork, 1 oz.	0	0	.10	.06	.89	.06	2.0	.25
Lung[1], 4 oz.:								
beef, braised	44	37	.04	.16	2.83	.02	9.1	2.94
pork, braised	0	9	.09	.37	2.15	.09	n.a.	2.30
Luxury loaf[2], pork, 1-oz. slice	0	6	.20	.08	.99	.09	m.q.	.39

1. *Prepared without added ingredients.*
2. *With added ascorbic acid or sodium ascorbate; vitamin C value for product without additives would be negligible.*

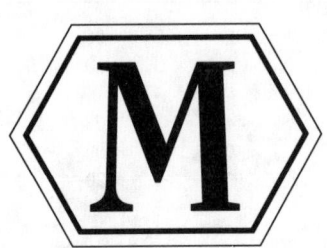

Food and Measure	A I.U.	C mg.	Thi mg.	Rib mg.	Nia mg.	B₆ mg.	Fol mcg.	B₁₂ mcg.
Macadamia nut, 1 oz.:								
dried	0	0	.10	.03	.61	n.a.	m.q.	0
oil-roasted	3	0	.06	.03	.57	n.a.	m.q.	0
Macaroni, dry, cooked:								
enriched, 4 oz.	0	0	.23	.11	1.90	.04	7.9	0
elbow, enriched, 1 cup	0	0	.29	.14	2.34	.05	10.0	0
protein-fortified, 4 oz.	0	0	.34	.18	2.08	.07	12.5	0
vegetable (tricolor), 4 oz.	60	0	.13	.07	1.21	.03	6.8	0
whole wheat, 4 oz.	0	0	.12	.05	.80	.09	5.7	0
Mace, ground, 1 tsp.	14	n.a.	.01	.01	.02	n.a.	n.a.	0
Mackerel, meat only:								
Atlantic, raw, 1 oz.	47	<1	.05	.09	2.57	.11	m.q.	2.47
Atlantic, baked, broiled, or								
microwaved[1], 4 oz.	204	<1	.18	.47	.78	.52	m.q.	21.54
king, raw, 1 oz.	206	(0)	.03	.14	2.43	.14	2.1	4.42
Pacific or jack, raw, 1 oz.	12	(0)	.03	.12	2.57	.09	.5	1.25
Mackerel, canned, jack, drained,								
4 oz.	492	1	.05	.24	7.01	.24	5.7	7.87
Malted milk:								
natural flavor, powder, ¾ oz. or								
2–3 heaping tsp.	68	0	.11	.14	1.07	.08	10.0	.16
natural flavor, prepared[2]	376	2	.20	.54	1.28	.18	22.0	1.04
chocolate flavor, powder, ¾ oz. or								
2–3 heaping tsp.	20	n.a.	.04	.04	.43	.03	5.0	.05
chocolate flavor, prepared[2]	326	2	.14	.43	.69	.13	17.0	.92
Mammy apple, peeled and seeded,								
1 oz.	65	4	.01	.01	.11	n.a.	n.a.	0
Mango:								
1 medium, approx 10.6 oz.	8060	57	.12	.19	1.21	.28	n.a.	0

1. *Without added ingredients.*
2. *1 cup whole milk and ¾ oz. powder.*

Food and Measure	A I.U.	C mg.	Thi mg.	Rib mg.	Nia mg.	B₆ mg.	Fol mcg.	B₁₂ mcg.
peeled and seeded, sliced, ½ cup ..	3213	23	.05	.05	.48	.11	n.a.	0
Marjoram, dried, 1 tsp.	48	<1	<.01	<.01	.03	n.a.	n.a.	0
Marmalade, citrus, 1 tbsp.	m.q.	1	tr.	tr.	tr.	n.a.	n.a.	n.a.
Melon, see specific listings								
Melon balls (cantaloupe and								
honeydew), frozen, ½ cup	1535	5	.14	.02	.55	.09	22.3	0
Milk, cow, fluid, 1 cup:								
buttermilk, cultured	81	2	.08	.38	.14	.08	m.q.	.54
whole:								
3.3% fat	307	2	.09	.40	.21	.10	12.0	.87
3.7% fat, producer	337	4	.09	.39	.21	.10	12.0	.87
low sodium	317	n.a.	.05	.26	.11	.08	m.q.	.88
lowfat 2%:								
1 cup	500	2	.10	.40	.21	.11	12.0	.89
nonfat milk solids added	500	2	.10	.42	.22	.11	13.0	.94
protein fortified	500	3	.11	.48	.25	.13	15.0	1.05
lowfat 1%:								
1 cup	500	2	.10	.41	.21	.11	12.0	.90
nonfat milk solids added	500	2	.10	.42	.22	.11	13.0	.94
protein fortified	500	3	.11	.47	.25	.12	15.0	1.05
skim:								
1 cup	500	2	.09	.34	.22	.10	13.0	.93
nonfat milk solids added	500	2	.10	.43	.22	.11	13.0	.95
protein fortified	500	3	.11	.48	.25	.12	15.0	1.10
Milk, canned, 1 cup:								
condensed, sweetened	1004	8	.28	1.27	.64	.16	34.0	1.36
evaporated, whole[1]	612	5	.12	.80	.49	.13	20.0	.41
evaporated, skim[1]	20	3	.11	.78	.44	.14	22.0	.61
Milk, dry, 1 oz.:								
buttermilk, sweet cream	62	2	.11	.45	.25	.10	13.3	1.08
whole	261	2	.08	.34	.18	.09	10.5	.92
nonfat:								
regular	10	2	.12	.44	.27	.10	14.2	1.14
calcium reduced	2	m.q.	.05	.47	.19	.08	m.q.	1.13
instant[1]	8	2	.12	.49	.25	.10	14.2	1.13
Milk, goat, fluid, whole, 1 cup	451	3	.12	.34	.68	.11	1.0	.16
Milk, human, fluid, whole, 1 cup ..	593	12	.03	.09	.44	.03	13.0	.11
Milk, Indian buffalo, fluid, whole,								
1 cup	434	5	.13	.33	.22	.06	14.0	.89
Milk, sheep, fluid, whole, 1 cup ..	360	10	.16	.87	1.02	m.q.	m.q.	1.74
Millet:								
raw, 1 oz.	n.a.	0	.12	.08	1.34	.11	n.a.	0
cooked, 1 cup	n.a.	0	.25	.20	3.19	.26	n.a.	0
Miso, ½ cup	120	0	.13	.35	1.19	.30	45.5	.29
Molasses, cane, blackstrap, 1 tbsp.	0	0	.02	.04	.40	n.a.	n.a.	0
Mortadella[2], beef and pork, 1 oz.	0	7	.03	.04	.76	.04	m.q.	.42

1. *Without added vitamin A.*
2. *With added ascorbic acid or sodium ascorbate; vitamin C value for product without additives would be negligible.*

Food and Measure	A I.U.	C mg.	Thi mg.	Rib mg.	Nia mg.	B6 mg.	Fol mcg.	B12 mcg.
Mother's loaf, pork, 1 oz.	0	0	.16	.05	.89	.05	m.q.	.30
Muffin, 1 piece:								
English, plain, 2 oz.	0	0	.26	.19	2.20	n.a.	m.q.	0
oat bran:								
almond and date (*Health Valley Fancy Fruit Muffins*)	54	2	.25	.14	.45	.20	17.0	0
blueberry (*Health Valley Fancy Fruit Muffins*)	36	5	.21	.13	.50	.13	13.8	0
raisin (*Health Valley Fancy Fruit Muffins*)	60	7	.20	.16	.85	.16	15.3	0
rice bran raisin (*Health Valley Fancy Fruit Muffins*)	2	5	.32	.08	3.60	.09	7.6	0
Muffin mix[1], 1.6-oz. piece:								
blueberry	50	tr.	.10	.17	1.10	n.a.	m.q.	n.a.
bran	100	0	.08	.12	1.90	n.a.	m.q.	n.a.
corn	90	tr.	.09	.09	.80	n.a.	m.q.	n.a.
Mulberry, ½ cup	18	26	.02	.07	.43	n.a.	n.a.	0
Mullet, striped, meat only:								
raw, 1 oz.	35	<1	m.q.	m.q.	m.q.	.12	2.4	m.q.
baked, broiled, or microwaved[2], 4 oz.	160	1	m.q.	m.q.	m.q.	.56	1.1	m.q.
Mung bean, mature seed, sprouted:								
raw, ½ cup	11	7	.04	.06	.39	.05	31.6	0
boiled, drained, ½ cup	8	7	.03	.06	.51	n.a.	m.q.	0
Mung bean, dried, boiled, ½ cup	24	1	.17	.06	.58	.07	160.3	0
Mushroom:								
raw, 1 medium, approx. .7 oz.	0	1	.02	.08	.74	.02	3.8	0
raw, pieces, ½ cup	0	1	.04	.16	1.44	.03	7.4	0
boiled, drained, pieces, ½ cup	0	3	.06	.23	3.48	.07	14.2	0
Mushroom gravy, canned, ¼ cup	0	0	.02	.04	.40	.01	n.a.	0
Mustard, prepared, yellow, 1 tsp.	0	tr.	tr.	.01	tr.	0	m.q.	0
Mustard greens, ½ cup:								
fresh, raw, chopped	1484	20	.02	.03	.22	m.q.	m.q.	0
fresh, boiled, drained, chopped	2122	18	.03	.04	.30	m.q.	m.q.	0
frozen, boiled, drained, chopped ...	3352	10	.03	.04	.19	.08	m.q.	0
Mustard seed, yellow, 1 tsp.	2	n.a.	.02	.01	.26	n.a.	n.a.	0

1. *Prepared according to package directions.*
2. *Without added ingredients.*

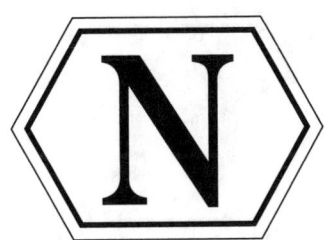

Food and Measure	A I.U.	C mg.	Thi mg.	Rib mg.	Nia mg.	B$_6$ mg.	Fol mcg.	B$_{12}$ mcg.
Natto, ½ cup	0	11	.14	.17	0	(0)	m.q.	0
Navy beans, dried, ½ cup:								
boiled	2	1	.18	.06	.48	.15	127.3	0
canned, w/liquid	2	2	.16	.08	.34	.13	146.2	0
Nectarine:								
pitted, sliced, ½ cup	508	4	.01	.03	.68	.02	2.6	0
1 medium, 2½″ diam., approx.								
5.3 oz.	1001	7	.02	.06	1.35	.03	5.1	0
New England Brand sausage[1],								
pork and beef, 1 oz.	n.a.	6	.18	.07	.99	.10	2.0	.38
New Zealand spinach, ½ cup:								
raw, chopped	1232	8	.01	.04	.14	n.a.	m.q.	0
boiled, drained, chopped	3260	14	.03	.10	.35	n.a.	m.q.	0
Noodle, egg, cooked, 1 cup:								
plain, enriched	32	0	.30	.13	2.38	.06	11.0	.14
spinach, enriched	165	0	.39	.20	2.36	.18	34.0	.22
Noodle, Chinese:								
cellophane or long rice, dehydrated,								
2 oz.	0	0	.09	0	.10	n.a.	n.a.	0
chow mein, 1 cup	38	0	.26	.19	2.68	.05	10.0	0
Noodle, Japanese, cooked:								
soba, 1 cup, approx. 4 oz.	n.a.	0	.11	.03	.58	.05	8.0	0
somen, 1 cup	n.a.	0	.03	.06	.17	.02	3.0	0
Nutmeg, ground, 1 tsp.	2	n.a.	.01	<.01	.03	n.a.	n.a.	0
Nuts, see specific listings								
Nuts, mixed, 1 oz.:								
dry-roasted, w/peanuts	4	<1	.06	.06	1.34	.08	14.3	0
oil-roasted, w/peanuts	6	<1	.14	.06	1.44	.07	23.6	0
oil-roasted, w/out peanuts	6	<1	.14	.14	.56	.05	16.0	0

1. *With added ascorbic acid or sodium ascorbate; vitamin C value for product without additives would be negligible.*

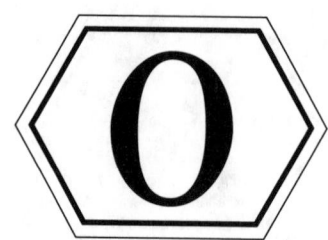

Food and Measure	A I.U.	C mg.	Thi mg.	Rib mg.	Nia mg.	B₆ mg.	Fol mcg.	B₁₂ mcg.
Oat (see also "Cereal"):								
whole grain, 1 cup	n.a.	0	1.19	.22	1.50	.19	87.0	0
rolled or oatmeal, dry, 1 oz.	29	0	.21	.04	.22	.03	9.1	0
rolled or oatmeal, cooked, 1 cup ...	38	0	.26	.05	.30	.05	9.0	0
Oat bran:								
raw, 1 oz.	n.a.	0	.33	.06	.26	.05	14.7	0
cooked, 1 cup	n.a.	0	.35	.07	.32	.06	14.0	0
Oat bran pilaf dinner, canned, w/garden vegetables (*Health Valley Fast Menu*), 7½ oz.	6174	5	.35	.11	.82	.15	44.8	0
Ocean perch, meat only:								
raw, 1 oz.	9	(0)	m.q.	.02	.43	m.q.	m.q.	.02
baked, broiled, or microwaved[1], 4 oz.	52	(0)	m.q.	.15	2.76	m.q.	m.q.	1.31
Oheloberry, ½ cup	581	4	.01	.03	.19	n.a.	n.a.	0
Oil, corn, olive, peanut, safflower, soybean (hydrogenated), soybean-cottonseed blend (hydrogenated), or sunflower, 1 tbsp.	0	0	0	0	0	n.a.	n.a.	0
Okra, ½ cup:								
fresh, raw, sliced	330	11	.10	.03	.50	.11	43.9	0
fresh, boiled, drained, sliced	460	13	.11	.04	.70	.15	36.5	0
frozen, boiled, drained, sliced	473	11	.09	.11	.72	.04	134.0	0
Olive, ripe, pitted, canned:								
Mission and Manzanilla:								
all sizes, 1 oz.	114	<1	tr.	(0)	.01	tr.	0	0
10 small, approx. 1.1 oz.	129	<1	tr.	(0)	.01	tr.	0	0

1. *Without added ingredients.*

Food and Measure	A I.U.	C mg.	Thi mg.	Rib mg.	Nia mg.	B₆ mg.	Fol mcg.	B₁₂ mcg.
10 large, approx. 1.6 oz.	177	<1	tr.	(0)	.02	tr.	0	0
Sevillano and Ascolano:								
all sizes, 1 oz.	98	<1	(0)	(0)	<.01	<.01	0	0
10 jumbo, approx. 2.9 oz.	287	1	(0)	.(0)	.02	.01	0	0
10 super colossal, approx. 5.4 oz.	526	2	(0)	(0)	.03	.02	0	0
Olive loaf[1], pork, 1-oz. slice	n.a.	2	.08	.07	.52	.07	m.q.	.36
Onion, mature, ½ cup:								
fresh, raw, chopped	0	5	.03	.02	.12	.09	15.0	0
fresh, boiled, drained, chopped	0	6	.05	.02	.17	.14	16.0	0
frozen, boiled, drained, chopped ...	36	3	.02	.03	.15	.07	14.1	0
Onion, green (scallion), w/top[2],								
chopped, ½ cup	193	9	.03	.04	.26	n.a.	32.0	0
Onion flakes, dehydrated,								
1 tbsp.	0	4	.03	.01	.05	.08	8.3	0
Onion powder, 1 tsp.	tr.	<1	.01	<.01	.01	n.a.	n.a.	0
Onion rings, breaded, frozen,								
heated, 2 rings or 1 oz.	45	<1	.06	.03	.72	.02	2.6	0
Orange:								
California navel:								
1 medium, 2⅞″ diam., approx.								
7.3 oz.	256	80	.12	.06	.41	.10	47.2	0
trimmed, sections w/out								
membrane, ½ cup	151	47	.07	.03	.24	.06	27.8	0
California Valencia:								
1 medium, 2⅝″ diam., approx.								
5.7 oz.	278	59	.11	.05	.33	.08	46.7	0
peeled and seeded, sections w/out								
membrane, ½ cup	207	44	.08	.04	.25	.06	34.8	0
Florida:								
1 medium, 2¹¹⁄₁₆″ diam., approx.								
7.2 oz.	302	68	.15	.06	.60	.08	26.1	0
peeled and seeded, sections w/out								
membrane, ½ cup	185	42	.09	.04	.37	.05	16.0	0
Mandarin, see "Tangerine, canned"								
Orange drink[3], canned, 1 cup	45	85	.01	.01	.08	.02	n.a.	0
Orange flavor drink[4], breakfast:								
frozen[5], w/orange pulp, 1 fl. oz.	0	22	.04	.01	0	0	n.a.	0
frozen[5], w/orange juice and pulp,								
1 fl. oz.	2	17	.03	.33	.08	.02	10.1	0
mix, 3 rounded tsp.	0	22	.04	.01	0	0	n.a.	0
Orange juice, 6 fl. oz.:								
fresh	372	93	.17	.06	.74	.07	m.q.	0
canned	330	64	.11	.05	.59	.16	m.q.	0
chilled	144	61	.21	.04	.52	.10	33.6	0
frozen[5]	144	73	.15	.04	.38	.08	81.6	0

1. *With added ascorbic acid or sodium ascorbate; vitamin C value for product without additives would be negligible.*
2. *Vitamin A value varies depending on proportion of bulb and top (leaves).*
3. *With added ascorbic acid.*
4. *With added nutrients.*
5. *Diluted according to package directions.*

Food and Measure	A I.U.	C mg.	Thi mg.	Rib mg.	Nia mg.	B_6 mg.	Fol mcg.	B_{12} mcg.
Orange peel, fresh, 1 tsp.	8	3	<.01	<.01	.02	<.01	n.a.	0
Orange-apricot juice drink,								
canned, 1 cup	1450	50	.05	.03	.50	n.a.	n.a.	0
Orange-grapefruit juice, canned,								
6 fl. oz.	222	54	.10	.05	.62	.04	m.q.	0
Oregano, ground, 1 tsp.	104	m.q.	.01	m.q.	.09	n.a.	n.a.	0
Oyster, meat only:								
Eastern:								
raw, 1 oz.	m.q.	(0)	n.a.	.05	.37	.01	2.8	5.42
raw, 6 medium, approx. 3 oz. ...	m.q.	(0)	n.a.	.14	1.10	.04	8.3	16.07
boiled, poached, or steamed[1],								
4 oz.	m.q.	(0)	n.a.	.38	2.82	.11	20.2	43.39
Pacific, raw, 1 medium, approx.								
1.75 oz.	m.q.	(0)	.03	.12	1.01	m.q.	m.q.	m.q.
Oyster, canned, Eastern, 4 oz. ..	m.q.	(0)	n.a.	.19	1.41	.11	10.1	21.70

1. *Without added ingredients.*

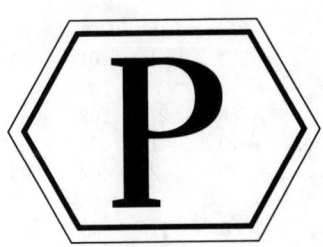

Food and Measure	A I.U.	C mg.	Thi mg.	Rib mg.	Nia mg.	B6 mg.	Fol mcg.	B12 mcg.
Pancake, frozen, microwave, 3.5 oz.:								
(*Aunt Jemima* Original)	0	0	.24	.26	2.10	.04	22.0	.27
blueberry (*Aunt Jemima*)	0	0	.21	.25	2.03	.04	46.0	.54
buttermilk (*Aunt Jemima*)	0	0	.24	.28	1.60	.04	27.0	.52
buttermilk (*Aunt Jemima* Lite)	0	0	.22	.25	2.00	m.q.	24.0	.48
Pancake batter, 3.6 oz.:								
(*Aunt Jemima* Original)	0	0	.27	.22	2.06	.04	15.0	.30
blueberry (*Aunt Jemima*)	0	0	.26	.20	1.99	.09	8.0	.73
buttermilk (*Aunt Jemima*)	0	0	.28	.25	2.16	.05	11.0	.23
Pancake mix[1], 3 cakes, 4″ each, except as noted:								
(*Aunt Jemima* Original)	0	0	.18	.09	1.11	.08	5.0	0
(*Aunt Jemima* Original Complete) ...	0	0	.33	.27	2.31	.09	9.0	.16
buckwheat (*Aunt Jemima*)	0	0	.22	.11	1.86	.07	16.0	n.a.
buttermilk:								
(*Aunt Jemima*)	0	0	.20	.15	1.33	.04	7.0	.13
(*Aunt Jemima* Complete)	0	0	.32	.31	2.06	.08	16.0	.21
(*Aunt Jemima* Lite)	0	0	.53	.34	3.00	.12	16.0	n.a.
(*Health Valley* Biscuit & Pancake Mix), 1 oz. dry	3	1	.15	.11	1.20	.08	13.5	0
whole wheat (*Aunt Jemima*)	0	0	.31	.44	3.64	.06	23.0	n.a.
Pancreas[2], 4 oz.:								
beef, braised	0	23	.20	.55	4.50	.20	m.q.	18.82
lamb, braised	0	23	.02	.24	2.90	.06	14.7	6.28
pork, braised	0	6	.10	.75	3.64	n.a.	m.q.	19.36
Papaya:								
1 medium, 3½″ × 5⅛″, 1 lb.	6122	188	.08	.10	1.03	.06	n.a.	0
peeled and seeded, cubed, ½ cup ..	1410	43	.02	.02	.24	.01	n.a.	0

1. *Prepared according to package directions, except as noted.*
2. *Prepared without added ingredients.*

Food and Measure	A I.U.	C mg.	Thi mg.	Rib mg.	Nia mg.	B₆ mg.	Fol mcg.	B₁₂ mcg.
Papaya nectar, canned, 6 fl. oz. . .	210	5	.01	.01	.28	.02	3.6	0
Paprika, 1 tsp.	1273	1	.01	.04	.32	n.a.	n.a.	0
Parsley:								
fresh, raw, chopped, ½ cup	1560	27	.02	.03	.21	.05	54.9	0
dried, 1 tsp.	70	<1	.01	.01	.02	<.01	m.q.	0
freeze-dried, ¼ cup	885	2	.02	.03	.15	.02	21.5	0
Parsnip, ½ cup:								
raw, sliced	0	11	.06	.03	.47	.06	44.8	0
boiled, drained, sliced	0	10	.07	.04	.57	.07	45.4	0
Passion fruit, purple, trimmed,								
1 oz.	198	9	n.a.	.04	.43	n.a.	n.a.	0
Passion fruit juice, fresh:								
purple, 6 fl. oz.	1332	55	n.a.	.24	2.71	n.a.	n.a.	0
yellow, 6 fl. oz.	4470	34	n.a.	.19	4.15	n.a.	n.a.	0
Pasta:								
dry, uncooked, 2 oz.:								
amaranth (*Health Valley* Spaghetti)	0	2	.23	.11	6.00	.17	27.5	0
oat bran (*Health Valley* Spaghetti)	9	1	.23	.07	1.00	.05	13.5	0
whole wheat (*Health Valley*								
Lasagna)	5	3	.53	.17	5.00	.21	38.9	0
whole wheat (*Health Valley*								
Spaghetti)	5	3	.53	.17	6.00	.20	37.6	0
whole wheat spinach (*Health Valley*								
Lasagna/Spaghetti)	2869	4	.53	.17	5.00	.28	119.0	0
dry, cooked, 1 cup:								
enriched	(0)	0	.29	.14	2.34	.05	10.0	0
protein-fortified	(0)	0	.42	.23	2.57	.09	15.0	0
corn	80	0	.07	.03	.78	.08	9.0	0
spinach	m.q.	0	.14	.14	2.14	.13	16.0	0
whole wheat	(0)	0	.15	.06	.99	.11	7.0	0
fresh, refrigerated, cooked:								
w/egg, 4 oz.	n.a.	0	.24	.17	1.12	.04	m.q.	.16
spinach, w/egg, 4 oz.	n.a.	0	.20	.15	1.15	.13	m.q.	.16
Pasta sauce, see "Tomato sauce"								
Pâté, canned, 1 tbsp.:								
chicken liver	94	1	.01	.18	.98	m.q.	m.q.	m.q.
liver	429	0	<.01	.08	.43	.01	8.0	.42
Peach, ½ cup, except as noted:								
fresh, 1 medium, 2½" diam., approx.								
4 per lb.	465	6	.02	.04	.86	.02	3.0	0
fresh, pulp, sliced	455	6	.01	.04	.84	.02	2.9	0
canned, halves or slices:								
in water, clingstone	649	4	.01	.02	.64	.02	4.1	0
in juice, clingstone or freestone . .	473	4	.01	.02	.72	m.q.	m.q.	0
in light syrup, clingstone	444	3	.01	.03	.74	.02	4.1	0
in heavy syrup, clingstone or								
freestone	425	4	.01	.03	.79	.02	4.1	0
canned, spiced, in heavy syrup,								
whole	384	6	.01	.04	.65	n.a.	n.a.	0

Food and Measure	A I.U.	C mg.	Thi mg.	Rib mg.	Nia mg.	B6 mg.	Fol mcg.	B12 mcg.
dehydrated, sulfured, uncooked	822	6	.02	.06	2.80	.09	3.8	0
dehydrated, sulfured, cooked	479	8	.01	.07	2.46	.07	3.4	0
dried, sulfured, halves:								
uncooked	1731	4	<.01	.17	3.50	.05	n.a.	0
cooked, unsweetened	254	5	.01	.03	1.96	.05	.1	0
cooked, sweetened	243	5	.01	.03	1.87	.22	.1	0
frozen, sweetened, sliced[1]	355	118	.02	.04	.82	.02	n.a.	0
Peach nectar, canned, 6 fl. oz.[2] ..	480	10	.01	.02	.54	n.a.	n.a.	0
Peanut, shelled, 1 oz.:								
raw:								
all types	0	0	.18	.04	3.38	.10	67.1	0
Spanish	0	0	.19	.04	4.46	.10	67.2	0
Valencia	0	0	.18	.08	3.61	.10	68.7	0
Virginia	0	0	.18	.04	3.47	.10	66.8	0
boiled, all types	0	0	.08	.02	1.68	.05	23.9	0
dry-roasted, all types	0	0	.12	.03	3.79	.07	40.7	0
oil-roasted:								
all types	0	0	.07	.03	4.00	.07	35.2	0
Spanish	0	0	.09	.02	4.18	.07	35.3	0
Valencia	0	0	.03	.04	4.02	.07	35.1	0
Virginia	0	0	.08	.03	4.12	.07	35.1	0
Peanut butter, 2 tbsp.:								
chunk style	0	0	.04	.04	4.38	.14	29.4	0
chunk or creamy (*Health Valley*)	0	6	.04	.04	4.80	.12	26.2	0
smooth style	0	0	.04	.03	4.19	.12	25.0	0
Peanut flour, defatted, 1 cup	0	0	.42	.29	16.20	.30	148.9	0
Pecan, shelled, dried, 1 oz.	36	1	.24	.04	.25	.05	11.1	0
Pear, ½ cup, except as noted:								
fresh, trimmed, w/skin, sliced	17	3	.02	.03	.08	.02	6.0	0
fresh, Bartlett, 2½" diam × 3½",								
approx. 2½ per lb.	33	7	.03	.07	.17	.03	12.1	0
canned, halves:								
in water	0	1	.01	.01	.07	.02	1.5	0
in juice	7	2	.01	.01	.25	m.q.	m.q.	0
in light syrup	0	1	.01	.02	.19	.02	1.5	0
in heavy or extra heavy syrup ...	0	2	.01	.03	.31	.02	1.5	0
dried, sulfured, halves:								
uncooked	3	6	.01	.13	1.24	n.a.	n.a.	0
cooked, unsweetened	54	5	.01	.03	.45	.04	0	0
cooked, sweetened	56	5	.01	.03	.47	.05	0	0
Pear nectar, canned, 6 fl. oz.[2]	2	2	.01	.02	.24	n.a.	n.a.	0
Peas, edible-podded, ½ cup:								
fresh, raw	105	43	.11	.06	.43	.12	m.q.	0
fresh, boiled, drained	104	38	.10	.06	.43	.12	m.q.	0
frozen, boiled, drained	133	18	.05	.10	.45	.14	m.q.	0
Peas, green, ½ cup:								
fresh, raw	461	29	.19	.10	1.51	.12	47.0	0

1. *With added ascorbic acid.*
2. *Without added ascorbic acid.*

Food and Measure	A I.U.	C mg.	Thi mg.	Rib mg.	Nia mg.	B₆ mg.	Fol mcg.	B₁₂ mcg.
Peas, green *(cont.)*								
fresh, boiled, drained	478	11	.21	.12	1.62	.17	50.7	0
canned, w/liquid	470	14	.14	.09	1.04	.08	35.4	0
canned, drained	653	8	.10	.07	.62	.05	37.7	0
frozen, boiled, drained	534	8	.23	.08	1.18	.09	46.9	0
Peas, split, boiled, ½ cup	7	<1	.19	.06	.87	.05	63.6	0
Peas, sprouted, mature seeds,								
raw, ½ cup	100	6	.14	.09	1.85	.16	86.4	0
Peas and carrots, ½ cup:								
canned, w/liquid	7386	8	.10	.07	.74	.11	23.5	0
frozen, boiled, drained	6209	7	.18	.05	.92	.07	20.8	0
Peas and onions, canned, w/liquid,								
½ cup	96	2	.06	.04	.77	m.q.	m.q.	0
Pepper, chili, hot:								
green, 1 medium, approx. 1.6 oz.	346	109	.04	.04	.43	.13	10.5	0
green, chopped, ½ cup	578	182	.07	.07	.71	.21	17.5	0
red, 1 medium, approx. 1.6 oz.	4838	109	.04	.04	.43	.13	10.5	0
red, chopped, ½ cup	8063	182	.07	.07	.71	.21	17.5	0
Pepper, ground, 1 tsp.:								
black	4	tr.	<.01	.01	.02	n.a.	n.a.	0
red or cayenne	749	1	.01	.02	.16	n.a.	n.a.	0
Pepper, jalapeño, canned,								
w/liquid, chopped, ½ cup	1156	9	.02	.03	.34	n.a.	n.a.	0
Pepper, sweet (bell):								
green:								
raw, 1 medium, approx. 3.2 oz. ..	468	66	.05	.02	.38	.18	16.0	0
raw, chopped, ½ cup	316	45	.03	.02	.26	.12	11.0	0
boiled, drained, chopped, ½ cup	403	51	.04	.02	.33	.16	11.0	0
red:								
raw, 1 medium, approx. 3.2 oz. ..	4218	141	.05	.02	.38	.18	16.0	0
raw, chopped, ½ cup	2850	95	.03	.02	.26	.12	11.0	0
boiled, drained, chopped, ½ cup	2557	116	.04	.02	.33	.16	11.0	0
Pepper sauce, hot (*Tabasco*),								
2 fl. oz.	1726	1	n.a.	n.a.	.20	.11	tr.	.04
Peppered loaf[1], pork and beef,								
1-oz. slice	0	7	.11	.09	.87	.08	m.q.	.56
Pepperoni, pork and beef, 1 oz. ...	0	n.a.	.09	.07	1.41	.07	m.q.	.71
Persimmon, Japanese:								
fresh, 1 medium, 2½" × 3½",								
approx. 1.1 oz.	3640	13	.05	.03	.17	n.a.	12.6	0
dried, 1 oz.	158	tr.	n.a.	.01	.05	n.a.	m.q.	0
Pheasant, raw, meat w/skin, 1 oz.	50	2	.02	.04	1.82	.19	m.q.	.22
Pickle, cucumber:								
dill, 1 medium, 3¾" long, approx.								
2.3 oz.	214	1	.01	.02	.04	.01	1.0	0
sour, 1 medium, 3¾" long, approx.								
2.3 oz.	51	<1	0	<.01	0	n.a.	n.a.	0

1. *With added ascorbic acid or sodium ascorbate; vitamin C value for product without additives would be negligible.*

Food and Measure	A I.U.	C mg.	Thi mg.	Rib mg.	Nia mg.	B_6 mg.	Fol mcg.	B_{12} mcg.
sweet, 1 large, 3″ long, approx.								
1.2 oz.	44	<1	<.01	.01	.06	.01	0	0
Pickle and pimiento loaf[1], pork,								
1-oz. slice	n.a.	4	.08	.07	.58	.05	m.q.	.33
Picnic loaf[1], pork and beef, 1-oz.								
slice	0	5	.11	.07	.65	.09	m.q.	.42
Pie, ⅙ of 9″-diam. pie:								
apple	50	2	.17	.13	1.60	n.a.	m.q.	n.a.
blueberry	140	6	.17	.14	1.70	n.a.	m.q.	n.a.
cherry	700	0	.19	.14	1.60	n.a.	m.q.	n.a.
custard	350	0	.14	.32	.90	n.a.	m.q.	n.a.
lemon meringue	240	4	.10	.14	.80	n.a.	m.q.	n.a.
peach	1150	5	.17	.16	2.40	n.a.	m.q.	n.a.
pecan	220	0	.30	.17	1.10	n.a.	m.q.	n.a.
pumpkin	3750	0	.14	.21	1.20	n.a.	m.q.	n.a.
Pie, frozen, baked, ⅙ of 8″-diam.								
pie:								
apple	10	1	.01	.01	.20	n.a.	m.q.	n.a.
cherry	280	2	.02	.02	.20	n.a.	m.q.	n.a.
coconut custard	160	tr.	.04	.16	.20	n.a.	m.q.	n.a.
Pie crust mix[2], 9″ crust	0	0	1.06	.80	9.90	n.a.	m.q.	n.a.
Pigeon pea, boiled, ½ cup	2	0	.12	.05	.66	.04	93.0	0
Pike, northern, meat only:								
raw, 1 oz.	20	1	.02	.02	m.q.	.03	m.q.	m.q.
baked, broiled, or microwaved[3],								
4 oz.	92	4	.08	.09	m.q.	.15	m.q.	m.q.
Pimiento, canned, 1 tbsp.	319	10	<.01	.01	.07	.03	1.0	0
Pine nut, shelled, 1 oz.:								
pignolias, dried	0	n.a.	.23	.05	1.01	n.a.	m.q.	0
piñons, dried	0	1	.35	.06	1.24	n.a.	m.q.	0
Pineapple, ½ cup:								
fresh, trimmed, diced	18	12	.07	.03	.33	.07	8.2	0
canned:								
in water, tidbits	19	10	.11	.03	.37	.09	6.0	0
in juice, chunks or tidbits	48	12	.12	.02	.36	m.q.	m.q.	0
in light syrup	19	10	.11	.03	.37	.09	6.0	0
in heavy syrup, chunks, tidbits or								
crushed	19	10	.12	.03	.37	.09	5.9	0
frozen, sweetened, chunks	37	10	.12	.04	.37	.09	m.q.	0
Pineapple juice, 6 fl. oz.:								
canned[4]	6	20	.10	.04	.48	.18	43.2	0
frozen[5]	18	22	.13	.04	.37	.14	m.q.	0
Pineapple-grapefruit juice								
drink[6], canned, 1 cup	88	115	.08	.04	.67	.11	26.2	0

1. *With added ascorbic acid or sodium ascorbate; vitamin C value for product without additives would be negligible.*
2. *Prepared according to package directions, with enriched flour and vegetable shortening.*
3. *Without added ingredients.*
4. *Without added ascorbic acid.*
5. *Diluted according to package directions.*
6. *With added ascorbic acid.*

Food and Measure	A I.U.	C mg.	Thi mg.	Rib mg.	Nia mg.	B_6 mg.	Fol mcg.	B_{12} mcg.
Pineapple-orange juice drink[1],								
canned, 1 cup	1328	56	.08	.05	.52	.12	27.2	0
Pinto bean, ½ cup:								
boiled	2	2	.16	.08	.34	.13	146.2	0
canned, w/liquid	1	1	.12	.08	.35	.09	72.7	0
Pistachio nut, shelled, dried, 1 oz.	66	n.a.	.23	.05	.31	n.a.	m.q.	0
Pitangua, trimmed, ½ cup	1298	23	.03	.03	.26	n.a.	n.a.	0
Pizza, frozen:								
cheese (*Celeste* Large), ¼ pie	779	0	.08	.39	1.11	.10	14.0	1.00
cheese (*Celeste* Pizza for One), 1 pie	927	0	.15	.44	1.23	.15	35.0	2.00
deluxe (*Celeste* Large), ¼ pie	950	0	.20	.55	2.65	.17	57.0	2.00
deluxe (*Celeste* Pizza for One), 1 pie	1226	0	.30	.82	3.53	.26	80.0	2.00
pepperoni (*Celeste* Large), ¼ pie ...	1343	0	.14	.57	1.63	.18	101.0	1.00
pepperoni (*Celeste* Pizza for One),								
1 pie	1316	0	.25	.71	2.58	.21	97.0	2.00
sausage (*Celeste* Large), ¼ pie	1048	0	.18	.51	1.95	.17	89.0	1.00
sausage (*Celeste* Pizza for One),								
1 pie	1359	0	.30	.77	2.85	.23	109.0	2.00
sausage and mushroom (*Celeste*								
Pizza for One), 1 pie	1200	0	.34	.87	3.93	.34	82.0	2.00
suprema (*Celeste* Large), ¼ pie	1167	0	.20	.68	2.20	.20	67.0	2.00
suprema (*Celeste* Pizza for One),								
1 pie	1943	0	.33	.92	3.72	.28	120.0	3.00
vegetable (*Celeste* Large), ¼ pie ...	750	0	.06	.17	1.20	m.q.	m.q.	m.q.
vegetable (*Celeste* Pizza for One),								
1 pie	1000	0	.09	.26	1.60	m.q.	m.q.	m.q.
Plantain:								
raw, 1 medium, approx. 9.7 oz.	2017	33	.09	.10	1.23	.54	39.4	0
raw, trimmed, sliced, ½ cup	834	14	.04	.04	.51	.22	16.3	0
cooked, sliced, ½ cup	700	8	.04	.04	.58	.19	20.0	0
Plum, ½ cup, except as noted:								
fresh, pitted, sliced	267	8	.04	.08	.41	.07	1.8	0
fresh, Japanese or hybrid, 1 medium,								
2⅛″ diam.	213	6	.03	.06	.33	.05	1.4	0
canned, purple:								
in water	1138	3	.03	.05	.46	.03	3.3	0
in juice	1271	4	.03	.07	.60	m.q.	m.q.	0
in light syrup	333	1	.02	.05	.37	.03	3.2	0
in heavy syrup	334	1	.02	.05	.38	.04	3.3	0
Poi, ½ cup	24	5	.16	.05	1.32	n.a.	n.a.	0
Polish sausage, pork, 1 oz.	0	0	.14	.04	.98	.05	m.q.	.28
Pollock, meat only:								
Atlantic, raw, 1 oz.	10	(0)	.01	.05	.93	.08	m.q.	.90
walleye, raw, 1 oz.	17	(0)	.02	.02	.33	.02	.8	.80
walleye, baked, broiled, or								
microwaved[2], 4 oz.	86	(0)	.08	.09	1.87	.08	4.1	4.76

1. *With added ascorbic acid.*
2. *Without added ingredients.*

Food and Measure	A I.U.	C mg.	Thi mg.	Rib mg.	Nia mg.	B6 mg.	Fol mcg.	B12 mcg.
Pomegranate, 1 medium, 3⅜″ × 3¾″, 9.7 oz.	tr.	9	.05	.05	.46	.16	n.a.	0
Popcorn, popped, 1 cup:								
air-popped, unsalted	10	0	.03	.01	.20	n.a.	n.a.	0
popped in vegetable oil, salted	20	0	.01	.02	.10	n.a.	n.a.	0
Poppy seed, 1 tsp.	tr.	tr.	.02	.01	.03	.01	n.a.	0
Pork[1], fresh, 4 oz., except as noted (see also "Ham"):								
loin, whole:								
braised, lean and fat	10	<1	.69	.34	6.77	.41	4.5	.90
braised, lean only	9	<1	.78	.40	7.87	.51	5.7	.95
broiled, lean and fat	10	<1	.95	.41	5.97	.43	5.7	1.11
broiled, lean only	9	<1	1.10	.48	6.75	.52	5.7	1.22
roasted, lean and fat	9	<1	.82	.36	6.11	.43	5.7	.99
roasted, lean only	8	<1	.91	.41	6.77	.51	6.8	1.05
loin, blade:								
braised, lean and fat	8	<1	.56	.31	5.44	.36	4.5	.86
braised, lean only	6	<1	.62	.37	6.29	.46	5.7	.93
broiled, lean and fat	10	<1	.75	.36	4.73	.39	4.5	1.07
broiled, lean only	9	<1	.86	.43	5.30	.49	5.7	1.18
pan-fried[2], lean and fat	11	<1	.69	.33	4.43	.33	1.1	.99
pan-fried[2], lean only	9	<1	.84	.42	5.13	.45	tr.	1.13
roasted, lean and fat	10	<1	.59	.33	4.80	.41	4.5	.86
roasted, lean only	9	<1	.65	.39	5.29	.50	5.7	.91
loin, center:								
braised, lean and fat	10	<1	.88	.27	6.79	.43	4.5	.69
braised, lean only	10	<1	1.00	.31	7.71	.51	5.7	.69
broiled, lean and fat	10	<1	1.13	.31	5.67	.45	5.7	.81
broiled, lean only	9	<1	1.30	.35	6.28	.53	6.8	.84
pan-fried[2], lean and fat	10	<1	1.16	.31	5.84	.44	5.7	.87
pan-fried[2], lean only	9	<1	1.42	.37	6.82	.57	6.8	.83
roasted, lean and fat	9	<1	.94	.27	5.72	.45	1.1	.68
roasted, lean only	9	<1	1.03	.30	6.19	.51	1.1	.68
loin, center rib:								
braised, lean and fat	11	<1	.60	.31	6.40	.36	6.8	.61
braised, lean only	10	<1	.66	.36	7.34	.44	9.1	.59
broiled, lean and fat	8	<1	.89	.32	5.35	.39	7.9	.77
broiled, lean only	7	<1	1.01	.37	5.93	.45	10.2	.79
pan-fried[2], lean and fat	10	<1	.72	.32	4.97	.37	6.8	.70
pan-fried[2], lean only	9	<1	.87	.40	5.85	.50	9.1	.70
roasted, lean and fat	9	<1	.67	.32	5.56	.40	9.1	.64
roasted, lean only	9	<1	.72	.35	6.07	.45	10.2	.62
loin, sirloin:								
braised, lean and fat	10	<1	.74	.34	5.69	.41	4.5	.75
braised, lean only	9	<1	.84	.39	6.42	.60	5.7	.76
broiled, lean and fat	10	<1	1.02	.39	4.92	.50	5.7	.91
broiled, lean only	9	<1	1.17	.46	5.40	.61	6.8	.95

1. *Prepared without added ingredients, except as noted.*
2. *In hydrogenated soybean and cottonseed oils.*

Food and Measure	A I.U.	C mg.	Thi mg.	Rib mg.	Nia mg.	B₆ mg.	Fol mcg.	B₁₂ mcg.
Pork, loin, sirloin *(cont.)*								
roasted, lean and fat	9	<1	.84	.35	5.89	.43	5.7	.86
roasted, lean only	8	<1	.90	.38	6.30	.48	6.8	.88
loin, top:								
braised, lean and fat	11	<1	.59	.30	6.25	.35	6.8	.61
braised, lean only	10	<1	.66	.36	7.34	.44	9.1	.59
broiled, lean and fat	9	<1	.87	.31	5.23	.39	7.9	.76
broiled, lean only	7	<1	1.01	.37	5.93	.45	10.2	.79
pan-fried,[1] lean and fat	10	<1	.72	.32	4.96	.37	6.8	.69
pan-fried,[1] lean only	9	<1	.87	.40	5.85	.50	9.1	.70
roasted, lean and fat	9	<1	.66	.31	5.48	.39	7.9	.64
roasted, lean only	9	<1	.72	.35	6.07	.45	10.2	.62
shoulder, whole:								
roasted, lean and fat	9	<1	.61	.36	4.52	.37	4.5	.94
roasted, lean only	8	<1	.66	.41	4.88	.45	5.7	1.00
shoulder, arm (picnic):								
braised, lean and fat	10	<1	.61	.35	5.92	.31	4.5	.78
braised, lean only	9	<1	.68	.41	6.74	.46	5.7	.81
roasted, lean and fat	9	<1	.59	.34	4.45	.32	4.5	.84
roasted, lean only	8	<1	.66	.40	4.89	.46	5.7	.88
shoulder, Boston blade:								
braised, lean and fat	11	<1	.57	.38	4.53	.26	1.1	.95
braised, lean only	10	<1	.63	.44	4.92	.31	5.7	1.02
broiled, lean and fat	10	<1	.76	.43	4.52	.31	4.5	1.18
broiled, lean only	9	<1	.85	.50	4.88	.35	5.7	1.28
roasted, lean and fat	9	<1	.62	.38	4.58	.31	4.5	1.03
roasted, lean only	8	<1	.67	.42	4.88	.34	5.7	1.09
spareribs, lean and fat, braised, 6.3 oz. (1 lb. raw w/bone)	18	n.a.	.72	.68	9.69	.62	7.0	1.91
tenderloin, lean only, roasted	8	<1	1.07	.44	5.34	.48	6.8	.62
Pork ear, frozen, simmered[2], 4 oz.	0	0	.02	.08	.64	m.q.	m.q.	m.q.
Pork jowl, raw, 1 oz.	3	n.a.	.11	.07	1.29	.03	0	.23
Potato, fresh or stored:								
raw, peeled, 1 medium, 2½" diam., 5.3 oz. w/skin	tr.	22	.10	.04	1.66	.29	14.3	0
baked in skin, 1 medium, 4¾" × 2⅓" diam., 7.1 oz.	tr.	26	.22	.07	3.32	.70	22.2	0
baked, pulp only, 4 oz.	tr.	15	.12	.02	1.58	.34	10.3	0
baked, skin only, 2 oz.	tr.	8	.07	.06	1.74	.35	12.2	0
boiled in skin, 1 medium, 2½" diam., 5.3 oz.	tr.	18	.14	.03	1.96	.41	13.6	0
boiled, w/out skin, pulp from 1 medium potato	tr.	10	.13	.03	1.77	.36	11.9	0
microwaved in skin, 1 medium, 4¾" × 2⅓" diam., 7.1 oz.	tr.	31	.24	.07	3.46	.70	24.2	0
mashed, w/whole milk, ½ cup	20	7	.09	.04	1.17	.25	8.6	.06
mashed, w/whole milk and margarine, ½ cup	177	6	.09	.04	1.13	.24	8.3	.05

1. *In hydrogenated soybean and cottonseed oils.*
2. *Without added ingredients.*

Food and Measure	A I.U.	C mg.	Thi mg.	Rib mg.	Nia mg.	B₆ mg.	Fol mcg.	B₁₂ mcg.
Potato, canned, drained:								
1"-diam. potato, 1.2 oz.	tr.	2	.02	.01	.32	.07	2.2	0
½ cup	tr.	5	.06	.01	.82	.17	5.6	0
Potato, frozen:								
french-fried, heated, 10 strips:								
1.75 oz.	tr.	6	.06	.02	1.15	.12	8.3	0
cottage cut, 1.75 oz.	tr.	5	.06	.02	1.21	.12	8.3	0
hash brown[1], ½ cup	n.a.	5	.09	.02	1.89	.10	m.q.	0
puffs, 1 piece, .25 oz.	1	<1	.01	.01	.15	.02	1.2	0
Potato, mix[2], ½ cup:								
mashed, flakes	189	10	.12	.05	.70	.01	7.8	.08
mashed, granules	195	6	.08	.08	.80	.14	8.0	0
Potato chip: 1 oz.:								
1 oz.	0	12	.04	.01	1.19	.14	12.8	0
all varieties (*Health Valley*)	n.a.	2	.04	.02	1.40	.14	12.9	0
Potato sticks, 1-oz. pkg.	0	13	.03	.03	1.36	.09	11.2	0
Poultry, see specific listings								
Poultry salad sandwich spread								
(chicken and turkey), 1 tbsp. ...	18	0	<.01	.01	.22	.01	1.0	.05
Poultry seasoning, 1 tsp.	39	<1	<.01	<.01	.05	n.a.	n.a.	0
Pretzels, 1 oz.	0	0	<.01	<.01	.20	n.a.	n.a.	0
Prickly pear, 1 medium, approx.								
4.8 oz.	53	14	.01	.06	.47	n.a.	n.a.	0
Prune, ½ cup, except as noted:								
canned, in heavy syrup	933	3	.04	.14	1.01	n.a.	n.a.	0
dehydrated, uncooked	1163	0	.08	.25	1.98	.49	1.3	0
dehydrated, cooked	732	0	.06	.04	1.38	.27	.2	0
dried, w/pits:								
uncooked	1600	3	.07	.13	1.58	.21	3.0	0
cooked, stewed, unsweetened ...	324	3	.03	.11	.77	.23	.1	0
cooked, stewed, sweetened	340	3	.03	.11	.80	.24	.1	0
dried, pitted, 4 oz.:								
uncooked	2253	4	.09	.18	2.22	.30	4.2	0
cooked, stewed, unsweetened ...	347	3	.03	.11	.82	.25	.1	0
cooked, stewed, sweetened	323	3	.02	.11	.77	.23	.1	0
Prune juice, canned, 6 fl. oz.	6	8	.03	.13	1.51	n.a.	.6	0
Pudding, ready to serve,								
5-oz. can:								
chocolate	100	tr.	.04	.17	.60	n.a.	n.a.	n.a.
tapioca	tr.	tr.	.03	.14	.40	n.a.	n.a.	n.a.
vanilla	tr.	tr.	.03	.12	.60	n.a.	n.a.	n.a.
Pudding mix[3], ½ cup:								
chocolate	140	1	.05	.20	.10	n.a.	n.a.	n.a.
chocolate, instant	130	1	.04	.18	.10	n.a.	n.a.	n.a.
rennet custard:								
caramel, fruit flavored, or vanilla	190	2	.04	.20	.15	n.a.	n.a.	n.a.
chocolate	180	2	.04	.19	.15	n.a.	n.a.	n.a.

1. *Prepared in vegetable oil.*
2. *Flakes and granules without milk; prepared according to package directions, with whole milk and butter.*
3. *Prepared according to package directions, with whole milk.*

Food and Measure	A I.U.	C mg.	Thi mg.	Rib mg.	Nia mg.	B$_6$ mg.	Fol mcg.	B$_{12}$ mcg.
Pudding mix *(cont.)*								
rice	140	1	.10	.18	.60	n.a.	n.a.	n.a.
vanilla	140	1	.04	.18	.10	n.a.	n.a.	n.a.
vanilla, instant	140	1	.04	.17	.10	n.a.	n.a.	n.a.
Pummelo, trimmed, sections,								
½ cup	0	58	.03	.03	.21	.03	n.a.	0
Pumpkin, ½ cup:								
fresh, boiled, drained, mashed	1320	6	.04	.10	.50	m.q.	m.q.	0
canned	26,908	5	.03	.07	.45	.07	15.0	0
Pumpkin pie mix[1] (*Libby's*), ⅙ pie	10,500	4	.09	.26	1.20	.26	n.a.	.30
Pumpkin pie spice, 1 tsp.	4	<1	<.01	<.01	.04	n.a.	n.a.	0
Pumpkin seeds, kernels, dried,								
1 oz.	108	n.a.	.06	.09	.50	n.a.	m.q.	0
Purslane, raw, ½ cup	284	5	.01	.02	.10	n.a.	n.a.	0

1. *Prepared according to package directions.*

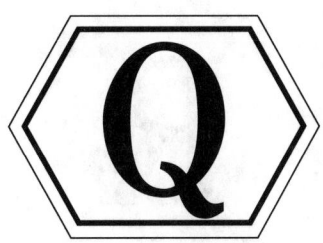

Food and Measure	A I.U.	C mg.	Thi mg.	Rib mg.	Nia mg.	B_6 mg.	Fol mcg.	B_{12} mcg.
Quail, raw, meat w/skin, 1 oz.	69	2	.07	.07	2.14	.17	2.3	m.q.
Quince, 1 medium, 5.3 oz.	37	14	.02	.03	.18	.04	n.a.	0

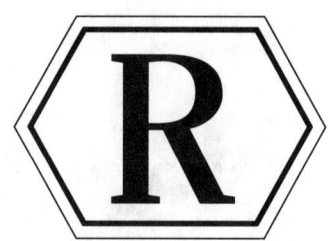

Food and Measure	A I.U.	C mg.	Thi mg.	Rib mg.	Nia mg.	B₆ mg.	Fol mcg.	B₁₂ mcg.
Rabbit¹, domesticated, meat only:								
roasted, 4 oz.	0	0	.08	.18	7.50	.42	10.2	7.38
stewed, 4 oz.	0	0	.07	.19	8.12	.39	10.2	7.38
Radish, raw, 10 medium, 1.75 oz.	3	10	<.01	.02	.14	.03	12.2	0
Radish, Oriental, raw, sliced,								
½ cup	0	10	.01	.01	.09	n.a.	m.q.	0
Radish, white icicle, raw, sliced,								
½ cup	0	15	.02	.01	.15	.04	7.0	0
Radish seeds, sprouted, raw,								
½ cup	74	6	.02	.02	.54	.05	18.0	0
Raisin:								
golden seedless, 1 oz.	12	1	<.01	.05	.32	.09	.9	0
golden seedless, ½ cup not packed	32	2	.01	.14	.83	.23	2.4	0
seeded, 1 oz.	0	2	.3	.5	.32	.05	.9	0
seeded, ½ cup not packed	0	4	.08	.13	.81	.14	2.4	0
seedless, 1 oz.	2	1	.04	.02	.23	.07	.9	0
seedless, ½ cup not packed	6	2	.11	.06	.59	.18	2.4	0
Raspberry, ½ cup, except as noted:								
fresh, 1 pint, 11.5 oz.	406	78	.09	.28	2.81	.18	m.q.	0
fresh, trimmed	80	15	.02	.06	.55	.04	m.q.	0
canned, red, in heavy syrup	43	11	.03	.04	.57	.05	13.4	0
frozen, red, sweetened	75	21	.02	.06	.29	.04	32.5	0
Red beans, canned (*Van Camp's*),								
1 cup	0	0	.10	.10	.61	n.a.	n.a.	n.a.
Refried beans, canned, ½ cup	0	8	.06	.07	.61	n.a.	m.q.	0
Relish, sweet, 1 tbsp.	20	1	tr.	tr.	0	m.q.	0	0
Rhubarb, ½ cup:								
fresh, trimmed, diced	61	5	.01	.02	.18	.02	4.3	0
frozen	73	3	.02	.02	.14	.02	5.6	0
frozen, cooked, sweetened	83	4	.02	.03	.24	.02	6.4	0

1. *Prepared without added ingredients.*

Food and Measure	A I.U.	C mg.	Thi mg.	Rib mg.	Nia mg.	B₆ mg.	Fol mcg.	B₁₂ mcg.
Rice, cooked, ½ cup (see also "Rice dishes, mix"):								
brown, long grain	0	0	.09	.02	1.50	.14	4.0	0
brown, medium grain	0	0	.10	.01	1.30	.15	4.0	0
white, enriched:								
long grain, regular	0	0	.17	.01	1.51	.10	3.0	0
long grain, parboiled	0	0	.22	.02	1.23	.02	3.0	0
long grain, precooked or instant . .	0	0	.06	.04	.72	.01	3.0	0
medium grain	0	0	.17	.02	1.87	.05	2.0	0
short grain	0	0	.17	.02	1.52	.06	2.0	0
Rice, glutinous, cooked, 1 cup . . .	0	0	.05	.03	.70	.06	3.0	0
Rice, Spanish, canned (*Van Camp's*), 1 cup	1228	1	.06	.10	1.24	m.q.	m.q.	n.a.
Rice, wild, see "Wild rice"								
Rice bran, crude, 1 cup	0	0	2.29	.24	28.22	3.38	52.0	0
Rice cakes, 1 piece:								
(*Mother's/Quaker*)	8	0	0	.01	.54	.01	2.0	0
(*Mother's/Quaker* Unsalted)	8	0	0	.01	.53	.01	2.0	0
corn (*Mother's/Quaker*)	8	0	0	.01	.42	.01	2.0	0
multigrain (*Mother's/Quaker*)	8	0	0	.01	.55	.01	1.0	0
sesame (*Mother's/Quaker*)	8	0	0	.01	.51	.01	2.0	0
sesame (*Mother's/Quaker* Unsalted)	8	0	0	.01	.51	.01	1.0	0
Rice dishes, mix, dry:								
broccoli au gratin (*Golden Grain/ Rice-A-Roni Savory Classics*), 1.12 oz.	110	0	.07	.06	1.10	.04	9.0	.11
cauliflower au gratin (*Golden Grain/ Rice-A-Roni Savory Classics*), 1.2 oz.	46	0	.21	.10	2.16	.04	8.0	.07
cheddar, zesty (*Golden Grain/Rice-A-Roni Savory Classics*), 1.3 oz.	87	0	.24	.10	2.50	.05	8.0	.14
chicken Florentine (*Golden Grain/ Rice-A-Roni Savory Classics*), 1.12 oz.	60	0	.19	.11	2.08	.06	23.0	0
green bean almondine (*Golden Grain/ Rice-A-Roni Savory Classics*), 1.25 oz.	87	1	.19	.12	2.03	.04	9.0	.14
Parmesan and herbs, creamy (*Golden Grain/Rice-A-Roni Savory Classics*), 1.22 oz.	55	0	.22	.11	2.40	.04	9.0	.11
pilaf, garden (*Golden Grain/Rice-A-Roni Savory Classics*), 1.12 oz.	262	0	.20	.08	2.46	.06	14.0	0
vegetables, spring, and cheese (*Golden Grain/Rice-A-Roni Savory Classics*), 1.22 oz.	54	n.a.	.21	.10	.04	.04	9.0	.08
Rice flour, 1 cup:								
brown	0	0	.70	.13	10.02	1.16	25.0	0
white	0	0	.22	.03	4.09	.69	6.0	0

Food and Measure	A I.U.	C mg.	Thi mg.	Rib mg.	Nia mg.	B₆ mg.	Fol mcg.	B₁₂ mcg.
Rockfish, Pacific, meat only:								
raw, 1 oz.	54	(0)	.01	.02	.91	n.a.	m.q.	m.q.
baked, broiled, or microwaved[1], 4 oz.	248	(0)	.05	.10	4.44	n.a.	m.q.	m.q.
Roll, 1 piece:								
brown and serve:								
dinner or pan, 1-oz. piece	tr.	tr.	.07	.06	.60	n.a.	m.q.	n.a.
Parkerhouse, 1-oz. piece	tr.	tr.	.06	.06	.60	n.a.	m.q.	n.a.
dinner, 1 oz.	tr.	tr.	.14	.09	1.10	n.a.	m.q.	n.a.
hard, 1.8 oz.	0	0	.20	.12	1.70	n.a.	m.q.	n.a.
hoagie or submarine, 11½″ long,								
4.8 oz.	0	0	.54	.33	4.50	n.a.	m.q.	n.a.
hot dog or hamburger, 1.4 oz.	tr.	tr.	.20	.13	1.60	n.a.	m.q.	n.a.
Roll mix[2], cloverleaf, 1.2-oz. piece	tr.	tr.	.02	.04	.20	n.a.	m.q.	n.a.
Rose apple, trimmed, 1 oz.	96	6	.01	.01	.23	n.a.	n.a.	0
Roselle, trimmed, 1 oz. or ½ cup	81	3	<.01	.01	.09	n.a.	n.a.	0
Rosemary, dried, 1 tsp.	38	1	.01	n.a.	.01	n.a.	n.a.	0
Rutabaga, ½ cup:								
raw, cubed	0	18	.06	.03	.49	.07	14.3	0
boiled, drained, cubed	0	19	.06	.03	.54	.08	13.2	0
boiled, drained, mashed	0	26	.09	.04	.76	.11	18.6	0
Rye flour, 1 cup:								
dark	0	0	.40	.32	5.47	.57	77.0	0
light	0	0	.34	.09	.82	.24	23.0	0
medium	0	0	.29	.12	1.76	.27	20.0	0

1. *Without added ingredients.*
2. *Prepared according to package directions, with water.*

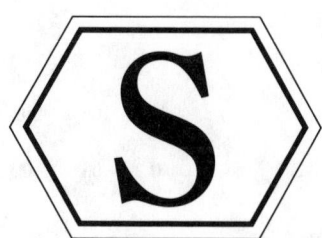

Food and Measure	A I.U.	C mg.	Thi mg.	Rib mg.	Nia mg.	B₆ mg.	Fol mcg.	B₁₂ mcg.
Sage, ground, 1 tsp.	41	<1	.01	<.01	.04	n.a.	n.a.	0
Salad dressing, 1 tbsp.:								
blue cheese	32	<1	tr.	.02	tr.	n.a.	n.a.	n.a.
French, regular or low-calorie	tr.	tr.	tr.	tr.	tr.	n.a.	n.a.	n.a.
Italian	30	tr.	tr.	tr.	tr.	n.a.	n.a.	n.a.
Italian, low-calorie	tr.	tr.	tr.	tr.	tr.	n.a.	n.a.	n.a.
mayonnaise type	32	0	tr.	tr.	tr.	n.a.	n.a.	n.a.
Thousand Island, regular or low-calorie	50	0	tr.	tr.	tr.	n.a.	n.a.	n.a.
vinegar and oil	0	0	0	0	0	n.a.	n.a.	0
Salami[1], 1 oz.:								
beef, cooked	n.a.	4	.04	.07	.97	.06	1.0	1.37
beef and pork, cooked	n.a.	3	.07	.11	1.01	.06	1.0	1.04
beer, beef	n.a.	4	.03	.03	.81	.06	.9	.60
beer, pork	n.a.	8	.16	.05	.92	.10	.9	.25
dry or hard, pork	n.a.	m.q.	.26	.09	1.59	.16	m.q.	.79
dry or hard, pork and beef	n.a.	7	.17	.08	1.38	.14	m.q.	.54
Salmon, meat only:								
Atlantic, raw, 1 oz.	11	(0)	.06	.11	2.23	.23	m.q.	.90
chinook, smoked, 4 oz.	100	(0)	.03	.11	5.35	.32	2.2	3.70
sockeye, raw, 1 oz.	54	(0)	.06	.04	1.64	.54	m.q.	.08
sockeye, baked, broiled, or microwaved[2], 4 oz.	237	(0)	.24	.19	7.56	.25	m.q.	6.58
Salmon, canned, 4 oz.:								
pink, w/bone and liquid	62	0	.03	.21	7.41	m.q.	17.5	m.q.
sockeye, w/bone, drained	200	0	.02	.22	6.21	m.q.	11.1	m.q.
Salsify, ½ cup:								
raw, sliced	0	5	.05	.15	.34	n.a.	m.q.	0
boiled, drained, sliced	0	3	.04	.12	.27	n.a.	m.q.	0

1. *With added sodium ascorbate; vitamin C value for product without additives would be negligible.*
2. *Without added ingredients.*

Food and Measure	A I.U.	C mg.	Thi mg.	Rib mg.	Nia mg.	B6 mg.	Fol mcg.	B12 mcg.
Salt, 1 tsp.	0	0	0	0	0	n.a.	n.a.	0
Salt, substitute or imitation								
(*Instead of Salt*), 1 tsp.	186	0	.01	0	.10	0	<.1	0
Salt pork, raw, 1 oz.	0	0	.06	.02	.46	.02	0	.08
Sandwich spread, pork and beef,								
1 tsp.	n.a.	0	.03	.02	.26	.02	n.a.	.17
Sapodilla:								
1 medium, 3″ × 2½″, approx.								
7.5 oz.	102	25	n.a.	.03	.34	.06	n.a.	0
trimmed, ½ cup	73	18	n.a.	.02	.24	.04	n.a.	0
Sapote, 1 medium, approx.								
11.2 oz.	923	45	.02	.05	4.05	n.a.	n.a.	0
Sardines, canned:								
Atlantic, in soybean oil, 2 medium,								
approx. .8 oz.	54	(0)	.02	.05	1.26	.04	2.8	2.15
Pacific, in tomato sauce, 1 medium,								
approx. 1.3 oz.	139	<1	.02	.09	1.60	.05	9.2	3.42
Sauerkraut, canned, w/liquid,								
½ cup	21	17	.03	.03	.17	.15	m.q.	0
Sausage (see also specific listings):								
Italian, pork, raw, 4-oz. link	0	3	.64	.19	3.67	.34	n.a.	1.03
Italian, pork, cooked, 3 oz. (4-oz.								
raw link)	0	1	.52	.19	3.46	.28	n.a.	1.08
pork, fresh:								
raw, 1 oz. or 1 link	0	<1	.16	.05	.80	.07	1.0	.32
raw, 1 patty, approx. 2 oz.	0	<1	.31	.09	1.62	.14	2.0	.64
cooked, 1 link, .5 oz. (1-oz. raw								
link)	0	0	.10	.03	.59	.04	n.a.	.22
cooked, 1 patty, approx. 1 oz.								
(2-oz. raw patty)	0	0	.20	.07	1.22	.09	n.a.	.47
pork and beef, fresh, cooked, .5 oz.								
(1-oz. raw link)	0	n.a.	.05	.02	.44	.01	n.a.	.06
pork and beef, fresh, cooked, 1 oz.								
(2-oz. raw patty)	0	n.a.	.10	.04	.91	.01	n.a.	.12
smoked, pork, 1 link, 4″ long ×								
1⅛″	0	1	.48	.18	3.08	.24	n.a.	1.11
smoked, pork and beef[1], 1 link,								
4″ long × 1⅛″	0	13	.18	.12	2.19	.12	n.a.	1.03
Sauce, see specific listings								
Scallop, mixed species, meat only,								
raw, 2 large or 5 small, 1.1 oz.	m.q.	(0)	<.01	.02	.35	m.q.	m.q.	.46
Scallop squash, ½ cup:								
raw, sliced	72	12	.05	.02	.39	.07	19.6	0
boiled, drained, sliced	77	10	.05	.02	.42	.08	18.6	0
Seaweed, 1 oz.:								
agar, dried	0	0	<.01	.01	<.01	n.a.	n.a.	0
kelp, raw	33	n.a.	<.01	.04	.13	n.a.	51.0	0
laver, raw	1474	11	.03	.13	.42	.05	n.a.	0

1. *With added sodium ascorbate; vitamin C value for product without additives would be negligible.*

Food and Measure	A I.U.	C mg.	Thi mg.	Rib mg.	Nia mg.	B$_6$ mg.	Fol mcg.	B$_{12}$ mcg.
wakame, raw	102	1	.02	.06	.45	n.a.	n.a.	0
Semolina, whole grain, enriched,								
1 cup	n.a.	0	1.35	.95	10.00	.17	120.0	0
Sesame butter, 1 tbsp.:								
paste, from whole seeds	8	0	.04	.03	1.07	n.a.	n.a.	0
tahini, from raw and stoneground								
kernels	n.a.	0	.19	.08	.89	n.a.	n.a.	0
Sesame flour, 1 oz.:								
high fat	20	0	.76	.08	3.80	.04	8.7	0
partially defatted	20	0	.72	.08	3.58	.04	8.2	0
lowfat	18	0	.72	.08	3.56	.04	8.2	0
Sesame meal, partially defatted,								
1 oz.	19	0	.73	.08	3.64	.04	8.4	0
Sesame seeds:								
whole, dried, 1 tbsp.	1	0	.07	.02	.41	.07	8.7	0
kernels, dried, 1 tbsp.	5	0	.06	.01	.38	n.a.	m.q.	0
decorticated, 1 tsp.	2	0	.02	<.01	.13	<.01	n.a.	0
Shallot, freeze-dried, ¼ cup	n.a.	1	.01	<.01	.04	.06	4.2	0
Shark, mixed species, meat only,								
raw, 1 oz.	66	(0)	.01	.02	.83	n.a.	m.q.	.42
Sherbet, orange, ½ cup	93	2	.02	.04	.07	.01	7.0	.08
Shortening, vegetable, 1 tbsp. ...	0	0	0	0	0	n.a.	n.a.	0
Shrimp, mixed species, meat only:								
raw, 1 oz.	m.q.	(0)	.01	.01	.72	.03	.8	.33
boiled, poached, or steamed[1], 4 oz.	m.q.	(0)	.04	.04	2.94	.14	4.0	1.69
Shrimp, canned, 4 oz.	m.q.	(0)	.03	.04	3.12	.13	2.0	1.37
Smelt, rainbow, meat only, raw,								
1 oz.	m.q.	(0)	n.a.	.03	.41	m.q.	m.q.	.97
Snack bar, 1 bar, except as noted:								
apple (*Health Valley Apple Bakes*) ...	4	3	.10	.12	.50	.27	15.3	0
date (*Health Valley Date Bakes*)	5	3	.08	.22	.60	.29	15.9	0
oat bran:								
almond and date (*Health Valley*								
Jumbo Fruit Bars)	30	3	.03	.06	.55	.06	20.3	0
apricot (*Health Valley Oat Bran*								
Apricot Bakes)	1	1	.14	.03	.66	.05	9.3	0
fig and nut (*Health Valley Oat Bran*								
Fig & Nut Bakes)	14	1	.08	.03	.62	.05	9.3	0
fruit and nut (*Health Valley Jumbo*								
Fruit Bars)	335	3	.03	.06	.60	.06	19.5	0
raisin and cinnamon (*Health Valley*								
Jumbo Fruit Bars)	3	7	.02	.05	.51	.16	19.5	0
raisin (*Health Valley Raisin Bakes*) ..	5	4	.10	.15	.50	.30	17.0	0
rice bran, almond, and date (*Health*								
Valley Rice Bran Jumbo Fruit								
Bars)	117	<1	.69	.45	4.00	.08	4.1	0

1. *Without added ingredients.*

Food and Measure	A I.U.	C mg.	Thi mg.	Rib mg.	Nia mg.	B₆ mg.	Fol mcg.	B₁₂ mcg.
Soft drinks and mixers, 12 fl. oz.:								
all flavors except grape, lemon-lime,								
orange, and low-calorie cola ...	0	0	0	0	0	0	0	0
cola, low-calorie[1]	0	0	.02	.08	0	0	0	0
grape or orange	0	0	0	0	n.a.	0	0	0
lemon-lime	0	0	0	0	.06	0	0	0
Sole, see "Flatfish"								
Soup, canned, ready to serve:								
bean, black (*Health Valley*), 7½ oz.	5112	5	.27	.27	.85	.19	77.1	0
beef, chunky, 1 cup	2611	7	.06	.15	2.71	.13	13.4	.61
beef broth (*Health Valley*), 7½ oz. ..	1	0	.04	.11	7.40	.01	3.6	0
chicken, chunky, 1 cup	1299	1	.09	.17	4.42	.05	4.6	.25
chicken broth (*Health Valley*),								
7½ oz.	<1	<1	.04	.05	2.10	.02	3.4	.15
clam chowder, Manhattan, 1 cup ...	3292	12	.06	.06	1.85	.26	9.3	7.92
clam chowder, Manhattan (*Health*								
Valley), 7½ oz.	5106	3	.04	.23	6.00	.42	16.1	30.10
chicken rice, chunky, 1 cup	5858	4	.02	.10	4.10	m.q.	3.8	n.a.
crab, 1 cup	505	0	.20	.07	1.34	.12	m.q.	.20
gazpacho, 1 cup	200	3	.05	.02	.93	.15	m.q.	0
lentil (*Health Valley*), 7½ oz.	255	2	.02	.13	5.20	.36	4.5	0
lentil, w/ham, 1 cup	360	4	.17	.11	1.35	.22	49.6	.30
minestrone (*Health Valley*), 7½ oz.	11,140	4	.04	.38	5.10	.17	8.5	0
mushroom barley (*Health Valley*),								
7½ oz.	5325	4	.15	.11	1.80	.19	37.2	0
pea, green, split (*Health Valley*),								
7½ oz.	5122	1	.32	.28	5.90	.47	22.6	0
pea, split, w/ham, chunky	4871	7	.12	.09	2.52	m.q.	4.7	n.a.
potato leek (*Health Valley*), 7½ oz.	4985	3	.19	.36	5.20	.29	23.6	0
tomato (*Health Valley*), 7½ oz.	4952	3	.12	.11	1.90	.26	7.0	0
turkey, chunky, 1 cup	7156	6	.04	.11	3.59	.31	11.1	2.12
vegetable:								
(*Health Valley*), 7½ oz.	14,700	3	.23	.08	2.10	.18	38.4	0
chicken, chunky (*Health Valley*),								
7½ oz.	3283	1	.26	.08	3.50	.22	15.5	.11
chunky, 1 cup	5877	6	.07	.07	1.20	.19	16.5	0
five bean, chunky (*Health Valley*),								
7½ oz.	11,970	3	.02	.17	3.10	.21	39.3	0
Soup, canned, condensed, 1 cup[2]:								
asparagus, cream of	445	3	.05	.08	.78	.01	m.q.	n.a.
asparagus, cream of[3]	599	4	.10	.28	.88	.06	m.q.	n.a.
bean, black	506	1	.08	.05	.53	.09	24.7	.02
bean w/bacon	889	2	.09	.03	.57	.04	31.9	n.a.
beef noodle	629	<1	.07	.06	1.07	.04	4.4	.20
celery, cream of	306	<1	.03	.05	.33	.01	2.4	n.a.
celery, cream of[3]	461	1	.07	.25	.44	.06	8.5	n.a.

1. *Aspartame sweetened.*
2. *Prepared according to package directions, with water, except as noted.*
3. *Prepared with whole milk.*

Food and Measure	A I.U.	C mg.	Thi mg.	Rib mg.	Nia mg.	B₆ mg.	Fol mcg.	B₁₂ mcg.
cheese	1088	0	.02	.14	.40	.03	m.q.	0
cheese[1]	1243	1	.06	.33	.50	.08	m.q.	.44
chicken:								
broth	0	0	.01	.07	3.35	.02	m.q.	.24
cream of	560	<1	.03	.06	.82	.02	1.6	m.q.
cream of[1]	715	1	.07	.26	.92	.07	7.7	m.q.
and dumplings	518	0	.02	.07	1.75	.04	m.q.	.16
gumbo	136	5	.02	.05	.66	.06	m.q.	m.q.
noodle	711	<1	.05	.06	1.39	.03	2.2	m.q.
rice	660	<1	.02	.02	1.13	.02	1.1	m.q.
vegetable	2656	1	.04	.06	1.23	.05	m.q.	m.q.
chili beef	1510	4	.06	.08	1.07	.16	m.q.	.32
clam chowder:								
Manhattan	963	4	.03	.04	.82	.10	10.0	4.06
New England	8	2	.02	.04	.96	.08	3.7	8.01
New England[1]	164	4	.07	.24	1.03	.13	9.7	10.25
consomme, w/gelatin	0	1	.02	.03	.71	.02	3.0	0
minestrone	2337	1	.05	.04	.94	.10	16.1	0
mushroom:								
barley	198	0	.02	.09	.88	m.q.	m.q.	0
w/beef stock	1255	1	.03	.10	1.21	.04	9.2	0
cream of	0	1	.05	.09	.73	.02	m.q.	.05
cream of[1]	154	2	.08	.28	.91	.06	m.q.	n.a.
onion	0	1	.03	.02	.60	.05	15.2	0
oyster stew	71	3	.02	.04	.23	.01	m.q.	2.19
oyster stew[1]	225	4	.07	.23	.34	.06	m.q.	2.63
pea:								
green	202	2	.11	.07	1.24	.05	1.8	0
green[1]	356	3	.16	.27	1.34	.10	7.9	.44
split, w/or w/out ham	444	1	.15	.08	1.48	.07	2.5	n.a.
pepper pot	865	1	.05	.05	1.22	.06	m.q.	.17
potato, cream of	288	0	.03	.04	.54	.04	3.0	n.a.
potato, cream of[1]	443	1	.08	.24	.64	.09	9.2	n.a.
Scotch broth	2180	1	.02	.05	1.16	.07	m.q.	.27
stockpot	3980	2	.04	.05	1.22	.09	m.q.	0
tomato:								
1 cup	688	67	.09	.05	1.42	.11	14.7	0
1 cup[1]	849	68	.13	.25	1.52	.16	20.9	.44
beef w/noodle	533	0	.08	.09	1.87	.09	m.q.	.19
bisque	721	6	.07	.07	1.15	.09	m.q.	0
bisque[1]	879	7	.11	.27	1.25	.14	m.q.	.44
rice	755	15	.06	.05	1.06	.08	m.q.	0
turkey noodle	292	<1	.07	.06	1.40	.04	m.q.	m.q.
vegetable:								
w/beef	1891	2	.04	.05	1.03	.08	10.6	.31
w/beef broth	2091	2	.05	.05	1.00	.06	m.q.	0
vegetarian	3005	1	.05	.05	.92	.06	10.6	0

1. *Prepared with whole milk.*

Food and Measure	A I.U.	C mg.	Thi mg.	Rib mg.	Nia mg.	B₆ mg.	Fol mcg.	B₁₂ mcg.
Soup mix, 1 cup[1]:								
beef noodle	9	1	.12	.06	.69	.04	1.6	n.a.
chicken noodle	63	<1	.07	.06	.88	.01	1.4	n.a.
chicken vegetable	14	1	.07	.05	.69	.09	n.a.	n.a.
onion	2	<1	.03	.06	.48	m.q.	1.5	n.a.
pea, green, split or w/ham	49	tr.	.22	.15	1.34	.05	15.0	n.a.
tomato, regular or cream of	832	5	.06	.05	.78	.10	6.7	n.a.
tomato vegetable	190	6	.06	.05	.79	m.q.	m.q.	n.a.
vegetable beef	238	n.a.	.03	.04	.46	.05	m.q.	n.a.
Soursop, trimmed, ½ cup	3	23	.08	.06	1.01	.07	m.q.	0
Soy beverage (*Soy Moo*), 1 cup ...	95	n.a.	.06	.03	0	n.a.	n.a.	0
Soy flour, 1 cup, stirred:								
full-fat	102	0	.49	.99	3.67	.39	293.3	0
full-fat, roasted	93	0	.35	.80	2.79	.30	193.3	0
defatted	40	0	.70	.25	2.61	.57	305.4	0
low-fat	35	0	.33	.25	1.90	.46	360.8	0
Soy milk, fluid, 1 cup	77	0	.39	.17	.35	.10	3.6	0
Soy sauce, 1 tbsp.:								
soy (tamari)	0	0	.01	.03	.71	.04	3.3	0
soy and wheat (shoyu)	0	0	.01	.02	.61	.03	2.8	0
Soybean, green, ½ cup:								
raw	230	37	.56	.22	2.11	n.a.	m.q.	0
boiled, drained	140	15	.23	.14	1.13	n.a.	m.q.	0
Soybean, dried, ½ cup:								
boiled	8	6	.13	.25	.34	.20	46.2	0
roasted	172	2	.09	.13	1.21	.18	181.5	0
dry-roasted	20	4	.37	.65	.91	.19	175.9	0
Soybean, sprouted, ½ cup:								
raw	4	5	.12	.04	.40	.06	60.1	0
steamed	5	4	.10	.03	.51	n.a.	m.q.	0
Soybean kernels, roasted and								
toasted, 1 oz.	57	1	.03	.04	.50	.09	64.0	0
Spaghetti squash, ½ cup:								
raw, cubed	25	1	.02	.01	.48	.05	6.0	0
baked or boiled, drained	86	3	.03	.02	.63	.08	6.2	0
Spinach, ½ cup, except as noted:								
fresh:								
raw, 10-oz. pkg.	13,699	57	.16	.39	1.48	.40	396.5	0
raw, chopped	1880	8	.02	.05	.20	.06	54.4	0
boiled, drained	7371	9	.09	.21	.44	.22	131.2	0
canned, w/liquid	7526	16	.02	.12	.32	.09	67.8	0
canned, drained	9390	15	.02	.15	.42	.11	104.6	0
frozen, boiled, drained, leaf	7395	12	.06	.16	.40	.14	102.1	0
Spleen[2], 4 oz.:								
beef, braised	0	57	.05	.34	6.31	.05	m.q.	5.69
pork, braised	0	13	.16	.29	6.73	.07	n.a.	3.13
Squash, see specific listings								

1. *Prepared according to package directions, with water.*
2. *Prepared without added ingredients.*

Food and Measure	A I.U.	C mg.	Thi mg.	Rib mg.	Nia mg.	B6 mg.	Fol mcg.	B12 mcg.
Squash seeds, see "Pumpkin seeds"								
Squid, mixed species, meat only:								
raw, 1 oz.	m.q.	1	.01	.12	.62	.02	m.q.	.37
dipped in flour, fried, 4 oz.	m.q.	5	.06	.52	2.95	.07	m.q.	1.39
Stomach, pork, raw, 1 oz.	0	n.a.	.10	.13	5.05	.05	n.a.	1.12
Straightneck squash, see "Crookneck squash"								
Strawberry, ½ cup, except as noted:								
fresh, 1 pint, approx. 12 oz.	87	182	.06	.21	.74	.19	56.6	0
fresh, trimmed	21	42	.02	.05	.17	.04	13.2	0
canned, in heavy syrup	33	40	.03	.04	.07	.06	35.6	0
frozen:								
unsweetened	33	31	.02	.03	.34	.02	12.5	0
sweetened, whole	35	50	.02	.10	.37	.04	4.9	0
sweetened, sliced	31	53	.02	.07	.51	.04	19.0	0
Strawberry flavor drink mix:								
powder, 2–3 heaping tsp.	n.a.	<1	<.01	.02	.02	tr.	n.a.	0
(*Carnation* Instant Breakfast), 1 pkt.	1750	27	.30	.17	5.00	.40	100.0	.60
Stuffing mix[1], 1 cup:								
dry type	910	0	.17	.20	2.50	n.a.	n.a.	n.a.
moist type	850	0	.10	.18	1.60	n.a.	n.a.	n.a.
Succotash, ½ cup:								
canned, w/liquid	187	6	.04	.07	.82	.06	40.5	0
canned, w/cream style corn	187	9	.04	.09	.81	.17	58.9	0
frozen, boiled, drained	196	5	.06	.06	1.11	.08	28.3	0
Sugar:								
brown, 1 cup packed	0	0	.02	.07	.20	n.a.	n.a.	n.a.
granulated or powdered, 1 tbsp. ...	0	0	0	0	0	0	0	0
Sugar apple:								
1 medium, 2⅞" × 3¼", approx. 9.9 oz.	9	56	.17	.18	1.37	.31	n.a.	0
trimmed, ½ cup	8	45	.14	.14	1.10	.25	n.a.	0
Sunflower seeds, kernels, dried, 1 oz.	14	0	.65	.07	1.28	m.q.	n.a.	0
Sweet potato, fresh:								
raw, 1 medium, 5" long, 6.3 oz.	26,082	30	.09	.19	.88	.33	18.0	0
baked in skin, peeled, 4 oz.	24,877	28	.08	.15	.69	.28	25.7	0
baked in skin, peeled, mashed, ½ cup	21,822	25	.07	.13	.60	.24	22.6	0
boiled w/out skin, mashed, ½ cup ..	27,968	28	.09	.23	1.05	.40	18.2	0
Sweet potato, canned, ½ cup:								
mashed	19,268	7	.03	.12	1.22	m.q.	m.q.	0
vacuum pack, pieces	7983	26	.04	.06	.74	.19	16.6	0
vacuum pack, mashed	10,178	34	.05	.07	.95	.24	21.2	0

1. *Prepared according to package directions.*

Food and Measure	A I.U.	C mg.	Thi mg.	Rib mg.	Nia mg.	B_6 mg.	Fol mcg.	B_{12} mcg.
Sweet potato, canned *(cont.)*								
syrup pack, w/liquid	6520	12	.03	.05	.52	.58	m.q.	0
syrup pack, drained	7014	11	.03	.04	.33	.06	m.q.	0
Sweet potato, frozen, boiled,								
drained, ½ cup	14,441	8	.06	.05	.49	.16	19.6	0
Swiss chard, chopped, ½ cup:								
raw	594	5	.01	.02	.07	n.a.	m.q.	0
boiled, drained	2762	16	.03	.08	.32	n.a.	m.q.	0
Swordfish, meat only:								
raw, 1 oz.	34	<1	.01	.03	.27	.09	m.q.	.50
baked, broiled, or microwaved[1],								
4 oz.	155	1	.05	.13	13.37	.43	m.q.	2.29
Syrup, table (corn and maple),								
2 tbsp.	0	0	0	0	0	0	0	0

1. *Without added ingredients.*

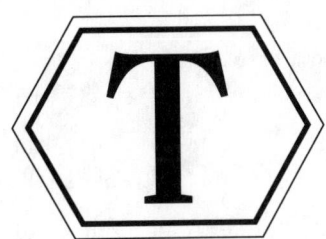

Food and Measure	A I.U.	C mg.	Thi mg.	Rib mg.	Nia mg.	B₆ mg.	Fol mcg.	B₁₂ mcg.
Tahini, see "Sesame butter"								
Tamale, canned (*Wolf* Brand), scant cup	2150	m.q.	.08	.49	1.94	.26	23.0	0
Tamarind, trimmed, ½ cup	18	2	.26	.09	1.16	.04	n.a.	0
Tangerine:								
fresh, 1 medium, 2⅜″ diam., approx. 4.1 oz.	773	26	.09	.02	.13	.06	17.1	0
fresh, sections w/out membrane, ½ cup	897	30	.10	.02	.16	.07	19.9	0
canned, in light syrup, ½ cup	1058	25	.07	.06	.56	m.q.	m.q.	0
Tangerine juice, 6 fl. oz.:								
fresh	780	58	.11	.04	.19	m.q.	m.q.	0
canned, sweetened	786	41	.11	.04	.19	.06	m.q.	0
frozen[1], sweetened	1038	44	.10	.04	.17	.08	8.4	0
Tapioca, pearl, dry, 1 oz.	n.a.	0	<.01	0	0	<.01	1.1	0
Taro, ½ cup:								
raw, sliced	0	2	.05	.01	.31	n.a.	n.a.	0
cooked, sliced	0	3	.07	.02	.34	n.a.	n.a.	0
Taro, Tahitian, ½ cup:								
raw, sliced	1268	60	.04	.15	.62	n.a.	n.a.	0
cooked, sliced	1200	26	.03	.14	.33	n.a.	n.a.	0
Taro leaves, steamed, ½ cup	3136	26	.10	.28	.94	n.a.	n.a.	0
Tarragon, ground, 1 tsp.	67	n.a.	<.01	.02	.14	n.a.	n.a.	0
Tartar sauce, 1 tbsp.	30	tr.	tr.	tr.	0	n.a.	n.a.	n.a.
Tea:								
brewed, 6 fl. oz.	0	0	0	.03	0	0	9.2	0
instant, powder:								
1 tsp.	0	0	tr.	.01	.09	.01	.7	0
lemon flavor, 1 rounded tsp.	0	0	0	.02	.09	n.a.	n.a.	0
lemon flavor, sugar sweetened, 3 rounded tsp.	0	0	0	.05	.09	n.a.	9.6	0

1. *Diluted according to package directions.*

Food and Measure	A I.U.	C mg.	Thi mg.	Rib mg.	Nia mg.	B₆ mg.	Fol mcg.	B₁₂ mcg.
Tea, instant powder *(cont.)*								
lemon flavor, saccharin sweetened, 2 tsp.	0	0	0	.01	.06	n.a.	4.6	0
Tea, herbal, brewed, 6 fl. oz.:								
all flavors, except chamomile	0	0	.02	.01	0	0	1.0	0
chamomile	36	0	.02	.01	0	0	1.0	0
Tempeh, ½ cup	569	0	.11	.09	3.84	.25	43.2	0
Teriyaki sauce, 1 tbsp.	0	0	.01	.01	.23	.02	3.6	0
Thirst quencher drink, bottled, 1 cup	0	0	.01	0	0	0	0	0
Thuringer cervelat[1], beef and pork, 1 oz.	0	7	.05	.09	1.16	.09	m.q.	1.31
Thyme, ground, 1 tsp.	53	n.a.	.01	.01	.07	n.a.	n.a.	0
Tofu, raw, ½ cup:								
firm	209	<1	.20	.13	.48	.12	36.9	0
regular	105	<1	.10	.06	.24	.06	18.6	0
Tomato, red, ripe:								
fresh:								
raw, 1 medium, 2⅗" diam., approx. 4.75 oz.	766	24	.07	.06	.77	.10	18.0	0
raw, chopped, ½ cup	561	17	.05	.04	.57	.07	13.5	0
boiled, ½ cup	892	27	.08	.07	.90	.11	16.0	0
canned, ½ cup:								
whole	725	18	.05	.04	.88	.11	m.q.	0
wedges, in tomato juice	757	19	.07	.04	.88	m.q.	m.q.	0
stewed	710	17	.06	.05	.91	m.q.	m.q.	0
w/green chilies	468	8	.04	.02	.77	m.q.	m.q.	0
Tomato, green, raw, 1 medium, 2⅗" diam., approx. 4.75 oz.	789	29	.07	.05	.62	m.q.	m.q.	0
Tomato juice, canned, 6 fl. oz.	1012	33	.09	.06	1.23	.20	36.1	0
Tomato paste, canned, ½ cup	3234	55	.20	.25	4.22	.50	m.q.	0
Tomato puree, canned, ½ cup	1701	44	.09	.07	2.14	.19	m.q.	0
Tomato sauce, canned, ½ cup, except as noted:								
½ cup	1195	16	.08	.07	1.40	n.a.	m.q.	0
(Health Valley), 1 cup	4916	<1	.11	.12	2.00	.24	1.9	0
marinara sauce	1202	16	.06	.07	1.99	n.a.	m.q.	0
w/mushrooms	1165	15	.09	.13	1.54	n.a.	m.q.	0
w/onions	1038	16	.09	.16	1.52	n.a.	m.q.	0
spaghetti or pasta sauce	1528	14	.07	.07	1.87	n.a.	m.q.	0
w/tomato tidbits	977	26	.09	.12	1.44	n.a.	m.q.	0
Tomato-beef cocktail, canned, 6 fl. oz.	234	2	tr.	.05	.30	n.a.	n.a.	n.a.
Tongue[2], 4 oz.:								
beef, simmered	n.a.	1	.03	.40	2.44	.18	5.7	6.69
lamb, braised	0	8	.09	.48	4.18	.19	3.4	7.14
pork, braised	0	2	.36	.58	6.06	.26	m.q.	2.71

1. *With added sodium ascorbate; vitamin C value for product without additives would be negligible.*
2. *Prepared without added ingredients.*

Food and Measure	A I.U.	C mg.	Thi mg.	Rib mg.	Nia mg.	B₆ mg.	Fol mcg.	B₁₂ mcg.
veal, braised	0	7	.08	.40	1.67	.17	10.2	6.01
Tripe, beef, raw, 1 oz.	0	1	<.01	.05	.02	n.a.	.6	.44
Triticale, whole grain, 1 cup	n.a.	0	.80	.26	2.75	.27	140.0	0
Triticale flour, whole grain, 1 cup	n.a.	0	.49	.17	3.72	.52	96.0	0
Trout, meat only:								
mixed species, raw, 1 oz.	16	<1	.10	.09	m.q.	m.q.	3.8	2.21
rainbow, raw, 1 oz.	18	1	.02	.05	m.q.	m.q.	m.q.	m.q.
rainbow, baked, broiled, or								
microwaved[1], 4 oz.	85	4	.10	.26	m.q.	m.q.	m.q.	m.q.
Tuna, meat only:								
bluefin, raw, 1 oz.	619	(0)	.07	.07	2.45	.13	m.q.	2.67
bluefin, baked, broiled, or								
microwaved[1], 4 oz.	2858	(0)	.32	.35	11.95	.60	n.a.	12.34
skipjack, raw, 1 oz.	15	(0)	.01	m.q.	m.q.	.24	m.q.	m.q.
yellowfin, raw, 1 oz.	17	(0)	.12	.01	2.78	m.q.	m.q.	m.q.
Tuna, canned, 4 oz.:								
light, in oil, drained	88	(0)	.04	m.q.	m.q.	.12	6.0	m.q.
white, in oil, drained	m.q.	(0)	.02	.09	13.27	m.q.	5.2	m.q.
Turbot, European, meat only, raw,								
1 oz.	10	(0)	.02	.02	.62	m.q.	m.q.	.62
Turkey, all classes, roasted[1], 4 oz.,								
except as noted:								
meat w/skin	0	0	.06	.20	5.77	.46	7.9	.40
meat only	0	0	.07	.21	6.17	.52	7.9	.42
skin only, 1 oz.	0	0	.01	.04	.75	.02	1.1	.07
dark meat w/skin	0	0	.07	.27	4.00	.36	10.2	.41
light meat w/skin	0	0	.06	.15	7.13	.53	6.8	.40
back, meat w/skin	0	0	.06	.25	3.91	.34	9.1	.39
breast, meat w/skin	0	0	.06	.15	7.22	.72	6.8	.41
leg, meat w/skin	0	0	.07	.27	4.04	.37	10.2	.41
wing, meat w/skin	0	0	.06	.15	6.50	.48	6.8	.39
Turkey, boneless and luncheon meat, breast, 1 oz.	0	0	.01	.03	2.36	.11	m.q.	.57
Turkey, canned, boned, w/broth,								
5-oz. can	0	3	.02	.24	9.40	m.q.	m.q.	m.q.
Turkey, frozen or refrigerated,								
prebasted w/broth, breast meat								
w/skin, roasted, 4 oz.	0	0	.06	.15	10.28	.36	m.q.	.36
Turkey, ground, cooked, 4 oz. ...	0	0	.06	.19	5.46	.44	7.9	.37
Turkey entree, frozen, gravy and,								
5-oz. pkg.	59	n.a.	.03	.18	2.56	.14	m.q.	m.q.
Turkey giblets, simmered[1], 4 oz.	6845	2	.05	1.03	5.11	.37	391.2	27.30
Turkey gizzard, simmered[1], 4 oz.	210	2	.04	.37	3.48	.14	59.0	2.20
Turkey heart, see "Heart"								
Turkey liver, see "Liver"								
Turmeric, ground, 1 tsp.	tr.	1	<.01	.01	.11	n.a.	n.a.	0

1. *Without added ingredients.*

Food and Measure	A I.U.	C mg.	Thi mg.	Rib mg.	Nia mg.	B_6 mg.	Fol mcg.	B_{12} mcg.
Turnip, ½ cup:								
raw, cubed	0	14	.03	.02	.26	.06	9.5	0
boiled, drained, cubed	0	9	.02	.02	.23	.05	7.1	0
Turnip greens, ½ cup:								
fresh, raw, chopped	2128	17	.02	.03	.17	.07	54.4	0
fresh, boiled, drained, chopped	3959	20	.03	.05	.30	.30	85.3	0
canned, w/liquid	4196	18	.01	.07	.42	.42	48.2	0
frozen, boiled, drained	6540	18	.04	.06	.38	.38	32.3	0

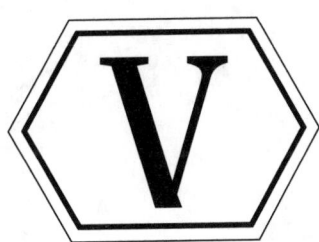

Food and Measure	A I.U.	C mg.	Thi mg.	Rib mg.	Nia mg.	B₆ mg.	Fol mcg.	B₁₂ mcg.
Vanilla flavor drink mix								
(*Carnation* Instant Breakfast),								
1 pkt.	1750	27	.30	.17	5.00	.40	100.0	.60
Veal¹, meat only, 4 oz.:								
cubed, for stew, leg and shoulder,								
braised, lean only	0	0	.08	.45	9.41	.43	18.1	1.89
ground, broiled	0	0	.08	.31	9.11	.44	12.5	1.44
leg (top round):								
braised, lean w/fat	0	0	.07	.40	11.98	.41	20.4	1.33
braised, lean only	0	0	.07	.41	12.16	.42	20.4	1.35
pan-fried in vegetable oil, lean								
w/fat	0	0	.07	.36	11.26	.35	18.1	1.33
pan-fried in vegetable oil, lean								
only	0	0	.07	.37	11.43	.35	18.1	1.34
roasted, lean w/fat	0	0	.08	.40	13.66	.56	17.0	1.64
roasted, lean only	0	0	.08	.42	14.33	.58	18.1	1.71
loin:								
braised, lean w/fat	0	0	.05	.34	10.24	.29	15.9	1.37
braised, lean only	0	0	.06	.39	11.40	.32	17.0	1.50
roasted, lean w/fat	0	0	.06	.32	10.05	.39	17.0	1.41
roasted, lean only	0	0	.07	.34	10.73	.42	18.1	1.49
rib:								
braised, lean w/fat	0	0	.06	.33	8.51	.36	18.1	1.64
braised, lean only	0	0	.07	.35	8.97	.39	18.1	1.74
roasted, lean w/fat	0	0	.06	.31	7.92	.28	14.7	1.66
roasted, lean only	0	0	.07	.33	8.51	.31	15.9	1.79
shoulder, whole:								
braised, lean w/fat	0	0	.07	.39	7.28	.28	17.0	2.09
braised, lean only	0	0	.07	.40	7.58	.29	18.1	2.20

1. *Prepared without added ingredients, except as noted.*

Food and Measure	A I.U.	C mg.	Thi mg.	Rib mg.	Nia mg.	B6 mg.	Fol mcg.	B12 mcg.
Veal, shoulder, whole *(cont.)*								
roasted, lean w/fat	0	0	.08	.39	7.18	.29	13.6	2.06
roasted, lean only	0	0	.08	.39	7.30	.29	14.7	2.11
shoulder, arm:								
braised, lean w/fat	0	0	.07	.35	11.43	.33	20.4	1.95
braised, lean only	0	0	.07	.37	12.15	.34	21.5	2.06
roasted, lean w/fat	0	0	.07	.36	9.09	.33	19.3	1.74
roasted, lean only	0	0	.08	.37	9.34	.34	19.3	1.78
shoulder, blade:								
braised, lean w/fat	0	0	.07	.40	6.24	.27	17.0	2.19
braised, lean only	0	0	.07	.41	6.44	.28	17.0	2.28
roasted, lean w/fat	0	0	.08	.40	6.50	.27	12.5	2.28
roasted, lean only	0	0	.08	.41	6.60	.27	12.5	2.34
sirloin:								
braised, lean w/fat	0	0	.06	.40	7.46	.40	17.0	1.68
braised, lean only	0	0	.07	.43	7.99	.43	18.1	1.80
roasted, lean w/fat	0	0	.07	.40	10.06	.36	17.0	1.61
roasted, lean only	0	0	.07	.42	10.58	.39	18.1	1.69
Vegetable juice cocktail, canned,								
6 fl. oz.	2130	50	.08	.05	1.32	.26	m.q.	0
Vegetables, see specific listings								
Vegetables, mixed, ½ cup:								
canned, w/liquid	6199	5	.04	.05	.59	.09	21.9	0
canned, drained	9551	4	.04	.04	.47	.07	19.4	0
frozen, boiled, drained	3892	3	.07	.11	.77	.07	17.3	0
Vienna sausage, canned, beef and								
pork, 1 oz.	0	0	.02	.03	.46	.03	m.q.	.29
Vinegar, cider, 1 tbsp.	0	0	0	0	0	n.a.	n.a.	0

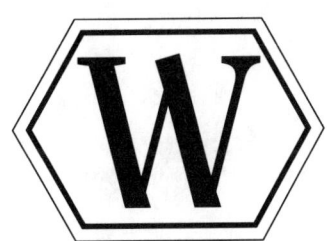

Food and Measure	A I.U.	C mg.	Thi mg.	Rib mg.	Nia mg.	B$_6$ mg.	Fol mcg.	B$_{12}$ mcg.
Waffle, frozen, 2.5 oz.:								
(*Aunt Jemina* Original)	0	0	.35	.34	3.74	.50	6.0	1.68
apple-cinnamon (*Aunt Jemima*)	0	0	.32	.29	3.21	.50	6.0	1.84
blueberry (*Aunt Jemima*)	0	0	.37	.38	3.78	.57	m.q.	2.11
buttermilk (*Aunt Jemima*)	0	0	.32	.34	3.42	.38	6.0	1.44
whole grain wheat (*Aunt Jemima*) . .	0	0	.36	.48	4.49	.74	m.q.	3.11
Walnut, shelled, 1 oz.:								
black, dried	84	tr.	.06	.03	.20	m.q.	m.q.	0
English or Persian, dried	35	1	.11	.04	.30	.16	18.7	0
Waterchestnuts, Chinese, canned,								
w/liquid, sliced, ½ cup	3	1	.01	.02	.25	n.a.	n.a.	0
Watercress, raw, chopped, ½ cup	799	7	.02	.02	.03	.02	n.a.	0
Watermelon:								
¹⁄₁₆ of 10″-diam. melon, 1″-thick slice	1762	47	.39	.10	.96	.69	10.4	0
trimmed, diced, ½ cup	293	8	.06	.02	.16	.12	1.7	0
Wheat, whole grain, 1 cup:								
durum	(0)	0	.81	.23	12.94	.81	m.q.	0
hard red spring	(0)	0	.97	.21	10.96	.64	83.0	0
hard red winter	(0)	0	.74	.22	10.49	.58	72.0	0
soft red winter	(0)	0	.66	.16	8.06	.46	68.0	0
hard white	(0)	0	.74	.21	8.41	.71	m.q.	0
soft white	(0)	0	.69	.18	8.01	.63	m.q.	0
Wheat, sprouted, 1 cup	(0)	3	.24	.17	3.33	.29	m.q.	0
Wheat bran, crude, 1 cup	(0)	0	.31	.35	8.15	.78	48.0	0
Wheat flour, 1 cup:								
whole grain	(0)	0	.54	.26	7.64	.41	52.0	0
white, enriched:								
all-purpose	(0)	0	.98	.62	7.38	.06	33.0	0
bread	(0)	0	1.11	.70	10.35	.05	40.0	0
cake	(0)	0	.97	.47	7.40	.04	21.0	0

Food and Measure	A I.U.	C mg.	Thi mg.	Rib mg.	Nia mg.	B6 mg.	Fol mcg.	B12 mcg.
Wheat flour, white, enriched *(cont.)*								
self-rising	(0)	0	.84	.52	7.29	.06	53.0	0
tortilla mix	(0)	0	.82	.55	6.46	.04	n.a.	0
Wheat germ:								
(*Kretschmer*), 1 oz. or ¼ cup	33	0	.48	.21	1.41	.16	106.0	.05
crude, 1 oz.	(0)	0	.53	.14	1.93	.37	79.7	0
honey crunch (*Kretschmer*), 1 oz. or								
¼ cup	0	0	.34	.18	1.16	.14	82.0	0
toasted, 1 oz., approx. ¼ cup	(0)	2	.47	.23	1.59	.28	100.0	0
Whelk, unspecified, meat only:								
raw, 1 oz.	24	(0)	.01	.03	.30	.10	1.8	2.57
boiled, poached, or steamed[1], 4 oz.	184	(0)	.06	.24	2.26	.74	12.9	20.57
Whey:								
acid, fluid, 1 cup	17	<1	.10	.34	.19	.10	5.0	.44
acid, dry, 1 oz.	16	<1	.18	.58	.32	.18	9.4	.71
sweet, fluid, 1 cup	39	<1	.09	.39	.18	.08	2.0	.68
sweet, dry, 1 oz.	12	<1	.15	.63	.36	.17	3.4	.67
Whiskey sour mix, bottled,								
1 fl. oz.	7	1	<.01	<.01	0	0	0	0
White bean, ½ cup:								
boiled	0	0	.11	.04	.13	.08	72.7	0
canned, w/liquid	0	0	.13	.05	.15	.10	85.6	0
Whitefish, mixed species, smoked,								
4 oz.	215	(0)	.04	.11	2.72	.44	8.3	3.70
Whiting, mixed species, meat only:								
raw, 1 oz.	28	(0)	.02	.01	.37	.04	3.7	.65
baked, broiled, or microwaved[1],								
4 oz.	129	(0)	.08	.07	1.89	.20	17.0	2.95
Wild rice, cooked, 1 cup	0	0	.09	.14	2.11	.22	43.0	0
Wine:								
dessert, 18.8% alcohol, 2 fl. oz. ...	0	0	.01	.01	.13	0	.2	0
table, 11.5% alcohol, 4 fl. oz.:								
red	0	0	<.01	.01	.02	.01	.6	0
rosé	0	0	<.01	.01	.02	.01	.3	0
white	0	0	<.01	<.01	.02	<.01	.1	0
Winged bean, ½ cup:								
raw, sliced	28	n.a.	.03	.02	.20	.03	n.a.	0
boiled, drained	27	3	.03	.02	.20	.03	n.a.	0
Winged bean, dried, boiled,								
½ cup	0	0	.25	.11	.71	.04	8.9	0

1. *Without added ingredients.*

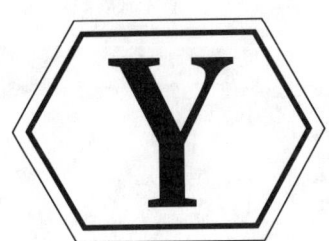

Food and Measure	A I.U.	C mg.	Thi mg.	Rib mg.	Nia mg.	B₆ mg.	Fol mcg.	B₁₂ mcg.
Yam, ½ cup:								
fresh, raw, cubed	0	13	.08	.02	.57	.22	17.3	0
fresh, boiled, drained, cubed	0	8	.07	.02	.38	.16	10.9	0
canned or frozen, see "Sweet potato"								
Yardlong bean, ½ cup:								
raw, sliced	394	86	.05	.05	.19	n.a.	n.a.	0
boiled, drained, sliced	234	8	.04	.05	.33	n.a.	n.a.	0
Yardlong bean, dried, boiled, ½ cup	14	<1	.18	.06	.47	.08	125.3	0
Yeast:								
baker's, active, dry, .2-oz. pkg.	tr.	tr.	.16	.38	2.60	m.q.	m.q.	0
brewer's, dry, 1 tbsp.	tr.	tr.	1.25	.34	3.00	m.q.	m.q.	0
Yellowtail, meat only, raw, 1 oz. . . .	27	1	.04	.01	1.93	.05	1.0	.37
Yogurt, 8 oz., except as noted:								
plain:								
whole milk	279	1	.07	.32	.17	.07	17.0	.84
lowfat	150	2	.10	.49	.26	.11	25.0	1.28
skim	16	2	.11	.53	.28	.12	28.0	1.39
(*Dannon* Lowfat)	145	tr.	.14	.68	tr.	m.q.	m.q.	1.30
(*Dannon* Nonfat)	tr.	tr.	.14	.68	tr.	m.q.	m.q.	1.30
all flavors (*Dannon* Extra Smooth), 4.4 oz.	110	tr.	.08	.38	tr.	m.q.	m.q.	.72
all flavors (*Dannon* Fruit-On-The-Bottom)	120	tr.	.11	.52	tr.	m.q.	m.q.	1.00
blueberry, raspberry, strawberry, or strawberry-banana (*Dannon* Fresh Flavors)	145	tr.	.13	.62	tr.	m.q.	m.q.	1.19
coffee, lemon, or vanilla (*Dannon* Fresh Flavors)	130	tr.	.13	.62	tr.	m.q.	m.q.	1.18
coffee or vanilla, lowfat	123	2	.10	.46	.24	.10	24.0	1.20

Food and Measure	A I.U.	C mg.	Thi mg.	Rib mg.	Nia mg.	B₆ mg.	Fol mcg.	B₁₂ mcg.
Yogurt *(cont.)*								
mixed berries or orchard fruit (*Dannon* Hearty Nuts & Raisins)	195	tr.	.10	.50	tr.	m.q.	m.q.	.95
vanilla (*Dannon* Hearty Nuts & Raisins)	100	tr.	.10	.47	tr.	m.q.	m.q.	.89
Yogurt drink, all flavors (*Dan'up*), 8 oz.	2	tr.	.08	.41	tr.	m.q.	m.q.	.78

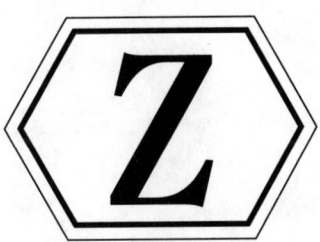

Food and Measure	A I.U.	C mg.	Thi mg.	Rib mg.	Nia mg.	B$_6$ mg.	Fol mcg.	B$_{12}$ mcg.
Zucchini, ½ cup:								
fresh, raw sliced	221	6	.05	.02	.26	.06	14.4	0
fresh, boiled, drained, sliced	216	4	.04	.04	.39	.07	15.1	0
canned, in tomato sauce	615	3	.05	.05	.60	m.q.	m.q.	0
frozen, boiled, drained, sliced	483	4	.05	.05	.43	.05	8.8	0

MINERALS

The importance of minerals in our diet has recently been receiving more attention. Fairly new and significant discoveries have resulted in further studies to ascertain the full impact these substances (at least the ones known at this time) have on our physical and mental well-being. What we do know for certain is that minerals work with vitamins and other nutrients—as well as with each other—to insure the efficient performance of vital processes in our bodies. As with vitamins, a shortage of one essential mineral may disrupt the balance of the others, and possibly render them ineffective altogether.

Minerals are inorganic substances, which the human body cannot manufacture. However, with few exceptions (notably iron) and depending on specific dietary limitations or physical disorders, we can generally get all the minerals we need through the food we eat. Even under conditions of great physical and emotional stress, which sap the body of nutrients, supplementing the missing minerals can frequently make up the loss.

Minerals generally fall into one of two categories: *macrominerals* (which include calcium, phosphorus, potassium, magnesium, and sodium), and *trace minerals* (including iron, zinc, manganese, selenium, and copper). Macrominerals, so called because they are found in body tissue in relatively high amounts, are measured in milligrams. Trace minerals, measured in micrograms, are present in *very* minute quantities, but they are no less vital for healthy body functioning.

Listed below is an overview of the major nutritional minerals.

Calcium
Though it is the most abundant mineral in the body, 99% of it is found in bones and teeth. The remaining 1%, which is scattered throughout the body,

is essential for a wide variety of important functions. Calcium is one of the two minerals most deficient in the diets of women in America (iron is the other). It is not easily absorbed (vitamin D aids in its absorption), and consistent shortages of this important mineral can lead to osteoporosis (brittle bones) and a host of other bone-related problems in adults.

Main Functions: works with phosphorus to build and strengthen bones and teeth; regulates heartbeat, alleviates insomnia (calcium is known to be a natural tranquilizer), and assists in blood clotting.

Best Natural Sources: milk and milk products, cheese, sardines, soybeans, salmon, peanuts, sunflower seeds, dried beans, and green leafy vegetables.

Recommended Daily Dosage: 800 milligrams for an average, healthy adult; 1200 milligrams for pregnant and lactating women. Higher doses are also suggested for the elderly—it appears that the body absorbs calcium less efficiently as we age.

Toxicity: high daily doses can result in bone and tissue calcification throughout the body, can interfere with the function of the nervous and muscular systems, and may cause drowsiness.

Copper
A trace mineral found in all body tissues, it is essential for the utilization of vitamin C.

Main Function: important in formation of red blood cells; boosts energy levels by enhancing iron absorption; involved in protein metabolism and healing; promotes healthy functioning of the central nervous system.

Best Natural Sources: dried beans and peas, whole wheat, prunes, calf and beef liver, shrimp and most seafood, green leafy vegetables, and almonds. Drinking tap water may be a good source if plumbing consists of copper piping.

Recommended Daily Dosage: 2 to 3 milligrams for adults.

Toxicity: rare, but excess copper in the body may accumulate in the blood and deplete the supply of zinc in the brain. Symptoms of toxicity include insomnia, depression, vomiting, diarrhea, hair loss, and irregular menstruation.

Iodine
This is a trace mineral, two-thirds of which is found in the thyroid gland.

Main Functions: promotes proper functioning of the thyroid gland, which in turn stimulates metabolism to assist in burning fat; enriches skin, hair, and nails.

Best Natural Sources: all seafood, seaweed or kelp, sea salt, and iodized salt.

Recommended Daily Dosage: 150 micrograms for adults; 175 micrograms during pregnancy and 200 micrograms during lactation.

Toxicity: none known from natural food or water sources; however, an excess can cause iodine sensitivity or poisoning in certain individuals. When prepared as a drug, iodine levels should be carefully monitored; overdoses can be serious.

Iron

Iron is a mineral concentrate in the blood that is present in all living cells. Along with calcium, iron is one of the minerals most often deficient in the diets of American women. Also, because less than 10% of our total iron intake is absorbed into the bloodstream, a condition called "iron-deficiency anemia" is one of our most common nutritional shortages.

Main Functions: builds up blood quality by aiding in the production of hemoglobin, which transports oxygen through the bloodstream; promotes efficient muscle contraction; works with other nutrients to improve respiratory function; increases resistance to stress and disease.

Best Natural Sources: liver and other organ meats, oysters, lean meat, green leafy vegetables, whole grains, dried fruits, molasses, egg yolks, oatmeal, and nuts. (*Note:* Iron from foods of animal origin is more easily absorbed than iron present in vegetable products.)

Recommended Daily Dosage: 10 milligrams for men and 15 for women, though 30 to 60 milligrams are suggested for pregnant women. The need for iron increases during periods of rapid growth, menstruation, surgery, and whenever there is a loss of blood.

Toxicity: rare in normal, healthy people; however, an overabundance, sometimes found in elderly men, may result in damage to the heart, liver, and pancreas. Coffee and tea in large quantities can contribute to the inhibition of proper iron absorption.

Magnesium

An essential mineral, 70% of magnesium is located in the bones and 30% in soft body tissues and fluids. Sometimes called the "antistress mineral" because of its beneficial effect on the nervous system. Deficiencies of magnesium are fairly common among alcoholics and in individuals with kidney disease, diabetes, and other physical disorders.

Main Functions: works most efficiently with calcium; important for proper functioning of nerves and muscles; can promote a healthy heart; aids in lessening depression; helps prevent calcium deposits, kidney stones, and gallstones; assists in bone formation.

Best Natural Sources: raw green leafy vegetables, almonds and cashews, soybeans, whole grains, milk, figs, corn, and apples.

Recommended Daily Dosage: 280 to 350 milligrams, the higher dosage suggested for men and pregnant and lactating women. Higher dosage recommended with use of alcohol and diuretics.

Toxicity: rare, but it can occur when there is a decrease in normal urinary function or when there is a marked increase in the body's absorption of the mineral. May result in depression of the central nervous system.

Manganese

This is a trace mineral that plays a vital part in activating numerous enzymes.

Main Functions: assists in the digestion of food and the utilization of vitamins and other minerals; helps maintain healthy bone structure; valuable in production of sex hormones; provides "food" for the brain and central nervous system.

Best Natural Sources: whole grains, nuts and seeds, egg yolks, green leafy vegetables, and fruits. A substantial portion of this mineral is generally lost in the processing of foods.

Recommended Daily Dosage: 2.5 to 5 milligrams are suggested for adults.

Toxicity: very high doses can result in inefficient storage and utilization of iron, weakness and motor coordination difficulties, or irritability.

Phosphorus

The second most abundant mineral in the body, phosphorus is found in every living cell.

Main Functions: works efficiently with calcium; important in the proper utilization of carbohydrates by the body for growth, maintenance, and repair of cells and for the production of energy; promotes regular heart function, bone growth, tooth development, and normal kidney function; important in the metabolism of many nutrients.

Best Natural Sources: high-protein foods, such as meat, fish, poultry, and eggs; whole grains, seeds, and nuts.

Recommended Daily Dosage: 800 to 1200 milligrams for adults.

Toxicity: none known, but if phosphorus intake is high, calcium may have to be increased to insure proper balance. (*Note:* Diets high in fat increase phosphorus absorption and lower calcium levels; adjustments must be made for proper balance.)

Potassium

Found mainly in intracellular fluid, it is an essential mineral. Potassium works with sodium, so a proper balance of these two minerals is very important.

Main Functions: helps regulate the body's water balance and heartbeat; important for normal growth; promotes healthy skin and proper kidney function to eliminate waste; sends oxygen to the brain (boosts clear thinking).

Best Natural Sources: citrus fruits, especially oranges; bananas, potatoes, all green leafy vegetables, whole grains, and sunflower seeds.

Recommended Daily Dosage: no official RDA established, but approximate recommended dosage ranges from 2000 to 5600 milligrams for adults.

Toxicity: excessive amounts in the blood may cause abnormal heartbeat. Certain medications, such as cortisone, deplete potassium supplies and can cause sodium retention; an adjustment may be necessary to maintain proper balance.

Selenium

Discovered less than twenty-five years ago, this essential mineral acts as an antioxidant and works closely with vitamin E. Deficiencies are rare, but some early studies indicate that a lack of selenium might result in infertility and premature aging.

Main Functions: helps to promote normal growth and fertility; functions as an antioxidant to prevent the breakdown of tissues, maintains elasticity, and delays aging.

Best Natural Sources: brewer's yeast, organ meats, egg yolks, dairy products, fish and shellfish, whole grains, and onions. (*Note:* selenium levels in food will vary depending on its presence in soil and in animal feed.)

Recommended Daily Dosage: 50 to 70 micrograms for adults; slightly higher amounts are recommended for lactating women.

Toxicity: very high levels can be toxic (possible symptoms are hair, tooth, and nail loss or dermatitis). Since the role of selenium in nutrition has not yet been fully explored, only moderate supplements are advised.

Zinc

This is an essential trace mineral. With the exception of iron, zinc is present in the body in larger amounts than any other trace mineral. It is a component of insulin and plays a major role in the efficiency of most bodily functions.

Main Functions: promotes growth and mental alertness; helps wounds heal; aids in cell formation.

Best Natural Sources: protein-rich foods, such as liver, meat, and eggs; natural unprocessed foods, such as whole grains, brewer's yeast, wheat bran, wheat germ, and raw seeds.

Recommended Daily Dosage: 12 to 15 milligrams for adults; slightly higher amounts for pregnant and lactating women.

Toxicity: excessive amounts may result in iron and copper losses; may cause nausea, vomiting, or diarrhea. Increased amounts of zinc in the diet may require the addition of vitamin A for balance.

THE MINERAL CONTENT OF FOOD

CALCIUM

◆

IRON

◆

MAGNESIUM

◆

PHOSPHORUS

◆

POTASSIUM

◆

ZINC

◆

COPPER

◆

MANGANESE

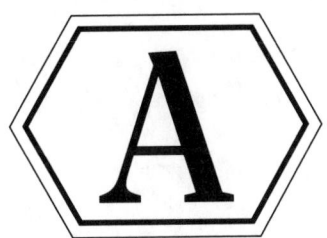

Food and Measure	Ca mg.	Fe mg.	Mag mg.	Pho mg.	Pot mg.	Zn mg.	Cop mcg.	Man mcg.
Abalone, mixed species, meat only,								
raw, 1 oz.	9	.90	14	m.q.	m.q.	.23	.06	.01
Acerola, trimmed, ½ cup	6	.10	9	6	72	n.a.	n.a.	n.a.
Acerola juice, fresh, 6 fl. oz.	18	.90	24	18	174	n.a.	n.a.	n.a.
Acorn squash, ½ cup:								
raw, cubed	23	.49	23	25	243	.09	.05	n.a.
baked, cubed	45	.95	43	46	446	.18	.09	n.a.
baked, mashed	32	.68	31	33	321	.13	.06	n.a.
Aduzi bean, boiled, ½ cup	32	2.30	60	193	612	2.03	.34	.66
Allspice, ground, 1 tsp.	13	.13	3	2	20	.02	.01	.06
Almond, 1 oz.:								
dried, unblanched	75	1.04	84	148	208	.83	.27	.65
dried, blanched	70	1.03	81	151	213	.90	.30	.41
dry-roasted, unblanched	80	1.08	86	156	219	1.39	.35	.56
oil-roasted, unblanched	66	1.09	86	155	194	1.39	.35	.56
oil-roasted, blanched	55	1.51	82	164	197	.40	.26	.42
toasted, unblanched	80	1.40	87	156	220	1.40	.35	.57
Almond butter, 1 tbsp.:								
plain	43	.59	48	84	121	.49	.14	.38
honey and cinnamon	43	.59	48	83	120	.48	.16	.37
Almond paste, 1 oz.	65	.90	73	127	184	.73	.24	.57
Amaranth, ½ cup:								
raw	30	.32	8	7	85	.13	.02	n.a.
boiled, drained	138	1.49	36	47	423	m.q.	n.a.	n.a.
Amaranth, whole grain, 1 cup ..	298	14.81	518	887	714	6.21	1.52	4.41
Amaranth dinner, canned, w/								
garden vegetables (*Health Valley*								
Fast Menu), 7½ oz.	43	4.90	25	81	102	.38	n.a.	n.a.
Anchovy, European, meat only,								
raw, 1 oz.	42	.92	12	49	108	.49	.06	n.a.

Food and Measure	Ca mg.	Fe mg.	Mag mg.	Pho mg.	Pot mg.	Zn mg.	Cop mcg.	Man mcg.
Anchovy, canned, in oil,								
5 medium	46	.93	14	50	109	.49	.07	n.a.
Anise seed, 1 tsp.	14	.78	6	7	48	.08	.02	.04
Apple, ½ cup, except as noted:								
fresh, cored, unpeeled:								
raw, 1 medium, 2¾″ diam.	10	.25	6	10	159	.05	.06	.06
raw, sliced	4	.10	3	4	63	.02	.02	.03
fresh, cored, peeled:								
raw, 1 medium, 2¾″ diam.	5	.09	4	9	144	.05	.04	.03
raw, sliced	2	.04	2	4	62	.02	.02	.01
boiled, sliced	4	.16	3	7	76	.04	.03	.10
microwaved, sliced	4	.14	3	7	79	.03	.04	.12
canned, sweetened, sliced:								
unheated	4	.23	2	6	69	.03	.05	.16
heated	4	.24	3	6	71	.05	.05	.17
dehydrated, sulfured:								
uncooked	6	.60	7	16	192	.09	.08	.04
cooked	4	.41	5	11	132	.06	.06	.03
dried, sulfured, uncooked	6	.61	7	17	194	.09	.08	.04
frozen, unsweetened, sliced:								
unheated	4	.16	3	7	67	.04	.05	.15
heated	5	.19	3	8	78	.05	.07	.15
Apple juice, 6 fl. oz.:								
canned or bottled	12	.66	6	12	222	.06	.04	.21
frozen[1]	12	.48	6	12	228	.06	.02	.11
Applesauce, canned, ½ cup:								
unsweetened	4	.15	4	9	91	.03	.03	.09
sweetened	5	.45	4	9	78	.05	.06	.10
Apricot, ½ cup, except as noted:								
fresh, 3 medium, approx. 4 oz.	15	.58	8	21	313	.28	.09	.08
fresh, pitted, halves	11	.84	12	30	458	.41	.14	.12
canned, unpeeled, halves:								
in water	10	.39	9	16	233	.14	.10	.06
in juice	15	.37	12	25	205	.14	.07	.06
in light syrup	14	.50	11	17	175	.14	.10	.07
in heavy syrup	11	.39	9	16	181	.14	.10	.07
canned, peeled, whole:								
in water	10	.62	11	19	175	.13	.08	.06
in heavy syrup	11	.55	10	17	173	.14	.08	.07
in extra heavy syrup	10	.77	10	18	155	.13	.08	.06
dehydrated, sulfured, uncooked	37	3.79	38	94	1110	.60	.35	.22
dehydrated, sulfured, cooked	30	3.08	31	77	902	.49	.28	.18
dried, sulfured, halves:								
uncooked	30	3.10	31	76	896	.49	.28	.18
cooked, unsweetened	20	2.08	21	52	611	.33	.19	.12
cooked, sweetened	20	2.05	20	51	598	.32	.19	.12
frozen, sweetened	12	1.09	11	23	277	.12	.08	.06

1. *Diluted according to package directions.*

Food and Measure	Ca mg.	Fe mg.	Mag mg.	Pho mg.	Pot mg.	Zn mg.	Cop mcg.	Man mcg.
Apricot nectar, canned, 6 fl. oz. ...	12	.72	12	18	216	.18	.14	n.a.
Arrowroot flour, 1 cup	51	.42	4	7	14	.09	.05	.60
Artichoke, globe, boiled, drained:								
fresh, 1 medium, approx. 10.6 oz. ...	54	1.55	72	103	425	.59	.28	.31
fresh, hearts, ½ cup	38	1.09	51	72	297	.41	.20	.22
frozen, ⅓ of 9-oz. pkg.	17	.45	25	49	211	.29	.05	.22
Asparagus, boiled, drained:								
fresh, 4 spears, ½″-diam. base	22	.59	17	54	279	.43	.09	.19
fresh, cuts and spears, ½ cup	15	.40	11	36	186	.29	.06	.13
canned, w/liquid, ½ cup	17	.71	11	46	186	.57	.13	.19
frozen, 4 spears	14	.38	8	33	131	.33	.10	.11
Avocado:								
California, 1 medium, approx. 8 oz.	19	2.04	70	73	1097	.73	.46	.42
California, pureed, ½ cup	13	1.36	47	49	729	.49	.31	.28
Florida, 1 medium, approx. 1 lb. ...	33	1.60	104	119	1484	1.28	.76	.52
Florida, pureed, ½ cup	13	.61	39	45	561	.49	.29	.20

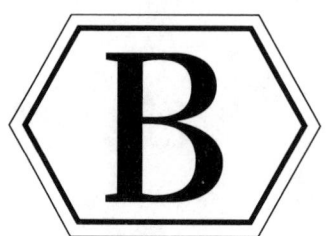

Food and Measure	Ca mg.	Fe mg.	Mag mg.	Pho mg.	Pot mg.	Zn mg.	Cop mcg.	Man mcg.
Bacon, cooked, 3 slices, 20 per lb.	2	.31	5	64	92	.62	.03	.01
Bacon, substitute:								
beef, cooked, 3 slices or 1.2 oz. ...	n.a.	1.07	9	80	140	2.17	n.a.	n.a.
pork, cured, cooked, 3 slices, 15 per 20-oz. pkg.	5	.67	9	90	158	1.25	.05	.02
turkey (*Louis Rich*), 1 heated slice	1	.19	3	41	36	.27	m.q.	m.q.
Bacon bits (*Oscar Mayer*), ¼ oz. ..	1	.14	2	41	38	.33	n.a.	n.a.
Bagel, plain or water, 3½"-diam. piece	29	1.80	m.q.	46	50	m.q.	m.q.	n.a.
Baked beans, canned, ½ cup, except as noted:								
plain or vegetarian	64	.37	41	132	376	1.78	.26	.44
Boston (*Health Valley*), 4 oz.	148	6.20	68	44	360	.25	m.q.	n.a.
w/beef	60	2.13	33	108	426	1.60	.40	.80
w/franks	61	2.22	35	133	301	2.39	.27	.54
w/pork	66	2.15	42	137	389	1.84	.27	.46
w/pork and sweet sauce	77	2.01	43	132	335	1.89	.13	.47
w/pork and tomato sauce	70	4.13	44	148	378	7.38	.32	.62
Baking powder, w/monocalcium phosphate monohydrate, 1 tsp.	58	0	n.a.	87	5	n.a.	n.a.	n.a.
Balsam pear, boiled, drained:								
leafy tips, ½ cup	12	.30	27	22	174	n.a.	n.a.	n.a.
pods, ½" pieces, ½ cup	6	.24	10	22	198	n.a.	n.a.	n.a.
Bamboo shoots, ½ cup:								
raw, ½" slices	10	.38	2	45	405	n.a.	n.a.	n.a.
boiled, drained, ½" slices..........	7	.15	2	12	320	n.a.	n.a.	n.a.
Banana:								
fresh, 1 medium, 8¾" × 1¹³⁄₃₂	7	.35	33	22	451	.19	.12	.17
fresh, mashed, ½ cup	7	.35	32	22	445	.19	.12	.17
dehydrated or powdered, 1 oz.	6	.33	31	21	423	.17	.11	.16
Barbecue loaf, pork and beef, 1 oz.	15	.33	5	38	93	.70	.02	.01

Food and Measure	Ca mg.	Fe mg.	Mag mg.	Pho mg.	Pot mg.	Zn mg.	Cop mcg.	Man mcg.
Barbecue sauce, 1 tbsp.	3	.14	m.q.	3	28	n.a.	n.a.	n.a.
Barley, 1 cup:								
raw	61	6.63	244	485	831	5.10	.92	3.58
pearled, raw	57	5.00	158	442	560	4.25	.84	2.64
pearled, cooked	17	2.09	35	85	145	1.29	.17	.41
Basil, ground, 1 tsp.	30	.59	6	7	48	.08	.02	.04
Bass, freshwater, mixed species,								
raw, 1 oz.	23	.42	9	57	101	.19	.03	.25
Bay leaf, crumbled, 1 tsp.	5	.26	1	1	3	.02	<.01	.05
Beans, see specific listings								
Beef[1], retail trim[2], meat only, 4 oz.,								
except as noted:								
brisket, whole, all grades, braised:								
lean and fat[3]	9	2.54	20	212	262	5.78	.11	.02
lean and fat[4]	8	2.87	24	245	294	6.76	.12	.02
lean only[5]	7	3.19	26	273	323	7.81	.13	.02
brisket, flat half, all grades, braised:								
lean and fat[3]	9	2.60	22	228	276	5.47	.11	.02
lean and fat[4]	6	3.12	27	281	328	6.93	.14	.02
lean only[5]	6	3.22	28	291	338	7.21	.14	.02
brisket, point half, all grades,								
braised:								
lean and fat[3]	10	2.49	19	198	251	6.07	.10	.02
lean and fat[4]	9	2.65	20	212	264	6.61	.11	.02
lean only[5]	7	3.16	25	256	310	8.38	.13	.02
chuck, arm pot roast, choice grade,								
braised:								
lean and fat[3]	11	3.46	22	245	276	7.60	.15	.02
lean and fat[4]	11	3.80	24	269	297	8.51	.16	.02
lean only[5]	10	4.30	27	304	328	9.82	.19	.02
chuck, arm pot roast, select grade,								
braised:								
lean and fat[3]	11	3.58	23	254	284	7.93	.16	.02
lean and fat[4]	11	3.90	25	276	303	8.75	.17	.02
lean only[5]	10	4.30	27	304	328	9.82	.19	.02
chuck, blade roast, choice grade,								
braised:								
lean and fat[3]	15	3.46	22	223	259	9.23	.14	.02
lean and fat[4]	15	3.58	23	230	265	9.64	.14	.02
lean only[5]	15	4.17	26	266	298	11.65	.17	.02
chuck, blade roast, select grade,								
braised:								
lean and fat[3]	15	3.58	23	230	265	9.64	.14	.02
lean and fat[4]	15	3.66	23	236	271	9.93	.15	.02
lean only[5]	15	4.17	26	266	298	11.65	.17	.02

1. *Prepared without added ingredients, except as noted.*
2. *Meat trimmed to 0" or ¼" fat refers to the amount of fat present during cooking. For "lean only" listings, all visible fat is trimmed after cooking. (Bear in mind that a small amount of fat is always present, even in meat trimmed to 0" fat before cooking.)*
3. *Trimmed to ¼" fat.*
4. *Trimmed to 0" fat.*
5. *Trimmed to ¼" or 0" fat.*

Food and Measure	Ca mg.	Fe mg.	Mag mg.	Pho mg.	Pot mg.	Zn mg.	Cop mcg.	Man mcg.
Beef *(cont.)*								
flank, choice grade[1]:								
braised, lean and fat	7	3.78	26	290	382	6.54	.13	.02
braised, lean only	7	3.93	27	303	398	6.86	.14	.02
broiled, lean and fat	8	2.85	26	261	456	5.28	.11	.02
broiled, lean only	8	2.91	27	268	469	5.44	.11	.02
ground, extra lean:								
raw, 1 oz.	2	.55	6	40	81	1.17	.02	.01
baked, medium	8	2.59	19	141	254	6.06	.09	.02
baked, well-done	10	3.36	25	184	330	7.87	.11	.02
broiled, medium	8	2.66	24	183	355	6.18	.08	.02
broiled, well-done	10	3.14	28	215	418	7.29	.09	.02
pan-fried, medium	8	2.68	24	181	354	6.15	.10	.02
pan-fried, well-done	9	3.10	27	210	408	7.11	.11	.02
ground, lean:								
raw, 1 oz.	2	.50	5	39	74	1.09	.02	<.01
baked, medium	10	2.37	19	145	254	5.78	.08	.02
baked, well-done	14	3.02	24	186	324	7.38	.10	.02
broiled, medium	12	2.39	24	179	341	6.08	.07	.02
broiled, well-done	14	2.78	27	206	396	7.03	.09	.02
pan-fried, medium	11	2.47	23	180	339	5.90	.09	.02
pan-fried, well-done	12	2.81	26	205	386	6.70	.10	.02
ground, regular:								
raw, 1 oz.	2	.49	4	37	65	1.01	.02	.01
baked, medium	11	2.73	17	155	251	5.55	.08	.02
baked, well-done	14	3.39	22	193	311	6.88	.10	.02
broiled, medium	12	2.77	23	193	331	5.87	.09	.02
broiled, well-done	14	3.11	25	217	371	6.59	.10	.02
pan-fried, medium	12	2.78	23	194	340	5.75	.09	.02
pan-fried, well-done	15	3.07	25	214	376	6.37	.10	.02
ground, frozen, patties, broiled,								
medium	12	2.38	23	179	333	6.12	.07	.02
Porterhouse steak (short loin),								
choice grade, broiled[2]:								
lean and fat	9	2.98	28	212	399	5.26	.14	.01
lean only	8	3.40	33	242	462	6.12	.16	.02
rib, whole (ribs 6–12), choice grade[2]:								
broiled, lean and fat	14	2.44	22	198	349	5.82	.09	.01
broiled, lean only	12	2.91	28	242	432	7.45	.11	.02
roasted, lean and fat	12	2.62	22	195	336	5.94	.09	.01
roasted, lean only	11	3.24	28	243	424	7.88	.11	.02
rib, whole (ribs 6–12), prime grade[2]:								
broiled, lean and fat	12	2.39	23	189	347	5.79	.09	.01
broiled, lean only	11	2.86	28	230	430	7.43	.11	.02
roasted, lean and fat	12	2.43	22	195	339	5.98	.09	.01
roasted, lean only	11	2.96	28	242	426	7.87	.11	.02

1. *Trimmed to 0" fat.*
2. *Trimmed to ¼" fat.*

Food and Measure	Ca mg.	Fe mg.	Mag mg.	Pho mg.	Pot mg.	Zn mg.	Cop mcg.	Man mcg.
rib, whole (ribs 6–12), select grade[1]:								
broiled, lean and fat	12	2.49	23	203	358	6.01	.09	.01
broiled, lean only	12	2.91	28	242	432	7.45	.11	.02
roasted, lean and fat	12	2.70	23	202	347	6.21	.10	.02
roasted, lean only	11	3.24	28	243	424	7.88	.11	.02
rib, large end (ribs 6–9), choice grade:								
broiled, lean and fat[1]	11	2.42	20	200	338	5.52	.09	.01
broiled, lean only[1]	10	2.91	26	246	422	7.12	.10	.02
roasted, lean and fat[1]	11	2.57	22	191	321	6.33	.10	.01
roasted, lean and fat[2]	11	2.64	23	195	329	6.52	.10	.01
roasted, lean only[3]	9	3.20	28	237	405	8.46	.12	.02
rib, large end (ribs 6–9), prime grade[1]:								
broiled, lean and fat	11	2.31	20	183	330	5.39	.09	.01
broiled, lean only	9	2.81	27	226	418	7.09	.10	.02
roasted, lean and fat	11	2.60	22	192	324	6.40	.10	.01
roasted, lean only	9	3.20	28	237	405	8.46	.12	.02
rib, large end (ribs 6–9), select grade:								
broiled, lean and fat[1]	11	2.48	22	206	349	5.74	.09	.01
broiled, lean only[1]	10	2.91	26	246	422	7.12	.10	.02
roasted, lean and fat[1]	11	2.68	23	197	335	6.67	.10	.02
roasted, lean and fat[2]	10	2.72	23	201	340	6.82	.10	.02
roasted, lean only[3]	9	3.20	28	237	405	8.46	.12	.02
rib, shortrib, choice grade:								
braised, lean and fat	14	2.62	17	184	254	5.53	.11	.01
braised, lean only	12	3.81	25	266	355	8.85	.12	.02
rib, small end (ribs 10–12), choice grade:								
broiled, lean and fat[1]	15	2.47	25	197	365	6.28	.10	.02
broiled, lean and fat[2]	15	2.59	26	208	388	6.72	.10	.02
broiled, lean only[3]	15	2.91	31	236	447	7.93	.11	.02
roasted, lean and fat[1]	15	2.66	22	202	356	5.41	.09	.01
roasted, lean only[1]	14	3.30	28	252	451	7.04	.10	.02
rib, small end (ribs 10–12), prime grade[1]:								
broiled, lean and fat	15	2.51	25	200	372	6.41	.10	.02
broiled, lean only	15	2.91	31	236	447	7.93	.11	.02
roasted, lean and fat	15	2.19	22	200	361	5.39	.09	.01
roasted, lean only	15	2.61	28	248	458	7.02	.10	.02

1. *Trimmed to 1/4" fat.*
2. *Trimmed to 0" fat.*
3. *Trimmed to 1/4" or 0" fat.*

Food and Measure	Ca mg.	Fe mg.	Mag mg.	Pho mg.	Pot mg.	Zn mg.	Cop mcg.	Man mcg.
Beef *(cont.)*								
rib, small end (ribs 10–12), select grade:								
broiled, lean and fat[1]	15	2.51	25	200	372	6.41	.10	.02
broiled, lean and fat[2]	15	2.61	26	209	390	6.78	.10	.02
broiled, lean only[3]	15	2.91	31	236	447	7.93	.11	.02
roasted, lean and fat[1]	15	2.73	23	208	366	5.57	.09	.01
roasted, lean only[1]	14	3.30	28	252	451	7.04	.10	.02
rib eye, small end (ribs 10–12), choice grade[2]:								
broiled, lean and fat	15	2.61	26	209	390	6.78	.10	.02
broiled, lean only	15	2.91	31	236	447	7.93	.11	.02
round, full cut, choice grade[1]:								
broiled, lean and fat	7	2.87	28	270	445	4.90	.11	.02
broiled, lean only	6	3.06	32	290	479	5.26	.12	.02
round, full cut, select grade[1]:								
broiled, lean and fat	7	2.88	29	270	445	4.91	.11	.02
broiled, lean only	6	3.07	32	290	480	5.28	.12	.02
round, bottom, choice grade:								
braised, lean and fat[1]	7	3.54	25	278	320	5.57	.14	.02
braised, lean and fat[2]	6	3.84	27	302	342	6.08	.15	.02
braised, lean only[3]	6	3.92	28	308	349	6.21	.15	.02
roasted, lean and fat[1]	7	3.24	28	247	403	4.76	.11	.02
roasted, lean and fat[2]	6	3.50	32	268	437	5.16	.12	.02
roasted, lean only[3]	6	3.55	32	271	443	5.24	.12	.02
round, bottom, select grade:								
braised, lean and fat[1]	7	3.57	26	280	321	5.61	.14	.02
braised, lean and fat[2]	6	3.87	28	304	345	6.12	.15	.02
braised, lean only[3]	6	3.92	28	308	350	6.21	.15	.02
roasted, lean and fat[1]	7	3.29	29	251	409	4.83	.12	.02
roasted, lean and fat[2]	6	3.53	32	270	440	5.21	.12	.02
roasted, lean only[3]	6	3.55	32	271	443	5.24	.12	.02
round, eye of, choice grade, roasted:								
lean and fat[1]	7	2.08	27	234	407	4.89	.11	.02
lean and fat[2]	6	2.20	31	254	445	5.34	.11	.02
lean only[3]	6	2.21	31	256	448	5.38	.11	.02
round, eye of, select grade, roasted:								
lean and fat[1]	7	2.10	28	237	414	4.96	.11	.02
lean and fat[2]	6	2.20	31	254	445	5.34	.11	.02
lean only[3]	6	2.21	31	256	448	5.38	.11	.02
round, tip, choice grade, roasted:								
lean and fat[1]	7	3.07	27	252	401	7.25	.13	.02
lean and fat[2]	6	3.24	29	267	425	7.76	.14	.02
lean only[3]	6	3.33	31	274	438	8.02	.14	.02
round, tip, prime grade, roasted[1]:								
lean and fat	7	3.06	27	249	398	7.18	.13	.02
lean only	6	3.33	31	274	438	8.02	.14	.02

1. *Trimmed to ¼" fat.*
2. *Trimmed to 0" fat.*
3. *Trimmed to ¼" or 0" fat.*

Food and Measure	Ca mg.	Fe mg.	Mag mg.	Pho mg.	Pot mg.	Zn mg.	Cop mcg.	Man mcg.
round, tip, select grade, roasted:								
lean and fat[1]	7	3.14	28	257	411	7.44	.13	.02
lean and fat[2]	6	3.27	29	269	429	7.82	.14	.02
lean only[3]	6	3.33	31	274	438	8.02	.14	.02
round, top, choice grade:								
braised, lean and fat[1]	6	3.50	27	239	354	4.81	.13	.05
braised, lean and fat[2]	5	3.71	28	253	374	5.10	.14	.06
braised, lean only[3]	5	3.76	29	256	379	5.17	.14	.06
broiled, lean and fat[1]	8	3.12	33	265	475	5.98	.13	.02
broiled, lean only[1]	7	3.27	35	279	501	6.32	.14	.02
pan-fried in vegetable oil, lean and fat[1]	7	3.31	36	304	533	4.84	.14	.02
pan-fried in vegetable oil, lean only[1]	6	3.57	40	331	582	5.24	.15	.02
round, top, prime grade[1]:								
broiled, lean and fat	7	3.21	34	273	490	6.17	.14	.02
broiled, lean only	7	3.27	35	279	501	6.32	.14	.02
round, top, select grade:								
braised, lean and fat[1]	6	3.56	27	243	359	4.89	.13	.05
braised, lean and fat[2]	5	3.71	28	253	374	4.50	.14	.06
braised, lean only[3]	5	3.76	29	256	379	5.17	.14	.06
broiled, lean and fat[1]	8	3.12	33	265	475	5.98	.13	.02
broiled, lean only[1]	7	3.27	35	279	501	6.32	.14	.02
shank crosscuts, choice grade[1]:								
simmered, lean and fat	34	3.97	31	271	458	10.56	.18	.02
simmered, lean only	36	4.38	34	298	507	11.90	.20	.02
sirloin, top, choice grade:								
broiled, lean and fat[1]	12	3.45	32	249	412	6.58	.15	.02
broiled, lean and fat[2]	12	3.65	34	265	438	7.04	.16	.02
broiled, lean only[3]	12	3.81	36	277	457	7.39	.17	.02
pan-fried in vegetable oil, lean and fat[1]	14	3.78	32	260	449	6.12	.15	.02
pan-fried in vegetable oil, lean only[1]	12	4.42	37	303	527	7.26	.17	.02
sirloin, top, select grade, broiled:								
lean and fat[1]	12	3.49	33	254	418	6.70	.15	.02
lean and fat[2]	12	3.72	35	271	446	7.20	.16	.02
lean only[3]	12	3.81	36	277	457	7.39	.17	.02
T-bone steak (short loin), choice grade[1]:								
broiled, lean and fat	9	3.01	28	209	403	5.31	.14	.01
broiled, lean only	8	3.40	33	236	462	6.12	.16	.02
tenderloin, choice grade:								
broiled, lean and fat[1]	9	3.55	29	237	414	5.49	.18	.02
broiled, lean and fat[2]	8	3.86	32	257	451	6.01	.19	.02
broiled, lean only[3]	8	4.06	34	270	475	6.34	.20	.02

1. *Trimmed to ¼" fat.*
2. *Trimmed to 0" fat.*
3. *Trimmed to ¼" or 0" fat.*

Food and Measure	Ca mg.	Fe mg.	Mag mg.	Pho mg.	Pot mg.	Zn mg.	Cop mcg.	Man mcg.
Beef, Tenderloin, Choice Grade *(cont.)*								
roasted, lean and fat[1]	10	3.47	29	263	454	4.50	.14	.02
roasted, lean only[1]	9	4.18	36	319	555	5.43	.16	.02
tenderloin, prime grade[1]:								
broiled, lean and fat	9	3.52	28	235	411	5.43	.17	.02
broiled, lean only	8	4.06	34	270	475	6.34	.20	.02
roasted, lean and fat	10	3.47	25	226	374	4.89	.16	.02
roasted, lean only	8	4.15	31	268	446	5.86	.19	.02
tenderloin, select grade:								
broiled, lean and fat[1]	9	3.63	29	243	424	5.62	.18	.02
broiled, lean and fat[2]	8	3.89	33	259	455	6.06	.19	.02
broiled, lean only[3]	8	4.06	34	270	475	6.34	.20	.02
roasted, lean and fat[1]	10	3.47	25	227	370	4.50	.14	.02
roasted, lean only[1]	8	4.18	31	271	443	5.43	.16	.02
top loin (short loin), choice grade, broiled:								
lean and fat[1]	10	2.52	26	218	392	5.14	.11	.02
lean and fat[2]	9	2.73	29	240	437	5.75	.12	.02
lean only[3]	9	2.80	31	247	449	5.92	.12	.02
top loin (short loin), prime grade[1]:								
broiled, lean and fat	10	2.52	26	218	392	5.14	.11	.02
broiled, lean only	9	2.80	31	247	449	5.92	.12	.02
top loin (short loin), select grade, broiled:								
lean and fat[1]	10	2.56	27	223	401	5.27	.11	.02
lean and fat[2]	9	2.76	29	243	440	5.79	.12	.02
lean only[3]	9	2.80	31	247	449	5.92	.12	.02
Beef, corned, brisket, cured, cooked, 4 oz.	9	2.11	14	142	164	5.19	.17	.02
Beef gravy, canned, ¼ cup	4	.41	n.a.	18	47	.58	.06	.12
Beef luncheon meat:								
loaf, 1-oz. slice	3	.66	4	34	59	.72	.03	.01
roast (*Oscar Mayer* Thin Sliced), .4-oz. slice	1	.22	2	34	39	.39	m.q.	m.q.
smoked (*Oscar Mayer*), .5-oz. slice	1	.37	2	31	50	.47	m.q.	m.q.
thin sliced, 5 slices, approx. ¾ oz.	n.a.	.45	4	35	86	.84	.02	.01
Beef stew, canned (*Wolf* Brand), scant cup	34	1.89	26	136	417	2.00	.11	0
Beer, 12 fl. oz.:								
regular	18	.18	23	44	89	.06	.03	.04
light	18	.12	17	43	64	.11	.09	.06
Beet, sliced, ½ cup:								
fresh, raw	11	.62	14	33	220	.25	.06	.24
fresh, boiled, drained	9	.53	31	26	266	.21	.05	.20
canned, w/liquid	17	.82	20	20	175	.28	.12	.30
Harvard, canned, w/liquid	13	.44	24	21	201	m.q.	m.q.	m.q.
pickled, canned, w/liquid	13	.47	18	20	169	.30	.13	m.q.

1. *Trimmed to ¼" fat.*
2. *Trimmed to 0" fat.*
3. *Trimmed to ¼" or 0" fat.*

Food and Measure	Ca mg.	Fe mg.	Mag mg.	Pho mg.	Pot mg.	Zn mg.	Cop mcg.	Man mcg.
Beet greens, ½ cup:								
raw, 1" pieces	23	.63	14	8	104	.07	.04	n.a.
boiled, drained, 1" pieces	82	1.37	49	29	654	.36	.18	n.a.
Berliner, pork and beef, 1 oz.	3	.33	4	37	80	.70	.02	.01
Biscuit, baking powder:								
mix[1], 2"-diam. piece	58	.70	m.q.	128	56	m.q.	n.a.	n.a.
refrigerated, 2"-diam. piece	4	.50	m.q.	79	18	m.q.	n.a.	n.a.
Black bean, boiled, ½ cup	24	1.80	60	120	306	.96	.18	.38
Black bean dinner, canned,								
western, w/garden vegetables								
(*Health Valley Fast Menu*),								
7½ oz.	179	4.40	55	124	276	.89	n.a.	n.a.
Black turtle soup bean, ½ cup:								
boiled	51	2.62	45	140	398	.70	.25	.30
canned, w/liquid	42	2.28	42	130	370	.65	.23	.28
Blackberry, ½ cup:								
fresh, trimmed	23	.41	14	15	141	.20	.10	.93
canned, in heavy syrup	27	.83	22	18	127	.23	.17	.89
frozen, unsweetened	22	.61	17	23	106	.19	.09	.92
Blueberry, ½ cup:								
fresh, trimmed	5	.12	4	8	65	.08	.04	.20
canned, in heavy syrup	7	.42	4	13	51	.09	.07	.26
frozen, unsweetened	6	.14	4	9	42	.06	.03	.11
frozen, sweetened	7	.45	3	8	69	.07	.05	.30
Bluefish, meat only, raw, 1 oz. ...	2	.14	9	64	105	.23	.02	.01
Bologna, 1 oz.:								
beef	3	.40	3	23	44	.57	.01	.01
beef and pork	3	.43	3	26	51	.55	.02	.01
Lebanon, beef	4	.67	4	42	87	1.11	.02	.02
pork	3	.22	4	39	80	.57	.02	.01
Bouillon, dehydrated, 1 cube:								
beef	n.a.	.08	2	8	15	.01	n.a.	.01
chicken	n.a.	.09	3	9	18	.01	n.a.	.02
Boysenberry, ½ cup:								
fresh, see "Blackberry"								
canned, in heavy syrup	23	.55	14	13	115	.24	.09	.32
frozen, unsweetened	18	.56	11	18	92	.15	.05	.36
Brains[2], 4 oz.:								
beef, pan-fried in vegetable oil	10	2.52	17	438	401	1.53	.25	.04
beef, simmered	10	2.51	16	399	272	1.42	.27	.04
lamb, braised	14	1.91	16	382	232	1.54	.24	.07
lamb, pan-fried in vegetable oil	24	2.31	25	561	406	2.27	.54	.08
pork, braised	10	2.06	14	249	221	1.68	.30	.10
veal, braised	18	1.89	18	437	243	1.83	.29	.04
veal, pan-fried in vegetable oil	11	1.21	20	492	535	2.06	.34	.05
Bran, unprocessed (*Quaker*),								
2 tbsp.	6	.98	42	110	121	.63	.09	.77

1. *Prepared according to package directions.*
2. *Prepared without added ingredients, except as noted.*

Food and Measure	Ca mg.	Fe mg.	Mag mg.	Pho mg.	Pot mg.	Zn mg.	Cop mcg.	Man mcg.
Bratwurst:								
pork, cooked, 1 oz.	13	.36	4	42	60	.65	.03	.01
pork and beef[1], 1 oz.	14	.29	4	38	80	.60	.02	.01
Braunschweiger, pork, 1 oz.	2	2.65	3	48	57	.80	.07	.04
Brazil nut, 1 oz.	50	.97	64	170	170	1.30	.50	.22
Bread, 1 slice or piece:								
Boston brown, canned, 1.6 oz.	41	.90	n.a.	72	131	n.a.	n.a.	n.a.
French, enriched, 1.2 oz.	39	1.10	m.q.	30	32	m.q.	n.a.	n.a.
Italian, enriched, 1.1 oz.	5	.80	m.q.	23	22	m.q.	n.a.	n.a.
mixed grain, 18 slices/lb.	27	.80	m.q.	55	56	m.q.	n.a.	n.a.
oatmeal, 18 slices/lb.	15	.70	m.q.	31	39	m.q.	n.a.	n.a.
pita, white, enriched, 6½" diam. . . .	49	1.40	m.q.	60	71	m.q.	n.a.	n.a.
pumpernickel, 1.1 oz.	23	.90	m.q.	71	141	m.q.	n.a.	n.a.
raisin, enriched, 18 slices/lb.	25	.80	m.q.	22	59	m.q.	m.q.	m.q.
rye, light, .9 oz.	20	.70	m.q.	36	51	m.q.	n.a.	n.a.
Vienna, enriched, .9 oz.	28	.80	m.q.	21	23	m.q.	n.a.	n.a.
wheat:								
cracked, 18 slices/lb.	16	.70	m.q.	32	34	m.q.	n.a.	n.a.
enriched, 18 slices/lb.	32	.90	m.q.	47	35	m.q.	n.a.	n.a.
whole, 16 slices/lb.	20	1.00	m.q.	74	50	m.q.	n.a.	n.a.
white, enriched:								
18 slices/lb.	32	.70	m.q.	27	28	m.q.	n.a.	n.a.
22 slices/lb.	25	.60	m.q.	21	22	m.q.	n.a.	n.a.
Bread, sweet, mix[2], cornbread,								
2½" × 2½" piece	133	.80	n.a.	209	61	n.a.	n.a.	n.a.
Bread cubes, white, 1 cup	38	.90	m.q.	32	34	m.q.	n.a.	n.a.
Breadcrumbs:								
dry, grated, 1 cup	122	4.10	m.q.	141	152	n.a.	n.a.	n.a.
soft, 1 cup	57	1.30	m.q.	49	50	n.a.	n.a.	n.a.
Breadfruit, trimmed, ½ cup	19	.60	28	33	539	.13	.09	.07
Breadsticks:								
regular, 7¾" long, 10 pieces	14	.50	m.q.	50	46	m.q.	n.a.	n.a.
Vienna, 6½" × 1¼", 1 piece	16	.30	n.a.	31	33	n.a.	n.a.	n.a.
Breakfast bar, 1 bar:								
chocolate chip (*Carnation*)	20	4.50	60	60	110	3.00	.50	.05
chocolate crunch (*Carnation*)	20	4.50	60	60	130	3.00	.50	.18
peanut butter, w/chocolate chips								
(*Carnation*)	20	4.50	60	60	110	3.00	.50	.18
peanut butter crunch (*Carnation*) . .	20	4.50	60	60	110	3.00	.50	.21
Broadbean, dried, ½ cup:								
boiled	31	1.27	36	106	228	.86	.22	.36
canned, w/liquid	34	1.28	41	101	310	.80	.14	.37
Broccoli:								
fresh:								
raw, 1 spear, 5.3 oz.	73	1.33	38	99	490	.60	.07	.35
boiled, drained, 1 spear, 6.3 oz.	82	1.50	43	107	526	.68	.08	.39
boiled, drained, chopped, ½ cup	36	.65	19	46	228	.30	.03	.17

1. *Nonfat dry milk added.*
2. *Prepared according to package directions, with egg and milk.*

Food and Measure	Ca mg.	Fe mg.	Mag mg.	Pho mg.	Pot mg.	Zn mg.	Cop mcg.	Man mcg.
frozen, boiled, drained, chopped, ½ cup	47	.56	19	51	166	.28	.04	.30
Brown gravy mix, ¼ cup[1]	17	.06	3	11	14	.08	.01	.02
Brownie:								
w/nuts, .9-oz. piece	13	.60	m.q.	26	50	m.q.	n.a.	n.a.
frozen, w/chocolate frosting, .9-oz. piece	10	.40	m.q.	31	44	m.q.	n.a.	n.a.
Brussels sprouts, boiled, drained:								
fresh, 1 sprout, .75 oz.	7	.25	4	12	67	.07	.02	.05
fresh, ½ cup	28	.94	16	44	247	.25	.07	.18
frozen, ½ cup	19	.58	19	42	254	.28	.06	.25
Buckwheat, whole grain, 1 cup ...	31	3.74	392	590	782	4.08	1.87	2.21
Buckwheat flour, 1 cup	49	4.88	301	404	692	3.75	.62	2.44
Buckwheat groats, roasted:								
dry, 1 oz.	5	.70	63	90	91	.69	.18	.46
cooked, 1 cup	14	1.58	101	139	175	1.21	.29	.80
Bulgur:								
dry, 1 oz.	10	.70	46	85	116	.55	.09	.86
cooked, 1 cup	18	1.75	58	73	124	1.04	.14	1.11
Burbot, meat only, raw, 1 oz.	14	.26	9	57	114	.21	.06	.20
Butter:								
regular, 1 stick	27	.18	2	26	29	.06	.02	<.01
regular, 1 tbsp.	3	.02	<1	3	4	.01	<.01	tr.
whipped, 1 stick	18	.12	2	17	20	.04	.01	<.01
whipped, 1 tbsp.	2	.02	<1	2	2	<.01	<.01	tr.
Butternut squash, ½ cup:								
fresh, raw, cubed	34	.49	24	23	246	.10	.05	n.a.
fresh, boiled, drained, cubed	42	.61	30	27	290	.13	.07	n.a.
frozen, boiled, mashed	23	.70	11	17	160	.14	.04	n.a.

1. *Prepared according to package directions, with water.*

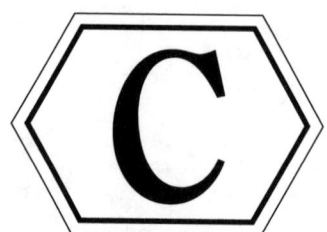

Food and Measure	Ca mg.	Fe mg.	Mag mg.	Pho mg.	Pot mg.	Zn mg.	Cop mcg.	Man mcg.
Cabbage:								
raw, 5¾"-diam. head	424	5.09	134	211	2231	1.66	.21	1.44
raw, shredded, ½ cup	16	.20	5	8	86	.06	.01	.06
boiled, drained, shredded, ½ cup ..	25	.29	11	18	154	.12	.02	.10
Cabbage, Chinese, shredded, ½ cup:								
bok-choy, raw	37	.28	7	13	88	m.q.	m.q.	m.q.
bok-choy, boiled, drained	79	.88	9	25	315	m.q.	m.q.	m.q.
pe-tsai, raw	29	.12	5	11	90	.09	.01	.07
pe-tsai, boiled, drained	19	.18	6	23	134	.11	.02	.09
Cabbage, red, ½ cup:								
raw, shredded	18	.17	5	15	72	.07	.03	.06
boiled, drained, shredded	28	.27	8	21	105	.11	.05	.10
Cabbage, savoy, ½ cup:								
raw, shredded	12	.14	10	15	81	m.q.	m.q.	m.q.
boiled, drained, shredded	22	.28	17	24	134	m.q.	m.q.	m.q.
Cake:								
cheesecake, ½₂ of 9"-diam. cake ...	52	.40	m.q.	81	91	m.q.	m.q.	n.a.
pound, 1-oz. slice	8	.50	m.q.	30	26	m.q.	n.a.	n.a.
white, w/white frosting, 2 layer, 2.5-oz. slice	33	1.00	m.q.	99	52	m.q.	n.a.	n.a.
yellow, w/chocolate frosting, 2 layer, 2.4-oz. slice	23	1.20	m.q.	117	123	m.q.	n.a.	n.a.
Cake, frozen, 1 piece:								
devil's food, w/chocolate frosting, ⅙ of 7½"-diam. cake	46	.70	m.q.	78	101	m.q.	m.q.	n.a.
devil's food, w/whipped cream filling and chocolate frosting, 2 layer, ⅙ of 7¼"-diam. cake	68	.50	m.q.	104	96	m.q.	m.q.	n.a.
Cake, snack, 1 piece:								
devil's food, w/creme filling, 1 oz. ..	21	1.00	m.q.	26	34	m.q.	m.q.	n.a.

Food and Measure	Ca mg.	Fe mg.	Mag mg.	Pho mg.	Pot mg.	Zn mg.	Cop mcg.	Man mcg.
sponge, w/creme filling, 1.5 oz.	14	.60	m.q.	44	37	m.q.	n.a.	n.a.
Cake mix[1], 1 piece:								
angel food, 1/12 of 9″-diam. tube	44	.20	m.q.	91	71	m.q.	n.a.	n.a.
coffee cake, crumb, 2.5 oz.	44	1.20	m.q.	125	78	m.q.	n.a.	n.a.
devil's food, w/chocolate frosting,								
2 layer, 2.4 oz.	41	1.40	m.q.	72	90	m.q.	n.a.	n.a.
gingerbread, 1/9 of 8″ square	57	1.20	m.q.	63	173	m.q.	n.a.	n.a.
yellow, w/chocolate frosting, 2 layer,								
2.4 oz.	63	1.00	m.q.	126	75	m.q.	n.a.	n.a.
Candy, 1 oz., except as noted:								
almond, chocolate coated	58	.80	m.q.	97	155	m.q.	m.q.	m.q.
almond, sugar coated	28	.50	m.q.	47	72	m.q.	m.q.	m.q.
(*Bar None*), 1.5-oz. bar	62	.51	31	85	166	.52	.11	.21
butterscotch	5	.40	n.a.	2	1	n.a.	n.a.	n.a.
candy corn	2	.10	n.a.	tr.	1	n.a.	n.a.	n.a.
caramel:								
plain or chocolate	42	.40	n.a.	35	54	m.q.	n.a.	n.a.
plain or chocolate, w/nuts	40	.40	n.a.	39	66	m.q.	n.a.	n.a.
chocolate coated (*Rolo*),								
1.93 oz.	73	.27	16	88	142	.38	.05	.11
(*Caramello*), 1.6-oz. bar	90	.50	19	73	m.q.	.43	.08	.07
cherry (*Y&S Nibs*)	18	.17	2	88	18	.05	.26	.04
chocolate, milk:								
plain	50	.40	16	61	96	m.q.	m.q.	n.a.
(*Hershey's*), 1.55-oz. bar	88	.48	29	136	180	.57	.18	.13
(*Hershey's Kisses*), 1.46 oz. or								
9 pieces	84	.54	27	128	170	.54	.17	.12
(*Symphony*), 1.4-oz. bar	10	.40	22	99	153	.45	.12	.07
w/almonds	65	.50	m.q.	77	125	m.q.	m.q.	m.q.
w/almonds (*Hershey's*), 1.45-oz.								
bar	108	.70	37	123	177	.66	.21	.25
w/crisps	48	.20	m.q.	57	100	m.q.	m.q.	m.q.
w/crisps (*Krackel*), 1.55-oz. bar ..	89	.31	26	105	149	.48	.18	.13
w/peanuts	49	.40	m.q.	83	138	m.q.	m.q.	m.q.
w/peanuts (*Mr. Goodbar*),								
1.75-oz. bar	55	.60	47	139	223	.89	.25	.40
chocolate, semisweet (*Hershey's*								
Special Dark), 1.45-oz. bar	8	.86	47	66	140	.62	.33	.33
chocolate chips, see "Chocolate,								
baking"								
chocolate disk, sugar coated	38	.40	m.q.	40	71	m.q.	n.a.	n.a.
chocolate flavor roll, 1 medium,								
2½″ long	5	.10	n.a.	10	10	n.a.	n.a.	n.a.
coconut, chocolate coated:								
1 oz.	14	.30	m.q.	22	47	m.q.	m.q.	m.q.
(*Mounds*), 1.9-oz. bar	12	1.13	36	65	m.q.	.55	.30	.40
w/almonds (*Almond Joy*),								
1.76-oz. bar	39	.60	33	70	m.q.	.40	.14	.28

1. *Prepared according to package directions.*

Food and Measure	Ca mg.	Fe mg.	Mag mg.	Pho mg.	Pot mg.	Zn mg.	Cop mcg.	Man mcg.
Candy *(cont.)*								
(5th Avenue), 2.1-oz. bar	42	.60	37	89	195	.64	.13	.22
fondant, mint	2	.10	n.a.	tr.	1	n.a.	n.a.	n.a.
fondant, mint, chocolate coated	16	.30	n.a.	15	26	n.a.	n.a.	n.a.
fudge:								
chocolate	22	.30	m.q.	24	42	m.q.	n.a.	n.a.
chocolate, w/nuts	22	.30	m.q.	32	50	m.q.	n.a.	n.a.
vanilla	32	.10	n.a.	24	36	n.a.	n.a.	n.a.
vanilla, w/nuts	31	.20	n.a.	32	32	n.a.	n.a.	n.a.
fudge, chocolate coated:								
chocolate	29	.40	m.q.	31	55	m.q.	n.a.	n.a.
chocolate, w/nuts	29	.40	m.q.	39	62	m.q.	n.a.	n.a.
w/caramel and peanuts	51	.40	m.q.	53	85	m.q.	m.q.	m.q.
w/peanuts and caramel	36	.30	m.q.	54	63	m.q.	m.q.	m.q.
(Golden Almond), 1.6 oz. or								
½ bar	149	.68	50	122	214	.77	.18	.38
(Golden III), 1.6 oz. or ½ bar	137	.27	30	100	206	.50	.13	.18
gum drops	2	.10	m.q.	tr.	1	n.a.	n.a.	n.a.
hard	tr.	.10	(0)	2	1	n.a.	n.a.	n.a.
honeycomb, w/peanut butter,								
chocolate coated	23	.50	m.q.	38	64	m.q.	n.a.	n.a.
jelly beans	1	.30	n.a.	1	11	n.a.	n.a.	n.a.
(Kit Kat), 1.625-oz. bar	101	.41	21	83	138	.46	.09	.14
marshmallow, all sizes	1	.50	m.q.	2	2	n.a.	n.a.	n.a.
nougat and caramel, chocolate								
coated	36	.50	m.q.	35	60	m.q.	n.a.	n.a.
peanut, chocolate coated	33	.40	m.q.	84	143	m.q.	m.q.	m.q.
peanut bar	12	.50	m.q.	77	127	m.q.	m.q.	m.q.
peanut brittle	10	.70	m.q.	27	43	m.q.	m.q.	m.q.
peanut butter, candy coated *(Reese's*								
Pieces), 1.85 oz. or 8 pieces ...	68	.79	42	121	231	.58	.07	.23
peanut butter, chocolate coated								
(Reese's Peanut Butter Cups),								
1.8 oz.	40	.56	43	122	204	.71	.20	.41
peppermint, chocolate coated *(York*								
Peppermint Pattie), 1.5 oz.	7	.64	27	40	m.q.	.33	.18	.17
raisin, chocolate coated	43	.70	m.q.	49	171	m.q.	m.q.	m.q.
(Solitaires), 1.6 oz. or ½ pkg.	163	.64	54	136	229	.83	.17	.38
toffee *(Skor)*, 1.4-oz. bar	44	.16	14	60	94	.30	.05	.06
vanilla creme, chocolate coated	36	.20	m.q.	31	50	n.a.	n.a.	n.a.
(Whatchamacallit), 1.8-oz. bar	62	.46	29	102	177	.57	.07	.22
Cantaloupe:								
½ of 5"-diam. melon	28	.57	28	45	825	.41	.11	.13
pulp, cubed, ½ cup	9	.17	9	14	247	.13	.03	.04
Carambola, trimmed, cubed,								
½ cup	3	.18	7	11	112	.08	.08	.06
Caraway seed, 1 tsp.	14	.34	5	12	28	.12	.02	.03
Cardamom, ground, 1 tsp.	8	.28	5	4	22	.15	.01	.56
Carissa, trimmed, sliced, ½ cup ..	9	.99	12	6	195	n.a.	.16	n.a.

Food and Measure	Ca mg.	Fe mg.	Mag mg.	Pho mg.	Pot mg.	Zn mg.	Cop mcg.	Man mcg.
Carob flour, 1 cup	359	3.03	56	81	852	.94	.59	.52
Carp, meat only:								
raw, 1 oz.	12	.35	8	117	94	.42	.02	n.a.
baked, broiled, or microwaved[1],								
4 oz.	59	1.80	43	602	484	2.15	.08	n.a.
Carrot, ½ cup, except as noted:								
fresh:								
raw, 7½″-long, approx. 2.5 oz. ..	19	.36	11	32	233	.14	.03	.10
raw, shredded	15	.27	8	24	178	.11	.03	.03
boiled, drained, sliced	24	.48	10	24	177	.23	.11	.59
canned, w/liquid, sliced	31	.75	11	25	213	.35	.13	.55
canned, drained, sliced	19	.47	6	17	131	.19	.08	.33
frozen, boiled, drained, sliced	21	.35	7	19	115	.18	.05	.30
Carrot juice, canned, 6 fl. oz.	44	.85	26	77	538	.33	.09	.24
Casaba, pulp, cubed, ½ cup	5	.34	7	6	179	n.a.	n.a.	n.a.
Cashew, 1 oz.:								
dry-roasted	13	1.70	74	139	160	1.59	.63	n.a.
oil-roasted	12	1.16	72	121	151	1.35	.62	.23
Cashew butter, 1 tbsp.	7	.80	41	73	87	.83	.35	n.a.
Catfish, channel, meat only, raw,								
1 oz.	11	.26	6	56	92	.17	.02	<.01
Catsup, 1 tbsp.	3	.10	3	6	72	.03	.03	.02
Cauliflower:								
fresh:								
raw, 3 flowerets, 5 oz.	16	.32	8	26	199	.10	.02	.11
raw, 1″ pieces, ½ cup	14	.29	7	23	178	.09	.02	.10
boiled, drained, 3 flowerets	14	.23	6	19	174	.13	.05	.10
boiled, drained, 1″ pieces,								
½ cup	17	.26	7	22	200	.15	.06	.11
frozen, boiled, drained, 1″ pieces,								
½ cup	15	.37	8	22	125	.12	.02	.14
Celery:								
raw, 7½″-long stalk, approx.								
1.6 oz.	16	.16	4	10	115	.05	.01	.04
raw, diced, ½ cup	24	.24	7	15	172	.08	.02	.06
boiled, drained, diced, ½ cup	32	.31	9	19	213	.10	.03	.08
Celery seed, 1 tsp.	35	.90	9	11	28	.14	.03	.15
Cereal, ready to eat, 1 oz., except								
as noted:								
amaranth:								
(*Health Valley* Flakes), ½ cup	5	.50	7	94	100	.07	n.a.	n.a.
w/bananas (*Health Valley*),								
½ cup	29	1.10	11	95	160	.10	n.a.	n.a.
w/raisins (*Health Valley Amaranth*								
Crunch), ¼ cup	20	1.40	47	150	65	.70	n.a.	n.a.

1. *Without added ingredients.*

Food and Measure	Ca mg.	Fe mg.	Mag mg.	Pho mg.	Pot mg.	Zn mg.	Cop mcg.	Man mcg.
Cereal, ready to eat *(cont.)*								
bran (see also "oat bran," "rice bran," and "wheat bran," below):								
(All Bran)	25	4.50	122	278	320	3.75	.34	n.a.
(All Bran Extra Fiber)	30	4.50	103	200	300	3.75	.26	n.a.
(Bran Buds)	20	4.50	107	248	310	3.75	.28	n.a.
(40+ Bran Flakes)	13	18.00	54	140	170	3.75	.17	n.a.
(Fruitful Bran), 1 oz. cereal w/ .3 oz. fruit	12	18.00	45	146	180	3.75	.26	n.a.
(Kellogg's Raisin Bran), 1 oz. cereal w/.4 oz. fruit	16	18.00	64	146	260	3.75	.21	n.a.
(Quaker Crunchy Bran)	23	8.66	13	38	54	3.28	.07	.39
w/apples and cinnamon *(Health Valley* 100% Natural), ¼ cup ...	13	.40	30	115	80	.41	n.a.	n.a.
w/raisins *(Health Valley* Flakes), ½ cup	19	1.40	63	174	110	1.30	n.a.	n.a.
w/raisins *(Health Valley* 100% Natural), ¼ cup	13	1.40	46	119	100	.74	n.a.	n.a.
corn:								
(Corn Pops)	2	1.80	2	8	20	1.50	.02	n.a.
(Health Valley Fruit Lites), ½ cup	3	.30	2	21	50	.01	n.a.	n.a.
(Health Valley Lites Puffed Corn), ½ cup	3	.40	0	36	35	0	n.a.	n.a.
(Kellogg's Corn Flakes)	3	4.50	8	28	35	3.75	.07	n.a.
(Kellogg's Frosted Flakes)	1	1.80	3	11	25	.19	.02	n.a.
(Nut & Honey Crunch)	4	1.80	6	16	40	.10	.04	n.a.
(Nut & Honey Crunch Biscuits) ..	11	4.50	27	90	95	1.50	.07	n.a.
(Nutri•Grain Corn)	1	.60	26	67	80	3.75	.08	n.a.
blue *(Health Valley* Corn Flakes), ½ cup	2	3.70	26	37	79	.65	n.a.	n.a.
granola, see "mixed grain and natural style," below								
mixed grain and natural style:								
(Apple Jacks)	3	4.50	8	28	30	3.75	.07	n.a.
(Apple Raisin Crisp), 1 oz. cereal w/.3 oz. fruit	10	1.80	7	59	115	1.50	.04	n.a.
(Cap'n Crunch)	6	4.81	10	30	36	2.37	.04	.19
(Cap'n Crunch's Crunchberries) ..	7	4.74	11	33	43	2.83	.01	.19
(Cap'n Crunch's Peanut Butter Crunch)	5	5.00	14	38	52	2.56	.05	.18
(Crispix)	3	1.80	7	26	30	1.50	.05	n.a.
(Crunchy Nut Oh!s)	10	5.78	14	41	46	3..02	.05	.26
(Health Valley Fiber 7 Flakes), ½ cup								
(Honey Graham Oh!s)	13	6.28	11	31	46	3.23	.04	.24
(Just Right w/Fiber Nuggets)	8	18.00	23	71	75	15.00	.06	n.a.
(King Vitaman)	6	8.10	14	40	50	.30	.04	.22

Food and Measure	Ca mg.	Fe mg.	Mag mg.	Pho mg.	Pot mg.	Zn mg.	Cop mcg.	Man mcg.
(*Müeslix* Bran), 1 oz. cereal w/ .4 oz. fruit and nuts	28	7.20	66	186	150	3.75	.19	n.a.
(*Müeslix* Five Grain), 1 oz. cereal w/.45 oz. fruit and nuts	19	4.60	42	112	180	3.87	.08	n.a.
(*Nutri•Grain* Nuggets)	10	.90	26	67	125	3.75	.03	n.a.
(*Nutrific*), 1 oz. cereal w/.5 oz. fruit and nuts	32	4.50	64	143	250	3.75	.17	n.a.
(*Product 19*)	4	18.00	12	37	45	15.00	.05	n.a.
(*Quaker* 100% Natural)	43	.79	31	101	134	.63	.12	.68
(*Special K*)	10	4.50	18	57	55	3.75	.12	n.a.
w/almonds (*Sun Country* 100% Natural Granola)	26	1.19	26	81	110	.57	.08	.76
almond date (*Health Valley Healthy Crunch*), ¼ cup	13	.70	37	70	75	.57	n.a.	n.a.
almond raisin (*Nutri•Grain*), 1 oz. cereal w/.4 oz. fruit and nuts ..	16	.80	11	77	130	3.75	.03	n.a.
apple cinnamon (*Health Valley Healthy Crunch*), ¼ cup	14	.60	31	70	70	.52	n.a.	n.a.
apple and cinnamon (*Quaker* 100% Natural)	34	1.00	30	71	143	.59	.12	.69
w/bananas and Hawaiian fruit (*Health Valley Sprouts 7*), ¼ cup	15	1.10	10	86	130	.08	n.a.	n.a.
fruit and nut (*Just Right*), 1 oz. cereal w/.3 oz. fruit and nuts ..	16	18.00	26	73	120	15.00	.07	n.a.
w/raisins (*Health Valley Sprouts 7*), ¼ cup	13	1.40	8	85	170	.09	n.a.	n.a.
w/raisins (*Sun Country* Granola)	25	1.15	24	79	114	.48	.09	.66
raisin and date (*Quaker* 100% Natural)	40	.83	29	99	145	.57	.11	.67
w/raisins and dates (*Sun Country* 100% Natural Granola)	23	1.07	24	72	121	.45	.08	.66
oat (*Life*)	93	8.10	46	162	171	.84	.17	1.03
oat, cinnamon (*Life*)	89	8.10	47	159	167	1.07	.16	1.30
oat bran:								
(*Common Sense*)	14	4.50	40	126	115	.15	.15	n.a.
(*Cracklin' Oat Bran*)	15	1.80	59	166	160	1.50	.19	n.a.
(*Health Valley* Flakes), ½ cup	11	1.00	47	142	85	.71	n.a.	n.a.
(*Oat Bran O's*), ¾ cup	12	1.80	25	88	110	.69	n.a.	n.a.
almond crunch (*Real*), ¼ cup	14	1.10	53	154	82	.91	n.a.	n.a.
w/almonds and dates (*Health Valley* Flakes), ½ cup	20	1.10	40	150	100	.60	n.a.	n.a.
fruit, Hawaiian (*Real*), ¼ cup	26	1.40	58	156	237	.95	n.a.	n.a.
fruit and nut (*Oat Bran O's*), ¾ cup	21	.50	36	111	110	.65	n.a.	n.a.
w/raisins (*Common Sense*), 1 oz. cereal w/.3 oz. fruit	18	4.50	40	129	170	3.75	.17	n.a.
w/raisins (*Health Valley* Flakes), ½ cup	17	1.30	43	130	100	.65	n.a.	n.a.

Food and Measure	Ca mg.	Fe mg.	Mag mg.	Pho mg.	Pot mg.	Zn mg.	Cop mcg.	Man mcg.
Cereal, ready to eat, oat bran *(cont.)*								
raisin nut *(Real)*, ¼ cup	14	1.20	54	159	82	.93	n.a.	n.a.
rice:								
(Cocoa Krispies)	6	1.80	11	30	45	1.50	.06	n.a.
(Frosted Krispies)	2	1.80	7	23	25	.28	.02	n.a.
(Health Valley Fruit Lites), ½ cup	5	.20	2	22	65	.02	n.a.	n.a.
(Health Valley Lites Puffed Rice),								
½ cup	5	.30	0	31	45	0	n.a.	n.a.
(Quaker Puffed Rice), .5 oz.	1	.35	4	17	18	.16	.13	.13
(Rice Krispies)	3	1.80	11	34	35	.38	.05	n.a.
rice bran *(Rice Bran O's)*, ¾ cup ...	11	1.60	43	93	183	.35	n.a.	n.a.
rice bran, w/almonds and dates								
(Health Valley), ½ cup	17	.90	49	122	85	.01	n.a.	n.a.
wheat:								
(Apple Cinnamon Squares)	11	8.10	25	79	85	3.75	.07	n.a.
(Blueberry Squares)	10	8.10	27	86	85	1.50	.06	n.a.
(Frosted Mini Wheats)	10	1.80	29	82	80	1.50	.10	n.a.
(Frosted Mini Wheats Bite Size) ..	9	1.80	27	76	100	1.50	.12	n.a.
(Health Valley Fruit Lites), ½ cup	6	.50	12	35	90	.17	n.a.	n.a.
(Health Valley Lites Puffed Wheat),								
½ cup	7	.70	16	50	75	.24	n.a.	n.a.
(Honey Smacks)	3	1.80	14	35	40	.31	.05	n.a.
(Nutri•Grain Biscuits)	13	1.20	42	103	115	3.75	.14	n.a.
(Nutri•Grain Wheat)	9	.70	30	92	90	3.75	.12	n.a.
(Nutri•Grain Wheat & Raisins),								
1 oz. cereal w/.4 oz. fruit	15	1.00	31	99	170	3.75	.13	n.a.
(Quaker Puffed Wheat), .5 oz. ...	3	.63	19	47	53	.44	.09	.28
(Quaker Shredded Wheat),								
2 biscuits	16	1.03	67	131	147	1.00	.20	1.22
(Raisin Squares)	10	8.10	25	82	110	1.50	.06	n.a.
(S.W. Graham)	11	.80	22	62	90	1.50	.10	n.a.
(S.W. Graham Cinnamon)	10	.70	18	52	80	1.50	.08	n.a.
(Strawberry Squares)	11	8.10	28	87	90	1.50	.07	n.a.
wheat bran, toasted *(Kretschmer)* ..	26	3.63	180	376	399	3.18	.31	4.93
Cereal, cooking, uncooked, 1 pkt.,								
except as noted:								
corn grits, yellow or white, enriched,								
regular or quick, 1 oz.	1	1.11	8	21	39	.12	.02	.03
oat and oatmeal:								
(Instant Quaker)	170	8.35	39	140	103	.88	.14	1.20
(Quaker Quick/Old Fashioned),								
⅓ cup or ⅔ cup cooked	15	1.08	38	130	109	.87	.09	1.22
(Quaker Extra)	222	18.00	n.a.	124	104	15.00	n.a.	n.a.
apple and cinnamon *(Instant*								
Quaker)	168	5.89	39	102	108	.66	.13	.01
apples and spice *(Quaker Extra)*	220	18.00	n.a.	118	116	15.00	n.a.	n.a.
cinnamon and spice *(Instant*								
Quaker)	178	8.08	40	143	117	.84	.13	1.10

Food and Measure	Ca mg.	Fe mg.	Mag mg.	Pho mg.	Pot mg.	Zn mg.	Cop mcg.	Man mcg.
maple and brown sugar (*Instant Quaker*)	170	8.35	42	149	116	.85	.14	1.15
peaches and cream (*Instant Quaker*)	146	5.71	35	123	140	.67	.11	.87
raisin, date, and walnut (*Instant Quaker*)	134	5.33	39	126	127	.77	.15	.96
raisins and cinnamon (*Quaker Extra*)	278	18.00	n.a.	111	139	15.00	n.a.	n.a.
raisins and spice (*Instant Quaker*)	165	6.23	39	135	152	.91	.15	1.20
strawberries and cream (*Instant Quaker*)	157	5.48	35	121	140	.67	.11	.99
oat bran (*Quaker/Mother's*), ⅓ cup or ⅔ cup cooked	22	1.84	69	212	169	1.19	.08	1.56
wheat, farina, enriched, 1 oz.	4	1.05	4	25	26	.15	.02	n.a.
wheat, whole (*Quaker/Mother's Natural*), ⅓ cup or ⅔ cup cooked	10	.96	31	99	125	.73	.12	.70
Chayote:								
raw, 1 medium, approx. 7.2 oz.	39	.81	28	53	305	n.a.	n.a.	n.a.
boiled, drained, 1″ pieces, ½ cup ...	10	.18	9	23	138	n.a.	n.a.	n.a.
Cheese, 1 oz., except as noted:								
American, pasturized process	174	.11	6	211	46	.85	.01	<.01
blue	150	.09	7	110	73	.75	.01	<.01
brick	191	.12	7	128	38	.74	.01	<.01
Brie	52	.14	m.q.	53	43	m.q.	.01	.01
Camembert	110	.09	6	98	53	.68	.01	.01
cheddar	204	.19	8	145	28	.88	.01	<.01
colby	194	.22	7	129	36	.87	.01	<.01
cottage, ½ cup not packed:								
creamed, large curd	68	.16	6	149	95	.42	.03	<.01
creamed, small curd	63	.15	5	139	88	.39	.03	<.01
creamed, w/fruit	54	.12	5	118	76	.33	.03	<.01
dry curd	23	.17	3	75	23	.34	.02	<.01
lowfat 2%	77	.18	7	170	109	.48	.03	<.01
lowfat 1%	69	.16	6	151	97	.43	.03	<.01
cream	23	.34	2	30	34	.15	.01	<.01
Edam	207	.12	8	152	53	1.06	.01	<.01
feta	140	.18	5	96	18	.82	.01	.01
fontina	156	.06	4	m.q.	m.q.	.99	.01	<.01
Gouda	198	.07	8	155	34	1.11	.01	<.01
Gruyère	287	m.q.	m.q.	172	23	n.a.	.01	.01
Limburger	141	.04	6	111	36	.60	.01	.01
mozzarella:								
whole milk	147	.05	5	105	19	.63	.01	<.01
low-moisture	163	.06	6	117	21	.70	.01	<.01
part skim	183	.06	7	131	24	.78	.01	<.01
part skim, low-moisture	207	.07	7	149	27	.89	.01	<.01
Muenster	203	.12	8	133	38	.80	.01	<.01

Food and Measure	Ca mg.	Fe mg.	Mag mg.	Pho mg.	Pot mg.	Zn mg.	Cop mcg.	Man mcg.
Cheese *(cont.)*								
Neufchâtel	21	.08	2	39	32	.15	<.01	<.01
Parmesan:								
grated	390	.27	14	229	30	.90	.01	.01
grated, 1 tbsp.	69	.05	3	40	5	.16	<.01	<.01
hard	336	.23	12	197	26	.78	.01	.01
pimiento, pasturized process	174	.12	6	211	46	.84	.01	<.01
provolone	214	.15	8	141	39	.92	.01	<.01
ricotta, whole milk, ½ cup	257	.47	14	196	130	1.40	.03	.01
ricotta, part skim, ½ cup	337	.55	18	226	155	1.70	.04	.01
Roquefort	188	.16	8	111	26	.59	.01	.01
Swiss	272	.05	10	171	31	1.11	.01	<.01
Swiss, pasturized process	219	.17	8	216	61	1.02	.01	<.01
Tilsit, whole milk	198	.06	4	142	18	.99	.01	<.01
Cheese food, 1 oz.:								
American, cold pack	141	.24	8	113	103	.85	.01	<.01
American, pasturized process	163	.24	9	130	79	.85	.01	<.01
Swiss, pasturized process	205	.17	8	149	81	1.01	.01	<.01
Cheese sauce mix, ½ cup[1]	285	.14	24	219	277	.49	n.a.	n.a.
Cheese spread, American,								
pasturized process, 1 oz.	159	.09	8	202	69	.73	.01	.01
Cheese stick or straw, 5″ long,								
10 pieces or 2.1 oz.	155	.40	n.a.	124	38	n.a.	n.a.	n.a.
Cherry, ½ cup, except as noted:								
fresh:								
sour, red, w/pits	8	.17	5	8	89	.05	.05	.06
sour, red, w/out pits	12	.25	7	12	134	.08	.08	.09
sweet, 10 medium, approx.								
2.6 oz.	10	.26	8	13	152	.04	.07	.06
sweet, trimmed, w/out pits	11	.28	8	14	163	.05	.07	.07
canned, sour, red:								
in water	13	1.67	7	12	120	.08	.09	.09
in light syrup	13	1.66	7	12	119	.08	.09	.09
in heavy syrup	13	1.66	7	12	119	.08	.08	.09
canned, sweet:								
in water	13	.45	11	19	162	.09	.09	.08
in juice	17	.73	16	27	163	.12	.09	.08
in light syrup	12	.45	11	23	186	.13	.18	.08
in heavy syrup	12	.46	11	23	187	.13	.18	.08
frozen, sour, red, unsweetened	10	.41	7	13	96	.08	.07	.04
frozen, sweet, sweetened	16	.45	13	21	257	.05	.03	.14
Chestnut, Chinese, shelled, 1 oz.:								
raw	5	.40	24	27	127	.25	.10	.46
roasted	5	.43	26	29	135	.26	.11	m.q.
Chestnut, European, shelled,								
1 oz.:								
raw, unpeeled	8	.29	9	26	147	.15	.13	.27
dried, unpeeled	19	.68	21	50	280	.10	.19	.37
roasted	8	.26	9	30	168	.16	.14	.34

1. *Prepared according to package directions, with whole milk.*

Food and Measure	Ca mg.	Fe mg.	Mag mg.	Pho mg.	Pot mg.	Zn mg.	Cop mcg.	Man mcg.
Chestnut, Japanese, shelled, 1 oz.:								
raw	9	.41	14	21	94	.31	.16	.45
boiled or steamed	3	.15	5	7	34	.11	.06	.16
dried	20	.96	33	48	218	.73	.37	1.05
roasted	10	.60	18	26	m.q.	.41	.21	.59
Chicken[1], fresh, 4 oz., except as noted:								
broiler-fryer, fried, flour coated, meat w/skin:								
4 oz.	19	1.56	28	217	265	2.31	.09	.04
dark meat	19	1.70	27	200	261	2.95	.10	.04
light meat	18	1.37	31	242	271	1.43	.07	.03
back	27	1.84	26	188	256	2.80	.10	.06
breast	18	1.35	34	264	294	1.25	.06	.03
drumstick, 1.7 oz. (2.6-oz. raw drumstick w/bone)	6	.66	11	86	112	1.42	.04	.01
leg, 4 oz. (5.5-oz. raw leg w/bone)	15	1.60	27	204	261	3.00	.10	.04
thigh, 2.2 oz. (2.9-oz. raw thigh w/bone)	8	.93	5	116	147	1.56	.06	.02
wing, 1.1 oz. (2.2-oz. raw wing w/bone)	5	.40	6	48	57	.56	.02	.01
broiler-fryer, roasted:								
meat w/skin	17	1.43	26	206	253	2.20	.07	.02
meat only	17	1.37	28	221	276	2.38	.08	.02
skin only, 1 oz.	4	.43	4	35	39	.35	.02	.01
dark meat w/skin	17	1.54	25	191	249	2.82	.09	.02
dark meat only	17	1.51	26	203	272	3.18	.09	.02
light meat w/skin	17	1.29	28	227	257	1.39	.06	.02
light meat only	17	1.20	31	245	280	1.39	.06	.02
roaster, roasted:								
meat w/skin	14	1.43	23	203	239	1.64	.07	.02
meat only	14	1.37	24	218	260	1.72	.06	.02
dark meat only	12	1.51	23	194	254	2.42	.08	.02
light meat only	15	1.22	26	246	268	.88	.05	.02
stewing, stewed:								
meat w/skin	15	1.55	23	204	206	2.01	.11	.02
meat only	15	1.62	25	231	229	2.34	.13	.02
dark meat only	14	1.86	25	212	231	3.54	.16	.03
light meat only	16	1.35	26	255	226	.94	.10	.02
capon, roasted, meat w/skin	16	1.69	27	279	289	1.97	.08	.02
Chicken, boneless and luncheon meat:								
breast, oven-roasted (*Oscar Mayer*), 1 oz.	2	.23	5	89	80	.13	m.q.	m.q.
breast, smoked (*Oscar Mayer*), 1 oz.	2	.18	5	80	79	.12	m.q.	m.q.
roll, light meat, 1 oz.	12	.28	5	45	65	.21	.01	m.q.

1. *Prepared without added ingredients, except as noted.*

Food and Measure	Ca mg.	Fe mg.	Mag mg.	Pho mg.	Pot mg.	Zn mg.	Cop mcg.	Man mcg.
Chicken giblets, broiler-fryer, simmered[1], 4 oz.	14	7.30	23	260	179	5.18	.29	.19
Chicken gizzard, broiler-fryer, simmered[1], 4 oz.	11	4.71	23	176	203	4.97	.12	.07
Chicken gravy, canned, ¼ cup ...	12	.28	n.a.	17	65	.48	.06	.12
Chicken heart, see "Heart"								
Chicken liver, see "Liver"								
Chick-pea, ½ cup:								
boiled	40	2.37	39	137	239	1.25	.29	.85
canned, w/liquid	39	1.62	35	108	206	1.27	.21	.73
Chicory, witloof, raw, 5–7″ head, approx. 2.1 oz.	n.a.	.26	7	11	96	n.a.	n.a.	n.a.
Chicory greens, raw, chopped, ½ cup	90	.81	27	42	378	n.a.	n.a.	n.a.
Chicory root, raw, 1″ pieces, ½ cup	18	.36	10	27	131	n.a.	n.a.	n.a.
Chili, canned:								
w/beans:								
(*Wolf* Brand), 1 cup	59	2.54	57	252	633	2.00	.23	0
extra spicy (*Wolf* Brand), scant cup	55	2.38	53	236	593	2.00	.22	0
vegetarian, mild (*Health Valley*), 4 oz.	3	1.60	98	59	410	.32	n.a.	n.a.
vegetarian, spicy (*Health Valley*), 4 oz.	3	1.60	82	52	460	.30	n.a.	n.a.
w/out beans (*Wolf* Brand), 1 cup ...	64	3.86	30	146	717	2.00	.13	0
w/out beans, extra spicy (*Wolf* Brand), scant cup	60	3.62	28	137	672	2.00	.12	0
w/lentils, vegetarian, mild (*Health Valley*), 7½ oz.	40	1.10	37	43	390	.24	n.a.	n.a.
w/macaroni (*Wolf* Brand Chili Mac), scant cup	28	1.87	28	136	337	2.00	.17	0
Chili powder, 1 tsp.	7	.37	4	8	50	.07	.01	.06
Chili sauce, hot dog (*Wolf* Brand), approx. ⅙ cup	16	.57	15	41	102	0	.07	0
Chitterlings, pork, simmered[1], 4 oz.	31	4.20	11	53	9	5.74	.26	n.a.
Chives, raw, chopped, 1 tbsp.	2	.05	2	2	8	n.a.	n.a.	n.a.
Chocolate, baking:								
chips, semi-sweet, ¼ cup	13	1.45	m.q.	45	148	n.a.	n.a.	n.a.
unsweetened, 1 oz.	22	1.90	83	109	235	n.a.	m.q.	n.a.
Chocolate flavor drink mix, powder:								
2–3 heaping tsp. or ¾ oz.	8	.68	21	28	128	.33	.15	.15
(*Carnation* Instant Breakfast), 1 pkt.	150	4.50	80	150	410	3.00	.50	n.a.
malt (*Carnation* Instant Breakfast), 1 pkt.	80	4.50	80	100	260	3.00	.50	n.a.

1. *Without added ingredients.*

Food and Measure	Ca mg.	Fe mg.	Mag mg.	Pho mg.	Pot mg.	Zn mg.	Cop mcg.	Man mcg.
Chocolate milk, 1 cup:								
whole	280	.60	33	251	417	1.02	.16	.19
lowfat 2%	284	.60	33	254	422	1.02	.16	.19
lowfat 1%	287	.60	33	256	426	1.02	.16	.19
Chocolate syrup, w/out added								
nutrients, 2 tbsp. or 1 fl. oz. ..	5	.79	24	48	84	.27	.19	.14
Cinnamon, ground, 1 tsp.	28	.88	1	1	11	.05	.01	.38
Cisco, smoked, 4 oz.	2	.05	2	14	27	.03	.02	<.01
Citrus fruit juice drink, frozen[1],								
6 fl. oz.	17	2.08	11	19	208	.09	.06	.14
Clam, mixed species, meat only:								
raw, 1 oz.	13	3.96	3	48	89	.39	.10	.14
raw, 9 large or 20 small, approx.								
6.3 oz.	83	25.16	17	304	565	2.46	.62	.90
boiled or steamed[2], 4 oz.	104	31.71	20	383	712	3.10	.78	n.a.
boiled or steamed[2], 20 small	83	25.16	17	304	565	2.46	.62	n.a.
Clam, canned, drained, 4 oz.	104	31.71	20	383	712	3.10	.78	n.a.
Clove, ground, 1 tsp.	14	.18	6	2	23	.02	.01	.63
Cocoa mix:								
w/out added nutrients, 1-oz. pkt. or								
3–4 heaping tsp.	93	.34	24	89	202	.41	.08	.08
w/added nutrients, 1.1-oz. pkt.	100	1.80	22	111	404	.22	.10	.09
(*Carnation* 70 Calorie), 1 pkt.	97	.43	20	82	220	.30	.01	n.a.
chocolate:								
fudge (*Carnation*), 1 pkt.	44	.63	20	66	260	.27	.24	n.a.
milk (*Carnation*), 1 pkt. or								
4 heaping tsp.	76	.43	20	90	260	.36	.15	n.a.
rich (*Carnation*), 1 pkt. or								
4 heaping tsp.	60	.45	20	84	260	.30	.15	tr.
w/marshmallows (*Carnation*), 1 pkt.	57	.45	19	80	240	.28	.15	tr.
Coconut, meat:								
raw, 1 piece, 2″ × 2″ × ½″, approx.								
1.6 oz.	6	1.09	14	51	160	.57	.23	.78
dried, unsweetened, 1 oz.	7	.94	26	59	154	.52	.09	.13
dried, sweetened, shredded, 1 oz.	4	.54	14	30	96	.68	.43	.57
Cod, Atlantic, meat only:								
raw, 1 oz.	4	.11	9	58	117	.13	.01	<.01
baked, broiled, or microwaved[2],								
4 oz.	16	.56	48	156	277	.66	.04	n.a.
dried, salted, 1 oz.	45	.70	37	266	408	.44	.05	n.a.
Cod, canned, w/liquid, 4 oz.	24	.56	46	295	599	.66	.04	n.a.
Coffee, brewed, 6 fl. oz.	3	.08	10	2	96	.03	.01	.05
Coffee, flavored, instant, 6 fl. oz.[3]:								
cappuccino flavor	7	.15	9	26	119	.08	.03	.03
mocha flavor[4]	7	.24	9	29	119	.15	.06	.05

1. *Diluted according to package directions.*
2. *Without added ingredients.*
3. *Prepared according to package directions.*
4. *With added calcium.*

Food and Measure	Ca mg.	Fe mg.	Mag mg.	Pho mg.	Pot mg.	Zn mg.	Cop mcg.	Man mcg.
Coffee, substitute, cereal grain								
beverage, 1 tsp. dry	1	.11	6	13	42	.01	.01	.03
Coffee flavor drink mix								
(*Carnation* Instant Breakfast),								
1 pkt.	150	4.50	80	150	340	3.00	.50	n.a.
Coffee liqueur, 1 fl. oz.	tr.	.02	1	2	10	.01	.01	n.a.
Coffee with cream liqueur,								
1 fl. oz.	5	.04	1	15	10	.05	.01	n.a.
Collards, ½ cup:								
fresh, raw, chopped	5	.03	2	2	30	.02	.01	.05
fresh, boiled, drained, chopped	15	.10	5	5	84	.07	.02	.15
frozen, boiled, drained, chopped ...	179	.95	26	23	214	.23	.05	.56
Cookie:								
almond date (*Health Valley Fruit*								
Jumbos), 1 piece	8	.40	11	36	40	.19	m.q.	m.q.
amaranth (*Health Valley Amaranth*								
Cookies), 1 piece	20	.40	11	42	40	.19	n.a.	n.a.
animal cracker, 10 pieces or .9 oz.	14	.10	n.a.	30	25	n.a.	n.a.	n.a.
animal cracker, oat bran (*Health*								
Valley), 7 pieces	13	.80	26	79	125	.50	n.a.	n.a.
apricot almond (*Health Valley Fancy*								
Fruit Chunks), 2 pieces	17	.70	20	57	135	.40	m.q.	m.q.
butter, thin, rich, 10 pieces or								
1.8 oz.	63	.30	n.a.	47	30	n.a.	n.a.	n.a.
chocolate chip, 4 pieces or 1.5 oz. ..	13	.80	m.q.	41	68	m.q.	n.a.	n.a.
chocolate sandwich, 4 pieces or								
1.4 oz.	12	1.40	m.q.	40	66	n.a.	n.a.	n.a.
coconut bar, 10 pieces or 3.2 oz. ...	65	1.30	m.q.	108	205	m.q.	m.q.	m.q.
date pecan (*Health Valley Fancy Fruit*								
Chunks), 2 pieces	21	.70	17	51	135	.40	m.q.	m.q.
fig bar, 4 pieces or 2 oz.	40	1.40	m.q.	34	162	m.q.	m.q.	m.q.
fruit:								
(*Fruit & Fitness*), 5 pieces	23	1.00	m.q.	111	193	m.q.	n.a.	n.a.
tropical (*Health Valley Fancy Fruit*								
Chunks), 2 pieces	16	.50	21	51	140	.40	n.a.	n.a.
tropical (*Health Valley Fruit*								
Jumbos), 1 piece	10	.40	11	42	63	.18	n.a.	n.a.
gingersnap, 10 pieces or 2.5 oz. ...	51	1.60	n.a.	33	323	n.a.	n.a.	n.a.
graham cracker:								
plain, 1 square piece	6	.40	7	20	36	m.q.	m.q.	n.a.
amaranth (*Health Valley Amaranth*								
Graham Crackers), 7 pieces ...	31	1.70	29	94	85	.48	n.a.	n.a.
chocolate coated, .5-oz. piece ...	15	.30	m.q.	27	42	m.q.	m.q.	n.a.
honey, fancy (*Health Valley*),								
7 pieces	5	.80	25	74	60	.68	n.a.	n.a.
oat bran (*Health Valley*), 7 pieces	18	1.20	30	102	84	.70	n.a.	n.a.
sugar honey, 2 square pieces	12	.20	m.q.	47	38	m.q.	m.q.	n.a.

Food and Measure	Ca mg.	Fe mg.	Mag mg.	Pho mg.	Pot mg.	Zn mg.	Cop mcg.	Man mcg.
honey:								
cinnamon (*Health Valley Honey Jumbos*), 1 piece	20	.70	9	36	40	.18	n.a.	n.a.
oat bran (*Health Valley Honey Jumbos*), 1 piece	8	.36	22	96	25	.16	n.a.	n.a.
peanut butter, crisp (*Health Valley Honey Jumbos*), 1 piece	5	.22	11	40	42	.20	m.q.	m.q.
ladyfinger, 4 pieces or 1.6 oz.	18	.70	m.q.	72	31	m.q.	n.a.	n.a.
macaroon, 2 pieces or 1.3 oz.	10	.30	m.q.	32	176	m.q.	m.q.	m.q.
molasses, 1 piece or 1.1 oz.	17	.70	m.q.	27	45	n.a.	m.q.	n.a.
oat bran (*Health Valley Fruit Jumbos*), 1 piece	6	.72	10	39	35	.23	n.a.	n.a.
oat bran, fruit and nut (*Health Valley*), 2 pieces	23	.80	32	84	150	.60	m.q.	m.q.
oatmeal raisin, 4 pieces or 1.8 oz.	18	1.10	m.q.	58	90	m.q.	m.q.	m.q.
peanut (*Health Valley Fancy Peanut Chunks*), 2 pieces	12	.68	20	56	93	.40	m.q.	m.q.
raisin nut (*Health Valley Fruit Jumbos*), 1 piece	8	.40	11	36	45	.19	m.q.	m.q.
raisin oat bran (*Health Valley Fancy Fruit Chunks*), 2 pieces	16	.60	17	51	120	.30	m.q.	m.q.
shortbread, 4 small or 1.1 oz.	13	.80	m.q.	39	38	m.q.	n.a.	n.a.
tofu (*The Great Tofu Cookie*), 2 pieces	9	1.80	3	18	24	.02	n.a.	n.a.
vanilla sandwich, 4 pieces or 1.4 oz.	12	1.40	n.a.	40	66	m.q.	n.a.	n.a.
vanilla wafer, 10 pieces or 1.4 oz.	16	.80	m.q.	36	50	n.a.	n.a.	n.a.
vanilla wafer, brown-edge, 10 pieces or 2 oz.	24	.20	n.a.	37	42	n.a.	n.a.	n.a.
wheat-free (*The Great Wheat Free Cookie*), 4 pieces	36	3.50	4	21	35	.03	n.a.	n.a.
Cookie, refrigerated:								
chocolate chip, 4 pieces or 1.7 oz.	13	1.00	m.q.	34	62	m.q.	n.a.	n.a.
sugar, 4 pieces or 1.7 oz.	50	.90	m.q.	91	33	m.q.	m.q.	n.a.
Coriander:								
fresh, raw, 9 plants, approx. .8 oz.	20	.39	5	7	108	n.a.	m.q.	m.q.
dried, leaf, 1 tsp.	7	.25	4	3	27	n.a.	.01	.04
Coriander seed, 1 tsp.	13	.29	6	7	23	.08	.02	.03
Corn, sweet, ½ cup, except as noted:								
fresh:								
raw, 3.2-oz. ear	2	.46	34	80	243	.41	.05	.15
boiled, drained, 3.2-oz. ear	2	.47	24	79	192	.37	.04	.15
boiled, drained	2	.50	26	84	204	.39	.04	.16
canned:								
w/liquid	5	.44	20	65	196	.46	.07	.04
cream style	4	.49	22	65	172	.68	.07	.05
vacuum pack	5	.44	24	67	195	.48	.05	.07
frozen, boiled, 4-oz. ear	2	.39	18	47	158	.40	.03	.09
frozen, boiled, drained	2	.25	15	39	114	.28	.03	.15
Corn, whole grain, 1 cup	12	4.50	211	349	476	3.66	.52	.81
Corn bran, crude, 1 cup	32	2.12	48	55	33	1.18	.19	.11

Food and Measure	Ca mg.	Fe mg.	Mag mg.	Pho mg.	Pot mg.	Zn mg.	Cop mcg.	Man mcg.
Corn chips and similar snacks, 1 oz.:								
(*Health Valley*)	6	.33	32	49	30	.44	n.a.	n.a.
(*Health Valley* No Salt Added)	4	.33	22	49	30	.44	n.a.	n.a.
w/cheddar (*Health Valley*)	18	.35	22	57	60	.44	n.a.	n.a.
tortilla (*Buenitos*)	6	.38	32	55	70	.44	n.a.	n.a.
tortilla (*Buenitos* No Salt Added) ...	4	.38	22	55	70	.44	n.a.	n.a.
Corn flour, 1 cup:								
whole grain	8	2.78	109	318	369	2.02	.27	.54
masa, enriched	161	8.22	125	255	340	2.03	.19	.55
Corn grits, enriched, cooked, 1 cup	1	1.55	11	29	54	.17	.03	.04
Cornbread, see "Bread, sweet, mix"								
Cornmeal, 1 cup:								
whole grain	7	4.21	155	294	350	2.21	.24	.61
degermed, enriched	7	5.70	56	116	224	.99	.11	.14
self-rising, enriched[1]:								
bolted	440	7.03	105	981	331	2.44	.18	n.a.
bolted, w/wheat flour	508	8.41	91	1106	352	2.36	.24	n.a.
degermed	482	6.53	68	859	235	1.38	.18	n.a.
Cornstarch, 1 cup	2	.61	3	16	4	.08	.06	.07
Cottonseed flour, lowfat, 1 oz. ...	135	3.57	203	451	500	3.30	.33	n.a.
Couscous, cooked, 1 cup	15	.69	15	39	104	.46	.07	.15
Cowpea, ½ cup:								
fresh, raw	90	.79	37	38	311	.73	.09	.40
fresh, boiled, drained	105	.92	42	42	342	.85	.11	.47
frozen, boiled, drained	20	1.80	42	104	319	1.21	.16	.67
Cowpea, dried, ½ cup:								
boiled	21	2.16	46	134	239	1.11	.23	.41
canned, w/liquid	24	1.17	33	83	206	.84	.14	.34
canned, w/pork	21	1.71	52	116	213	1.24	.20	.47
Crab, meat only:								
Alaska king, raw, 1 oz.	13	.17	m.q.	62	58	1.68	.26	.01
blue, raw, 1 oz.	25	.21	10	65	93	1.00	.19	.04
blue, boiled or steamed[2], 4 oz.	118	1.03	37	234	367	4.79	.73	n.a.
dungeness, raw, 1 oz.	13	.10	13	52	100	1.21	.19	.02
Crab, canned, blue, 4 oz.	115	.95	44	295	424	4.56	.86	n.a.
Crabapple, w/skin, sliced, ½ cup	10	.20	4	9	107	n.a.	.04	.06
Cracker:								
butter, 10 round or 1.2 oz.	49	.20	n.a.	86	37	n.a.	n.a.	n.a.
cheese, plain, 1″ square, 10 pieces	11	.30	m.q.	17	17	m.q.	n.a.	n.a.
cheese-peanut butter sandwich, .3-oz. piece	7	.30	m.q.	25	17	m.q.	n.a.	n.a.

1. *With added nutrients.*
2. *Without added ingredients.*

Food and Measure	Ca mg.	Fe mg.	Mag mg.	Pho mg.	Pot mg.	Zn mg.	Cop mcg.	Man mcg.
graham, see "Cookie"								
melba toast, plain, .2-oz. piece	6	.10	n.a.	10	11	n.a.	n.a.	n.a.
rice bran (*Health Valley*), 7 pieces ..	22	1.60	31	108	190	.25	n.a.	n.a.
rye wafer, whole grain, 2 pieces or								
.5 oz.	7	.50	m.q.	44	65	m.q.	n.a.	n.a.
saltine, 10 pieces or 1 oz.	6	.30	m.q.	26	34	m.q.	n.a.	n.a.
snack type, 1 round or .1 oz.	3	.10	n.a.	6	4	n.a.	n.a.	n.a.
soda biscuit, 10 pieces or 1.8 oz. ...	11	.80	m.q.	45	60	n.a.	m.q.	n.a.
soup or oyster, 10 pieces	2	.10	m.q.	7	9	n.a.	n.a.	n.a.
wheat:								
(*Health Valley* Stoned Wheat),								
13 pieces	14	1.10	44	87	95	.52	m.q.	n.a.
(*Health Valley* Stoned Wheat No								
Salt Added), 13 pieces	9	1.10	26	85	40	.52	m.q.	n.a.
herb (*Health Valley* Stoned Wheat),								
13 pieces	3	.90	44	85	100	.52	m.q.	n.a.
herb (*Health Valley* Stoned Wheat								
No Salt Added), 13 pieces	3	1.10	26	87	35	.52	m.q.	n.a.
sesame (*Health Valley* Stoned								
Wheat), 13 pieces	2	1.20	48	90	80	.62	m.q.	n.a.
sesame (*Health Valley* Stoned								
Wheat No Salt Added),								
13 pieces	2	1.20	31	91	75	.62	m.q.	n.a.
thin, 4 pieces or .3 oz.	3	.30	m.q.	15	17	m.q.	m.q.	n.a.
vegetable, seven grain (*Health								
Valley* Stoned Wheat), 13 pieces	17	.70	37	95	65	.57	m.q.	n.a.
vegetable, seven grain (*Health								
Valley* Stoned Wheat No Salt								
Added), 13 pieces	2	1.10	37	95	50	.57	m.q.	n.a.
whole, 2 pieces or .3 oz.	3	.20	m.q.	22	31	m.q.	m.q.	n.a.
Cranberry, fresh, ½ cup:								
whole	4	.10	3	4	34	.06	.03	.07
chopped	4	.11	3	5	39	.07	.03	.09
Cranberry bean, boiled, ½ cup ..	44	1.84	44	119	340	1.00	.20	.33
Cranberry juice cocktail,								
6 fl. oz.:								
bottled	7	.28	4	4	34	.14	.03	.37
frozen[1]	9	.17	4	3	27	.07	.02	.08
Cranberry sauce, canned,								
sweetened, ½ cup	5	.30	4	8	35	.07	.03	.08
Cranberry-apple juice drink,								
bottled, 6 fl. oz.	13	.11	3	5	50	.08	.01	n.a.
Cranberry-apricot juice drink,								
bottled, 6 fl. oz.	17	.28	6	10	113	.07	.03	n.a.
Cranberry-grape juice drink,								
bottled, 6 fl. oz.	15	.02	6	7	44	.07	.01	n.a.
Cranberry-orange relish, canned,								
½ cup	15	.28	6	11	53	m.q.	.06	n.a.

1. *Diluted according to package directions.*

Food and Measure	Ca mg.	Fe mg.	Mag mg.	Pho mg.	Pot mg.	Zn mg.	Cop mcg.	Man mcg.
Crayfish, mixed species, meat only:								
raw, 1 oz.	7	.69	7	73	78	.37	.12	n.a.
boiled or steamed[1], 4 oz.	34	3.56	35	374	398	1.91	.63	n.a.
Cream:								
half and half, 1 cup	254	.17	25	230	314	1.23	.02	<.01
half and half, 1 tbsp.	16	.01	2	14	19	.08	<.01	tr.
light, coffee or table, 1 cup	231	.10	21	192	292	.65	.02	<.01
light, coffee or table, 1 tbsp.	14	.01	1	12	18	.04	<.01	tr.
medium (25% fat), 1 cup	216	.10	20	169	274	.62	.02	<.01
medium (25% fat), 1 tbsp.	14	.01	1	11	17	.04	<.01	tr.
whipping:								
light, 1 cup, approx. 2 cups								
whipped	166	.07	17	146	231	.60	.02	<.01
light, 1 tbsp.	10	tr.	1	9	15	.04	<.01	tr.
heavy, 1 cup, approx. 2 cups								
whipped	154	.07	17	149	179	.55	.01	<.01
heavy, 1 tbsp.	10	tr.	1	9	11	.03	tr.	tr.
whipped topping, pressurized, 1 cup	61	.03	6	54	88	.22	.06	tr.
whipped topping, pressurized,								
1 tbsp.	3	tr.	tr.	3	4	.01	<.01	tr.
Cream, sour, cultured:								
1 cup	268	.14	26	195	331	.62	.04	.01
1 tbsp.	14	.01	1	10	17	.03	<.01	tr.
half and half, 1 tbsp.	16	.01	2	14	19	.08	<.01	tr.
Cream, sour, nondairy, 1 oz. ...	1	n.a.	n.a.	13	46	n.a.	.02	.03
Cream topping, nondairy,								
1 tbsp.:								
frozen, semisolid	tr.	tr.	tr.	tr.	1	tr.	<.01	<.01
powdered[2]	4	tr.	tr.	3	6	.01	tr.	tr.
pressurized	tr.	tr.	tr.	1	1	tr.	<.01	<.01
Creamer, nondairy, liquid (*Coffee-mate*), ½ fl. oz.	<1	.01	<.01	7	20	.01	0	n.a.
Creme de menthe, 1 fl. oz.	0	.02	0	0	0	n.a.	.03	.01
Cress, garden, raw, ½ cup	20	.33	m.q.	19	152	n.a.	n.a.	n.a.
Croaker, Atlantic, meat only, raw, 1 oz.	4	.10	11	60	98	.12	.01	<.01
Croissant, 2-oz. piece	20	2.10	n.a.	64	68	n.a.	n.a.	n.a.
Crookneck squash, ½ cup:								
fresh, raw, sliced	14	.31	14	21	138	.19	.07	.10
fresh, boiled, drained, sliced	24	.32	22	35	173	.35	.09	.19
canned, drained, sliced	13	.7	14	22	104	.32	.09	.11
frozen, boiled, drained, sliced	19	.49	26	40	243	.32	.07	.25
Cucumber, w/peel:								
1 medium, 8¼" long, 10.9 oz.	42	.84	33	51	448	.69	.12	.18
sliced, ½ cup	7	.14	6	9	78	.12	.02	.07
Cumin seed, 1 tsp.	20	1.39	8	10	38	.10	.02	.07

1. *Without added ingredients.*
2. *Prepared with whole milk.*

Food and Measure	Ca mg.	Fe mg.	Mag mg.	Pho mg.	Pot mg.	Zn mg.	Cop mcg.	Man mcg.
Currant, ½ cup:								
black European, fresh	31	.86	14	33	180	.15	.05	.14
red and white, fresh	18	.56	7	24	154	.13	.06	.10
Zante, dried	62	2.34	30	90	642	.47	.34	.34
Curry powder, 1 tsp.	10	.59	5	7	31	.08	.02	.09
Custard apple, trimmed, 1 oz. ...	9	.20	5	6	108	n.a.	n.a.	n.a.
Cuttlefish, mixed species, meat only, raw, 1 oz.	26	1.70	m.q.	110	105	.49	.17	n.a.

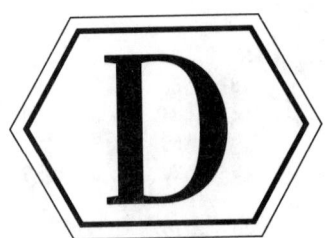

Food and Measure	Ca mg.	Fe mg.	Mag mg.	Pho mg.	Pot mg.	Zn mg.	Cop mcg.	Man mcg.
Danish pastry:								
plain, 2-oz. round piece	60	1.10	n.a.	58	53	m.q.	n.a.	n.a.
w/fruit, 2.3-oz. round piece	17	1.30	n.a.	80	57	m.q.	n.a.	n.a.
Date, domestic, natural and dry:								
pitted, 10 dates, 2.9 oz.	27	.96	29	33	541	.24	.24	.25
pitted, chopped, ½ cup	29	1.03	32	35	581	.26	.26	.27
Dill, 1 tsp.:								
seed	32	.34	5	6	25	.11	.02	.04
weed, dried	18	.49	5	5	33	.03	<.01	.04
Dolphin fish, meat only, raw, 1 oz.	m.q.	.32	m.q.	m.q.	118	.13	.01	<.01
Donut, 1 piece:								
cake type, 3¼″ diam.	22	1.00	n.a.	111	58	m.q.	n.a.	n.a.
yeast type, glazed, 3¼″ diam.	17	1.40	n.a.	55	64	m.q.	n.a.	n.a.
Drum, freshwater, meat only, raw,								
1 oz.	17	.26	9	51	78	.19	.07	.20
Duck[1]:								
domesticated, roasted, meat w/skin,								
4 oz.	12	3.06	18	177	231	2.11	.26	n.a.
domesticated, roasted, meat only,								
4 oz.	14	3.06	23	230	286	2.95	.26	n.a.
wild, raw, meat w/skin, 1 oz.	1	1.18	6	48	71	.22	.09	n.a.
Dutch brand loaf, pork and beef,								
1-oz. slice	24	.35	6	46	107	.49	.02	.01

1. *Cooked meats are prepared without added ingredients.*

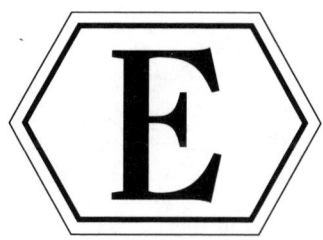

Food and Measure	Ca mg.	Fe mg.	Mag mg.	Pho mg.	Pot mg.	Zn mg.	Cop mcg.	Man mcg.
Eel, mixed species, meat only:								
raw, 1 oz.	6	.14	m.q.	61	77	.46	<.01	.01
baked, broiled, or microwaved[1],								
4 oz.	29	.73	m.q.	314	396	2.36	.03	(0)
Egg, chicken:								
raw:								
whole, fresh or frozen, 1 large,								
approx. 1.75 oz.	25	.72	5	89	60	.55	.01	.01
white, fresh or frozen, from								
1 large egg	2	.01	4	4	48	0	<.01	<.01
yolk, fresh, from 1 large egg	23	.59	1	81	16	.52	<.01	.01
yolk, frozen[2], 1 oz.	33	.86	3	118	28	.75	.01	.02
yolk, frozen, sugared, 1 oz.	31	1.11	3	101	24	.67	n.a.	n.a.
cooked, 1 large egg:								
fried[3]	25	.72	5	89	61	.55	.01	.01
hard boiled	25	.60	5	86	63	.52	.01	.01
omelet[4]	26	.73	5	90	62	.56	.01	.01
poached	25	.72	5	89	60	.55	.01	.01
scrambled[5]	44	.73	7	104	84	.61	.01	.01
dried, 1 oz.:								
whole	60	2.23	13	192	139	1.53	.08	.04
whole, stabilized[6]	63	2.35	14	203	146	1.62	.08	.04
white, stabilized[6], flakes	24	.07	19	24	295	.04	.07	.02
white, stabilized[6], powder	25	.07	20	25	316	.05	.05	.01
yolk	80	2.94	8	268	48	1.74	.08	.03

1. *Without added ingredients.*
2. *Includes approximately 17% white.*
3. *Recipe: 95% egg, 5% margarine, and salt.*
4. *Recipe: 74% egg, 22% water, 4% margarine, and salt.*
5. *Recipe: 74% egg, 22% whole milk, 4% margarine, and salt.*
6. *Glucose reduced.*

Food and Measure	Ca mg.	Fe mg.	Mag mg.	Pho mg.	Pot mg.	Zn mg.	Cop mcg.	Man mcg.
Egg, chicken, substitute or imitation, 1 oz.:								
frozen	21	.56	n.a.	20	60	.28	.01	<.01
liquid	15	.60	n.a.	34	94	.37	.01	<.01
powder	92	.90	n.a.	136	211	n.a.	.06	.02
Egg, duck, fresh, whole, raw, 1 egg, approx. 2.5 oz.	45	2.70	12	154	156	.99	.04	.03
Eggnog, dairy, 1 cup	330	.51	47	278	420	1.17	m.q.	m.q.
Eggplant, ½ cup:								
raw, 1" pieces	15	.22	5	13	90	.06	.05	.06
boiled, drained, cubed	3	.17	6	11	119	.07	.05	.07
Endive, raw:								
1 head, approx. 1.3 lbs.	267	4.23	74	145	1611	4.05	.51	2.16
chopped, ½ cup	13	.21	4	7	79	.20	.03	.11

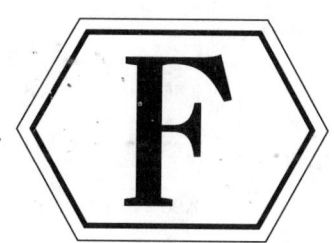

Food and Measure	Ca mg.	Fe mg.	Mag mg.	Pho mg.	Pot mg.	Zn mg.	Cop mcg.	Man mcg.
Farina, whole grain, enriched,								
cooked, 1 cup	4	1.16	4	28	30	.16	.03	n.a.
Fast foods, unspecified:								
breakfast:								
biscuit, plain, 2.6 oz.	90	1.63	9	260	86	.29	.04	.30
biscuit, w/egg:								
4.8 oz.	154	3.13	20	184	160	1.10	.08	.30
and bacon, 5.3 oz.	189	3.73	23	238	250	1.64	.11	.28
and ham, 6.8 oz.	221	4.55	30	317	319	2.23	.14	.30
and sausage, 6.3 oz.	155	3.96	25	490	319	2.16	.10	.32
and steak, 5.2 oz.	138	5.30	24	225	306	2.80	.11	.25
cheese and bacon, 5.1 oz.	164	2.55	20	459	230	1.54	.08	.26
biscuit, w/ham, 4 oz.	161	2.73	22	554	197	1.65	.04	.36
biscuit, w/sausage, 4.4 oz.	128	2.59	20	446	198	1.56	.05	.36
biscuit, w/steak, 5 oz.	115	4.31	27	205	233	2.66	.12	.42
croissant, w/egg and cheese:								
4.5 oz.	244	2.20	22	349	174	1.76	.09	.23
and bacon, 4.6 oz.	151	2.19	23	276	201	1.90	.10	.22
and ham, 5.4 oz.	144	2.13	26	336	272	2.17	.13	.22
and sausage, 5.6 oz.	144	3.04	25	290	283	2.15	.11	.25
danish pastry:								
cheese, 3.2 oz.	70	1.85	16	80	116	.63	.09	.35
cinnamon, 3.1 oz.	37	1.80	14	74	96	.49	.08	.37
fruit, 3.3 oz.	22	1.40	14	69	110	.48	.06	.19
eggs, scrambled, 2 eggs	54	2.43	13	228	138	1.56	.06	.04
English muffin:								
w/butter, 2.2 oz.	103	1.59	13	85	69	.42	.06	.21
w/cheese and sausage,								
4.1 oz.	168	2.25	24	186	215	1.68	.08	.22
w/egg, cheese, and Canadian								
bacon, 5.1 oz.	207	3.28	33	319	213	1.80	.13	.26

Food and Measure	Ca mg.	Fe mg.	Mag mg.	Pho mg.	Pot mg.	Zn mg.	Cop mcg.	Man mcg.
Fast foods, breakfast, English muffin *(cont.)*								
w/egg, cheese, and sausage,								
5.8 oz.	196	3.46	30	288	294	2.36	.12	.30
French toast, w/butter, 2 slices,								
4.8 oz.	73	1.89	16	146	177	.60	.07	.21
French toast sticks, 5 sticks,								
5 oz.	78	2.96	26	123	126	.93	.27	.22
pancakes, w/butter, and syrup,								
3 cakes, 8.2 oz.	128	2.61	48	476	250	1.03	.15	.32
potatoes, hashed brown, ½ cup ..	7	.48	16	69	267	.22	.07	.11
sausage, 1-oz. patty	9	.34	5	50	97	.68	.04	.02
sausage, .5-oz. link	4	.16	2	24	47	.33	.02	.01
entrees:								
chicken, breaded, fried:								
dark meat, 5.2 oz. or 1 thigh								
and 1 drumstick	36	1.60	37	240	446	3.24	.12	.13
light meat, 5.7 oz. or								
2 pieces	60	1.49	38	307	566	1.55	.10	.16
chicken, breaded, fried, boneless,								
6 pieces:								
plain, 3.6 oz.	16	1.27	20	204	251	1.06	.17	.13
w/barbecue sauce, 4.6 oz.	21	1.46	25	214	319	1.11	.17	.16
w/honey, 4.1 oz.	17	1.32	20	203	255	1.09	.17	.14
w/mustard sauce, 4.6 oz.	25	1.48	25	219	280	1.14	.17	.17
w/sweet and sour sauce,								
4.6 oz.	20	1.48	23	211	277	1.10	.17	.15
chili con carne, 1 cup	67	5.19	45	198	691	3.56	.60	.40
clams, breaded and fried, ¾ cup	21	3.04	31	239	265	1.63	.10	.31
crab, baked, 2.1-oz. cake	228	.76	45	185	329	3.86	.59	.43
crab, soft shell, fried,								
4.4-oz. crab	55	1.81	25	132	163	1.06	.19	.31
crab cake, 3.8-oz. cake	367	2.03	46	412	295	3.86	.67	.51
fish, battered or breaded, fried,								
3.2-oz. fillet	17	1.92	22	156	292	.40	.04	.17
oysters, battered or breaded,								
fried, 6 pieces, 4.9 oz.	27	4.46	24	195	182	15.64	.80	.42
pizza, ⅛ of 12″ pie:								
w/cheese	90	.45	12	88	85	.63	.06	.18
w/cheese, meat, vegetables ...	83	1.26	15	108	147	.92	.10	.10
w/pepperoni	48	.70	6	56	114	.39	.05	.07
scallops, breaded, fried, 6 pieces,								
5.1 oz.	18	2.04	32	292	294	1.08	.22	.30
shrimp, breaded, fried, 6–8								
pieces, 5.8 oz.	84	2.94	39	345	184	1.21	.14	.33
Mexican foods:								
burrito, w/beans, 2 pieces:								
7.7 oz.	113	4.52	86	97	653	1.53	.38	.87
and cheese, 6.6 oz.	214	2.27	80	180	496	1.64	.35	.43
and chilies, 7.2 oz.	100	4.54	72	114	580	3.40	.33	.78

Food and Measure	Ca mg.	Fe mg.	Mag mg.	Pho mg.	Pot mg.	Zn mg.	Cop mcg.	Man mcg.
and meat, 8.1 oz.	105	4.89	83	142	656	3.84	.38	.83
cheese and beef, 7.2 oz.	131	3.73	50	140	410	2.35	.33	.40
cheese and chilies, 11.9 oz. ...	288	7.68	99	286	810	6.07	.59	.81
burrito, w/beef, 2 pieces:								
7.8 oz.	84	6.09	81	175	739	4.73	.41	.79
and chilies, 7.1 oz.	87	4.43	60	141	499	4.32	.32	.75
cheese and chilies, 10.7 oz. ...	223	7.81	69	316	667	7.91	.36	.61
chimichanga, w/beef, 1 piece:								
6.1 oz.	63	4.55	62	123	587	4.95	.42	.56
and cheese, 6.5 oz.	238	3.84	60	187	203	3.37	.35	.49
and red chilies, 6.7 oz.	71	4.18	65	113	613	3.03	.28	.62
cheese and red chilies,								
6.3 oz.	218	3.14	41	146	330	4.63	.56	.39
enchilada, w/cheese, 1 piece:								
5.7 oz.	324	1.31	50	133	240	2.51	.26	.24
and beef, 6.8 oz.	228	3.08	82	168	574	2.69	.52	.58
enchirito, w/cheese, beef, and								
beans, 1 piece, 6.8 oz.	217	2.39	71	224	560	2.75	.27	.38
frijoles, w/cheese, 1 cup	188	2.24	85	175	605	1.73	.34	.50
nachos, w/cheese, 6–8 pieces:								
4 oz.	272	1.27	55	276	172	1.78	.14	.22
and jalapeños, 7.2 oz.	620	2.45	109	394	293	2.90	.17	.44
beans, ground beef, and								
peppers, 9 oz.	384	2.78	97	389	451	3.65	.75	.42
taco, 1 small, 6 oz.	221	2.42	71	203	473	3.93	.21	.44
taco, 1 large, 9.3 oz.	339	3.72	109	313	728	6.05	.32	.68
taco salad[1], 1½ cup	192	2.28	52	143	416	2.68	.22	.33
taco salad, w/chili[2], 1½ cup	246	2.67	52	154	393	3.29	.30	.34
tostada, 1 piece:								
w/beans and cheese, 5.1 oz. ..	211	1.88	59	116	403	1.90	.21	.37
w/beans, beef, and cheese,								
7.9 oz.	190	2.45	68	173	490	3.18	.32	.36
w/beef and cheese, 5.7 oz.	217	2.86	64	180	572	3.68	.26	.50
w/guacamole, 4.6 oz.	212	.82	37	117	325	2.03	.13	.18
sandwiches, 1 piece:								
cheeseburger, single meat patty:								
plain, 3.6 oz.	140	2.44	21	196	165	2.37	.09	.23
w/condiments[3], 4 oz.	111	2.43	21	177	223	2.09	.10	.18
w/condiments and vegetables[4],								
5.4 oz.	182	2.65	26	216	229	2.62	.12	.29
cheeseburger, double meat patty:								
plain, 5.5 oz.	232	3.41	33	374	308	4.96	.13	.23
w/condiments and vegetables[4],								
5.9 oz.	171	3.42	31	242	335	3.49	.15	.30
double-decker bun, plain								
5.6 oz.	224	3.70	33	338	285	4.35	.14	.30

1. *Recipe: lettuce, tomato, chili sauce, ground beef, cheese, and taco shell.*
2. *Recipe: chili con carne, lettuce, tomato, cheese, and taco shell.*
3. *Condiments include catsup, mustard, pickles, and onions.*
4. *Condiments and vegetables include catsup, mustard, mayonnaise-style dressing, pickles, onions, lettuce, and tomatoes.*

Food and Measure	Ca mg.	Fe mg.	Mag mg.	Pho mg.	Pot mg.	Zn mg.	Cop mcg.	Man mcg.
Fast foods, cheeseburger, double meat patty *(cont.)*								
double-decker bun, w/ condiments and vegetables[1], 8 oz.	169	4.71	36	350	389	4.13	.16	.27
cheeseburger, large, single meat patty:								
plain, 6.5 oz.	91	5.47	38	423	644	5.54	.16	.31
w/bacon and condiments[2], 6.9 oz.	162	4.73	44	399	331	6.82	.16	.33
w/condiments and vegetables[1], 7.7 oz.	205	4.66	43	312	445	4.60	.19	.31
ham, w/condiments and vegetables[1], 9 oz.	301	5.04	51	530	539	6.63	.25	.37
cheeseburger, large, double meat patty, w/condiments and vegetables[1], 9.1 oz.	240	5.91	52	396	596	6.68	.21	.32
chicken fillet sandwich:								
plain, 6.4 oz.	60	4.68	35	233	353	1.87	.23	.47
w/cheese, 8 oz.	258	3.63	43	407	334	2.90	.17	.38
fish sandwich, w/tartar sauce:								
5.6 oz.	84	2.60	33	212	339	.99	.19	.37
and cheese, 6.5 oz.	185	3.50	37	312	353	1.17	.12	.36
hamburger, single meat patty:								
plain, 3.2 oz.	63	2.41	19	102	145	2.00	.09	.21
w/condiments[2], 3.8 oz.	52	2.46	23	110	215	2.05	.12	.21
w/condiments and vegetables[1], 3.9 oz.	63	2.62	22	125	227	2.06	.10	.25
hamburger, double meat patty:								
plain, 6.2 oz.	87	4.55	36	234	363	5.71	.17	.28
w/condiments[2], 7.6 oz.	92	5.55	44	284	527	5.80	.19	.33
hamburger, large, single meat patty:								
plain, 4.8 oz.	74	3.57	28	176	268	4.11	.13	.24
w/condiments and vegetables[1], 7.7 oz.	96	4.92	43	233	479	4.98	.20	.35
hamburger, large, double meat patty, w/condiments and vegetables[1], 8 oz.	102	5.85	49	314	569	5.68	.22	.25
ham and cheese, 5.1 oz.	130	3.25	16	152	290	1.38	.18	.14
ham, egg, and cheese, 5 oz.	212	3.11	26	346	209	1.99	.12	.24
hot dog:								
plain, 3.5 oz.	24	2.31	13	97	143	1.98	.08	.09
w/chili, 4 oz.	19	3.29	10	192	166	.78	.10	.11
coated (corn dog), 6.2 oz.	101	6.18	17	166	262	1.31	.25	.19
roast beef, plain, 4.9 oz.	54	4.23	31	239	316	3.39	.10	.13
roast beef, w/cheese, 6.2 oz.	183	5.05	40	401	345	5.37	.20	.31

1. *Condiments and vegetables include catsup, mustard, mayonnaise-style dressing, pickles, onions, lettuce, and tomatoes.*
2. *Condiments include catsup, mustard, pickles, and onions.*

Food and Measure	Ca mg.	Fe mg.	Mag mg.	Pho mg.	Pot mg.	Zn mg.	Cop mcg.	Man mcg.
steak, chopped, w/lettuce,								
tomato, mayonnaise, 7.2 oz. ..	91	5.17	49	297	525	4.54	.22	.37
submarine:								
w/cold cuts[1], 8 oz.	189	2.51	68	287	394	2.58	.30	.53
w/roast beef[2], 7.6 oz.	41	2.81	67	193	330	4.39	.36	.43
w/tuna salad[3], 9 oz.	74	2.65	79	219	335	1.88	.43	.51
salad, w/out dressing, 1½ cup:								
plain[4]	26	1.30	22	80	356	.43	.10	.31
w/added cheese and egg[5]	100	.68	24	132	371	.99	.09	.27
w/added chicken[6]	37	1.09	33	169	447	.90	.09	.25
w/added pasta and seafood[7]	73	3.16	50	204	600	1.68	.36	.67
w/added shrimp[8]	60	.91	38	159	404	1.27	.16	.14
chef, w/added turkey, ham, and								
cheese[9]	235	1.96	48	401	402	3.15	.17	.36
side dishes:								
coleslaw, ¾ cup	34	.73	9	36	177	.19	.04	.12
corn on cob, w/butter, 1 ear	5	.88	42	108	360	.90	.07	.20
hush puppies, 5 pieces, 2.8 oz. ..	69	1.43	16	190	188	.43	.21	.27
onion rings, 8–9 rings, 2.9 oz. ...	73	.85	15	86	129	.35	.07	.30
potato, baked, 1 potato:								
topped w/cheese sauce:								
10.4 oz.	310	3.02	66	320	1167	1.88	.63	.52
and bacon, 10.5 oz.	309	3.15	68	347	1179	2.16	.65	.51
and broccoli, 12 oz.	334	3.33	77	347	1440	2.03	.65	.80
and chili, 13.9 oz.	409	6.13	111	498	1570	3.78	.83	.68
topped w/sour cream and								
chives, 10.1 oz.	105	3.13	70	185	1383	.90	.69	.58
potato, french-fried:								
regular, 2.7 oz.	12	1.02	25	101	541	.39	.10	.19
large, 4.1 oz.	18	1.55	38	153	819	.60	.16	.29
potato, mashed, ⅓ cup	17	.37	15	44	236	.25	.08	.09
potato chips, 1 oz.	7	.34	17	43	369	.30	.06	.13
potato salad, ⅓ cup	13	.69	7	53	256	.19	.08	.07
desserts:								
animal crackers, 2.4-oz. box	11	1.47	11	64	57	.30	.05	.33
brownie, 1 piece, 2.1 oz.	25	1.29	16	87	83	.55	0	.11
chocolate chip cookies, 1.9-oz.								
box	20	1.47	17	52	82	.33	.18	.24
fruit pie[10], fried, 3-oz. pie	12	.89	8	38	51	.17	.04	.17
ice milk cone, vanilla, soft-serve,								
3.6 oz.	153	.15	16	139	169	.57	.02	.02

1. *Recipe: bread, lettuce, cheese, salami, ham, tomato, onion, and oil.*
2. *Recipe: bread, beef, tomato, lettuce, and mayonnaise.*
3. *Recipe: tuna salad, bread, lettuce, oil.*
4. *Recipe: lettuce, cabbage, cucumber, green pepper, tomatoes, radish, and carrot.*
5. *Recipe: lettuce, tomato, egg, cheese, celery, cucumber, and radish.*
6. *Recipe: lettuce, chicken, celery, tomato, green pepper, and carrot.*
7. *Recipe: lettuce, macaroni, salad dressing, pollock, sweet pepper, carrot, celery, crab, turbot, olives, and onion.*
8. *Recipe: lettuce, shrimp, celery, tomato, green pepper, and carrot.*
9. *Recipe: lettuce, tomatoes, turkey, ham, cheese, egg, celery, cucumber, radish, and carrot.*
10. *Apple, cherry, or lemon.*

Food and Measure	Ca mg.	Fe mg.	Mag mg.	Pho mg.	Pot mg.	Zn mg.	Cop mcg.	Man mcg.
Fast foods, desserts *(cont.)*								
sundae:								
caramel, 5.5 oz.	189	.22	28	217	318	.82	.08	.09
hot fudge, 5.6 oz.	207	.58	34	228	395	.95	.13	.13
strawberry, 5.4 oz.	161	.32	25	154	270	.66	.08	.17
beverages:								
beer, regular, 12 fl. oz.	1	.01	2	4	7	0	<.01	<.01
beer, light, 12 fl. oz.	1	.01	1	4	5	.01	.01	.01
coffee, brewed, 6 fl. oz.	1	.01	2	0	16	0	<.01	.01
coffee, instant, decaffeinated,								
6 fl. oz.	6	.08	7	5	63	.05	.01	.02
hot chocolate, 6 fl. oz.	96	.35	25	89	203	.46	.09	.08
juice, 6 fl. oz.:								
grapefruit	15	.25	20	26	252	.09	.06	.04
orange	17	.19	19	30	355	.09	.08	.03
tomato	16	1.06	20	34	400	.26	.18	.14
lemonade, 8 fl. oz.	8	.41	5	5	38	.09	.05	.01
orange drink, 6 fl. oz.	12	.53	3	3	33	.16	.01	.03
shake, 10 fl. oz.:								
chocolate	319	.88	47	288	567	1.15	.18	.11
strawberry	320	.30	36	283	516	1.00	.06	.04
vanilla	344	.26	35	289	492	1.01	.14	.04
soda, 12-fl.-oz. can:								
cola	9	.13	3	46	4	.05	.04	.13
ginger ale	12	.66	3	1	5	.18	.07	n.a.
lemon-lime	9	.25	2	1	4	.18	.04	.05
orange	19	.23	4	4	9	.38	.06	n.a.
pepper type	12	.14	1	41	2	.15	.02	n.a.
root beer	19	.18	4	2	3	.26	.03	n.a.
tea, brewed, 6 fl. oz.	0	.04	5	1	66	.04	.02	n.a.
tea, iced, instant, sugar-								
sweetened, lemon flavor,								
12 fl. oz.	8	.08	8	4	74	.12	.03	1.01
Fat, see specific listings								
Fennel seed, 1 tsp.	24	.37	8	10	34	.07	.02	.13
Fenugreek seed, 1 tsp.	6	1.24	7	11	28	.09	.04	.05
Fig, ½ cup, except as noted:								
fresh, 1 medium, approx. 1.8 oz. ...	18	.18	8	7	116	.07	.04	.06
canned:								
in water	35	.37	13	13	128	.15	.14	.11
in light syrup	35	.37	13	13	128	.14	.14	.11
in heavy syrup	35	.37	13	13	129	.15	.14	.11
dried:								
uncooked, 10 figs, approx. 6.6 oz.	269	4.18	111	128	1332	.94	.59	.73
uncooked	143	2.23	59	68	709	.50	.31	.39
cooked	79	1.23	33	38	391	.28	.17	.21
Filbert, dried, unblanched, 1 oz. ..	53	.93	81	89	126	.68	.43	.57
Fish, see specific listings								
Fish fillet, breaded, fried, frozen,								

Food and Measure	Ca mg.	Fe mg.	Mag mg.	Pho mg.	Pot mg.	Zn mg.	Cop mcg.	Man mcg.
2-oz. piece, 4″ × 2″ × ½″	11	.42	14	103	149	.38	.06	.14
Fish stick, breaded, fried, frozen,								
1-oz. stick, 4″ × 1″ × ½″	6	.21	7	51	73	.19	.03	.07
Flatfish, meat only:								
raw, 1 oz.	5	.10	9	52	102	.13	.01	<.01
baked, broiled, or microwaved[1],								
4 oz.	20	.39	66	328	390	.71	.03	(0)
Flounder, see Flatfish								
Frankfurter:								
bacon and cheddar (*Oscar Mayer*),								
1.6-oz. link	18	.43	6	88	86	.81	m.q.	m.q.
beef, 1 link, 5″ long × 7⅛″, approx.								
2 oz.	7	.76	6	47	90	1.21	.03	.03
beef and pork, 1 link, 5″ long ×								
7⅛″, approx. 2 oz.	6	.66	6	49	95	1.05	.05	.02
cheese (cheesefurter or cheese								
smokie), 1 oz.	16	.30	4	50	58	.64	.02	.01
French toast, frozen, 3 oz.:								
(*Aunt Jemima* Original)	96	2.04	15	99	120	.60	.05	n.a.
cinnamon swirl (*Aunt Jemima*)	95	1.97	15	112	122	.60	.07	.20
raisin (*Aunt Jemima*)	94	2.13	17	100	156	.78	.10	.23
Frosting mix[2], fudge, 1 cup:								
chocolate	50	3.10	n.a.	205	195	n.a.	n.a.	n.a.
creamy[3]	96	2.70	n.a.	218	238	n.a.	n.a.	n.a.
creamy[4]	91	2.50	n.a.	198	218	n.a.	n.a.	n.a.
Fruit, see specific listings								
Fruit, mixed:								
canned, in heavy syrup, ½ cup	1	.46	6	13	100	.09	.07	n.a.
dried, pitted, 1 oz.	11	.77	11	22	226	.14	.11	.06
frozen, sweetened, ½ cup	9	.35	7	15	164	.06	.04	.08
Fruit cocktail, canned, ½ cup:								
in water	6	.31	8	14	115	.11	.09	n.a.
in juice	10	.26	9	17	118	.11	.08	n.a.
in light syrup	8	.37	7	14	112	.11	.09	n.a.
in heavy or extra heavy syrup	8	.36	7	14	112	.11	.09	n.a.
Fruit punch drink, 1 cup:								
canned	20	.15	5	2	62	.30	.13	.50
frozen[5]	9	.22	6	2	31	.09	.07	.25
Fruit punch flavor drink mix,								
2 rounded tsp.	36	.13	0	52	1	.03	.03	.01
Fruit punch juice drink, frozen[5],								
1 cup	18	.57	9	n.a.	191	.54	.06	.15
Fruit salad, canned, ½ cup:								
in water	8	.36	7	11	95	.09	.08	n.a.
in juice	14	.31	10	18	144	.18	.06	n.a.

1. *Without added ingredients.*
2. *Prepared according to package directions.*
3. *Prepared with water.*
4. *Prepared with water and table fat.*
5. *Diluted according to package directions.*

Food and Measure	Ca mg.	Fe mg.	Mag mg.	Pho mg.	Pot mg.	Zn mg.	Cop mcg.	Man mcg.
Fruit salad *(cont.)*								
in light syrup	8	.36	7	11	104	.09	.08	n.a.
in heavy syrup	8	.36	7	12	103	.09	.08	n.a.
tropical, in heavy syrup[1]	17	.66	17	10	168	.14	.10	n.a.

1. *With added calcium chloride.*

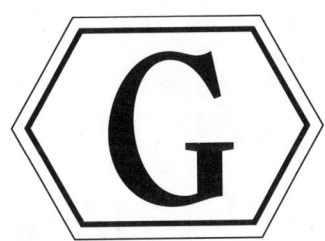

Food and Measure	Ca mg.	Fe mg.	Mag mg.	Pho mg.	Pot mg.	Zn mg.	Cop mcg.	Man mcg.
Garlic, raw, 1 clove	5	.05	1	5	12	n.a.	n.a.	n.a.
Garlic powder, 1 tsp.	2	.08	2	12	31	.07	<.01	.02
Gefilte fish, in jars, sweet,								
w/broth, 1.5-oz. piece	10	1.04	4	31	38	.35	.08	.03
Gelatin, unflavored, powder, dry,								
.2-oz. pkt.	1	0	n.a.	0	2	n.a.	n.a.	n.a.
Ginger:								
root, raw, sliced, ¼ cup	4	.12	10	7	100	n.a.	n.a.	n.a.
ground, 1 tsp.	2	.21	3	3	24	.08	.01	.48
Ginkgo nut, 1 oz.:								
raw	1	.28	8	35	145	.10	.08	.03
dried	6	.45	15	76	283	.19	.15	.06
Goose[1], domesticated, 4 oz.:								
roasted, meat w/skin	15	3.21	25	306	373	m.q.	.30	n.a.
roasted, meat only	16	3.25	28	350	440	m.q.	.31	n.a.
Gooseberry, ½ cup:								
fresh, trimmed	19	.24	8	20	149	.09	.05	.11
canned, in light syrup	20	.42	8	9	97	.14	.27	.22
Gourd, dishcloth, boiled, drained,								
1″ slices, ½ cup	8	.32	18	28	403	n.a.	n.a.	n.a.
Granola and cereal bars, 1 bar:								
caramel nut (*Quaker Granola Dipps*)	31	.50	16	51	84	.37	.08	.20
chocolate chip (*Quaker Chewy*)	27	.70	22	65	94	.43	.11	.37
chocolate chip (*Quaker Granola*								
Dipps)	29	.75	19	56	89	.37	.10	.26
chocolate fudge (*Quaker Granola*								
Dipps)	52	.40	2	15	101	.09	0	n.a.
honey and oats (*Quaker Chewy*)	30	.68	21	65	92	.43	.08	.43
nut and raisin, chunky (*Quaker*								
Chewy)	24	.62	26	68	111	.45	.11	.34

1. *Prepared without added ingredients.*

Food and Measure	Ca mg.	Fe mg.	Mag mg.	Pho mg.	Pot mg.	Zn mg.	Cop mcg.	Man mcg.
Granola and cereal bars *(cont.)*								
peanut butter:								
(*Quaker Chewy*)	26	.59	24	71	100	.53	.19	.40
(*Quaker Granola Dipps*)	27	.68	10	45	110	.09	n.a.	n.a.
chocolate chip (*Quaker Chewy*) ...	23	.55	25	74	107	.48	.11	.38
chocolate chip (*Quaker Granola Dipps*)	37	.46	10	44	120	.08	n.a.	n.a.
raisin and cinnamon (*Quaker Chewy*)	29	.67	20	62	101	.37	.08	.36
S'mores (*Quaker Chewy*)	25	.73	20	57	78	.37	.08	.36
Grape:								
fresh:								
American type, 10 medium, approx. 1.4 oz.	3	.07	1	2	46	.01	.01	.17
American type, peeled and seeded, ½ cup	7	.14	3	5	88	.02	.02	.33
European type, 10 medium, ⅝″ × ⅞″, approx. 1.75 oz.	5	.13	3	6	93	.03	.05	.03
European type, seedless or seeded, ½ cup	9	.21	5	11	148	.05	.07	.05
canned, Thompson seedless:								
in water, ½ cup	13	1.19	8	22	131	.06	.07	.05
in heavy syrup, ½ cup	13	1.20	8	22	132	.06	.07	.05
Grape juice, 6 fl. oz.:								
canned or bottled	18	.48	18	18	252	.12	.05	.68
frozen[1]	6	.18	6	6	42	.06	.02	.33
Grapefruit:								
pink and red, all areas:								
½ of 3¾″-diam. fruit, approx. 8.5 oz.	13	.15	10	11	158	.09	.05	.01
sections w/juice, ½ cup	13	.14	9	10	148	.08	.05	.01
white, all areas:								
½ of 3¾″-diam. fruit, approx. 8.5 oz.	14	.07	11	9	175	.08	.06	.02
sections w/juice, ½ cup	14	.07	11	9	170	.08	.06	.02
canned or in jars, ½ cup:								
in water	18	.50	12	12	161	.11	.08	.01
in juice	19	.26	13	15	209	.09	.05	.01
in light syrup	18	.51	13	13	164	.11	.08	.01
Grapefruit juice, 6 fl. oz.:								
fresh	17	.37	23	28	300	.10	.06	.04
canned, unsweetened	12	.36	18	18	282	.18	.07	.04
canned, sweetened	12	.66	18	18	306	.12	.09	.04
frozen[1]	12	.24	18	24	252	.12	.06	.04
Great northern bean, ½ cup:								
boiled	60	1.87	44	145	344	.77	.22	.46
canned, w/liquid	69	2.05	67	178	459	.85	.21	.53
Green bean, ½ cup:								
fresh, raw	21	.57	14	21	115	.13	.04	.12

1. *Diluted according to package directions.*

Food and Measure	Ca mg.	Fe mg.	Mag mg.	Pho mg.	Pot mg.	Zn mg.	Cop mcg.	Man mcg.
fresh, boiled, drained	29	.79	16	24	185	.23	.06	.18
canned, drained	18	.61	9	13	74	.20	.03	.14
frozen, boiled, drained	31	.56	15	16	76	.42	.05	.25
Grouper, meat only:								
raw, 1 oz.	8	.25	9	46	137	.14	.01	<.01
baked, broiled, or microwaved[1],								
4 oz.	24	1.29	42	162	539	.58	.05	.01
Guava, trimmed, ½ cup:								
common	17	.09	9	21	235	.19	.09	.12
strawberry	26	.27	21	34	357	n.a.	n.a.	n.a.
Guava sauce, cooked, ½ cup	8	.21	8	13	268	.20	.09	.13

1. *Without added ingredients.*

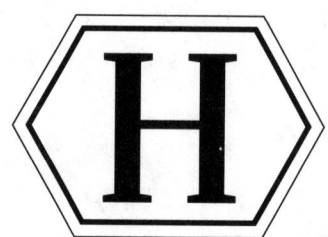

Food and Measure	Ca mg.	Fe mg.	Mag mg.	Pho mg.	Pot mg.	Zn mg.	Cop mcg.	Man mcg.
Haddock, meat only:								
raw, 1 oz.	9	.30	11	53	88	.11	.01	.01
baked, broiled, or microwaved[1],								
4 oz.	48	1.53	57	273	452	.54	.04	(0)
smoked, 4 oz.	56	1.59	61	285	471	.57	.05	(0)
Halibut, meat only:								
Atlantic and Pacific, raw, 1 oz.	13	.24	24	63	127	.12	.02	<.01
Atlantic and Pacific, baked, broiled,								
or microwaved[1], 4 oz.	68	1.21	121	323	653	.60	.04	n.a.
Greenland, raw, 1 oz.	1	.17	m.q.	46	76	m.q.	m.q.	n.a.
Ham, patty[2], grilled, 4 oz.	10	1.83	11	115	227	2.15	.11	n.a.
Ham, fresh, roasted[1], 4 oz. (see								
also "Ham, cured"):								
whole leg, lean and fat	7	1.13	25	280	373	3.24	.11	.04
whole leg, lean only	8	1.27	28	319	423	3.70	.12	.04
rump half, lean and fat	8	1.19	29	295	404	3.11	.12	.03
rump half, lean only	8	1.29	33	323	443	3.41	.12	.03
shank half, lean and fat	7	1.10	24	271	352	3.32	.11	.03
shank half, lean only	8	1.26	28	315	408	3.91	.12	.04
Ham, cured[2], whole:								
lean and fat, unheated, 1 oz.	2	.20	4	57	88	.50	.02	.01
lean and fat, roasted, 4 oz.	8	.99	22	243	324	2.63	.09	.02
lean only, unheated, 1 oz.	2	.23	5	66	105	.58	.02	.01
lean only, roasted, 4 oz.	8	1.07	25	257	358	2.91	.10	.02
Ham, cured[2], boneless:								
regular (approx. 11% fat):								
unheated, 1-oz. slice	2	.28	5	70	94	.61	.03	.01
roasted, 4 oz.	9	1.52	25	319	464	2.80	.16	.05

1. *Without added ingredients.*
2. *Fully cooked as purchased.*

Food and Measure	Ca mg.	Fe mg.	Mag mg.	Pho mg.	Pot mg.	Zn mg.	Cop mcg.	Man mcg.
extra lean and regular:								
unheated, 1-oz. slice	2	.26	5	67	84	.58	.03	.01
roasted, 4 oz.	9	1.59	22	281	411	2.98	.13	.05
extra lean (approx. 5% fat):								
unheated, 1-oz. slice	2	.22	5	62	99	.55	.02	.01
roasted, 4 oz.	9	1.68	16	222	325	3.27	.09	.06
steak, extra lean, unheated, 1 oz. ...	1	.28	5	74	92	.57	.28	.01
Ham, canned:								
regular (approx. 13% fat):								
unheated, 1 oz.	2	.23	4	49	90	.47	.02	.01
roasted, 4 oz.	9	1.55	19	276	405	2.84	.15	.03
extra lean and regular:								
unheated, 1 oz.	2	.26	5	59	95	.52	.02	.01
roasted, 4 oz.	8	1.21	23	251	398	2.63	.09	.03
extra lean (approx. 4% fat):								
unheated, 1 oz.	2	.27	5	63	103	.55	.02	.01
roasted, 4 oz.	7	1.04	24	237	395	2.53	.06	.03
chopped, 1 oz.	2	.27	4	39	81	.52	.01	.01
Ham luncheon meat, 1 oz.:								
boiled (*Oscar Mayer*), .7-oz. slice ...	1	.19	4	65	60	.40	m.q.	m.q.
chopped	2	.24	4	44	91	.55	.02	.01
cooked, sliced, regular (11% fat) ...	2	.28	5	70	94	.61	.03	.01
cooked, sliced, extra lean (5% fat) ..	2	.22	5	62	99	.55	.02	.01
honey (*Oscar Mayer*), .7-oz. slice ..	1	.23	4	56	61	.38	.m.q.	m.q.
minced	3	.22	5	44	88	.54	.02	.01
pepper, black, cracked (*Oscar*								
Mayer), .7-oz. slice	1	.22	4	58	63	.39	m.q.	m.q.
smoked (*Oscar Mayer*), .7-oz. slice	1	.19	4	58	66	.37	m.q.	m.q.
Ham salad spread, 1 tbsp.	1	.09	1	18	22	.17	.01	(0)
Ham and cheese loaf or roll,								
1 oz.	16	.26	5	72	83	.57	.02	.01
Ham and cheese spread, 1 tbsp.	33	.11	3	74	24	.34	.01	.01
Hazelnut, see "Filbert"								
Head cheese, pork, 1-oz. slice ...	4	.33	3	17	9	.37	.03	.01
Heart[1], 4 oz.:								
beef, simmered	7	8.52	28	284	264	3.55	.84	.07
chicken, broiler-fryer, simmered ...	22	10.24	23	226	150	8.28	.57	.12
lamb, braised	16	6.26	27	288	213	4.17	.69	.06
pork, braised	8	6.61	27	202	234	3.50	.58	.08
turkey, simmered	15	7.81	25	232	208	5.98	.71	.10
veal, braised	9	4.90	20	284	226	2.54	.49	m.q.
Herring, Atlantic, meat only:								
raw, 1 oz.	16	.31	9	67	93	.28	.03	.01
baked, broiled, or microwaved[1],								
4 oz.	84	1.60	46	344	475	1.44	.13	n.a.
kippered, 4 oz.	95	1.71	52	369	507	1.54	.15	n.a.
pickled, 4 oz.	87	1.38	9	101	78	.60	.12	.05

1. *Prepared without added ingredients.*

Food and Measure	Ca mg.	Fe mg.	Mag mg.	Pho mg.	Pot mg.	Zn mg.	Cop mcg.	Man mcg.
Hominy, canned, white or yellow,								
½ cup	8	.50	13	28	7	.84	.02	.06
Honey, 1 tbsp.	1	.10	n.a.	1	11	n.a.	n.a.	n.a.
Honey loaf, pork and beef, 1 oz. ..	5	.38	5	41	97	.69	.02	.01
Honey roll sausage, beef, 1 oz. ..	3	.62	4	39	83	.92	.03	.01
Honeydew:								
¹⁄₁₀ of 7"-diam. melon, 2" slice,								
approx. 8 oz.	8	.09	9	13	350	n.a.	.05	.02
pulp, cubed, ½ cup	5	.06	6	9	231	n.a.	.04	.02
Hubbard squash, ½ cup:								
raw, cubed	8	.23	11	12	186	.07	.04	n.a.
baked, cubed	17	.48	22	23	365	.15	.05	n.a.
boiled, mashed	12	.33	16	17	252	.11	.06	n.a.
Hyacinth bean, ⅜ cup:								
raw	20	.30	16	19	101	m.q.	m.q.	n.a.
boiled, drained	18	.33	18	22	115	m.q.	m.q.	n.a.
Hyacinth bean, dried, boiled,								
½ cup	39	4.44	80	117	327	2.77	.33	n.a.

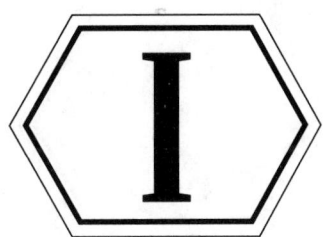

Food and Measure	Ca mg.	Fe mg.	Mag mg.	Pho mg.	Pot mg.	Zn mg.	Cop mcg.	Man mcg.
Ice cream, vanilla, ½ cup:								
hardened, 10% fat	88	.06	9	67	129	.71	.01	<.01
hardened, 16% fat	76	.05	8	58	111	.61	.01	<.01
French, soft-serve	118	.22	13	100	169	1.00	.02	.01
nuggets, chocolate coated:								
dark chocolate (*Carnation Bon Bons*), 5 pieces	55	.10	m.q.	49	80	m.q.	n.a.	n.a.
milk chocolate (*Carnation Bon Bons*), 5 pieces	75	.22	m.q.	65	110	m.q.	n.a.	n.a.
Ice milk, vanilla, ½ cup:								
hardened	88	.09	10	65	133	.28	.02	.01
soft-serve	137	.14	15	101	206	.43	.02	.01
Italian sausage, pork, cooked, 1 link, approx. 3 oz. (4 oz. raw)	20	1.24	15	141	253	1.98	.06	.07

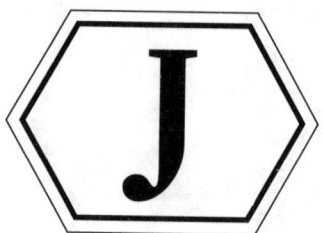

Food and Measure	Ca mg.	Fe mg.	Mag mg.	Pho mg.	Pot mg.	Zn mg.	Cop mcg.	Man mcg.
Jackfruit, trimmed, 1 oz.	10	.17	10	10	86	.12	.05	.06
Jam and preserves, all flavors, 1 tbsp.	4	.20	n.a.	2	18	n.a.	n.a.	n.a.
Java plum, seeded, ½ cup	13	.13	11	12	53	n.a.	n.a.	n.a.
Jelly, all flavors, 1 tbsp.	4	.30	tr.	1	14	n.a.	n.a.	n.a.
Jerusalem artichoke, raw, sliced, ½ cup	10	2.55	13	58	n.a.	n.a.	n.a.	n.a.
Jujube, 1 oz.:								
raw, seeded	6	.14	3	7	71	.01	.02	.02
dried	22	.51	10	28	151	.05	.08	.09

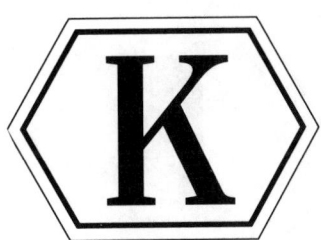

Food and Measure	Ca mg.	Fe mg.	Mag mg.	Pho mg.	Pot mg.	Zn mg.	Cop mcg.	Man mcg.
Kale, ½ cup:								
fresh, raw, chopped	46	.58	12	19	152	.15	.10	.26
fresh, boiled, drained, chopped	47	.59	12	18	148	.15	.10	.27
frozen, boiled, drained, chopped ...	90	.61	12	18	209	.12	.03	.29
Kale, Scotch, ½ cup:								
raw, chopped	70	1.02	30	21	153	.13	.08	.22
boiled, drained, chopped	86	1.25	37	25	178	.15	.10	.27
Kidney bean, red, ½ cup:								
boiled	25	2.58	40	125	355	.94	.21	.42
canned, w/liquid	31	1.61	36	120	329	.70	.19	.31
Kidneys[1], 4 oz.:								
beef, simmered	19	8.29	20	347	203	4.79	.77	.21
lamb, braised	20	14.06	23	329	202	4.31	.42	.16
pork, braised	15	6.00	20	272	162	4.71	.77	.17
veal, braised	33	3.45	27	422	180	4.82	.41	.14
Kielbasa, pork and beef[2], 1 oz. ...	12	.41	5	42	77	.57	.03	.01
Kiwifruit, 1 medium, approx.								
3.1 oz.	20	.31	23	31	252	n.a.	n.a.	n.a.
Knockwurst, pork and beef, 1 oz.	3	.26	3	28	57	.47	.02	n.a.
Kohlrabi, ½ cup:								
raw, sliced	17	.28	13	32	245	n.a.	m.q.	m.q.
boiled, drained, sliced	20	.33	16	37	279	n.a.	m.q.	m.q.
Kumquat, seeded, 1 oz.	12	.11	4	5	55	.02	.03	.02

1. *Prepared without added ingredients.*
2. *Nonfat dry milk added.*

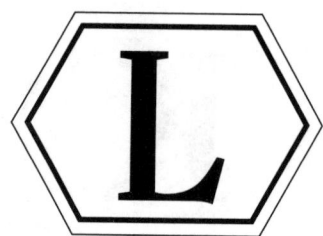

Food and Measure	Ca mg.	Fe mg.	Mag mg.	Pho mg.	Pot mg.	Zn mg.	Cop mcg.	Man mcg.
Lamb[1], domestic, meat only, 4 oz.:								
cubed for stew or kabob, leg and								
shoulder:								
braised, lean only	17	3.18	32	232	295	7.46	.16	.04
broiled, lean only	14	2.65	35	254	380	6.54	.17	.03
foreshank, braised:								
lean w/fat	23	2.43	25	188	291	8.72	.14	.03
lean only	23	2.57	26	198	303	9.82	.15	.03
ground, broiled	25	2.03	27	228	384	5.30	.15	.03
leg, roasted:								
whole, lean w/fat	12	2.25	27	217	355	4.99	.13	.03
whole, lean only	9	2.40	29	234	383	5.60	.14	.03
shank half, lean w/fat	11	2.25	28	225	370	5.28	.13	.03
shank half, lean only	9	2.34	29	236	388	5.69	.14	.03
sirloin, lean w/fat	12	2.27	25	208	341	4.68	.13	.02
sirloin, lean only	9	2.49	28	230	378	5.50	.13	.03
loin:								
broiled, lean w/fat	23	2.05	27	222	371	3.95	.15	.02
broiled, lean only	22	2.27	32	256	426	4.68	.16	.03
roasted, lean w/fat	20	2.40	26	204	279	3.87	.13	.02
roasted, lean only	19	2.77	31	234	303	4.60	.14	.03
rib:								
broiled, lean w/fat	22	2.13	26	202	306	4.54	.14	.02
broiled, lean only	18	2.51	33	242	355	5.98	.16	.03
roasted, lean w/fat	25	1.81	23	188	307	3.96	.13	.02
roasted, lean only	24	2.01	34	221	357	5.07	.15	.03
shoulder, whole:								
braised, lean w/fat	28	2.72	27	211	281	7.22	.14	.03
braised, lean only	29	3.03	31	231	296	8.53	.15	.04
broiled, lean w/fat	24	2.30	29	225	341	6.49	.15	.03

1. *Prepared without added ingredients.*

Food and Measure	Ca mg.	Fe mg.	Mag mg.	Pho mg.	Pot mg.	Zn mg.	Cop mcg.	Man mcg.
broiled, lean only	24	2.48	33	246	367	7.48	.16	.03
roasted, lean w/fat	23	2.23	26	209	285	5.93	.12	.02
roasted, lean only	22	2.42	28	227	301	6.85	.13	.03
shoulder, arm:								
braised, lean w/fat	28	2.71	29	234	347	6.89	.16	.03
braised, lean only	29	3.06	33	263	383	8.28	.17	.03
broiled, lean w/fat	20	2.37	29	223	350	5.54	.15	.03
broiled, lean only	19	2.62	34	248	386	6.50	.16	.03
roasted, lean w/fat	20	2.30	26	208	294	5.08	.13	.02
roasted, lean only	18	2.53	29	229	314	5.95	.14	.03
shoulder, blade:								
braised, lean w/fat	31	2.66	27	210	276	7.78	.14	.03
braised, lean only	32	2.95	29	229	288	9.14	.15	.04
broiled, lean w/fat	27	1.95	27	225	381	6.37	.14	.03
broiled, lean only	27	2.05	29	245	417	7.35	.15	.03
roasted, lean w/fat	24	2.18	25	208	279	6.33	.12	.02
roasted, lean only	24	2.35	28	226	293	7.35	.12	.03
Leek:								
raw, 1 medium, approx. 9.9 oz.	73	2.60	35	43	223	n.a.	m.q.	m.q.
boiled, drained, chopped, ½ cup ...	16	.58	8	8	46	n.a.	m.q.	m.q.
Lemon:								
w/peel, 1 medium, 2⅛″ diam.,								
3.9 oz.	66	.76	13	16	157	.11	.28	n.a.
w/peel, 1-oz. wedge, ¼ medium ...	16	.19	3	4	39	.03	.07	n.a.
w/out peel, 1 medium, 2⅛″ diam.,								
3.9 oz.	15	.35	n.a.	9	80	.04	.02	n.a.
Lemon juice, 1 fl. oz.:								
fresh	2	.01	2	2	38	.02	.01	<.01
canned or bottled	3	.04	3	3	31	.02	.01	.01
frozen, single strength	2	.04	3	3	27	.02	.01	.01
Lemon peel, fresh, 1 tsp.	3	.02	tr.	tr.	3	n.a.	n.a.	n.a.
Lemonade:								
frozen[1], 1 cup	8	.41	5	5	38	.09	.05	.01
mix, 2 tbsp. or 1 scoop	66	.14	0	34	33	.04	n.a.	n.a.
Lemonade flavor drink mix,								
2 tbsp.[2]	24	.03	0	3	1	.01	.01	n.a.
Lentil dinner, canned, hearty, w/								
garden vegetables (*Health Valley*								
Fast Menu), 7½ oz.	87	4.70	24	103	361	.59	n.a.	n.a.
Lentils, dried, boiled, ½ cup	19	3.30	35	178	366	1.25	.25	.49
Lentils, sprouted, raw, ½ cup ...	9	1.22	14	66	122	.57	.13	.19
Lettuce:								
bibb, Boston, or butterhead, 5″-								
diam. head, approx. 7.75 oz. ..	m.q.	.49	m.q.	m.q.	416	.28	.04	.22
cos or romaine, shredded, ½ cup ..	10	.31	2	13	81	m.q.	m.q.	m.q.
iceberg, 6″-diam. head, 1.25 lbs. ...	102	2.70	48	108	852	1.19	.15	.81
iceberg, 1 leaf, approx. .7 oz.	4	.10	2	4	32	.04	.01	.03

1. *Diluted according to package directions.*
2. *With added nutrients.*

Food and Measure	Ca mg.	Fe mg.	Mag mg.	Pho mg.	Pot mg.	Zn mg.	Cop mcg.	Man mcg.
Lettuce *(cont.)*								
looseleaf, shredded, 1 oz. or ½ cup	19	.39	3	7	74	m.q.	m.q.	m.q.
Lima bean, ½ cup:								
fresh, boiled, drained	27	2.08	63	111	485	.67	.26	1.06
canned, w/liquid	35	1.97	42	88	334	.79	.20	.87
frozen, baby, boiled, drained	25	1.76	50	101	370	.50	.18	.73
frozen, Fordhook, boiled, drained ..	19	1.16	29	54	347	.37	.05	.26
Lima bean, dried, ½ cup:								
large, boiled	16	2.25	41	104	478	.89	.22	.49
large, canned, w/liquid	25	2.17	47	89	264	.78	.22	.44
baby, boiled	26	2.18	49	116	365	.93	.20	.53
Lime, 1 medium, 2″ diam., approx.								
2.8 oz.	22	.40	m.q.	12	68	.07	.04	m.q.
Lime juice, 1 fl. oz.:								
fresh	3	.01	2	2	34	.02	.01	<.01
canned or bottled	4	.07	2	3	23	.02	.01	<.01
Ling, meat only, raw, 1 oz.	10	.18	18	56	107	n.a.	n.a.	n.a.
Lingcod, meat only, raw, 1 oz.	4	.09	7	57	124	.13	<.01	<.01
Liquor, pure distilled, 1 fl. oz.[1] ...	0	.01	0	1	0	.01	.01	.01
Litchee:								
fresh, shelled and seeded, ½ cup ..	5	.30	10	30	163	.06	.14	.05
dried, 1 oz.	9	.48	12	51	315	.08	.18	.07
Liver[2], 4 oz., except as noted:								
beef, braised	8	7.68	23	458	266	6.88	5.12	.47
beef, pan-fried in vegetable oil	12	7.12	26	523	413	6.18	5.06	.48
chicken, simmered	16	9.60	24	354	159	4.92	.42	.34
goose, raw, 1 oz.	12	m.q.	7	74	65	m.q.	2.13	m.q.
lamb, braised	9	9.39	25	476	251	8.95	8.02	.59
lamb, pan-fried in vegetable oil	10	11.57	26	484	399	6.38	11.15	.67
pork, braised	11	20.32	16	273	170	7.62	.72	.34
turkey, simmered	12	8.85	17	308	220	3.50	.64	.29
veal (calf), braised	8	2.97	22	362	232	10.80	9.02	.13
veal (calf), pan-fried in vegetable oil	14	5.93	29	498	497	8.92	11.21	.23
Liver cheese, pork, 1 oz.	2	3.07	3	59	64	1.05	.11	.06
Liver pâté, see "Pâté"								
Lobster, northern, meat only,								
boiled or steamed[3], 4 oz.	69	.44	40	210	399	3.31	2.20	.07
Loganberry, frozen, ½ cup	19	.47	16	19	107	.03	.09	.92
Longan, 1 oz.:								
fresh, shelled and seeded	<1	.04	3	6	75	.01	.05	.01
dried	13	1.53	13	56	187	.06	.23	.07
Loquat, peeled and seeded, 1 oz.	5	.08	4	8	75	.01	.01	.04
Luncheon meat, pork and beef:								
pork and beef, 1-oz. slice	3	.24	4	24	57	.47	.01	.01
pork and beef, sausage, 1 oz.	4	.40	4	34	70	.69	.02	.01
canned, pork, 1 oz.	2	.20	3	23	61	.42	.01	.01

1. *Includes gin, rum, vodka, whiskey, and others, with insignificant variations in mineral content depending on type of liquor.*
2. *Prepared without added ingredients, except as noted.*
3. *Without added ingredients.*

Food and Measure	Ca mg.	Fe mg.	Mag mg.	Pho mg.	Pot mg.	Zn mg.	Cop mcg.	Man mcg.
Lungs, braised[1], 4 oz.:								
beef	12	6.12	11	202	196	1.86	.25	.02
pork	9	18.61	14	211	171	2.78	n.a.	n.a.
Luxury loaf, pork, 1-oz. slice	10	.30	6	52	107	.86	.03	.01

1. *Without added ingredients.*

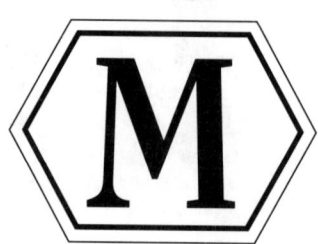

Food and Measure	Ca mg.	Fe mg.	Mag mg.	Pho mg.	Pot mg.	Zn mg.	Cop mcg.	Man mcg.
Macadamia nut, 1 oz.:								
dried	20	.68	33	39	104	.49	.08	n.a.
oil-roasted	13	.51	33	57	94	.31	.09	n.a.
Macaroni, dry, cooked:								
enriched, 4 oz.	8	1.59	20	61	35	.60	.11	.32
elbow, enriched, 1 cup	10	1.96	25	76	44	.74	.14	.40
protein fortified, 4 oz.	11	.82	34	57	48	.57	.10	.47
vegetable (tricolor), 4 oz.	12	.56	22	57	35	.50	.10	1.12
whole wheat, 4 oz.	17	1.20	34	101	50	.92	.19	1.56
Mace, ground, 1 tsp.	4	.24	3	2	8	.04	.05	.03
Mackerel, meat only:								
Atlantic, raw, 1 oz.	3	.46	21	61	89	.18	.02	<.01
Atlantic, baked, broiled, or								
microwaved[1], 4 oz.	17	1.78	110	315	455	1.07	.11	(0)
king, raw, 1 oz.	9	.50	9	70	123	.16	.01	<.01
Pacific and jack, raw, 1 oz.	6	.33	8	35	115	.19	.03	<.01
Spanish, raw, 1 oz.	3	.12	9	58	126	.14	.02	<.01
Spanish, baked, broiled, or								
microwaved[1], 4 oz.	15	.84	43	307	628	.70	.07	.01
Mackerel, canned, jack, drained,								
4 oz.	273	2.31	42	341	220	1.16	.17	.05
Malted milk:								
natural flavor, powder, ¾ oz., or								
2–3 heaping tsp.	56	.16	20	79	159	.21	.06	.09
natural flavor, prepared[2]	347	.29	52	307	529	1.14	.08	.09
chocolate flavor, powder, ¾ oz. or								
2–3 heaping tsp.	13	.38	15	37	130	.19	.13	.13
chocolate flavor, prepared[2]	304	.50	48	265	500	1.11	.16	.14

1. *Without added ingredients.*
2. *1 cup whole milk and ¾ oz. powder.*

Food and Measure	Ca mg.	Fe mg.	Mag mg.	Pho mg.	Pot mg.	Zn mg.	Cop mcg.	Man mcg.
Mango:								
1 medium, approx. 10.6 oz.	21	.26	18	22	322	.07	.23	.06
peeled and seeded, sliced, ½ cup ..	9	.11	8	9	129	.03	.09	.02
Marjoram, dried, 1 tsp.	12	.50	2	2	9	.02	.01	.03
Marmalade, citrus, 1 tbsp.	7	.10	tr.	2	7	n.a.	n.a.	n.a.
Melon balls (cantaloupe and								
honeydew), frozen, ½ cup	9	.25	12	11	242	.15	.05	.03
Milk, cow, fluid, 1 cup:								
buttermilk, cultured	285	.12	27	219	371	1.03	.03	.01
whole:								
3.3% fat	291	.12	33	228	370	.93	.02	.01
3.7% fat, producer	290	.12	33	227	368	.93	.02	.01
low sodium	246	n.a.	12	209	617	n.a.	.02	.01
lowfat 2%:								
1 cup	297	.12	33	232	377	.95	.02	.01
nonfat milk solids added	313	.12	35	245	397	.98	.02	.01
protein fortified	352	.15	40	276	447	1.11	.02	.01
lowfat 1%:								
1 cup	300	.12	34	235	381	.95	.02	.01
nonfat milk solids added	313	.12	35	245	397	.98	.02	.01
protein fortified	349	.15	39	273	444	1.11	.02	.01
skim:								
1 cup	302	.10	28	247	406	.98	.03	.01
nonfat milk solids added	316	.12	36	255	418	1.00	.03	.01
protein fortified	352	.15	40	275	446	1.11	.03	.01
Milk, canned, 1 cup:								
condensed, sweetened	868	.58	78	775	1136	2.88	.05	.02
evaporated, whole	658	.48	60	510	764	1.94	.04	.02
evaporated, skim	738	.74	68	496	846	2.30	.04	.02
Milk, dry, 1 oz.:								
buttermilk, sweet cream	336	.09	31	265	451	1.14	.03	.01
whole	259	.13	24	220	377	.94	.02	.01
nonfat:								
regular	356	.09	31	274	509	1.16	.01	.01
calcium reduced	79	n.a.	17	287	193	n.a.	.01	<.01
instant	349	.09	33	279	483	1.25	.01	.01
Milk, goat, fluid, whole, 1 cup	326	.12	34	270	499	.73	.11	.04
Milk, human, fluid, whole, 1 cup	79	.07	8	34	126	.42	.13	.06
Milk, imitation, fluid, 1 cup	79	.95	16	181	279	2.88	.12	.23
Milk, Indian buffalo, fluid, whole,								
1 cup	412	.29	76	286	434	.54	.11	.04
Milk, sheep, fluid, whole, 1 cup ..	474	.24	45	387	334	n.a.	.11	.04
Millet:								
raw, 1 oz.	2	.85	32	81	55	.48	.21	.46
cooked, 1 cup	8	1.51	105	240	148	2.18	.39	.65
Miso, ½ cup	92	3.78	58	211	226	4.58	.60	1.19
Molasses, cane, blackstrap, 1 tbsp.	137	5.05	n.a.	17	586	n.a.	n.a.	n.a.
Monkfish, meat only, raw, 1 oz. ..	2	.09	6	m.q.	m.q.	.12	<.01	<.01
Mortadella, beef and pork, 1 oz. ..	5	.40	3	27	46	.60	.02	.01

Food and Measure	Ca mg.	Fe mg.	Mag mg.	Pho mg.	Pot mg.	Zn mg.	Cop mcg.	Man mcg.
Mother's loaf, pork, 1 oz.	12	.38	4	37	64	.41	.03	.02
Muffin, 1 piece:								
English, plain, 2 oz.	96	1.70	m.q.	67	331	m.q.	n.a.	n.a.
oat bran:								
almond and date (*Health Valley*								
Fancy Fruit Muffins)	41	4.00	67	159	210	101.00	n.a.	n.a.
blueberry (*Health Valley Fancy*								
Fruit Muffins)	62	4.50	70	159	213	102.00	n.a.	n.a.
raisin (*Health Valley Fancy Fruit*								
Muffins)	58	3.30	61	176	187	101.00	n.a.	n.a.
rice bran, raisin (*Health Valley Fancy*								
Fruit Muffins)	47	3.10	90	225	399	.95	n.a.	n.a.
Muffin mix[1], 1.6-oz. piece:								
blueberry	15	.90	m.q.	90	54	m.q.	n.a.	n.a.
bran	27	1.70	m.q.	182	50	m.q.	n.a.	n.a.
corn	30	1.30	m.q.	128	31	m.q.	n.a.	n.a.
Mulberry, ½ cup	28	1.30	13	27	136	n.a.	n.a.	n.a.
Mullet, striped, meat only:								
raw, 1 oz.	11	.29	8	63	101	.15	.01	<.01
baked, broiled, or microwaved[2],								
4 oz.	35	1.60	37	277	519	1.00	.16	.02
Mung bean, dried, boiled, ½ cup	27	1.42	48	100	268	.85	.16	.30
Mung bean, sprouted, ½ cup:								
raw	7	.47	11	28	77	.21	.09	.10
boiled, drained	7	.40	9	17	63	.29	.08	.09
Mushroom:								
raw, 1 medium, approx. .7 oz.	1	.22	2	19	67	.13	.09	.02
raw, pieces, ½ cup	2	.43	4	36	130	.17	.04	.04
boiled, drained, pieces, ½ cup	4	1.36	10	68	277	.68	.39	.09
Mushroom gravy, canned, ¼ cup	4	.39	n.a.	9	63	.42	.06	.18
Mussel, blue, meat only:								
raw, 1 oz.	7	1.12	10	56	91	.45	.03	n.a.
boiled or steamed[2], 4 oz.	37	7.62	42	323	304	3.03	.17	n.a.
Mustard, prepared, yellow, 1 tsp.	4	.10	m.q.	4	7	m.q.	n.a.	n.a.
Mustard greens, ½ cup:								
fresh, raw, chopped	29	.41	9	12	99	m.q.	m.q.	m.q.
fresh, boiled, drained, chopped	52	.49	10	29	141	m.q.	m.q.	m.q.
frozen, boiled, drained, chopped ...	75	.84	10	18	104	.15	.04	.22
Mustard seed, yellow, 1 tsp.	17	.33	10	28	23	.19	.01	.06

1. *Prepared according to package directions, with eggs and water.*
2. *Without added ingredients.*

Food and Measure	Ca mg.	Fe mg.	Mag mg.	Pho mg.	Pot mg.	Zn mg.	Cop mcg.	Man mcg.
Natto, ½ cup	191	7.57	101	153	642	2.67	.59	1.35
Navy bean, ½ cup:								
boiled	64	2.25	53	143	335	.97	.27	.51
canned, w/liquid	62	2.42	61	176	378	1.01	.27	.49
Nectarine:								
1 medium, 2½″ diam., approx.								
5.3 oz.	6	.21	11	22	288	.12	.10	.06
pitted, sliced, ½ cup	3	.11	6	11	146	.06	.05	.03
New England brand sausage,								
pork and beef, 1 oz.	2	.27	4	39	91	.77	.03	.01
New Zealand spinach, ½ cup:								
raw, chopped	16	.22	11	8	36	n.a.	n.a.	n.a.
boiled, drained, chopped	43	.59	29	20	92	n.a.	n.a.	n.a.
Noodle, egg, cooked, 1 cup:								
plain, enriched	19	2.55	31	110	45	1.00	.14	.42
spinach, enriched	30	1.74	38	91	59	1.01	.13	.51
Noodle, Chinese:								
cellophane or long rice, dehydrated,								
2 oz.	14	1.23	2	18	6	n.a.	n.a.	n.a.
chow mein, 1 cup	9	2.13	23	72	54	.63	.08	.61
Noodle, Japanese, cooked:								
soba, 1 cup, approx. 4 oz.	4	.55	11	29	40	.14	.01	n.a.
somen, 1 cup	14	.92	4	47	51	.39	.05	.44
Nutmeg, ground, 1 tsp.	4	.07	4	5	8	.05	.02	.06
Nuts, see specific listings								
Nuts, mixed, 1 oz.:								
dry-roasted, w/peanuts	20	1.05	64	124	169	1.08	.36	.55
oil-roasted, w/peanuts	31	.91	67	132	165	1.44	.47	.54
oil-roasted, w/out peanuts	30	.73	71	127	154	1.32	.51	.44

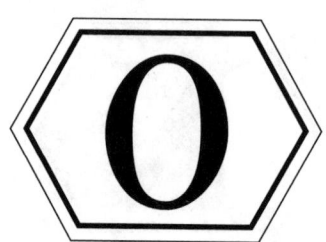

Food and Measure	Ca mg.	Fe mg.	Mag mg.	Pho mg.	Pot mg.	Zn mg.	Cop mcg.	Man mcg.
Oat (see also "Cereal"):								
whole grain, 1 cup	84	7.37	276	816	669	6.19	.98	7.67
rolled or oatmeal, dry, 1 oz.	15	1.19	42	134	99	.87	.10	1.03
rolled or oatmeal, cooked, 1 cup . . .	20	1.59	56	178	132	1.15	.13	1.37
Oat bran:								
raw, 1 oz.	16	1.53	67	208	160	.88	.11	1.60
cooked, 1 cup	22	1.93	88	262	202	1.17	.14	2.11
Oat bran pilaf dinner, canned, w/garden vegetables (*Health Valley Fast Menu*), 7½ oz.	51	2.40	76	224	373	1.40	n.a.	n.a.
Ocean perch, meat only:								
raw, 1 oz.	23	.20	6	46	58	.10	.01	<.01
baked, broiled, or microwaved[1], 4 oz.	155	1.34	44	314	397	.69	.04	n.a.
Octopus, meat only, raw, 1 oz. . . .	15	1.50	m.q.	53	m.q.	.48	.12	<.01
Oil, corn, olive, peanut, safflower, soybean (hydrogenated), soybean-cottonseed blend (hydrogenated), and sunflower, 1 tbsp.	0	0	(0)	0	0	n.a.	n.a.	n.a.
Okra, ½ cup:								
fresh, raw, sliced	41	.40	28	32	151	.30	.05	.50
fresh, boiled, drained, sliced	50	.36	46	45	257	.44	.07	.73
frozen, boiled, drained, sliced	88	.62	47	42	215	.57	.09	.94
Old fashioned loaf (*Oscar Mayer*), 1 oz.	28	.29	6	49	95	.49	n.a.	n.a.
Olive, ripe, pitted, canned:								
Mission and Manzanilla:								
all sizes, 1 oz.	25	.94	1	1	2	.06	.07	<.01
10 small, approx. 1.1 oz.	28	1.06	1	1	3	.07	.08	<.01
10 large, approx. 1.6 oz.	39	1.45	2	1	4	.10	.11	.01

1. *Without added ingredients.*

Food and Measure	Ca mg.	Fe mg.	Mag mg.	Pho mg.	Pot mg.	Zn mg.	Cop mcg.	Man mcg.
Sevillano and Ascolano:								
all sizes, 1 oz.	27	.94	n.a.	n.a.	3	n.a.	.06	n.a.
10 jumbo, approx. 2.9 oz.	78	2.76	n.a.	n.a.	7	n.a.	.19	n.a.
10 super colossal, approx. 5.4 oz.	143	5.05	n.a.	n.a.	14	n.a.	.34	n.a.
Olive loaf, pork, 1-oz. slice	31	.15	5	36	84	.39	.01	.01
Onion, ½ cup:								
fresh, raw, chopped	16	.17	8	27	125	.15	.05	.11
fresh, boiled, drained, chopped	23	.26	11	37	174	.22	.07	.16
frozen, boiled, drained, chopped ...	17	.32	7	20	114	.07	.02	.08
Onion, green (scallion), w/top,								
chopped, ½ cup	36	.74	10	18	138	.20	.04	.08
Onion flakes, dehydrated, 1 tbsp.	13	.08	5	15	81	.09	.02	.07
Onion powder, 1 tsp.	8	.05	3	7	20	.05	.04	.01
Onion rings, breaded, frozen,								
heated, 2 rings, .7 oz.	6	.34	4	16	26	.08	.02	.08
Orange:								
California navel:								
1 medium, 2⅞" diam., approx.								
7.3 oz.	56	.17	15	27	250	.08	.08	.04
trimmed, sections w/out								
membrane, ½ cup	33	.10	9	16	147	.05	.05	.02
California Valencia:								
1 medium, 2⅝" diam., approx.								
5.7 oz.	48	.11	12	21	217	.07	.05	.03
peeled and seeded, sections w/out								
membrane, ½ cup	36	.08	9	16	161	.06	.03	.02
Florida:								
1 medium, 2¹¹⁄₁₆" diam., approx.								
7.2 oz.	65	.13	15	18	254	.12	.06	.04
peeled and seeded, sections w/out								
membrane, ½ cup	40	.08	10	11	156	.08	.04	.02
Mandarin, see "Tangerine, canned"								
Orange drink, canned, 1 cup	15	.69	5	2	45	.22	.01	.04
Orange flavor drink, breakfast:								
mix, 3 rounded tsp.	46	.16	0	31	40	.04	.02	.01
Orange juice, 6 fl. oz.:								
fresh	20	.38	20	32	372	.10	.08	.03
canned	18	.84	18	24	324	.12	.11	.02
chilled	18	.30	18	24	354	.06	.07	.04
frozen[1]	18	.18	18	30	354	.12	.08	.02
Orange-grapefruit juice, canned,								
6 fl. oz.	18	.84	18	24	294	.12	.14	.03
Orange peel, fresh, 1 tsp.	3	.02	tr.	tr.	4	n.a.	n.a.	n.a.
Oregano, ground, 1 tsp.	24	.66	4	3	25	.07	.01	.07
Oyster, meat only:								
Eastern:								
raw, 1 oz.	13	1.90	15	39	65	25.78	1.26	.13
raw, 6 medium, approx. 3 oz. ...	38	5.63	46	117	192	76.40	3.75	.38

1. *Diluted according to package directions.*

Corinne T. Netzer

Food and Measure	Ca mg.	Fe mg.	Mag mg.	Pho mg.	Pot mg.	Zn mg.	Cop mcg.	Man mcg.
Oyster, Eastern *(cont.)*								
boiled, poached, or steamed[1],								
4 oz.	101	15.20	124	315	519	206.29	10.12	m.q.
Pacific, raw, 1 medium, approx.								
1.75 oz.	4	2.56	11	81	84	8.31	.79	.32
Oyster, canned, Eastern, 4 oz. ..	51	7.60	61	158	260	103.14	5.06	m.q.

1. *Without added ingredients.*

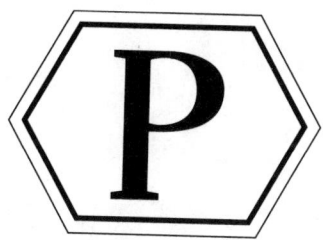

Food and Measure	Ca mg.	Fe mg.	Mag mg.	Pho mg.	Pot mg.	Zn mg.	Cop mcg.	Man mcg.
Pancake, frozen, microwave, 3.5 oz.:								
(*Aunt Jemima* Original)	146	1.97	18	312	119	.49	.07	.25
blueberry (*Aunt Jemima*)	157	1.99	19	327	113	.54	.09	.27
buttermilk (*Aunt Jemima*)	72	2.09	19	318	150	.57	.08	.27
buttermilk (*Aunt Jemima* Lite)	200	1.80	16	450	50	.60	.08	m.q.
Pancake batter, 3.6 oz.:								
(*Aunt Jemima* Original)	53	1.82	15	311	101	.43	.08	.20
blueberry (*Aunt Jemima*)	46	1.71	15	186	96	.44	.08	.23
buttermilk (*Aunt Jemima*)	60	1.84	16	316	126	.55	.08	.19
Pancake mix[1], 3 cakes, 4" each, except as noted:								
(*Aunt Jemima* Original)	150	1.43	22	280	67	.35	.06	.34
(*Aunt Jemima* Original Complete) ...	111	2.45	31	466	190	.69	.13	.37
buckwheat (*Aunt Jemima*)	215	2.91	74	438	161	.77	.17	.70
buttermilk:								
(*Aunt Jemima*)	171	1.50	16	263	91	.36	.07	.25
(*Aunt Jemima* Complete)	280	2.34	34	400	223	.61	.12	.33
(*Aunt Jemima* Complete Lite)	350	2.70	40	400	100	.90	.16	m.q.
(*Health Valley* Biscuit & Pancake Mix), 1 oz. dry	20	.70	29	109	250	.62	m.q.	m.q.
whole wheat (*Aunt Jemima*)	216	4.38	62	415	243	1.22	.25	1.37
Pancreas, braised[2], 4 oz.:								
beef	18	2.60	24	514	279	5.22	.10	.24
lamb	14	2.40	22	489	330	3.04	m.q.	.05
pork	18	3.05	26	330	191	4.86	.12	.22
Papaya:								
1 medium, 3½″ × 5⅛″, 1 lb.	72	.30	31	16	780	.22	.05	.03
peeled and seeded, cubed, ½ cup ..	17	.07	7	4	180	.05	.01	.01
Papaya nectar, canned, 6 fl. oz. ..	18	.66	6	1	60	.30	.02	.02

1. *Prepared according to package directions, except as noted.*
2. *Without added ingredients.*

Food and Measure	Ca mg.	Fe mg.	Mag mg.	Pho mg.	Pot mg.	Zn mg.	Cop mcg.	Man mcg.
Paprika, 1 tsp.	4	.50	4	7	49	.08	.01	.02
Parsley:								
fresh, raw, chopped, ½ cup	39	1.86	13	12	161	.22	.02	.05
dried, 1 tsp.	4	.29	1	1	11	.01	<.01	.03
freeze-dried, ¼ cup	2	.75	5	8	88	.09	.01	.02
Parsnip, ½ cup:								
raw, sliced	24	.39	19	47	251	.40	.08	.38
boiled, drained, sliced	29	.45	23	54	287	.20	.11	.23
Passion fruit, purple, trimmed,								
1 oz.	3	.45	8	19	99	n.a.	n.a.	n.a.
Passion fruit juice, yellow, fresh,								
6 fl. oz.	6	.66	30	48	516	n.a.	n.a.	n.a.
Pasta:								
dry, uncooked, 2 oz.:								
amaranth (*Health Valley* Spaghetti)	20	2.70	58	216	240	1.20	n.a.	n.a.
oat bran (*Health Valley* Spaghetti)	15	1.30	40	133	126	.68	n.a.	n.a.
whole wheat (*Health Valley*								
Lasagna)	20	4.50	70	232	240	1.80	n.a.	n.a.
whole wheat (*Health Valley*								
Spaghetti)	20	4.50	67	232	240	1.70	n.a.	n.a.
whole wheat spinach (*Health Valley*								
Lasagna/Spaghetti)	20	4.50	100	243	240	1.90	n.a.	n.a.
dry, cooked, 1 cup:								
enriched	10	1.96	25	76	44	.74	.14	.40
protein fortified, enriched	14	1.01	42	70	58	.70	.12	.58
corn	2	.34	50	106	43	.88	.09	.21
spinach	42	1.46	87	151	81	1.51	.29	2.11
whole wheat	21	1.49	42	124	61	1.13	.23	1.93
fresh, refrigerated, cooked:								
w/egg, 4 oz.	7	1.29	20	71	27	.64	.11	.25
spinach, w/egg, 4 oz.	20	1.26	27	65	42	.71	.09	.36
Pasta sauce, see "Tomato sauce"								
Pastrami (*Oscar Mayer*), .6-oz. slice	1	.43	3	35	53	.51	m.q.	m.q.
Pâté, liver, 1 tbsp.	9	.72	2	26	18	m.q.	.05	.02
Peach, ½ cup, except as noted:								
1 medium, 2½" diam., approx.								
4 per lb.	5	.10	6	11	171	.12	.06	.04
pulp, sliced	5	.10	6	11	167	.12	.06	.04
canned, halves or slices:								
in water, clingstone	3	.39	6	13	121	.11	.07	.06
in juice, clingstone or freestone ..	8	.33	9	22	159	.13	.06	m.q.
in light syrup, clingstone	5	.45	6	14	122	.11	.07	.06
in heavy syrup, clingstone or								
freestone	4	.35	7	15	118	.11	.07	.06
canned, spiced, in heavy syrup,								
whole	8	.35	8	12	103	.10	.12	m.q.
dehydrated, sulfured, uncooked	22	3.20	33	94	783	.45	.29	.24
dehydrated, sulfured, cooked	19	2.74	28	80	671	.39	.24	.21

Food and Measure	Ca mg.	Fe mg.	Mag mg.	Pho mg.	Pot mg.	Zn mg.	Cop mcg.	Man mcg.
dried, sulfured, halves:								
uncooked	23	3.25	34	96	797	.46	.29	.24
cooked, unsweetened	12	1.69	18	50	413	.24	.15	.13
cooked, sweetened	11	1.62	17	47	395	.23	.14	.12
frozen, sliced, sweetened	3	.47	6	14	163	.07	.03	.04
Peach nectar, canned, 6 fl. oz. ...	12	.36	6	12	78	.12	.13	.04
Peanut, shelled, 1 oz.:								
raw:								
all types	26	1.28	47	105	197	.91	.32	.54
Spanish	30	1.09	53	109	208	.59	.25	.74
Valencia	17	.59	52	94	93	.94	.33	.55
Virginia	25	.71	48	106	193	1.24	.31	.48
boiled, all types	18	.32	33	63	58	.59	.16	.33
dry-roasted, all types	15	.63	49	100	184	.93	.19	.58
oil-roasted:								
all types	25	.51	52	145	191	1.86	.36	.58
Spanish	28	.64	47	108	217	.56	.19	.66
Valencia	15	.46	45	89	171	.86	.24	.48
Virginia	24	.47	53	142	183	1.85	.36	.56
Peanut butter, 2 tbsp.:								
chunk style	13	.61	51	101	239	.89	.17	.60
chunk or creamy (*Health Valley*)	10	.60	52	120	190	.94	m.q.	m.q.
smooth style	11	.53	50	103	231	.80	.18	.49
Peanut flour, defatted, 1 oz.	84	1.26	222	456	774	3.06	1.08	2.94
Pear, ½ cup, except as noted:								
fresh, w/skin, sliced	10	.21	5	9	104	.10	.09	.06
fresh, Bartlett, 2½″ diam. × 3½″,								
approx. 2½ per lb.	19	.41	9	18	208	.20	.19	.13
canned:								
in water	5	.26	5	9	65	.11	.06	.04
in juice	11	.36	9	15	119	.11	.07	n.a.
in light syrup	7	.35	6	9	83	.11	.06	.04
in heavy syrup	6	.28	6	9	83	.11	.06	.04
dried, sulfured, halves:								
uncooked	30	1.89	30	53	480	.35	.33	.29
cooked, unsweetened	21	1.30	21	37	330	.24	.23	.20
cooked, sweetened	22	1.36	22	38	344	.25	.24	.21
Pear nectar, canned, 6 fl. oz.	6	.48	6	6	24	.12	.13	.05
Peas, edible-podded, ½ cup:								
fresh, raw	31	1.50	17	38	144	m.q.	m.q.	m.q.
fresh, boiled, drained	33	1.58	21	44	192	.30	.06	.13
frozen, boiled, drained	48	1.92	22	46	173	.39	m.q.	m.q.
Peas, green, ½ cup:								
fresh, raw	18	1.06	24	77	176	.89	.13	.30
fresh, boiled, drained	22	1.24	31	94	217	.95	.14	.42
canned, w/liquid	22	1.37	21	66	108	.86	.13	.33
canned, drained	17	.81	15	57	147	.60	.07	.26
frozen, boiled, drained	19	1.26	23	72	134	.75	.11	.33
Peas, split, boiled, ½ cup	13	1.26	36	97	355	.98	.18	.39

Food and Measure	Ca mg.	Fe mg.	Mag mg.	Pho mg.	Pot mg.	Zn mg.	Cop mcg.	Man mcg.
Peas, sprouted, mature seeds,								
raw, ½ cup	21	1.35	34	99	229	.63	.16	.26
Peas and carrots, ½ cup:								
canned, w/liquid	29	.97	18	58	128	.74	.13	.46
frozen, boiled, drained	18	.75	13	39	127	.36	.06	.16
Peas and onions, canned, w/liquid,								
½ cup	10	.52	10	30	57	.35	.06	m.q.
Pecan, shelled, dried, 1 oz.	10	.60	36	83	111	1.55	.34	1.28
Pepper, chili, hot, green and red:								
raw, 1 medium, approx. 1.6 oz.	8	.54	11	20	153	.14	.08	.11
raw, chopped, ½ cup	13	.90	19	34	255	.23	.13	.18
Pepper, ground, 1 tsp.:								
black	9	.61	4	4	26	.03	.02	.11
red or cayenne	3	.14	3	5	36	.05	.01	.04
white	6	.34	2	4	2	.03	.02	.10
Pepper, jalapeño, canned,								
w/liquid, chopped, ½ cup	18	1.90	8	12	92	.13	.10	n.a.
Pepper, sweet (bell), green and red:								
raw, 1 medium, approx. 3.2 oz.	7	.34	7	14	131	.09	.05	.09
raw, chopped, ½ cup	5	.23	5	10	89	.06	.03	.06
boiled, drained, chopped, ½ cup ...	6	.31	7	12	113	.08	.04	.08
Pepper sauce, hot (*Tabasco*),								
2 fl. oz.	6	.40	6	11	79	.07	.07	n.a.
Peppered loaf, pork and beef,								
1-oz. slice	15	.30	6	48	112	.92	.03	.02
Pepperoni, pork and beef, 1 oz. ...	3	.40	5	34	98	.71	.02	n.a.
Perch, mixed species, meat only:								
raw, 1 oz.	23	.26	9	57	76	.31	.04	.20
baked, broiled, or microwaved[1],								
4 oz.	116	1.32	43	291	390	1.62	.22	n.a.
Persimmon, Japanese:								
fresh, 1 medium, 2½″ × 3½″,								
approx. 7.1 oz.	13	.26	15	28	270	.18	.19	.60
dried, 1 oz.	7	.21	9	23	227	.12	.13	.39
Pheasant, raw, meat w/skin, 1 oz.	3	.33	6	61	69	.27	.02	<.01
Pickle, cucumber:								
dill, 1 medium, 3¾″ long, approx.								
2.3 oz.	6	.35	7	14	75	.09	.05	.01
sour, 1 medium, 3¾″ long, approx.								
2.3 oz.	0	.14	1	5	8	.01	.03	m.q.
sweet, 1 large, 3″ long, approx.								
1.2 oz.	1	.21	1	4	11	.03	.04	.01
Pickle and pimiento loaf, pork,								
1-oz. slice	27	.29	5	40	96	.40	.04	.01
Picnic loaf, pork and beef,								
1-oz. slice	13	.29	4	36	76	.62	.02	.01

1. *Without added ingredients.*

Food and Measure	Ca mg.	Fe mg.	Mag mg.	Pho mg.	Pot mg.	Zn mg.	Cop mcg.	Man mcg.
Pie, ⅙ of 9″-diam. pie:								
apple	13	1.60	m.q.	35	126	n.a.	n.a.	n.a.
blueberry	17	2.10	m.q.	36	158	n.a.	n.a.	n.a.
cherry	22	1.60	m.q.	40	166	n.a.	n.a.	n.a.
custard	146	1.50	m.q.	172	208	n.a.	n.a.	n.a.
lemon meringue	20	1.40	m.q.	69	70	n.a.	n.a.	n.a.
peach	16	1.90	m.q.	46	235	n.a.	n.a.	n.a.
pecan	65	4.60	m.q.	142	170	n.a.	n.a.	n.a.
pumpkin	78	1.40	m.q.	105	243	· n.a.	n.a.	n.a.
Pie crust mix[1], 9″-diam. crust	131	9.30	m.q.	272	179	n.a.	n.a.	n.a.
Pigeon peas, dried, boiled, ½ cup	36	.93	38	100	322	.76	.23	.42
Pike, meat only:								
northern, raw, 1 oz.	16	.16	m.q.	62	73	.19	.01	n.a.
northern, baked, broiled, or								
microwaved[2], 4 oz.	83	.81	m.q.	320	375	.98	.07	n.a.
walleye, raw, 1 oz.	31	.37	9	60	110	.18	.05	.23
Pimiento, canned, 1 tbsp.	1	.20	1	2	19	.02	.01	.01
Pine nut, shelled, dried, 1 oz.:								
pignolias	7	2.61	m.q.	144	170	1.21	.29	n.a.
piñons	2	.87	67	10	178	1.22	.29	n.a.
Pineapple, ½ cup:								
fresh, trimmed, diced	6	.29	11	6	88	.06	.09	1.28
canned:								
in water, tidbits	19	.49	22	5	157	.15	.13	1.38
in juice, chunks or tidbits	17	.35	18	8	152	.12	.11	m.q.
in light syrup	18	.49	20	9	133	.15	.13	1.38
in heavy syrup, chunks, tidbits, or								
crushed	18	.49	20	9	132	.15	.13	1.38
frozen, sweetened, chunks	11	.49	12	5	122	.14	.12	1.30
Pineapple juice, 6 fl. oz.:								
canned	30	.48	24	12	252	.24	.17	1.86
frozen[3]	18	.54	18	12	252	.24	.17	1.85
Pineapple-grapefruit juice								
drink, canned, 1 cup	18	.77	15	14	154	.15	.11	1.03
Pineapple-orange juice drink,								
canned, 1 cup	13	.67	14	10	116	.14	.10	.90
Pinto bean, ½ cup:								
boiled	41	2.22	47	136	398	.92	.22	.47
canned, w/liquid	44	1.93	32	110	362	.83	.17	.28
Pistachio nut, shelled, 1 oz.:								
dried	38	1.92	45	143	310	.38	.34	.09
dry-roasted	20	.90	37	135	275	.39	.34	.10
Pitangua, trimmed, ½ cup	8	.18	11	10	89	n.a.	n.a.	n.a.
Pizza, frozen:								
cheese (*Celeste* Large), ¼ pie	204	1.00	30	226	268	3.0	.14	n.a.
cheese (*Celeste* Pizza for One), 1 pie	375	1.36	48	386	342	4.0	.24	n.a.

1. *Prepared according to package directions.*
2. *Without added ingredients.*
3. *Diluted according to package directions.*

Food and Measure	Ca mg.	Fe mg.	Mag mg.	Pho mg.	Pot mg.	Zn mg.	Cop mcg.	Man mcg.
Pizza, frozen *(cont.)*								
deluxe (*Celeste* Large), ¼ pie	267	1.85	38	357	352	3.0	.22	n.a.
deluxe (*Celeste* Pizza for One), 1 pie	332	2.57	61	480	498	5.0	.35	n.a.
pepperoni (*Celeste* Large), ¼ pie ...	186	1.42	39	386	284	4.0	.16	n.a.
pepperoni (*Celeste* Pizza for One),								
1 pie	336	2.04	53	443	416	4.0	.29	n.a.
sausage (*Celeste* Large), ¼ pie	322	1.52	40	385	311	3.0	.18	n.a.
sausage (*Celeste* Pizza for One),								
1 pie	371	2.28	60	505	456	n.a.	.34	n.a.
sausage and mushroom (*Celeste*								
Pizza for One), 1 pie	362	2.41	60	504	459	5.0	.34	n.a.
suprema (*Celeste* Large), ¼ pie	295	1.78	41	408	342	3.0	.23	n.a.
suprema (*Celeste* Pizza for One),								
1 pie	454	2.73	64	602	528	5.0	.36	n.a.
vegetable (*Celeste* Large), ¼ pie ...	300	1.10	m.q.	m.q.	100	m.q.	m.q.	n.a.
vegetable (*Celeste* Pizza for One),								
1 pie	500	1.44	m.q.	m.q.	170	m.q.	m.q.	n.a.
Plantain:								
raw, 1 medium, approx. 9.7 oz.	5	1.07	66	61	893	.25	.15	n.a.
raw, trimmed, sliced, ½ cup	2	.45	28	25	370	.11	.06	n.a.
cooked, sliced, ½ cup	2	.45	25	22	358	.10	.05	n.a.
Plum, ½ cup, except as noted:								
pitted, sliced, ½ cup	3	.09	2	4	57	.03	.01	.02
Japanese or hybrid, 1 medium, 2⅛″								
diam., approx. 2.5 oz.	2	.07	4	7	113	.06	.03	.03
canned, purple:								
in water	9	.20	7	17	157	.10	.05	.04
in juice	13	.42	10	20	195	.14	.07	m.q.
in light syrup	12	1.08	7	17	117	.10	.05	.04
in heavy syrup	12	1.09	7	17	117	.10	.05	.04
Poi, ½ cup	19	1.06	29	47	220	n.a.	n.a.	n.a.
Polish sausage, pork, 1 oz.	3	.41	4	39	67	.55	.03	.01
Pollock, meat only:								
Atlantic, raw, 1 oz.	17	.13	19	63	101	.13	.01	<.01
walleye, raw, 1 oz.	1	.06	m.q.	m.q.	84	.11	.01	<.01
walleye, baked, broiled, or								
microwaved[1], 4 oz.	7	.32	m.q.	m.q.	439	.68	.06	(0)
Pomegranate, 1 medium, 3⅜″								
diam. × 3¾″ high, 9.7 oz.	5	.46	n.a.	12	399	n.a.	n.a.	n.a.
Pompano, Florida, meat only:								
raw, 1 oz.	6	.17	8	55	108	.20	.01	<.01
baked, broiled, or microwaved[1],								
4 oz.	49	.76	35	387	721	.78	.09	.03
Popcorn, popped, 1 cup:								
air-popped, unsalted	1	.20	n.a.	22	20	n.a.	n.a.	n.a.
popped in vegetable oil, salted	3	.30	n.a.	31	19	n.a.	n.a.	n.a.
Poppy seed, 1 tsp.	41	.26	9	24	20	.29	.05	.19

1. *Without added ingredients.*

Food and Measure	Ca mg.	Fe mg.	Mag mg.	Pho mg.	Pot mg.	Zn mg.	Cop mcg.	Man mcg.
Pork[1], fresh, 4 oz., except as noted (see also "Ham"):								
loin, whole, lean and fat:								
braised	9	1.32	23	226	391	3.44	.12	.02
broiled	8	.92	28	266	398	2.78	.10	.01
roasted	9	1.15	22	251	361	2.97	.12	.02
loin, whole, lean only:								
braised	11	1.59	27	271	475	4.22	.14	.02
broiled	8	1.05	33	316	474	3.31	.11	.01
roasted	10	1.30	25	288	416	3.45	.11	.02
loin, blade, lean and fat:								
braised	16	1.47	19	200	379	4.37	.12	.01
broiled	12	1.03	24	229	376	3.46	.10	.01
pan-fried[2]	11	.93	22	206	337	3.07	.09	.01
roasted	14	1.21	17	196	332	3.39	.10	.01
loin, blade, lean only:								
braised	19	1.84	23	243	473	5.59	.15	.02
broiled	15	1.22	28	278	463	4.30	.11	.01
pan-fried[2]	15	1.18	27	269	447	4.16	.11	.01
roasted	16	1.42	19	228	392	4.07	.11	.01
loin, center, lean and fat:								
braised	7	.94	22	244	359	2.80	.11	.03
broiled	5	.92	28	239	407	2.19	.09	.01
pan-fried[3]	6	.95	29	243	412	2.22	.09	.01
roasted	6	1.12	22	222	365	2.31	.09	.02
loin, center, lean only:								
braised	7	1.08	25	285	422	3.30	.12	.04
broiled	6	1.04	34	277	476	2.53	.09	.01
pan-fried[2]	6	1.13	36	301	516	2.73	.10	.01
roasted	7	1.24	24	248	411	2.59	.09	.02
loin, center rib, lean and fat:								
braised	11	1.21	23	238	468	2.66	.10	.01
broiled	15	.82	28	257	421	2.30	.09	.02
pan-fried[2]	8	.72	24	236	399	1.84	.08	.01
roasted	11	1.01	22	254	417	2.22	.08	.01
loin, center rib, lean only:								
braised	14	1.43	26	284	568	3.20	.11	.01
broiled	17	.92	34	302	498	2.70	.09	.02
pan-fried[2]	10	.91	32	307	527	2.34	.09	.01
roasted	12	1.13	24	290	480	2.52	.09	.01
loin, sirloin, lean and fat:								
braised	7	1.28	26	222	418	2.90	.13	.02
broiled	6	.88	33	256	416	2.30	.11	.01
roasted	10	1.13	25	260	382	2.57	.11	.03
loin, sirloin, lean only:								
braised	8	1.51	32	263	502	3.48	.15	.02

1. *Prepared without added ingredients, except as noted.*
2. *In hydrogenated soybean and cottonseed oils.*

Food and Measure	Ca mg.	Fe mg.	Mag mg.	Pho mg.	Pot mg.	Zn mg.	Cop mcg.	Man mcg.
Pork, loin, sirloin, lean only *(cont.)*								
broiled	6	1.01	39	301	492	2.68	.12	.01
roasted	11	1.24	27	286	420	2.82	.12	.03
loin, top, lean and fat:								
braised	11	1.17	22	231	452	2.59	.10	.01
broiled	14	.79	27	248	405	2.23	.08	.02
pan-fried[1]	8	.75	24	235	397	1.84	.08	.01
roasted	11	1.00	20	248	407	2.18	.08	.01
loin, top, lean only:								
braised	14	1.43	26	284	568	3.20	.11	.01
broiled	17	.92	34	302	498	2.70	.09	.02
pan-fried[1]	10	.91	32	307	527	2.34	.09	.01
roasted	12	1.13	24	290	480	2.52	.09	.01
shoulder, whole, lean and fat,								
roasted	8	1.49	20	227	345	4.07	.13	.02
shoulder, whole, lean only, roasted	9	1.72	23	262	399	4.81	.15	.03
shoulder, arm (picnic):								
lean and fat, braised	8	1.83	20	217	381	4.58	.16	.02
lean and fat, roasted	9	1.35	19	234	332	3.75	.13	.04
lean only, braised	9	2.21	25	256	459	5.64	.18	.02
lean only, roasted	10	1.61	23	280	398	4.62	.15	.05
shoulder, Boston blade, lean and fat:								
braised	8	1.95	22	209	395	5.23	.16	.01
broiled	6	1.33	27	239	398	4.11	.13	.01
roasted	7	1.61	20	221	355	4.33	.13	.01
shoulder, Boston blade, lean only:								
braised	9	2.32	25	243	467	6.32	.19	.02
broiled	7	1.53	32	277	464	4.84	.15	.01
roasted	8	1.81	23	248	400	4.96	.15	.02
spareribs, lean and fat, braised,								
6.3 oz. (1 lb. raw w/bone)	38	3.28	43	463	566	8.15	.25	.03
tenderloin, lean only, roasted	10	1.75	28	327	610	3.40	.18	.04
Potato, fresh or stored:								
raw, peeled, 2½"-diam. potato,								
5.3 oz. w/skin	8	.85	24	52	608	.44	.29	.30
baked in skin, 1 medium, 4¾" ×								
2⅓" diam., 7.1 oz.	20	2.75	55	115	844	.65	.62	.46
baked, pulp only, 4 oz.	6	.40	28	57	443	.32	.24	.18
baked, skin only, 2 oz.	19	3.99	24	57	325	.28	.46	.35
boiled in skin, 1 medium, 2½" diam.,								
5.3 oz.	7	.42	30	60	515	.41	.26	.19
boiled, w/out skin, pulp from								
2½"-diam. potato	10	.42	26	54	443	.37	.23	.19
microwaved in skin, 1 medium,								
4¾" × 2⅓" diam., 7.1 oz.	22	2.50	54	212	903	.73	.68	.59
mashed, w/whole milk, ½ cup	28	.29	19	50	314	.30	.15	.12
mashed, w/whole milk and butter,								
½ cup	27	.28	19	49	303	.29	.14	.12

1. *In hydrogenated soybean and cottonseed oils.*

Food and Measure	Ca mg.	Fe mg.	Mag mg.	Pho mg.	Pot mg.	Zn mg.	Cop mcg.	Man mcg.
Potato, canned, drained:								
1"-diam. potato, approx. 1.2 oz. ...	2	.44	5	10	80	.10	.02	.03
½ cup	5	1.13	12	25	206	.25	.05	.09
Potato, frozen:								
french fried[1], oven-heated, 10 strips,								
1.75 oz.	4	.67	11	43	229	.21	.08	.15
cottage-cut, 1.75 oz.	5	.75	11	33	240	.21	.10	.15
hash brown[2], ½ cup	12	1.17	13	56	340	.25	.12	.17
puffs[1], 1 piece, approx. .25 oz.	2	.11	1	3	27	.02	<.01	.02
Potato, mix[3], ½ cup:								
mashed, flakes	52	.23	19	59	245	.18	.02	n.a.
mashed, granules	37	.20	20	63	152	.26	.02	<.01
Potato chips, 1 oz.:	7	.34	17	43	369	.30	.06	.13
all varieties (*Health Valley*), 1 oz. ...	7	.50	14	44	320	.23	n.a.	n.a.
Potato sticks, 1-oz. pkg.	3	.41	12	31	223	.18	.06	.08
Poultry, see specific listings								
Poultry seasoning, 1 tsp.	15	.53	3	3	10	.05	.01	.10
Pout, ocean, meat only, raw, 1 oz.	3	.01	4	m.q.	m.q.	.29	.01	<.01
Prickly pear, 1 medium, approx.								
4.8 oz.	58	.31	88	25	226	n.a.	n.a.	n.a.
Pretzels, 1 oz.	6	.43	n.a.	37	37	n.a.	n.a.	n.a.
Prune:								
canned, in heavy syrup, ½ cup	20	.48	17	30	264	.22	.14	.11
dehydrated, uncooked, ½ cup	48	2.32	43	74	699	.50	.40	.21
dehydrated, cooked, ½ cup	34	1.64	30	52	494	.35	.29	.15
dried, w/pits, ½ cup:								
uncooked	41	2.00	37	64	600	.43	.35	.18
cooked, stewed, unsweetened ...	24	1.18	21	37	354	.25	.21	.10
cooked, stewed, sweetened	25	1.24	22	39	371	.26	.21	.11
dried, pitted, 4 oz.:								
uncooked	58	2.81	51	90	845	.60	.49	.25
cooked, stewed, unsweetened ...	26	1.26	23	40	379	.27	.22	.11
cooked, stewed, sweetened	24	1.18	22	37	354	.25	.20	.10
Prune juice, canned, 6 fl. oz.	23	2.27	27	48	530	.40	.13	.29
Pudding, ready to serve,								
5-oz. can:								
chocolate	74	1.20	n.a.	117	254	n.a.	n.a.	n.a.
tapioca	119	.30	n.a.	113	212	n.a.	n.a.	n.a.
vanilla	79	.20	n.a.	94	155	n.a.	n.a.	n.a.
Pudding mix[4], ½ cup:								
chocolate	146	.20	n.a.	120	190	n.a.	n.a.	n.a.
chocolate, instant	130	.30	n.a.	329	176	n.a.	n.a.	n.a.
rennet custard:								
caramel or vanilla	147	tr.	n.a.	115	160	n.a.	n.a.	n.a.
chocolate	156	tr.	n.a.	123	160	n.a.	n.a.	n.a.
raspberry or strawberry	296	tr.	n.a.	206	160	n.a.	n.a.	n.a.

1. *Par-fried in vegetable oil.*
2. *Prepared in vegetable oil.*
3. *Flakes and granules without milk; prepared according to package directions, with whole milk and butter.*
4. *Prepared according to package directions, with whole milk.*

Food and Measure	Ca mg.	Fe mg.	Mag mg.	Pho mg.	Pot mg.	Zn mg.	Cop mcg.	Man mcg.
Pudding mix *(cont.)*								
rice	133	.50	n.a.	110	165	n.a.	n.a.	n.a.
tapioca	131	.10	n.a.	103	167	n.a.	n.a.	n.a.
vanilla	129	.10	n.a.	273	164	n.a.	n.a.	n.a.
vanilla, instant	132	.10	n.a.	102	166	n.a.	n.a.	n.a.
Pummelo, trimmed, sections,								
½ cup	4	.11	6	16	206	.08	.05	.02
Pumpkin, ½ cup:								
fresh, boiled, drained, mashed	18	.70	11	37	281	m.q.	m.q.	m.q.
canned	32	1.70	28	42	251	.21	.13	m.q.
Pumpkin pie mix[1] (*Libby's*), ⅙ pie	100	2.70	36	165	290	.82	.10	n.a.
Pumpkin pie spice, 1 tsp.	12	.34	2	2	11	.04	.01	.27
Pumpkin seed kernels, dried,								
1 oz.	12	4.25	152	333	229	2.12	.39	n.a.
Purslane, raw, ½ cup	14	.43	15	10	107	n.a.	n.a.	n.a.

1. *Prepared according to package directions.*

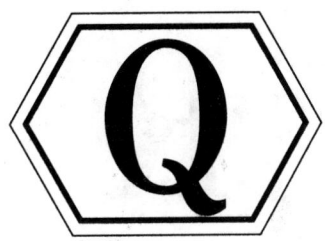

Food and Measure	Ca mg.	Fe mg.	Mag mg.	Pho mg.	Pot mg.	Zn mg.	Cop mcg.	Man mcg.
Quail, raw, meat w/skin, 1 oz.	4	1.13	n.a.	78	61	m.q.	.14	n.a.
Quince, 1 medium, 5.3 oz.	10	.64	7	16	181	n.a.	.12	n.a.
Quinoa, 1 cup	102	15.73	357	697	1258	5.61	1.39	n.a.

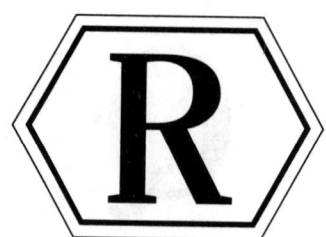

Food and Measure	Ca mg.	Fe mg.	Mag mg.	Pho mg.	Pot mg.	Zn mg.	Cop mcg.	Man mcg.
Rabbit[1], domesticated, meat only:								
roasted, 4 oz.	17	2.02	19	234	340	2.02	.17	.03
stewed, 4 oz.	23	2.69	23	256	340	2.69	.20	.04
Radish, raw, 10 medium, 1.75 oz.	9	.13	4	8	104	.13	.02	.03
Radish, Oriental, raw, sliced,								
½ cup	12	.18	7	10	100	n.a.	n.a.	n.a.
Radish, white icicle, raw, sliced,								
½ cup	14	.40	5	14	140	m.q.	n.a.	n.a.
Radish seeds, sprouted, raw,								
½ cup	10	.16	8	21	16	.11	.02	.05
Raisin:								
golden seedless, 1 oz.	15	.51	10	33	211	.09	.10	.09
golden seedless, ½ cup not packed	38	1.30	26	84	541	.24	.26	.22
seeded, 1 oz.	8	.73	9	21	234	.05	.09	.08
seeded, ½ cup not packed	21	1.88	22	55	599	.13	.22	.19
seedless, 1 oz.	14	.59	9	27	213	.08	.09	.09
seedless, ½ cup not packed	36	1.51	24	70	545	.19	.22	.22
Raspberry, ½ cup, except as noted:								
fresh, 1 pint, 11.5 oz.	69	1.78	55	37	474	1.44	.23	3.16
fresh, trimmed	14	.35	11	8	94	.29	.05	.62
canned, red, in heavy syrup	14	.54	16	12	120	.20	.07	.30
frozen, red, sweetened	19	.81	16	21	143	.23	.13	.81
Refried beans, canned, ½ cup	59	2.22	49	106	495	1.72	.52	n.a.
Relish, sweet, 1 tbsp.	3	.10	m.q.	2	30	m.q.	m.q.	m.q.
Rhubarb, ½ cup:								
fresh, trimmed, diced	52	.14	7	9	175	.06	.01	.12
frozen	132	.20	12	8	73	.07	.02	.07
frozen, cooked, sweetened	174	.25	15	10	115	.10	.03	.09
Rice, cooked, ½ cup (see also "Rice dishes, mix"):								
brown, long grain	10	.41	42	81	42	.62	.10	.89

1. *Prepared without added ingredients.*

Food and Measure	Ca mg.	Fe mg.	Mag mg.	Pho mg.	Pot mg.	Zn mg.	Cop mcg.	Man mcg.
brown, medium grain	10	.52	43	76	77	.61	.08	1.08
white, enriched:								
long grain, regular	12	1.12	13	47	40	.47	.07	.48
long grain, parboiled	17	.99	10	37	33	.27	.08	.23
long grain, precooked or instant ..	6	.52	4	12	3	.20	.05	.19
medium grain	3	1.52	13	38	30	.43	.04	.38
short grain	1	1.49	9	33	27	.41	.07	.37
Rice, glutinous, cooked, 1 cup ...	2	.17	6	9	12	.49	.06	.31
Rice, wild, see "Wild rice"								
Rice bran, crude, 1 cup	47	15.38	648	1392	1232	5.02	.60	11.79
Rice cake, 1 piece:								
corn (*Quaker*)	1	.13	10	29	24	.20	.04	.46
multigrain (*Quaker*)	3	.23	13	34	31	.24	.04	.50
sesame (*Quaker*)	1	.13	12	33	25	.23	.04	.55
sesame (*Quaker* Unsalted)	1	.12	12	34	26	.22	.03	.45
Rice dishes, mix, dry:								
broccoli au gratin (*Golden Grain/ Rice-A-Roni Savory Classics*), 1.12 oz.	43	.57	9	77	93	.36	.10	.20
cauliflower au gratin (*Golden Grain/ Rice-A-Roni Savory Classics*), 1.2 oz.	40	1.25	14	82	105	.46	.08	.24
cheddar, zesty (*Golden Grain/Rice-A-Roni Savory Classics*), 1.3 oz.	46	1.82	10	87	77	.43	.11	.20
chicken florentine (*Golden Grain/ Rice-A-Roni Savory Classics*), 1.12 oz.	30	1.53	23	50	92	.37	.11	.32
green bean almondine (*Golden Grain/ Rice-A-Roni Savory Classics*), 1.25 oz.	49	1.28	17	106	101	.52	.09	.24
Parmesan and herbs, creamy (*Golden Grain/Rice-A-Roni Savory Classics*), 1.22 oz.	47	1.27	14	93	98	n.a.	.08	.22
pilaf, garden (*Golden Grain/Rice-A-Roni Savory Classics*), 1.12 oz.	11	1.45	11	63	87	.36	.11	.22
vegetables, spring, and cheese (*Golden Grain/Rice-A-Roni Savory Classics*), 1.22 oz.	40	1.29	14	83	107	.45	.10	.24
Rice flour, 1 cup:								
brown	18	3.13	177	533	456	3.87	.36	6.34
white	16	.55	55	155	120	1.26	.21	1.90
Rockfish, Pacific, meat only:								
raw, 1 oz.	3	.12	7	50	115	.12	.01	<.01
baked, broiled, or microwaved[1], 4 oz.	14	.60	39	259	588	.60	.04	(0)
Roll, 1 piece:								
brown and serve, unbaked:								
dinner or pan, 1-oz. piece	20	.50	m.q.	23	25	n.a.	n.a.	n.a.

1. *Without added ingredients.*

Food and Measure	Ca mg.	Fe mg.	Mag mg.	Pho mg.	Pot mg.	Zn mg.	Cop mcg.	Man mcg.
Roll, brown and serve *(cont.)*								
Parkerhouse, 1-oz. piece	9	.50	m.q.	21	23	n.a.	n.a.	n.a.
dinner, 1 oz.	33	.80	n.a.	44	36	n.a.	n.a.	n.a.
hard, 1.8 oz.	24	1.40	m.q.	46	49	n.a.	n.a.	n.a.
hoagie or submarine, 11½" long,								
4.8 oz.	100	3.80	m.q.	115	128	n.a.	n.a.	n.a.
hot dog or hamburger, 1.8 oz.	54	1.20	m.q.	44	56	n.a.	n.a.	n.a.
Roll mix[1], cloverleaf, 1.2-oz. piece	20	.20	m.q.	34	43	n.a.	n.a.	n.a.
Rose apple, trimmed, 1 oz.	8	.02	1	2	35	.02	<.01	.01
Roselle, trimmed, 1 oz. or ½ cup	62	.42	15	11	59	n.a.	n.a.	n.a.
Rosemary, dried, 1 tsp.	15	.35	3	1	11	.04	.01	.02
Rutabaga, ½ cup:								
raw, cubed	33	.36	16	41	236	.24	.03	.12
boiled, drained, cubed	36	.40	18	42	244	.26	.03	.13
boiled, drained, mashed	50	.56	25	59	344	.36	.04	.18
Rye, whole grain, 1 cup	56	4.51	204	632	446	6.30	.76	4.53
Rye flour, 1 cup:								
dark	72	8.26	318	809	934	7.19	.96	8.61
light	21	1.84	72	198	238	1.78	.26	2.01
medium	24	2.16	77	211	347	2.03	.29	5.57

1. *Prepared according to package directions, with water.*

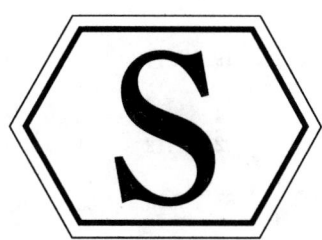

Food and Measure	Ca mg.	Fe mg.	Mag mg.	Pho mg.	Pot mg.	Zn mg.	Cop mcg.	Man mcg.
Sage, ground, 1 tsp.	12	.20	3	1	7	.03	.01	.02
Salad dressing, 1 tbsp.:								
blue cheese	12	tr.	n.a.	11	6	n.a.	n.a.	n.a.
French	2	tr.	2	1	2	n.a.	n.a.	n.a.
French, low-calorie	6	tr.	n.a.	5	3	n.a.	n.a.	n.a.
Italian	1	tr.	n.a.	1	5	n.a.	n.a.	n.a.
Italian, low-calorie	1	tr.	n.a.	1	4	n.a.	n.a.	n.a.
mayonnaise type	2	tr.	n.a.	4	1	n.a.	n.a.	n.a.
Thousand Island	2	.10	n.a.	3	18	n.a.	n.a.	n.a.
Thousand Island, low-calorie	2	.10	n.a.	3	17	n.a.	n.a.	n.a.
vinegar and oil	0	0	n.a.	0	1	n.a.	n.a.	n.a.
Salami, 1 oz.:								
beer, beef	3	.39	3	30	52	.75	.01	n.a.
beer, pork	2	.22	4	29	72	.49	.01	.01
cooked, beef	2	.57	4	29	64	.61	.03	.01
cooked, beef and pork	4	.76	4	33	56	.61	.06	.02
dry or hard, pork	4	.37	6	65	n.a.	1.19	.05	.02
dry or hard, pork and beef	2	.43	5	40	107	.92	.02	.01
Salmon, meat only:								
chinook, smoked, 4 oz.	12	.96	20	186	198	.35	.26	.02
chum, raw, 1 oz.	3	.02	m.q.	80	122	.13	.02	<.01
sockeye, raw, 1 oz.	2	.13	7	61	111	.15	.01	<.01
sockeye, baked, broiled, or microwaved[1], 4 oz.	8	.62	35	313	425	.58	.08	(0)
Salmon, canned, 4 oz.:								
pink, w/bone and liquid	242	.95	39	373	370	1.04	.12	n.a.
sockeye, w/bone, drained	271	1.16	33	370	428	1.16	.10	(0)
Salsify, ½ cup:								
raw, sliced	40	.47	15	50	255	m.q.	n.a.	n.a.
boiled, drained, sliced	32	.37	12	38	192	m.q.	n.a.	n.a.
Salt, 1 tsp.	14	tr.	7	3	tr.	n.a.	n.a.	n.a.

1. *Without added ingredients.*

Food and Measure	Ca mg.	Fe mg.	Mag mg.	Pho mg.	Pot mg.	Zn mg.	Cop mcg.	Man mcg.
Salt, substitute or imitation,								
(*Instead of Salt*), 1 tsp.	19	.77	7	13	40	.14	n.a.	n.a.
Sandwich spread:								
(*Oscar Mayer*), 1 oz.	4	.26	3	18	30	.27	m.q.	m.q.
pork and beef, 1 tbsp.	2	.12	1	9	16	.15	.02	<.01
Sapote, 1 medium, approx.								
11.2 oz.	88	2.25	68	63	773	n.a.	n.a.	n.a.
Sardine, canned:								
Atlantic, in soybean oil, 2 medium,								
approx. .8 oz.	92	.70	9	118	95	.31	.05	.03
Pacific, in tomato sauce, 1 medium,								
approx. 1.3 oz.	91	.87	13	139	130	.53	.10	.08
Sauerkraut, canned, w/liquid,								
½ cup	36	1.73	15	23	201	.22	.11	n.a.
Sausage (see also specific listings):								
beef, smoked (*Oscar Mayer*								
Smokies), 1.5-oz. link	4	.70	6	102	76	1.32	m.q.	m.q.
cheese, smoked (*Oscar Mayer*								
Smokies), 1.5-oz. link	18	.46	7	126	80	.84	m.q.	m.q.
pork:								
fresh, cooked, .5 oz. (1-oz. raw								
link)	4	.16	2	24	47	.33	.02	.01
fresh, cooked, 1 oz. (2-oz. raw								
patty)	9	.34	5	50	97	.68	.04	.02
smoked, 1 link, 4″ long × 1⅛″,								
approx. 2.4 oz.	20	.79	13	110	228	1.92	.05	m.q.
pork and beef:								
fresh, cooked, .5 oz. (1-oz. raw								
link)	m.q.	.15	1	14	m.q.	.24	tr.	m.q.
fresh, cooked, 1 oz. (2-oz. raw								
patty)	m.q.	.31	3	29	m.q.	.50	.01	m.q.
smoked, 1 link, 4″ long × 1⅛″,								
approx. 2.4 oz.	7	.99	8	73	129	1.44	.04	.03
Savory, ground, 1 tsp.	30	.53	5	2	15	.06	.01	.09
Scallop, mixed species, meat only,								
raw, 2 large or 5 small, 1.1 oz.	7	.09	17	66	97	.29	.02	.03
Scallop squash, ½ cup:								
raw, sliced	12	.26	15	23	118	.19	.07	.10
boiled, drained, sliced	14	.29	17	25	126	.22	.08	.12
Scup, meat only, raw, 1 oz.	11	.15	7	m.q.	81	.14	.01	.01
Sea bass, mixed species, meat								
only:								
raw, 1 oz.	3	.08	12	55	73	.10	<.01	<.01
baked, broiled, or microwaved[1],								
4 oz.	15	.42	60	281	372	.59	.03	n.a.
Sea trout, mixed species, meat								
only, raw 1 oz.	5	.08	9	71	97	.13	.01	<.01

1. *Without added ingredients.*

Food and Measure	Ca mg.	Fe mg.	Mag mg.	Pho mg.	Pot mg.	Zn mg.	Cop mcg.	Man mcg.
Seaweed, 1 oz.:								
agar, dried	177	6.07	218	15	319	n.a.	n.a.	1.20
Irish moss, raw	20	2.52	n.a.	45	18	.55	.04	.10
kelp, raw	48	.81	34	12	25	.35	.04	.06
laver, raw	20	.51	<1	16	101	.30	.07	.28
wakame, raw	43	.62	30	23	14	.11	.08	.40
Semolina, whole grain, enriched, 1 cup	29	7.28	78	226	311	1.75	.32	1.03
Sesame butter, 1 tbsp.:								
paste, from whole seeds	154	3.07	58	105	93	1.17	.67	.41
tahini, from raw and stoneground kernels	63	.38	14	113	62	.70	.24	m.q.
Sesame flour, 1 oz.:								
high fat	45	4.31	102	229	120	3.03	n.a.	n.a.
partially defatted	43	4.06	103	230	121	3.04	n.a.	n.a.
lowfat	42	4.04	96	215	113	2.84	n.a.	n.a.
Sesame meal, partially defatted, 1 oz.	43	4.13	98	220	115	2.91	n.a.	n.a.
Sesame seed:								
whole, dried, 1 tbsp.	88	1.31	32	57	42	.70	.37	.22
kernels, dried, 1 tbsp.	10	.62	28	62	33	.82	m.q.	m.q.
decorticated, 1 tsp.	4	.21	9	21	11	.28	.04	.04
Shad, American, meat only, raw, 1 oz.	13	.27	9	77	109	.10	.02	.01
Shallot, freeze-dried, ¼ cup	7	.22	4	11	59	.07	.02	.05
Shark, mixed species, meat only, raw, 1 oz.	10	.24	14	60	45	.12	.01	<.01
Sheepshead, meat only:								
raw, 1 oz.	6	.13	9	89	115	.11	.01	<.01
baked, broiled, or microwaved[1], 4 oz.	42	.76	40	397	581	.71	.14	.02
Sherbet, orange, ½ cup	52	.16	8	37	99	.67	.03	.01
Shortening, vegetable, 1 tbsp. ...	0	0	n.a.	0	0	n.a.	n.a.	n.a.
Shrimp, mixed species, meat only:								
raw, 1 oz.	15	.67	10	58	52	.31	.07	.01
boiled, poached, or steamed[1], 4 oz.	44	3.50	38	155	206	1.77	.22	.05
Shrimp, canned, mixed species, 4 oz.	67	3.11	46	264	238	1.43	.34	m.q.
Smelt, rainbow, meat only:								
raw, 1 oz.	17	.26	9	65	82	.47	.04	.20
baked, broiled, or microwaved[1], 4 oz.	87	1.30	43	335	422	2.40	.20	n.a.
Snack bar (see also "Granola and cereal bar"), 1 bar, except as noted:								
apple (*Health Valley Apple Bakes*) ...	15	1.50	22	72	137	.65	n.a.	n.a.
date (*Health Valley Date Bakes*)	12	1.00	3	106	175	.68	n.a.	n.a.

1. *Without added ingredients.*

Food and Measure	Ca mg.	Fe mg.	Mag mg.	Pho mg.	Pot mg.	Zn mg.	Cop mcg.	Man mcg.
Snack bar *(cont.)*								
oat bran:								
almond and date (*Health Valley Jumbo Fruit Bars*)	25	3.00	43	139	111	.90	n.a.	n.a.
apricot (*Health Valley Oat Bran Apricot Bakes*)	9	.56	28	57	94	.47	n.a.	n.a.
fig and nut (*Health Valley Oat Bran Fig & Nut Bakes*)	11	.61	n.a.	53	102	.47	n.a.	n.a.
fruit and nut (*Health Valley Jumbo Fruit Bars*)	25	3.10	40	134	114	.80	n.a.	n.a.
raisin and cinnamon (*Health Valley Jumbo Fruit Bars*)	58	3.90	61	136	123	1.10	n.a.	n.a.
raisin (*Health Valley Raisin Bakes*) ..	14	3.20	20	110	150	.71	n.a.	n.a.
rice bran, almond and date (*Health Valley Jumbo Fruit Bars*)	67	n.a.	94	217	178	1.40	n.a.	n.a.
Snapper, mixed species, meat only:								
raw, 1 oz.	9	<.01	9	56	118	.10	.01	<.01
baked, broiled, or microwaved[1], 4 oz.	45	.27	42	228	592	.50	.05	.02
Soft drinks and mixers, 12 fl. oz., except as noted:								
club soda	17	n.a.	4	0	6	.36	n.a.	n.a.
cola	9	.13	3	46	4	.05	.04	.13
cola, low-calorie[2]	12	.11	4	30	0	.28	n.a.	n.a.
cream	19	.19	3	0	4	.24	.03	n.a.
ginger ale	12	.66	3	1	5	.18	.07	n.a.
grape	12	.31	4	0	3	.26	.08	n.a.
lemon-lime	9	.25	2	1	4	.18	.04	.05
mineral water (*Perrier*), 8 fl. oz.	32	0	1	0	0	0	0	0
orange	19	.23	4	4	9	.38	.06	n.a.
pepper type	12	.14	1	41	2	.15	.02	n.a.
root beer	19	.18	4	2	3	.26	.03	n.a.
Sole, see "Flatfish"								
Soup, canned, ready to serve:								
bean, black (*Health Valley*), 7½ oz.	57	11.30	46	108	311	.80	n.a.	n.a.
beef, chunky, 1 cup	31	2.32	n.a.	120	336	2.64	.24	.24
beef broth (*Health Valley*), 7½ oz. ..	21	1.50	1	19	80	.01	n.a.	n.a.
chicken, chunky, 1 cup	24	1.73	n.a.	113	176	1.00	.25	.25
chicken broth (*Health Valley*), 7½ oz.	7	.35	2	47	120	.16	n.a.	n.a.
clam chowder, Manhattan (*Health Valley*), 7½ oz.	53	3.80	28	102	298	.99	m.q.	m.q.
clam chowder, Manhattan, chunky, 1 cup	67	2.64	n.a.	84	384	1.68	.24	.24
lentil (*Health Valley*), 7½ oz.	53	4.70	47	100	360	1.60	n.a.	n.a.
minestrone (*Health Valley*), 7½ oz.	53	2.10	34	93	255	1.10	n.a.	n.a.
mushroom barley (*Health Valley*), 7½ oz.	21	8.70	23	72	332	.29	n.a.	n.a.

1. *Without added ingredients.*
2. *Aspartame sweetened.*

Food and Measure	Ca mg.	Fe mg.	Mag mg.	Pho mg.	Pot mg.	Zn mg.	Cop mcg.	Man mcg.
pea, green, split (*Health Valley*),								
7½ oz.	53	2.10	58	143	404	2.00	n.a.	n.a.
potato leek (*Health Valley*), 7½ oz.	32	2.30	23	57	276	1.20	n.a.	n.a.
tomato (*Health Valley*), 7½ oz.	26	1.60	32	55	550	.46	n.a.	n.a.
turkey, chunky, 1 cup	50	1.91	n.a.	104	361	2.12	.24	.24
vegetable:								
(*Health Valley*), 7½ oz.	33	11.30	26	72	296	.39	n.a.	n.a.
chicken, chunky (*Health Valley*),								
7½ oz.	36	.99	27	99	383	.49	n.a.	n.a.
chunky, 1 cup	56	1.63	n.a.	72	396	3.12	.24	.48
five bean, chunky (*Health Valley*),								
7½ oz.	43	1.90	26	74	298	.81	n.a.	n.a.
Soup, canned, condensed[1], 1 cup:								
asparagus, cream of	29	.80	4	39	173	.88	.12	.38
asparagus, cream of[2]	175	.87	20	153	359	.93	.14	.38
bean, black	45	2.16	42	107	273	1.41	.39	.64
bean w/bacon	81	2.05	44	132	403	1.03	.40	.67
bean w/frankfurters	86	2.34	49	166	477	1.18	.40	.79
beef noodle	15	1.10	6	46	99	1.54	.14	.27
celery, cream of	40	.62	6	37	123	.15	.14	.25
celery, cream of[2]	186	.69	22	151	309	.20	.15	.25
cheese	142	.75	4	136	154	.64	.13	.26
cheese[2]	288	.81	20	250	340	.69	.14	.26
chicken:								
broth	9	.51	2	73	210	.25	.12	.25
cream of	34	.61	3	38	87	.63	.12	.38
cream of[2]	180	.67	18	152	273	.68	.14	.38
and dumplings	15	.62	4	61	116	.37	.12	.49
gumbo	24	.89	4	25	75	.38	.12	.25
noodle	17	.78	5	36	55	.40	.20	.29
rice	17	.75	1	21	100	.26	.12	.37
vegetable	18	.87	6	41	154	.37	.12	.37
chili beef	43	2.13	30	148	515	1.40	.40	1.05
clam chowder:								
Manhattan	26	1.64	11	41	188	.97	.13	.38
New England	43	1.48	7	54	146	.75	.12	.25
New England[2]	187	1.48	23	157	300	.80	.14	.25
consomme, w/gelatin	8	.53	0	32	153	.37	.25	.37
minestrone	34	.92	7	56	312	.74	.12	.37
mushroom:								
w/beef stock	10	.84	9	36	158	1.38	.25	.38
cream of	46	.51	5	50	101	.59	.12	.25
cream of[2]	178	.59	20	156	270	.64	.14	.25
onion	26	.67	2	11	69	.61	.12	.25
oyster stew	22	.98	5	48	49	10.29	1.59	.37
oyster stew[2]	167	1.04	21	162	235	10.34	1.61	.37

1. *Prepared according to package directions, with water, except as noted.*
2. *Prepared with whole milk.*

Food and Measure	Ca mg.	Fe mg.	Mag mg.	Pho mg.	Pot mg.	Zn mg.	Cop mcg.	Man mcg.
Soup, canned, condensed *(cont.)*								
pea:								
green	27	1.95	39	124	190	1.71	.38	.66
green[1]	173	2.01	55	238	377	1.76	.39	.66
split, w/ham	22	2.28	48	213	399	1.32	.37	.67
pepper pot	23	.89	5	42	152	1.22	.12	.61
potato, cream of	20	.48	1	46	137	.63	.25	.38
potato, cream of[1]	166	.54	17	160	323	.68	.26	.38
Scotch broth	15	.83	4	55	159	1.59	.25	.37
stockpot	22	.87	4	54	238	1.16	.13	.26
tomato:								
1 cup	13	1.76	8	34	263	.24	.25	.25
1 cup[1]	159	1.82	23	148	450	.29	.26	.25
beef, w/noodle	18	1.12	8	56	221	.75	.12	.25
bisque	40	.82	9	60	417	.59	.13	.26
bisque[1]	186	.88	25	174	604	.63	.14	.26
rice	23	.79	5	33	330	.51	.13	.39
turkey noodle	12	.94	5	48	75	.58	.12	.25
turkey vegetable	17	.76	4	40	175	.61	.12	.25
vegetable:								
beef	17	1.11	6	40	173	1.55	.18	.32
w/beef broth	18	.97	7	39	192	.80	.15	.34
vegetarian	21	1.08	7	35	209	.46	.12	.46
Soup mix, 1 cup[2]:								
beef broth or bouillon	10	n.a.	6	26	36	n.a.	n.a.	.04
beef noodle	5	.33	9	40	81	.10	n.a.	n.a.
chicken:								
broth or bouillon	15	.08	4	13	25	.01	n.a.	n.a.
noodle	32	.50	7	32	31	.20	.04	.02
vegetable	n.a.	.59	21	32	68	.21	.03	n.a.
mushroom	67	n.a.	n.a.	77	199	.09	.03	n.a.
onion	13	.14	6	31	63	.06	.02	.06
pea, green, split, or w/ham	22	1.01	46	134	238	.59	.19	.27
tomato, regular or cream of	54	.42	15	66	295	.21	.09	n.a.
tomato vegetable[3]	8	.63	20	29	103	.17	.03	n.a.
Sour cream sauce mix, ½ cup[4]	273	.31	n.a.	n.a.	367	.69	.04	n.a.
Soursop, trimmed, ½ cup	16	.68	23	31	313	n.a.	n.a.	n.a.
Soy beverage (*Soy Moo*), 1 cup	40	.72	n.a.	115	120	m.q.	m.q.	m.q.
Soy flour, 1 cup, stirred:								
full-fat, raw	175	5.42	364	420	2138	3.33	2.48	1.93
full-fat, roasted	160	4.94	314	405	1734	3.04	1.89	1.77
defatted	241	9.24	290	674	2384	2.46	4.07	3.02
low-fat	165	5.27	202	522	2262	1.04	4.47	2.71
Soy milk, fluid, 1 cup	10	1.38	45	117	338	.54	.29	.41
Soy sauce, 1 tbsp.:								
soy	3	.49	8	38	64	.04	.02	0

1. *Prepared with whole milk.*
2. *Prepared according to package directions, with water.*
3. *Includes Italian vegetable and spring vegetable.*
4. *Prepared according to package directions, with whole milk.*

Food and Measure	Ca mg.	Fe mg.	Mag mg.	Pho mg.	Pot mg.	Zn mg.	Cop mcg.	Man mcg.
soy (tamari)	4	.43	7	23	38	.08	.02	n.a.
soy and wheat (shoyu)	3	.36	6	20	32	.07	.02	n.a.
Soybean, green, raw, ½ cup	131	2.25	m.q.	142	m.q.	m.q.	m.q.	m.q.
Soybean, dried, ½ cup:								
boiled	88	4.42	74	211	443	.99	.35	.71
dry-roasted	232	3.40	196	558	1173	4.10	.93	1.88
roasted	119	3.35	125	312	1264	2.70	.71	1.86
Soybean, sprouted, ½ cup:								
raw	24	.74	25	57	169	.41	.15	.25
steamed	28	.62	28	64	167	.49	.16	.33
Soybean kernels, roasted and toasted, 1 oz.	39	1.26	49	103	417	1.03	.30	n.a.
Spaghetti squash, ½ cup:								
raw, cubed	11	.16	6	6	54	.09	.02	n.a.
baked or boiled and drained	17	.26	8	11	91	.16	.03	n.a.
Spinach:								
fresh:								
raw, 10-oz. pkg.	202	5.52	161	100	1139	1.09	.27	1.83
raw, chopped, ½ cup	28	.76	22	14	156	.15	.04	.24
boiled, drained, ½ cup	122	3.21	79	50	419	.69	.16	.84
canned, w/liquid, ½ cup	97	1.85	66	37	269	.49	.14	.58
canned, drained, ½ cup	135	2.46	81	47	370	.49	.19	.64
frozen, boiled, drained, leaf, ½ cup	139	1.44	65	46	283	.66	.13	.90
Spleen, braised[1], 4 oz.:								
beef	14	44.63	22	346	322	3.16	1.05	.09
pork	15	25.21	n.a.	321	257	4.01	.15	.05
Spot, meat only, raw, 1 oz.	4	.09	12	53	141	.14	.01	.01
Squash, see specific listings								
Squash seed, see "Pumpkin seed"								
Squid, mixed species, meat only:								
raw, 1 oz.	9	.19	9	63	70	.43	.54	.01
dipped in flour, fried, 4 oz.	44	1.15	43	285	316	1.97	2.40	(0)
Stomach, pork, raw, 1 oz.	3	.62	n.a.	44	57	.57	.10	n.a.
Straightneck squash, see "Crookneck squash"								
Strawberry, ½ cup, except as noted:								
fresh, 1 pint, approx. 12 oz.	45	1.23	34	60	530	.40	.16	.93
fresh, trimmed	11	.29	8	14	124	.10	.04	.22
canned, in heavy syrup	16	.62	11	15	109	.12	.08	.25
frozen:								
unsweetened	12	.56	8	10	110	.10	.04	.22
sweetened, whole	15	.61	8	16	125	.07	.02	.32
sweetened, sliced	14	.75	9	16	125	.07	.03	.32
Strawberry flavor drink mix (*Carnation* Instant Breakfast), 1 pkt.	150	4.50	80	150	300	3.00	.50	n.a.
Stroganoff sauce mix, ½ cup[2] ...	261	.67	n.a.	151	336	.55	.04	n.a.

1. *Without added ingredients.*
2. *Prepared according to package directions, with whole milk and water.*

Food and Measure	Ca mg.	Fe mg.	Mag mg.	Pho mg.	Pot mg.	Zn mg.	Cop mcg.	Man mcg.
Stuffing mix[1], 1 cup:								
dry type	92	2.20	n.a.	136	126	n.a.	n.a.	n.a.
moist type	81	2.00	m.q.	134	118	m.q.	n.a.	n.a.
Succotash, ½ cup:								
canned, w/liquid	14	.68	24	71	209	.64	.14	.47
canned, w/cream style corn	15	.73	1	78	243	n.a.	.24	.86
frozen, boiled, drained	13	.76	19	59	225	.38	.05	.24
Sucker, white, meat only, raw,								
1 oz.	20	.37	9	60	108	.21	.06	.17
Sugar:								
brown, 1 cup packed	187	4.80	n.a.	56	757	n.a.	n.a.	n.a.
granulated, 1 tbsp.	tr.	tr.	0	tr.	tr.	0	n.a.	n.a.
powdered, 1 tbsp.	0	tr.	n.a.	0	tr.	n.a.	n.a.	n.a.
Sugar apple, trimmed, ½ cup	30	.75	27	41	310	n.a.	n.a.	n.a.
Sunfish, pumpkinseed, meat only,								
raw, 1 oz.	23	.34	9	51	99	.44	.09	.20
Sunflower seed kernels, dried,								
4 oz.	33	1.92	100	200	196	1.44	.50	.57
Sweet potato, fresh:								
raw, 1 medium, 5″ long, 6.3 oz.	29	.76	14	37	265	.36	.22	.46
baked in skin, peeled, 4 oz.	32	.52	23	62	397	.33	.24	.64
baked in skin, peeled, mashed,								
½ cup	28	.45	20	55	348	.29	.21	.56
boiled w/out skin, mashed, ½ cup	35	.92	16	44	301	.43	.26	.55
Sweet potato, canned, ½ cup:								
mashed	38	1.70	31	67	268	.27	.35	1.26
vacuum pack, pieces	22	.89	23	49	313	.18	.14	.46
vacuum pack, mashed	28	1.13	29	63	398	.23	.18	.08
syrup pack, w/liquid	18	.92	15	31	212	.21	.14	.58
syrup pack, drained	16	.93	12	25	189	.16	.16	.60
Sweet potato, frozen, baked,								
cubed, ½ cup	31	.47	18	39	332	.26	.16	.59
Sweet and sour sauce mix,								
½ cup[2]	21	.81	n.a.	n.a.	33	.05	.01	n.a.
Swiss chard, ½ cup:								
raw, chopped	9	.32	15	8	68	m.q.	n.a.	m.q.
boiled, drained, chopped	51	2.00	76	29	483	m.q.	n.a.	m.q.
Swordfish, meat only:								
raw, 1 oz.	1	.23	8	75	82	.32	.04	.01
baked, broiled, or microwaved[3],								
4 oz.	7	1.18	39	382	418	1.67	.18	(0)
Syrup, table (corn and maple),								
2 tbsp.	1	tr.	n.a.	4	7	n.a.	n.a.	n.a.

1. *Prepared according to package directions.*
2. *Prepared according to package directions, with water and vinegar.*
3. *Without added ingredients.*

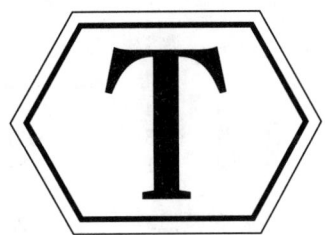

Food and Measure	Ca mg.	Fe mg.	Mag mg.	Pho mg.	Pot mg.	Zn mg.	Cop mcg.	Man mcg.
Tamale, canned (*Wolf* Brand), scant cup	68	2.19	43	141	279	2.00	.11	0
Tamarind, trimmed, ½ cup	45	1.68	55	68	377	n.a.	n.a.	n.a.
Tangerine, ½ cup, except as noted:								
fresh, 1 medium, 2⅜″ diam., approx. 4.1 oz.	12	.09	10	8	132	m.q.	.02	.03
fresh, sections w/out membrane ...	14	.10	12	10	153	m.q.	.03	.03
canned, in juice	14	.33	14	13	165	.63	.04	m.q.
canned, in light syrup	9	.46	10	12	99	.30	.06	m.q.
Tangerine juice, 6 fl. oz.:								
fresh or canned, sweetened	36	.36	12	24	330	.06	.05	.07
frozen, sweetened	12	.18	12	18	204	.06	.05	.07
Tapioca, pearl, dry, 1 oz.	6	.45	<1	2	3	.03	.01	.03
Taro, ½ cup:								
raw, sliced	22	.29	17	43	307	n.a.	n.a.	n.a.
cooked, sliced	12	.48	20	50	319	n.a.	n.a.	n.a.
Taro, Tahitian, ½ cup:								
raw, sliced	80	.81	29	28	376	n.a.	n.a.	n.a.
cooked, sliced	101	1.06	34	45	423	n.a.	n.a.	n.a.
Taro leaves, steamed, ½ cup	63	.87	15	20	240	n.a.	n.a.	n.a.
Taro shoots, cooked, sliced, ½ cup	9	.29	6	18	240	n.a.	n.a.	n.a.
Tarragon, ground, 1 tsp.	18	.52	6	5	48	.06	.01	.13
Tartar sauce, 1 tbsp.	3	.10	n.a.	4	11	n.a.	n.a.	n.a.
Tea:								
brewed, 6 fl. oz.	0	.04	5	1	66	.04	.02	n.a.
instant, powder:								
1 tsp.	0	.03	3	3	46	.02	.01	.52
lemon flavor, 1 rounded tsp.	0	.01	2	1	48	.02	.01	.43
lemon flavor, sugar sweetened, 3 rounded tsp.	1	.04	3	3	49	.02	.01	.67

Food and Measure	Ca mg.	Fe mg.	Mag mg.	Pho mg.	Pot mg.	Zn mg.	Cop mcg.	Man mcg.
Tea, instant powder *(cont.)*								
lemon flavor, saccharin sweetened, 2 tsp.	0	.14	2	2	41	.01	<.01	.49
Tea, herbal, brewed, 6 fl. oz.[1]	4	.14	2	0	15	.06	.03	.08
Tempeh, ½ cup	77	1.88	58	171	305	1.50	.56	1.19
Teriyaki sauce, 1 tbsp.	4	.31	11	28	41	.02	.02	0
Thirst quencher drink, bottled, 1 cup	0	.12	1	22	26	.05	.05	0
Thuringer cervelat, beef and pork, 1 oz.	2	.58	3	28	65	.57	.02	.01
Thyme, ground, 1 tsp.	26	1.73	3	3	11	.09	.01	.11
Tilefish, meat only:								
raw, 1 oz.	7	.07	8	53	123	.10	.01	<.01
baked, broiled, or microwaved[2], 4 oz.	29	.35	37	268	581	.60	.06	.02
Tofu, raw, ½ cup:								
firm	258	13.19	118	239	298	1.98	.48	.49
regular	130	6.65	127	120	150	1.00	.24	.75
Tomato, red, ripe:								
fresh:								
raw, 1 medium, 2⅗″ diam., approx. 4.75 oz.	6	.55	13	30	273	.11	.09	.13
raw, chopped, ½ cup	4	.40	10	22	200	.08	.07	.09
boiled, ½ cup	7	.67	16	37	335	.13	.11	.16
canned, ½ cup:								
whole	32	.73	14	23	265	.19	.13	m.q.
wedges, in tomato juice	34	.61	15	31	329	.21	.14	m.q.
stewed	42	.93	15	25	307	.21	.14	m.q.
w/green chilies	24	.31	13	17	129	.16	.11	m.q.
Tomato, green, raw, 1 medium, 2⅗″ diam., approx. 4.75 oz.	16	.63	13	35	251	.09	.11	.12
Tomato juice, canned, 6 fl. oz.	16	1.06	20	34	400	.26	.18	.14
Tomato paste, canned ½ cup	46	3.91	67	104	1221	1.05	.78	m.q.
Tomato puree, canned, ½ cup	19	1.16	30	50	526	.54	.41	m.q.
Tomato sauce, canned, ½ cup, except as noted:								
½ cup	17	.94	23	39	452	.30	.24	m.q.
(*Health Valley*), 1 cup	25	1.80	33	53	594	.50	m.q.	m.q.
marinara sauce	22	1.00	30	44	531	.34	.18	m.q.
w/mushrooms	16	1.08	23	39	464	.25	.24	m.q.
w/onions	20	1.13	23	48	504	.28	.22	m.q.
spaghetti or pasta sauce	35	.81	30	45	479	.27	.14	m.q.
w/tomato tidbits	13	.83	24	51	455	.23	.02	.27
Tongue[3], 4 oz:								
beef, simmered	8	3.84	19	161	204	5.44	.25	.03
lamb, braised	11	2.98	18	152	179	3.39	.24	.04

1. *Prepared with distilled water.*
2. *Without added ingredients.*
3. *Prepared without added ingredients.*

Food and Measure	Ca mg.	Fe mg.	Mag mg.	Pho mg.	Pot mg.	Zn mg.	Cop mcg.	Man mcg.
pork, braised	22	5.66	23	197	269	5.14	n.a.	n.a.
veal, braised	10	2.37	20	188	184	5.11	.24	.05
Tripe, beef, raw, 1 oz.	n.a.	.55	2	22	77	.70	.03	n.a.
Triticale, whole grain, 1 cup	72	4.93	250	686	637	6.63	.88	6.16
Triticale flour, whole grain, 1 cup	45	3.37	199	417	605	3.46	.73	5.44
Trout, meat only:								
mixed species, raw, 1 oz.	12	.42	6	69	102	.19	.05	.24
rainbow, raw, 1 oz.	19	.54	9	71	140	.31	.03	.20
rainbow, baked, broiled, or								
microwaved[1], 4 oz.	98	2.77	44	364	719	1.58	.16	n.a.
Tuna, meat only:								
bluefin, raw, 1 oz.	m.q.	.29	m.q.	m.q.	71	.17	.24	<.01
bluefin, baked, broiled, or								
microwaved[1], 4 oz.	m.q.	1.49	m.q.	m.q.	366	.87	.12	(0)
skipjack, raw, 1 oz.	8	.35	10	63	115	.23	.02	<.01
yellowfin, raw, 1 oz.	5	.21	m.q.	54	m.q.	.15	.02	<.01
Tuna, canned, 4 oz.:								
light, in oil, drained	15	1.58	35	353	235	1.02	.08	.02
white, in oil, drained	5	.74	39	303	378	.53	.15	n.a.
Turbot, European, meat only, raw,								
1 oz.	5	m.q.	15	36	67	.06	.01	n.a.
Turkey, all classes, roasted[1], 4 oz.,								
except as noted:								
meat w/skin	29	2.03	28	230	318	3.36	.11	.02
meat only	28	2.02	29	242	338	3.52	.11	.02
skin only, 1 oz.	10	.51	5	39	45	.59	.02	.01
dark meat w/skin	37	2.57	26	222	311	4.72	.18	.03
light meat w/skin	24	1.60	29	236	323	2.31	.05	.02
back, meat w/skin	37	2.48	25	214	295	4.45	.16	.03
breast, meat w/skin	24	1.59	31	238	327	2.30	.05	.02
leg, meat w/skin	36	2.61	26	226	318	4.84	.17	.03
wing, meat w/skin	27	1.66	28	223	302	2.38	.06	.02
Turkey, boneless and luncheon								
meat, 1 oz., except as noted:								
breast:								
1 oz.	2	.11	6	65	79	.32	.01	m.q.
honey-roasted (*Louis Rich*)	3	.28	6	70	78	.37	m.q.	m.q.
smoked (*Oscar Mayer*), .7-oz. slice	2	.15	4	70	69	.18	m.q.	m.q.
roll, light meat	11	.36	5	52	71	.44	.01	m.q.
roll, light and dark meat	9	.38	5	48	77	.57	.02	m.q.
Turkey, frozen and refrigerated:								
breast w/skin[2], roasted, 4 oz.	10	.75	24	243	281	1.74	.05	m.q.
breast tenderloins, cooked[1] (*Louis*								
Rich), 1 oz.	1	.30	10	74	119	.46	m.q.	m.q.
thigh w/skin[2], roasted, 4 oz.	9	1.71	19	194	273	4.67	.16	m.q.
white and dark meat, roasted,								
seasoned, 4 oz.	6	1.85	25	277	338	2.88	.07	m.q.

1. *Without added ingredients.*
2. *Prebasted with broth.*

Food and Measure	Ca mg.	Fe mg.	Mag mg.	Pho mg.	Pot mg.	Zn mg.	Cop mcg.	Man mcg.
Turkey, ground, cooked, 4 oz. ...	28	2.19	27	222	306	3.24	.10	.02
Turkey bologna, 1 oz.	24	.43	4	37	56	.49	.01	n.a.
Turkey entree, frozen, gravy and,								
5-oz. pkg.	20	1.31	12	114	m.q.	.99	m.q.	m.q.
Turkey frankfurter:								
(Louis Rich), 1.6-oz. link	66	.73	7	85	87	.87	m.q.	m.q.
cheese (Louis Rich), 1.6-oz. link ...	55	.71	7	97	83	.87	m.q.	m.q.
Turkey giblets, simmered[1], 4 oz. .	15	7.61	19	231	227	4.17	.44	.20
Turkey gizzard, simmered[1], 4 oz. .	17	6.17	22	145	239	4.72	.20	.11
Turkey ham (Louis Rich), 1 oz. ...	2	.37	6	82	82	.75	m.q.	m.q.
Turkey heart, see "Heart"								
Turkey pastrami (Louis Rich),								
1 oz.	2	.40	6	83	79	.73	m.q.	m.q.
Turkey salami, cooked, 1 oz.	6	.46	4	30	69	.51	.01	n.a.
Turkey sausage:								
(Louis Rich Kielbasa), 1 oz.	3	.29	4	59	55	.47	m.q.	m.q.
breakfast, cooked (Louis Rich), 1 oz.	5	.52	6	55	83	.91	m.q.	m.q.
Turkey summer sausage (Louis								
Rich), 1 oz.	4	.59	5	73	70	.63	m.q.	m.q.
Turmeric, ground, 1 tsp.	4	.91	4	6	56	.10	.01	.17
Turnip, ½ cup:								
raw, cubed	20	.20	7	18	124	m.q.	n.a.	n.a.
boiled, drained, cubed	18	.17	6	15	106	m.q.	n.a.	n.a.
Turnip greens, ½ cup:								
fresh, raw, chopped	53	.31	9	12	83	.05	.10	.13
fresh, boiled, drained, chopped	99	.57	16	21	146	.10	.18	.24
canned, w/liquid	138	1.77	24	24	165	.27	.10	.32
frozen, boiled, drained	125	1.59	21	27	184	.34	.12	.39

1. *Without added ingredients.*

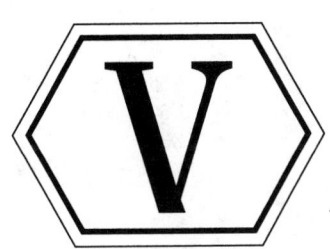

Food and Measure	Ca mg.	Fe mg.	Mag mg.	Pho mg.	Pot mg.	Zn mg.	Cop mcg.	Man mcg.
Vanilla flavor drink mix								
(*Carnation* Instant Breakfast),								
1 pkt.	150	4.50	80	150	300	3.00	.50	n.a.
Veal[1], meat only, 4 oz.:								
cubed for stew, leg and shoulder,								
braised, lean only	33	1.63	32	271	388	6.82	.17	.05
ground, broiled	19	1.12	27	246	382	4.39	.12	.04
leg (top round):								
braised, lean w/fat	9	1.50	33	282	434	4.49	.16	.04
braised, lean only	10	1.50	34	286	439	4.57	.16	.05
pan-fried in vegetable oil, lean								
w/fat	7	1.00	35	316	482	3.66	.07	.04
pan-fried in vegetable oil,								
lean only	8	1.00	36	329	501	3.83	.07	.04
roasted, lean w/fat	7	1.03	32	265	441	3.45	.15	.03
roasted, lean only	7	1.02	32	268	446	3.49	.15	.04
loin:								
braised, lean w/fat	32	1.24	27	249	318	4.12	.10	.04
braised, lean only	36	1.25	31	269	337	4.64	.11	.04
roasted, lean w/fat	22	.99	28	240	369	3.44	.12	.03
roasted, lean only	24	.96	29	252	386	3.67	.13	.03
rib:								
braised, lean w/fat	25	1.60	28	238	347	6.32	.15	.04
braised, lean only	27	1.64	29	247	361	6.78	.16	.05
roasted, lean w/fat	12	1.10	25	223	335	4.64	.11	.03
roasted, lean only	14	1.09	27	235	353	5.09	.12	.04
shoulder, whole:								
braised, lean w/fat	40	1.61	31	284	350	7.47	.17	.04
braised, lean only	42	1.64	32	295	362	7.94	.18	.04
roasted, lean w/fat	31	1.17	28	244	365	5.81	.16	.03
roasted, lean only	31	1.17	28	247	371	5.95	.16	.03

1. *Prepared without added ingredients, except as noted.*

Food and Measure	Ca mg.	Fe mg.	Mag mg.	Pho mg.	Pot mg.	Zn mg.	Cop mcg.	Man mcg.
Veal *(cont.)*								
shoulder, arm:								
braised, lean w/fat	32	1.56	33	298	378	6.59	.15	.04
braised, lean only	34	1.60	34	313	393	7.08	.15	.04
roasted, lean w/fat	29	1.30	29	251	395	4.74	.16	.03
roasted, lean only	31	1.32	31	356	404	4.90	.17	.03
shoulder, blade:								
braised, lean w/fat	43	1.63	29	277	337	7.94	.19	.04
braised, lean only	45	1.67	32	286	346	8.38	.19	.04
roasted, lean w/fat	32	1.13	27	240	347	6.33	.16	.03
roasted, lean only	32	1.13	27	244	352	6.49	.16	.03
sirloin:								
braised, lean w/fat	19	1.36	31	276	364	4.90	.15	.04
braised, lean only	22	1.39	33	294	384	5.39	.16	.04
roasted, lean w/fat	15	1.04	29	253	398	3.80	.15	.03
roasted, lean only	16	1.03	31	262	414	4.01	.15	.03
Vegetable juice cocktail,								
canned, 6 fl. oz.	13	.51	13	20	234	.24	.24	.12
Vegetables, mixed, ½ cup:								
canned, w/liquid	26	.79	19	46	169	.63	.13	.52
canned, drained	22	.86	13	34	239	.34	.06	m.q.
frozen, boiled, drained	22	.75	20	46	154	.45	.08	.35
Vienna sausage, canned, beef and								
pork, 1 oz.	3	.25	2	14	29	.45	.01	.01
Vinegar, cider, 1 tbsp.	1	.10	n.a.	1	15	n.a.	n.a.	n.a.